ENCYCLOPEDIA OF BIOETHICS

ENCYCLOPEDIA OF
BIOETHICS

REVISED EDITION

Warren Thomas Reich

EDITOR IN CHIEF

Georgetown University

Volume 2

MACMILLAN LIBRARY REFERENCE USA

SIMON & SCHUSTER MACMILLAN

NEW YORK

SIMON & SCHUSTER AND PRENTICE HALL INTERNATIONAL

LONDON   MEXICO CITY   NEW DELHI   SINGAPORE   SYDNEY   TORONTO

Copyright © 1995 by Warren T. Reich

Simon & Schuster Macmillan
866 Third Avenue, New York, NY 10022

PRINTED IN THE UNITED STATES OF AMERICA

printing number
  2   3   4   5   6   7   8   9   10

LIBRARY OF CONGRESS CATALOG-IN-PUBLICATION DATA
Encyclopedia of bioethics / Warren T. Reich, editor in chief. — Rev.
  ed.
    p. cm.
    Includes bibliographical references and index.
    ISBN 0-02-897355-0 (set)
    1. Bioethics—Encyclopedias.   2. Medical ethics—Encyclopedias.
  I. Reich, Warren T.
  QH332.E52   1995
  174′.2′03—dc20   94-38743
                                                    CIP

Lines from the poem "The Scarred Girl" by James Dickey, quoted in the entry on "Interpretation," originally appeared in *Poems, 1957–1967,* © 1978 by James Dickey, Wesleyan University Press, and have been reprinted here by permission of the University Press of New England.

The paper used in this publication meets the minimum requirements of American National Standard for Information Sciences—Permanence of Paper for Printed Library Materials, ANSI Z39.48-1984.

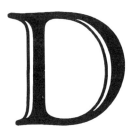

(Continued)

DECISION MAKING, MEDICAL

See MEDICINE, ART OF. *See also* LIFE, QUALITY OF, *article on* QUALITY OF LIFE IN MEDICAL DECISION MAKING.

DEEP ECOLOGY

See ENVIRONMENTAL ETHICS, *article on* DEEP ECOLOGY. *See also* ANIMAL WELFARE AND RIGHTS, *article on* ETHICAL PERSPECTIVES ON THE TREATMENT AND STATUS OF ANIMALS.

DEFINITION OF DEATH

See DEATH, DEFINITION AND DETERMINATION OF.

DENMARK

See MEDICAL ETHICS, HISTORY OF, *section on* EUROPE, *subsection on* CONTEMPORARY PERIOD, *article on* NORDIC COUNTRIES.

DENTISTRY

The ills that can befall the human mouth can be prevented and remedied far more effectively through the expertise of the dentist than through self-care alone.

Therefore, those who suffer from oral pain or dysfunction or who wish to prevent it desire to make use of dentists' expertise. In the United States, most dentists practice, individually or in small groups, as independent entrepreneurs. Nevertheless, dental care is not generally viewed as an ordinary commodity in the marketplace. Instead, the vast majority of dentists and the vast majority of the larger community have long considered dentistry a profession. That is, the larger community considers dentists to be expert in relevant knowledge and skills and committed individually and collectively to giving priority to their patients' well-being in the practice of that expertise. Consequently, when someone becomes a dentist, he or she makes a commitment to the larger community and accepts the norms and obligations of the profession. These norms and obligations are the subject matter of the subdiscipline called "dental ethics."

Many people are surprised that the professional obligations of dentists need careful study, in that dentists rarely deal with life-and-death decisions. But important human values are at stake in dental care: relieving and preventing intense pain; relieving and preventing less intense pain and discomfort; preserving and restoring patients' oral function, on which both nutrition and speech depend; preserving and restoring patients' physical appearance; and preserving and restoring patients' control over their bodies. These matters are important, and dentists who are committed to responding to them in accord with professional norms often face complex ethical questions as a result.

Ethical dilemmas like these are regularly faced by almost every dentist:

1. When examining a new patient, a dentist finds evidence of poor dental work. What should the dentist say to the patient? Should the dentist contact the previous dentist to discuss the matter? Should the dentist contact the local dental society?

2. May a dentist ethically advertise that his or her practice will produce "happy smiles" as well as quality dental care, or is such advertising false or significantly misleading?

3. May a dentist tell a patient that his or her teeth are unattractive, with a view to recommending aesthetic treatment, when the patient has not asked for this opinion and has indicated no displeasure with his or her appearance?

4. Can a dentist justify manipulating data on an insurance form in order to secure a better or more timely therapy for a patient who could otherwise not afford it? May a dentist ethically refrain from recommending a superior kind of therapy to a capitation patient (a patient whose insurance provides the dentist with a fixed payment per year for all the treatment the patient might need), and recommend instead a clinically acceptable but minimal form of therapy because the dentist knows that payment will cover only the minimal therapy, and the patient may well need still more care during the payment period? How much loss of income is a dentist professionally obligated to bear in order to provide needed but non-emergency treatment to a patient?

5. May a dentist ethically decline to treat a patient with a highly infectious disease? What obligations does the dentist have regarding the information that such a patient is a carrier of infection?

6. How ought a dentist deal with an adult patient who cannot fully participate in deciding about care? Do treatment considerations depend on the reason for this inability? What should a dentist do when the guardian of a minor or an incompetent adult patient refuses to approve the best kind of therapy for the patient? What may a dentist do to obtain cooperative behavior from a young or developmentally disabled patient who needs dental care but is uncontrollable in the chair?

7. Do dentists have an obligation to warn their patients, even when patients don't want to hear it, about the dangers of smoking or other substance dependencies?

8. What obligations does a dentist have, and to whom, when the dentist learns that another dentist is substance dependent in a manner that likely affects the care he or she is providing?

The specific requirements of the dentist's professional commitment in any particular aspect of professional practice will depend upon the specific facts and circumstances of the situation. But the principle categories of dentists' professional obligations can be conveniently surveyed under these eight headings: (1) Who are dentistry's chief clients? (2) What is the ideal relationship between a dentist and the patient? (3) What are the central values of dental practice? (4) What are the norms of competence for dental practice? (5) What sacrifices is the dentist professionally committed to, and in what respects do obligations to the patient take priority over other morally relevant considerations? (6) What is the ideal relationship between dentists and coprofessionals? (7) What is the ideal relationship between dentists, both individually and collectively, and the larger community? (8) What are members of the dental profession obligated to do to preserve the integrity of their commitment to its professional values and to educate others about them?

Issues and themes in dental ethics

The chief client.   For every profession there is a person or set of persons whose well-being the profession and its members are chiefly committed to serving. The patient in the dental chair is certainly the most obvious of a dentist's chief clients. But dentists also have professional obligations to the patients in the waiting room and to all their patients of record, and arguably to the whole larger community, especially in matters of public health. The relative weight of a dentist's obligations to each of these, when these obligations come into conflict, is ordinarily taken to favor the patient in the chair over the others, but sometimes the patient in the chair has already received his or her due in comparison with other patients. Comparative judgments of patients' degrees of need are also involved. This is a topic that has not been discussed much in the dental ethics literature and that deserves careful attention.

An ideal relationship between professional and patient.   What is the proper relationship between the dentist and the patient in the chair as they make judgments and choices about the patient's care? There are a number of different ways of conceiving this ideal relationship when it is a relationship between the dentist and a fully competent adult: with the dentist alone making the judgment that determines action; with the judgment resting with the patient alone; or with that judgment shared in various ways by both parties.

Since the late 1960s, the accepted norm of dental practice in the United States has shifted toward the third model, of shared judgment and choice regarding treatment. The legal doctrine of informed consent identifies a minimum standard of such shared decision making for dentists and their patients. But it is still worth asking whether informed consent fully expresses the ideal relationship between dentist and fully capable patient (Segal and Warner, 1979; Ozar, 1985; Hirsch and Gert, 1986).

In addition, what is the proper relationship between the dentist and a patient who cannot fully participate in treatment decisions? What is the dentist's proper role in this relationship? What is the role of the patient, up to the limit of the patient's capacity to participate? What is the proper role of other parties?

In practice, most dentists depend on the choices of the parents and guardians of such patients when they are available and when these parties' choices are not harmful to patients' oral or general health. But there is no clear consensus, within dentistry or in the larger community, about how dentistry should proceed when these conditions fail. The dental ethics literature is just beginning careful discussion of the dentist's relationship with patients of diminished capacity for decision making or no capacity for decision making at all (Bogert and Creedon, 1989).

A hierarchy of central values.   Regardless of many professions' rhetoric on the subject, no profession can actually be expert in fostering the complete well-being of its clients. There is instead a certain set of values that are the appropriate focus of each profession's particular expertise. These values can be called the central values of that profession. They determine and/or establish parameters for most aspects of a professional's judgments in practice. They are the criteria by which a client is judged to have need of professional assistance in the first place, and by which such needs are judged to have been met by the professional's intervention.

What then are the central values of dentistry and dental practice? In addition, if there is more than one, how are the several central values ranked? One proposal is that the central values of the dental profession are, in this order: (1) the patient's life and general health; (2) the patient's oral health, understood as appropriate and pain-free oral functioning; (3) the patient's autonomy, to the extent he or she is capable of it, over what happens to his or her body (including the patient's ranking of health, comfort, cost, esthetic considerations, and other values); (4) preferred patterns of practice on the part of the dentist (including differing philosophies of dental practice); (5) aesthetic considerations from the point of view of skilled dental practice; (6) considerations of efficiency, which may include considerations of cost, from the dentist's point of view (Ozar and Sokol, 1994).

A particular dental intervention may achieve each of these values to a greater or lesser degree, and each of these values will be more or less urgent for a particular patient. The dentist strives to take the details of each situation into account and to maximize dentistry's central values, in accord with their ranked priority, in every encounter with every patient.

Competence.   Every professional is obligated to both acquire and maintain the expertise needed to undertake his or her professional tasks; every professional is obligated to undertake only those tasks that are within his or her competence. In practice, every dentist is therefore required to make subtle determinations about whether he or she has sufficient competence to make a particular diagnosis or to perform a particular procedure for a patient in a given set of clinical circumstances, especially when this involves something nonroutine.

Of necessity, the dental community, not the community at large, determines the details of standards of competence because doing so requires dental expertise. But the larger community can justifiably demand to understand the reasoning involved, especially regarding the trade-offs between quality of care and access to care that the setting of such standards inevitably involves.

Sacrifice and the relative priority of the patient's well-being.   Most sociologists who study professions, and most of the literature of professions about themselves, speak of "commitment to service" or "commitment to the public" as one of the characteristic features of a profession. Dentistry's self-descriptions are similar in this respect. But these expressions admit many different interpretations with different implications for actual practice concerning, for example, the sorts of sacrifices dentists are professionally committed to make for the sake of their patients, or the sorts of risks to life and health, financial well-being, or reputation that a dentist may be obligated to face.

The related question of the proper relationship between entrepreneurship and commitment to the patient and the sacrifices of self-interest this involves has been discussed in every age of the dental profession. The consensus is certainly that, especially in emergency situations, the patient's oral and general health require significant sacrifices of personal convenience and financial interest on the part of a dentist. Since the arrival of HIV and AIDS, even more urgent implications of the obligation to give priority to the patient, including accepting an increased risk of infection, have also become part of this discussion.

Relations with coprofessionals.   Each profession has norms, usually largely implicit and unstated, concerning the proper relationship between members of the profession. For example, a dentist could relate to other dentists as competitors in the marketplace, or as cobeneficiaries in the monopoly that their exclusive expertise gives them in the marketplace, or in other ways.

What is the ideal relationship between dentists and how is it connected with the fact that they are members of the same profession, and not only entrepreneurs in the same marketplace?

How should a dentist deal with another dentist's inferior work when its consequences are discovered in the mouth of a new patient or a patient referred for specialty care? The discovering dentist could inform the patient of his or her judgment that bad work has been done, or could hide this judgment from the patient. The discovering dentist can contact the dentist whose work had a bad outcome or possibly the local dental society. What is the proper balance between obligations to this and other patients, and obligations to one's fellow dentist? As in other professions, obligations to the patient ordinarily take preeminence in dentistry, but this principle does not yield automatic answers to the complexities of such situations.

To take another example: As more and more graduating dentists find themselves financially unable to establish solo practices, what is the proper relationship between an employing dentist and an employed dentist? These relationships are sometimes very beneficial on both sides, and sometimes ethically problematic, as when internal performance standards push an employed dentist to provide care that is below the level of quality that he or she judges appropriate. The professional literature is just beginning to discuss these relationships as ethical matters, rather than merely practical or business matters.

Another area of coprofessional relations concerns race and gender discrimination within the profession. Until the 1970s, dentistry in the United States was almost exclusively the domain of white males. The last quarter of the century saw increasing numbers of women and minorities accepted to dental schools and moving into professional practice. But by 1993, still only about 10 percent of the country's 150,000 practicing dentists were women, although women made up more than a third of the dental school population that year.

There are also situations in which members of different professions are caring for the same patients. Many dentists, for example, work very closely with dental hygienists, whose professional skills and central professional values are closely related to, but significantly distinct from, those of dentists. In the best relationships, their differences complement one another to the benefit of the patient. But in other situations, the skills of the dental hygienist may be demeaned or dental hygiene's status as a profession challenged. Implicit in each profession's ethical commitments is an obligation to develop a relationship that is most conducive to mutual respect and to the well-being of its patients.

Relations between dentists and the larger community. The activities of every profession involve numerous relationships with the larger community as a whole and with important subgroups of it. Both the dental profession and individual dentists have obligations to monitor the quality of dental work and practice, and to report and address instances of inferior work and unethical practice. They also relate to the community as dental-health educators, both by direct educational efforts and by monitoring the dependability and effectiveness of dental-care products offered to the public. Dentists' relationships with the larger community bring responsibilities regarding the proper standards for professional advertising. Dentists have an important role in public-health efforts, both in preserving public oral health and also in regard to serious epidemic diseases like HIV infection in the larger community. Individual dentists and the dental profession as a whole also have responsibilities regarding access to dental care for people with unmet dental needs. Dentists also may be obligated to be educationally and politically active when policies are being made to determine how the society will distribute its health-care resources.

Organized dentistry

Ultimately, the content of a profession's obligations is the product of a dialogue between the profession and the larger community that entrusts it and its members with a high degree of autonomy in practice, including the power of self-regulation. In the case of dentistry, this dialogue is often subtle and informal. Codes of ethics formulated by professional organizations and in state dental-practice acts never articulate more than a small part of its content. If the larger community had no part in this dialogue, its trust of a profession would make no sense, but the community exercises its role more often by passive tolerance than by active articulation. So the initiative ordinarily falls first to the members of the profession to articulate, in word and action, the current understanding of the profession's ethical commitments within a given society.

While the dental profession, properly speaking, includes every dentist who practices competently and ethically, those who speak for the profession most articulately and are heard most widely are dentistry's professional organizations. Therefore, these organizations have a special responsibility to foster reflection on and contribute to discussion of dental ethics. Dental organizations, such as the American Dental Association (ADA) and the American College of Dentists (ACD), have been quite active in regard to ethical issues. There have also been issues that temporarily focused many dentists' attention on dentistry's ethical commitments, for example, when the ADA's Council on Dental Therapeutics first awarded its Seal of Approval to a commercial dentifrice (Dummett and Dummett, 1986) and when the ADA first issued a policy statement regarding dentists' obligation to treat HIV-positive patients (Ozar, 1993).

But until the late 1970s, most dental organizations fulfilled this responsibility chiefly through editorials and other hortatory articles in their journals and through a published code of conduct. Detailed, carefully reasoned discussions of ethical issues, in which assumptions were explicit and alternative points of view were accounted for, or that carefully reflected on the profession and its specific features, or that examined ethical issues as they arose in particular cases, were few and far between. Even the published codes of conduct, significant as they have been as representative articulations of dentistry's professional commitments, did not exhaust the contents of dental ethics or effectively address all the issues as they arose.

Since the late 1970s, however, the level of interest in and sophisticated discussion of ethical issues within organized dentistry has increased steadily. Responding to newly significant ethical issues in a rapidly changing social climate, the ADA's Council on Ethics, Bylaws, and Judicial Affairs has prepared, after considerable debate in print and other forums, a number of revisions and amendments of the ADA's *Principles of Ethics and Code of Professional Conduct* (1992). The ADA and its Council have also sponsored national workshops and other educational programs on specific ethical issues facing the dental community. The *Journal of the American Dental Association* initiated a regular feature on dental ethics, "Ethics at Chairside," which moved to the American Academy of General Dentistry's journal, *General Dentistry,* in 1991.

The ACD sponsored several national workshops and a national grass-roots educational program to train dentists in more sophisticated forms of reflection on ethical issues. Many other dental organizations have incorporated programs on dental ethics into their meetings and published scholarly and popular articles on these topics in their journals. A number of them also undertook major revisions of their codes of ethics. A new organization, the Professional Ethics in Dentistry Network (PEDNET), founded in 1982 by a group of dental school faculty members, grew into a national and international organization with members in full-time practice as well as representatives from organized dentistry, dental schools, dental hygiene, and the larger health-care ethics community.

Dental education

The changing climate of dental practice from the late 1970s into the 1980s and a much-heightened awareness of ethical issues throughout the dental profession during that period also brought about changes in dental schools. Until then, few dental schools had formal programs in dental ethics. Inspirational lectures by respected senior faculty or local or national heroes were the standard fare (Odom, 1982). But with prompting from the American Association of Dental Schools (AADS), the ACD, and the ADA, dental schools began offering formal programs in dental ethics. They identified faculty with interest in dental ethics who began to develop curricular materials and to network with faculty in other institutions. The University of Minnesota pioneered an innovative four-year curriculum in dental ethics in the early 1980s. A new scholarly journal, the *Journal of Law and Ethics in Dentistry,* was founded. PEDNET grew into a major resource for dental-ethics educators and, at its national meetings, a locus for scholarly discussion of issues in dental ethics.

The work of the 1980s culminated in a joint project of the AADS, ADA, and ACD to produce "Curriculum Guidelines on Ethics and Professionalism in Dentistry." In the early 1990s, several new textbooks were published, the number of scholarly articles on issues in dental ethics increased, and additional educational programs and materials were developed for use in the classroom, in the clinic, and in continuing education programs.

Dentistry as a profession has always taken dental ethics seriously. But as a field of study, a subdiscipline within the study of moral theory and professional ethics, dental ethics is still quite young. Nevertheless, as this work is taken more seriously and participated in more widely by practicing dentists, dental school faculty and students, and leaders of organized dentistry, the dental profession's norms and their implications for daily practice will be understood more clearly, and creative dialogue about the ethical practice of dentistry will grow more widespread and sophisticated.

DAVID T. OZAR

Directly related to this entry are the entries PROFESSION AND PROFESSIONAL ETHICS; ALLIED HEALTH PROFESSIONS; *and* LICENSING, DISCIPLINE, AND REGULATION IN THE HEALTH PROFESSIONS. *For a further discussion of topics mentioned in this article, see the entries* AIDS; AUTONOMY; BENEFICENCE; COMPETENCE; HEALTH-CARE FINANCING, *article on* HEALTH-CARE INSURANCE; *and* INFORMED CONSENT, *article on* MEANING AND ELEMENTS OF INFORMED CONSENT. *Other relevant material may be found under the entries* CLINICAL ETHICS, *article on* ELEMENTS AND METHODOLOGIES; PROFESSIONAL–PATIENT RELATIONSHIP, *article on* ETHICAL ISSUES; *and* TEAMS, HEALTH-CARE. *See also the* APPENDIX (CODES, OATHS, AND DIRECTIVES RELATED TO BIOETHICS), SECTION III: ETHICAL DIRECTIVES FOR OTHER HEALTH-CARE PROFES-

SIONS, PRINCIPLES OF ETHICS *of the* AMERICAN DENTAL ASSOCIATION.

Bibliography

AMERICAN ASSOCIATION OF DENTAL SCHOOLS. 1989. "Curriculum Guidelines on Ethics and Professionalism in Dentistry." *Journal of Dental Education* 53, no. 2:144–148.

AMERICAN DENTAL ASSOCIATION. 1992. *ADA Principles of Ethics and Code of Professional Conduct, with Official Advisory Opinions.* Chicago: Author. (Revised periodically.)

BEBEAU, MURIEL J. 1991. "Ethics for the Practicing Dentist: Can Ethics be Taught?" *Journal of the American College of Dentists* 58, no. 1:5, 10–15.

BEBEAU, MURIEL J.; SPIDEL, THOMAS M.; and YAMOOR, CATHERINE M. 1982. *A Professional Responsibility Curriculum for Dental Education.* Minneapolis: University of Minnesota Press.

BOGERT, JOHN, and CREEDON, ROBERT, eds. 1989. *Behavior Management for the Pediatric Dental Patient.* Chicago: American Academy of Pediatric Dentistry.

BURNS, CHESTER R. 1974. "The Evolution of Professional Ethics in American Dentistry." *Bulletin of the History of Dentistry* 22, no. 2:59–70.

CHIODO, GARY T., and TOLLE, SUSAN W. 1992. "Diminished Autonomy: Can a Person with Dementia Consent to Dental Treatment?" *General Dentistry* 40, no. 5:372–373.

DUMMETT, CLIFTON O., and DUMMETT, LOIS DOYLE. 1986. *The Hillenbrand Era: Organized Dentistry's "Glanzperiode."* Bethesda, Md.: American College of Dentists.

HIRSCH, ALLAN C., and GERT, BARNARD. 1986. "Ethics in Dental Practice." *Journal of the American Dental Association* 113, no. 4:599–603.

HOROWITZ, HERSCHELL S. 1978. "Overview of Ethical Issues in Clinical Studies." *Journal of Public Health Dentistry* 38, no. 1:35–43.

JONG, ANTHONY, and HEINE, CAROLE SUE. 1982. "The Teaching of Ethics in the Dental Hygiene Curriculum." *Journal of Dental Education* 46, no. 12:699–702.

McCULLOUGH, LAURENCE B. 1993. "Ethical Issues in Dentistry." In *Clark's Clinical Dentistry,* rev. ed., vol. 1, pp. 1–17. Edited by James W. Clark and Jefferson F. Hardin. Philadelphia: Lippincott.

ODOM, JOHN G. 1982. "Formal Ethics Instruction in Dental Education." *Journal of Dental Education* 46, no. 9:553–557.

OZAR, DAVID T. 1985. "Three Models of Professionalism and Professional Obligation in Dentistry." *Journal of the American Dental Association* 110, no. 2:173–177.

———. 1993. "AIDS, Ethics, and Dental Care." In *Clark's Clinical Dentistry,* rev. ed., vol. 3, pp. 1–21. Edited by James W. Clark and Jefferson Hardin. Philadelphia: Lippincott.

OZAR, DAVID T., and SOKOL, DAVID J. 1994. *Dental Ethics at Chairside: Professional Principles and Practical Applications.* St. Louis, Mo.: Mosby-Yearbook.

PROFESSIONAL ETHICS IN DENTISTRY NETWORK. 1993. *The PEDNET Bibliography, 1993.* Chicago: Author.

RULE, JAMES T., and VEATCH, ROBERT M. 1993. *Ethical Questions in Dentistry.* Chicago: Quintessence.

SEGAL, HERMAN, and WARNER, RICHARD. 1979. "Informed Consent in Dentistry." *Journal of the American Dental Association* 99, no. 6:957–958.

WEINSTEIN, BRUCE D., ed. 1993. *Dental Ethics.* Philadelphia: Lea and Febiger.

DEONTOLOGICAL ETHICS

See ETHICS, *article on* NORMATIVE ETHICAL THEORIES.

DIALYSIS

See KIDNEY DIALYSIS.

DISABILITY

I. ATTITUDES AND SOCIOLOGICAL PERSPECTIVES

"Americans with disabilities are the largest, poorest, least employed, and least educated minority in America" (West, 1991, p. xi). Until the advent of a civil rights movement of people with disabilities in the last part of the twentieth century, no medical professional, educator, or policymaker would have found such an observation noteworthy or indicative of any situation amenable to remediation. Government, medicine, and people with and without disabilities generally assumed that disabled people would be impoverished, poorly educated, unemployed, and uninvolved in most recreational or civic activities. Illness, injury, or "deformity" rendered them too physically or mentally incapacitated to perform the tasks of ordinary life.

The characterization with which this article began, and the U.S. law enacted as one effort to change this grim picture, signal reinterpretation of the situation of people with disabilities in light of scholarship and activism that has flourished since the late 1960s. During these years, people with disabilities and other advocates have argued that a substantial portion of the difficulties disabled people face can be explained by social stigma and practices that reflect and perpetuate discrimination and exclusion.

Despite the simultaneous emergence of the field of bioethics and of the movement for change in the perception of people with disabilities, bioethics has paid scant attention to the perspective that attributes most of their disadvantaged status to nonphysiological characteristics. Bioethics has largely reflected what some term the medical model of disability (Gliedman and Roth, 1980). The following discussion contrasts the major sociological perspectives on the situation of disabled people and then examines their implications for bioethics.

Health, normality, and disability

Members of a given society and historical era share a perception of what is typical physical functioning and role performance for children and adults. One commentator describes this consensus in terms of a "normal opportunity range": "The normal opportunity range for a given society is the array of life plans reasonable persons in it are likely to construct for themselves" (Daniels, 1985, p. 33). Individual physical characteristics are evaluated with reference to a standard of normality, health, and "species-typical functioning" (Boorse, 1987; Daniels, 1985).

Christopher Boorse's (1987) discussion of what signifies less than optimal health focuses on typical capacities rather than on the etiology of any problem:

> A condition of a part or process in an organism is pathological when the ability of the part or process to perform one or more of its species-typical biological functions falls below some central range of the statistical distribution for that ability. . . . (Boorse, 1987, p. 370)

Ethicists and policymakers discuss the importance of health care, urge accident prevention, and promote healthy lifestyles because they perceive a certain level of health not only as intrinsically desirable, but as prerequisite for an acceptable life.

In itself, there may be nothing to question about these descriptions of the statistical norm for or the desirability of health. Whether an individual's impaired functioning stems from prenatal injury, genetic transmission, acquired illness, or traumatic accident, people with such conditions experience difficulties in typical functioning and thus require medical treatment (and sometimes rehabilitation and other services) to cure or reduce their physiological limitations. Social, ethical, and policy questions arise in considering the connection

that does or should exist between health and the range of opportunities open to people in the population who do not meet that standard of species-typical functioning, estimated to be one-sixth of the United States population (Americans with Disabilities Act, 1990, P.L. 101–336, Section 2). People with disabilities contend not only with their physiological conditions, but also with the perceptions that they and others have about how their impairments affect their lives.

Disability as difference: The medical model

The socially accepted notion of what is typical for human beings and the level of health that has been deemed necessary for a satisfying life help to explain the social consequences for people who differ from the norm. Physicians, the academy, and charitable and governmental social welfare systems have all interpreted limitations and problems of people with disabilities as the inevitable consequences of their diagnosed physiological impairments. (See Albrecht, 1992; Gliedman and Roth, 1980, for summaries and critiques.) Despite its drawbacks, this medical view of disability resonates with nearly universal, transcultural, and transhistorical valuations of health and of a typical physical appearance and level of functioning (Albrecht, 1992; Hahn, 1988; Scheer and Groce, 1988). Unaccustomed weakness, lack of energy, acute and unrelieved pain, or sudden loss of capacity to move freely temporarily impede usual activity. The socially approved stance toward someone who has experienced an acute illness or a traumatic accident is that the individual should be excused from customary activities until recovered, and that during the recuperative process, he or she should surrender control to knowledgeable professionals whose direction should be uncritically obeyed (Parsons, 1951).

Although someone recovering from such transitory conditions as dental surgery, the flu, or a broken leg may welcome this social prescription and time to rest and heal, those with conditions that will not be totally cured discover that this same social prescription leads to long-lasting custodialization and isolation. Even specialists in rehabilitation services who adapt the medical model to those with chronic or permanent conditions (see Albrecht, 1992; Caplan et al., 1987, for discussions of rehabilitation's approach) believe that the professional is the expert in the situation and should mediate between the disabled individual and the rest of the community: "Indeed, the attitudes of these professionals may strongly influence the attitudes of members of the first social circle [family and significant associates] . . . as well as the attitudes exhibited within . . . the society at large" (Antonak and Livneh, 1988, pp. 14–15).

According to the rehabilitation medicine framework, the disabled individual should use available means to adapt and function in the community, recognizing that the disability will always impose some limits on activity. This model accepts what the disability rights movement (exemplified by Fine and Asch, 1988) works to modify: namely that the person with the condition must understand that it is he or she who diverges from the majority and he or she who must function as well as possible in a world that assumes a level of physical capability the disabled person does not possess (Fine and Asch, 1988).

Attitudes about disability and disabled persons

Perhaps because health is highly prized and illness or disability is feared, people who are atypical in appearance or function are themselves frequently feared, devalued, and excluded from ordinary social life. To the extent that medical professionals and social institutions perceive the man with a heart condition or the woman with sickle-cell disease as permanently and solely sick and in need of professional care, they will reject those who, in spite of their impairments, seek to participate in work and community life.

Confronted by another's atypical physical appearance, weakness, or pain, nondisabled people are reported to be anxious, fearful, sad, or repulsed (Livneh, 1988; Siller, 1988). Beatrice Wright (1983, 1988) points out that when those who have never known a disabled person encounter someone with a disability, they may react strongly and negatively to the person because the condition distresses or offends them. Were people exclusively rational, the nondisabled person could appreciate the norm of two arms without rejecting the person with only one; unfortunately, the negative reaction to this atypical appearance often spills over into rejecting the person with the salient characteristic. Until people have sufficient exposure to and information about a disabled person to recognize that the disability is only one among his or her myriad attributes, people may be overwhelmed and see only the physical deviation.

Nondisabled people have equated incapacity in one area with incapacity in all areas (Wright, 1983, 1988). On his way to meet a friend for lunch, the man who is blind is literally shoved into a seat on the subway because other passengers unthinkingly equate the inability to see with the inability to stand. The proprietor ignores the woman who walks with crutches and expects her nondisabled friend to give the order for both women. The fourth-grader with cystic fibrosis may have to convince her classmates and teachers that even if she takes pills, she is not too sick or weak to play soccer or go on a camping trip.

Imputing global incapacity to someone with a disability engenders strained interactions between disabled and nondisabled people. Many nondisabled people assume that they display a "positive" attitude toward those with disabilities by what Elaine Makas (1988) describes as "give the disabled person a break" behavior—for example, giving a blind person a second chance after making a mistake in a word game. Like the man who is shoved into a subway seat or the woman who is ignored by the store proprietor, the player is likely to find such behavior patronizing and insulting. Similarly offensive because it suggests that a physical condition transforms moral character is the so-called "disabled as saint" view (Makas, 1988). According to Makas's attitude survey, disabled people loathe being viewed as saintly and courageous simply for living their lives.

In contrast to the view that disabled people are saintly, other stereotypes sometimes equate physical incapacity with cognitive, psychological, and moral deficits. Some nondisabled people are reported to consider those with disabilities as morally blemished, viewing the disability as punishment for some transgression (Siller, 1988). Daniel Wikler (1987) points out, and Wright (1983) and Esther Zernitzky-Shurka (1988) confirm, that moral disapproval of disabled people is especially likely if others believe that the disability has resulted from questionable behavior such as smoking, drug use, or reckless driving. Conversely, individuals with disabilities may be excused or forgiven if their disabilities are the result of heroic endeavors, as is the case with male war veterans. Although *attitudes* toward disabled people may vary based on the origin of the disability, patronizing and discriminatory *behavior* are part of the life of virtually every disabled person.

Students of encounters between those with and without disabilities report that nondisabled people anticipate that they will not know how to handle themselves when with a disabled person. They will help too much or too little, either overemphasizing disability or failing to consider it when the disabled person expects them to do so. The disabled person will not be able to join them in any of their typical social, work, or leisure activities (Davis, 1961; Gliedman and Roth, 1980). The nondisabled person may fear that time spent with disabled persons will be unrewarding at best and emotionally (if not financially) costly (Stroman, 1982).

All these psychological mechanisms may explain why, as Erving Goffman describes it, stigmatized people are treated by others as "not quite human" (Goffman, 1963, p. 5). Persons whose disabilities are visible may arouse more stigma than those with nonvisible impairments (Hahn, 1988; Richardson, 1976), but as Goffman takes pains to make clear, when people with nonvisible differences reveal them to others, they often encounter hostility, aversion, and discomfort. People with epilepsy (even if it does not result in a visible seizure) frequently meet rejection when others find out about their condition (Schneider and Conrad, 1983).

Attitude researchers note that expressed negative

views decrease with higher levels of education; that being female correlates with being more accepting of people with disabilities; and that more frequent contact with disabled people increases the positive views of the nondisabled (Antonak and Livneh, 1988). Rehabilitation professionals, who are often women with advanced education and specialized training and who work closely with disabled persons, might be expected to display relatively positive attitudes and serve to dispel public prejudice. Reviews of attitude literature, however, reveal that rehabilitation and other medical personnel are not markedly more accepting of disabled people than others are (Geskie and Salasek, 1988). In order for contact with disabled and other disadvantaged people to alleviate prejudices and stereotypes, the interaction needs to be equal-status, and should take place outside of medical settings (Antonak and Livneh, 1988; Wright, 1988). In fact, the interaction between rehabilitation professionals and disabled patients replicates one of the most common (and potentially detrimental) stereotypes in the literature about disability, namely, that the disabled individual is always the recipient of help rather than sometimes the recipient, at other times, the provider, and at still other times, simply a collaborating equal group member (Fine and Asch, 1988).

Disability as difference: The minority group model

"Society's negative attitudes toward its members who are disabled create real obstacles to the fulfillment of their roles and the attainment of their life goals" (Antonak and Livneh, 1988, p. 14). Proponents of the view that people with disabilities constitute a disadvantaged social minority focus on attitudes and practices that preclude their full participation in society. Although there is no accurate estimate of the size of what has become known as the disability rights movement (Scotch, 1989), nearly three-fourths of disabled United States residents surveyed by Louis Harris in 1986 said they felt a common identity with other disabled people, irrespective of impairment, and nearly half compared disability to a racial or ethnic minority status (Harris, 1986).

This minority-group view is compatible with that portion of the medical and rehabilitation perspective that supports the disabled in acquiring any treatment, skills, methods, or technology that will ensure maximum functioning. However, those who hold this perspective believe that the person with the disability, and not the rehabilitation professional, must remain in charge of the goals, if not the means, of treatment and service. Furthermore, the minority-group approach rejects the notion that those with disabilities are the only people who must adapt. Adherents argue that people with physical disabilities could participate fully in family, civic, economic, and political life in a society truly

committed to including them (Gliedman and Roth, 1980; Hahn, 1983).

Contrary to the medical and social science literature that construes people as "victims" of spinal cord injury or multiple sclerosis, the minority perspective contends that disabled people are victimized primarily by society's treatment of people with atypical, "different" bodies (Fine and Asch, 1988). While acknowledging that, regardless of social arrangements, some disabilities will restrict or preclude some highly desirable activities (hearing music if one is deaf, or viewing a sunset if one is blind), the minority-group approach claims that disability is a natural human experience that society should accommodate. As Martha Minow argues, "difference—whether of disability, sex, or race—is a problem only if the majority maintains its conviction that the existing social and economic arrangements are natural and neutral" (Minow, 1990, p. 52).

Official United States law partly endorses this perspective in some of its policy, as can be seen in the following excerpt from the Americans with Disabilities Act:

> Congress finds that . . . individuals with disabilities are a discrete and insular minority who have been faced with restrictions and limitations, subjected to a history of purposeful unequal treatment, and relegated to a position of political powerlessness in our society, based on characteristics that are beyond the control of such individuals and resulting from stereotypic assumptions not truly indicative of the individual ability of such individuals to participate in, and contribute to, society. . . . (Americans with Disabilities Act, 1990, P.L. 101–336, Section 2)

Implications for bioethics

Susan Wendell has characterized the way bioethics literature discusses disability as follows: "Under what conditions is it morally permissible/right to kill/let die a disabled person and how potentially disabled does a fetus have to be before it is permissible/right to prevent its being born?" (Wendell, 1989, p. 104).

Along with the paradigm of patient autonomy and self-determination, the disability-rights movement argues for consumer control of medical decision making and for detailed, individualized procedures for a genuinely informed consent. Despite this significant philosophical similarity between the disability rights movement and bioethics, however, bioethicists approach disability issues from a largely medicalized, rather than minority-group, vantage point. Perhaps because bioethics has concentrated on acute-care medicine (Caplan et al., 1987), and because philosophical and clinical bioethics have been influenced by the values and norms of the medical profession, bioethicists show little awareness of the minority-group, social-problem approach to life with disability.

Daniel Callahan, for example, approaches disability from within the medical model. In a 1988 article on families with disabled members, he framed the problem as one of finding a way for nondisabled relatives to flourish and not to be "burdened" with the care of a spouse, parent, or child with a disability. Callahan's analysis assumes that a family member's disability inevitably hinders the life plans of nondisabled family members. The article omits any discussion of the life plans of people with disabilities and portrays the disabled member as solely and inevitably draining the physical and emotional resources of others, rather than as at times draining, at times contributing, by virtue of all their qualities.

Callahan, Earl Shelp (1986), and many other philosophical ethicists make two assumptions that needlessly undermine the position of disabled people and those involved with them. First, they conclude that relying on others for certain physical assistance renders the disabled person "dependent" and "helpless," even if it is the disabled person who directs the assistant to perform the task. Framing physical incapacity with cognitive and psychological incapacity is false and demeaning and contributes to the stigma and isolation of people with disabilities. Furthermore, by failing to differentiate emotional nurturance from physical assistance (described as "care"), they conclude that the same people who provide emotional and intellectual companionship are the only ones who can, should, or will render physical assistance. Such assumptions demonstrate that—at least with respect to people with disabilities—many bioethicists operate within an ethics that values individualism, control, and perfection; values that, instead, they should join others in challenging (Asch, 1992; Minow, 1990; Sherwin, 1992). Approaches like those of Martha Minow (1990), Susan Sherwin (1992) and many writers with a disability-movement perspective (Hahn, 1987; Biklen, 1987; Asch, 1989, 1992) explore what sorts of changes in society would benefit the flourishing of all its members.

Whether they caution against prenatal diagnosis and selective abortion (Kass, 1985) or endorse it as a means of reducing suffering (Bayles, 1984; Elias and Annas, 1987; Steinbock, 1986, 1988), many other bioethics commentators do so without challenging existing social arrangements. Leon Kass, for example, argues for halting prenatal diagnoses and selective abortion primarily because he believes that nondisabled people learn compassion from caring for those with disabilities, not because he believes disabled people can lead lives that are meaningful and valuable for themselves and others. Conversely, Bonnie Steinbock supports claims for "wrongful life" on behalf of those born with disabilities:

We owe it to our children to see that they are not born with such serious impairments that their most basic interests will be doomed in advance. If being born to a surrogate is a handicap of this magnitude, comparable to being born blind or deaf or severely mentally retarded, then surrogacy can be seen as wronging the offspring. (Steinbock, 1988, p. 49)

A bioethics view informed by a disability analysis contends that people with impairments may contribute to their families and their society by virtue of all their characteristics, of which impairment is only one (Asch, 1989). Such a view recognizes that even in an inhospitable social milieu, many people with disabilities already lead lives that satisfy them and contribute to the lives of others, with interests that are not "doomed in advance."

The disability perspective on treatment of disabled newborns, physician-assisted suicide, and prenatal diagnosis and selective abortion shares nothing with the "right-to-life" analysis, with which it is often linked in bioethics discussion (Robertson, 1990). Although this disability perspective acknowledges that some disabled people may exercise self-determination in deciding to end their lives, it departs from much of traditional bioethics (Beauchamp and Childress, 1994) by pointing out that often these decisions occur in a context of prejudice and discrimination and before disabled people have gained access to community supports that might ease their difficulties. (Compare essays in Kliever, 1989, with Biklen, 1987; Fine and Asch, 1988; and Herr et al., 1992.) When people informed by a disability-rights analysis discuss these subjects, they argue that people with disabilities are as worthy of life and as able to benefit from and contribute to it as those who do not have disabilities; they then call for bioethics to honor the validity of a disabled person's claim for life and to endorse social changes that would improve life as vigorously as bioethics upholds the decisions of the disabled to end their lives (Asch, 1989; Biklen, 1987; Hahn, 1987).

ADRIENNE ASCH

Directly related to this article are the other articles in this entry: PHILOSOPHICAL AND THEOLOGICAL PERSPECTIVES, HEALTH CARE AND PHYSICAL DISABILITY, *and* LEGAL ISSUES. *For a further discussion of topics mentioned in this article, see the entries* GENETIC TESTING AND SCREENING, *articles on* PREIMPLANTATION EMBRYO DIAGNOSIS *and* PRENATAL DIAGNOSIS; HEALTH AND DISEASE, *articles on* SOCIOLOGICAL PERSPECTIVES, ANTHROPOLOGICAL PERSPECTIVES, *and* THE EXPERIENCE OF HEALTH AND ILLNESS; *and* REHABILITATION MEDICINE. *For a discussion of related ideas, see the entries* AUTHORITY; CHRONIC CARE; DEATH AND DYING: EUTHANASIA AND SUSTAINING LIFE, *article on* ETHICAL ISSUES; GENE THERAPY, *article on* STRATEGIES FOR GENE THERAPY; INFORMED

CONSENT, *article on* MEANING AND ELEMENTS OF IN-FORMED CONSENT; PERSON; PROFESSIONAL–PATIENT RE-LATIONSHIP, *articles on* HISTORICAL PERSPECTIVES, *and* SOCIOLOGICAL PERSPECTIVES; *and* SUICIDE.

Bibliography

ALBRECHT, GARY L. 1992. *The Disability Business: Rehabilitation in America.* Newbury Park, Calif.: Sage.

ANTONAK, RICHARD F., and LIVNEH, HANOCH. 1988. *The Measurement of Attitudes Toward People with Disabilities: Methods, Psychometrics, and Scales.* Springfield, Ill.: Charles C. Thomas.

ASCH, ADRIENNE. 1989. "Reproductive Technology and Disability." In *Reproductive Laws for the 1990s,* pp. 69–124. Edited by Sherrill Cohen and Nadine Taub. Clifton, N.J.: Humana.

———. 1993. "Abused or Neglected Clients—Or Abusive or Neglectful Service Systems?" In *Ethical Conflicts in the Management of Home Care: The Case Manager's Dilemma,* pp. 113–121. Edited by Rosalie A. Kane and Arthur L. Caplan. New York: Springer.

BAYLES, MICHAEL D. 1984. *Reproductive Ethics.* Englewood Cliffs, N.J.: Prentice-Hall.

BEAUCHAMP, TOM L., and CHILDRESS, JAMES F. 1994. *Principles of Biomedical Ethics.* 4th ed. New York: Oxford University Press.

BIKLEN, DOUGLAS. 1987. "Framed: Print Journalism's Treatment of Disability Issues." In *Images of the Disabled, Disabling Images,* pp. 79–93. Edited by Alan Gartner and Tom Joe. New York: Praeger.

BOORSE, CHRISTOPHER. 1987. "Concepts of Health." In *Health Care Ethics: An Introduction,* pp. 359–393. Edited by Donald VanDeVeer and Tom Regan. Philadelphia: Temple University Press.

CALLAHAN, DANIEL. 1988. "Families as Caregivers: The Limits of Morality." *Archives of Physical Medicine and Rehabilitation* 69, no. 5:323–328.

CAPLAN, ARTHUR L.; CALLAHAN, DANIEL; and HAAS, JANET. 1987. "Ethical and Public Policy Issues in Rehabilitation Medicine." *Hastings Center Report* 17, no. 4 (spec. suppl.): 1–20.

DANIELS, NORMAN. 1985. *Just Health Care.* New York: Cambridge University Press.

DAVIS, FRED. 1961. "Deviance Disavowal: The Management of Strained Interaction by the Visibly Handicapped." *Social Problems* 9, no. 2:120–132.

ELIAS, SHERMAN, and ANNAS, GEORGE J. 1987. *Reproductive Genetics and the Law.* Chicago: Year Book Medical.

FINE, MICHELLE, and ASCH, ADRIENNE. 1988. "Disability Beyond Stigma: Social Interaction, Discrimination, and Activism." *Journal of Social Issues* 44, no. 1:3–21.

GESKIE, MARY ANNE, and SALASEK, JAMES L. 1988. "Attitudes of Health Care Personnel Toward Persons with Disabilities." In *Attitudes Toward Persons with Disabilities,* pp. 187–200. Edited by Harold E. Yuker. New York: Springer.

GLIEDMAN, JOHN, and ROTH, WILLIAM. 1980. *The Unexpected Minority: Handicapped Children in America.* New York: Harcourt Brace Jovanovich.

GOFFMAN, ERVING. 1963. *Stigma: Notes on the Management of Spoiled Identity.* Englewood Cliffs, N.J.: Prentice-Hall.

HAHN, HARLAN. 1983. "Paternalism and Public Policy." *Society* 20, no. 3:36–46.

———. 1987a. "Civil Rights for Disabled Americans: The Foundation of a Political Agenda." In *Images of the Disabled: Disabling Images,* pp. 181–204. Edited by Alan Gartner and Tom Joe. New York: Praeger.

———. 1987b. "Public Policy and Disabled Infants: A Sociopolitical Perspective." *Issues in Law and Medicine* 3, no. 1:3–27.

———. 1988. "The Politics of Physical Differences: Disability and Discrimination." *Journal of Social Issues* 44, no. 1:39–47.

HARRIS, LOUIS, and ASSOCIATES. 1986. *The ICD Survey of Disabled Americans: Bringing Disabled Americans into the Mainstream, A Nationwide Survey of 1,000 Disabled People.* New York: Author.

HERR, STANLEY S.; BOSTROM, BARRY A.; and BARTON, REBECCA S. 1992. "No Place to Go: Refusal of Life-Sustaining Treatment by Competent Persons with Physical Disabilities." *Issues in Law and Medicine* 8, no. 1:3–36.

KASS, LEON R. 1985. *Toward a More Natural Science: Biology and Human Affairs.* New York: Free Press.

KLIEVER, LONNIE D., ed. 1989. *Dax's Case: Essays in Medical Ethics and Human Meaning.* Dallas, Tex.: Southern Methodist University Press.

LIVNEH, HANOCH. 1988. "A Dimensional Perspective on the Origin of Negative Attitudes Toward Persons with Disabilities." In *Attitudes Toward Persons with Disabilities,* pp. 35–46. Edited by Harold E. Yuker. New York: Springer.

MAKAS, ELAINE. 1988. "Positive Attitudes Toward Disabled People: Disabled and Non-Disabled Persons' Perspectives." *Journal of Social Issues* 44, no. 1:49–61.

MINOW, MARTHA. 1990. *Making All the Difference: Inclusion, Exclusion, and American Law.* Ithaca, N.Y.: Cornell University Press.

PARSONS, TALCOTT. 1951. *The Social System.* Glencoe, Ill.: Free Press.

RICHARDSON, STEPHEN A. 1976. "Attitudes and Behavior Toward the Physically Handicapped." *Birth Defects: Original Article Series* 12, no. 4:15–34.

ROBERTSON, JOHN A. 1990. "Procreative Liberty and Human Genetics." *Emory Law Journal* 39, no. 3:697–719.

SCHEER, JESSICA, and GROCE, NORA. 1988. "Impairment as a Human Constant: Cross-Cultural and Historical Perspectives on Variation." *Journal of Social Issues* 44, no. 1:23–37.

SCHNEIDER, JOSEPH W., and CONRAD, PETER. 1983. *Having Epilepsy: The Experience and Control of Illness.* Philadelphia: Temple University Press.

SCOTCH, RICHARD K. 1989. "Politics and Policy in the History of the Disability Rights Movement." *Milbank Quarterly* 67, suppl. 2, pt. 2:380–400.

SHELP, EARL E. 1986. *Born To Die?: Deciding the Fate of Critically Ill Newborns.* New York: Free Press.

SHERWIN, SUSAN. 1992. *No Longer Patient: Feminist Ethics and Health Care.* Philadelphia, Pa.: Temple University Press.

SILLER, JEROME. 1988. "Intrapsychic Aspects of Attitudes Toward Persons with Disabilities." In *Attitudes Toward Per-*

sons with Disabilities, pp. 58–67. Edited by Harold E. Yuker. New York: Springer.

STEINBOCK, BONNIE. 1986. "The Logical Case for 'Wrongful Life.'" Hastings Center Report 16, no. 2:15–20.

———. 1988. "Surrogate Motherhood as Prenatal Adoption." Law, Medicine and Health Care 16, nos. 1–2:44–50.

STROMAN, DUANE F. 1982. The Awakening Minorities: The Physically Handicapped. Washington, D.C.: University Press of America.

WENDELL, SUSAN. 1989. "Toward a Feminist Theory of Disability." Hypatia 4, no. 2:104–124.

WEST, JANE, ed. 1991. The Americans with Disabilities Act: From Policy to Practice. New York: Milbank Memorial Fund.

WIKLER, DANIEL. 1987. "Personal Responsibility for Illness." In Health Care Ethics: An Introduction, pp. 326–358. Edited by Donald VanDeVeer and Tom Regan. Philadelphia: Temple University Press.

WRIGHT, BEATRICE A. 1983. Physical Disability: A Psychosocial Approach. 2d ed. New York: Harper & Row.

———. 1988. "Attitudes and the Fundamental Negative Bias: Conditions and Corrections." In Attitudes Toward Persons with Disabilities, pp. 3–21. Edited by Harold E. Yuker. New York: Springer.

ZERNITZKY-SHURKA, ESTHER. 1988. "The Impact of Cultural, Ethnic, Religious, and National Variables on Attitudes Toward Persons with a Physical Disability: A Review." In Attitudes Toward Persons with Disabilities, pp. 96–106. Edited by Harold E. Yuker. New York: Springer.

II. PHILOSOPHICAL AND THEOLOGICAL PERSPECTIVES

How we understand what it means to be "normal" shapes our understanding of what it is to be "disabled." In a particular society, those who describe and name what it is to be normal have the power also to shape that society's treatment of and response to those considered to be "disabled." The values that supply the criteria for defining "normal" and "disabled" reflect and reveal what that society believes about what causes a disability, and what meaning disability has.

What is normal, then—and what is not—is defined by the social, cultural context. Historically, disabling conditions are social phenomena. Society not only selects which characteristics are to be considered normal, but also constructs a description of what is a disability. For example, in the case of mental retardation, there have always been persons whose marked cognitive impairments have made it almost impossible for them to meet the demands of their communities. What has changed throughout time is "our understanding of the nature of the construct to explain limited intellectual functioning and its consequence—social incompetence" (Vitello and Soskin, 1985, p. 1).

As late as 1983, the American Association on Mental Deficiency (AAMD) described mental retardation as a condition whereby one's intellectual, cognitive functioning was seen as significantly subaverage, existing concurrently with other deficits in one's adaptive skills. However, in 1992, this same organization, renamed the American Association on Mental Retardation (AAMR), no longer defined mental retardation as an intellectual impairment, but as a social dysfunction. Yet this dysfunction was still characterized by subaverage intellectual functioning, existing concurrently with other related limitations in social skills. There have been nine revisions of the definition of mental retardation in the United States since 1921. What is consistent in all these definitions is that this disability questions the full use of one's mind, a highly valued characteristic of being human. That is the reason we refer to such a condition as "mental" retardation.

Not only do the labels and categories within a disabling condition change, but more labels and categories that try to explain the cause, nature, and symptoms of various conditions are added. For example, the American Psychiatric Association's (APA) fourth Diagnostic and Statistical Manual of Mental Disorders, DSM-IV, widely used by health-service professionals for both diagnosis and prognosis of all psychologically based disabilities, describes 292 possible diagnoses of mental problems, up from the 106 disorders named in 1952 when the DSM-I was published (APA, 1994).

The existence of different, changing, and growing numbers of definitions of disabling conditions reflects the various, often contradictory perspectives present in society, which have implications for clinical practice, research, administration of programs, and educational and religious programs. What were once universally accepted definitions and descriptions of normality and disabling conditions have been continually deconstructed and reconstructed by various groups who vie for power in determining how society perceives and names what is normal and disabled. Such clashes affect people with disabilities and their families.

For example, consider three contrasting perspectives, each having powerful professional associations to advocate for a particular perception: (1) the medical-scientific model; (2) the ecological-social model; and (3) the religious-moral model.

Medical-scientific model. This perspective on disabling conditions defines the etiology and subsequent treatment of a disabling condition as physiological in nature. For example, in the earlier part of the twentieth century, the scientist H. H. Goddard, director of research at the Vineland Training School for Feeble-Minded Girls and Boys in New Jersey, developed the hereditarian theory of mental retardation; he called those with developmental disabilities "morons." He maintained that a single gene was the cause of mental retardation and that if this one gene could be traced and located, then it could be bred out of existence (Gould, 1981).

Later in the century, ethicist Joseph Fletcher, author of *Situation Ethics* (1966), questioned if anyone with an I.Q. below twenty is a person: "*Homo* is indeed *sapiens*, in order to be home. . . . Mere biological life, before minimal intelligence is achieved or after it is lost irretrievably, is without personal status. This has bearing, obviously, on decision making in gynecology, obstetrics and pediatrics, as well as in general surgery and medicine" (Fletcher, 1974, p. 4).

Social-ecological model.   This model advocates the view that many of the disability labels and categories, such as "learning disabled," are themselves modern phenomena invented, not discovered, through social and political forces. The label "learning disabled" was not listed as a disability in the Mental Retardation Facilities and Community Mental Health Centers Construction Act of 1963 (P.L. 88–164). Instead, educator-historian James Carrier understands special education itself as responsible for inventing such labels as "learning disabled" and applying them to the "have-nots" in society, which usually meant poor families with children marked for life in menial, service-oriented positions (Carrier, 1986).

There have also been theories of how the environment creates disabling conditions. Consider sociocultural retardation, which has been associated with low income, crowding, poor housing, and large families in which the mothers held unskilled jobs prior to marriage. The I.Q. of these children has been measured to be between 55 and 69. The label "six-hour retarded child" acknowledges another form of sociocultural retardation, describing the child who is unable to perform well academically but who excels once he or she leaves/finishes school (Edgerton, 1979).

Religious-moral model.   Ever since the disciples of Jesus asked the question, "Who sinned, this man or his parents that he was born blind?" (John 9:2), some people in the Christian church have drawn a direct causal relationship between one's moral life and a disabling condition. Even though Jesus explained that his healing of the man was primarily a way to reveal his relationship with the Creator, people have failed to read this part of the passage. Instead, the position has been taken that a disabling condition is associated with sin, and an equally erroneous position is taken that the disability will be miraculously cured if the sin is confessed, with the burden on the people with disabilities to rid themselves of their sin.

In 1652, the Reformation leader Martin Luther was to have said that people with mental retardation should be drowned, for "such changelings were merely a mass of flesh, a *massa carnis*, with no soul. For it is in the Devil's power that he corrupts people who have reason and souls, when he possesses them. The Devil sits in such changelings where their soul should have been" (Scheerenberger, 1987, p. 32). There are still many congregations and parishes that associate one's disabling condition, or the disability of a member, with the sinful condition of one's moral character.

There have been religious groups who have approached disabling conditions as another agenda of "liberation theology," calling God a "Disabled God," as well as those who have called themselves "evangelical," establishing separate churches and organizations just for Christians with certain disabling conditions. A "liberation theology of disability" is based on the understanding that people with disabilities are an oppressed, disenfranchised group of people who wish to be known as individuals, not as a disabling condition (Cooper, 1992).

There are various competing, often contradictory, perceptions of disabilities that professionals and disabled people alike name, and subsequently use, in treating others who have disabilities. Our understanding of what is normal and what is disabled is determined and taught by the primary community in which we are members. This community itself has been formed by either the theological or philosophical narratives and treatises that somehow provide people with a common viewpoint, particularly of disabling conditions. The philosopher Stephen Crites writes that these fundamental stories, be they sacred or secular, provide people with a sense of self and of the world that is created through them. Using such fundamental stories, and the authority ascribed to them, people can understand their own stories (Crites, 1989).

We depend upon these theological and philosophical narratives to provide the perspective necessary in explaining the unexplainable: Why are some people different from other people? As will be covered in the following section, this is as true today as it has been in various human communities throughout history; groups of people try to come to terms with differences in the human condition and search for meaning for disabling conditions.

Theological perspectives on disabilities

Religion has always shaped human understanding of what is normal and abnormal. For example, anthropologist Mary Douglas tells the story of the Nuer in Africa, who would throw their deformed babies into the river because they believed that the gods gave them the wrong babies and these disabled infants really belonged to the hippopotamuses. Their religious narrative, which formed their community, explained not only the condition of the infant but also the course of action in treating the child's disability—return the child to the rightful parents, the hippopotamuses (Douglas, 1966). Historian

Robert Scheerenberger writes that the power of a religious community's narrative in naming disabling conditions and proposed treatments can be traced back as far as 7000 B.C.E., when primitive people called upon the help of the spiritual authority, a shaman, to cure those who were ill. Often the cure consisted of exorcising evil spirits that were afflicting people. In the Babylonian Empire (1700–560 B.C.E.), a disability was perceived as punishment by a god because of someone's sin (Scheerenberger, 1987).

The theological narrative, as recorded in the Old and New Testaments, has also shaped the practices of how the people of God perceived, treated, and lived with people with disabilities.

The Old Testament and people with disabilities. While in other civilizations people were shunned or ostracized because of their disabling conditions, this was not naturally so in ancient Jewish society. According to the Genesis account of the exile of Adam and Eve from the Garden, enmity, strife, and pain became a part of the human condition (Gen. 3:14–24). In Jewish society, a disabling condition was not a reason for ostracism from the community as a whole. Granted, men with disabilities could not perform in temple worship. For example, consider this proclamation in Leviticus regarding temple worship:

> No one of your offspring throughout their generations who has a blemish may approach to offer the food of his God. For no one who has a blemish shall draw near, one who is blind, or lame, or one who has a mutilated face or a limb too long, or one who has a broken foot or a broken hand, or a hunch back, or a dwarf, or a man with a blemish in his eyes or an itching disease to scabs or crushed testicles. (Lev. 21:17–20, NRSV)

While this rule covered temple worship, which also excluded women and children, it is important to understand that one's "blemish" did not mean that one was to be excluded from being part of Jewish ritualistic life in total. Consider this verse: "He [the one with a disability] may eat of the food of his God, of the most holy as well as of the holy" (Lev. 21:22). Such exhortations to provide care for people with disabilities can be found throughout the Old Testament. In Deuteronomy, it is written that no one should make it harder for one who is blind: "Cursed be anyone who misleads a blind person on the road" (Deut. 27:18). Or again, in Leviticus (19:14): "You shall not revile the deaf or put a stumbling block before the blind; you shall fear your God: I am the Lord."

The stories of the Old Testament relate God's great concern for how neighbors were treated and cared for, especially neighbors with disabilities. People were to care for each other just as God loved and cared for his creation in spite of its sinful condition. In Isaiah

(43:8), God is bringing back the people of Israel from their Babylonian exile; the promise includes those with disabilities: "Bring forth the people who are blind, yet have eyes, who are deaf, yet have ears! You are my witnesses . . . and my servant whom I have chosen, so that you may know and believe me and understand that I am he."

Certain leaders of the children of Israel had what could be considered disabling conditions. For example, Jacob, the son of Isaac, wrestled with an angel, and even though he received a blessing from the angel, his hip was put out of joint, and he was left with a distinct limp (Gen. 32:31). Moses was thought to have had a speech impairment: "I am slow of speech and slow of tongue" (Exod. 4:10). But God did not reserve his missions for those who could only walk or speak well: "Who gives speech to mortals? Who makes them mute or deaf, seeing or blind? Is it not I, the Lord? Now go, and I will be with your mouth and teach you what you are to speak" (Exod. 4:12–13). Throughout the Old Testament, people with disabilities were thought to be disabled not because of a wrathful, avenging God; they were to have a secure place among the children of Israel. This tradition was continued in the ministry of Jesus Christ.

The New Testament and people with disabilities. Although some Christian communities maintain that they have the power to heal those with disabilities who have the "proper" faith, and although people with disabilities are cast in some Christian stories as objects of charity to be pitied, these approaches are not promoted in the Gospel accounts of Jesus of Nazareth's ministry on Earth. Instead, the image of God who sided with those who were oppressed, barely living on the margins of society, was given new expression in the ministry of Jesus.

According to all four Gospel accounts, Jesus kept company with the outcasts of Jewish society, including those with disabilities. Jesus even incorporated people with disabilities in stories about the kingdom of God, such as the parable of the Great Banquet Feast, at which those who finally came were not the able-bodied but people with disabilities (Luke 14:15–24), or the story of the woman with internal hemorrhaging who faithfully believed that Jesus alone could heal her affliction (Mark 5:34). Jesus' intimate relationship with the Creator was revealed in restoring sight to the man who was blind when the Pharisees and disciples thought that the condition was a situation of divine retribution for some past sin committed by the person in question (John 9:1–34).

It was this close identification with people, including people with disabilities, that became the model of ministry for others who were interested in following Jesus. First, Christians believed that Jesus not only preached the Good News but was the Good News incarnate, able to identify and meet the material and spiritual needs of people. Second, Christians believed that Jesus healed people physically and spiritually by literally and figuratively taking on the wounds of humanity, fulfilling the words of Isaiah: "He took our infirmities and bore our diseases" (Matt. 8:17). Finally, Jesus was able to administer this *agape*, love, because it was God in Christ who was working wonders, bringing forth a sense of new hope in the lives of those who believed in God, regardless of their abilities or limitations. God's gracious love was offered to all, not because of what we can do but because of who we are: God's children (Webb-Mitchell, 1994).

The Apostle Paul also was concerned with disease and infection of his body. Paul regarded his infirmities, "a thorn in the flesh," some kind of physical malady, as a "messenger" of Satan. He prayed to God three times for it to be taken away. His request was denied and he was told that God's grace should be sufficient for him, "For strength is completed [made perfect] in disease [weakness]" (2 Cor. 12:7–9). The lesson for Paul was that the disease was not a result of sin but instead a lesson for him: The weaker people are, the more manifest is the power of God when it works through them (O'Rourke, 1968).

From these earliest times of the Christian church, people with disabilities have either been cared for or abused by many within the church. For example, in terms of care, since the early medieval ages, a disability was often seen as a sign of grace by some Christians. They believed that as Christ healed many of their illnesses and disabilities, so sickness became a way to be purified of one's sins. Disease was suffering, and it was believed that through suffering, humanity could be completed by God's saving grace. As the person with a disability became an agent of God's grace, so, too, in caring for the disabled in one's home, a person fulfilled a Christian obligation. The person with a disability became a living symbol of the wounded Christ who called for his followers to care for the afflicted: "I was sick and you took care of me. . . . [J]ust as you did it to one of the least of these who are members of my family, you did it to me" (Matt. 25:36,40). With this rationale, monasteries established hospices that extended and formalized Christian service to those who were ill. In 436, the Council of Carthage urged the bishops to begin Christian hospices in close proximity to cathedrals (Sigerist, 1977).

However, such Christian care was not widely practiced in medieval Europe. In terms of abuse, some people with disabilities, such as mental retardation, were also considered playthings of the wealthy. For example, Pope Leo X's dinner was noted for fine food and for entertainment consisting of people with mental retardation who were "buffoons and jesters . . . where the guests were encouraged to laugh at their antics and at the cruel jokes which were played on them" (Scheerenberger, 1987).

In the sixteenth century during the Protestant Reformation, the plight of persons with disabilities may have reached one of its lowest periods. With the collapse of the church's authority, this period has been called the Age of Anxiety. People were anxious about the dramatic changes in their world, concerned that the upheavals were a possible condemnation by God. They tried various means of assuaging their anxiety: pilgrimages to holy places, increased devotion to relics, and the ceaseless drive to find some way to appease the wrath of God. Their fears were augmented by a rise in diseases, the Black Death plague, crop failures, waves of famine and pestilence, and upheaval within the Catholic Church itself, which meant the closing of many hospices.

As cited earlier, Martin Luther's own theological narrative blamed a child's mental retardation on Satan. This is not surprising in this period of reformation, as is evident in writings of the monks Johann Sprenger and Heinrich Kraemer who published *Malleus Maleficarum* (Hammer Against Witches). Sprenger and Kraemer stated that people with mental retardation should be considered witches: "If the patient can be relieved by no drugs, but rather seems to be aggravated by them, then the disease is caused by the Devil" (Scheerenberger, 1987, p. 32).

It is apparent that the perception was common that disability resulted from sinful acts; an encounter with evil in some demonic form was predominant. Yet there are also accounts of acts of compassion extended by the Christian community. For example, reformer-theologian John Calvin wrote that God implanted in all people an understanding of God's divine majesty. No nation was so barbarous and no people so savage that they could not have a deep-seated conviction that there was a God. Because all people had this conviction, no one could endure life without religion because religion was not crafted by human beings but by God. Even those who in other respects appeared to differ little from "brutes" were capable of knowing God (Calvin, 1960).

Philosophical perspectives on disabilities

The ancient Greek philosophers Plato and Aristotle were part of a culture that had certain high ideals of physical beauty and healthy bodies; soundness of mind and body were of great importance in this culture. For example, even earlier, in the Homeric period, 1300–1100 B.C.E., Odysseus observed that a "bad man is not one [who] drinks too much, murders, and betrays; he is one that is cowardly, stupid, or weak (Scheerenberger, 1987, p. 11)." Plato supposedly said that the "best of either sex should be united with the best as often, and the inferior with the inferior as seldom, as possible. . . . The proper officers will take the offspring of the good parents to the pen or fold, and then they will deposit them with certain nurses who will dwell in a separate quarter; but the offspring of the inferior, or of the better when they chance to be deformed, will be put away (Scheerenberger, 1987, p. 12)." In *Politics*, Aristotle wrote, "As to the exposure and rearing of children, let there be a law that no *deformed* child shall live" (Scheerenberger, 1987, p. 12).

Overall, the philosophical view of the body in the ancient Greco-Roman culture more or less connected mind (soul), body, matter, and pneuma (spirit). Biblical scholar Dale Martin has written that the different human elements of the body were viewed as being interconnected, "each acting on and reacting to one another . . . a confused commingling of substances. . . . The human body was of a piece with its environment . . . perceived as a location in a continuum of cosmic movement. The body—or the 'self'—is an unstable point of transition, not a secure essence of individualistic solidity" (Martin, 1994, p. 38). Thus a disabling of any part of the body would affect the other parts of the self, and the causes of such impairment may be from a variety of sources—physical, environmental, or spiritual.

However, this perception of the body or self as a "confused commingling of substances" was irrevocably changed by what the philosophical outlook of the Enlightenment brought into eighteenth-century Europe. While the church was in turmoil, European society was caught up by the Enlightenment's fundamental principles—autonomy, reason, natural law—that radically changed the way people understood God, the human condition, and the world in general.

During the Enlightenment, God was placed on trial, to be judged by the new faith people had in the ability to use their rational minds, thereby replacing what some considered the idiosyncratic and antiquated eccentricities of the authoritative traditions of the church. While John Calvin may have thought that religion was crafted by God, the philosophers of the Enlightenment believed that God was crafted by human beings; a product of imaginative, yet rational, minds (MacIntyre, 1988). The existence of God could be shown, proven, or known not by faith but by philosophical means (Hauerwas, 1990).

One of the results of the Enlightenment in the church was the question of theodicy: what happens to the loving goodness of an all-powerful God in the midst of people's suffering (Hall, 1986). People with disabilities were judged to be "suffering victims" by the able-bodied in the church. However, this notion of suffering victimization was the result of persons who were able-bodied projecting what they would feel like if they had disabling conditions.

In the rational mind of the Enlightenment thinkers, God had not moved quickly to solve the apparent problem of such suffering. If God would not and could not eliminate suffering, even though God may have the power to do so, "then [people] will have to do God's task to insure that God can remain God" (Hauerwas, 1990, p. 48). Since the Enlightenment, that is exactly what people have been trying to do: They have taken upon themselves the obligation to do God's task to eliminate suffering, such as disabilities, with the great benefit of their rational, just, and enlightened minds, all done in the name of the good of humanity.

Central to the philosophical thinking of the Enlightenment philosophers was the power of the mind, the most valued characteristic of the human condition, which was necessary in order to control the world. In the seventeenth century, philosopher Francis Bacon proposed that we understand the natural world best by empirical investigation of the phenomenal world, or the modern scientific experimental method, rather than by philosophical constructs and theological dogmas. The role of philosophy was to "serve the state of human beings, giving power to people to call the creatures by their true name"; this included the labeling of disabling conditions (Smith, 1992, p. 26).

In the seventeenth century, philosopher René Descartes redrew the boundary lines between mind and body, which had been viewed by ancient Greco-Roman philosophers as a "confused commingling of substances." There was the body, embracing the category of "nature," which involved those parts of the universe that could be "scientifically" observed. The body was seen as having no faculty of self-motion; it was a machine, a clock, and could be studied and fixed like a machine (Martin, 1994).

The other realm was "supernatural," the mind or soul. The mind "is in the body only like a pilot in a vessel. All [the] sensations of hunger, thirst, pain, etc., are nothing more than certain confused modes of thinking, arising from the union and *apparent* fusion of mind and body (Martin, 1994)." Descartes was fascinated by the nature of the mind, and he saw the self as an organizing mental entity: "I think, therefore I am." Philosopher John Locke echoed this thought, defining a person as a "thinking intelligent being, that has reason and reflection, and can consider itself the same thinking thing in different times and places" (Locke, 1975, p. 335).

These philosophical ideas—Bacon's primacy of being empirically human, Descartes's rational mind over the mechanics of the body, and Locke's supremacy of the human mind capable of resolving problems presented in life—were foundational to more current practices that aim to help those with disabilities. Born out of this faith in the powers of the mind to conquer the ills of the mind or the dysfunctional mechanical body were the social-science disciplines and

> [the belief] that the study of human behavior, when conducted according to the rigorous principles established by the physical and biological sciences, will produce objective facts, testable theories, and profound understandings of the human condition. Perhaps even universal laws. (Postman, 1992, p. 145)

The natural sciences provided the basis for the social sciences, with the belief that first, methods of the natural sciences can be applied to the study of human behavior; second, social science generates specific principles that can be used to organize society on a rational, humane basis; and third, "faith in science can serve as a comprehensive belief system that gives meaning to life, as well as a sense of well-being, morality, and even immortality" (Postman, 1992, p. 147). No longer did the church hold the "truth" of life: The mind and scientific methods were about the discovery of universal truth in general, and people's disabling conditions in particular.

However, while these philosophers were constructing their theories of truth, reason, and definitions of what was normal, philosopher Michel Foucault was correct in insisting that they were also constructing theories of unreason, of madness, and of abnormality. Foucault noted that, since the seventeenth century, people who were considered "mad," insane, or those with disabilities from mental retardation, and people with hearing and visual impairments, were increasingly segregated from sane and normal, able-bodied society, both categorically and physically. In fact, the institutionalization of the insane has continued unabated for the past three centuries. He called this move to shut difficult, dangerous, or merely different people away as "the Great Confinement" (Foucault, 1970). But even in institutions for people with mental illnesses, it appeared that power—the power of mastery and that of madness—resided in the mind, for the mind could control the actions of the body, for, as Descartes said, "the mind is the pilot of the vessel."

Today's response to people with disabilities is not necesssarily to put them into institutions but to provide for their care in and through community-based services whenever possible. Nonetheless, be it in such community-based programs, asylums, hospitals for the mentally retarded, or institutions for the deaf or blind, the task of caring for people with disabilities has been framed in a Cartesian mind–body dualism. Either we gain control of the complex mind, which has power over the body, or the obverse: We control the body through rigorous behavior modification programs as advocated by scientist B. F. Skinner, which gives us control over the mind. Meanwhile, psychiatrist Thomas Szaz wrote that there was no such thing as "mental illness," and that it is all myth-making at its best.

Consequences of theological and philosophical perspectives

The ideals of the Enlightenment are central in social-science disciplines, which have had the power to shape society's thinking about the cause and effect, care and treatment of disabling conditions. More important, these disciplines have defined what it is to be a normal or a disabled human being and have continued to separate disabilities of the mind from impairments of the body as if the two were separate entities.

Evidence of this philosophical view that separates mind and body and discounts spirit, resulting in the further segmentation of the human condition, is displayed in the growing cacophony of voices of health-service professionals that clamor to treat people with disabilities per their own worldview: People with disabilities have a problem to be medically cured, therapeutically resolved, behaviorally modified, educationally unlearned, socially reconstructed, or spiritually healed, with the intended result that no one should have any problem and thus be like everyone else: normal.

With this goal in mind, medicine has gone beyond the cautionary precept of the Hippocratic Oath, "First, do no harm," to finding ways of "curing" truly crippling conditions, such as plastic surgery for children with Down syndrome so they don't look disabled. Even though AAMR may recognize that the disabling condition of mental retardation may be more a functional impairment than an intellectual one, many people still understand it as essentially biological, advocating abortion of a fetus with mental retardation, renaming such procedures "foreordained pregnancy interruption" (Crocker, 1992, p. 307). Finally, there is the Human Genome Project, which is designed to decipher the more than 100,000 genes in the human body. Its goal is to screen out the genetic "defects" with hopes that it will better identify "the really smart kids." For the first time in history, parents may be enabled to decide what kind of children they will bear or to discard those seen as imperfect or defective (Kimbrell, 1993). This is the promotion of genetic essentialism, the idea that beings are essentially their genetic makeup, their bodies.

With the collapse of neighborhoods, religious communities, and loss of friendships, people now pay therapists to become hired friends. Mechanistic psychologists who practice behaviorism deny the existence of human free will and believe that once the body is controlled, life is totally predictable in a restrictive environment. Educationally, teachers believe either that many disabilities that impair learning are either learned and need to be unlearned or that new methods of instruction need to be incorporated in order that individual persons with disabling conditions will be able to function independently in the world. Legally, the Americans with Disabilities Act of 1990 allows legislators to enact federal and state laws, society's rules, and to control people's hearts and minds concerning how people with disabilities are cared for and treated in society.

Meanwhile, as the professionals differ among themselves in treating people with disabilities, there is also an emerging, rancorous voice of self-advocacy in the community of people with disabilities. No longer does the deaf community accept hearing impairment as a disability; hearing impairment is part of their culture as Deaf Americans. Yet even with the passage of the Americans with Disabilities Act and with the disabled community's voice increasing in terms of political clout and legal power, U.S. states like Oregon are rationing health-care services, which will adversely affect people with disabilities.

In conclusion, being "normal" means to be more or less like everyone else, with little tolerance for exceptions. People are still frightened and angered by the mere presence of people with disabilities, given all the "marvels" of modern medicine and psychology, and ask politely, "Why are they still here?" People still attribute disability to some past sin in the family, the work of the devil, or nature and the body gone awry, responses that are informed by the theological and/or philosophical narratives that formed their primary community.

BRETT WEBB-MITCHELL

Directly related to this article are the other articles in this entry: ATTITUDES AND SOCIOLOGICAL PERSPECTIVES, HEALTH CARE AND PHYSICAL DISABILITY, *and* LEGAL ISSUES. *For a further discussion of topics mentioned in this article, see the entries* JUDAISM; MENTAL HEALTH; MENTAL-HEALTH SERVICES; MENTAL ILLNESS; PROTESTANTISM; *and* ROMAN CATHOLICISM. *This article will find application in the entries* COMMITMENT TO MENTAL INSTITUTIONS; *and* COMPETENCE. *For a discussion of related ideas, see the entry* VALUE AND VALUATION. *Other relevant material may be found under the entries* EUGENICS; GENETIC ENGINEERING; GENETICS AND HUMAN BEHAVIOR; HEALTH AND DISEASE; MENTALLY DISABLED AND MENTALLY ILL PERSONS; *and* REHABILITATION MEDICINE.

Bibliography

AMERICAN MEDICAL ASSOCIATION ON MENTAL RETARDATION. 1992. *Mental Retardation: Definition, Classification, and Systems of Supports.* Washington, D.C.: Author.

AMERICAN PSYCHIATRIC ASSOCIATION. 1994. *Diagnostic and Statistical Manual of Mental Disorders (DSM-IV).* Washington, D.C.: Author.

CALVIN, JOHN. 1960. *Institutes of the Christian Religion.* Edited by John T. McNeill. London: SCM.

CARRIER, JAMES G. 1986. *Learning Disability: Social Class and the Construction of Inequality in American Education.* New York: Greenwood Press.

COOPER, BURTON. 1992. "The Disabled God." *Theology Today* 49:173–82.

CRITES, STEPHEN. 1989. "The Narrative Quality of Experience." In *Why Narrative? Readings in Narrative Theology,* pp. 65–88. Edited by Stanley Hauerwas and Gregory Jones. Grand Rapids, Mich.: William B. Eerdmans.

CROCKER, ALLEN. 1993. "Data Collection for the Evaluation of Mental Retardation Prevention Activities: The Fateful Forty-Three." *Mental Retardation* 30, no. 6:303–317.

DOUGLAS, MARY. 1966. *Purity and Danger: An Analysis of Concepts of Pollution and Taboo.* London: Routledge & Kegan Paul.

EDGERTON, ROBERT B. 1979. *Mental Retardation.* Cambridge, Mass.: Harvard University Press.

FLETCHER, JOHN. 1974. "Attitudes Toward Defective Newborns." *Hastings Center Studies* 2, no. 1:21–32.

FLETCHER, JOSEPH F. 1966. *Situation Ethics: The New Morality.* Philadelphia: Westminster.

FOUCAULT, MICHEL. 1970. *The Order of Things: An Archaeology of the Human Sciences.* New York: Vintage.

GOULD, STEPHEN JAY. 1981. *The Mismeasure of Man.* New York: W. W. Norton.

HALL, DOUGLAS J. 1986. *God and Human Suffering: An Exercise in the Theology of the Cross.* Minneapolis, Minn.: Augsburg.

HAUERWAS, STANLEY. 1990. *Naming the Silences: God, Medicine, and the Problem of Suffering.* Grand Rapids, Mich.: William B. Eerdmans.

KIMBRELL, ANDREW. 1993. *The Human Body Shop: The Engineering and Marketing of Life.* New York: HarperCollins.

LOCKE, JOHN. 1975. *An Essay Concerning Human Understanding.* Edited by P. H. Nidditch. Oxford: At the Clarendon Press.

MACINTYRE, ALASDAIR C. 1988. *Whose Justice? Which Rationality?* Notre Dame, Ind.: University of Notre Dame Press.

MARTIN, DALE. 1994. *The Corinthian Body.* New Haven, Conn.: Yale University Press. [Manuscript to be published by 1995].

O'ROURKE, JOHN J. 1968. "The Second Letter to the Corinthians." In *The New Testament and Topical Articles,* pp. 267–290. Edited by Raymond E. Brown, Joseph A. Fitzmeyer, and Roland E. Murphy. Englewood Cliffs, N.J.: Prentice-Hall.

POSTMAN, NEIL. 1992. *Technopoly: The Surrender of Culture to Technology.* New York: Knopf.

SCHEERENBERGER, ROBERT C. 1987. *A History of Mental Retardation: A Quarter Century of Promise.* Baltimore: Paul H. Brookes.

SIGERIST, HENRY ERNST. 1977. "The Special Position of the Sick." In *Culture, Disease, and Healing: Studies in Medical*

Anthropology, pp. 388–394. Edited by David Landy. New York: Macmillan.

SMITH, HARMON. 1992. "Genetic Technologies: Can We Do Responsibly Everything We Can Do Technologically?" *National Forum* 72, no. 1:26–29.

VITELLO, STANLEY J., and SOSKIN, RONALD M. 1985. *Mental Retardation: Its Social and Legal Context.* Englewood Cliffs, N.J.: Prentice-Hall.

WEBB-MITCHELL, BRETT. 1994. *Unexpected Guests at God's Banquet: Welcoming People with Disabilities into the Church.* New York: Crossroad.

III. HEALTH CARE AND PHYSICAL DISABILITY

The allocation and provision of health-care services for people with physical disabilities present special challenges to Western thinking about ethics and health care. These challenges stem in large part from societal attitudes about people with disabilities and from the changing social and political context that people with disabilities have helped to create.

This article outlines the changing social context of disability in Western society, the emergence of a "disability perspective" with regard to health care, and some of the leading issues in the provision and allocation of health-care services for people with physical disabilities. The discussion here is limited to health- and long-term-care services as they pertain to people with physical disabilities. Many of the issues that affect people with disabilities also affect older people generally, since a disproportionate number of older people have physical conditions that limit one or more major life activities.

The changing social context

Western society has witnessed a material shift in how people with disabilities view themselves and how they wish to be viewed by others. People with disabilities no longer want to be viewed as objects warranting charitable and paternalistic intervention, but rather as self-directed individuals willing and able to take their rightful place in the mainstream of community life. People with disabilities in many countries have organized to demand more sensitive and just approaches to eliminating various legal, economic, and physical barriers to education, employment, housing, transportation, and various public accommodations.

This movement of people with disabilities has come to its clearest expression in the United States, a society strongly committed to an ethic that encourages people to take responsibility for their own well-being. The movement also has surfaced, albeit less forcefully, in many other Western societies where welfare-state institutions enjoy greater public support and where there is a more organized response to individual needs.

The movement for independent living (IL) and disability rights (DR), as it is commonly known in North America, is perhaps best reflected in (1) the creation of more than 400 self-help centers or "independent-living centers" in the United States and Canada, and (2) the passage of the Americans with Disabilities Act (ADA) in 1990 that extends a variety of civil-rights protections to people with disabilities. The IL/DR movement shares many of the same self-help values that have characterized other social movements of the last few decades (e.g., the women's movement). Thus, one can find many similarities between the disability movement and other movements organized by people who have felt disfranchised in their respective societies.

While people with physical disabilities encounter many of the same issues in health care as do other disadvantaged groups, their interaction with the health-care system is somewhat different, in part because their impairments may require medical management and may alter the course of treatment for health conditions unrelated to their impairments. This interaction with the medical-care system, which could occur throughout the life of the individual, has made medical care a special object of concern for people with disabilities.

A disability perspective

In the United States, Canada, and to a lesser extent in other countries, a distinct disability perspective has emerged with respect to the provision of health-care services. Though dominant, it is not the only perspective that people with disabilities bring to health-care services. The disability perspective can be best understood by the response of independent-living adherents to two concepts from the sociology of medicine, namely the concept of the medical model and the concept of the sick role (Parsons, 1951; DeJong, 1979). Central to both concepts is the idea that the physician or health-care provider is the technically competent expert, and the patient is to assume a passive and compliant role in which he or she does everything possible to get better by following the provider's instructions. In the sick role, patients are exempt from everyday responsibilities while they are sick. The problem this model presents for people with disabilities is that their conditions are not of the temporarily limiting or incapacitating variety typical of the sick role. Consequently, to define their conditions as chiefly medical in nature is to confine disabled people to a lifetime of passivity and noninvolvement in social life.

As a result, people in the vanguard of the IL/DR movement have attempted vigorously to distance themselves from much of the formal health-care system, which, in their view, seriously undermines their capacity for self-direction and self-determination. In short, the disability perspective places a high value on autonomy and the provision of information that enables people with disabilities to make informed choices about their health care. The disability perspective includes a strong presumption of competence. At the same time, the disability perspective emphasizes the fiduciary responsibility and accountability of the health-care provider. It strongly favors a "user–provider" relationship that is voluntary, contractual, and informed. The disability perspective abhors paternalism.

As to the allocation of health- and long-term-care resources, the disability perspective has, for the most part, favored a vigorous societal response in which resources are distributed or, more accurately, redistributed to meet the needs of people with disabilities. The disability perspective tends to view health-care and personal-care services as rights, not as commodities to be distributed based on an individual's ability to pay. The disability-rights community in the United States has argued strongly that access to community-based services, such as personal care or "personal assistance," are tantamount to a right. Such services are said to be vital to people's ability to participate in the life of the community and their ability to exercise the rights accorded them in the ADA.

Leading issues in the provision of health-care services for people with disabilities

Five sets of issues have come to dominate health-care issues related to disability:

1. Issues related to autonomy, competence, and guardianship;
2. Issues related to justice and resource allocation;
3. Issues related to quality of life and the refusal of life-prolonging treatment;
4. Issues related to family and societal duties; and
5. Issues related to health-care priority setting or rationing.

These five sets of issues are highly interrelated and are presented in an order that allows each set of issues to set the stage for the next.

Autonomy, competence, and guardianship

Autonomy.   Autonomy, or self-direction, is the single most-prized value in the DR/IL movement and as such tends to trump most other competing considerations in the design of public policy and the provision of health-care services. Autonomy considerations for people with disabilities involve the extent to which the disability and social reactions to that disability have interfered with their taking charge of their lives, evolving a self and an identity that are meaningful and acceptable, and making choices and decisions that are congruent with that self (Banja, 1992).

Informed consent in an acute-care context tokens a person's agreeing or refusing to undergo some clinical procedure after having been informed about it. In a disability context, however, informed consent functions more as a metaphor for the disabled person's willingness to engage the world in a productive and meaningful way, along with his or her possession of and capacity to use certain information and strategies to do so successfully.

A number of factors affect the extent to which persons with disabilities are autonomous. First are the autonomy limitations that arise from social attitudes and practices, for example, negative stereotyping, architectural barriers, and discriminatory employment practices. These factors are independent of any functional limitation, but they impede or "handicap" the realization of autonomy for persons with disabilities. Second are the autonomy limitations that can arise from neurological impairment involving the cognitive or judgmental ability of a disabled person to manage his or her life. These impairments, insofar as they compromise the ability to understand, reason about, or use information and to have insight into the meaning and implications of decisions, obviously compromise one's judgmental ability. The stroke patient with severe aphasia, the morbidly depressed person with spinal-cord injury, or the memory-impaired individual with serious brain injury, all might be unable or "incompetent" to contribute to planning their own welfare.

Serious autonomy problems emerge when a person with a disability demands to have his or her decisions or preferences accommodated, but the health-care provider, family member, or some significant other believes that doing so would imperil the individual or others. Often it is unclear whether the disabled person's preferences can justifiably be overridden. Those who say they can will invariably argue that significant harm will result from accommodating what they perceive as the problematic choice. Yet such arguments may be extremely speculative. The anticipation that harm may result may be exaggerated by the provider's fear of legal liability (Meisel, 1991), or the provider's unwillingness to share decision-making power with the individual (Mullins, 1989). However, many persons with disabilities manifest blatantly unsafe or dangerous behaviors and require paternalistic interventions to ensure that they do not injure themselves or others. Consequently, when autonomous function is highly attractive but the disabled person's ability to function responsibly and without excessive risk is unclear, wrenching dilemmas may occur.

A classic rehabilitation problem, for example, involves the professional's uncertainty about whether a client's neurological impairment excessively interferes with his or her ability to drive an automobile. On the one hand, the professional's taking steps to prevent the individual from driving anticipates a considerable handicap and is antithetical to the interests of functional independence. On the other hand, a failure to protect the individual or others from an authentically menacing situation is equally serious and ethically trumps preserving whatever desire the individual has in maintaining the right to drive. In such situations, the professional's ethical obligation is to perform a careful risk assessment of the functional domain (in this case, driving) to determine whether or not the individual meets the prevailing standard of safety. If it is determined that the individual poses a risk to safety, the professional is ethically obligated to take appropriate measures—which frequently involve notifying third parties of the need for precautions.

Competence.   Competence has traditionally been associated with a variety of mental disorders that are so disabling (e.g., severe retardation, severe neurosis, psychosis) that a guardian or some form of institutionalization is required (Hommel et al., 1990). Obviously, persons with neurological disabilities may be "incompetent" due to some psychiatric morbidity ranging from depression to florid schizophrenia. But because the disabilities under consideration here are not of psychiatric but organic origin, "functional capacity" is a term that better captures the variety of domains in which persons with disability might or might not function autonomously. Thus, a person with aphasia might be able to execute a will but not operate a business; someone with a serious visual-perceptual deficit from brain injury might be able to raise a family but not drive an automobile; persons with information-processing impairments might be able to perform self-care tasks but not manage finances or deliberate about medical treatment. In sum, persons with disabilities may be functional or autonomous in one domain but not in another (Buchanan and Brock, 1989). When it has been determined that persons with disabilities are incompetent in some domain, caretakers may need to consider and initiate guardianship proceedings.

Guardianship.   Traditional approaches to competence tended to conceive incompetence as an "all-or-nothing" phenomenon, resulting in the "incompetent" person's requiring a guardian with plenary powers (i.e., making all decisions). This approach, however, eliminated the right of the ward to function autonomously in those domains where capacity might be preserved. Because of this obvious injustice, certain jurisdictions, beginning in 1989, began to revise their guardianship statutes so as to emphasize the idea of limited guardianship. This approach relies much more on a functional or "domain-specific" competence evaluation that insists that guardianship appointments respect the proposed

ward's right to retain as much autonomy as possible (Hommel et al., 1990).

Justice and resource allocation.   While there is considerable consensus in the disability community on the importance of issues related to autonomy and competence, there is less consensus on issues related to justice and resource allocation. Views of justice are frequently characterized as existing on a continuum, with libertarian views on one end and egalitarian views on the other. In the United States, and less so elsewhere, disability-rights advocates can be found along the entire libertarian–egalitarian continuum. Some in the disability-rights movement have their roots in more libertarian traditions where personal autonomy and individual liberty are the most important values. Other, and perhaps more visible, participants in the movement have their roots in the more egalitarian impulses that came with the social activism of the 1960s.

These two strands in the U.S. disability-rights movement converged for a period in the late 1980s and early 1990s to help make possible the passage of the ADA mainly because the ADA was not perceived as a resource-allocation issue but as a human-rights issue. The divergent strains in the disability-rights movement are more evident in resource-allocation issues such as health-care reform and long-term-care policy. Those on the more libertarian end of the spectrum shun direct government intervention and favor private-sector initiatives and public policies (e.g., income tax credits) that augment consumer choices by enabling individuals to secure their own services; those on the more egalitarian end of the spectrum want government funding and favor policies that augment consumer choices by increasing financial access for all income groups. In the health-care-reform debate of the early 1990s, for example, both groups believed that the health-care system was discriminatory (e.g., excluding from coverage people with preexisting conditions) and unjust. However, those toward the libertarian end favored tax credits and vouchers that would enable disabled individuals to secure their own health insurance while those at the egalitarian end favored government-sponsored, single-payer solutions that would guarantee disabled individuals access to health services. The latter group did not fully trust mid-spectrum market-based solutions such as "managed competition" to provide equal access to health care.

These divergent views of justice and resource allocation also characterized the debate about community-based, long-term-care services commonly known as "personal-assistance services" among disability advocates. Both groups wanted a service system that maximized their opportunity for autonomy and consumer choice. The one group, however, preferred indirect methods of funding such as tax credits while the other preferred direct government cash subsidies.

Quality of life and the refusal of life-prolonging treatment. While there are many conceptions about meaning and quality of life (Emanuel, 1987), much of the public debate has been framed as a polarity in terms of the "sanctity-of-life" versus the "quality-of-life" positions (Gilmore, 1984; Taylor, 1985). Oversimplified, the sanctity-of-life position holds that life itself, regardless of its limitations, is worth preserving. The quality-of-life position holds that life has meaning to the extent to which a person has some capacity for human interaction, emotional relationships, and self-determination. Quality-of-life considerations also typically include the ability to live active and productive lives outside of an institution.

The sanctity-of-life–quality-of-life debate has surfaced in two types of cases involving people with disabilities. The first are cases in which families and providers are attempting to decide for a newly injured or impaired person whether he or she should be allowed to live or die in the face of a greatly diminished capacity for living. Second are cases in which a disabled person is deciding for him- or herself whether he or she wants to live or die in the face of difficult circumstances that severely limit the quality of life.

A variant of the first case was the 1983 Baby Doe case in New York, in which parents declined corrective surgery for their newborn who had a combination of disorders that included meningomyelocele (a form of spina bifida), hydrocephaly, and microcephaly. With corrective surgery, her parents were told, Baby Doe would live up to twenty years albeit with severe retardation, epilepsy, and paralysis that would have left her bedridden with the threat of constant urinary-tract and bladder infections (Steinbock, 1984; Brown, 1986).

During the presidential administration of Ronald Reagan, the Baby Doe case became a disability issue when the Justice Department intervened to determine whether the decision not to perform corrective surgery constituted discrimination against a "handicapped newborn" under Section 504 of the 1973 Rehabilitation Act, which prohibited discrimination on the basis of handicap in any program or organization receiving federal funds. Invoking Section 504 was an unusual step, because Section 504 had been designed to address a very different set of discriminatory practices (e.g., access to employment, access to public buildings), and because the administration previously had been hostile to disability-rights issues. The administration's intervention responded to pressures from the anti-abortion community which strongly favored a sanctity-of-life position.

The response of the disability-rights community entailed both value-of-life and quality-of-life arguments. Disability advocates were outraged that an infant deemed handicapped had a life valued less than that of a nonhandicapped infant. The issue had been framed in terms that were perceived as a challenge to the worth of life for all people with disabilities. Disability advocates were equally outraged at the administration's inconsistency as evidenced by its determination to do everything possible to save the life of a handicapped infant (sanctity of life) while it sought to cut programs and gut civil-rights protections (e.g., Section 504 regulations) that made such lives, once saved, more meaningful (quality of life).

Examples of the second type of cases are the cases of Elizabeth Bouvia and Larry McAfee; both sought to refuse life-prolonging treatment. In 1983, Elizabeth Bouvia, a California woman with cerebral palsy, wanted Riverside County Hospital to assist her in her plan to starve herself to death by discontinuing her nasogastric tube feeding, because she believed that her quality of life had diminished to the point where it was no longer worth living (Kane, 1985; Longmore, 1987). In 1989, Larry McAfee, a Georgia man with high spinal-cord injury, wanted to end his life because his quadriplegia and need for a ventilator, in the absence of funding for community-based personal care services, had confined him to living in a nursing home.

Disability-rights advocates did not regard these cases as personal autonomy or as right-to-die cases as argued in the courts and depicted in the media, but primarily as justice or resource-allocation cases. The decisions of Bouvia and McAfee issued from the failure of society to make programs and resources available that would provide them with authentic options to enhance their quality of life. In the case of Larry McAfee, the absence of funding for community-based personal-care services—that made nursing-home living his only option—became a battle cry in the disability-rights community for more adequate funding for personal-assistance services.

Since 1975, about sixty cases involving an individual's right to have life-prolonging treatment withheld have reached the appellate level (Meisel, 1991). Self-referential requests to terminate life-sustaining treatments by persons with disabilities such as Elizabeth Bouvia and Larry McAfee have been rare (*McKay v. Bergstedt*, 1990). Nevertheless, when confronted with a disabled adult's request to have life-sustaining treatment discontinued, courts have employed a traditional competency approach that examines whether or not the individual possesses adequate understanding, reasoning, and insight into the elements, implications, and ramifications of his or her request.

While these discussions will fuel debates over the extent of society's duties to people with disabilities, one must also recognize a political agenda at stake in the form of how a request to discontinue life-prolonging treatment may appear to reinforce society's already negative stereotype of people with disabilities and how the perpetuation of that stereotype compromises the politics of disability. To the extent, however, that these discussions precipitate a greater awareness of the issues of justice affecting people with severe disabilities, it should insist in advancing society's moral sensitivity and willingness to accommodate their needs.

Family and societal duties.   There is considerable confusion about the proper scope of family responsibility to care for a family member who is dependent because of a physical disability. On the one hand, moral expectations about caregiving remain strong as a cultural ideal of what it means to be a good family member. On the other hand, there is increased recognition that today's needs are likely to exceed family care-giving capacities. These needs are often greater and of longer duration than in the past when people with disabilities were less likely to survive serious disease or injury and were more likely to succumb to secondary conditions if they did survive. Moreover, family caregiving capacities have diminished owing to geographic mobility and the changing character of today's family (Jennings et al., 1988; Callahan, 1988; DeJong and Batavia, 1989; DeJong et al., 1990).

Western societies differ greatly in defining the boundaries between family and societal responsibility. Western European countries, for example, support a high level of publicly funded, formal home care while the United States relies more heavily on voluntary family care. There has been a great fear in the United States that formal home care will displace family efforts to care for kin.

The ongoing debate about the distribution of family and societal responsibilities in caring for disabled family members often overlooks an important variable, namely, the age and time in one's life span at which one becomes, or is, disabled. Caregiving needs change depending on whether the family member with a disability is a child, an adolescent, a young or middle-aged adult, or an elder. The IL/DR movement has been especially attuned to this concern. Many in the vanguard of this movement acquired their disability in the awkward transition from adolescence to young adulthood. Arguing from experience, they observe that the imposition of traditional caregiving expectations can sometimes perpetuate the parent–child relationship into early adulthood and thus frustrate the transition to psychological and emotional independence.

The distribution of family and societal responsibilities in caring for persons with disabilities will remain a vexing issue, especially if society refuses to reflect seriously on the nature of familial obligations relative to new technologies that preserve life, albeit with increased disablement. Daniel Callahan (1988) argues that when cultural ideals are translated into "unlimited self-sacrifice," burdens may become excessive and result in a collapse of the family's care-giving capacity.

Framing the issue as family responsibility versus societal responsibilities obscures another important issue for people with disabilities. In most instances, societal responsibility for in-home care entails professionally supervised, agency-sponsored care in which the person with the disability is viewed as a patient or client. The IL/DR movement strongly advocates a user-directed model of personal assistance in which the person with a disability hires and directs an assistant to accomplish those daily tasks, including bodily care and home maintenance, that would otherwise be done by the disabled person if he or she did not have a disability (DeJong and Wenker, 1979; Litvak et al., 1987; Batavia et al., 1990). Personal autonomy is the central value in the user-directed model of personal assistance.

Formal health-care priority setting or rationing.   All the leading health issues in disability mentioned to this point (autonomy, justice, quality of life) are joined in the issue of health-care priority setting, commonly referred to as rationing. Disability and health-care priority setting became a public issue in the United States in 1992. At that time, the State of Oregon requested that the presidential administration of George Bush allow Oregon to waive provisions in its Medicaid program and limit particular kinds of health services. Community groups judged the outcome of these services to be of questionable value and believed Medicaid funds should be expanded to include a wider segment of the state's low-income population.

The Bush administration rejected Oregon's waiver request on the grounds that the plan discriminated against people with disabilities and was therefore in violation of the ADA. The administration argued that the statewide telephone survey used to rate various quality-of-life scenarios was "based in substantial part on the premise that the value of life of a person with a disability is less than the value of a life of a person without a disability" (*Oregonian*, 1992). In 1993, following several revisions in the Oregon plan, the Clinton administration approved the plan for a five-year period.

At the core of most formal health-care priority setting is some measure of outcome or quality of life that can be used to rank various interventions or treatments, which, in the Oregon case, led to the rankings of some 709 condition–treatment pairs. From a disability perspective, there are two main concerns: (1) quality of life as an intellectual construct, and (2) the method or procedure by which various quality-of-life states are ranked, weighted, or valued.

As to the first concern, people with disabilities do

not necessarily view their impairments or functional limitations as something that diminishes their quality of life. Some argue, as they did in the McAfee and Bouvia cases noted earlier, that quality of life is as much a function of societal accommodation as it is a function of the disabled state. Many people with disabilities argue that their quality of life is not something inherent in their physical impairments or functional limitations—a notion seldom grasped by the able-bodied world. The drawback to this view is that, if various disability states are not differentially valued, medical treatments designed to increase functional independence, for example, may not be considered particularly worthwhile (Hadorn, 1992). Although some might differ, most disabled persons, if given a choice, would prefer to be in nondisabled states.

As to the second concern, people with disabilities argue that people like themselves may not be adequately represented in the surveys used to rank or weight the quality of life of various condition–states. More important, they argue, is that quality-of-life ratings of condition–states are biased if they are made by people who know little or nothing about a particular condition–state or do not anticipate being in that state at some future time—a case of people rating other people's quality of life. This was a major criticism of the Oregon plan. Some go even further and argue that only those who have a particular condition are in a position to judge quality of life associated with that condition. This argument calls into question whether any community quality-of-life assessment of various condition–states is possible.

The principal rejoinder to this argument is that the rankings of condition–states made by people with disabilities are not materially different from those made by people without disabilities (Hadorn, 1992; Menzel, 1992; Doughtery, 1994). Data from the Oregon survey indicate that those who had experience with a particular condition–state did tend to view the condition–state somewhat more favorably than those who had not. In the twelve instances, where there were significant differences in preference scores by condition–state experience, the U.S. Congress Office of Technology Assessment found in its analysis of the Oregon data that the resulting preference weights were highly correlated ($r = .96$) between those who did and did not have experience with the twelve conditions (U.S. Congress, 1992).

Regardless of the empirical findings about preferences, a compelling moral question remains about the merits of nondisabled people making quality-of-life judgments of condition–states about which they have little knowledge and thus may be prone to impute various stereotypic or biased assumptions. The solution, according to Paul Menzel, is as follows:

[T]o insure that those who initially contribute the preferences are both reasonably knowledgeable about the conditions they are asked to rank and that they realize the utter personal seriousness of their responses—that their rankings may contribute to either others' or their own disadvantage in later allocations. (Menzel, 1992, p. 23)

Even this solution, as Menzel acknowledges, has its limitations (as in the case of congenital disabilities that survey respondents know they will never experience). These limitations point to the need to develop ranking methodologies that can incorporate both the wisdom of experience and the preferences of an informed citizenry.

Another possible solution is to consider improvement in quality of life as the outcome test for determining whether a person or group qualifies for a particular medical intervention. The improvement test would diminish the need to value various condition–states and would place people with disabilities on a more equal footing with their nondisabled counterparts. The improvement standard could disadvantage people with degenerative disabling conditions. For such individuals or groups, maintenance of quality of life might become the standard.

The collision between health-care priority setting and disability rights in the Oregon plan was an accident waiting to happen. It brought into question whether any health-care-rationing scheme might be considered inherently discriminatory against people with disabilities and whether a society such as the United States, committed to individual and minority-group rights, will be able to achieve the consensus it needs to limit the availability of marginally effective health-care interventions.

Conclusion

As noted at the outset of this article, the IL/DR movement has significantly changed much of Western thinking about disability. Central to this change is the shift from a medical model of thinking in which the pathology is centered in the individual to a sociopolitical model in which the pathology is located in the dependency-inducing features of the larger social, political, and physical environment. One unanswered question is whether traditional categories in biomedical ethics are adequate to address the moral and ethical challenges presented by the growing, politically active population of people with disabilities. In biomedical ethics, categories used to describe the social role of the disabled person include patient, client, and victim. Corresponding categories in the IL/DR movement would include consumer, voter, participant, and leader. The language used carries a great deal of cultural baggage. A question that remains is whether traditional biomedical ethics, by virtue of the language and categories used, is an unintended carrier of cultural baggage that limits our ability to think about the needs and concerns of people with disabilities in allocating and providing health-care and long-term-care services.

GERBEN DEJONG
JOHN BANJA

Directly related to this article are the other articles in this entry: ATTITUDES AND SOCIOLOGICAL PERSPECTIVES, PHILOSOPHICAL AND THEOLOGICAL PERSPECTIVES, *and* LEGAL ISSUES. *For a further discussion of topics mentioned in this article, see the entries* AGING AND THE AGED, *article on* HEALTH-CARE AND RESEARCH ISSUES; AUTONOMY; COMPETENCE; DEATH AND DYING: EUTHANASIA AND SUSTAINING LIFE, *article on* ETHICAL ISSUES; FAMILY; HEALTH-CARE FINANCING, *especially the articles on* MEDICARE, *and* MEDICAID; HEALTH-CARE RESOURCES, ALLOCATION OF, *article on* MACROALLOCATION; INFORMED CONSENT; JUSTICE; LIFE, QUALITY OF; LONG-TERM CARE; *and* PATERNALISM. *For a discussion of related ideas, see the entry* RIGHTS, *article on* RIGHTS IN BIOETHICS; *and* VALUE AND VALUATION. *Other relevant material may be found under the entries* CHILDREN, *article on* HEALTH-CARE AND RESEARCH ISSUES; HEALTH AND DISEASE; MENTAL-HEALTH SERVICES; MENTALLY DISABLED AND MENTALLY ILL PERSONS; *and* REHABILITATION MEDICINE.

Bibliography

BANJA, JOHN D. 1988. "Independence and Rehabilitation: A Philosophic Perspective." Commentary. *Archives of Physical Medicine and Rehabilitation* 69, no. 5:381–382.

———. 1992. "Ethics in Rehabilitation." *Rehabilitation Medicine: Contemporary Clinical Perspectives,* pp. 269–298. Edited by Gerald F. Fletcher, John D. Banja, Brigitte B. Jann, and Steven L. Wolf. Philadelphia: Lea and Febiger.

BATAVIA, ANDREW I. 1991. "A Disability Rights-Independent Living Perspective on Euthanasia." *Western Journal of Medicine* 154, no. 5:616–617.

BATAVIA, ANDREW I.; DEJONG, GERBEN; and McKNEW, LOUISE BOUSCAREN. 1991. "Toward a National Personal Assistance Program: The Independent Living Model of Long-Term Care for Persons with Disabilities." *Journal of Health Politics, Policy and Law* 16, no. 3:523–545.

BROWN, LAWRENCE D. 1986. "Civil Rights and Regulatory Wrongs: The Reagan Administration and the Medical Treatment of Handicapped Infants." *Journal of Health Politics, Policy and Law* 11, no. 2:231–254.

BUCHANAN, ALLEN E., and BROCK, DAN W. 1989. *Deciding for Others: The Ethics of Surrogate Decisionmaking.* New York: Cambridge University Press.

CALLAHAN, DANIEL. 1988. "Families as Caregivers: The Limits of Morality." *Archives of Physical Medicine and Rehabilitation* 69, no. 5:323–328.

DEJONG, GERBEN. 1979. "Independent Living: From Social Movement to Analytic Paradigm." *Archives of Physical Medicine and Rehabilitation* 60, no. 10:435–446.

DEJONG, GERBEN, and BATAVIA, ANDREW I. 1989. "Societal Duty and Resource Allocation for Persons with Severe Traumatic Brain Injury." *Journal of Head Trauma Rehabilitation* 4, no. 1:1–12.

DEJONG, GERBEN; BATAVIA, ANDREW I.; and WILLIAMS, JANET M. 1990. "Who Is Responsible for the Lifelong Well-Being of a Person with a Head Injury?" *Journal of Head Trauma Rehabilitation* 5, no. 1:9–22.

DEJONG, GERBEN, and WENKER, TEG. 1979. "Attendant Care as a Prototype Independent Living Service." *Archives of Physical Medicine and Rehabilitation* 60, no. 10:477–482.

DOUGHTERY, CHARLES J. 1994. "Quality-Adjusted Life Years and the Ethical Values of Health Care." *American Journal of Physical Medicine and Rehabilitation* 73, no. 1:61–65.

EMANUEL, EZEKIEL J. 1987. "A Communal Vision of Care for Incompetent Patients." *Hastings Center Report* 17, no. 5:15–20.

GILMORE, ANNE. 1984. "Sanctity of Life Versus Quality of Life—The Continuing Debate." *Canadian Medical Association Journal* 130, no. 2:180–181.

HADORN, DAVID C. 1992. "The Problem of Discrimination in Health Care Priority Setting." *Journal of the American Medical Association* 268, no. 11:1454–1459.

HOMMEL, PENELOPE A.; WANG, LU-IN; and BERGMAN, JAMES A. 1990. "Trends in Guardianship Reform: Implications for the Medical and Legal Professions." *Law, Medicine and Health Care* 18, no. 3:213–226.

JENNINGS, BRUCE; CALLAHAN, DANIEL; and CAPLAN, ARTHUR L. 1988. "Ethical Challenges of Chronic Illness." *Hastings Center Report* 18, no. 1 (suppl.):1–16.

KANE, FRANCIS I. 1985. "Keeping Elizabeth Bouvia Alive for the Public Good." *Hastings Center Report* 15, no. 6:5–8.

LITVAK, SIMI; ZUKAS, HAL; and HEUMANN, JUDITH. 1987. *Attending to America: Personal Assistance for Independent Living.* Berkeley, Calif.: World Institute on Disability.

LONGMORE, PAUL K. 1987. "Elizabeth Bouvia, Assisted Suicide and Social Prejudice." *Issues in Law and Medicine* 3, no. 2:141–168.

McKay v. Bergstedt. 1990. 801 P.2d 617 (Nev.).

MEISEL, ALAN. 1991. "Legal Myths About Terminating Life Support." *Archives of Internal Medicine* 151, no. 8:1497–1502.

MENZEL, PAUL T. 1992. "Oregon's Denial: Disabilities and Quality of Life." *Hastings Center Report* 22, no. 6:21–25.

MULLINS, LARRY L. 1989. "Hate Revisited: Power, Envy, and Greed in the Rehabilitation Setting." *Archives of Physical Medicine and Rehabilitation* 70, no. 10:740–744.

PARSONS, TALCOTT. 1951. *The Social System.* New York: Free Press.

State v. McAfee. 1989. 385 S.E.2d 651 (Ga.).

STEINBOCK, BONNIE. 1984. "Baby Jane Doe in the Courts." *Hastings Center Report* 14, no. 1:13–19.

TAYLOR, SUSAN G. 1985. "Ethics: The Effect of Quality of Life

and Sanctity of Life on Clinical Decision Making."
AORN Journal 41, no. 5:924–928.

U.S. Congress, Office of Technology Assessment. 1992.
Evaluation of the Oregon Medicaid Proposal. OTA–H–531.
Washington, D.C.: Author.

Veatch, Robert M. 1980. "Voluntary Risks to Health: The
Ethical Issues." *Journal of the American Medical Association*
243, no. 1:50–55.

IV. LEGAL ISSUES

Persons with disabilities daily face challenges beyond
their individual disabilities. Social prejudice and physical barriers often pose far greater hindrances. Prejudice
takes the form of the myths, stereotypes, and irrational
fears that many people in society associate with impaired
functioning. Barriers are those environmental factors,
both physical and social, that limit the meaningful involvement of persons with disabilities in normal life activities (West, 1993). While a corpus of law has been
developed in the United States to protect persons with
disabilities, the passage of the Americans with Disabilities Act (ADA) of 1990 (42 U.S.C. 112101–12213
[Supp. II 1990]) marks the most important federal anti-
discrimination legislation since the Civil Rights Act of
1964.

The social situation of persons with disabilities

The ADA was enacted in response to profound inequities and injustice for persons with disabilities. Disabled Americans are typically poorer, less educated, less
likely to be employed, and less likely to participate in
social events than other groups in society. Social attitudes toward persons with disabilities add to their burdens. Persons with disabilities may be ignored, treated
with pity or fear, adulated as "inspirations" for their efforts to overcome their disabilities, or expected to be as
"normal" as possible. Moreover, disabled Americans
have historically lacked a subculture from which to derive a collective strength, primarily due to the disparity
of their disabilities and backgrounds. Disability interest
groups, offshoots of civil rights groups, are slowly filling
this void (West, 1993).

Such prejudice and barriers raise a number of legal
issues, most notably discrimination. In employment, in
education, and in mobility, society often fails in its efforts to effectively accommodate persons with disabilities.

Legal responses to disability

Legal responses to disability issues range from application of constitutional theory to statutory initiatives. It
would be comforting to believe that the U.S. Consti-

tution provides meaningful protection to persons with
disabilities. Sadly, the Constitution has little to offer
persons with disabilities except in egregious cases. The
Bill of Rights is applicable to the state or those acting
under color of state law. Since most forms of discrimination take place in the private sector, the Constitution
is of limited applicability.

Even where state action can be demonstrated, the
Supreme Court has never enunciated a coherent and
compelling constitutional doctrine to protect persons
with disabilities against discrimination. The Court, for
example, has never found disability to be a "suspect classification," and most government activities do not deprive persons with disabilities of a "fundamental freedom
such as liberty" (*City of Cleburne*, 1985). Accordingly,
the Court might be expected to uphold a state discriminatory action, provided the government could show a
reasonable basis for its policy.

The Supreme Court, in one of its few decisions concerning discrimination against persons with disabilities,
did suggest that it would not tolerate clear instances of
prejudice or animus in government policies. In *City of
Cleburne, Texas v. Cleburne Living Center* (1985), the
Court struck down a city zoning ordinance that excluded group homes for persons with mental retardation.
The Court, in a particularly thorough search of the record, found no rational basis to believe that mentally retarded people would pose a special threat to the city's
legitimate interest (Gostin, 1987).

A convincing constitutional argument could be
made that persons with disabilities should have the same
level of constitutional protection as African-Americans
due to their similar history of exclusion and alienation
by the wider society. In the field of race, the Court has
fashioned its principle of the least restrictive alternative.
That doctrine requires government policies to achieve
their objectives in ways that are least intrusive on individual rights and liberties. Although the ADA does not
expressly use the phrase "least restrictive alternative," it
clearly embraces the concept. If a person's disabilities
truly disqualify him or her from a job, or make him or
her ineligible for a public service, reasonable accommodations should be designed to provide the least con-
straining opportunity for the person.

Statutory initiatives in disability law fall into three
general categories: (1) programs and services, (2) income maintenance, and (3) civil rights. Such statutes
incrementally have sought the legislative goals of full
participation and independence for persons with disabilities. While state laws vary in scope and effect, at the
federal level three main acts shaped the corpus of disability law prior to enactment of the ADA.

The federal Rehabilitation Act (29 U.S.C. 791–
794 [1988 and Supp. I 1989]), enacted in 1973, covered
federally funded entities (and continues to cover all fed-

eral employees). Section 504 of this act (broadened by amendments in 1987) prohibits discrimination against otherwise qualified disabled persons in any federally funded program, executive agency, or the Postal Service. Sections 501 and 503 require affirmative-action hiring plans in the federal government and certain large federal contractors.

The Individuals with Disabilities Education Act (IDEA) (42 U.S.C. 6000–6081 [1975]; 20 U.S.C. 1400 et seq. [1991]), enacted in 1975 and amended in 1990, mandates a free and appropriate education for all children with disabilities, encouraging integration ("mainstreaming") whenever possible.

The Fair Housing Amendments Act of 1988 (42 U.S.C. 3601–3619 [1988]) ensures that persons with disabilities are a protected class in housing discrimination cases, and mandates access requirements for new housing and adaptation requirements for existing housing to ensure that the housing needs of disabled persons are met. This act continues to cover housing discrimination in place of specific provisions in the ADA.

The Americans with Disabilities Act of 1990

While these initiatives were a start, they failed to address cohesively the needs and rights of persons with disabilities. The ADA is a definitive response to the needs and rights of persons with disabilities, needs and rights articulated by the growing voice of disability interest groups in America.

More specifically, as an outgrowth of civil rights law, the ADA serves as a premier legal tool because of its broad scope and unique ability to adopt the visions of both equality and special treatment. The ADA recognizes that a person's disabilities often have little to do with his or her inabilities. Often it is society's reactions to the person with disabilities or society's structural barriers that disable the person. The mandate of civil rights law is to destroy those negative reactions and dismantle those barriers in order to restore equal opportunity and full participation in daily life activities with dignity, not charity. The ADA strives to achieve this objective.

The act prohibits discrimination against qualified persons with disabilities in employment, public services, public accommodations, and telecommunications. The principal change in federal law is that the ADA applies to all covered entities, whether or not they receive federal funding. The ADA states that nothing in the act can be construed so as to apply a lesser standard than is already required under existing law (sec. 501). This means that the case law precedents under existing disability law are the minimum standards required by the ADA.

The impact of the ADA on public-health departments and communicable-disease law (Gostin, 1991b)

and on the health-care system (Gostin and Beyer, 1993) is significant. It will also have a significant impact on other important areas of bioethics, including the duty to treat, the right to health-benefit coverage, and medical testing and examinations by employers (Parmet, 1990).

Although the specific titles of the ADA have slightly different provisions, a finding of discrimination is based on adverse treatment of a person (1) with a "disability" who is (2) "qualified" or who (3) would be qualified if "reasonable accommodations" or modifications were made available (Feldblum, 1991).

Disability is defined broadly to mean "a physical or mental impairment that substantially limits one or more of the major life activities," a record of such impairment, or being regarded as having such impairment (sec. 3). The definition of disability covers a wide range of medical conditions. Congress and the courts have recognized disabilities that are both genetic (e.g., Down syndrome [Bowen v. American Hospital Association (1986)], muscular dystrophy [S. Rep. no. 116 (1989)]); or cystic fibrosis [Gerben v. Holsclaw (1988)] and multifactorial (e.g., heart disease, schizophrenia, or arthritis [S. Rep. no. 116 (1989)]). Disability includes diseases that are communicable (e.g., tuberculosis [School Bd. of Nassau County, Fla. v. Arline (1987)], hepatitis [New York State Assn. of Retarded Children v. Carey (1979)], or syphilis); as well as those that are not (e.g., cerebral palsy [Alexander v. Choate (1985)], or diabetes [S. Rep. no. 116 (1989)]).

The ADA covers most patients who are not seen as "deserving" by some segments of society, such as persons with HIV/AIDS (Benjamin R. v. Orkin Exterminating Co. [1990]), alcoholism (Traynor v. Turnage [1988]), and epilepsy (Reynolds v. Brock [1987]). However, a person who is currently using illegal drugs is not considered disabled, but is covered once he or she has been successfully rehabilitated and is no longer using drugs (sec. 510). Similarly, a range of socially disapproved behavior disorders are excluded from protection, such as most gender-identity disorders, pedophilia, exhibitionism, voyeurism, compulsive gambling, kleptomania, pyromania, and psychoactive drug-use disorders (sec. 511).

Moreover, a person is disabled if he or she has a "record" of, or is "regarded" as, being disabled, even if there is no actual disability (Southeastern Community College v. Davis [1979]). A "record" indicates that a person has, for example, a history of disability, thus protecting persons who have recovered from a disability or disease, such as cancer survivors.

The term "regarded" includes individuals who do not have disabilities but are treated as if they did. This concept protects people who are discriminated against in the false belief that they are disabled. It would be inequitable for a defendant who intended to discriminate on the basis of disability to successfully raise the defense that the person claiming discrimination was not, in fact, disabled. This provision is particularly important for individuals who are perceived to have stigmatizing or disfiguring conditions such as HIV, leprosy, or severe burns (S. Rep. no. 116 [1989]).

The fact that a perception of disability is included in the ADA is vitally important in determining whether a pure carrier of disease should be regarded as disabled. Congress expressly signaled its intention to include asymptomatic infection such as HIV, and this has been affirmed by the courts (*Doe v. Centinela Hosp.* [1988]).

A person is "qualified" if he or she is capable of meeting the essential performance or eligibility criteria for the particular position, service, or benefit. Thus, a person with a disability is not protected unless he or she is otherwise qualified to hold the job or to receive the service or benefit.

Qualification standards can include a requirement that the person with a disability does "not pose a direct threat to the health or safety of others" (secs. 103[b], 302 [b][3]). The "direct threat" standard means that persons can be excluded from jobs, public accommodations, or public services if necessary to prevent a "significant risk" to others (*School Bd. of Nassau County* [1987]). The "significant risk" standard originally applied only to persons with infectious disease. However, it was extended by the House Judiciary Committee to all persons with disabilities (H.R. Conf. Rep. no. 101-596 [1990]).

In order to determine, for example, that a person with mental illness poses a significant risk to others, evidence of specific dangerous behavior must be presented. In the context of infectious diseases such as tuberculosis, the Supreme Court laid down four criteria to determine significant risk: (1) the mode of transmission, (2) the duration of infectiousness, (3) the probability of the risk, and (4) the severity of the harm (*School Bd. of Nassau County* [1987]). These criteria would apply to HIV as well.

The ADA requires reasonable accommodations or modifications for otherwise qualified individuals unless it would pose an undue hardship (secs. 102[b][5], 302[b][2][A][ii]). This requires adaptation of facilities to make them accessible, modification of equipment to make it usable, and job restructuring to provide more flexible schedules for persons who need medical treatment (sec. 101[9]). To accommodate otherwise qualified persons with infectious conditions, an entity might have to reduce or eliminate the risk of transmission. Employers, for example, might be required to provide infection control and training to reduce nosocomial (disease or condition acquired in the hospital) or blood-borne infections. An employer, however, is not forced to endure an undue hardship that would alter the fundamental nature of the business or would be disproportionately costly. The Eighth Circuit Court of Appeals, for exam-

ple, held that a school for persons with mental retardation was not obliged to vaccinate employees in order reasonably to accommodate a student who was an active carrier of hepatitis B virus (*Kohl v. Woodhaven Learning Center* [1989]).

Conceptual foundations of the ADA

Conceptually, the ADA follows two distinct traditions. First, it is the culmination of the aforementioned series of federal statutes prohibiting discrimination against persons with disabilities. The ADA does not replace, but supplements, the large body of disability law that already exists.

The ADA treats persons with disabilities as if their disabilities do not matter by requiring businesses, public accommodations, public services, transportation, and communications authorities not to discriminate. This concept of equal treatment is powerfully articulated in the law. At the same time disability law also requires special treatment. The law requires the aforementioned entities to adopt a concept of affirmative action that *focuses* on the person's disabilities, as well as on societal barriers to equal treatment (Feldblum, 1993). The ADA requires reasonable accommodations or modifications designed to enable or empower the person with disabilities to take his or her rightful place in society. The law, therefore, insists on special treatment when that is necessary to allow a person to perform a job, enter a public building, or receive public service. As the Supreme Court observed over two decades ago, "Sometimes the greatest discrimination can lie in treating things that are different as though they were exactly alike" (*Jenness et al. v. Fortson* [1971] at 442).

Disability law, however, does not take the special treatment principle to its logical extension. It does not allocate tax dollars to enable the person to participate equally in society, beyond use of government funds for "reasonable accommodations" in such areas as public transportation. Nor does it require covered entities to spend unlimited amounts to provide equal access and opportunities for persons with disabilities. The law allows employers and others to avoid the burden of reasonable accommodations or modifications if they can demonstrate an undue hardship.

The ADA arises out of a second distinct tradition: civil rights law. Like civil rights law, the ADA views disabled persons as unique individuals with strengths and weaknesses, but also with inherent worth, equal to all others. The act, therefore, perceives discrimination on the basis of disability in much the same way that civil rights law views African-Americans, women, and religious minorities. In each case the law will not allow different treatment based upon a status or immutable condition.

Disability law, therefore, views discrimination by examining the motivation of the bigot. The question asked is whether the person is treating an individual differently because of prejudice, irrational fear, or stereotype. Nor can the person who discriminates hide behind the fears or prejudices of others. It may, for example, seem unfair for the law to require a restaurant to hire a food worker with AIDS or a disfiguring condition that will drive the owner out of business. If the reason for discrimination is not bigotry but business necessity, should not the law be more flexible? If the reason for discrimination is the refusal of fellow employees to work with the person or the refusal of customers to patronize the establishment, should not the law have sympathy for the owner?

If disability law is to follow the precedent of civil rights law, the answer is that no flexibility can be shown. One might ask whether civil rights law can or should excuse a restaurant owner from hiring an African-American because white people would not enter the establishment. The tradition of civil rights law is that client preference or the prejudice or irrational fears of others can never excuse discrimination.

Disability law stands for this proposition. The only basis for treating persons with disabilities differently is that they are not qualified for the job or eligible for the service. Even if their disability renders them unqualified or ineligible, they must be provided accommodations, modifications, or services reasonably necessary to them to perform their job or become eligible for the service.

The ADA promises to replace a great deal of constitutional analysis. It does so because, unlike the Constitution, it reaches deep into the private sector. It delivers a promise of true equal protection of the law in a way that the Constitution as construed by the Supreme Court has never done. That promise of equal protection goes beyond equal treatment. It promises special treatment.

Conclusion: A new vision

The ADA may revolutionize the way we view the law's protection and empowerment of persons with disabilities. No longer will we see persons with disabilities through the lens of charity, sympathy, or benign discretion. Now we must see persons with disabilities through the lens of civil rights law. Under civil rights law persons with disabilities need not ask for societal favors. They can demand an equal place in a society that has long been structured—physically and sociologically—by and for the able-bodied.

LAWRENCE O. GOSTIN
BARBARA L. LOONEY

Directly related to this article are the other articles in this entry: ATTITUDES AND SOCIOLOGICAL PERSPECTIVES, PHILOSOPHICAL AND THEOLOGICAL PERSPECTIVES, *and* HEALTH CARE AND PHYSICAL DISABILITY. *For a further discussion of topics mentioned in this article, see the entries* LAW AND BIOETHICS; RACE AND RACISM; *and* SEXISM. *For a discussion of related ideas, see the entries* COMPETENCE; JUSTICE; *and* RIGHTS. *Other relevant material may be found under the entries* AGING AND THE AGED; AIDS; HEALTH-CARE FINANCING, *especially the articles on* MEDICARE, *and* MEDICAID; HEALTH-CARE RESOURCES, ALLOCATION OF, *article on* MACROALLOCATION; HEALTH AND DISEASE; LAW AND MORALITY; LIFE, QUALITY OF; MENTAL ILLNESS; MENTALLY DISABLED AND MENTALLY ILL PERSONS; PATIENTS' RIGHTS, *article on* ORIGIN AND NATURE OF PATIENTS' RIGHTS; *and* REHABILITATION MEDICINE.

Bibliography

Alexander v. Choate. 469 U.S. 287 (1985).

Americans with Disabilities Act of 1990. 42 U.S.C. 12101–12213 (Supp. II 1990).

Benjamin R. v. Orkin Exterminating Co. 390 S.E.2d 148 (W.Va.S.Ct. 1990).

Bowen v. American Hospital Association. 476 U.S. 610 (1986).

City of Cleburne, Texas v. Cleburne Living Center, Inc. 473 U.S. 432 (1985).

Civil Rights Act of 1964, codified as amended in scattered sections of 42 U.S.C. (1988).

Doe v. Centinela Hosp. 57 USLW 2034 (C.D. Cal. 1988).

Education for All Handicapped Children Act of 1975. 20 U.S.C. 1400 et seq. (1975).

Fair Housing Amendments Act of 1988. 42 U.S.C. 3601–3619 (1988).

FELDBLUM, CHAI R. 1991. "The Americans with Disabilities Act: Definition of Disability." *Labor Lawyer* 7, no. 1:11–26.

———. 1993. "Anti-Discrimination Requirements of the ADA." In *Implementing the Americans with Disabilities Act: Rights and Responsibilities of All Americans*, pp. 35–56. Edited by Lawrence O. Gostin and Henry Beyer. Baltimore: Paul H. Brooks.

Gerben v. Holsclaw. 692 F.Supp. 557 (E.D.Pa. 1988).

GOSTIN, LAWRENCE O. 1987. "The Future of Public Health Law." *American Journal of Law and Medicine* 12, nos. 3–4:461–490.

———. 1991a. "Genetic Discrimination: The Use of Genetically Based Diagnostic and Prognostic Tests by Employers and Insurers." *American Journal of Law and Medicine* 17, nos. 1–2:109–144.

———. 1991b. "Public Health Powers: The Imminence of Radical Change." *Milbank Memorial Fund Quarterly* 69 (suppl. 1–2):268–290.

———. 1993. "Impact of the ADA on the Health Care System: Genetic Discrimination in Employment and Insurance." In *Implementing the Americans with Disabilities Act: Rights and Responsibilities of All Americans*, pp. 175–187.

Edited by Lawrence O. Gostin and Henry Beyer. Baltimore: Paul H. Brooks.

GOSTIN, LAWRENCE O., and BEYER, HENRY, eds. 1993. *Implementing the Americans with Disabilities Act: Rights and Responsibilities of All Americans.* Baltimore: Paul H. Brooks.

H.R. Conf. Rep. no. 101-596. 102nd Cong., 1st Sess. (1990).

Individuals with Disabilities Education Act of 1992. 20 U.S.C. 1400 et seq. (1991).

Jenness et al. v. Fortson. 403 U.S. 431 (1971).

Kohl v. Woodhaven Learning Center. 865 F.2d 930 (8th Cir. 1989).

New York State Assn. of Retarded Children v. Carey. 612 F.2d 644 (2d Cir. 1979).

PARMET, WENDY E. 1990. "Discrimination and Disability: The Challenges of the ADA." *Law, Medicine and Health Care* 18, no. 4:331–344.

Rehabilitation Act of 1973. 29 U.S.C. 791–794. (1988 and Supp. I 1989).

Reynolds v. Brock. 815 F.2d 571 (9th Cir. 1987).

School Bd. of Nassau County, Fla. v. Arline. 480 U.S. 273 (1987).

Southeastern Community College v. Davis. 442 U.S. 397 (1979).

S. Rep. no. 116. 101st Cong., 1st Sess. (1989).

Traynor v. Turnage. 485 U.S. 535 (1988).

WEST, JANE. 1993. "The Evolution of Disability Rights." In *Implementing the Americans with Disabilities Act: Rights and Responsibilities of All Americans,* pp. 3–15. Edited by Lawrence O. Gostin and Henry Beyer. Baltimore: Paul H. Brooks.

DISABILITY FOR PUBLIC OFFICE

A person's claim to aspire to, or resist expulsion from, a particular public office depends largely on his or her physical and mental capacities to perform the duties of that office. Beyond the general principle that a person holding an office has a duty to be able to execute the demands of the office because the public trust resides precisely in an elected or appointed person's competence, the legal and ethical grounds for exclusion may vary dramatically from office to office ((Robins and Rothschild, 1988). A disability per se is not a disqualification for public office. People who are physically limited by accidents or congenital anomalies, for example, may execute superbly the duties of a particular office.

More subtle forms of disability, however, such as mental and emotional impairments, may be incapacitating enough to be disqualifying. Ironically, they are often the least evident characteristic of an officeholder or candidate. Depression, delusional syndromes, and cognitive disabilities, for example, may impair officeholders to the point that they place the common welfare in peril. Does a public official have a responsibility to divulge sensitive medical information that might have bearing on his performance? What is the role of the medical profession in monitoring the behavior of patients who are entrusted with the public welfare? How should a physician discern when—if ever—he or she should break confidence with a patient whose illness is having an impact on public affairs?

History provides instances in which illness and power have converged to highlight these questions. This article examines: (1) the cases of three U.S. presidents; (2) the constitutional response to an incapacitated president; and (3) the ethical challenges such situations offer to society and to health professionals in particular.

Illness and the American presidency

Woodrow Wilson. By the time Woodrow Wilson assumed the office of president of the United States in 1912, he was already suffering from the aftereffects of a series of strokes (Weinstein, 1970, 1981; L'Etang, 1970; Park, 1986). The symptoms that followed these neurologic events included sudden changes in mood, severe headaches, numbness, transient blindness in one eye, and, toward the end of Wilson's life, total paralysis of the affected limbs and periods of unconsciousness.

Wilson led the United States into World War I in the midst of what would eventually become a picture of evolving neurologic devastation and later directed his country's effort during the Versailles Peace Conference. While at the Versailles Conference in April of 1919, Wilson began to exhibit irrational, even paranoid behavior (Crispell and Gomez, 1988). Following his return to the United States that summer, the president embarked on an arduous, cross-country trip to enlist public support for the Versailles Treaty. At the end of this trip, he collapsed with a massive stroke, which resulted in complete paralysis of his left side.

Despite the president's severely compromised state, he remained in office. When Wilson's secretary of state, Robert Lansing, tentatively raised the issue of the president's disability—and of a possible transfer of power to the vice president—the president's physician, Cary Grayson, became incensed and accused the secretary of state of disloyalty. Dr. Grayson declared that he would never certify that the president was disabled. In this debilitated, paralyzed condition, the president of the United States waited out the completion of his term in 1920.

Franklin Roosevelt. The political career of Franklin D. Roosevelt, who was crippled by polio as a young adult, provides a powerful reminder that obvious signs of disability (e.g., the need for a wheelchair) do not constitute grounds for exclusion from public office. Despite his physical limitations, Roosevelt governed with an energy and vigor that astounded even his most ardent critics (L'Etang, 1970). Yet Roosevelt was eventually more seriously and insidiously disabled by a quiet disease, hypertension. Its chronic, unremitting course had devastating effects on the rest of his cardiovascular system.

The president and his advisers were aware of the problem, though they went to great lengths to hide it from the public. As early as December 1941, shortly after election to his unprecedented third term, Roosevelt began making clandestine visits to Bethesda Naval Hospital under assumed names. James D. Elliott, Ralph Frank, Rolphe Frank, and Mr. Delano were some of the aliases the ailing President used as he sought help from a young naval cardiologist, Howard Bruenn, for his worsening congestive heart failure (Crispell and Gomez, 1989). Hampered by what was then a very limited therapeutic armamentarium, Bruenn nevertheless managed to sustain his patient through four arduous years as commander in chief (Bruenn, 1970).

The case has been made that the United States was being served by an extremely unhealthy president throughout a period of enormous challenge to the republic and its allies. By February of 1945, for example, during the Yalta negotiations, observers at the conference were struck by the president's appearance: his ashen face, gaunt figure, and shaking hands betrayed the gravity of his condition (L'Etang, 1970). That the Yalta conference did not go as well as the Allies had hoped was, according to some, more a function of wartime planning than of the president's illness at the conference. Yet the same argument can be made to suggest that it was precisely this lack of foresight during the war—the planning of which devolved on an ailing president—that changed the nature of postwar Europe.

John F. Kennedy.   If the case of Franklin Roosevelt shows the potential damage of having medical practice taken over by political concerns, John F. Kennedy's story raises even more perplexing questions about the medical profession's responsibility to a patient who holds high public office.

Despite his public image as a youthful, vigorous leader, John Kennedy had been chronically sick since birth, and had been administered the last rites of the Catholic Church at least twice by the time he reached the White House in 1960 (Blair and Blair, 1976). As early as 1948, Kennedy had been diagnosed with Addison's disease, which is the endpoint of a gradual deterioration of the adrenal glands. Symptoms include hypotension, anorexia, lethargy, and general malaise. If left untreated, it is fatal. Fortunately for Kennedy, by the time he had his first documented Addisonian crisis, cortisone had been synthesized and was just starting to be used successfully in patients with adrenal insufficiency.

As a relatively obscure senator, John Kennedy could hope to live out a normal life, taking cortisone supplementation and altering his life's stresses to meet his physical needs. As a candidate for president, however, he faced not only enormous new stresses, but an additional political problem as well: His medical history had been published (without naming Kennedy specifically) in 1954 when he underwent back surgery (Nicholas et al., 1955; Nichols, 1967). During the 1960 campaign, the candidates' health problems were, for the first time, front-page news. Kennedy faced the embarrassing prospect of having his Addison's disease discovered.

Kennedy's private physician, Janet Travell, and his press secretary issued a series of public statements designed to quell speculation about the future president's health. Noting that the disease first described by Thomas Addison involved tuberculous destruction of the adrenal glands, Kennedy's campaign spokesperson stated that the candidate did not have the ailment "described classically as Addison's disease." He failed to mention that most twentieth-century cases of Addison's disease, including Kennedy's, were not infectious but autoimmune in origin (Lattimer, 1980). Press releases went on to note that though Kennedy might have had "mild adrenal insufficiency" as a result of the trauma of his wartime experiences, he had been "rehabilitated" from "a depletion of adrenal function," conveniently ignoring the fact that his "rehabilitation" involved daily dosing of steroids, with their potential for serious side effects, including overwhelming infections and changes in mental status (Blair and Blair, 1976).

These statements, issued under a physician's authority, helped to defuse successfully a potentially awkward revelation for the nascent Kennedy campaign. Whether or not President Kennedy was any the worse for his illness, however well compensated, is still debated. Nevertheless, it was an issue neither the future president nor his physicians wanted debated in public.

Constitutional response

The Kennedy presidency itself provided an impetus for constitutional reform for transfer of presidential power. Following President Kennedy's assassination in November 1963, Congress conducted a series of hearings, chaired by then Senator Birch Bayh, which eventually led to the passage in 1964 of the Twenty-fifth Amendment, with final ratification in 1967 (Feerick, 1976).

Of the amendment's four sections, the last section attempts to deal with the most troublesome cases of presidential inability—those in which the president cannot or will not declare himself or herself unable to serve. In such instances, the vice president and a majority of the cabinet are to inform Congress, in writing, of the president's disability. With that, the vice president becomes acting president. The president may subsequently declare to Congress that the inability has ceased to exist. The vice president and the cabinet then have four days to respond, either by returning power to the president, or by issuing a challenge to the declaration. In the latter event, Congress is required to convene within forty-eight hours and decide the matter within twenty-one days. If the twenty-one–day period expires and Congress fails to act, or the challenge is not upheld by a two-thirds majority vote in both houses, the president resumes office.

Despite the detailed provisions of the amendment, it has been criticized for being too unwieldy and unworkable. Yet even a more tightly written constitutional amendment would still fail to respond adequately to the delicate situation created by an impaired officeholder. The case histories of the presidents outlined above illustrate this point.

Physician's response

The physician, in particular, is placed in an awkward situation: How does one decide when a particular ailment or handicap disqualifies a patient from public office? In some instances, the burden of disease obviously seems beyond the patient's capacity to hide and still function in office. In other instances however, the decision seems less obvious. In 1972, for example, revelations about Senator Thomas Eagleton's history of recurrent depression were sufficient to make him untenable as Senator George McGovern's running mate. Would Abraham Lincoln's tendency toward depression have disqualified him from modern presidential politics?

More to the point, the greater difficulty ultimately may lie not in deciding what disqualifies a person from public office, but in discerning the responsibilities and duties physicians and the rest of society have when an officeholder refuses to disqualify himself or herself from office despite a handicap that impairs the ability to perform duties.

In accepting the limitations of the law and the restrictions on physicians by canons of professional conduct, the following general rules might help protect the rights and needs of both the patient and the public:

1. Physicians should not lie on behalf of the officeholder-patient. It is one thing to remain silent about a patient's illness, but quite another to lie publicly about it. Physicians may have an obligation to hold fast to the first stipulation but should rarely (if ever) engage in the second. Moreover, they should make this plain to patients at the outset of the relationship.

2. Physicians should exercise medical judgment. In other words, physicians should exercise that capacity for which they have been trained. That the patient in question is also an officeholder may enter into consideration, but only as it relates to the patient's medical condition.

3. Physicians should not confuse professional roles. The cases of the presidents' physicians discussed in this article all share, to some extent, the common failing of physicians' falling into a political role. Not only could one argue that in doing so, they failed to serve the public's interest; perhaps more importantly, they also failed to serve their patient's interests. Medical practice was subordinated to political exigencies. The particular psychological demands of a patient in public office may make this a difficult line to draw, but that is all the more reason to draw it sharply.

4. Physicians should appeal to the patients' sense of professional responsibility. Any patient is entitled to privacy and confidentiality, but that entitlement is not an absolute right. Moreover, any person, whether disabled or not at the outset, should be prepared either to surrender part of his or her privacy (allow the public to be informed of the malady and to judge its impact on the office) or, alternatively, to surrender the office should he or she be unable to discharge its duties.

CARLOS F. GOMEZ

For a further discussion of topics mentioned in this article, see the entries CONFIDENTIALITY; CONFLICT OF INTEREST; EXPERT TESTIMONY; *and* PRIVILEGED COMMUNICATIONS. *Other relevant material may be found under the entries* COMPETENCE; DIVIDED LOYALTIES IN MENTAL-HEALTH CARE; *and* RESPONSIBILITY.

Bibliography

BLAIR, JOAN, and BLAIR, CLAY. 1976. *The Search for JFK.* New York: Beckley.

BROWNELL, HERBERT. 1958. "Presidential Inability: The Need for a Constitutional Amendment." *Yale Law Journal* 68, no. 2:189–231.

BRUENN, HOWARD G. 1970. "Clinical Notes on the Illness and Death of President Franklin D. Roosevelt." *Annals of Internal Medicine* 72, no. 4:579–591.

CRISPELL, KENNETH R., and GOMEZ, CARLOS F. 1988. *Hidden Illness in the White House.* Durham, N.C.: Duke University Press.

CURRAN, WILLIAM J. 1986. "Presidential Inability to Function: The Medicolegal Issues." *New England Journal of Medicine* 132, no. 5:301–302.

FEERICK, JOHN D. 1976. *The Twenty-Fifth Amendment: Its Complete History and Earliest Applications.* New York: Fordham University Press.

LATTIMER, JOHN K. 1980. *Kennedy and Lincoln: Medical and Ballistic Comparisons of Their Assassinations.* New York: Harcourt, Brace, Jovanovich.

L'ETANG, HUGH. 1970. *The Pathology of Leadership.* New York: Hawthorn.

NICHOLAS, JAMES A.; BURSTEIN, CHARLES L.; UMBERGER, CHARLES J.; and WILSON, PHILIP D. 1955. "Management of Adrenocortical Insufficiency During Surgery." *Archives of Surgery* 71:737–742.

NICHOLS, JOHN. 1967. "President Kennedy's Adrenals." *Journal of the American Medical Association* 201, no. 2:115–116.

PARK, BERT E. 1986. *The Impact of Illness of World Leaders.* Philadelphia: University of Pennsylvania Press.

ROBINS, ROBERT S., and ROTHSCHILD, HENRY. 1988. "Ethical Dilemmas of the President's Physician." *Politics and Life Sciences* 7, no. 1:3–10.

SIEGLER, MARK. 1982. "Confidentiality in Medicine: A Decrepit Concept." *New England Journal of Medicine* 307, no. 1:1518–1521.

WEINSTEIN, EDWIN A. 1970. "Woodrow Wilson's Neurological Illness." *Journal of American History* 57, no. 2:324–351.

———. 1981. *Woodrow Wilson: A Medical and Psychological Biography.* Princeton, N.J.: Princeton University Press.

DISEASE

See HEALTH AND DISEASE.

DIVIDED LOYALTIES IN MENTAL-HEALTH CARE

In many situations in mental-health care, professionals face conflicts between obligation to the patient and obligation to another individual or organization. These conflicts are referred to as "double-agent" or divided-loyalty dilemmas and are most dramatic when the health professional is employed by a prison, the armed forces, or a government agency. Regardless of the size or character of the institution or agency, doctors are faced with a critical question: Whom do they serve? The institution or agency that employs them or the individual patient? What are the moral claims on the doctor in such situations? Whose claims should take precedence when these claims are in conflict?

Ruth Macklin contends that from the moral point of view most double-agent situations are best seen as cases of conflicting loyalty or clashing duties. The doctor must choose one loyalty or duty over another (Macklin, 1982). On what basis should he or she make this choice?

Thomas Murray has written that it is appropriate to analyze divided-loyalty dilemmas in a way that will link them with the social conditions that nurture them and to examine their ethical implications in the light of an adequate conceptual understanding of them. He states further that divided-loyalty dilemmas permit four generalizations (Murray, 1986): They are often linked with the need to perform a social control function; they must be understood in terms of the moral values served by the medical profession; significant in their creation and resolution are patients' expectations of their doctors; and understanding the complex nature of the doctor–patient relationship is essential in making sense out of divided-loyalty dilemmas.

The doctor–patient relationship is generally understood to rest on a contract, with duties and compensations spelled out, or as a covenant implying the trusting and reciprocal nature of the relationship. No matter how the doctor–patient relationship is described, patients' expectations are crucial. Patients expect that their needs will be the doctor's first consideration, and that the doctor will be their advocate.

The nature of the doctor–patient relationship and the expectations of the patient define the conduct of medical practice. The belief that the doctor's responsibility is to the patient and to no other is a value like informed consent and confidentiality, and arises from a commitment to the individual. When this belief or value is in conflict with the interests and needs of another person, family, institution, or organization, the divided-loyalty dilemma emerges.

A doctor may work directly for individual patients or as an employee of others such as family, industry, school, courts, prison system, the armed forces, or health maintenance organizations (HMOs). Under some circumstances, the doctor may retain an autonomous role and act as an agent for patients. In other circumstances, the organization that has employed the doctor may encroach on the doctor's role in serving first and foremost the interests and needs of the patient. An example may be a university who has a student evaluated by the psychiatrist employed in the university's health service (Arnstein, 1986). The student has emotional problems that he believes can be dealt with while remaining in school. The psychiatrist evaluates the student and makes recommendations to the university. The student may assume that the psychiatrist is working on his behalf, and maybe she is. At the same time, she is working for the university and may be strongly influenced by a loyalty to the university and how the university wants the problem with the student resolved. The psychiatrist has been forced into a double-agent situation, in part because of who has hired her. Thus, Thomas Szasz insists that this question must always be asked: In a given situation, whose side does the psychiatrist take, the individual's or another party's? (Szasz,

1970). If the answer is not clarified, then the psychiatrist is functioning as a double agent, with a loyalty divided between the two.

Divided-loyalty dilemmas may be created by an effort to subvert the goals or ends of medicine. The athlete who wants the sports physician to permit him to compete despite injuries that might well become aggravated into chronic disabilities, or to take drugs like anabolic steroids that the athlete believes will enhance his competitive abilities, may create a conflict or disagreement about values. The conflict is between the importance of success in a sport and the value of conserving health. A physician asked to help someone in risking his health is in a divided-loyalty dilemma, because he is torn between loyalty to his patient's interests, as the patient sees or defines them, and loyalty to the ends of medicine, including the pursuit of health and the avoidance of potential harm.

Double-agent or divided-loyalty dilemmas linked with the need to perform a social control function have had a long history in mental-health care, ranging in complexity from coercive forms of behavior control to expanding the diagnostic categories of mental illness so as to cover behaviors not usually considered deviant.

Background and history

Divided-loyalty dilemmas have been most blatant in efforts at social control. Since mental-health care often deals with deviance in behavior, its conceptions run parallel to society's conceptions of social behavior, personal worth, and morality. Thus, in certain situations, there may be great pressure for mental-health professionals to label patients on the basis of social, ethical, or legal norms and not on clearly established clinical or laboratory evidence of psychopathology.

As David Mechanic emphasizes, doctors are influenced in their activity and judgment by the sociocultural context, by the ideology implicit in their professional training, and by the economic and organizational constraints of the setting in which they practice. Their practice involves multiple and, at times, competing professional roles with different social and ethical requirements, but often with no clear definition of boundaries (Mechanic, 1981). In the middle of any of these contexts, with claims from many sides, the practitioner must always ask the crucial question: Whom do I represent and whom do I serve? History is replete with cases showing that the patient is not always the primary one represented.

The problem of divided or dual loyalties reached a surrealistic dimension in the Nazi death camps where physicians who were committed by professional oath to heal the sick carried out government orders and initiated acts that dehumanized, maimed, and destroyed people they were dedicated to save (Drob, 1992; Lifton, 1986). Nazi doctors acted completely contrary to their own moral and professional commitments, serving the state and not their patients. These historic lessons make more urgent the need to examine divided loyalties.

The use of psychiatry as an instrument of social control has had a long history among the former Soviets. Soviet authorities chose to have dissenters from official governmental policy labeled with mental-illness designations, such as schizophrenia or paranoid development of the personality. The labeling of persons as mentally ill is an effective way to discredit their beliefs and actions, past or present, while maintaining control over those persons of whom the government disapproves. These dissenters were given therapy with little or no intention of addressing their needs and wishes but rather to make them less angry and thereby more satisfied with the political and social system as it existed.

Certain practices in Soviet psychiatry resulted in extreme forms of divided loyalties in mental-health professionals, and there is little comparison between the practices of Soviet psychiatry and those of psychiatry in the United States. It remains instructive, however, to compare the differences in the moral and political realm between behavior control in a totalitarian regime and behavior control in a free society (Macklin, 1982).

Activities in our country have at times shown how an agency or family in a free society may use psychiatry to serve its interests and not those of the patient. One notorious example is the case of Frances Farmer. Institutionalized by her mother for political nonconformism, the actress received electroshock treatments and finally a lobotomy (Arnold, 1978). In cases of socially controversial new religious movements, distressed families may request that a psychiatrist assess the mental state of recruits to such groups, often labeled cults. The psychiatrist may be caught in a divided-loyalty dilemma between family values and religious liberties, possibly medicalizing religious conversions and then treating them as illnesses (Post, 1993).

Double agentry can occur when the mental-health professional has written an article about a patient, a research subject, or the subject of a forensic examination. The dilemma in these situations involves a conflict between respecting patient confidentiality and the professional's own interest or sense of obligation to disseminate scientific knowledge.

Marketing and advertising strategies in medicine, and particularly in psychiatry, have contributed to double-agentry problems. The conflict here is between what is best for the patient and what is the most profitable course of action for the professional or the institution. Charles Dougherty describes this long-standing problem:

"There is money to be made in the creation of new psychological diseases, in defining behavioral problems as mental disorders, and in cultivating a false desire for the elusive ideal or perfect mental health" (Dougherty, 1988, p. 18).

The question of divided loyalty can readily arise in matters of confidentiality. Do mental-health professionals owe confidentiality to patients who reveal plans or acts that endanger others? This question came dramatically to public attention in 1974 in the murder of a college student, Tatiana Tarasoff, and the subsequent lawsuits brought by the student's parents against the university, the campus police, and the psychotherapist who had failed to warn her of threats against her life by her murderer, a homicidal patient (*Tarasoff* v. *Regents of the University of California,* 1976). The therapist had alerted campus police to the danger the patient posed; they arrested him but found him harmless and released him. Later, on her return to the university from a vacation, Tarasoff was murdered by the patient.

The courts have now imposed on mental-health professionals a legal duty to warn and to take action in case of a patient's posing a danger to third persons. Many professionals believe that this judicial mandate to warn has resulted in the impairment of the therapeutic relationship, the one avenue of intervention most likely to help patients establish control over their aggression, and has caused an erosion of public confidence in the psychiatrist's ability to assure confidentiality. Actually, this double-agentry dilemma could be avoided if warnings were discretionary rather than mandatory. This would allow the psychiatrist first to use his clinical resources to seek help if needed from the patient's family and relevant authorities in instituting hospitalization. If efforts at a rescue intervention in the face of realistic danger fail, then the duty to warn a specific victim becomes the priority.

The military is an organization whose needs and interests may compete with those of the patient. In the military, mental-health professionals are committed to serving society by supporting their commanders in carrying out military operations (Howe, 1986). The psychiatrist who returns a soldier to mental health may return him to a battlefield where he could be killed. Robert Jay Lifton highlights the ethical-psychological conflict by showing that the soldier's very sanity in seeking escape from the environment via a psychiatric judgment of instability renders him eligible for the continuing madness of killing and dying (Lifton, 1976). Even in military situations, mental-health professionals retain obligations to their profession. Further, their clinical effectiveness requires that they give high priority to the needs and interests of the military personnel they treat. In most cases, the mental-health professional's

ambiguous position in military medicine as double agent allows the mental-health professional to believe that he or she is participating in both the care of patients and the public interest (Howe, 1986).

The prison system has been the setting for a variety of divided-loyalty dilemmas. The professional may be called upon to restore the prisoner's sanity in order that the prisoner can go to trial. In a more extreme situation a prisoner is on death row awaiting execution, but his psychosis is causing the execution to be delayed. The prison authorities request treatment for the prisoner so he will be well enough to be executed. What does the prisoner want? Is informed consent obtained? Are such endeavors related in any way to the healing role of health professionals?

Conflicting obligations can easily arise in situations where doctors simultaneously deliver medical care to patients and use them as research subjects. While most doctors comply with their primary obligation to deliver the best possible care to their patients, the demands of adhering to a strict research design can create obligations that compete with those of giving good medical care. The rewards for doing research and publishing the results of a successful project are great, especially in the academic medical center. The research-oriented physician can be seduced into switching his or her primary obligation from the patient to the research.

Ethical analysis and resolution

James Dwyer states that a beginning step in resolving divided loyalties is to think of loyalty as an attachment or allegiance to a person or cause and to see it as expressing a coherent meaning that unifies one's personal and professional conduct. Loyalties develop with the assumption of roles and relationships inside as well as outside professional practice (Dwyer, 1992). The professional's identity is connected with the primary role of restoring the patient to health. In approaching a divided-loyalty dilemma, it is necessary to articulate and reflect on the meaning of one's commitments in order to determine how these commitments ought to be ordered or reconciled in a particular case.

A basic principle of medical practice is that health professionals should be loyal to their patients and be advocates for them. This commitment does not always avoid conflict. For example, even when health professionals devote themselves exclusively to the good of the patient and show no allegiance to other persons or causes, conflicts still may arise between what the professional sees as good treatment and what the patient wants and sees as good treatment.

The roots of the confidentiality concept are essentially ethical and not legal, and from the earliest days of medical practice, respect for the patient's confidences was considered an important part of the obligation owed by the physician to the patient. Communications told in secret and in trust were guarded and respected. In a situation such as the *Tarasoff* case, while acknowledging the desirability of maintaining patients' confidences, one sees a strong competing ethical obligation. When a patient intends harm to another person or when information is required for the adjudication of a dispute in court, physicians are faced with the claim that societal interests should take precedence. Today, while absolute confidentiality is no longer the expectation, arguments for protecting and extending confidentiality, even in the face of competing demands, remain strong. The arguments usually rest on both ethical and utilitarian grounds and center on the moral good reflected in protecting private utterances. The arguments relate to the belief that confidentiality promotes desirable goals, such as encouraging potential patients to seek medical care and allowing patients to unburden themselves while giving all information essential for the doctor to help them.

In a health-care system such as that in the United States, the practitioner's relationship to the patient is fiduciary, that is, he or she acts for the benefit of the patient. Can modifications be made that do not compromise the fiduciary relationship? Can the doctor–patient relationship be extended to support affirmative duties not only to the patient but also for the benefit of third parties? Ralph Slovenko, an attorney-psychologist, answers yes to this question, stating that a psychiatrist's loyalty to the patient and responsibility for treating the professional relationship with respect and honor do not negate responsibility to third parties, to the rest of the profession, to science, or to society. Slovenko goes on to say, however, that how these other duties are accepted, how the patient is kept informed, and how the patient is cared for when other duties are carried out can introduce or avoid a divided-loyalty dilemma (Slovenko, 1975).

Joan Rinas and Sheila Clyne-Jackson recommend a forthright stance in preventing double-agentry dilemmas. They argue that the mental-health professional has obligations to all parties with whom he or she has a relationship (Rinas and Clyne-Jackson, 1988). These duties include notifying all parties of their rights, the professional's specific obligations to each party, potential and realistic conflicts that may arise, and limitations in knowledge and therefore service. If on exchange of this information the mental-health professional concludes that he or she is not the appropriate one to provide the requested service, the patient or the third party should be referred to a professional appropriate and qualified to perform the desired function. Participants in a Hastings Center symposium on double agentry made a similar set of recommendations for addressing divided-loyalty dilemmas (Steinfels and Levine, 1978).

The answer to what appears to be a divided-loyalty dilemma in court cases may rest on a particular type of disclosure. Where the psychiatrist is functioning as a friend of the court, the primary loyalty is not to the patient but to society as embodied in the judicial system. In such settings, the doctor–patient relationship does not exist in the traditional sense, and both doctor and patient must understand this from the outset. Divided-loyalty dilemmas are prevented when the psychiatrist advises all parties involved that the relevant materials they provide will be used in the court proceedings and that the doctor is functioning as a consultant to the court (Goldzband, 1992).

Divided loyalties are becoming prevalent in relation to cost containment and rationing of health services. Society is demanding that health-care costs be controlled. In response, careful protocols are being developed as to what services can be given, how much, and for how long. These cost-containment methods may interfere with what patients realistically need to remedy their health problems and compromise the ethical principle of doctor as patient advocate. Macklin emphasizes that whether doctors are used to cut costs voluntarily in treating their patients, or are required to adhere to policies instituted by others, their ability to advocate vigorously for their patients' medical needs is weakened (Macklin, 1987). When rationing becomes a factor in physicians' treatment decisions, such as which of their patients will be admitted to the hospital and for how long, physicians are forced into a divided-loyalty conflict. Further, the care obligation embraced by medical ethics cannot be accomplished without permitting a physician to strive for "a robust patient–physician relationship, patient well-being, and avoidance of harm" (Wolf, 1994, p. 38).

Conclusion

Conflicting responsibilities, contradictory goals, hidden scenarios, and unsigned contracts existing in the changing world of both the patient and the professional remind us each day that ideal resolutions may be unattainable in many divided-loyalty dilemmas. Professionals must be very sensitive to the possibility that they may become double agents in the routines of their everyday practice with its many ambiguities and subtleties. Further, review and examination of double-agent issues should be a continuing obligation of mental-health professionals, according to Allen Dyer, for that is one way to prevent these issues from disrupting the doctor-patient relationship. He states that a function of professional ethics is to keep these reminders alive through education, codes, and professional discipline (Dyer, 1988).

JAMES ALLEN KNIGHT

Directly related to this entry are the entries CONFLICT OF INTEREST; MENTAL HEALTH; *and* MENTAL ILLNESS. *For a further discussion of topics mentioned in this entry, see the entries* CONFIDENTIALITY; FAMILY; FIDELITY AND LOYALTY; HARM; NATIONAL SOCIALISM; PRISONERS; PROFESSIONAL–PATIENT RELATIONSHIP; PSYCHIATRY, ABUSES OF; RESEARCH, UNETHICAL; *and* SPORTS. *For a discussion of related ideas, see the entries* COMMITMENT TO MENTAL INSTITUTIONS; FRAUD, THEFT, AND PLAGIARISM; HEALTH OFFICIALS AND THEIR RESPONSIBILITIES; HOMOSEXUALITY; MEDICAL EDUCATION; MENTAL-HEALTH SERVICES; MENTAL-HEALTH THERAPIES; MENTALLY ILL AND MENTALLY DISABLED PERSONS; MILITARY PERSONNEL AS RESEARCH SUBJECTS; MINORITIES AS RESEARCH SUBJECTS; *and* PSYCHOANALYSIS AND DYNAMIC THERAPIES. *See also the* APPENDIX (CODES, OATHS, AND DIRECTIVES RELATED TO BIOETHICS), SECTION II: ETHICAL DIRECTIVES FOR THE PRACTICE OF MEDICINE, *and* SECTION III: ETHICAL DIRECTIVES FOR OTHER HEALTH PROFESSIONS.

Bibliography

ARNOLD, WILLIAMS. 1978. *Shadowland.* New York: McGraw-Hill.

ARNSTEIN, ROBERT L. 1986. "Divided Loyalties in Adolescent Psychiatry: Late Adolescence." *Social Science and Medicine* 23, no. 8:797–802.

DOUGHERTY, CHARLES J. 1988. "Mind, Money, and Morality: Ethical Dimensions of Economic Change in American Psychiatry." *Hastings Center Report* 18, no. 3:15–20.

DROB, SANFORD L. 1992. "The Lessons from History: Physicians' Dual Loyalty in the Nazi Death Camps." *Review of Clinical Psychiatry and the Law,* 3:167–171.

DWYER, JAMES. 1992. "Conflicting Loyalties in the Practice of Psychiatry: Some Philosophical Reflections." *Review of Clinical Psychiatry and the Law* 3:157–166.

DYER, ALLEN R. 1988. *Ethics and Psychiatry: Toward Professional Definition.* Washington, D.C.: American Psychiatric Press.

GOLDZBAND, MELVIN G. 1992. "Dual Loyalties in Custody Cases and Elsewhere in Child and Adolescent Psychiatry." *Review of Clinical Psychiatry and the Law* 3:201–207.

HOWE, EDMUND G. 1986. "Ethical Issues Regarding Mixed Agency of Military Physicians." *Social Science and Medicine* 23, no. 8:803–815.

LIFTON, ROBERT JAY. 1976. "Advocacy and Corruption in the Healing Professions." *International Review of Psycho-Analysis* 3, no. 4:385–398.

———. 1986. *The Nazi Doctors: Medical Killing and the Psychology of Genocide.* New York: Basic Books.

MACKLIN, RUTH. 1982. *Man, Mind, and Morality: The Ethics of Behavior Control.* Englewood Cliffs, N.J.: Prentice-Hall.

———. 1987. *Mortal Choices: Bioethics in Today's World.* New York: Pantheon.

MECHANIC, DAVID. 1981. "The Social Dimension." In *Psychiatric Ethics,* pp. 46–60. Edited by Sidney Bloch and Paul Chodoff. New York: Oxford University Press.

MURRAY, THOMAS H. 1986. "Divided Loyalties for Physicians: Social Context and Moral Problems." *Social Science and Medicine* 23, no. 8:827–832.

POST, STEPHEN P. 1993. "Psychiatry and Ethics: The Problematics of Respect for Religious Meanings." *Culture, Medicine and Psychiatry* 17, no. 3:363–383.

RINAS, JOAN, and CLYNE-JACKSON, SHEILA. 1988. *Professional Conduct and Legal Concerns in Mental Health Practice.* Norwalk, Conn.: Appleton and Lange.

SLOVENKO, RALPH. 1975. "Psychotherapy and Confidentiality." *Cleveland State Law Review* 24:375–396.

STEINFELS, MARGERET O'BRIEN, and LEVINE, CAROL, eds. 1978. "In the Service of the State: The Psychiatrist as Double Agent." *Hastings Center Report* 8, no. 2 (spec. supp.):1–24.

SZASZ, THOMAS S. 1970. *Ideology and Insanity: Essays on the Psychiatric Dehumanization of Man.* New York: Anchor.

WOLF, SUSAN M. 1994. "Health Care Reform and the Future of Physician Ethics." *Hastings Center Report* 24, no. 2: 28–41.

DIVORCE AND CUSTODY

See CHILDREN, *article on* CHILD CUSTODY.

DNA TYPING

DNA typing is a technique for identifying people through their genetic constitution. It involves comparing small portions of DNA from different sources—a child and an alleged father; a bloodstain and a criminal suspect—and determining whether those portions match. DNA typing can discriminate among people almost as accurately as fingerprinting, and it can be used in a far wider range of circumstances, since DNA is found in virtually all human cells; can be extracted from blood, semen, saliva, or hair roots; and is highly resistant to decay and contamination.

Since its introduction in the mid-1980s, DNA typing has been employed in thousands of cases of disputed identity, including criminal, paternity, immigration, and other proceedings. It is a versatile technology that can help to implicate or clear a criminal suspect, distinguish serial from copycat crimes, resolve parentage disputes, identify remains, and help parents locate missing children. This article will focus on its use in criminal cases and will address the principal issues that have been raised about its reliability, its impact on the legal system, its threat to privacy, and its regulation.

In theory, we could identify people with absolute certainty by examining their entire genetic sequence, or genome, since each person's genome is unique. But because the genome is spread over forty-six chromosomes, each containing millions of smaller molecules, this is not a practical procedure. DNA identification became feasible with the discovery of small regions of DNA, or loci, that vary from person to person in length and in other respects. Using standard techniques of molecular genetics, investigators can compare these variable loci in DNA taken from different sources. But since the range of possible variants, or alleles, found at any given locus is relatively small, it is necessary to compare several loci to make an accurate identification.

Consider a case in which a semen stain is found on the clothing of a rape victim. Through DNA typing, investigators can ascertain whether the stain may have come from the suspect by comparing DNA from his blood with DNA extracted from the stain. The failure to obtain a match excludes the suspect as a source of the semen; the discovery of a match includes the suspect in a subpopulation of potential sources. The more loci at which matches are obtained, the smaller this subpopulation will be, and thus the smaller the probability that someone besides the suspect contributed the semen.

Admissibility and evidential weight

The controversy over the admissibility of DNA typing has focused in part on the *criteria for declaring a match.* The standard way to measure the length of DNA segments is to measure the extent of their "migration" down an electronically charged gel. But a wide range of field and laboratory conditions may cause fragments of equal length to migrate at different rates—a phenomenon known as band-shifting. And even without band-shifting, there is room for error and bias in comparing DNA segments. These problems have been partially resolved, however, by standardizing match criteria, developing controls for band-shifting, and adopting new typing technologies that do not use electrophoresis.

A second focus of controversy involves the *statistical interpretation of a match.* In calculating the probability that someone other than the suspect was the source of the semen, we need to know the frequency of the matched alleles in the population of potential offenders. At present, geneticists sharply disagree about the extent to which allele frequencies differ among subgroups in the population. If there are significant differences, it becomes a matter of some importance how we define the class of alternative offenders. If a criminal suspect is

Dominican, should the statistical interpretation of a match be based on the frequency of the matching alleles among white males, Hispanic males, or Dominican males? If the suspect in a Harlem assault case is white, should the class of alternative offenders be white males, black males, male Harlem residents, or some other subpopulation? Should the resolution of such questions depend on the evidence in the specific case, or should there be a general rule?

In 1992, the National Research Council issued a report that called for using the highest allele frequency for any population subgroup if there were any significant differences among groups. Under this ceiling principle, the probability that someone besides the suspect in the rape case contributed the semen stain would be assessed using the frequency for the subgroup in which the matched alleles were most common, even if there were no reason to think that someone from that subgroup was involved in the incident. This proposal remains controversial—seen by some forensic scientists as excessively conservative, and by some population geneticists as excessively speculative.

Proper testing procedures are no less critical to the accuracy of DNA typing evidence than are valid statistical inferences. Sample-switching and contamination may be at least as significant a source of error as misjudgments about band matches and allele frequency. Blind tests of the laboratories that perform DNA typing have not been totally reassuring; they highlight the need for regular proficiency testing and quality control.

Even if DNA typing is reliably performed and analyzed, some critics are concerned that juries and judges will exaggerate its relevance or misunderstand its significance. For example, a finding that the suspect was the source of semen on the victim's clothing will have only limited inculpatory value if the issue in the case is not identity but consent. Similarly, a finding that the suspect was not the source of the semen will have only limited exculpatory value if the victim had been gang-raped.

Social impact and regulation

Forensic DNA typing may have a significant effect not only in solving crimes, where its impact will be limited to cases where there are bodily residues, but also in fostering a healthy skepticism about other forms of identification evidence. The laboratories performing forensic DNA typing on suspects report exclusion rates of one-third or more; in some of these cases, the suspect had been implicated by an eyewitness or other conventional evidence. While exclusion does not always mean innocence, these findings suggest a high rate of error, and they may increase the sensitivity of law enforcement officials to the risk of mistaken accusations. The attention given to DNA typing may also promote the more frequent and careful utilization of other forensic evidence, which should further enhance the accuracy of criminal adjudication.

The threat to privacy from DNA typing arises from two sources: the ease with which DNA can be obtained and the amount of data it can yield. Usable DNA can be extracted not just from blood and semen (which may be taken only with probable cause and a court order) but also from trace amounts of tissue and saliva. The courts have yet to decide what constraints should govern the "seizure" of such material, or whether people have constitutionally protected privacy interests in such material once it leaves their bodies.

Furthermore, DNA data banks are being developed that will facilitate the broader investigative use of DNA profiles. By 1992, more than a dozen states required DNA samples from all convicted sexual or violent felony offenders. In the future, such data banks may be augmented by other types of information, such as fingerprints, criminal records, and behavioral profiles, and by DNA from other groups, such as military personnel and employees in positions requiring security clearance. It may soon be technically possible to screen a large portion of the population for involvement in any crime where testable body residues are found.

The DNA molecule itself is becoming an increasingly rich source of personal information. Thousands of medical conditions have already been mapped to specific regions of the genome, and genetic markers are likely to be found for many physical traits and psychiatric conditions. While most of the loci used in typing do not appear to have functional significance, the mapping of the human genome may place some of these loci in close proximity to the genes associated with significant traits. Access to personal data could be limited by storing only DNA profiles, but there are reasons for preserving the DNA itself—for example, to allow reanalysis by an independent laboratory or with a new technique. While it is important to develop safeguards to prevent abuse with respect to DNA data banks, it is first necessary to determine what constitutes abuse.

Much of the debate over the acceptance of forensic DNA typing concerns the issue of who should make that determination. Scientists do not want the fate of new technologies to depend on the findings of judges and juries or the vagaries of adversarial justice; lawyers are reluctant to entrust the review of these technologies to scientists, whom they regard as insensitive to values besides accuracy and as inclined to exaggerate the precision of techniques resting on fallible judgment. There has been a promising attempt to bridge the divide between these two cultures in the creation of special panels of scientists and lawyers, most notably the National Research Council's commission on forensic DNA typing.

Though these panels have sometimes divided on the very conflicts they were created to resolve, they may serve as prototypes for the cautious reception of other powerful but risky technologies.

DAVID WASSERMAN

For a discussion of topics mentioned in this entry, see the entries: CONFIDENTIALITY; GENOME MAPPING AND SEQUENCING; HOMICIDE; *and* LAW AND BIOETHICS. *For a discussion of related ideas, see the entries* BIOMEDICAL ENGINEERING; *and* EXPERT TESTIMONY.

Bibliography

ANNAS, GEORGE J. 1990. "DNA Fingerprinting in the Twilight Zone." *Hastings Center Report* 20, no. 2:35–37.
———. 1992. "Setting Standards for the Use of DNA-Typing Results in the Courtroom—The State of the Art." *New England Journal of Medicine* 326, no. 24:1641–1644.
BARINGA, MARCIA. 1989. "DNA Fingerprinting: Pitfalls Come to Light." *Nature* 339, no. 6220:89.
BURK, DAN L. 1988. "DNA Fingerprinting: Possibilities and Pitfalls of a New Technique." *Jurimetrics Journal* 28, no. 3:455–471.
———. 1990. "DNA Identification: Possibilities and Pitfalls Revisited." *Jurimetrics Journal* 31, no. 1:53–85.
CASKEY, C. THOMAS. 1991. "Comments on DNA-Based Forensic Analysis." *American Journal of Human Genetics* 49, no. 4:893–895.
CHARKRABORTY, RANAJIT. 1991. "Statistical Interpretation of DNA-Typing Data." *American Journal of Human Genetics* 49, no. 4:895–897.
DAIGER, STEPHEN P. 1991. "DNA Fingerprinting." *American Journal of Human Genetics* 49, no. 4:897.
DEVLIN, B.; RISCH, NEIL; and ROEDER, KATHRYN. 1993. "Statistical Evaluation of DNA Fingerprinting: A Critique of the NRC's Report." *Science* 259, no. 5096:748–749.
EVETT, I. W. 1992. "DNA Statistics: Putting the Problems into Perspective." *Jurimetrics Journal* 33, no. 1:139–145.
GILL, PETER; JEFFREYS, ALEC J.; and WERRETT, DAVID J. 1985. "Forensic Applications of DNA 'Fingerprints.'" *Nature* 318, no. 6046:577–579.
HOEFFEL, JANET C. 1990. "The Dark Side of DNA Profiling: Unreliable Scientific Evidence Meets the Criminal Defendant." *Stanford Law Review* 42:465–538.
JACOBY, JOAN E.; MELLON, LEONARD, R.; RUTLEDGE, EDWARD C.; and HUNTER, STANLEY H. 1982. *Prosecutorial Decisionmaking: A National Study.* Washington, D.C.: U.S. Government Printing Office.
JEFFREYS, ALEC J.; WILSON, VICTORIA; and THEIN, SWEE LAY. 1985. "Hypervariable 'Minisatellite' Regions in Human DNA." *Nature* 314, no. 6006:67–73.
KAYE, D. H. 1991. "The Admissibility of DNA Testing." *Cardozo Law Review* 13, nos. 2-3:353–360.
LANDER, ERIC S. 1989. "DNA Fingerprinting on Trial." *Nature* 339, no. 6025:501–505.
———. 1991a. "Lander Reply." *American Journal of Human Genetics* 49, no. 4:899–903.

———. 1991b. "Research on DNA Typing Catching up with Courtroom Application." *American Journal of Human Genetics* 48, no. 5:819–823.

———. 1992. "DNA Fingerprinting: Science, Law, and the Ultimate Identifier." In *The Code of Codes: Scientific and Social Issues in the Human Genome Project*, pp. 191–211. Edited by Daniel J. Kevles and Leroy E. Hood. Cambridge, Mass.: Harvard University Press.

LEMPERT, RICHARD. 1991. "Some Caveats Concerning DNA as Criminal Identification Evidence: With Thanks to the Reverend Bayes." *Cardozo Law Review* 13, nos. 2–3:303–341.

LEWIN, ROGER. 1989. "DNA Typing on the Witness Stand." *Science* 244, no. 4908:1033–1035.

LEWONTIN, RICHARD C., and HARTL, DANIEL L. 1991. "Population Genetics in Forensic DNA Typing." *Science* 254, no. 5039:1745–1750.

MARX, JEAN L. 1988. "DNA Fingerprinting Takes the Witness Stand." *Science* 240, no. 4859:1616–1618.

MAYS, G. LARRY; PURCELL, NOREEN; and WINFREE, L. THOMAS. 1992. "DNA (Deoxyribonucleic Acid) Evidence, Criminal Law, and Felony Prosecutions: Issues and Prospects." *Justice System Journal* 16, no. 1:111–122.

MOENSSENS, ANDRE A. 1990. "DNA Evidence and Its Critics—How Valid are the Challenges?" *Jurimetrics Journal* 31, no. 1:87–108.

NEUFELD, PETER J., and COLMAN, NEVILL. 1990. "When Science Takes the Witness Stand." *Scientific American* 262, no. 5:46–55.

NORMAN, COLIN. 1989. "Maine Case Deals Blow to DNA Fingerprinting." *Science* 246, no. 4937:1556.

PETERSON, JOSEPH L. 1989. "Impact of Biological Evidence on the Adjudication of Criminal Cases: Potential for DNA Technology." In *DNA Technology and Forensic Science*, pp. 55–70. Edited by Jack Ballantyne, George Sensabaugh, and Jan A. Witkowske. Banbury Report no. 32. Cold Spring Harbor, N.Y.: Cold Spring Harbor Laboratory Press.

RISCH, NEIL J., and DEVLIN, B. 1992. "On the Probability of Matching DNA Fingerprints." *Science* 255, no. 5045: 717–720.

SCHMITZ, ANTHONY. 1988. "Murder on Black Pad." *Hippocrates* 2, no. 1:48–58.

THOMPSON, WILLIAM C., and FORD, SIMON. 1989. "DNA Typing: Acceptance and Weight of the New Genetic Identification Tests." *Virginia Law Review* 75, no. 1:45–107.

U.S. CONGRESS, OFFICE OF TECHNOLOGY ASSESSMENT. 1988. *Criminal Justice: New Technologies and the Constitution.* OTA-CIT-366. Washington, D.C.: U.S. Government Printing Office.

———. 1990. *Genetic Witness: Forensic Uses of DNA Tests.* OTA-BA-438. Washington, D.C.: U.S. Government Printing Office.

WASSERMAN, DAVID, and WEEDN, VICTOR. 1992. "Forensic DNA Typing: Consensus and Controversy." *Scientific Evidence Review* 1:32–36.

WEEDN, VICTOR, and ROBY, RHONDA K. 1993. "Forensic DNA Testing." *Archives of Pathology and Laboratory Medicine* 117, no. 5:486–491.

WOOLEY, JAMES R. 1991. "A Response to Lander: The Courtroom Perspective." *American Journal of Human Genetics* 49, no. 4:892–893.

DOMESTIC ANIMALS AND PETS

See ANIMAL WELFARE AND RIGHTS, *articles on* PET AND COMPANION ANIMALS, *and* ANIMALS IN AGRICULTURE AND FACTORY FARMING. *See also* VETERINARY ETHICS; *and* ANIMAL WELFARE AND RIGHTS, *articles on* ETHICAL PERSPECTIVES ON THE TREATMENT AND STATUS OF ANIMALS, *and* ZOOS AND ZOOLOGICAL PARKS.

DOMESTIC PARTNERSHIPS

See MARRIAGE AND OTHER DOMESTIC PARTNERSHIPS.

DOMESTIC VIOLENCE

See ABUSE, INTERPERSONAL.

DO NOT RESUSCITATE (DNR) ORDERS

See DEATH AND DYING: EUTHANASIA AND SUSTAINING LIFE. *See also* ARTIFICIAL ORGANS AND LIFE-SUPPORT SYSTEMS.

DOUBLE EFFECT

Roman Catholic moral theology traditionally includes a form of reasoning called the doctrine of double effect. (The term "doctrine" is technically inaccurate because the highest Catholic authorities have never explicitly taught it.) According to double effect, actions and omissions are permissible only when their gravely bad effects are allowed for good reason ("proportional reason") and are unintended. The tradition of double effect developed out of Thomas Aquinas's (1224–1274) discussion of self-defense to help deal with a host of quandaries including warfare, deception, and cooperation in evil (*Summa Theologiae*, pt. II-II, p. 64, art. 7). The recent bioethical discussion has focused on cases involving the foreseen death of medical patients or of the unborn.

Certain contrasting cases have become standard illustrations of the application of double effect in medical ethics. The first involves abortifacient procedures. In one case, a physician aims to save the life of a pregnant woman by removing from her body a diseased and life-threatening uterus or Fallopian tube containing a fetus. The physician recognizes that the procedure is sure to cost the fetus's life when the latter is not yet viable. The tradition considered this at worst only an "indirect abortion," that is, one in which there is no specific intent to end the life or development of the fetus, although the physician expects them to end. Double effect, as traditionally applied, normally permitted such a medical procedure if there was no other way to secure the woman's survival. (The Catholic tradition holds that a human being is alive in the womb from conception. In the contrasting case, a physician strives to save a woman's life by performing a craniotomy on a fetus, the emergence of whose head will otherwise likely cause a fatal hemorrhage in the mother. According to traditional discussions, this latter physician intends grave harm, even death, to the fetus, and the procedure is therefore impermissible. (However, Joseph Boyle, an influential interpreter of double effect, thinks double effect need not rule out the craniotomy in this situation. See Flannery, 1993.)

The second example contrasts two situations in which life-shortening doses of chemicals are administered. In one case, a physician seeks to alleviate a patient's pain by administering the painkiller morphine but recognizes that the dosage is likely to shorten the patient's life. The physician regrets this result but can avoid it only by so reducing the dosage that the chemical will not have sufficient painkilling effect. According to traditional expositions of double effect, in this situation the physician expects to kill but does not intend to do so (does not kill "directly"), and the action may well be justified by the proportionately grave reason for administering the treatment.

In the contrasting case, a mercy killer administers strychnine to a patient in order to shorten the patient's life and thereby spare him or her the pain that would otherwise be experienced. In this latter situation, according to the traditional discussions, the agent intends the evil of causing the patient's death as a means to the good of relieving the pain, and the action is therefore impermissible. (The tradition presupposed that causing the death even of the most afflicted was an evil; of course, this is widely denied today, but this dispute must be resolved independently of double effect and its application.)

While no exact formulation has become standard, in the theological literature certain principal elements of double effect emerge. A course of behavior (whether an active intervention or an omission) is immoral in any of these circumstances: (1) the behavior belongs to a class of actions (e.g., adultery, blasphemy, and lying) that are wrong even aside from their bad effects; (2) one or more of the evil effects is not merely expected but is intended either as means or as an ultimate end; (3) an

evil effect results from one of the good effects; or (4) the evil effects are disproportionate to the good effects.

These are best understood only as sufficient conditions, not necessary ones, for the agent to behave immorally in adopting the course of behavior. A course of medical treatment that meets none of these criteria, and thus "passes" the moral test that double effect proposes, might still be illicit for other reasons. For example, it might violate the autonomy of a patient who has not consented, or break a promise made to the patient.

While discussion here will concentrate on the second condition, the others require some consideration. The types of actions that those who developed double effect reasoning had in mind as wrong in themselves were thought to be wrong partly because anyone who commits them is acting with certain evil intentions. It is probably better to interpret the first condition as holding that a course of action is immoral if it is of a type that is wrong regardless of its good and bad effects; for instance, blasphemy is wrong whether or not it causes grave harm. Joseph Boyle and others have persuasively argued that the third condition serves only to specify certain circumstances in which it is not plausible to deny that a bad effect is intended, that is, cases when the agent brings about a good effect by means of the bad effect (Boyle, 1980). The fourth condition does not presuppose that the goodness or badness of every effect can be sensibly compared with that of every other effect. Indeed, some prominent advocates of double effect have insisted that certain fundamental values are not "commensurable" in that way (Finnis, 1991). The point of the fourth condition is only that, when the values at stake can be compared as greater, lesser, or equal, then, if an action's bad effects are out of proportion to its good ones (e.g., much greater than them), then the act is illicit. Within double effect, "proportional reason" is never merely a matter of counting heads.

Function

It has not always been made clear whether the function of double effect is (1) to distinguish more culpable from less culpable agents or (2) to distinguish permissible from impermissible actions. If the latter, a further question arises: Is double effect supposed to provide (2a) a procedure for agents to use in decision making or (2b) a criterion of wrongfulness for moral judges to use in determining wrongdoing? Double effect has sometimes been employed to address all these questions, but (2b) is central (Boyle, 1980).

Bioethics and moral theology after the Second Vatican Council

Attempting more clearly to vindicate certain intrusive new medical procedures (such as organ transplantation) and to defend the morality of artificial contraception, after the Second Vatican Council (1962–1965), a "revisionist" Catholic moral theology arose. In the new view, only moral evil (sin itself) was always immoral to intend. Revisionists dubbed such ills as death and amputation "premoral" or "ontic" evils, contending that they were undersirable in the abstract, but allowing that an action involving such an evil may, in a particular situation, be morally justified. They taught that it was permissible for agents intentionally to cause or allow a "premoral" evil, provided "proportional reason" held the promise of some compensating good. This new movement began as a reinterpretation of double effect, emphasizing the fourth condition's ban on acting with disproportionately bad results, and depreciating the first condition's distinction between what was intended and what was foreseen. Eventually, the revisionists effectively rejected the methodology of double effect for a different, "proportionalist" one that, like utilitarianism, focused on the comparison of those goods and evils that agents realize in or as a result of their behavior (see Hoose, 1987; Curran and McCormick, 1979).

Pope John Paul II's 1993 encyclical *Veritatis splendor* carefully and explicitly criticized proportionalist method as a distortion of traditional Catholic moral thought rather than a revision of it and cast doubt over the movement's future. Having lost favor among Catholic theologians during the 1960s and 1970s, the tradition of double effect also won little support among either secular or Protestant bioethicists. (Paul Ramsey was an important exception; see his debate with Richard McCormick in McCormick and Ramsey, 1978.) However, often critics of double effect either misunderstood it so profoundly that their criticisms were misdirected or else they wound up relying on the same distinctions. In the United States, for example, the U.S. President's Commission for the Study of Ethical Problems in Medicine and Biomedical and Behavioral Research explicitly rejected reliance on the moral significance of the difference between cases in which medical personnel intended patients to die (as in mercy killing) and those in which they merely expected the patient to die as a result of palliative treatment.

However, the Commission went on to affirm that death may be tolerated in medical treatment only as a "risk" and only in pursuit of proper professional goals (U.S. President's Commission, 1983). These claims reintroduced, in different language, the same distinctions that double effect employs. The mercy killer, unlike the physician trying to reduce the intensity of the patient's pain, cannot be said merely to "risk" causing the patient's death. He or she is trying to cause it. Moreover, in excluding euthanasia as incompatible with the medical profession's goals while accepting treatment whose likely side effects include shortening the patient's life,

the U.S. President's Commission implicitly relied upon a distinction between adopting illegitimate goals, either ultimate or subsidiary, and merely accepting certain unfortunate side effects of pursuing legitimate goals. This is precisely the distinction that plays a central role in double effect: that between "direct" and "indirect" intention or, in more straightforward language, the distinction between results that are merely expected and those that are intended.

Several influential moral philosophers and theorists of human action have defended modified versions of some principal elements in double effect, especially its claim that certain effects, which may be morally impermissible to allow or bring about intentionally, may licitly result from an agent's actions or omissions, provided they are only foreseen but not intended (Devine, 1978; Nagel, 1986; Bratman, 1987; Quinn, 1989). During the 1980s, ethicists working on nuclear deterrence devoted substantial attention to the morality of intentions, an issue central to double effect.

Challenges

One major question that arises in applying double effect is, "When does an agent intend to kill somebody as a means?" Donald Marquis helpfully suggests that we best understand double effect if we construe this as a question about what situations an agent plans and how the agent means them to be related (Marquis, 1991). Following this line, we can answer that question by saying that an agent intends to kill person Smith as a means to his or her objective only if the agent plans for that objective to result precisely from killing Smith. (Normally, the killer would mean for it to result from Smith's death.) Contrast physician A, who prescribes morphine to lessen the intensity of a patient's pain, with physician B, who administers strychnine so that death will end the patient's misery. Only physician B kills as a means. The good that physician A seeks is not meant to be achieved as a result of the patient's death. The mercy killer, physician B, aims at deriving the supposed good of pain relief from the evil of death, contrary to the second and third conditions of double effect.

Critics have subjected each element of double effect to close scrutiny, but the second condition has drawn the most attention. There are three main lines of criticism. First, critics charge that the supposed distinction between what an agent intends to result from behavior and what the agent merely expects to result marks no real difference in mental states (Lackey, 1987). Second, some contend that the distinction in mental states, even if legitimate, makes little or no difference to the moral permissibility of the agent's behavior, either because it is an irrational basis for discriminating among actions or because consideration of intentions has no place in moral deliberation (Bennett, 1981). Third, some maintain that the distinction does not sort cases in the way that proponents of double effect have thought. For example, it fails to explain why euthanasia is morally wrong when life-shortening doses of painkiller may not be, or why a fetal craniotomy is forbidden while hysterectomy on a pregnant woman might be permissible. While secular moral philosophers usually condemn double effect as too restrictive, some criticize it for being too permissive, claiming that it exonerates actions a moral code ought to forbid (Bole, 1991).

Analytical work in the philosophy of mind and in the philosophy of action substantially undermines the first line of criticism. What one intends to do, many theorists have urged, is what one means and plans to do, and what one plans to do is normally what one takes steps to accomplish, what one normally does in order to accomplish something further (i.e., for the sake of some result). What one intends is something whose doing makes one and one's behavior at least a partial success, and whose nonachievement makes one and one's action at least a partial failure (Bratman, 1987).

It is highly implausible to maintain that in this sense agents intend every result they foresee, or even every result whose occurrence matters to them. To take one of our standard illustrations, the mercy killer plans to kill, takes steps (administers the strychnine) in order to kill, kills for the sake of a purported good (release from pain) that results from the death, and is a success if he or she kills and a partial failure if he or she doesn't, even if things take such a turn (e.g., a miraculous recovery) that there is little or no disappointment about the failure. None of these claims is true of the physician who gives the morphine to lessen the pain that the patient feels prior to death. We can explain the latter physician's behavior very well without claiming that he or she intends to kill. Unlike the mercy killer, the latter physician does not plan to kill; he or she seeks to derive no good as a result of the death; and if the patient survives, that fact does not imply failure in anything the physician was doing.

Several philosophers suggest responses to the second line of criticism. Intentions may matter in morals because:

1. It is chiefly through them that virtues are expressed.
2. In adopting them, agents reflexively shape their own character.
3. They help determine the quality of our conduct within the relationships we have with other people.
4. They are part of treating others with the respect their dignity demands.
5. They are an appropriate way of responding to the value embodied in people and their well-being (Nagel, 1986; Finnis, 1991; Garcia, 1993).

The third line of criticism does nothing to show the essential aims of double effect to be false. At most, it would show that its proponents have misapplied it. Still, critics have a point when they say, for example, that a physician need not intend to kill the fetus in performing a craniotomy, because the plan to save the woman's life does not require that the fetus die but only that the physician do something (i.e., remove the fetus from the womb) that it is known will likely lead to a death. They also have a point that this concession threatens the usefulness of double effect reasoning. Some argue, for example, that even agents who shield themselves from harm by throwing others on top of live grenades, or who remove vital organs from unwilling victims, need intend only that the victims' bodies be blown up or vivisected, not that the victims die. These critics worry that the agent can escape the strictures of double effect by intending these other results without intending the person's death. Double effect reasoning does not by itself justify these actions, since it does not provide a complete set of conditions sufficient for moral permissibility. But these cases seem to be just the sort double effect is supposed to address. Warren Quinn helpfully proposes that in the above cases the agent wrongs the victim by involving him or her as an "intentional object" in the agent's plans even though the victim cannot reasonably share those plans (Quinn, 1989).

What is crucial to the application of double effect is not that the agent intends death, but simply that the agent intends some means that constitutes a substantial injury to the person affected (Sullivan and Atkinson, 1994). Defenders of the doctrine of double effect can say that the gruesome injuries that the agent undeniably intends for the victims in the above cases—that their bodies be destroyed, that they be deprived of healthy and vital organs, and so on—are things it is never permissible to will. Ultimately, of course, we want to be able to explain why it is wrong to intend them, but the defense of double effect requires only that intending them is always wrong.

Prospects

In the 1970s it appeared that the only promise for double effect lay in developing the fourth condition's emphasis on proportional reason and playing down the first condition's distinction between intent and expectation, so as to bring the tradition closer to sophisticated consequentialist moral analyses. However, later work in the theory of human action and in philosophical moral theory indicates new directions for research. Future work may build on the writings of Michael Bratman and others in understanding the nature of intent and developing rigorous and reliable tests to determine just which results a given agent intends in certain circumstances and which are unintended, even though foreseen (Bratman, 1987).

A different project may focus on the justification of the claim that the distinction between what is intended and what is merely expected (or "permitted") can bear the conclusive moral weight that double effect assigns it. Some secular philosophers who defend elements of versions of double effect claim only that it is harder to justify a course of action that is intended to result in serious evils than one that is meant only to bring good results but is expected to have significant bad effects as well (Foot, 1985; Quinn, 1989). They reject the absolutist claim of traditional Catholic moral theology that one may never will an innocent person serious injury.

An inquiry especially needed, one to which Jonathan Glover's work directs our attention, would identify which actions and effects are such that intending to realize them is wrong in all circumstances, which ones are such that intending them can be justified by the agent's reasonable and freely given consent, and which might be justified simply by appeal to the needs of others (Glover, 1977). The goal of this investigation would be to justify and explain the claims that not only is it always immoral to intend to kill innocent people but it is also wrong to intend to crush their heads or to blow up their bodies. This investigation also needs to clarify why removing certain organs may sometimes be permitted when the patients give consent and when the organs are either dangerously diseased or needed for saving others' lives.

There are several sources on which the researcher can build in this last project. Thomas Nagel suggests that it is especially repugnant for an agent to subordinate the will to the sort of "guidance" by evil involved in intending to bring evil about. He also proposes that intending and thus actively pursuing evil, even as a means, is contrary to the nature of evil as something to be avoided (Nagel, 1986). Warren Quinn claims that it is manipulative and disrespectful to plan to bring harm to another person when that person cannot properly assent to those plans (Quinn, 1989). Some work in virtue-based moral theory may prove useful to future defenders of double effect. Such accounts of the moral justification of action turn inward and backward, seeking the source of an action's immorality not in its total effects but in the quality of the sensitivities, decisions, and plans it embodies and in how it fits or deforms the human relationship between caregiver and patient (Garcia, 1993). Finally, John Finnis, Joseph Boyle, and Germain Grisez, in arguing for the importance of intentions, emphasize the "reflexive" character of action, whereby acting shapes not only the world but also the character of the agents (Finnis, 1991; Finnis et al., 1987).

JORGE L. A. GARCIA

Directly related to this entry is the entry ROMAN CATHOLICISM. *For a further discussion of topics mentioned in this entry, see the entries* AUTONOMY; DEATH; ETHICS, *especially the article on* RELIGION AND MORALITY; FETUS; HARM; LIFE; OBLIGATION AND SUPEREROGATION; PAIN AND SUFFERING; PROTESTANTISM; REPRODUCTIVE TECHNOLOGIES; TECHNOLOGY; UTILITY; *and* VIRTUE AND CHARACTER. *This entry will find application in the entries* ABORTION, *especially the section on* RELIGIOUS TRADITIONS, *article on* ROMAN CATHOLIC PERSPECTIVES; BIOETHICS; *and* DEATH AND DYING: EUTHANASIA AND SUSTAINING LIFE, *especially the article on* ETHICAL ISSUES. *For a discussion of related ideas, see the entries* BENEFICENCE; CARE; CASUISTRY; COMPASSION; EASTERN ORTHODOX CHRISTIANITY; JUDAISM; NATURAL LAW; *and* ORGAN AND TISSUE PROCUREMENT, *especially the article on* ETHICAL AND LEGAL ISSUES REGARDING CADAVERS.

Bibliography

ASHLEY, BENEDICT M., and O'ROURKE, KEVIN D. 1982. *Health Care Ethics: A Theological Analysis.* Ch. 8. 2d ed. St. Louis, Miss.: Catholic Health Care Association of the United States.

BENNETT, JONATHAN. 1981. "Morality and Consequences." In *Tanner Lectures on Human Values* 2:45–116.

BOLE, THOMAS J., ed. 1991. *Journal of Medicine and Philosophy* 16, no. 5. Special issue, "Double Effect: Theoretical Function and Bioethical Implications."

BOYLE, JOSEPH M., JR. 1980. "Toward Understanding the Principle of Double Effect." *Ethics* 90, no. 4:527–538.

BRATMAN, MICHAEL. 1987. *Intention, Plans, and Practical Reason.* Cambridge, Mass.: Harvard University Press.

Catechism of the Catholic Church. 1994. Vatican City: Libreria Editrice Vaticana. Part Three, Section Two, Article Five.

CURRAN, CHARLES E, and MCCORMICK, RICHARD A., eds. 1979. *Moral Norms and Catholic Tradition.* New York: Paulist Press.

DEVINE, PHILIP E. 1978. *Ethics of Homicide.* Ithaca, N.Y.: Cornell University Press.

FINNIS, JOHN. 1991. *Moral Absolutes: Tradition, Revision, and Truth.* Washington, D.C.: Catholic University of America Press.

FINNIS, JOHN; BOYLE, JOSEPH M.; and GRISEZ, GERMAIN G. 1987. *Nuclear Deterrence, Morality, and Realism.* Oxford: Oxford University Press.

FLANNERY, KEVIN L. 1993. "What Is Included in a Means to an End?" *Gregorianum* 74, no. 3:499–513.

FOOT, PHILIPPA. 1985. "Morality, Action, and Outcome." In *Morality and Objectivity: A Tribute to J. L. Mackie,* pp. 23–38. Edited by Ted Honderich. London: Routledge & Kegan Paul.

GARCIA, JORGE L. A. 1993. "The New Critique of Anti-Consequentialist Moral Theory." *Philosophical Studies* 71, no. 1:1–32.

GLOVER, JONATHAN. 1977. *Causing Death and Saving Lives.* New York: Penguin.

HOOSE, BERNARD. 1987. *Proportionalism: The American Debate and Its European Roots.* Washington, D.C.: Georgetown University Press.

KAGAN, SHELLY. 1989. *The Limits of Morality.* Oxford: Oxford University Press.

KUHSE, HELGA. 1987. *The Sanctity-of-Life Doctrine in Medicine: A Critique.* Oxford: Oxford University Press.

LACKEY, DOUGLAS. 1987. "The Moral Irrelevance of the Counterforce/Countervalue Distinction." *The Monist* 70, no. 3:255–275.

MANGAN, JOSEPH T. 1949. "Historical Analysis of the Principle of Double Effect." *Theological Studies* 10:41–61.

MARQUIS, DONALD B. 1991. "Four Versions of Double Effect." *Journal of Medicine and Philosophy* 16, no. 5:515–544.

MAY, WILLIAM E., ed. 1980. *Principles of Catholic Moral Life.* Chicago: Franciscan Herald Press.

MCCORMICK, RICHARD A. 1981. "The Principle of the Double Effect." In his *How Brave a New World? Dilemmas in Bioethics,* pp. 413–429. Washington, D.C.: Georgetown University Press.

———. 1988. "Consistent Ethics of Life: Is There an Historical Soft Underbelly?" In *The Consistent Ethic of Life,* pp. 96–122. Edited by Thomas G. Feuchtmann. Kansas City, Mo.: Sheed & Ward.

MCCORMICK, RICHARD A., and RAMSEY, PAUL, eds. 1978. *Doing Evil to Achieve Good.* Chicago: Loyola University Press.

NAGEL, THOMAS. 1986. *The View from Nowhere.* Oxford: Oxford University Press.

QUINN, WARREN S. 1989. "Actions, Intentions, and Consequences: The Doctrine of Double Effect." *Philosophy and Public Affairs* 18, no. 4:334–351.

SMITH, JANET E. 1991. *"Humanae Vitae": A Generation Later.* Washington, D.C.: Catholic University of America Press.

SULLIVAN, THOMAS D., and ATKINSON, GARY. 1993. "*Malum Vitandum:* The Role of Intentions in First-Order Morality." *International Journal of Philosophical Studies* 1, no. 1:99–110.

UGORJI, LUCIUS IWEJURU. 1985. *The Principle of Double Effect.* Frankfurt au Main: Peter Lang.

U.S. PRESIDENT'S COMMISSION FOR THE STUDY OF ETHICAL PROBLEMS IN MEDICINE AND BIOMEDICAL AND BEHAVIORAL RESEARCH. 1983. *Deciding to Forgo Life-Sustaining Treatment: A Report on the Ethical, Medical, and Legal Issues in Treatment Decisions.* Washington, D.C.: Author.

DRUG AND ALCOHOL ABUSE

See SUBSTANCE ABUSE.

DRUG INDUSTRY

See PHARMACEUTICS, *article on* PHARMACEUTICAL INDUSTRY.

DRUGS, PRESCRIPTION OF

See PHARMACEUTICS, *article on* ISSUES IN PRESCRIBING.

DURABLE POWER OF ATTORNEY FOR HEALTH CARE

See DEATH AND DYING: EUTHANASIA AND SUSTAINING LIFE, *articles on* ADVANCE DIRECTIVES, *and* PROFESSIONAL AND PUBLIC POLICIES.

DYNAMIC THERAPIES

See PSYCHOANALYSIS AND DYNAMIC THERAPIES; *and* MENTAL-HEALTH THERAPIES.

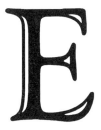

EASTERN EUROPE

See MEDiCAL ETHICS, HISTORY OF, *section on* EUROPE, *subsection on* CONTEMPORARY PERIOD, *article on* CENTRAL AND EASTERN EUROPE.

EASTERN ORTHODOX CHRISTIANITY

The Eastern Orthodox church considers itself identical with the Church established by Jesus Christ and believes itself to be guided by the Holy Spirit, continuing that ecclesial reality into the present age as an organic historical, theological, liturgical continuity and unity with the apostolic Church of the first century. Historically, it sees itself as identical with the "One, Holy, Catholic, and Apostolic Church" that suffered the "Great Schism" in 1054 that led to the division of Christendom into Eastern and Western Christianity.

The Orthodox church is organized hierarchically, with an ordained clergy and bishops. A number of national and ethnic Orthodox churches, under the leadership of patriarchs, are united by tradition, doctrine, and spirit rather than by authority, although the Ecumenical Patriarch of Constantinople is accorded a primacy of honor. The church's identity is rooted in the experience of the Holy Spirit in all aspects of its life and in a doctrinal perspective that serves as a matrix for its ethical teachings (Ware, 1964; Pelikan, 1974). In the sphere of bioethics, this theological matrix forms a co-

herent source of values for bioethical decision making. At its center is the view that life is a gift of God that should be protected, transmitted, cultivated, cared for, fulfilled in God, and considered a sacred reality. Consequently, there is a high regard for the concerns usually identified with the field of bioethics.

Doctrine and ethics

In Orthodox belief, the teaching of the church is found in the Old and New Testaments, the writings of the church fathers, and all aspects of the synodical, canonical, liturgical, and spiritual tradition of faith as lived, experienced, and reflected upon in the consciousness of the church, for which the general name "holy tradition" is used.

The Eastern Orthodox church understands ultimate reality to be the Holy Trinity, or God who is a triune unity of persons: the Father, source of the other two fully divine persons; the Son, forever born of the Father; and the Holy Spirit, forever proceeding from the Father. Thus, ultimate uncreated and uncontingent reality is a community of divine persons living in perpetual love and unity.

This divine reality created all else that exists, visible and invisible, as contingent reality. Human beings are created as a composite of body and spirit, as well as in the "image and likeness" of the Holy Trinity. "Image" refers to those characteristics that distinguish humanity from the rest of the created world: intelligence, creativity, the ability to love, self-determination, and moral perceptivity. "Likeness" refers to the potential open to such a creature to become "God-like." This potential for deification, or *theosis,* has been lost through the choice of human beings to separate themselves from communion with God and their fellow human beings; that is to say, sin is a part of the human condition. Though weakened and distorted, the "image" remains and differentiates human existence from the rest of creation.

The work of redemption and salvation is accomplished by God through the Son, the second person of the Holy Trinity who took on human nature (except for sin) in the person of Jesus Christ. He taught, healed, gave direction, and offered himself upon the cross for the sins of humanity, and conquered the powers of death, sin, and evil through his resurrection from the dead. This saving work, accomplished for all humanity and all creation, is appropriated by each human person through faith and baptism, and manifested in continuous acts of self-determination in communion with the Holy Spirit. This cooperation between the human and divine in the process of growth toward the fulfillment of God-likeness is referred to as *synergy.*

The locus for this appropriation is the Church—specifically, its sacramental and spiritual life. The sacraments, or "mysteries," use both material and spiritual elements, as does the life of spiritual discipline known as "struggle" and "asceticism" (*agona* and *askesis*). Both foster a communion of love between the Holy Trinity and the human being, among human beings, and between humans and the nonhuman creation, making possible continuous growth toward God-likeness, which is full human existence.

Though in this earthly life growth toward God-likeness can be continuous, it is never completed. In the Eastern Orthodox worldview, the eternal Kingdom of God provides a transcendent referent for everything. The Kingdom is not only yet to come in the "last days," but is now a present reality through Christ's resurrection and the presence of the Holy Spirit. Within this spiritual reality, the goal of human life is understood to be an ongoing process of increasing communion with God, other persons, and creation. This forms the matrix for Orthodox Christian ethics and provides it with the materials and perspectives for articulating the "ought" dimensions of the church's teaching (Mantzaridis, 1993).

Among the more important aspects of these teachings for bioethics are (1) the supreme value of love for God and neighbor; (2) an understanding that sees nature fallen but also capable of providing basic norms for living through a foundational and elementary natural moral law; (3) the close relationship of material and spiritual dimensions of human existence and their appropriate relationship and integration; (4) the capacity for self-determination by human beings to make moral decisions and act on them; and (5) the criterion of movement toward God-likeness—all within a framework that is both this and other-world focused.

In practice, ethical norms are arrived at in holy tradition and by contemporary Orthodox ethicists by defining moral questions within this context of faith in a search for ethical guidelines that embody the good, the right, and the fitting (Harakas, 1983).

Bodily health

Concern for the health of the body, though not central, has a significant place in Eastern Orthodox ethics (Harakas, 1986a). Orthodox Christian ethics calls for "a healthy mind and a healthy spirit with a healthy body." The body is neither merely an instrument nor simply a dwelling place of the spirit. It is a constituent part of human existence, and requires attention for the sake of the whole human being. Thus, in its sinful condition, the body can also be a source of destructive tendencies that need to be controlled and channeled. This is one of the works of asceticism, which seeks to place the body under control of the mind and the spirit. But asceticism is never understood as a dualistic condemnation of the body. As a good creation, under the direction of the proper values, the body is seen as worthy of nurturing care. Thus, everything that contributes to the well-being of the body should be practiced in proper measure, and whatever is harmful to the health of the body ought to be avoided. The Eastern Christian patristic tradition is consistent in this concern (Constantelos, 1991; Darling, 1990).

Practices that contribute to bodily health and well-being are ethically required. Adequate nourishment, proper exercise, and other good health habits are fitting and appropriate, while practices that harm the body are considered not simply unhealthful, but also immoral. Abuse of the body is morally inappropriate. Both body and mind are abused through overindulgence of alcohol and the use of narcotics for nontherapeutic purposes. Orthodox teaching holds that persons who might be attracted to these passions need to exercise their ethical powers in a form of ascetic practice to overcome their dependence upon them as part of their growth toward God-likeness.

Healing illness

When illness occurs, Orthodox Christianity affirms an ethical duty to struggle against sickness, which if unaddressed can lead to death. The moral requirement to care for the health of the body indicates it is appropriate to use healing methods that will enhance health and maintain life. Two means are used concurrently: spiritual healing and different forms of medicine. The first is embodied in nearly all services of the church, in particular, the sacrament of healing, or holy unction. There is also a continuing tradition of multiple forms of prayer and saintly intercessions for the healing of body and soul.

The church does not see spiritual healing as exclusive nor as competitive with scientific medicine. In the fourth century, Saint John Chrysostom, one of the great church fathers, frequently referred to his need for medical attention and medications. In his letters to Olympias, he not only speaks of his own use of medications but advises others to use them as well. Saint Basil, another great fourth-century church father, underwent various forms of therapy for his illnesses. In fact, both of these church fathers had studied medicine. Basil offers a classic Christian appreciation of the physician and the medical profession:

> Truly, humanity is the concern of all of you who follow the profession of medicine. And it seems to me that he who would prefer your profession to all other life pursuits would make a proper choice, not straying from the right, if really the most precious of all things, life, is painful and undesirable unless it can be possessed with health. And your profession is the supply vein of health. (Basil, *Epistle 189*, *To Eustathius, the Court Physician* fourth century, p. 228)

Recent studies have highlighted the Eastern Orthodox church's concern with healing, both in its medical and spiritual dimensions. Orthodox monks established the hospital as a place of healing, a tradition maintained by Orthodox monasticism for almost a thousand years, until it was taken over by the medical establishment (Miller, 1985; Scarborough, 1985; Harakas, 1990).

Bioethical concerns and methods

Bioethics as a distinct discipline is only a few decades old, but some topics now included in the discipline, such as abortion, have been addressed by the Christian tradition over the centuries. Many bioethical issues are new, however, and the Orthodox church's views concerning them have yet to be officially stated. The method contemporary Orthodox ethicists use to determine Eastern Orthodox perspectives on bioethical questions is the same as the general method used to make ethical decisions. The general doctrinal stance and ethos of the church form the larger context, delineating basic perspectives. The church requires further study, however, to assess the moral dimensions of newly created bioethical questions.

The ethicist concerned with bioethical questions then consults the tradition, which embodies the mind of the church: Scripture, patristic writings, decisions of the ecumenical councils and other synods, the received doctrinal teachings of the church, canon law, ascetical writings, monastic *typika* (constitutions of monastic establishments), liturgical texts and traditions, *"exomologetaria"* (penitential books), the exercises of *economia* (a process of judgment that allows for consideration of circumstances in a particular case, but without setting precedents for future normative decision making), and theological studies, for specific references that exhibit the mind of the church in concrete ethical situations. The "mind of the church" is understood as the consciousness of the people of God, together with the formulation of theological opinion, in conjunction with the decisions of the church in local, regional, and ecumenical synods, conceived and experienced as arising from the guidance of the Holy Spirit. It is a mindset, rather than a set of rules or propositions. The purpose of examining these sources is to determine whether these sources speak either directly, or indirectly, or by analogy, to new questions of bioethics. The historical contexts of these specific sources are kept in mind, and will serve to condition contemporary judgments.

Both general and specific applications can then be made and expressed as theological opinion on topics in bioethics. These views, however, are tentative, until the mind of the church specifically decides. Wherever this has already occurred, it will be noted below. Otherwise, what follows should be understood as thoughtfully considered theological opinion, subject to correction by the mind of the church (Harakas, 1980; Harakas, 1986b).

The protection of life

Orthodox thought holds that life is a gift from God, given to creation and to human beings as a trust to be preserved and protected. Just as the care for one's health is a moral duty for the individual, society's concern for public health is also a moral imperative. The first large division of concern is that existing life be protected. This can be expressed in a number of ethical positions characteristic of an Orthodox perspective.

The protection of life has been a value pursued throughout history by the church. During the early days of the rise and spread of Christianity, abortion was widely practiced in the Roman Empire. The Church, based on its respect for life, condemned this practice in its canon law as a form of murder. The Church considered abortion particularly heinous because of the defenseless and innocent condition of the victim (Kowalczyk, 1977). Of course, no moral stance is absolute. In Orthodox traditional teaching, however, abortion is nearly always judged to be wrong. There can be unusual circumstances, such as an ectopic pregnancy that threatens the life of the mother, that might be judged prudentially as calling for an abortion, but such situations are rare.

Historically related to the rejection of abortion was a condemnation of the exposure of infants, that is, their abandonment, a practice that caused their death or led to their exploitation by unscrupulous persons who profited from forcing children into prostitution or begging. These are severe examples of child abuse that unfortunately have continued into the modern age. Every such case, historic or contemporary, violates the moral requirement that adults care for children in a loving and supportive manner.

Modern medical technology and ethics

The development of medical science and technology has raised many new issues, however. Studying these issues from within the mind of the church has produced a body of positions that are expressive of the church's commitment to the protection of life. Some of these follow.

Allocation of medical resources. A bioethical question that finds a response in the concern for the protection of life is the issue of the allocation of scarce medical resources. A health-care system that fosters the widest possible distribution of health-care opportunities is the most morally responsible, since it reflects the common human situation before God.

Professional–patient relationships. In the area of the relationships of providers and recipients of health care, the church affirms the existence of patients' rights and requires that the medical profession honor them. The full human dignity of every person under treatment should be among the controlling values of health-care providers, manifested in their concern to maintain the patient's privacy, obtain informed consent for medical procedures, develop wholesome personal contacts between the patient and the medical team members, and treat the patient as a total human being rather than an object of medical procedures.

Human experimentation. Because of the role it plays in the development of medical therapies and the possible cure of individual persons, human experimentation must be conducted and is morally justified by an appeal to the value of the protection of life. Wherever possible, however, such experimentation should fulfill the following minimal conditions: The patient should be informed of the risks involved and should accept participation in the experiment freely and without coercion, and the experiment should have potential benefit for the patient. Increased knowledge should be secondary to the welfare of the patient.

Organ transplantation. Protection of life finds intense application in the area of organ transplantation. This topic may serve as a somewhat more extensive example of Orthodox bioethical reflection. Organ transplantation was unknown in the ancient world. Some Orthodox Christians consider it wrong, a violation of the integrity of the body. Significant as this consideration is, it does not outweigh the value of concern for the welfare of the neighbor, especially since organs for transplants are generally donated by persons who are philanthropically motivated for the protection of life. The sale of organs is seen as commercializing human body parts and therefore unworthy, and is prohibited by a concern for the protection of life and its dignity.

There are two categories of potential donors: the living and the dead. Usually, the potential living donor of a duplicated organ is a relative. In such cases, concern for the well-being of the patient may place undue pressure upon the potential donor. No one has an absolute moral duty to give an organ. Health-care professionals must respect the integrity of the potential donor as well as the potential recipient. Yet it is certainly an expression of God-likeness for a person to give an organ when motivated by caring concern and love for the potential recipient. Ethical consideration must be given to the physical and emotional consequences upon both donor and recipient and weighed in conjunction with all other factors. When these are generally positive, the option for organ donation by a living person has much to commend it.

In the case of donation of organs from the dead, some of the same considerations hold, while several new issues arise. Organs can be donated in anticipation of death. Some states, for example, encourage people to declare their donation of particular organs (liver, kidney, cornea) in conjunction with the issuance of auto licenses. There do not appear to be serious objections to this practice; many Orthodox consider it praiseworthy. When no expressed wish is known, permission of donation should be sought from relatives. Their refusal should be respected.

Persons may donate organs through bequests associated with their wills. This choice should be made known to responsible survivors before death. In 1989, for example, the Greek Orthodox Archbishop of Athens announced in the press that he had made provision for the donation of his eyes after his death.

Body donation to science. Similarly connected with the protection of life is the issue of donating one's body to science. Much of the answer from an Orthodox Christian perspective has to do with what the representatives of science will do with it. Giving one's body to science means, in nearly all cases, that it will be used for the education of medical students. There has been a bias against this practice in many countries because at the same time that the personal identity of the body is destroyed, the body itself is treated without respect. The alternative to using donated bodies for medical education, however, is that medical students and young physicians will learn surgical skills on living patients. The concern for the protection of life could not, thus, totally disapprove of the practice of body donation. In principle, then, giving one's body for medical education cannot be ethically prohibited. But medical schools should strive to create an atmosphere of reverence and respect for the bodily remains of persons given for this purpose. In some medical schools, this already takes place; in most, it has not. Potential donors of their bodies should inquire about procedures and refuse to donate their bodies to schools that do not show adequate respect for the body. Usually this means making arrangements for ecclesial burial of the remains after their educational use.

The aged.   The protection of life covers the whole life span. The Orthodox church has always had a special respect and appreciation for the aged. Industrial society, with its smaller, nuclear families, has tended to isolate the aged from the rest of society. The aging themselves ought not to accept such marginalization passively. They should continue to live active and fulfilling lives, with as much independence of movement and self-directed activity as possible. Spiritually, growth in the life of Christ continues to be important. Repentance, prayer, communion with God, service to others, and loving care for others are important in this and every age bracket.

Children and relatives should do everything possible to enhance the quality of life for their aging parents and relatives. But in cases of debilitating conditions and illnesses, it may be necessary to institutionalize them. Many Orthodox Christians feel that this is an abandonment of their moral responsibilities to their parents. If institutionalization is a way of abdicating one's responsibilities to parents for the sake of convenience, then it is wrong. However, it is often the best solution. Even when it is morally indicated, the important values remain; in a nursing home or outside of it, children still have the obligation to express love, care, and respect for their parents.

Death.   Concern for the protection of life is also present at the end of life. Death should come of itself, without human intervention. God gives us life; God should be allowed to take it away. Proponents of so-called euthanasia hold that persons should be allowed and may even be obliged to end their earthly lives when "life is not worth living." In the church's judgment, this is a form of suicide, which the church condemns. If one does this to another person, it is a case of murder. Orthodox Christian ethics rejects euthanasia as morally wrong.

Modern medical practice has raised some related issues, however. The possibility that vital signs can be maintained artificially, even after death has occurred, raises the complex question of turning off "life-sustaining" machines after brain death is diagnosed. The tradition has never supported heroic intervention in situations where death is imminent and no further ther-apies exist. It has been Eastern Orthodox practice not only to allow a person to die but also to actively pray for it when, according to the best medical judgment available, a person is struggling to die. If a person is clinically dead but his or her vital organs are kept functioning by mechanical means, turning off the machines is not considered euthanasia. Until the determination of clinical death, both physician and family should seek to maintain the comfort of the patient. Spiritually, all should provide the dying person opportunities for repentance and reconciliation with God and with his or her fellows (Breck, 1989).

Suffering.   In all serious medical situations, suffering should be relieved as much as possible; this is especially true for the Orthodox patient who has participated in the sacraments of Holy Confession and Holy Communion. Pain that cannot be relieved should be accepted in as redemptive a way as possible. For the church, a "good death" (in Greek, *euthanasia*) is one in which the human being accepts death with hope and confidence in God, in communion with him, as a member of his kingdom, and with a conscience that is at peace. Genuine humanity is achievable even on the deathbed.

The transmission of life

The Eastern Orthodox approach to marriage provides the context for discussing procreative and sexual issues. The church sees marriage as a sacramental dimension of human life, with ecclesial and interpersonal dimensions and purposes (Guroian, 1988). The Orthodox church sees both men and women as equal before God as human beings and as persons called to grow toward God-likeness. Both men and women are persons in their own right before God and may be endowed with many potentialities that ought to be developed as part of their human growth. Yet the special sacramental relationship of marriage, procreation, and child rearing gives to women, in the mind of the church, a special role. Accompanying it is the role of husband and father in constituting a marriage and creating a family. Most of the bioethical issues regarding the transmission of life arise out of this marital and familial perspective in Orthodox thought.

Reproductive technologies.   Artificial insemination assists spouses to procreate when they cannot conceive through normal sexual intercourse. In such cases, the sperm of the husband is artificially introduced into the wife's child-bearing organs. There are differences of opinion in the Orthodox church regarding this procedure. A major objection is that this is a totally unnatural practice. But since other "unnatural practices" such as cooking food, wearing clothes, using technical devices such as eye-glasses and hearing aids, and performing or undergoing surgery are considered morally acceptable, this argument loses much of its force.

More cogent is the argument that artificial insemination separates "baby-making" from "love-making," which is a way of emphasizing the unity of the spiritual and bodily dimensions of marriage. In the case of artificial insemination by husband (AIH), the personal, social, and spiritual context seems to indicate that AIH is morally acceptable. The opposite holds true when the semen of a donor is used (AID). The intrusion of a third party in providing the semen violates the psychosomatic unity of the marital couple.

The same pattern of ethical reflection applies to other procedures, such as artificial inovulation and in vitro fertilization. If the sperm and ovum come from the spouses themselves, and the wife bears the child to term, ethical objections to these procedures are lessened. Often, however, fertilized ova are discarded in the procedures. The majority of Orthodox consider this a form of abortion. Others hold that for abortion to take place, implantation in the womb must have previously occurred. Nevertheless, surrogate mothers, egg donation, and sperm donation from parties outside the marriage find no place in an ethical approach that places heavy emphasis on the wholeness and unity of the bodily and spiritual aspects of human life, and of the marital relationship in particular.

Sterilization.   Where sterilization is intended to encourage promiscuous sexual living, Orthodox Christianity disapproves. A strong ethical case can be made for it when there are medical indications that a pregnancy would be life-threatening to the wife. An as yet unexplored ethical area is the case of almost all older, yet still fertile, married couples, for whom there is a significant likelihood that the children of their mature love would be bearers of serious genetic diseases.

Genetics.   Genetic counseling seeks to provide information to a couple before they conceive children so that potentially serious conditions in newborns can be foreknown. Genetic counseling is also related to genetic screening of population groups that might be carriers of particular genetic illnesses. Genetic screening refines and makes more accurate the earlier practices of the church and of society that sought to reduce the incidence of deformed and deficient children, through the restriction of marriages between persons closely related genetically.

As a procedure that would reduce the number of persons entering into marriages with dangerously high chances for the transmission of genetic illnesses, these procedures ought to be strongly encouraged. Premarital genetic screening of young people with Mediterranean backgrounds, where there is a relatively high incidence of thalessemia B and Tay-Sachs disease, might guide them in the selection of spouses. Once a child is conceived and growing in the womb, however, the church could not consider the termination of the pregnancy as anything other than abortion. An impaired child is still the image of God with a right to life (Harakas, 1982). Since the church strenuously opposes abortion, prenatal diagnostic information indicating the prospective birth of a genetically deformed child cannot justify ending the life of the baby in the womb. Instead, this information serves to prepare the parents to receive their child with the love, acceptance, and courage required to care for such an exceptional baby.

Genetic engineering.   Concern with genetic engineering as an aspect of the transmission of life provokes a conflicting reaction among Orthodox Christian ethicists. Some Orthodox ethicists value the potential therapeutic possibilities of genetic engineering. In this case, the treatment of the genome to correct deficiencies is looked at positively, as a form of medical therapy. Nevertheless, there is concern when these same techniques are thought of as means for eugenic goals. The potential for misuse and abuse make Orthodox Christian reactions very cautious (Breck, 1991).

Conclusion

The common denominator in all these issues is the high regard and concern of the church for human life as a gift of God. Eastern Orthodox Christianity takes a conservative approach to these issues, seeing in them a dimension of the holy and relating them to transcendent values and concerns. Only an intense respect for human life can curb the modern tendencies to destroy human life both before birth and as it approaches its end. The human person, from the very moment of conception and implantation in the womb, is dependent upon others for life and sustenance. It is in the community of the living—especially as it relates to the source of life, God in Trinity—that life is conceived, nurtured, developed, and fulfilled in communion with God. The trust that each person has in others for the continued well-being of his or her own life forms a basis for generalization. Eastern Orthodox ethics, consequently, functions with a pro-life bias that honors and respects the life of each person as a divine gift that requires protection, transmission, development, and enhancement.

Stanley S. Harakas

Directly related to this entry is the entry Roman Catholicism. *Also directly related is the entry* Population Ethics, *section on* religious traditions, *article on* eastern orthodox christian perspectives. *For a further discussion of topics mentioned in this entry, see the entries* Abortion; Abuse, Interpersonal, *especially the article on* child abuse; Aging and the Aged; Bioethics; Body; Death; Death, Definition and Deter-

MINATION OF, *especially the article on* PHILOSOPHICAL AND THEOLOGICAL PERSPECTIVES; DEATH AND DYING: EUTHANASIA AND SUSTAINING LIFE; ETHICS, *especially the article on* RELIGION AND MORALITY; FAMILY; GENETIC COUNSELING; GENETIC ENGINEERING; GENETIC TESTING AND SCREENING; HEALING; HEALTH-CARE RESOURCES, ALLOCATION OF; HUMAN NATURE; LIFE; LIFESTYLES AND PUBLIC HEALTH; LOVE; MARRIAGE AND OTHER DOMESTIC PARTNERSHIPS; MEDICAL EDUCATION; NATURE; ORGAN AND TISSUE PROCUREMENT; ORGAN AND TISSUE TRANSPLANTS; PERSON; PROFESSIONAL–PATIENT RELATIONSHIP; REPRODUCTIVE TECHNOLOGIES; RESEARCH, HUMAN: HISTORICAL ASPECTS; RIGHTS; SUBSTANCE ABUSE; *and* TECHNOLOGY. *For a discussion of related ideas, see the entries* AUTHORITY; DEATH, ATTITUDES TOWARD; ENVIRONMENT AND RELIGION; EUGENICS AND RELIGIOUS LAW, *article on* CHRISTIANITY; FETUS; GENE THERAPY; MEDICAL ETHICS, HISTORY OF, *section on* EUROPE, *subsection on* CONTEMPORARY PERIOD, *article on* SOUTHERN EUROPE; PASTORAL CARE; *and* PROTESTANTISM.

Bibliography

BASIL, SAINT. 1968. "Epistle 189." Letters. *A Select Library of Nicene and Post-Nicene Fathers of the Christian Church.* Edited by Philip Schaff and H. Wace. Grand Rapids, Mich.: Eerdmans.

BRECK, JOHN. 1989. "Selective Nontreatment of the Terminally Ill: An Orthodox Moral Perspective." *St. Vladimir's Theological Quarterly* 33, no. 3:261–273.

———. 1991. "Genetic Engineering: Setting the Limits." In *Health and Faith: Medical, Psychological and Religious Dimensions,* pp. 51–56. Edited by John Chirban. Lanham, Md.: University Press of America.

CONSTANTELOS, DEMETRIOS J. 1991. *Byzantine Philanthropy and Social Welfare.* 2d rev. ed. New Rochelle, N.Y.: A. D. Caratzas.

DARLING, FRANK C. 1990. *Christian Healing in the Middle Ages and Beyond.* Boulder, Colo.: Vista Publications.

GUROIAN, VIGEN. 1988. *Incarnate Love: Essays in Orthodox Ethics.* Notre Dame, Ind.: University of Notre Dame Press.

HARAKAS, STANLEY S. 1980. *For the Health of Body and Soul: An Eastern Orthodox Introduction to Bioethics.* Brookline, Mass.: Holy Cross Orthodox Press.

———. 1983. *Toward Transfigured Life: The Theoria of Eastern Orthodox Ethics.* Minneapolis, Minn.: Light and Life.

———. 1986a. "The Eastern Orthodox Church." In *Caring and Curing: Health and Medicine in the Western Religious Traditions,* pp. 146–172. Edited by Ronald L. Numbers and Darel W. Amundsen. New York: Macmillan.

———. 1986b. "Orthodox Christianity and Bioethics." *Greek Orthodox Theological Review* 31:181–194.

———. 1990. *Health and Medicine in the Eastern Orthodox Tradition: Faith, Liturgy and Wholeness.* New York: Crossroad.

KOWALCZYK, JOHN. 1977. *An Orthodox View of Abortion.* Minneapolis, Minn.: Light and Life.

MANTZARIDIS, GEORGIOS. 1993. "How We Arrive at Moral Judgements: An Orthodox Perspective." *Phronema* 3: 11–20.

MILLER, TIMOTHY S. 1985. *The Birth of the Hospital in the Byzantine Empire.* Baltimore: Johns Hopkins University Press.

PELIKAN, JAROSLAV. 1974. Vol. 2, *The Spirit of Eastern Christendom (600–1700). The Christian Tradition: A History of the Development of Doctrine.* Chicago: University of Chicago Press.

SCARBOROUGH, JOHN, ed. 1985. *Symposium on Byzantine Medicine: Dumbarton Oaks Papers, Number 38.* Washington, D.C.: Dumbarton Oaks Research Library and Collection.

WARE, KALLISTOS. 1964. *The Orthodox Church.* Baltimore: Penguin.

ECOFEMINISM

See ENVIRONMENTAL ETHICS, *article on* ECOFEMINISM. *See also* ANIMAL WELFARE AND RIGHTS, *article on* ETHICAL PERSPECTIVES ON THE TREATMENT AND STATUS OF ANIMALS.

ECOLOGY AND ECOSYSTEMS

See ENDANGERED SPECIES AND BIODIVERSITY; ENVIRONMENTAL ETHICS; *and* ENVIRONMENTAL HEALTH.

ECONOMIC CONCEPTS IN HEALTH CARE

Health care has always been an economic activity; people invest time and other resources in it, and they trade for it with each other. It is thus amenable to economic analysis—understanding the demand for it, its supply, its price, and their interrelationship. Economic analysis, of course, does not merely discern what the supply, demand, and price for health care in private or public markets are. It also attempts to understand why those are what they are: What behavior on the part of suppliers affects the demand for health care? How does a particular insurance framework affect supply and demand? And so on. Beyond its descriptive and explanatory functions, economic analysis is indispensable in the larger attempt to improve health care—to make it more efficient, for example, so that people can accomplish more with their investment in health care, or more in life generally with the resources they have.

The economics of health care, in fact, has grown into an established specialty within professional economics. Though virtually every good is in some sense an "economic good," economists have been quick to notice some differences between most health care and ordinary market commodities. Final demand seems to be more supplier-created in the case of health care than it is with most goods; both the shape of health services and their price are very directly influenced by providers. Other forms of what economists call "market failure" also occur in health care—for example, when people with a considerable demand for health care do not receive services because their high risk to insurers drives prices for even the most basic insurance to unaffordable levels. Other economic distinctions and concepts are important for understanding health care: the respective, different roles of price inflation and real increases in services in raising both unit price and aggregate cost; the hidden costs of further tests necessitated by "false positive" results that emerge in initial screening or diagnosis; and the hidden savings of an effective service in avoiding later costs. Routine though not always undisputed concepts in economics, such as the discounting of future costs and benefits back to present value, increase the sophistication of our understanding of health care.

As we have become more and more concerned about rising cost, economic concepts have gained greater general currency in people's consideration of health care. Price is seldom "no object," and the search for efficiency is vigorous. This article on economic concepts in health care will (1) clarify the differences between two important forms of efficiency analysis in health care; (2) articulate some of the difficulties in devising and using a common unit of health benefit; (3) examine the monetary evaluation of one health benefit, life extension; (4) focus on some of the fundamental moral difficulties that the demand for efficiency poses for clinical practice; and (5) briefly explore the notions of "externality" and "public good" and their role in health policy.

Throughout it will be important to keep in mind that economists, qua economists, usually think of their primary task as describing the world, not saying what it ought to be. The relationship of economic concepts to ethical concerns pursued in this discussion, however, will tend to pick out those economic elements that often raise ethical issues when they become the basis of someone's normative judgments about health care.

One should also note that although many economic concepts may appear to be more at home in capitalist than in centralized, collectivist, or socialist economies, they virtually always have a role to play in those other economies. For example, cost-effectiveness and cost–benefit analysis are used at least as much in socialist as in more capitalist health-care systems. While the economic concepts developed here may not be ideology-free, they are hardly confined to free-market frameworks.

Cost-effectiveness, cost–benefit, and risk–benefit analysis

Efficiency involves the basic economic concept of "opportunity cost": the value from alternatives that we might have pursued with the same resources. When the value of any alternative use is less than the value of the current service, the current one is efficient; when the value of some alternative is greater, the current service is inefficient. In thinking of the possible alternative uses, our sights can be set either narrowly or broadly. If we focus just on other options in health care, wondering whether we can get more benefit for our given health-care dollars, or whether we can get the same health benefit more cheaply, we are engaged in cost-effectiveness analysis (CEA). If, on the other hand, we are comparing an investment in health care with all the other things we might have done with the same time, effort, and money, we are engaged in cost–benefit analysis (CBA). CEA asks whether the money spent on a particular program or course of treatment could produce healthier or longer lives if it were spent on other forms of care. CBA involves an even more difficult query: whether the money we spend on a particular portion of health care is "matched" by the benefit; we determine that by asking whether it could produce greater value, not just healthier or longer lives, were it devoted to other things.

Both kinds of analysis are important. We want to get the most health and life for our investment in health care (CEA), but we also want neither to be so occupied with other investments that we ignore improvements in health that would really be worth more to us, nor to pass up other, better things in life because we are investing too much in relatively unproductive health care (CBA). CEA is the less difficult, less ambitious enterprise: We compare different health-care services, detecting either final differences in expense to achieve the same health benefit or differences in some health benefit (added years of life, reductions in morbidity, etc.). That itself is a tall order, but it is less daunting than CBA, which must compare the value of the longer life and better health achieved by health care with the value of the other possible improvements in human life achievable by other investments of equivalent resources.

CBA as an economic concept puts no a priori restrictions on what sorts of things' value might be compared with health care. CBA is difficult, of course, because the advantages gained from those other uses of resources so often seem incommensurable with health and longevity. But improvements *within* health care often seem terribly incommensurable, too: How do we really compare the values of non–life-extending hip replacement and life-extending dialysis or transplants?

At this point our understanding of economic analysis is aided greatly by a formal statement of what constitutes CBA. Formal, economic CBA puts into common *monetary* terms the various benefits of the endeavors in life that are being compared—a life saved with health care is seen to have a value, let us say, of $1 million. With the benefits thus monetarized, the conceptual package of resource trading is tied together; we are able to compare the benefits of health-care and non–health-care endeavors with each other in the same (monetary) terms. Without any comparison with other investments, in fact, we can ascertain whether the benefits are worth the costs, since costs have been stated from the beginning in monetary terms. If, for example, it will likely take three $500,000 liver transplants to get one lifesaving success, and if a life saved has a monetary value of $1 million, then the transplants cost more than the life they save is worth. Whether we are achieving actual "value for money," which is the focus of efficiency judgments, now gets explicit answers. (Superficial answers, critics will say, doubting that we can ever sustain the judgment that a life saved had a monetary value of $1 million, not the $1.5 million that would make the transplants in this example a costworthy bargain.)

Another, less formalized kind of analysis is "risk–benefit analysis": One compares the probabilities of harm presented by a certain course of action with its likely benefits. If another procedure is likely to produce similar benefits with less risk, the latter is obviously preferable. It is not always clear, however, when one risk is "less" than another; the two may be risks of different things—one perhaps of paralysis and the other, say, of chronic pain. Moreover, one procedure may harbor lower risk but also promise fewer health benefits; again we are left with a nonquantifiable final trade-off. Unlike CEA, the beneficial effects in risk–benefit analysis are not all measured on a common scale, and unlike CBA, the benefits are not put in the same terms as the costs or risks. The analysis only helps us see what risks we incur in the pursuit of what benefits.

We use the economic tools of CEA and CBA to discern potential improvements in cases of market failure (frequent in health care) where efficiency is not achieved. The existence of a potential efficiency improvement, however, does not by itself tell us that we should pursue it. Efficiency is only one goal; we might also need to consider the fairness of distributing goods and resources in the most efficient way. Economists, though, will be quick to note efficiency's especially great moral force in two sorts of circumstances: where the new, more efficient distribution is "Pareto superior" (some gain and no one loses), or where the gain to some is sufficient to allow them to compensate the "losers" back to their reference point and still retain some net benefit for themselves. If, for example, so many people gain from water fluoridation that they are still better off when taxed to provide an ample compensation fund for those who suffer some side effect, then everyone, even the "losers," gains by fluoridation of the water supply.

Health benefit units: Well-years or quality-adjusted life years (QALYs)

CEA, unlike CBA, does not venture answers to the question of how much money to spend for a given health benefit. It does, however, attempt ambitious as well as modest comparisons within health care. All that it needs to be able to do this is a common unit of health benefit. In some contexts this will quite naturally be present; suppose we are comparing the respective prolongations of life provided by bypass grafts and "medical management" (drug therapy) for a certain kind of coronary problem. The more difficult task for CEA comes in translating widely different health benefits into a common conceptual currency. The notion developed for this purpose by economists and health-policy analysts goes by various labels: a "well-year," a "quality-adjusted life year" (QALY, pronounced to rhyme with "holly"), or "health-state utility." In any case, the essential idea is a unit that combines mortality with quality of life considerations—"a year of healthy life," as one defender of QALYs puts it. We can then compare not only life-prolonging measures with each other but also measures that enhance quality with those that prolong life—hip replacements with kidney dialysis, for example. And we could also, in public-health terms, track the health of a population, calculating increases (or decreases) in per capita "years of healthy life."

Having available a unit that combines mortality and morbidity will be immensely useful if we are trying to maximize the "health benefit" of a given amount of resources invested in health care. Suppose dialysis patients' self-stated quality of life is 0.7 (where 0 is death and 1.0 is normal healthy life). They would gain 7.0 QALYs from 10 years on $35,000-a-year dialysis, a cost/benefit ratio of $50,000 per QALY. Suppose hip replacements improve 15 years of life from 0.9 quality ranking to 0.99. That will be a 1.35 QALY gain for the $8,000 operation, a cost of less than $6,000 per QALY. To achieve greater efficiency, we apparently should solidify or even expand the use of hip replacements in our total complement of health services, and look much harder at dialysis.

A sizable literature of CEA has developed, not only studies of particular procedures but also discussions about the construction of common units of health benefit. Take the QALY. Questions abour.d. Whom does one ask to discern quality-of-life rankings for different sorts of health states—patients with the problems, or other citizens and subscribers who are less dominated by their desire to escape their immediate health need? What questions do we ask them? Those building the

QALY and well-year frameworks have used "time trade-off" (how much shorter a life in good health would you still find preferable to a longer lifetime with the disability or distress you are ranking?), "standard gamble" (what risk of death would you accept in return for being assured that if you did survive, you would be entirely cured?), and several others. Whatever question people are asked, it should convey as accurately as possible what might be called the "QALY bargain": their exposure to a greater risk of being allowed to die should they have an incurable, low-ranking condition, in return for a better chance of being helped to significant recovery or saved for prospectively normal health.

The moral argument for using some such common health benefit unit is more than just some narrow focus on aggregate economic efficiency per se. The major moral argument for using both quality adjustment and longevity extension in a serious attempt to maximize the benefit that a plan or an entire health care system produces is that it is people themselves who implicitly quality-rank their own lives and thus consent to the allocation priorities that QALYs or well-years generate. Critics charge, however, that maximizing years of healthy life in our lifesaving policies systematically fails to respect the individual with an admittedly lower quality of life. To what interpersonal trade-offs have people consented, even when it might involve themselves? Suppose you yourself now prefer, as you did previously, a shorter, healthier life to a longer, less healthy one. You are now an accident victim who could survive, though paraplegic, while someone else could be saved for more complete recovery. Admittedly, you yourself prefer a life with recovery to one with paraplegia, and you would be willing to take a significant risk of dying from a therapy that promised significant recovery if it succeeded. You do not admit, though (and you never have admitted), that when life itself is on the line, a life with paraplegia is any less valuable to the person whose life it is than life without that disability. Compared with death, your paraplegic life could still be as valuable to you as anyone else's "better" life is to them—that is, you want to go on living as fervently as the nondisabled person does.

Similar puzzles attend what people would see themselves as consenting to in the way of interpersonal trade-offs between improving the quality of life and saving life itself. Perhaps those doubts and ambiguities about what people are really conveying when they quality-rank their own lives can be clarified or resolved, and the use of well-years or QALYs can be made consistent with our moral common sense. At least that might be possible for the vast bulk of citizens who are not relegated to a more difficult life for large and predetermined segments of their lives. For people with congenital or long-standing illnesses and disabilities, however, the moral problem is undoubtedly more stubborn. It seems more dubious to

claim that at some time they have consented, or would have consented, to a set of trade-offs between themselves and others whom they know are chronically better off.

Common health benefit units will undoubtedly continue to be developed and used. They are very important to the attempt to bring any kind of overall efficiency to a health-care system. Their contested character only indicates that the process of economic analysis into which they fit, systemwide CEA, is itself a morally contested vision for health care.

The monetary value of life

CBA, in contrast to CEA, demands the assignment of monetary value to the benefits of the program or procedure being assessed. The health benefit whose monetarization has received the most explicit attention in the literature of CBA is life itself. Such economic evaluation of life, as superficial and distorting as it may sound, is in one sense an innocent and unremarkable phenomenon in modern life. Now that a great number of effective but often costly means of preserving life are available, we inevitably and repeatedly pass up potential lifesaving measures for other good things, and money mediates those trade-offs. In CBA, however, we not only need to speak of life as having economic or monetary value; we also need to assign a particular monetary value, or range of monetary value, to it. Is that value $200,000 or $2,000,000? Is the monetary value of a relatively short remaining segment of life (a year, say) simply an arithmetic proportion of the whole life's value? If we assume that the length of different people's lives that remains to be saved or preserved is equal, is the economic value of their lives the same, or does it vary—for example, with income level, wealth, or future earning power, and therefore, perhaps, with race and gender? And if it does vary, should we still use those varying values or instead some common average in doing CBA of health care?

Independent of the debate about how those questions are to be resolved, economists have developed two main models for translating empirical data into an economic value of life: discounted future earnings (DFE), also known as the "human capital" model, and willingness to pay (WTP). DFE looks at the future earnings forgone when a person dies. In the economy, those earnings are what is lost when a person dies, so that from the perspective of the "whole economy" (if we can speak of any such thing), it would be self-defeating to refuse to save a life for $200,000 if the value of the person's earnings (after discounting the future figures back to present value) was more than that. While such DFE calculations continue to be used in some CBAs in health care, DFE has been largely surpassed in the work of economists by WTP. Here the value of life is taken to be a direct function of people's willingness to use resources to increase their chances of survival. Suppose one annually demands an extra $500, and only $500 extra, to work in an occupation that runs an additional 1-in-1000 risk of dying. Then according to WTP, $500,000 (1000 × $500) is the monetary value one puts on one's life. Within the context of CBA, this would mean it would be inefficient to devote more than $500,000 per life saved to health care that eliminates moderate prospective risks of death.

In economic theory, WTP is generally regarded as the superior model; it captures the range of life's subjective, intangible values that DFE seems to ignore. Generally people spend money for reasons of subjective preference satisfaction quite independent of monetary return. That is, economic value incorporates consumption values, not just investment. Despite that firm basis in underlying economic theory, WTP has raised a host of objections. For one thing, questions arise similar to those that afflict DFE. For example, just as with wide variations in persons' DFEs, there are wide variations in willingness to pay—largely based on people's wealth and income. Should we see those variations in value as legitimately affecting what is spent on lifesaving measures? If their effect is legitimate, is that only for services privately purchased, or also for those funded through public programs? Defenders of WTP have articulated a whole battery of refinements and responses to handle these and a host of other critical questions, but the model may still seem suspicious. "It was efficient not to save his life [now lost]—it was worth only $500,000" is not easily accepted. Consequently, despite its popularity in professional CBA, WTP has hardly gained widespread moral acceptance as a conceptual tool for health-policy decisions.

The basic problem is simply that in the end the world is such a different place for a loser than it is for a winner. Suppose one refuses to pay more than $500 (when one could) for a CAT scan or magnetic resonance image (MRI) that one knows is likely to eliminate a 1-in-1000 portion of the risk of dying from one's malady, and that one later dies because of that decision. Of course one has in some sense consented to what happened, but one never thought anything remotely like "$500,000—no more—is the value of my life," the life that after the fact is irretrievably lost. The move that economists make in WTP to get from an initial trade-off between money and risk and the value of a real, irreplaceable life is puzzling. One critic has claimed that in principle only valuations of life made directly in the face of death are correct reflections of the actual economic value of life (Broome, 1982). But as another contributor to this discussion has noted, we do not know of anyone "who would honestly agree to accept any sum of money to enter a gamble in which, if at the first toss of a coin

it came down heads, he would be summarily executed" (Mishan, 1985, pp. 159–160). Some conclude from this that CBA can set no rational limit on what to spend to save a life because no particular finite amount of money is adequate to represent the real value of life.

Even if this point about the actual value of a life is correct, however, it may not render the sort of thing that is going on in WTP estimates of the value of life irrelevant for use in CBA affecting health policy. In the context of setting policy about whether to include a certain service in our package of insurance, we cannot assume that the later perspective of an individual immediately in the face of death is the correct one from which to make decisions. The in-the-face-of-death perspective may be proper for the legal system to adopt in awarding compensation for wrongful death, where we are trying to compensate people for the losses actually incurred. But perhaps health-care decisions ought to be made from an earlier perspective. In modern medical economies, after all, most people either subscribe to insurance plans or are covered by public health-care spending. Once insured, whether in private or public arrangements, subscribers and patients as well as providers find themselves with strong incentive to overuse care and a marked tendency to underestimate opportunity costs. Why should we not address the problem of controlling the use of care in the face of these value-distorting incentives at the point in the decision process, insuring, where the cost-expansion trouble fundamentally starts? For the use of CBA in devising health policy, justification of a willingness-to-risk model as showing us the "value of life" may not be necessary; it is appropriate to use in any case. Perhaps what is important in decisions to invest resources in health care is only that what we refer to in CBA as "the monetary value of the benefits" should be derived from people's decisions to bind themselves in advance to certain restrictions on the provision of care. Perhaps many of the "values of life" generated by WTP are not sufficiently close to actual decisions of the persons affected to limit their own investment in lifesaving; that would make any resulting particular CBAs that used them crude and morally ungrounded, but would not necessarily seal the fate of all CBA.

The monetary value of other health benefits, such as freedom from morbidity, has received much less empirical work than the monetary value of life. Those benefits too, however, are crucial to monetarize if CBA is going to contribute greatly to decisions on health-care policy. It is possible that as a formal method of analysis, CBA will thus not have great influence in the future. Even if that is true, however, the larger enterprise of less formal CBA will remain an active and crucial dimension of the broader attempt to find the proper place of health care in our lives overall. We will still be concerned about whether the marginal dollar we invest in health care provides sufficient value.

The difficulties that economic concepts pose for clinical practice

Suppose that economic efficiency analysis, of the CEA, CBA, or some other less formalized sort, lays the groundwork for subsequent recommendations about the kind and amount of health care to use—fewer diagnostic MRIs in certain low-yield situations, less use of dialysis and intensive care, and very cautious introduction of new, expensive drugs like Cyntoxin, for example, and more hip replacements, much more assertive and widely diffused prenatal care, and more frequent use of angiograms and contingent follow-up coronary bypass operations for patients with certain combinations of heart symptoms. The former, service-reducing steps would not constitute the elimination of merely wasteful procedures that generate no net health benefit; they would constitute much harder, genuine rationing in which some patients did not get what for them would be optimal care. How does such rationing for efficiency relate to the ethical obligations of practicing health-care providers? The traditional (at least traditionally professed) ethic of physicians is one of loyalty to individual patients. Generally, in turn, that loyalty is interpreted to mean beneficence within the limits of respect for patient autonomy: doing whatever benefits a patient the most, within the limits of what the competent patient willingly accepts. If health care is to be rationed to control the resources it consumes from the rest of our lives, will the basic clinical ethic have to change? If it will, is the achievement of efficiency worth its moral cost? This potential clash between traditional ethical obligations and the economic and social demands of the "new medicine" in an age of scarcity is one of the central foci of ethical controversies in medicine as we enter the twenty-first century.

One can divide the potential views here into "incompatibilist" and "reconciliationist" camps: those who think that the demands of societywide (or at least large-group) efficiency cannot be reconciled with the ethical obligations of practitioners, and those who think they can be. The incompatibilists will end up in two different positions: (1) the "well, then, to hell with morality" view in which one is willing to pursue economic efficiency anyhow; and (2) the anti-efficiency stance that opposes rationing in the name of a morality of strict beneficence toward individual patients. Reconciliationist views will also come in distinctly different sorts: (1) the view that the clash was more apparent than real all along, for providers have always shaped the lengths to which they would go to benefit individual patients by considerations of their effective overall practices; (2) the separation-of-roles position, which insists that parties more distant from the patient than clinicians make all rationing decisions and that clinicians then ration within determined practice guidelines; (3) the view that as a provider, one's proper loyalty to a patient, though not dominated by efficiency, is to the patient as a member of a just society, a condition that then enables the clinician to participate in rationing with a clean conscience when it is based on considerations of fairness and justice; and (4) the view that takes its cue from the autonomous choices of patients as longer-lived persons and sees rationing to be grounded in the consent of the prepatient subscriber to restrictions on his or her later care (why would the patient consent?—to reserve resources for other, more value-producing activities in life).

The strength of the incompatibilist views may seem to be that they call a spade a spade, but their abiding weakness is that instead of truly eliminating one side or the other of the conflict, they just dam up the conflict and create later, greater explosions between economic efficiency and other moral considerations in contemporary medicine. The last three reconciliationist views, on the other hand, deal directly and constructively with the conflict, allowing conscientious clinical medicine still to find roots in a more cost-controlled, socially acceptable aggregate of health-care practice. Their weakness may be the great difficulties they face in actually being used; the separate-roles view requires extremely clear formulation of detailed care-rationing practice guidelines in abstraction from the medically relevant particulars of individual patients, the patient-in-a-just-society model requires a great degree of agreement on what constitutes a just society, and the prior-consent-of-patients solution must involve not only accurate readings of what restrictions people are actually willing to bind themselves to beforehand but also a willingness of subscribers and citizens to think seriously about resource trade-offs beforehand and abide honestly by the results even when that places them on the short end of rationing's stick.

Undoubtedly this discussion is not about to reach immediate resolution in societies that are enamored of the ever-expanding technological armamentarium of medicine, see themselves as respectful of individual patients, and are determined to steward their resources wisely.

Externalities and public goods

Externalities and public goods play a prominent role in economics-informed discussions of public policy. Externalities are costs or benefits of a behavior not borne by or accruing to the actor, but by or to others. They pose a distinct problem for the achievement of efficiency in market exchanges. If I am making and selling an item whose production involves harms or burdens to others for which I do not have to pay, I will be able to price the product under its true cost and sell it more easily. Also, if I am buying a product whose use harms or burdens others, I will be willing to pay more for it than its true net worth; that, in turn, will entice more production of the good than its true cost and benefit would efficiently warrant. The solution to these distortions is to correct producers' and buyers' incentives by imposing a tax on the item equivalent to its external cost (or a subsidy equivalent to its external benefit). Even better, one could give the proceeds of that tax to the parties harmed by the item's use or production. Externalities, then, immediately propel us into public-policy decisions about taxes and subsidies.

Public goods also directly raise questions of public regulation and taxation. A "public good" in the economist's sense is one whose benefits accrue even to those who do not buy it. If you clean up your yard, I benefit from a somewhat better appearance on the block regardless of whether I clean up my own or help you clean up yours. Or if a large number of people contribute to an educational system in the community, I get some of the benefits of the more civilized culture and productive economy that results even if I never contribute anything. The benefit is thus public and nonexclusive: Once a certain mass of contributors is in place, it is difficult if not impossible to exclude from the benefits of these enterprises an individual who chooses not to contribute. Standard examples of public goods on the large social scale include many of the basic functions of the modern state (public safety, national defense, education, public health, and the reduction of pollution). That is no accident, for the public goods dimension of these functions is itself a primary justification of the state's coercive power. If I contribute not a penny to a police force, for example, I will still receive most of its benefits of public safety; I will thus "free-ride" on others' willingness to fund police. The obvious solution to this unfairness on my part is for the collective to tax me my fair share.

The use of both public goods and externalities is undoubtedly on the rise in our analysis of certain issues in health care. Note just a few examples of the interesting contexts in which these concepts come up.

One is the taxing of health-complicating products such as tobacco and alcohol. Smoking and excessive drinking undoubtedly increase certain costs to others—health-care expenditures for smoking- and drinking-related diseases; lost work time; displeasure, sadness, and pain in dealing with others' destruction of their social and biological lives; and even direct loss of life (from passive smoking, drunk driving, etc.). These externalities provide part of the momentum behind the movement to increase taxes on tobacco and alcohol; as societies look for ways to deal with rising health-care costs, a fair source of revenue would be special taxes on the activities of those who increase the health-insurance premiums and taxes of others through their own originally voluntary behavior. Note, however, that the empirical picture can be much more complicated, and in the case of tobacco it certainly is. First-impression, informal cost analysis of smoking (and many published academic studies as well) tells us that smokers cost nonsmokers a great deal of money. That conclusion ignores, however, two hidden "savings" of smoking that accrue to others: Because smokers die earlier, and generally near the end of their earning years or shortly thereafter, they save others the pension payouts and unrelated health-care expenditures they would have incurred had they lived longer, without losing that saving through reduced earnings and the taxes thereon. One leading study, in fact, concludes that the average 1989-level U.S. cigarette tax of $.37 per pack is adequate to cover all the costs that smokers impose on others, including losses from fires and the costs of the U.S. tobacco subsidies (Manning et al., 1989; 1991). Subsequent increases may thus not be justifiable by any empirically well-informed externalities argument. This is not the last word on the net external costs of smoking, but it illustrates the subtleties and hidden costs that increasingly sophisticated economic analyses reveal. Such studies may turn up equally surprising results in the future as we turn more and more to prevention in the hope of controlling health-care costs; prevention that saves health-care expense in one respect may lose those gains as its longer-living beneficiaries draw more pension payouts and end up incurring high costs of illness in their longer lives.

A second example might be paying for one person's life extension that others would never buy for themselves. Suppose the family of a permanently comatose patient insists on continued life support, and that such care will incur considerable insurer-paid expense (for example, see Cranford, 1991). Should others in the insurance pool (private subscribers or public taxpayers) who think that such comatose life is worth no investment of valuable resources have to pay for that family's or patient's decision? Greater efficiency (getting costs in line with the real value of benefits) would be achieved were we to arrange things in our health-care system so that people somehow had to pay for their beliefs about the value of life. The argument against doing this claims there is something objectionable about making people pay for their moral beliefs, not just their consumption habits and lifestyle choices. The argument for it, however, is that people ought to face up to the necessity to allocate scarce resources only for those benefits of sufficient value to justify the expense. Even a person who believes that comatose life is worth living may not believe it is worth enough, when put to the test, to pull large amounts of resources away from other things.

A third example is sharing in the costs of a health-care system that provides access to those who otherwise cannot pay. Suppose that most people think a good society provides basic care to those who cannot afford it. Suppose, furthermore, that in addition to that proposition about the relative responsibilities of the poor and those who are better off, most people believe that in a good society, the financial burdens of medical misfortunes that people cannot have been expected to control by their own choices ought to be shared equally by well and ill. It is then possible to analyze the situation in terms of public goods and the prevention of free-riding. If a considerable amount of charity care is provided and thus improves access, I gain both the security of knowing that I will be helped if I become poor or sick, and the satisfaction of knowing that I live in a society that does not neglect its poor and ill. If I do not contribute to make this more secure and better society possible, I am free-riding on the largess of others. This may provide the justification for requiring people to pay into an insurance pool even when they think they are safe.

Many other interesting and controversial instances of the use of these and other economic concepts in the analysis of health care could be cited. Without being targeted accurately on identifiable pockets of market failure, tax breaks for health-insurance premiums would seem to create incentives for inefficient overinvestment in health care. If physicians significantly create demand for their own services, their incomes will need to be regulated either by the government or by market forces at work among health plans using salary or capitation payments (as distinct from fee for service) to compensate physicians. And so on and so forth. More generally, how to discern what constitutes efficiency in the investment of resources in health care, how to arrange incentives to stimulate efficient use of care, and how the achievement of efficiency is to be compared with the realization of other values central to the whole health-care enterprise constitute the challenge that economic concepts bring to health care as we move into the twenty-first century.

PAUL T. MENZEL

Directly related to this entry are the entries HEALTH-CARE FINANCING, *the* INTRODUCTION, *and articles on* HEALTH-CARE INSURANCE, *and* PROFIT AND COMMERCIALISM; HEALTH-CARE RESOURCES, *articles on* MACROALLOCATION, *and* MICROALLOCATION; *and* LIFE, QUALITY OF, *article on* QUALITY OF LIFE IN HEALTH-CARE ALLOCATION. *For a further discussion of topics mentioned in this entry,* *see the entries* HARM; JUSTICE; RISK; UTILITY; *and* VALUE AND VALUATION. *Other relevant material may be found under the entries* COMMERCIALISM IN SCIENTIFIC RESEARCH; CONFLICT OF INTEREST; HEALTH-CARE DELIVERY; HEALTH POLICY, *article on* POLITICS AND HEALTH CARE; LIFE, QUALITY OF, *article on* QUALITY OF LIFE IN CLINICAL DECISIONS; PUBLIC POLICY AND BIOETHICS; *and* TECHNOLOGY, *article on* TECHNOLOGY ASSESSMENT.

Bibliography

BELL, JOHN M., and MENDUS, SUSAN, eds. 1988. *Philosophy and Medical Welfare.* Cambridge: At the University Press. A collection of valuable papers, many on QALYs and the various ethical and philosophical problems of measuring and maximizing the value of health benefits.

BRENNAN, TROYEN A. 1991. *Just Doctoring: Medical Ethics in the Liberal State.* Berkeley: University of California Press. A comprehensive statement of the view that a physician's loyalty to individual patients must be placed in the context of the justice of the entire health-care system.

BRONZINO, JOSEPH D.; SMITH, VINCENT H.; and WADE, MAURICE L. 1990. "Economics of Medical Technology." In their *Medical Technology and Society: An Interdisciplinary Perspective,* pp. 38–86. New York: McGraw-Hill. An introductory economic analysis of health care generally and the impact of medical technology in particular.

BROOME, JOHN. 1982. "Uncertainty in Welfare Economics and the Value of Life." In *The Value of Life and Safety: Proceedings of a Conference Held by the "Geneva Association,"* pp. 201–217. Edited by Michael W. Jones-Lee. Amsterdam: North-Holland. One of the most vigorous and challenging responses to the WTP model for valuing life.

CRANFORD, RONALD E. 1991. "Helga Wanglie's Ventilator." *Hastings Center Report* 21, no. 4:23–24. This short description, together with articles by Felicia Ackerman, Daniel Callahan, and Michael Rie in the same issue, presents various sides of a famous case involving familial insistence on life support for a permanently comatose patient that the attending physicians wish to withdraw.

DANIELS, NORMAN. 1986. "Why Saying No to Patients in the United States Is So Hard." *New England Journal of Medicine* 314, no. 21:1381–1383. A classic example of the view that the physician's role in rationing for efficiency should be contingent on the constructive place of rationing in ensuring justice in the overall health-care system.

FELDSTEIN, PAUL. 1988. *Health Care Economics.* 3d ed. New York: John Wiley & Sons. A highly respected, comprehensive text.

FUCHS, VICTOR R. 1986. "Health Care and the United States Economic System." In his *The Health Economy,* pp. 11–31. Cambridge, Mass.: Harvard University Press. A helpful analysis of the particular features of the U.S. economy that affect our understanding of its health-care system.

GROSSMAN, MICHAEL. 1972. *The Demand for Health: A Theoretical and Empirical Investigation.* New York: Columbia

University Press. A distinctive study pursuing the notion of investment in health as a case of investment in human capital.

HARRIS, JOHN. 1987. "QALYfying the Value of Life." *Journal of Medical Ethics* 13, no. 3: 117–123. A clear, concise attack on the attempt to quantify the value of health benefits and to maximize that value.

JENNETT, BRYAN. 1986. *High Technology Medicine: Benefits and Burdens.* New ed. Oxford: Oxford University Press. An often skeptical examination of the actual medical benefits of modern medical technologies.

KAPLAN, ROBERT M., and ANDERSON, JOHN P. 1990. "The General Health Policy Model: An Integrated Approach." In *Quality of Life Assessments in Clinical Trials,* pp. 131–149. Edited by Bert Spilker. New York: Raven. A useful and comprehensive description and defense of measuring advances in a health-care system in terms of well-years.

MANNING, WILLARD G.; KEELER, EMMETT B.; NEWHOUSE, JOSEPH P.; SLOSS, ELIZABETH M.; and WASSERMAN, JEFFREY. 1989. "The Taxes of Sin: Do Smokers and Drinkers Pay Their Way?" *Journal of the American Medical Association* 261, no. 11:1604–1609. A comprehensive assessment of the economic impact of tobacco and alcohol use on others and a succinct analysis of the role of externalities in tax policy.

———. 1991. *The Costs of Poor Health Habits.* Cambridge, Mass.: Harvard University Press. This further details and expands the authors' 1989 work.

MENZEL, PAUL T. 1990. *Strong Medicine: The Ethical Rationing of Health Care.* New York: Oxford University Press. A critical discussion of the economic valuation of life, the role of economic efficiency in a physician's obligations to patients, measurement of health benefits (QALYs), long-term net costs of smoking, and the problem that many economists see in providing equal care for rich and poor.

MISHAN, EZRA J. 1985. "Consistency in the Valuation of Life: A Wild Goose Chase?" In *Ethics and Economics,* pp. 152–167. Edited by Ellen Frankel Paul, Jeffrey Paul, and Fred D. Miller, Jr. Oxford: Basil Blackwell. A revealing reexamination of the author's classic statement fourteen years earlier of the WTP model for valuing life.

MORREIM, E. HAAVI. 1991. *Balancing Act: The New Medical Ethics of Medicine's New Economics.* Dordrecht, Netherlands: Kluwer. A detailed case for incorporating limited rationing of care, for economic efficiency, into physicians' conceptions of their moral obligations.

NORD, ERIK. 1992. "An Alternative to QALYs: The Saved Young Life Equivalent (SAVE)." *British Medical Journal* 305, no. 6858:875–877. An interesting proposal for an alternative benefit unit, to replace QALYs, that would elicit less public resentment.

PELLEGRINO, EDMUND D., and THOMASMA, DAVID C. 1988. *For the Patient's Good: The Restoration of Beneficence in Health Care.* New York: Oxford University Press. A defense of the view that fidelity to the individual patient's best interest is still the proper heart of medical ethics.

RHOADS, STEVEN E., ed. 1980. *Valuing Life: Public Policy Dilemmas.* Boulder, Colo.: Westview. A useful anthology on economic valuation of life that includes some of the classic articles by economists, including Ezra J. Mishan, on

the DFE and WTP models, and responses by noneconomist critics.

RICE, DOROTHY P.; HODGSON, THOMAS A.; SINSHEIMER, PETER; BROWMER, WARREN; and KOPSTEIN, ANDREA N. 1986. "The Economic Costs of the Health Effects of Smoking, 1984." *Milbank Quarterly* 64, no. 4:489–547. A detailed assessment of the costs of smoking that omits the savings in later pension payouts and unrelated health-care expenditures that Manning et al. (above) includes.

ROBINSON, JAMES C. 1986. "Philosophical Origins of the Economic Valuation of Life." *Milbank Quarterly* 64, no. 1:133–155. A qualified defense of the now relatively unpopular DFE model for valuing life.

RUSSELL, LOUISE B. 1986. *Is Prevention Better Than Cure?* Washington, D.C.: Brookings Institution. An empirical examination, and a presentation of the conceptual framework for that examination, of the relative efficiency of selected preventive health-care measures.

SCHMID, A. ALLAN. 1989. *Benefit-Cost Analysis: A Political Economy Approach.* Boulder, Colo.: Westview. A comprehensive presentation of cost–benefit analysis as a method for assessing economic efficiency.

TORRANCE, GEORGE W. 1986. "Measurement of Health State Utilities for Economic Appraisal: A Review." *Journal of Health Economics* 5:1–30.

VEATCH, ROBERT M. 1986. "DRGs and the Ethical Allocation of Resources." *Hastings Center Report* 16, no. 3:32–40. A clear statement of the view that the proper role of the physician is never to engage in active judgments to ration care.

WARNER, KENNETH E., and LUCE, BRYAN R. 1982. *Cost-Benefit and Cost-Effectiveness Analysis in Health Care: Principles, Practice, and Potential.* Ann Arbor, Mich.: Health Administration Press. A comprehensive, textlike presentation of economic efficiency analysis in health care.

WILLIAMS, ALAN. 1985. "Economics of Coronary Artery Bypass Grafting." *British Medical Journal* 291, no. 6491:326–329. A notable article, using and defending QALYs for use in health-care policy, by one of the economists most influential in developing the QALY concept.

EGYPT

See MEDICAL ETHICS, HISTORY OF, *section on* NEAR AND MIDDLE EAST, *articles on* ANCIENT NEAR EAST, *and* CONTEMPORARY ARAB WORLD.

ELECTRICAL STIMULATION OF THE BRAIN

The central nervous system (CNS), which consists of the brain and spinal cord, forms the bridge between the sensory and motor functions of the peripheral nervous system. It is specialized to interpret nerve impulses and functions together with the endocrine system to coordinate the activities of all the other body systems. The CNS also can store experience in memory and learn by establishing patterns of responses based on prior experiences.

The spinal cord has two principal functions: It integrates simple responses to certain types of stimuli, and it carries information (such as touch, position, pain, and temperature) to the brain and the response to such information from the brain. The brain integrates the information presented to it by the nerve fibers located in the spinal cord and by the cranial nerves for smell, sight, taste, and facial sensation. This integration results in responses to the information—the output of the brain—known as behavior. The CNS receives and transmits all this information by means of complex electrochemical interactions that can be affected by direct electrical stimulation (Ackerman, 1992).

Development of electrical stimulation

The basic electrical nature of the nervous system has been suspected since the beginning of recorded history. Scientific work in this field probably dates from the observations of Luigi Galvani in 1791 that electrical stimulation of the frog's spinal cord resulted in leg movement (McHenry, 1969). During the nineteenth and twentieth centuries optimistic reports of healing by electrical stimulation were reported by Benjamin Franklin, Michael Faraday, and André Ampère. Neurology, neurological surgery, and psychiatry began to emerge, and with them the development of modern, consistent, and understandable uses of electrical brain stimulation (ESB) to alter the responses of the brain or spinal cord. It was observed that when a specific area of the brain or spinal cord is electrically stimulated, there results an excitation or inhibition of the usual response of that area. Early ESB was used as a method of mapping cerebral cortical function, matching the site of stimulation of the brain's surface with the patient's response during operations under local anesthesia. This procedure continues today, with more electronic sophistication, for cortical mapping to avoid injury to critical areas, such as those associated with speech or movement, during operations on the brain and to precisely localize areas of the brain involved with epilepsy, occasionally by stimulating to provoke seizures. An important observation concerning stimulation is that the effects are reversible: When stimulation is discontinued, its effects cease.

Stimulation of various regions of the brain or the spinal cord has been performed in attempts to relieve symptoms produced by brain diseases and brain trauma. Electrical stimulation does not result in any proven curative effect. In 1947, a technique called stereotaxic surgery became available to localize targets within the brain precisely so that those areas could be stimulated or destroyed. Stereotaxic techniques are the basis for the most common applications of ESB, the relief of chronic pain and the symptoms due to tremor or increased muscle tone in certain degenerative diseases of the nervous system, such as Parkinson's disease.

The most common use of central nervous system stimulation, the control of chronic pain, was first described in 1954 (Heath, 1954). In 1969, David Reynolds described the phenomenon of analgesia produced by stimulating the gray matter in the region of the midbrain. In the 1970s deep stimulation of other selected targets within the brain was demonstrated to relieve pain (Young, 1990). An associated technique for pain relief, called epidural spinal cord stimulation, involves stimulating the spinal cord from the space between the covering over the spinal cord, the dura mater, and the overlying bone of the spinal column. This treatment has been demonstrated to be effective in relieving certain nerve injury–related pain and pain due to lack of circulation in an extremity.

Current application

Currently ESB includes therapeutic applications for pain control and relief of symptoms in disorders such as Parkinson's disease, as a diagnostic adjunct in the diagnosis and treatment of epilepsy, as a tool for localizing specific brain areas in order to avoid injury during surgical procedures, and as a means of documenting the position of electrodes placed within the brain. Experimental work is progressing on the use of stimulation for specific sensory (visual, aural) and motor (phrenic nerve stimulation for breathing, sacral nerve stimulation for bladder continence) prosthetic devices whose purpose is to mimic as accurately as possible a lost neurologic function (Girvin, 1985). Electrical stimulation in the neck of the vagus nerve, a cranial nerve known to assist regulation of the heart, lungs, and gastrointestinal tract, has been demonstrated to reduce epileptic seizures. Studies are currently being undertaken in humans to assess the efficacy of this modality in reducing seizures (Hammond et al., 1992). A peripherally related emerging field of investigation utilizes the induction of electrical currents by an applied magnetic field to stimulate areas of the brain (Geddes, 1991).

Although in the 1960s concerns were voiced regarding suggested use of electrical stimulation to control behavior, there has been no evidence suggesting that ESB has been utilized specifically for that purpose (Delgado, 1969). Speculation about this application was offered on the basis of experimentally observed influences of ESB on the behavior of animals and observations on a restricted number of patients experiencing stimulation during operations for other reasons, such as for the treatment of epilepsy (Valenstein, 1973). Such speculation was enhanced by such popular novels as Michael Crichton's *Terminal Man*, whose main character becomes violent under the influence of a stimulator placed in the brain to control epileptic seizures (Crichton, 1972).

Technical considerations

Stereotaxis is used to stimulate the brain at a precise location: A special head frame is attached to the skull under local anesthesia, and electrodes are implanted, using internal brain targets located with reference to anatomical landmarks determined by brain scanning or by injecting air into the fluid space of the brain as a radiographic contrast material. Since the mid-1980s, computed tomographic imaging (CAT scanning) or magnetic resonance imaging technology (MRI) has been used to guide the placement of electrodes within the brain. A hole is drilled in the skull, the outer covering of the brain is opened, and the electrode is inserted. Preselected target points are then stimulated electrically while the patient's response is monitored. When the desired response—for example, a tingling sensation in the appropriate body part—is produced, the electrode wires are attached to disposable lead wires that are brought out through the scalp to allow a trial of stimulation—monitoring electrode combinations and pain relief, or production of the desired effect. A successful trial, with relief of the appropriate symptoms, such as pain or tremor, results in a return to the operating theater and placement of a transmitting or receiving device under the skin that activates the appropriate electrodes. Inadequate relief results in electrode removal.

Small electrodes may be placed around peripheral nerves, outside the brain and spinal cord, as a means of using stimulation to relieve symptoms of pain or epilepsy. In the evaluation of epilepsy and in research situations for a visual prosthesis, large arrays of electrodes may be placed, via openings in the skull, to record electrical activity or stimulate the brain surface to produce visual responses (Girvin, 1985). Small wires have been implanted in the cochlea to allow a microphone input designed to stimulate the ear to perceive sound in certain cases of deafness (Girvin, 1985).

Risk

The primary risk of ESB is that attendant on stereotaxic or brain surgery in general. The effects of stimulation itself are reversible, and thus permanent complications due to the stimulation itself are unusual. Stereotaxic implantation of an electrode into the brain or opening the skull to implant electrodes carries with it the risks of infection, hemorrhage within the brain, or neurologic injury. Epidural spinal cord electrodes are subject to

these risks as well as to spinal fluid leakage. The overall incidence of complications is on the order of 5 percent (Young, 1990). Long-term complications are primarily involved with lead wire breakage and or movement from the desired location. This can occur in 10 percent or more of the cases, especially with spinal cord stimulation.

Ethical issues

Informed consent. Given the ongoing investigational nature of many stimulation procedures, especially deep-brain stimulation for Parkinson's disease or other diseases involving abnormal movement, guidelines protecting patient autonomy by requiring informed consent are critical. At the outset, the experimental or nonexperimental nature of the intended procedure should be made clear to the patient. The potential patient should be fully informed of the balance of efficacy versus risk, and his or her decision recognized and respected.

Many afflicted with chronic intractable pain or abnormal motor control, such as cerebral palsy or Parkinson's disease, fall into a category of patients who, due to the chronicity of their illness and frustration with their disease or to disease-related cognitive impairment, may consent to almost any proposition of treatment promising symptomatic relief. Acute-care medicine aims to restore to the patient freedom from illness, while the goal in chronic care, as is the case here, is to sustain some meaning in a life lived with illness (Jennings et al., 1988). ESB attempts to alleviate symptoms to the extent that quality of life is improved. The ethical burden then lies with the clinician to involve caregivers, family, guardians, and decision makers. Treatment should not, however, be imposed on the patient by others if the patient is capable of deciding autonomously. If the patient cannot decide for himself or herself, the improvement in the patient's self-control, freedom, and dignity as a result of treatment should be assessed in decision making.

Experimental vs. therapeutic treatment. The decision to opt for a treatment offering some relief of symptoms may be compelling in spite of high or unknown risk. Two situations present themselves: the experimental and the therapeutic. Truly informed consent may not be possible in the experimental situation, for the outcomes presumably are unknown (Laforet, 1976; Donagan, 1977). Whether in the experimental or the therapeutic situation, the primary function of informed consent is to enable and protect individual autonomous choice.

In many ESB techniques, especially those associated with pain relief, it is important to determine when the procedure is no longer considered experimental. The boundary between therapeutic and experimental usage has historically been determined when the treatment is demonstrated to relieve the symptoms it is intended to relieve and when a significant proportion of physicians, especially those working in the field, are convinced that the intended outcome will appear without adverse long- or short-term effects outweighing the benefits. Definition of "long-term" may be somewhat arbitrary, but it implies a sufficient follow-up to separate effects of the treatment from the natural history of the disease. Formal mechanisms are in place to codify the transition of a procedure or treatment from experimental to accepted therapy. The Food and Drug Administration has assumed this role for products such as electrical stimulation devices. Its procedures are designed to establish the effectiveness of treatment modalities based on scientific and medical studies and judgment. Some believe that without the FDA's blessing, a procedure remains experimental.

Others argue that its requirements for convincing evidence, its safeguards to protect both animals and humans, and its bureaucratic slowness make it difficult to assess the experimental status of technology. The FDA does provide a relatively independent forum for decision making. Decisions as to the experimental or therapeutic use of ESB may be aided by assessing FDA comments. However, the ethical justification for the use of a treatment must always be determined by the clinical judgment that the chance of benefit outweighs the hazards (Merskey, 1991).

The question of experimental or therapeutic status for ESB is of concern because the implementation of these therapies is often denied or approved according to their "experimental" status. Intent is crucial after devices—for example, stimulators with FDA approval—are no longer considered experimental. When the physician intends to use a particular therapy to increase knowledge of the therapy, whether regarding safety or efficacy, such intervention should be experimental, thus requiring special consent. If the intent is to produce effects generally beneficial to the patient that have previously been demonstrated in similar cases, the intervention is therapeutic.

Monetary cost as a reason to deny treatment

With ESB procedures there comes a high procedural and equipment cost. Does the expected benefit to this individual justify the cost in resources to the community? Proof of efficacy is critical to demonstrate that resources are not wasted by using ineffective measures. For example, spinal cord stimulation has been shown to be routinely effective in relieving pain due to injured nerves and to be more effective than repeat operations for leg pain persisting after spinal disk surgery (Meyerson,

1990). Yet some insurance systems have chosen not to authorize the use of this treatment, primarily because of the cost, although the denial is occasionally justified by the label "experimental." Patients covered under these policies who have severe and intractable pain are unable to obtain a potentially beneficial therapy. The problem is the extent to which expensive technologies that do bring some benefit should be used when the benefit is considered disproportionate to the cost. The insurance carrier may consider the cost of implant plus maintenance too high unless the patient returns to work or stops using medication. The patient may feel that stimulation is worthwhile if 30 percent of the pain is relieved, even if he or she remains disabled and continues to take supplementary medications. The population of patients with chronic disabling pain represents a group that has, by and large, been ignored at the stage where curative interventions have failed to give relief. Further treatment is often seen as futile. If no other care plan is available and efficacy has been demonstrated in similar cases, then treatment should be considered worthwhile.

Behavioral control

Modern ESB has little to do with psychosurgery, brain surgery whose primary intent is to alter behavior. ESB should not be equated with electroconvulsive therapy (ECT), which uses scalp-applied external electric shock to produce seizurelike discharges in the brain, as used in the treatment of depression. Progress in ESB has not demonstrated applications in this area. It is entirely possible, however, given appropriate investigations, that behavioral alteration, if not control, may be feasible (Delgado, 1969). At present, insufficient experimental and clinical information exists for one to comment on current use in altering behavior. The initial flurry of interest in the 1960s was quenched largely by concerns over potential abuse and the development of effective psychotropic medications—medications designed to treat psychiatric disease, such as antidepressant medication. The necessary results of disciplined research in the use of ESB for behavior control are not available in a form to allow adequate decision making and judgment in its application. ESB should not be judged in this highly sensitive area by the abuses to which it might lead, however. We need to acquire much more information than is currently available. ESB is known to affect behavior; it is unknown whether it might be used as therapy for patients with psychiatric disease. It is unlikely that it might be employed to affect the behavior of large numbers of normal persons.

If ethical questions arise in the medical use of ESB, it is because the techniques deal with the direct stimulation of the brain. No other organ is so closely involved with concepts of mind or person. The brain is the organ of behavior, and presumably interventions involving its structure risk alteration in behaviors that determine personhood. These interventions *may* alter behavior and must be diligently observed for abuses, but the history of the implementation of ESB in medical treatments has thus far not demonstrated the feared problems of behavioral control or personality alteration.

JOHN C. OAKLEY

Directly related to this entry are the entries LIFE, QUALITY OF, *article on* QUALITY OF LIFE IN CLINICAL DECISIONS; PAIN AND SUFFERING; ELECTROCONVULSIVE THERAPY; *and* PSYCHOSURGERY. *For a further discussion of topics mentioned in this entry, see the entries* INFORMATION DISCLOSURE, *article on* ETHICAL ISSUES; *and* INFORMED CONSENT, *articles on* MEANING AND ELEMENTS OF INFORMED CONSENT, *and* CLINICAL ASPECTS OF CONSENT IN HEALTH CARE. *Other relevant material may be found under the entries* ALTERNATIVE THERAPIES; RISK; *and* TECHNOLOGY, *article on* PHILOSOPHY OF TECHNOLOGY.

Bibliography

ACKERMAN, SANDRA. 1992. *Discovering the Brain.* Washington, D.C.: National Academy Press. An introduction to the basic electrochemical nature of the brain.

CRICHTON, MICHAEL. 1972. *Terminal Man.* New York: Knopf.

COOPER, IRVING S., ed. 1978. *Cerebellar Stimulation in Man.* New York: Raven Press. An example of a technique that enjoyed a brief period of enthusiasm.

DELGADO, JOSÉ M. R. 1969. *Physical Control of the Mind: Toward a Psychocivilized Society.* New York: Harper & Row.

DONAGAN, ALAN. 1977. "Informed Consent in Therapy and Experimentation." In *Ethical Issues in Modern Medicine,* pp. 94–102. Edited by John Arras and Robert Hunt. Palo Alto, Calif.: Mayfield.

GARRISON, FIELDING H., and MCHENRY, LAWRENCE C., JR. 1969. *History of Neurology,* pp. 185–214. Edited by Sidney Bloch and Paul Chodoff. Springfield, Ill.: Charles C. Thomas. The early history of electricity and the nervous system.

GEDDES, LAWRENCE A. 1991. "History of Magnetic Stimulation of the Nervous System." *Journal of Clinical Neurophysiology* 8, no. 1:3–9.

GIRVIN, JOHN P. 1985. "Neural Prostheses." In *Neurosurgery,* pp. 2543–2545. Edited by Robert H. Wilkins and Setti S. Rengachary. New York: McGraw-Hill.

HAMMOND, EDWARD J.; UTHMAN, BASIM M.; REID, STEVEN A.; and WILDER, B. JOE. 1992. "Electrophysiological Studies of Cervical Vagus Nerve Stimulation in Humans: I. EEG Effects." *Epilepsia* 33, no. 6:1013–1020.

HEATH, RICHARD C. 1954. *Studies in Schizophrenia.* Cambridge, Mass.: Harvard University Press. The earliest description of the use of ESB to control pain.

JENNINGS, BRUCE; CALLAHAN, DANIEL; and CAPLAN, ARTHUR. 1988. "Ethical Challenges of Chronic Illness." *Hastings Center Report* 18, no. 1:(spec. suppl.)1–16.

LAFORET, EUGENE G. 1976. "The Fiction of Informed Consent." *Journal of the American Medical Association* 235, no. 15:1579–1585.

MERSKEY, HAROLD. 1991. "Ethical Aspects of Physical Manipulation of the Brain." In *Psychiatric Ethics,* 2d ed. Oxford: Oxford University Press.

MEYERSON, BJORN A. 1990. "Electrical Stimulation of the Spinal Cord and Brain." In *The Management of Pain,* pp. 1862–1877. Edited by John Bonica. Philadelphia: Lea and Febiger. A fairly technical review of this most common use of ESB.

REYNOLDS, DAVID V. 1969. "Surgery in the Rat During Electrical Analgesia Induced by Focal Brain Stimulation." *Science* 164, no. 878:444–445.

VALENSTEIN, ELLIOT S. 1973. *Brain Control: A Critical Examination of Brain Stimulation and Psychosurgery.* New York: Wiley.

YOUNG, RONALD F. 1990. "Brain Stimulation." *Neurosurgery Clinics of North America* 1, no. 4:865–879. A review of the use of ESB primarily for pain relief.

ELECTROCONVULSIVE THERAPY

Electroconvulsive therapy (ECT) is a highly efficacious treatment in psychiatry (Crowe, 1984), and yet there is ethical controversy about its use. Some have claimed that ECT should be outlawed because it seriously impairs memory; others, that ECT is best viewed as a crude form of behavior control that psychiatrists frequently coerce patients to accept. Still others claim that, even if coercion is not employed, depressed patients are rarely, if ever, capable of giving a valid consent to the treatment (Breggin, 1979). The complaint is also sometimes voiced that ECT is given more frequently to women patients than to men. There is also ample evidence that, in earlier years, ECT was given in ways that are not used today: higher amounts of electrical current, and sometimes daily or several-times-daily treatments. Undoubtedly, this harmed some patients (Breggin, 1979). Probably because of concerns like these, one state, California, has passed legislation making it difficult for psychiatrists to employ ECT without satisfying many administrative regulations (California Welfare and Institutions Code, 1979).

The nature of the treatment itself understandably frightens some persons, and there have been gruesome depictions of it in popular films and novels (Kesey, 1962). The notion of passing an electrical current through the brain, stimulating a cerebral seizure and causing unconsciousness, may seem forbidding, particularly in view of the fact that ECT's therapeutic mechanism of action remains largely unknown. There are, however, many effective treatments in medicine whose mechanisms are unknown, and there are probably many surgical treatments that would seem equally forbidding if they were observed by a layperson. In appraising the ethical legitimacy of ECT as a treatment, it is important to ask the same questions about ECT that are asked about any treatment: Of what does it consist, what is the likelihood that it will help, and what kinds of harm can it cause?

ECT treatment

There are several excellent reviews of the history, clinical indications, and likely harms and benefits of ECT (Abrams, 1992; American Psychiatric Association, 1990; Crowe, 1984; Kendell, 1981; Ottosson, 1985). The essential feature of the treatment is the induction of a cerebral seizure (which is easily measured via concomitant electroencephalography) by means of electrodes attached to the scalp, through which current is applied for a fraction of a second. The electrodes may be attached to both sides of the head (bilateral ECT), inducing a seizure in both hemispheres of the brain, or to only one side (unilateral ECT), limiting the seizure to that side. Patients are premedicated with a muscle relaxant and anesthetized with a short-acting barbiturate general anesthetic. Patients remain unconscious after the treatment for about five minutes and are usually mildly confused for an hour or so after they awaken. They have no memory of the treatment itself. Treatments are usually given two or three times weekly for two to four weeks.

ECT was used originally as a treatment for schizophrenia on the basis of the now-discredited hypothesis that epilepsy, which ECT was thought to mimic, and schizophrenia did not occur in the same persons. It is now used almost entirely with patients suffering from severe depression; most psychiatrists suggest its use to patients only when drug treatment and/or psychotherapy have not helped. ECT is used occasionally with patients suffering from a life-threatening degree of manic excitement, or from a catatonic stupor, when these conditions do not improve with drug therapy.

The effectiveness of ECT in reversing severe depression seems beyond dispute (Crowe, 1984; Kendell, 1981): Many large studies show a significant recovery from depression in 75 to 85 percent of patients who receive ECT, as compared with 50 to 60 percent of depressed patients who respond to antidepressant medication. Patients who do not respond to drugs show the same high response rate to ECT as do patients in general. ECT also works more quickly than drugs: Patients who improve typically begin to do so after about one week; drugs, if they work, typically take three to four weeks, sometimes longer, to have a significant effect.

Most studies show that unilateral and bilateral ECT are equally effective treatments, although a minority have found unilateral ECT to be on average less effective.

Although ECT can cause death, it does so so seldom that it is difficult to estimate a mortality rate. The largest modern report (Heshe and Roeder, 1976) studied 3,438 courses of treatment (22,210 ECTs), and only one death occurred. When ECT does cause death, it is usually cardiovascular in origin and is related to the use of a general barbiturate anesthesia.

The principal adverse effect of ECT on some patients is on memory. ECT causes two limited kinds of memory deficit. During the two to three weeks that treatments are given, memory and other cognitive functions are usually mildly to moderately impaired because of the ongoing seizures. Moreover, in later years patients are unable to recall many events that took place shortly before, during, and shortly after the two- to three-week course of treatment. Neither of these effects bothers most patients, as long as they understand ahead of time that they will occur.

The more important and controversial question is how often ECT causes an ongoing, permanent deficit in memory function. If and when it does, it is possible that the treatment has damaged parts of the brain underlying memory function. This has proven to be an elusive research problem, despite dozens of studies, many quite sophisticated, that have been carried out (Taylor et al., 1982). Among the many methodological problems involved in doing this research (Strayhorn, 1982), depression itself often causes cognitive impairment, including memory dysfunction.

A small minority of patients—the exact percentage seems unknown—do notice mild, ongoing, permanent memory problems after ECT; nearly all of them rate the memory problem as annoying but not serious (Strayhorn, 1982). However, when patients treated with ECT are compared with appropriate control groups, no deterioration in performance on objective tests of memory ability has been found. What is most troublesome is that a very small number of patients, perhaps 1 to 2 percent, complain of serious ongoing memory problems. Memory complaints occur more frequently after bilateral than unilateral ECT, which has led many commentators to recommend that unilateral treatment be given, and that bilateral treatment be used only in serious conditions and when unilateral ECT has failed.

Ethical issues

Is ECT so harmful that it should be outlawed? Very few persons maintain this position. ECT has an extremely small risk of causing death. It also has a small risk of causing chronic mild memory impairment, and a very small risk of causing chronic serious memory impairment. It is frequently used, however, in clinical settings where it is the only available treatment and where the patient is suffering intensely and may be at risk of dying. Severe depression is a miserable and a serious illness: The three-year death rate in untreated or undertreated patients is about 10 percent, while in treated patients, it is about 2 percent (Avery and Winokur, 1976). Even if the risks of ECT were substantially greater than they are, it would still be rational in the clinical setting of severe depression for patients to consent to ECT.

As with all other treatments in medicine, the possible harms and benefits of ECT should be explained to the patient during the consent process. The risk of death and of chronic memory dysfunction should be mentioned specifically. The patient's understanding of the data presented should be appraised, questions should be encouraged, and ample time for decision making should be allowed. Patients should be free to change their minds about receiving ECT, either before the treatments start or once they are under way.

ECT is often suggested to patients only after other treatments have failed. However, although it has slight risks, ECT has several advantages over other treatments: It works more quickly, in a higher percentage of cases, and it does not have the annoying and, for some cardiac patients, dangerous side effects of many antidepressant drugs. Following the general notion that part of an adequate valid consent process is to inform patients of any available rational treatment options (Culver and Gert, 1982; Group for the Advancement of Psychiatry, 1990), a strong argument can be made that from the outset of treatment, seriously depressed patients should be offered ECT as one therapeutic option (Culver et al., 1980).

Do psychiatrists often coerce patients into receiving ECT? This seems doubtful, but there are no data addressing this question. In the overwhelming majority of cases, psychiatrists should not force any treatment on a patient. Nonetheless, there are very rare clinical situations in which it is ethically justified to give ECT to patients who refuse it (Group for the Advancement of Psychiatry, 1990): for example, patients in danger of dying from a severe depression that has not been responsive to other forms of treatment (Merskey, 1991). But this is a special instance of the general ethical issue of justified paternalistic treatment, and no special rules should apply to psychiatric patients or to ECT (Group for the Advancement of Psychiatry, 1990).

There seems no reason to believe that the consent or the refusal depressed patients give to ECT is not in most cases valid. If a patient is given adequate information about the treatment, if he or she understands and appreciates this information, and if the patient's choice is not forced, then the decision is valid and, in almost all cases, should be respected. Most psychiatrists would assert that the great majority of depressed patients

are like the great majority of all patients: They feel bad, they would like to feel better, and if presented with information about available treatment options, they try to make a rational choice.

Is ECT disproportionally and unjustly given to women patients? There are no data that address this question, and it would be useful to obtain them. However, given the fact that women suffer from clinically significant depression two to three times more frequently than men (Willner, 1985), the critical question is not whether more women in total receive ECT, as would be expected, but whether ECT is given at a higher rate to women than to equally depressed men.

CHARLES M. CULVER

Directly related to this entry are the entries MENTAL-HEALTH THERAPIES; MENTALLY DISABLED AND MENTALLY ILL PERSONS, *article on* HEALTH-CARE ISSUES; PSYCHOSURGERY; *and* ELECTRICAL STIMULATION OF THE BRAIN. *For a further discussion of topics mentioned in this article, see the entries* BEHAVIOR CONTROL; BEHAVIOR MODIFICATION THERAPIES; COMPETENCE; INFORMED CONSENT, *article on* ISSUES OF CONSENT IN MENTAL-HEALTH CARE; *and* PSYCHOPHARMACOLOGY. *Other relevant material may be found under the entries* MENTAL HEALTH; MENTAL-HEALTH SERVICES; MENTAL ILLNESS; *and* PSYCHIATRY, ABUSES OF.

Bibliography

ABRAMS, RICHARD. 1992. *Electroconvulsive Therapy.* 2d ed. New York: Oxford.
AMERICAN PSYCHIATRIC ASSOCIATION. TASK FORCE ON ELECTROCONVULSIVE THERAPY. 1990. *The Practice of Electroconvulsive Therapy: Recommendations for Treatment, Training, and Privileging.* Washington, D.C.: Author.
AVERY, DAVID, and WINOKUR, GEORGE. 1976. "Mortality in Depressed Patients Treated with Electroconvulsive Therapy and Antidepressants." *Archives of General Psychiatry* 33, no. 9:1029–1037.
BREGGIN, PETER ROGER. 1979. *Electroshock: Its Brain-Disabling Effects.* New York: Springer.
California Welfare and Institutions Code. 1979. §§5325.1, 5326.7, 5326.8, 5434.2.
CROWE, RAYMOND R. 1984. "Electroconvulsive Therapy—A Current Perspective." *New England Journal of Medicine* 311, no. 3:163–167.
CULVER, CHARLES M.; FERRELL, RICHARD B.; and GREEN, RONALD M. 1980. "ECT and Special Problems of Informed Consent." *American Journal of Psychiatry* 137: 586–591.
CULVER, CHARLES M., and GERT, BERNARD. 1982. *Philosophy in Medicine: Conceptual and Ethical Issues in Medicine and Psychiatry.* New York: Oxford.
GROUP FOR THE ADVANCEMENT OF PSYCHIATRY. COMMITTEE ON MEDICAL EDUCATION. 1990. *A Casebook in Psychiatric Ethics.* New York: Brunner/Mazel.

HESHE, JOERGEN, and ROEDER, ERICK. 1976. "Electroconvulsive Therapy in Denmark." *British Journal of Psychiatry* 128:241–245.

KENDALL, ROBERT E. 1981. "The Present Status of Electroconvulsive Therapy." *British Journal of Psychiatry* 139: 265–283.

KESEY, KEN. 1962. *One Flew over the Cuckoo's Nest.* New York: New American Library.

MERSKEY, HAROLD. 1991. "Ethical Aspects of the Physical Manipulation of the Brain." In *Psychiatric Ethics*, 2d ed., pp. 185–214. Edited by Sidney Bloch and Paul Chodoff. Oxford: Oxford University Press.

OTTOSSON, JAN-OTTO. 1985. "Use and Misuse of Electroconvulsive Treatment." *Biological Psychiatry* 20, no. 9: 933–946.

STRAYHORN, JOSEPH M., JR. 1982. *Foundations of Clinical Psychiatry.* Chicago: Year Book Medical Publishers.

TAYLOR, JOHN R.; TOMPKINS, RACHEL; DEMERS, RENÉE; and ANDERSON, DALE. 1982. "Electroconvulsive Therapy and Memory Dysfunction: Is There Evidence for Prolonged Defects?" *Biological Psychiatry* 17, no. 10:1169–1193.

WILLNER, PAUL. 1985. *Depression: A Psychobiological Synthesis.* New York: Wiley.

EMBODIMENT

See BODY, *article on* EMBODIMENT: THE PHENOMENOLOGICAL TRADITION; *and* HEALTH AND DISEASE, *article on* EXPERIENCE OF HEALTH AND ILLNESS.

EMBRYO BANKING

See REPRODUCTIVE TECHNOLOGIES, *article on* CRYOPRESERVATION OF SPERM, OVA, AND EMBRYOS.

EMBRYOS

For a discussion of human embryonic development, the moral standing of the human embryo, and research on human embryos, see the entry FETUS.

EMBRYO TRANSFER

See REPRODUCTIVE TECHNOLOGIES, *article on* IN VITRO FERTILIZATION AND EMBRYO TRANSFER.

EMOTIONS

The place of emotions in morality

In bioethics as in ethics more generally, there is much debate about the significance of emotions in an account of moral character. Intuitively speaking, emotions are important because as moral beings we care not only about how we act but also about how we feel—what our moods are, as well as our attitudes and affects. Within the practice of health care, the emotions of compassion and empathy seem to have a particularly important place in a full description of decent and ethical treatment of a patient. The general point is not that emotion is internal and action external, for both action and emotion have exterior moments that point to deeper interior states, commonly thought of as character. Rather, emotions are important as modes of sensitivity that record what is morally salient and that then communicate those concerns to self and others. Thus, to grieve, pity, show empathy, or love is to focus on an aspect of self or other and to grasp information to which purer cognition or thought may not have access. Additionally, it is to express those concerns in a way that more bland or affectless action fails to do. Thus, emotion is distinct from both thought and action. More specifically, emotions are sensitive to particular kinds of salience. In the case of grief, what is salient is that humans suffer and face loss; in the case of pity, that they sometimes fail through blameless ignorance, duress, sickness, or accident; in the case of empathy, that they need the expressed support and union of others who can understand and identify with them; in the case of love, that they find certain individuals attractive and worthy of their time and attention.

In relations where caring for others is definitive, emotional sensitivity has an important place. In choosing a physician, for example, we tend to value medical skill and ability, but also character and judgment. And part of what we look for in character and judgment is not only reliable and principled action but also a certain range of emotional responsiveness. Medical care ministered without human gesture may not be received in the same way as that conveyed with compassion and empathy. While in some cases emotional tone is neither here nor there—urgency requires other priorities—in other cases, it matters deeply. A physician's sensitivity to a patient's needs, worries, and fears may be relevant to diagnosis and treatment, just as the physician's communication of emotions may be relevant to how a patient confronts illness and recovery. As in any relationship, emotional interaction is part of the exchange. In more intimate friendships, we hope that loved ones will be able to respond to our joy and suffering in more than merely intellectual ways, and will communicate feelings through spontaneous affect and gesture as well as more deliberate action.

The inclusion of emotions as part of what is ethically important faces notorious problems, however. In a familiar series of objections, often embodied in a traditional reading of Immanuel Kant, emotions are viewed as the enemy of both reason and morality. First, there is the problem of partiality: Emotions may respond to what is morally salient, but in a very partial and selective way; for instance, emotions can be unresponsive to more circumspect judgment. In addition, there is the alleged unreliability of emotions; they sometimes emerge on the scene strong and impetuous, only to peter out into a whimper. They cannot be relied on as motives, and nature and nurture cannot be counted on to distribute emotions evenly in all persons. For these sorts of reasons, emotions are sometimes thought to be an unreliable foundation for virtue. Furthermore, as passions (states that we undergo and suffer; from the Greek *paschein*, to be affected or suffer), emotions come to be construed as involuntary happenings that we endure with little intervention or consent. They come over us like the weather. Unlike action or belief, they appear to be exempt from direct willing. We cannot will to feel in the same way we can will to believe or will to act. Finally, emotions are typically attached to objects and events that are beyond our control. Through emotions, we invest importance in what we cannot control or master or make permanent: loved ones die, friends turn on us, attachment to status and security come undone by sickness and old age. When caregivers experience the death of patients to whom they feel especially attached, fear of loss can generate fear of attachment in future cases. Often emotions are investments in what is impermanent, and thus investments that make us vulnerable to loss.

These are familiar objections well entrenched in the literature. But increasingly they are being countered by philosophers of various stripes (Williams, 1973; Blum, 1980; Sherman, 1989; Nussbaum, 1990), including contemporary expositors of Kant (Herman, 1985). Against the various objections, it can be argued that emotions may sometimes show irrationality, perhaps of a more stubborn sort than beliefs; but even so, as is clear in the Aristotelian tradition, emotions have firm cognitive foundations. That emotions are sometimes irrational is not incompatible with the more basic fact that they seem to rest on appraisals or evaluations of situations that involve cognition. Again, through the emotions, we sometimes attend to situations in a partial and uneven way that does not always befit more universal principle and duty. Where partiality involves inappropriate emotions of bias and parochialism, then, like prejudiced beliefs, these emotions need to be controlled or transformed. But sometimes partiality is permissible and even encouraged. Contemporary Kantian views, for example, emphasize that the positive duty of beneficence must always be carried out by humans who by their nature are finite and subject to limitations of time and resources. Deliberation about the particulars, for example, of whom to help and when and where, must rely materially on emotions and the information they provide us about urgency and moral salience. Here, as suggested above, the report of the emotions may not be final or decisive.

But it is an important way to begin to mark a moral occasion. In medical decisions, similar sorts of judgments about the particulars of the case may rely on initial readings of need and urgency conveyed through emotional sensitivity.

Taking up the next objection, certain emotions may be involuntary, being more similar to compulsion and physical disease than to intention. And these may warrant pardon or pity. But emotions are varied and complex phenomena. Passivity need not imply involuntarism. Indeed, many emotions involve their own kind of assent and susceptibility to regulation, even though control and transformation are part of a slow and imperfect process. Though individuals typically cannot will to feel certain emotions at a moment's notice, they can choose to cultivate certain emotional dispositions over time as a significant part of developing moral character.

The vulnerability of the emotional life to contingent events and objects—to the vicissitudes of accident and loss—is a more complex matter. Traditional Kantians do not worry about the contingent aspects of the moral life, viewing them as problems for happiness and not morality. That is, the fulfillments and satisfactions of desire and emotional investment affect one's chances for happiness, not the goodness of one's moral will. More contemporary Kantians, who take emotions to be helpful and important allies to duty, hold that duty must still be on guard as regulator of emotion. Thus, where depression or anger stands in the way of professional or moral requirements to help, duty stands ready to fill the void and in all cases remains the only morally worthy motive.

For the Aristotelian, in contrast, moral motives are partially constituted by emotions, and goodness as well as happiness can be irreversibly affected by the state of one's emotions. There is no separate source of motive, such as Kant's pure practical reason, from which morality issues. Tragic loss can deprive one of happiness, and also of goodness, as in the case of Medea's evil pawning of her own children because of her jealous rage against Jason.

What are emotions?

We have talked in a general way about reasons for including emotions in an account of morality. But what are emotions? What kind of account can we give of them? There are a number of possibilities that it is important to review.

The first is the commonsense view in which emotion is thought to be an irreducible quality of feeling or sensation. It may be caused by a physical state, but the emotion itself is the sensation we feel when we are in that state. It is a felt affect, a distinctive feeling, but not something dependent upon thought content or appraisal of a situation. This is roughly David Hume's view, 1739.

The view quickly falters, however, when we realize that in this view emotions become no more than private states and feel like itches and tickles that have little to do with what the emotions are about and how one construes or represents those states of affairs.

A second view, associated with William James (James and Gurney, 1884) and Carl Lange, is that emotions are an awareness of bodily changes in the peripheral nervous system. We are afraid because we tremble or flee, not the other way around; angry because of the knots in our stomachs. The view, though rather counterintuitive, nonetheless captures the idea that emotions, more than other mental states, seem to have conspicuous physiological and kinesthetic components. These often dominate children's and adults' reports of their emotional experiences. They dominate literary accounts as well. Consider in this vein the lines of the Greek poet Sappho, composed about 600 B.C.E.:

> When I see you, my voice fails,
> my tongue is paralyzed,
> a fiery fever runs through my whole body
> my eyes are swimming,
> and can see nothing
> my ears are filled with a throbbing din
> I am shivering all over . . .

Literary history, social convention, and perhaps evolution conspire to tell us this is love. But even here it is not hard to imagine that what is described could be dread or awe or, perhaps, mystical inspiration. Even well-honed physiological feelings do not easily identify specific emotions. An awareness of our skin tingling or our chest constricting or our readiness to flee or fight does not specify exactly what emotion we are feeling. Many distinct emotions share these features, and without contextual clues and thoughts that focus on those clues, we are in the dark about what we are experiencing (Schacter and Singer, 1962). The chief burden of the work of Walter Cannon (1929) was to show that emotional affects are virtually identical across manifestly different states.

A third view with some kinship to the James–Lange view holds that emotions are felt action tendencies (Arnold, 1960). They are modes of readiness to act or, in the different idiom of psychoanalysis, discharge impulses. Support for this view comes from the fact that we tend to describe emotions in terms of dispositions to concrete behavior: "I felt like hitting him," "I could have exploded," "I wanted to spit," "I wanted to be alone with him, wrapped in his embrace." Yet, the action tendency view seems at best a partial account of emotion. The basic issue here is not that some emotions, such as apathy, inhibition, and depression, seem to lack activation modes while others are more a matter of the rich movement of thought so well depicted, for example, in Henry James's novels. It is, rather, that emotions are about something (internal or external) that we represent in thought. As such they have propositional or cognitive content. They are identified by that content, by what we dwell on, whether fleetingly or with concentrated attention.

This takes us to the fourth and final view of the emotions, which is, in some respects, the most plausible approach. This is the view that emotions are thought-dependent and are constituted by appraisals. (It is the view that Aristotle develops in the *Rhetoric*.) Such an account need not exclude other features of emotion, such as awareness of physiological and behavioral responses or felt sensations. But these, when present, are dependent on the appraisals of circumstances that capture what the emotion is about. Moreover, it is compatible with this view that emotions have neuropsychological structures that can be investigated by science.

More precisely, the appraisal is a belief about or evaluation of the goodness or badness of some perceived or imagined event. Anger requires an evaluation that one has been unjustly slighted by another; fear, that there is present harm or danger; grief, that something valuable has been lost; love, that one values a person as supremely important in one's life. Typically, the evaluation is experienced with pleasure or pain. In some cases the emotion includes a reactive desire not unlike what was referred to earlier as an action tendency. "Anger," Aristotle says, "is a desire (*orexis*) accompanied by pain toward the revenge of what one regards as a slight toward oneself or one's friends that is unwarranted" (*Rhetoric*, 1378a 30–32).

An account of the emotions needs to include evaluations that are weaker than strict belief (Greenspan, 1988). Many of the thoughts that ground emotions are not judgments to which we would give assent but are thoughts, perceptions, imaginings, construals, and fantasies that we nonetheless dwell on in a compelling way without concern about "objective truth." In these cases, there may be a certain laxity in the standards of evidence, or a partiality in what an agent takes to be relevant. There are familiar sorts of examples that illustrate the point. I may fear spiders even though I know that most spiders I am likely to encounter are harmless; or Clarissa may know that Joe is a no-good lover for her but still finds her heart yearning for him. In these cases emotions have thought contents or appraisals, though ones that are at odds with more circumspect judgment. They are mental states that seem to lag behind what we are ready to grasp by belief. The Aristotelian notion of *phantasia*, the capacity by which things appear to us or are seen interpretatively, is helpful here. So, too, is Ludwig Wittgenstein's notion of "seeing as." These notions make clear that emotions are not blind urges but thought-dependent responses that nevertheless can be irrational. Their recalcitrance to reason may reveal, on the one hand, that they are in need of tutoring or at least of the slow healing of time; it may also reveal, on the other hand, a clear view of what we really care about or fear, however irrational that reaction may be and whatever our more public beliefs or postures.

The notion of objectless emotions is sometimes presented as a counterexample to a thought-dependent account, according to which emotions are perceived to have an object. It is true that emotions such as depression seem to be about nothing in particular. The world just goes sour, infecting everything with its bile, without any direct focus. But even here, though the evaluation is indefinite, it still is about something—that something may harm one or in some way disappoint, even if one cannot specify the object. Further specification may simply await reflection, including deep reflection that may unmask what has long been repressed or forgotten.

Another element to review is the pleasant and painful feelings that are a part of emotions. As has been said, pleasure or pain is directed at evaluation. But some emotions have only a slight affective feel. In such cases, there is only a faint stirring in the heart and only mild disquiet of a pleasurable or painful sort. So, for example, a patient reflecting on his or her illness may have fears that all may not turn out well, even though he or she never feels any strong or noticeable tension when focusing on that thought. The thought has a clear negative value. But the person does not feel it with the sort of intensity characteristic of episodes of fear experienced before. Accordingly, a plausible account of the emotions must allow for variations in intensity of felt affect of this sort. There is no one strength that all emotions must have to qualify. Some are more intense, others are more subdued.

The felt affect of emotion may be a mixture of both pleasure and pain. According to Aristotle, anger involves felt pain at perceived injury but also the pleasure that comes from focusing on the prospect of revenge or reparation. In its simplest moments love can be bittersweet, infused with the giddy pleasure of vertiginous romance and the pain of vulnerability. A single emotion may thus have different "feels" in subtle mixtures. Even a "flash" of emotion may switch from one affective pole to another. Specific emotions may best be thought of as complex phenomena made up of an array of component emotions with felt affects that vary across them.

It is also important to examine the motivational aspect of emotion. In what sense is an emotion a desire to act? In what sense does emotion involve a reason or motive for action? Again, recognition of the diversity and variety of emotions is crucial here. Some emotions, such as calmness, confidence, and equanimity, do not in an obvious way involve a desire for action. In contrast, anger often involves a desire for revenge, just as envy seems to involve a desire to thwart others from having various goods. These sorts of desires can go on to constitute a motive or reason for full-fledged action, although often we train ourselves not to act and not to take all our impulses and desires as a motive for action. In some cases, we act out our emotions only in our minds, as when, out of anger, we slay the old bugger in our fantasy life. Here there are certainly impulses and urgings, but they are not taken up as reasons for action.

At yet other times we do externally act out our emotions, but in a way that still seems to fall short of that emotion constituting a full-fledged reason or motive for action. In anger, we sometimes act impulsively, slamming the door and storming out of the room. It is a venting, a way of letting out tension, not a strategy for sweet revenge. Defiling a photograph of an ex-lover comes closer to the mark, for here at least there is a symbolic aim. But still, these cases of anger do not really aim at effective revenge. They are more reactive than purposive. And yet, they seem to be voluntary. They are certainly not the involuntary responses of the viscera. In stroking a patient's brow or tousling a child's hair, emotion motivates the action. These two actions are likely done out of compassion and affection. But it seems strained, at least in some of the cases cited, to say that one does these actions in order to show compassion or affection—which is the common pattern a demand for reasons often takes. The gesture just expresses compassion or affection. The explanation stops there. It is not like drinking in order to slake thirst, where drinking strategically promotes that end (Hursthouse, 1991).

Still other cases of emotional motivation might seem more like acting on emotion than acting out of emotion, and in this sense might more fully constitute a case of taking up the emotion as a reason for action. In such cases, there is often control and strategy, as the result of either deliberation or habituation or both. In the case of annoyance or disappointment, the felt desire to respond may be viewed as an opportunity for acting constructively in praiseworthy or socially adaptive ways. One works out ways of dealing with one's emotions— ways, as an agent, of responding to one's more impulsive urgings. Here the idea of a practical syllogism, as a schematizing reason for action, makes good sense. Desires such as those for revenge join with beliefs about how best to act on those desires. The conclusion is a reasoned decision. "Best" may have a moral flavor, but not necessarily; it may simply refer to some notion of what is efficient or effective. One may act on one's anger in ways that deflect it, or in ways that sweeten and deepen it. The point now is that one responds with some deliberateness. One creates an agenda of what to do when in the grip of an emotion. One becomes a practical agent who can exercise a certain amount of choice about how to act on emotions, and how in general to stand toward them. When we stand well toward our emotions, Aristotle would claim, we express virtue.

In this section, we have seen that a thought-dependent account of emotion typically has three components: an appraisal, feelings of pleasure and pain, and a desire for action. We can now turn to further consideration about how we stand well toward our emotions. More specifically, how do we exercise agency in the shaping and cultivation of emotions? In what sense are we agents, not merely with regard to action but also with regard to the experiencing of emotions over a lifetime?

Control and responsibility

One way of posing this question is to ask, To what degree can we be held responsible for our emotions? In what sense are they within our control? Emotions are often sources of excuses for the actions they explain. Remarks such as "I couldn't help it, I was fuming with anger" and "Ignore his actions, he was overcome with passion" focus on emotions as largely involuntary responses. But emotions are a heterogeneous breed. Some occurrences or episodes of emotion, but by no means all, may be involuntary. Setting out to cultivate certain kinds of emotional dispositions is often something within our control, even if a given display falls short because of compulsion or weakness. Aristotle is helpful here. Both action and emotion, he holds, are subject to choice in that we choose to develop a state of character that stabilizes certain dispositions to action and emotion. In this sense, how we feel (and act) may be less a matter of choice at the moment than a product of choice over time. In the case of emotion, especially, there are few shortcuts. For unlike action, emotion does not seem to engage choice (or will) in each episode. At a given moment, we may simply not be able to will to feel a certain way even though we can will to act in a given way. Cultivation of appropriate ways of standing toward our emotions, that is, of dispositions or character states, is our best preparation for those moments.

Both upbringing and genetic inheritance—nurture and nature—have profound effects on how these dispositions are cultivated. But an individual's own contribution, which will vary from one stage to another, is no less important. Also, how a person develops the capacity to respond emotionally will depend in no small measure on the kind and quality of his or her most important relationships and the attachments that are formed.

But more specifically, how do character states involving emotions come to be habituated and controlled? How do we refine emotional states, and make them more discriminating and less impulsive? How do they come to be organized into stable states that can be relied upon for moral motivation?

Common parlance includes many expressions that presume emotions are "up to us" in various ways. We exhort ourselves and others by such phrases as "pull yourself together," "snap out of it," "put on a good face," "lighten up," "be cheerful," "think positive," "keep a stiff upper lip." In many of these cases, we are being implored to assume the semblance of an emotion so that it can "take hold" and rub off on our inner state. Practice as if you believe, and you will believe. As Ronald de Sousa puts it, "Earnest pretense is the royal road to sincere faith" (de Sousa, 1988, p. 324). Sometimes we "pretend" through behavioral changes—changes in facial expressions, body gestures, and vocalizations that evoke in us a changed mood. If we are fuming, relaxing our facial muscles, ungnarling our fingers, breathing deeply and slowly may put us in the frame of mind to see things in a calmer light. We try to inhibit the present emotion by inhibiting the physiognomic or physiological responses that typically accompany it. Conversely, we can fuel the flames of an emotion by allowing it bodily expression. To weep may intensify our grief, or simply bring us to acknowledge its presence. The James–Lange theory may be in the background here, with its notion of proprioceptive feedback from expression. Sometimes it is a matter of shaping an emotional state from outside in—trying on broader smiles as a way of trying to become more loving. By the same token, a newly felt affect may demand a new look, a concrete and stable realization for oneself and others to behold. Here the nudging works from inside out, though it is still the facial or gestural expression that is aimed at coaching the emotion. There are other sorts of actions one might take that are not a matter of body language or putting on a new face. One may try to talk oneself out of love, but discover that only when one changes locales do the old ways begin to lose their grip. Other times, it is more trial by fire: staying put and exposing oneself to what is painful in order to become inured. The process involves desensitization.

Sometimes changing one's mood may be more a matter of mental or perceptual strategy than facial or gestural alteration or action. It may be a matter of bringing oneself to focus on different objects and thoughts. One tries to see things under a new gestalt or to recompose the scene. Exhortation and persuasion play an important role here. A patient depressed by the possibility of relapse might be reminded of the favorable statistics and the steady progress he or she has made to date. Seeing things in a new light, with new emphases and stresses, helps to allay the fear. In a different vein, anger at a child may subside when one focuses less on minor annoyances and more on admirable traits. One may work on a more forgiving attitude in general by choosing to downplay others' perceived faults or foibles. In certain cases, experiencing emotions is a matter of giving inner assent—of allowing oneself to feel angry or giving the green light to a new interest or love. It is as if something grabs hold, and then it is one's turn to have some influence.

Mental training can of course follow a more methodical and introspective model. An individual can learn to take more careful note of the onset of certain emotions and the movement of mind from one perceived object of importance to another. He or she can label the kind of mood or emotional experience that is occurring and note how it disposes him or her to others, even when the emotional experience is only a transient flash. He or she can watch how emotions begin to accelerate to clingy attachments or dependencies, and try to disengage from those cravings. What is cultivated is a watchful mindfulness, an intensification of consciousness such that through awareness and knowledge, he or she comes to be more in charge (Nyanoponika, 1986).

There are other methods of effecting emotional change that depend upon "depth" psychology. In psychoanalysis, the recapitulation of patterns of emotional response through transference onto an analyst is intended to be a way of seeing at a detached level. The patient relives an emotional experience at the same time he or she watches and interprets it. This is the putative advantage of an empathic, clinical setting: A patient can come to see an emotional pattern in a detached way, free from judgment and accusation, and the crippling emotions that are often involved. In some cases, a patient tries to relieve the pain of present disabling emotions, such as anger, anxiety, or shame, by coming to see their roots in primitive conflicts and frustrations that may have long been repressed. The goal is not to remove the patient from the vulnerabilities of emotion but to make possible a way of experiencing emotions, including shame and anger, that is less crippling and self-destructive.

It is important to grasp the moral dimensions of psychoanalytic therapy, even though these are often not emphasized and are even thought to be at odds with the notion of the clinical hour as a haven from moral judgment. At the most basic level, therapy is a form of deep self-knowledge about emotions and their role in one's life. But it is not merely self-knowledge. On the Socratic model, it is self-knowledge that leads to character change. Depth psychology is meant to be a way of transforming the emotions. To the extent that virtuous character is a way of standing well toward the emotions, psychoanalytic therapy becomes one way of engaging in this process of emotional transformation. Therapy, in general, as a way of taking charge of one's self, including one's emotional self, has an important role in moral development.

More radical extirpation or removal of emotions

Because emotions are valued as modes of attention, motivation, communication, and knowledge, we tend to put up with their messiness while attempting their re-

form. But there are venerable traditions in which moderating through transformation and education is viewed as an inadequate therapy and an inadequate way of training moral character and agency. The Stoic view, which influenced later Kantian views and bears rough similarities to certain Eastern traditions, argues that the surges and delusions of emotions warrant their extirpation. Investment in objects and events we cannot control is the source of our suffering, and modification of our beliefs about these values is the source of our cure. In Stoic theory, according to Chrysippus and Zeno, as well as to such later Roman writers as Cicero and Seneca, virtue comes to be rooted in reason alone, for it is reason that is most appropriate to our nature and is under our true dominion. Since this line of argument has had a powerful influence on the history of moral thought, we would do well briefly to review it.

According to Stoic doctrine, emotion is judgment. It is a cognitive assent, an embracing or a commitment to a presentation, typically expressed linguistically, through a proposition. However, for the Stoics, emotions become by definition defective and in error. They are vicious and faulty states of character in need of extirpation if the equanimity of virtuous living is to prevail. Extirpation works on the assumption that emotions can be treated by radical changes of belief through persuasion and philosophical enlightenment. For if emotions are no more than false beliefs, then they should be treatable by a method that works essentially at the level of belief. Persuasion and argument should be able to grab hold of those beliefs entirely—without remainder. Accordingly, the Stoics propose philosophy as itself a spiritual therapy that cures the diseases or passions of the soul. Its practice involves a thoroughgoing denial of judgments to which voluntary but faulty assent was formerly given. Most fundamentally, what is required is to come to believe that what lies outside the self, and is external to one's true nature or reason, is not a proper object of importance. Attachments to wealth, fame, friends, health, noble birth, beauty, strength, and so on must be severed and these objects recognized as having no intrinsic value in morality or happiness. "The man who would fear losing any of these things cannot be happy. We want the happy man to be safe, impregnable, fenced and fortified, so that he is not just largely unafraid, but completely" (Cicero, 1945, V.40–41).

The attraction of the Stoic view rests in its powerful description of the anguish of the engaged emotional life. Many emotions (though not all) lead to attachment, but objects of attachment are never perfectly stable. Abandonment, separation, failure, and loss are the constant costs of love, effort, and friendship. The more tightly we cling to our investments, the more dependent we become upon what is uncontrolled and outside our own mastery. Self-reproach and self-persecution are often responses to lack of control. In our relations with others, the same clinginess of emotions can lead to overstepping what is appropriate, just as it can lead to exclusionary preferences and partialities. Provincialism can grow out of stubborn preference for what is familiar and comfortable according to class lines or other restrictive values.

This is a reasonable portrait of some moments of the life lived through emotion. Detachment and watchful awareness directed toward the emotions are important therapeutic stances in such a life. In addition, detachment and watchful awareness should be directed toward reason itself and its own tendencies toward egoism and imperious control. This is clearly at odds with Stoic practice and more in line with Eastern practices such as Buddhism. But it is difficult to see how a thoroughgoing rejection of the emotions can be compatible with what is a human life. Emotions, for all their selectivity, intensity, and stirring, enable us, through those very vulnerabilities, to attend, see, know, and experience in a way that pure cognition cannot. Some of that way of knowing and being known anguishes beyond words. Poetry and literature can only begin to express the reality. But even if at times unruled by reason's measure, emotion must not, on that account, be an outlawed feature of human life. Nor must it be an outlawed feature of morality. How we care for others and what we notice and reveal both depend greatly on the subtlety, fineness, and often deep truth of our emotional readings of the world.

Conclusion

From the above remarks, we can begin to see the importance of emotions in the moral life. Emotions are valued as modes of attention, communication, motivation, and self-knowledge. Each of these modes is a way we express moral character. As modes of attention, they help us discern moral salience in ways that would not be accessible to the cold eye of reason. Such discernment is a crucial preparatory moment for moral judgment and choice. Using them as modes of communication, we interact with others and express our engagement and involvement in ways that go well beyond affectless or bland action. As modes of motivation, emotions involve desires or impulses that can come to constitute more deliberate reasons for action. As modes of self-knowledge, present emotions can be used to relive and awaken past emotions that have been repressed. By looking squarely at such emotions, we begin to relieve the pain involved in repression and self-deception. In all these ways, emotions become a resource for moral agency and an important part of moral character. They help to constitute a notion of moral character in which the capacities for self-knowledge and candid engagement with others become crucial.

We can also begin to see that emotions will play an expanded role within bioethics and within the moral practices of health-care professionals. Emotional sensitivity will be important for discerning the complexity of situations, and for appreciating the competing needs and interests of various parties. A simple matter of noticing a patient's distress or displeasure, perhaps by attending to his or her facial expressions and bodily gestures, could figure importantly in assessing a case. But by the same token, it is important to communicate one's own emotions and not just record those of others. Conveying compassion to a patient can be a significant part of therapeutic treatment, and in general an important part of establishing a relationship in which medical counsel can be trusted and followed. Again, emotions figure in deliberation of choices. Compassion toward a patient can ground a reason for telling a patient the truth of his or her condition in a tone that respects the patient's fragile emotional state. The relevant choice a caretaker faces may not be whether to withhold the truth but how to tell the truth in a way that respects a patient's autonomy and feelings. It is here that a health-care provider's own feelings of compassion and sympathy can importantly ground the specific choices he or she makes. Finally, a health-care provider, as a morally responsible agent, needs to have ready access to his or her own emotions, so that emotions help rather than hinder effective care. Where, for example, fears and prejudice cloud more circumspect judgment, the health-care provider must recognize these as emotional impediments to delivering quality care. In general, a reflective stance toward one's own emotions becomes an important part of caring for others.

NANCY SHERMAN

Directly related to this entry are the entries LOVE; COMPASSION; CARE; VIRTUE AND CHARACTER; CONSCIENCE; ETHICS, *articles on* MORAL EPISTEMOLOGY, *and* NORMATIVE ETHICAL THEORIES; OBLIGATION AND SUPEREROGATION; ACTION; *and* VALUE AND VALUATION. *For a discussion of related ideas, see the entries* AUTONOMY; BENEFICENCE; FEMINISM; FRIENDSHIP; HUMAN NATURE; INTERPRETATION; JUSTICE; LITERATURE; METAPHOR AND ANALOGY; NARRATIVE; PAIN AND SUFFERING; PERSON; PSYCHOANALYSIS AND DYNAMIC THERAPIES; *and* TRAGEDY. *The topics in this entry will find application in the entries* FAMILY; MARRIAGE AND OTHER DOMESTIC PARTNERSHIPS; *and* MATERNAL–FETAL RELATIONSHIP.

Bibliography

ARISTOTLE. 1984. *The Complete Works of Aristotle: The Revised Oxford Translation.* Edited by Jonathan Barnes. Princeton, N.J.: Princeton University Press.

ARNOLD, MAGDA B. 1960. *Emotion and Personality*. 2 vols. New York: Columbia University Press.

BLUM, LAWRENCE A. 1980. *Friendship, Altruism and Morality*. Boston: Routledge & Kegan Paul.

CALHOUN, CHESHIRE, and SOLOMON, ROBERT C., eds. 1984. *Classic Readings in Philosophical Psychology*. New York: Oxford University Press.

CANNON, WALTER B. 1927. *Bodily Changes in Pain, Hunger, Fear and Rage: An Account of Researches into the Function of Emotional Excitement*. 2d ed. New York: Appleton.

CICERO, MARCUS ILLIUS. 1943. *Tusculan Disputations*. Translated by John Edward King. Rev. ed. Cambridge, Mass.: Harvard University Press.

DAVIS, WAYNE A. 1987. "The Varieties of Fear." *Philosophical Studies* 51, no. 2:287–310.

DE SOUSA, RONALD. 1987. *The Rationality of Emotion*. Cambridge, Mass.: MIT Press.

———. 1988. "Emotion and Self-Deception." In *Perspectives on Self-Deception*, pp. 324–344. Edited by Brian P. McLaughlin and Amélie Oksenberg Rorty. Berkeley: University of California Press.

FRIJDA, NICO H. 1986. *The Emotions*. Cambridge: At the University Press.

GORDON, ROBERT M. 1987. *The Structure of Emotions: Investigations in Cognitive Philosophy*. Cambridge: At the University Press.

GREENSPAN, PATRICIA S. 1988. *Emotions and Reasons: An Inquiry into Emotional Justification*. New York: Routledge.

GREENSPAN, STANLEY I. 1989. *The Development of the Ego: Implication for Personality Theory, Psychopathology, and the Psychotherapeutic Process*. Madison, Conn.: International Universities Press.

HERMAN, BARBARA. 1985. "The Practice of Moral Judgment." *Journal of Philosophy* 82, no. 8:414–436.

HURSTHOUSE, ROSALIND. 1991. "Arational Actions." *Journal of Philosophy* 88, no. 2:57–68.

JAMES, WILLIAM and GURNEY, EDMUND. 1884. "What Is an Emotion?" *Mind* 19:188–204.

NUSSBAUM, MARTHA C. 1987. "The Stoics on the Extirpation of the Passions." *Apeiron* 20:129–177.

———. 1990. *Love's Knowledge: Essays on Philosophy and Literature*. New York: Oxford University Press.

NYANOPONIKA, THERA. 1986. *The Vision of Dhamma*. London: Rider.

PARROT, W. GERROD. 1988. "The Role of Cognition in Emotional Experience." In *Recent Trends in Theoretical Psychology: Proceedings of the Second Biannual Conference of the International Society for Theoretical Psychology, April 20–27, 1987, Banff, Alberta, Canada*, pp. 327–337. Edited by William J. Baker, Leendert P. Mos, Hans V. Rappard, and Hendrikus J. Stam. New York: Springer-Verlag.

RORTY, AMÉLIE OKSENBERG, ed. 1980. *Explaining Emotions*. Berkeley: University of California Press.

SCHACTER, STANLEY, and SINGER, JEROME. 1962. "Cognitive, Social, and Physiological Determinants of Emotional State." *Psychological Review* 69, no. 5:379–399.

SHERMAN, NANCY. 1989. *The Fabric of Character: Aristotle's Theory of Virtue*, pp. 13–50, 118–200. New York: Oxford University Press.

———. 1990. "The Place of Emotions in Kantian Morality."

In *Identity, Character, and Morality: Essays in Moral Psychology*, pp. 149–170. Edited by Owen Flanagan and Amélie Oksenberg Rorty. Cambridge, Mass.: MIT Press.

WILLIAMS, BERNARD. 1973. "Morality and the Emotions." In his *Problems of the Self: Philosophical Papers, 1956–1972*, pp. 207–229. Edited by Bernard Williams. Cambridge: At the University Press.

ENDANGERED SPECIES AND BIODIVERSITY

Although projections vary, reliable estimates are that about 20 percent of Earth's species may be lost within a few decades, if present trends go unreversed. These losses will be about evenly distributed through major groups of plants and animals in both developed and developing nations, with special concerns over tropical forests (Ehrlich and Ehrlich, 1981; Wilson, 1988).

The United Nations at the 1992 Earth Summit in Rio de Janeiro launched the Convention on Biological Diversity, signed by 153 nations that are "concerned that biological diversity is being significantly reduced by certain human activities" and who are "conscious of the intrinsic value of biological diversity and of the ecological, genetic, social, economic, scientific, educational, cultural, recreational and aesthetic values of biological diversity," and "conscious also of the importance of biological diversity for evolution and for maintaining life sustaining systems of the biosphere" (United Nations, 1992, Preamble).

The U.S. Congress has lamented the lack of "adequate concern [for] and conservation [of]" species, and has sought to protect species through the Endangered Species Act, as well as through the Convention on International Trade in Endangered Species (U.S. Congress, 1973, Sec. 2(a) (1)). About five hundred species, subspecies, and varieties of fauna have been lost since 1600 in what is now the continental United States. The natural rate would have been about ten (Opler, 1976). In Hawaii, of sixty-eight species of birds unique to the islands, forty-one are extinct or virtually so. Half of the twenty-two hundred native plants are endangered or threatened. A candidate list for all states contains over two thousand taxa (species and significant subspecies and forms) considered to be endangered, threatened, or of concern, three categories used to rank degree of jeopardy (U.S. Fish and Wildlife Service, 1990). Human-caused extinctions threaten to approach and even exceed the catastrophic extinction rates of the geological past.

Even where species are not endangered, almost all inhabited lands are impoverished of their native fauna and flora, owing to development, loss of habitat, hunting, collection, trade in fauna and flora, toxic pollutants, introduction of exotic species, and other disturbances produced by humans. Sustainable biodiversity, the use of biotic resources so as to leave them unimpaired for future generations, is an increasing concern. Another concern is the loss of wetlands, permanently or periodically flooded or wet areas, which today in many areas are less than 10 percent of their original area. There is hardly a forest, grassland, or desert system in the developed world that is not impoverished of its once-native fauna and flora. Old-growth or pristine forests have been cut rapidly, as have tropical rain forests. Island ecosystems, often with species peculiar to that location and found nowhere else, are particularly at risk.

In the conservation of endangered species and biodiversity, bioethics in principle and in practice involves an unprecedented mix of science and conscience, especially since the species and ecosystem levels seldom figured in earlier ethical deliberations. A rationale for saving species that centers on their worth to persons is anthropocentric; a rationale that includes their intrinsic and ecosystemic values, in addition to or independently of persons, is naturalistic.

On an anthropocentric account, the duties involved are to persons; there are no duties to endangered species, though duties may concern species. Persons have a strong duty of nonmaleficence—not to harm others—and a weaker, though important, duty of beneficence—to help others. Many endangered species—which ones we may not now know—are expected to have agricultural, industrial, and medical benefits. They may be of scientific value, serve as indicators of ecosystem health, or provide genetic breeding stock for improvement of cultivated plants. Humans ought to conserve their global resources, a matter of prudence and enlightened self-interest in general, but a matter of moral concern when some persons threaten the benefits of these resources for other persons. Nonrenewable resources may have to be mined and consumed, but biological resources can be perennially renewable.

A developing concern between the species-rich, often underdeveloped countries and the developed countries, which are frequently responsible in part for environmental degradation, is who should bear the costs of saving species relative to benefits gained. Historically, native plant species, seeds, and germ plasm have been considered not to be owned by any nation. Developing nations are now claiming ownership by the country of origin, arguing that these resources cannot be used by those in other nations without negotiating compensation. At the same time, developing nations claim that their biological resources are being conserved for the benefit of other nations, and that the developed nations ought to pay developing nations not only for new con-

servation measures put into effect there but also for the lost opportunity costs of development in such conserved areas.

The Convention on Biological Diversity states: "States have sovereign rights over their own biological resources" (United Nations, 1992, Preamble) and continues, "Recognizing the sovereign rights of States over their natural resources, the authority to determine access to genetic resources rests with the national governments and is subject to national legislation" (Art. 15). Nevertheless, the problem of reconciling biodiversity as a common heritage of humankind with biodiversity as a national resource remains unresolved. States may control access to biodiversity, but this does not imply ownership. The United States refused to sign the Convention over questions of ownership, both of the wild biodiversity and of beneficial technology derived from it.

On the harm side, the loss of a few species may have no evident results now, but the loss of many species imperils the resilience and stability of the ecosystems on which humans depend. The danger increases with subtractions from the ecosystem, a slippery slope into serious troubles. Many species that have no direct value to humans are part of the biodiversity that keeps ecosystems healthy. On the benefits side again, there are less tangible benefits. Species that are too rare to play roles in ecosystems can have recreational and aesthetic value—even, for many persons, religious value. Species can be curiosities. They can be clues to understanding natural history. Destroying species is like tearing pages out of an unread book, written in a language humans hardly know how to read, about the place where they live. Humans need insight into the full text of natural history.

Such anthropic reasons are pragmatic and impressive. They are also moral, since persons are benefited or hurt. But can all duties concerning species be analyzed as duties to persons? Many endangered species have no resource value, nor are they particularly important for the other reasons given above. Are there worthless species? As curiosities and relics of the past, perhaps all species can be given an umbrella protection by saying that humans ought to preserve an environment adequate to match their capacity to wonder. Nature is a kind of wonderland. But this introduces the question of whether preserving resources for wonder is not better seen as preserving a remarkable natural history that has objective worth—an evolutionary process that has spontaneously assembled millions of species. A naturalistic account values species and speciation directly.

A further rationale is that humans of decent character will refrain from needless destruction of all kinds, including destruction of any species. Such a prohibition seems to depend, however, on some value in the species as such, for there need be no prohibition against destroying a valueless thing. The deeper problem with the anthropocentric rationale is that its justifications are less than fully moral, fundamentally exploitive, and self-serving, even if subtly so. This is not true intraspecifically among humans, when out of a sense of duty an individual defers to the values of other persons. But it is true interspecifically, since *Homo sapiens* treats all other species as resources. Ethics has always involved partners with entwined destinies. But ethics has never been very convincing when pleaded as enlightened self-interest (that one ought always to do what is in one's intelligent self-interest), including class self-interest, even though in practice altruistic ethics often needs to be reinforced by self-interest. To value all other species only in terms of human interests is rather like a nation's arguing all its foreign policy in terms of national self-interest. Neither seems to be completely moral.

It is safe to say that in the decades ahead, the quality of life will decline in proportion to the loss of biotic diversity, though it is often thought that one must sacrifice that diversity to improve human life. So there is a sense in which humans will not be losers if we save endangered species. Humans who protect endangered species will, if and when they change their value priorities, be better persons for their admiring respect for other forms of life. But this should not obscure the fact that humans can be short-term losers. Sometimes we do have to make genuine sacrifices, at least in terms of what we presently value, to preserve species. If, for instance, Americans wish to save the spotted owl, they will have to pay higher prices for timber and accept some job losses and relocations.

Dealing with a problem correctly requires an appropriate way of thinking about it. On the scale of evolutionary time, humans appear late and suddenly. Even later and more suddenly they increase the extinction rate dramatically. What is offensive in such conduct is not merely the loss of resources but also the maelstrom of killing and insensitivity to forms of life. What is required is not prudence but principled responsibility to the biospheric Earth.

There are problems at two levels when considering duties to species; one is about facts (a scientific issue), and one is about values (an ethical issue). First, what sort of biological entity is a species? Indeed, do species exist at all? No one doubts that individual organisms exist, but species can have a more controversial factual reality. Taxonomists regularly revise species designations and routinely put after a species the name of the "author" who, they say, "erected" the taxon. If a species is only a category or class, boundary lines may be arbitrarily drawn, and the species is nothing more than a convenient grouping of its members, an artifact of taxonomists. Some natural properties are used—reproductive structures, bones, teeth. But which properties are selected and where the lines are drawn vary with taxonomists.

If this approach is pressed, species can become a conventional concept, a mapping device, that is only theoretical, something like the lines of longitude and latitude. Sometimes endangered species designations have altered when taxonomists have decided to lump or split previous groupings. To whatever degree species are artifacts of taxonomists, duties to save them seem unconvincing. No one proposes duties to genera, families, orders, phyla; biologists concede that these do not exist in nature.

On a more realist account, a biological species is not just a class; it is a living historical form (Latin *species*, a natural kind), propagated in individual organisms, that flows dynamically over generations. Species are dynamic natural kinds, historically particular lineages. A species is a coherent, ongoing form of life expressed in organisms, encoded in gene flow, and shaped by the environment. In this sense, species are objectively there as living processes in the evolutionary ecosystem—found, not made, by taxonomists. The claim that there are specific forms of life historically maintained in their environments over time does not seem arbitrary but, rather, as certain as anything else we believe about the empirical world, even though at times scientists revise the theories and taxa with which they map these forms.

Species are not so much like lines of latitude and longitude as like mountains and rivers, phenomena objectively there to be mapped. The edges of such natural kinds will sometimes be fuzzy, to some extent discretionary. We can expect that one species will slide into another over evolutionary time. But it does not follow from the fact that speciation is sometimes in progress that species are merely made up, instead of found as evolutionary lines articulated into diverse forms, each with its more or less distinct integrity, breeding population, gene pool, and role in its ecosystem (Rojas, 1992).

Having recognized what a species is, the next question is why species ought to be protected. The naturalistic answer is that humans ought to respect these dynamic life forms preserved in historical lines, vital informational processes that persist genetically over millions of years, overleaping short-lived individuals. It is not *form* (species) as mere morphology, but the *formative* (speciating) process that humans ought to preserve, although the process cannot be preserved without its products. Endangered "species" is a convenient and realistic way of tagging this process, but protection can be interpreted (as the Endangered Species Act permits) in terms of subspecies, variety, or other taxa or categories that point out the diverse forms of life.

A consideration of species is both revealing and challenging because it offers a biologically based counterexample to the focus on individuals—typically sentient and usually persons—so characteristic in Western ethics. In an evolutionary ecosystem, it is not mere individuality that counts; the species is also significant because it is a dynamic life form maintained over time by an informed genetic flow. The individual represents (re-presents) a species in each new generation. It is a token of a type, and the type is more important than the token. A biological identity—a kind of value—is here defended. The dignity resides in the dynamic form; the individual inherits this, exemplifies it, and passes it on.

A species lacks moral agency, reflective self-awareness, sentience, and organic individuality. Some have been tempted to say that species-level processes cannot count morally. But each ongoing species defends a form of life, and these diverse species are, on the whole, good kinds. Such speciation has achieved all the planetary richness of life. All ethicists say that in *Homo sapiens* one species has appeared that not only exists but also ought to exist. A naturalistic ethic refuses to say this exclusively of a late-coming, highly developed form, and extends this duty more broadly to the other species—though not with equal intensity over them all, in view of varied levels of evolutionary achievement. Only the human species contains moral agents, but conscience ought not to be used to exempt every other form of life from consideration, with the resulting paradox that the sole moral species acts only in its collective self-interest toward all the rest.

Extinction shuts down the generative processes. The wrong that humans are doing, or allowing to happen through carelessness, is stopping the historical gene flow on which the vitality of life is based, and which, viewed at another level, is the same as the flow of natural kinds. Every extinction is an incremental decay in this stopping of life. Every extinction is a kind of superkilling. It kills forms (species) beyond individuals. It kills "essences" beyond "existences," the "soul" as well as the "body." It kills collectively, not just distributively. We do not merely lament the loss of potential human information; we lament the loss of biological information, present independently of instrumental human uses of it. A shutdown of the life stream on Earth is the most destructive event possible. Each human-caused extinction edges us further in this direction; already the rate may be catastrophic.

A consideration of species strains any ethic fixed on individual organisms, much less on sentience or persons. But the result can be biologically sounder, though it revises what was formerly thought to be logically permissible or ethically binding. When ethics is informed by this kind of biology, it is appropriate to attach duty dynamically to the specific form of life. The species line is the more fundamental living system, the whole of which individual organisms are the essential parts. The species, too, has its integrity, its individuality; and it is more important to protect this than to protect individual integrity. The appropriate survival unit is the appropriate level of moral concern.

A species is what it is inseparably from the environmental niche into which it fits. Particular species may not be essential in the sense that the ecosystem can survive the loss of individual species without adverse effect. But habitats are essential to species, and an endangered species typically means an endangered habitat. Species play lesser or greater roles in their habitats. This leads to an enlarged concern for the preservation of species in the system. It is not merely *what* they are, but *where* they are that one must value correctly. This limits the otherwise important role that zoos and botanical gardens can play in the conservation of species. They can provide research, a refuge for species, breeding programs, aid for public education, and so forth, but they cannot simulate the ongoing dynamism of gene flow over time under the selection pressures in a wild ecosystem. They amputate the species from its habitat.

Extinction is a quite natural event, but there are important theoretical and practical differences between natural and anthropogenic (human-caused) extinctions. Artificial extinction, caused by human encroachments, is radically different from natural extinction. Relevant differences make the two as morally distinct as death by natural causes is from murder. Though harmful to a species, extinction in nature is seldom an evil in the system. It is, rather, the key to tomorrow. The species is employed in, but abandoned to, the larger historical evolution of life. There are replacements. Such extinction is normal turnover in ongoing speciation.

Anthropogenic extinction differs from evolutionary extinction in that hundreds of thousands of species will perish because of culturally altered environments that are radically different from the spontaneous environments in which such species are naturally selected and in which they sometimes go extinct. In natural extinction, nature takes away life when it has become unfit in habitat, or when the habitat alters, and typically supplies other life in its place. Artificial extinction shuts down tomorrow, because it shuts down speciation. Natural extinction typically occurs with transformation, either of the extinct line or of related or competing lines. Artificial extinction is without issue. One opens doors; the other closes them. In artificial extinctions, humans generate and regenerate nothing; they only dead-end these lines.

Through evolutionary time nature has provided new species at a net higher rate than the extinction rate; hence the accumulated global diversity. There have been infrequent catastrophic extinction events, anomalies in the record, each succeeded by a recovery of previous diversity. Although natural events, these extinctions so deviate from the normal trends that many paleontologists look for causes external to the evolutionary ecosystem—supernovas or collisions with asteroids. Typically, however, the biological processes that characterize Earth are both prolific and have considerable powers of recovery after catastrophe. Uninterrupted by accident, or even interrupted so, they steadily increase the numbers of species.

An ethicist has to be circumspect. An argument may commit what logicians call the genetic fallacy in supposing that present value depends upon origins. Species judged today to have intrinsic value may have arisen anciently and anomalously from a valueless context, akin to the way in which life arose mysteriously from nonliving materials. But in an ecosystem, what a thing is differentiates poorly from the generating and sustaining matrix. The individual and the species have their value inevitably in the context of the forces that beget them. There is something awesome about an Earth that begins with zero and runs up toward five to ten million species in several billion years, setbacks notwithstanding.

Several billion years' worth of creative toil, several million species of teeming life, have been handed over to the care of the late-coming species in which mind has flowered and morals have emerged. On the humanistic account, such species ought to be saved for their benefits to humans. On the naturalistic account, the sole moral species has a duty to do something less self-interested than count all the products of an evolutionary ecosystem as human resources; rather, this host of species has a claim to care in its own right. There is something Newtonian, not yet Einsteinian, as well as something morally naive, about living in a reference frame where one species takes itself as absolute and values everything else relative to its utility.

In addition to the deeper ethical principles at issue in conservation of species, questions of pragmatic strategy arise. One strategy proposed when there are limited resources is to sort jeopardized species into three groups: those that are probably going extinct even if we try hard to save them, those that will probably survive without our help, and those that will probably go extinct unless we intervene. This strategy is called triage. An alternative, or complementary, strategy is to focus more on endangered ecosystems than on single species, an approach that may result both in more effective management and in more efficient use of resources. Another strategy discourages claiming biodiversity as a national resource while thinking of conservation in other nations in terms of foreign policy, for if biodiversity is the common heritage of humankind, all nations share duties to protect it.

HOLMES ROLSTON, III

Directly related to this entry are the entries ANIMAL WELFARE AND RIGHTS, *articles on* ETHICAL PERSPECTIVES ON THE TREATMENT AND STATUS OF ANIMALS, *and* WILDLIFE CONSERVATION AND MANAGEMENT; ENVIRONMENTAL ETHICS, *articles on* DEEP ECOLOGY, *and* LAND ETHIC; ENVIRONMENTAL POLICY AND LAW; *and* HAZARDOUS WASTES AND TOXIC SUBSTANCES. *For a discussion of related ideas, see the entries* ENVIRONMENT AND RELIGION; FUTURE GENERATIONS, OBLIGATIONS TO; *and* RIGHTS, *article on* RIGHTS IN BIOETHICS. *Other relevant material may be found under the entries* AGRICULTURE; BIOETHICS; CLIMATIC CHANGE; ENVIRONMENTAL ETHICS, *the* OVERVIEW, *and article on* ECOFEMINISM; EVOLUTION; NATIVE AMERICAN RELIGIONS; *and* SUSTAINABLE DEVELOPMENT. *See also the* APPENDIX (CODES, OATHS, AND DIRECTIVES RELATED TO BIOETHICS), Section VI: ETHICAL DIRECTIVES PERTAINING TO THE ENVIRONMENT.

Bibliography

EHRLICH, PAUL, and EHRLICH, ANNE. 1981. *Extinction: The Causes and Consequences of the Disappearance of Species.* New York: Random House.

NORTON, BRYAN G., ed. 1986. *The Preservation of Species: The Value of Biological Diversity.* Princeton, N.J.: Princeton University Press.

OPLER, PAUL A. 1976. "The Parade of Passing Species: A Survey of Extinctions in the U.S." *The Science Teacher* 43, no. 9:30–34.

ROJAS, MARTHA. 1992. "The Species Problem and Conservation: What Are We Protecting?" *Conservation Biology* 6, no. 2:170–178.

ROLSTON, HOLMES, III. 1985. "Duties to Endangered Species." *Bioscience* 35:718–726.

———. 1988. "Life in Jeopardy: Duties to Endangered Species." Chap. 4 in his *Environmental Ethics: Duties to and Values in the Natural World.* Philadelphia: Temple University Press.

UNITED NATIONS ENVIRONMENT PROGRAM. 1992. *Convention on Biological Diversity, 5 June 1992.*

UNITED STATES CONGRESS. 1973. Endangered Species Act of 1973. 87 Stat. 884. Public Law 93-205.

UNITED STATES FISH AND WILDLIFE SERVICE. 1990. List in 55 *Federal Register* no. 35 (February 21): 6184–6229.

WILSON, EDWARD O., ed. 1988. *Biodiversity.* Washington, D.C.: National Academy Press.

ENGLAND

See MEDICAL ETHICS, HISTORY OF, *section on* EUROPE, *subsection on* CONTEMPORARY PERIOD, *article on* UNITED KINGDOM.

ENVIRONMENTAL ETHICS

I. OVERVIEW

The magnitude and urgency of contemporary environmental problems—collectively known as the environmental crisis—form the mandate for environmental ethics: a reexamination of the human attitudes and values that influence individual behavior and government policy toward nature. The principal approaches to environmental ethics are "anthropocentrism," or the human-centered approach; "biocentrism," or the life-centered approach; and "ecocentrism," or the ecosystem-centered approach. Variously related to these main currents of environmental ethics are "ecofeminism" and "deep ecology." Moral "pluralism" in environmental ethics urges that we endorse all of these approaches and employ any one of them as circumstances necessitate.

Anthropocentrism

An anthropocentric environmental ethic grants moral standing exclusively to human beings and considers nonhuman natural entities and nature as a whole to be only a means for human ends. In one sense, any human outlook is necessarily anthropocentric, since we can apprehend the world only through our own senses and conceptual categories. Accordingly, some advocates of anthropocentric environmental ethics have tried to preempt further debate by arguing that a non-anthropocentric environmental ethic is therefore an oxymoron. But the question at issue is not, "Can we apprehend nature from a nonhuman point of view?" Of course we cannot. The question is, rather, "Should we extend moral consideration to nonhuman natural entities or nature as a whole?" And that question, of course, is entirely open.

In the mainstream of the Western cultural tradition, only human beings have been treated morally. Thus—at least for those working in that tradition—anthropocentrism is the most conservative approach to environmental ethics. Nevertheless, anthropocentric environmental ethicists have had to assume a more reactive than proactive posture and devote considerable effort to defending traditional Western moral philosophy against calls by bolder thinkers to widen the purview of ethics to encompass nonhuman natural entities and nature as a whole.

John Passmore and Kristin Shrader-Frechette were among the first to advocate a strictly anthropocentric approach to environmental ethics. Shrader-Frechette finds it "difficult to think of an action which would do irreparable harm to the environment or ecosystem, but which would not also threaten human well-being" (Shrader-Frechette, 1981, p. 17). Since many of the anthropocentric ethics in the Western canon censure behavior that threatens human well-being (utilitarianism, most directly), she argues that there is therefore no need to develop a newfangled non-anthropocentric environmental ethic.

Some of the damage that people have done to the environment certainly does threaten human well-being. Global warming and the depletion of the ozone layer are notorious examples. But it is easy to think of other instances of environmental vandalism that do not materially threaten human well-being. David Ehrenfeld asks us to contemplate the probable demise of the endangered Houston toad, a victim of urban sprawl, that "has no demonstrated or conjectural resource value to man" (Ehrenfeld, 1976, p. 650). But, as Ehrenfeld points out, the Houston toad is not unique in this respect. Thousands of other species in harm's way are nondescript "non-resources."

To morally censure the extinction of such species and other kinds of environmental destruction that do not materially threaten human well-being, must we abandon anthropocentrism? Amplifying the work of Mark Sagoff (1988) and Eugene C. Hargrove (1989), Bryan Norton (1987), the leading contemporary apologist for anthropocentric environmental ethics, argues that we should enlarge our conception of human well-being instead. In addition to goods (energy, foods, medicines, raw materials for manufacture) and services (crop pollination, oxygen replenishment, water purification), an undegraded natural environment contributes to human well-being in important psychological, spiritual, and scientific ways. Scenery unmarred by strip mines or clear cuts and undimmed by dirty air is important to human aesthetic satisfaction. Clean air and water, open spaces and green belts, complex and diverse landscapes, national parks and wilderness playgrounds are important human "amenities." Experiencing the solitude of wilderness and the otherness of wild things is an important aspect of human religious experience. Even if no one will be materially worse off after the extinction of "non-resource" species before science has a chance to discover and study them, important subject matter for pure, disinterested human knowledge will nevertheless have been irredeemably lost. Norton (1987) also suggests that contact with and care for the integrity of the natural environment can also be "transformative"; it can make better people of us.

Additionally, Norton argues that we should, as a matter of intergenerational justice, ensure that future human beings will be able to enjoy bountiful natural resources, a whole and functioning ecosystem, the full spectrum of environmental amenities, and the opportunity to partake of the psycho-spiritual experiences afforded by nature and to explore ecology and taxonomy intellectually. If we make our conception of human well-being both wide and long, he thinks that we may ground an adequate and effective environmental ethic without sailing off into the unfamiliar and treacherous waters of non-anthropocentrism.

The principal reason Norton offers for preferring an anthropocentic approach to environmental ethics is pragmatic. Anthropocentrism and non-anthropocentrism, he argues, support the same environmental policies. Norton (1991) calls this practical equivalence of anthropocentrism and non-anthropocentrism the "convergence hypothesis." Why then advocate non-anthropocentrism? Most people, including most environmentalists, he claims, accept the familiar and venerable idea that human beings are ends-in-themselves deserving moral standing. On the other hand, the suggestion that all living beings (and species and ecosystems) ought to be granted a similar status is unfamiliar and controversial. If we rest environmental ethics on as broad and firm a foundation as possible, we can best ensure its rapid implementation. Indeed, Norton suggests that the vigorous philosophical effort to develop non-anthropocentric approaches to environmental ethics has actually done the beleaguered environment a disservice. The environmental movement, as a result, has been divided over purely intellectual issues that have little if any practical import.

Norton's empirical claim that most people and even most environmentalists are anthropocentrists is supported only anecdotally. But opinion polls and the outcome of political contests suggest that most people probably have narrower allegiances—to self-interest, to institutional interests, to class interests, or to national interests—than to present and future collective or general human interests, very broadly construed. On the other hand, a growing minority of environmentalists seem to doubt the philosophical foundations of anthropocentrism. Are human beings really created in the image of God—the idea upon which anthropocentrism in Western religious ethics is founded? Are we uniquely self-conscious, rational, autonomous (some of the foundations of anthropocentrism in Western moral philosophy)? Must every being possess such characteristics

to qualify for moral treatment? One may agree with the convergence hypothesis—that practical environmental goals are as well served by anthropocentric as by non-anthropocentric environmental ethics—but disagree that anthropocentrism is philosophically defensible. Hence, the question of the philosophical merits—the truth, as it were, of anthropocentrism—remains open.

Norton's convergence hypothesis, furthermore, overlooks an important difference between the way anthropocentric and non-anthropocentric environmental ethics support the same environmental policies. Suppose, as non-anthropocentrists variously argue, that the environment is "intrinsically" as well as "instrumentally" valuable—that is, that the environment is valuable for its own sake as well as for all the benefits, tangible and intangible, that it provides human beings. Warwick Fox decisively argues that such a supposition would shift the burden of proof from those who would disinterestedly preserve the environment to those who would destroy it for personal gain:

> If the nonhuman world is only considered to be instrumentally valuable then people are permitted to use and otherwise interfere with it for whatever reasons they wish. . . . If anyone objects to such interference then, within this framework of reference, the onus is clearly on the person who objects to justify why it is *more useful* to humans to leave that aspect of the nonhuman world alone. If, however, the nonhuman world is considered intrinsically valuable then the onus shifts to the person who would want to interfere with it to justify why they should be allowed to do so; anyone who wants to interfere with any entity that is intrinsically valuable is morally obliged to be able to offer *sufficient justification* for their actions. (Fox, 1993, p. 101)

Norton, for example, might object to lumber companies cutting down redwood forests because the remaining redwood forests are of greater benefit to present and future human generations as amenities than as raw material for decks and hot tubs. But to preserve the remaining redwood forests, Norton would have to persuade a court to issue an injunction preventing lumber companies from harvesting redwoods, based on the assertion that the trees, while living, are more useful to human beings as psycho-spiritual and transformative resources than cut down and sawed up as consumptive resources. If, on the other hand, the trees were regarded as being intrinsically valuable, then a lumber company would have to make a case in court that the utility of redwood forests as raw material is so enormous as to justify their destruction. Thus, although Norton may be correct in claiming that a long and wide anthropocentric environmental ethic supports the same policies as non-anthropocentric environmental ethics—in the case at hand, the policy of preserving redwood forests—he cannot correctly claim that it would do so as forcefully.

Biocentrism

At first, theories of environmental ethics that morally enfranchise both individual living beings and natural wholes, such as species and ecosystems, were called "biocentric." Then, Paul W. Taylor (1986) commandeered the term to characterize his militantly individualistic theory of environmental ethics. Not only in deference to Taylor's influence and authority, but in deference to the literal sense of the term ("life-centered"), "biocentrism" in this discussion refers to theories of environmental ethics that morally enfranchise living beings only. Since species and ecosystems are not, per se, living beings, a biocentric theory would not accord them any moral standing.

Although animal welfare ethics and environmental ethics are by no means the same, biocentrism is launched from a platform provided by animal welfare ethics. Both attempt to extend our basic anthropocentric ethics—which, generally speaking, prohibit harming human "others" or violating their rights—to a more inclusive class of individuals: animal welfare ethics to various kinds of animals, biocentric environmental ethics to all living beings.

Peter Singer and Tom Regan, the principal architects of contemporary animal welfare ethics, exposed anthropocentric ethics to a dilemma. If the criterion for moral standing is pitched high enough to exclude all nonhuman beings, it will also exclude some human beings; but if it is pitched low enough to include all human beings, it will also include a large and diverse group of nonhuman animals.

An anthropocentrist may follow such philosophers as René Descartes and Immanuel Kant and proffer some highly esteemed and peculiarly human capacity—such as the capacity to reason, to speak, or to be a moral agent—as the qualification a being must possess to deserve ethical consideration. However, if practice is to be consistent with theory, anthropocentrism, so justified, should permit people who cannot reason or speak or who are not morally accountable for their behavior—human infants, the severely retarded, and the abjectly senile, for example—to be treated in the same ways that it permits animals to be treated: used as experimental subjects in painful biomedical research, hunted for sport, slaughtered and processed into dog food, and so on. To obviate these repugnant implications, Singer (1975) suggests that we follow Jeremy Bentham, the founder of utilitarian ethics, and settle upon sentience, the capacity to experience pleasure and pain, as a less hypocritical—and arguably a more relevant—qualification for moral consideration. That standard would secure the ethical standing of the so-called marginal cases, since irrational, unintelligent, or irresponsible people are all capable of experiencing pleasure and pain. But it would open membership in the moral community to all other sentient beings as well. If, as Bentham asserted, pleasure is good and pain is evil, and if, as Bentham also asserted, we should try to maximize the one and minimize the other irrespective of who experiences them, then animal pleasure and pain should count equally with human pleasure and pain in all our moral deliberations.

Singer vigorously advocates vegetarianism. Ironically, however, Singer's Benthamic animal welfare ethic is powerless to censure raising animals in comfort and slaughtering them painlessly to satisfy human dietary preferences. Indeed, one might even deduce from Singer's premises that people have a positive moral obligation to eat meat, provided that the animals bred for human consumption experience a greater balance of pleasure over pain during their short lives. For if everyone became a vegetarian, many fewer cows, pigs, chickens, and other domestic animals would be kept and thus many fewer animals would have the opportunity, for a brief time, to pursue happiness.

Recognizing these (and other) inadequacies of Singer's theory in relation to the moral problems of the treatment of animals, Tom Regan (1983) advocates a "rights approach." He argues that some individual animals have "inherent value" because they are, like ourselves, not only sentient but "subjects of a life"—beings that are self-conscious, experience desire and frustration, and that anticipate future states of consciousness—that from their point of view can be better or worse. Inherent value, in turn, may be the grounds for basic moral rights.

Neither Singer's nor Regan's prototype of animal welfare ethics will also serve as environmental ethics. For one thing, neither provides moral standing for plants and all the many animals that may be neither sentient nor, more restrictively still, subjects of a life—let alone for the atmosphere and oceans, species and ecosystems. Moreover, concern for animal welfare, on the one hand, and concern for the larger environment, on the other, often lead to contradictory indications in practice and policy. Examples follow: Advocates of animal liberation and rights frequently oppose the extermination of feral animals competing with native wildlife and degrading plant communities on the public ranges; they characteristically demand an end to hunting and trapping, whether environmentally benign or necessary; and they may prefer to let endangered plant species become extinct, rather than save them by killing sentient or subject-of-a-life animal pests.

On the other hand, animal welfare ethics and environmental ethics lead to convergent indications on other points of practice and policy. Both should resolutely oppose "factory farming": animal welfare ethics because of the enormous amount of animal suffering and killing involved; environmental ethics because of the enormous amount of water used and soil eroded in meat production. Both should staunchly support the preservation of wildlife habitat: animal welfare ethics because nature reserves provide habitat for sentient subjects; environmental ethics because many other forms of life, rare and endangered species, and the health and integrity of ecosystems are accommodated as well.

Despite the differences, animal welfare ethics may be regarded as "on the way to becoming" full-fledged environmental ethics, according to Regan (1982, p. 187). Animal welfare ethicists went the first leg of the philosophical journey by plausibly lowering the qualifying attribute for moral consideration. Albert Schweitzer (1989), Kenneth Goodpaster (1978), Robin Attfield (1983), and Paul Taylor (1986) variously suggest pitching it lower still—from being sentient to being alive.

Schweitzer, writing long before the efflorescence of contemporary animal welfare and environmental ethics literature, appears to ground his "reverence for life" ethic in the voluntarism of Arthur Schopenhauer:

> Just as in my own will-to-live there is a yearning for more life . . . so the same obtains in all the will-to-live around me, equally whether it can express itself to my comprehension or whether it remains unvoiced.
>
> Ethics consists in this, that I experience the necessity of practising the same reverence for life toward all will-to-live, as toward my own. (Schweitzer, 1989, pp. 32–33)

Contemporary biocentrism appears to have been inspired by Joel Feinberg's observations about the moral importance of interests and the range of entities to which interests may be attributed. The foundational role of the concept of "conation" (an often unconscious striving, reified by Schopenhauer as the "will-to-live") in Feinberg's characterization of interests unifies contemporary Anglo-American biocentric environmental ethics with Schweitzer's version. According to Feinberg:

> A mere thing, however valuable to others, has no good of its own . . . [because] mere things have no conative life: no conscious wishes, desires, and hopes; or urges or impulses; or unconscious drives, aims, and goals; or latent tendencies, directions of growth, and natural fulfillments. Interests must be compounded somehow out of conations; hence mere things have no interests, A fortiori, they have no interests to be protected by legal or moral rules. Without interests a creature can have no "good" of its own the achievement of which can be its due. Mere things are not loci of value in their own right, but rather their value consists entirely in their being objects of other beings' interests. (Feinberg, 1974, pp. 49–50)

The clear implication of this passage is that the "insuperable line," as Bentham called the boundary separating beings who qualify for moral consideration from those who do not, falls between living beings and nonliving things, not between sentient animals and insentient animals and plants. Why? Because even plants have "unconscious drives, aims, and goals; or latent tendencies, directions of growth, and natural fulfillments." Feinberg, nevertheless, goes on to deny that plants have interests of their own. His reasons for doing so, however, appear to be less clear and decisive than his derivation of interests from conations and his argument that beings who have interests deserve moral consideration.

Kenneth Goodpaster (1978) argues that all living beings, plants as well as animals, have interests. And he argues, appealing to Feinberg as an authority, that beings who have interests deserve "moral considerability"—a term that Goodpaster uses to indicate precisely the ethical status of moral patients (those on the receiving end of an action), as distinct from moral agents (those who commit an act). Goodpaster agrees with Singer that their sentience is a sufficient condition for extending moral considerability to animals, but he disagrees that it is a necessary one, because sentience evolved to serve something more fundamental—life: "Biologically, it appears that sentience is an adaptive characteristic of living organisms that provides them with a better capacity to anticipate, and so avoid, threats to life. . . . [T]he capacities to suffer and enjoy are ancillary to something more important, rather than tickets to considerability in their own right" (Goodpaster, 1978, p. 316).

Goodpaster's life-principle ethic is modest. All living beings are morally considerable, but all may not be of equal moral "significance." He leaves open the question of how much weight we should give to a plant's interests when they conflict with a sentient creature's or with our own. Paul Taylor (1987) has struck a much stronger and bolder stance and argued that all living beings are of equal "inherent worth."

Taylor bases a living being's inherent worth on the fact that it has a good of its own, quite independent of our anthropocentric instrumental valuation of it and quite independent of whether the organism is sentient or cares. Light, warmth, water, and rich soil are good for a sprig of poison ivy, though poison ivy may not be good for us. Unlike machines and other purposeful artifacts that we design to serve our own ends, organisms are ends-in-themselves. Most generally, they strive to reach a state of maturity and to reproduce. Therefore, just as we insist that others not interfere with our own striving and thriving, so, Taylor urges, expressly patterning his reasoning on Kant's, we should respect the striving and thriving of all other "teleological centers of life." Kant argued that we should respect, as individuals-in-themselves, all rational, autonomous beings equally.

And Taylor argues that we should respect equally all living beings because they too are ends-in-themselves.

Because biocentrism is concerned exclusively with biological individuals, not biological wholes, it is an approach to environmental ethics that seems at once so restrictive that it would be impossible to practice, and an approach that has scant relevance to the set of problems constituting the environmental crisis. How can we do anything at all, if, before we act, we are obliged to consider the interests of each and every living being that we might affect? Why should we feel compelled to do so for the sake of the environment? Environmental concern focuses primarily on the current spasm of abrupt massive species extinction and the loss of biodiversity generally, on rapid global warming and the erosion of stratospheric ozone, on soil erosion, water pollution, and the like; not on the welfare of individual grubs, bugs, and shrubs.

Schweitzer and Goodpaster frankly acknowledge the difficulty in practicing biocentrism. Schweitzer writes, "It remains a painful enigma how I am to live by the rule of reverence for life in a world ruled by creative will which is at the same time destructive will" (Schweitzer, 1989, p. 35). And Goodpaster writes:

> The clearest and most decisive refutation of the principle of respect for life is that one cannot *live* according to it, nor is there any indication in nature that we were intended to. We must eat, experiment to gain knowledge, protect ourselves from predation. . . . To take seriously the criterion being defended, all these things must be seen as somehow morally wrong. (Goodpaster, 1978, p. 310)

Both reasonably suggest that we can at least respect the interests of other living beings when they do not conflict with our own. According to Goodpaster, biocentrism is not suicidal. It requires only that we use living beings considerately and sensitively. Schweitzer thinks that biocentrism permits us to injure or destroy other forms of life, but only when doing so is necessary and unavoidable.

Taylor's egalitarianism renders the practicability problem of biocentrism virtually insurmountable (Wenz, 1988). Starting with any individual's right to self-defense, he rationalizes our annihilating disease organisms with medicines and goes on from there to defend our killing and eating other living beings to feed ourselves. But the satisfaction of any "nonbasic" human interest, according to Taylor, must be forgone if it violates the basic interests of another teleological center of life. So it would seem that strict adherence to biocentric egalitarianism would require one to live a life of sacrifice that would make a monk's life appear opulent.

Writing before the advent of the environmental crisis, Schweitzer was not intending to address its problems. He seems genuinely concerned, rather, with the welfare of individual living beings. Thus, it would be unfair and anachronistic to criticize his reverence-for-life ethic for being largely irrelevant to the set of problems constituting the environmental crisis. Taylor, on the other hand, represents his biocentric ethic as an environmental ethic. And he is clearly aware that contemporary environmental concerns focus on such things as species loss and ecosystem deterioration. But he remains antagonistic to the holistic environmental ethics crafted in response to such concerns. He prefers to think of the extinction of species and destruction of ecosystems in anthropocentric, rather than in biocentric or ecocentric terms. Goodpaster, on the other hand, invokes "concern felt by most person about 'the environment'" as a reason for trying to extend moral considerability to all living beings (Goodpaster, 1975, p. 309). He seems, moreover, to be aware that to actually reach the concern felt by most persons about the environment, biocentrism would have to "admit of application to . . . systems of entities heretofore unimagined as claimants on our moral attention (such as the biosystem itself)" (Goodpaster, 1975, p. 310). Having once mentioned systems of entities, however, Goodpaster lavishes all his attention on individual living beings and has nothing at all to say about how biocentrism might actually admit of application to species, ecosystems, and the biosphere as a whole.

Biocentrism may be not only irrelevant to actual environmental concerns, it could aggravate them. Biocentrism can lead its proponents to a revulsion toward nature—giving an ironic twist to Taylor's title, *Respect for Nature*—because nature seems as indifferent to the welfare of individual living beings as it is fecund. Schweitzer, for example, comments that

> the great struggle for survival by which nature is maintained is a strange contradiction within itself. Creatures live at the expense of other creatures. Nature permits the most horrible cruelties. . . . Nature looks beautiful and marvelous when you view it from the outside. But when you read its pages like a book, it is horrible. (Schweitzer, 1969, p. 120)

Ecocentrism

Though the term "ecocentrism" is a contradiction of the phrase "ecosystem-centered," ecocentrism would provide moral considerability for a spectrum of nonindividual environmental entities, including the biosphere as a totality, species, land, water, and air, as well as ecosystems. The various ecologically informed holistic environmental ethics that may appropriately be called ecocentric are less closely related, theoretically, than either the anthropocentric or biocentric families of environmental ethics.

Lawrence E. Johnson has attempted to generate an environmental ethic that reaches species and ecosystems by a further extension of the biocentric approach. He does this not by making the criterion for moral considerability more inclusive but by attributing interests to species and ecosystems. Extensively developing the line of thought that Feinberg (1974) tentatively and ambiguously initiated, Johnson concludes that we should "give *due* respect to all the interests of all beings that have interests, in proportion to their interests" (Johnson, 1991, p. 118). As this, his summary moral principle, suggests, Johnson follows Goodpaster in allowing that all interests are not equal and thus that all interested beings, though morally considerable, are not of equal moral significance. Johnson, however, provides no principle or method for hierarchically ordering interests and the beings who possess them; nor does he provide an ethical procedure for adjudicating conflicts of interest between people, animals, and plants, and, more difficult still, between all such individuals and environmental wholes.

In arguing that species have interests, Johnson exploits the fact that some biologists and philosophers of biology regard species not as classes of organisms but as spatially and temporally protracted individuals. To plausibly assign them interests, in other words, Johnson assimilates species to individual organisms. During the first quarter of the twentieth century, ecosystems (though then they were not so denominated) were represented in ecology as supraorganisms. Johnson adopts this characterization of ecosystems, as doing so allows him to attribute interests to ecosystems by assimilating them to individual organisms, just as in the case of species. Finally, Johnson points out that James Lovelock (1979) has suggested that the Earth as a whole is an integrated living being (named Gaia); if so, it (she) too may have interests and thus may be morally considerable. Adopting nonstandard, obsolete, or highly controversial scientific models of species, ecosystems, and the biosphere is the price Johnson pays to purchase moral considerability for these natural wholes. His attempt to add an ecocentric dimension to his essentially biocentric approach to environmental ethics is thus seriously compromised.

Holmes Rolston's ecocentric environmental ethic, like Johnson's, is launched from a biocentric platform. Rolston (1988) endorses the central tenet of biocentrism that each living being has a good of its own and that having a good of its own is the ground of a being's intrinsic value. And upon the existence of intrinsic value in nature he founds our duties to the natural world in all its aspects.

Rolston's biocentrism, in sharp contrast to Taylor's, is inegalitarian. Rolston finds more intrinsic value in beings that sense their own good, that feel hurt when harmed, than in those that lack consciousness. And Rolston finds the most intrinsic value of all in normal adult human beings because we are rational and fully self-conscious as well as conative and sentient.

Rolston avoids the scientifically suspect route that Johnson takes to enfranchise ethically such environmental wholes as species and ecosystems. Rolston argues instead that since the most basic telos of a teleological center of life is to be "good of its kind" and to reproduce its species, then its kind or species is its primary good. Species per se do not have a good of their own, but as the most basic good of beings that do have a good of their own, they too can be said to possess intrinsic value. The myriad natural kinds or species, however, evolved not in isolation but in a complex matrix of relationships—that is, in ecosystems. Thus, though not themselves teleological centers of life, either, some intrinsic value rubs off on ecosystems in Rolston's theory of environmental ethics. Rolston coins a special term, "systemic value," to characterize the value of ecosystems.

Systemic value does not seem to be entirely parallel, logically or conceptually speaking, to intrinsic value in Rolston's theory of environmental ethics. Rather, it seems that a necessary condition for the existence of the things that he believes do have intrinsic value—beings with a good of their own and the goods (their kinds or species) that such beings strive to actualize and perpetuate—is the existence of their natural contexts or matrices. Like the moon that shines by a borrowed light, systemic value seems to be a kind of reflected intrinsic value. Rolston finds a similar sort of derivative intrinsic value, "projective value," in elemental and organic evolutionary processes going all the way back to the Big Bang, since such processes eventually produced (or "projected") living beings with goods of their own.

Rolston's theory of environmental ethics hierarchically orders intrinsically valuable individuals in a familiar and conventional way. Human beings are at the pinnacle of the value hierarchy, followed by the higher animals, and so on, pretty much as in the Great Chain of Being envisioned by many Western philosophers of yore. Rolston is prepared to invoke his hierarchical arrangement of intrinsically valuable kinds of beings to resolve biocentric moral conundrums. For example, he expressly argues that it is morally permissible for people to kill and eat animals and for animals to kill and eat plants. Though such a hierarchical ordering of intrinsically valuable beings jibes with tradition and uncultivated common sense, it may not always jibe with, and hence may not adequately justify, our considered environmental priorities. Most environmentalists, faced with the hard choice of saving a sensitive, subjective dog or an unconscious, merely conative thousand-year-old redwood tree, would probably opt for the tree—and not only because redwoods are becoming rare. Pressed for good reasons for making this choice, Rolston might answer that an environmentally ethical agent is perfectly free, in reaching a decision to give priority to the redwood over the dog, to add to their intrinsic value the way standing redwoods are valued anthropocentrically and the way they serve the systemic value of ecosystems. The ethical agent can legitimately add the redwood's economic value to its systematic value, intrinsic value, aesthetic value, or religious value. How the intrinsic value of species and the systemic value of ecosystems fits into Rolston's value hierarchy is not entirely clear. Is a plant species more or less intrinsically valuable than a specimen of *Homo sapiens,* or than a specimen of *Ovis aries* (domestic sheep)?

According to Regan (1981) the very possibility of an environmental ethic turns on constructing a plausible theory of intrinsic (or "inherent") value in nature. He argues that anthropocentric environmental ethics are "management ethics," ethics for the "use" of the environment, not environmental ethics proper. Regan sets clear and stringent conditions for such value: first, it must be strictly objective, independent of any valuing consciousness; second, it must attend some property or set of properties that natural entities possess; and third, it must be normative, it must command ethical respect or moral considerability.

Rolston's basing a being's intrinsic value on its having a good of its own seems to meet the first two of these conditions, but possibly not the third. Before consciousness evolved, living beings had goods of their own; they could be harmed if not hurt; they had interests, whether they cared or not. The move, however, from the hardly disputable fact that living beings objectively possess goods of their own to the assertion that they have objective intrinsic value may turn on an ambiguity in the meaning of "good."

The word "good" has a teleological as well as a normative sense. All living beings have goods of their own in the teleological sense. They have, in other words, ends that were not imposed upon them—as the goods or ends of machines and other artifacts are—by beings other than themselves. But it is still possible to ask if such teleological goods generate normative goods. At this point in the argument, the smallpox and AIDS viruses are usually invoked as examples of organisms that have goods of their own in the teleological sense of the term, but organisms that one would be loath to say are good in the normative sense of the term.

However this particular conceptual issue may be resolved, another, moral general one casts a very large and dark shadow on Rolston's claim of finding objective intrinsic value in nature. While Rolston is very careful not to buck prevailing scientific opinion on the sort of reality possessed by species, ecosystems, and evolutionary processes, his argument that intrinsic value exists objectively in nature does buck more general assumption of modern science. From the modern scientific point of view, nature is value-free. Goodness and badness, like beauty and ugliness, are in the eye of the beholder. According to this entrenched dogma of modern science, there can be no valuees without valuers. Nothing under the sun—no rational self-conscious person, no sentient animal, no vegetable, no mineral—has value of any kind, either as a means or an end, unless it is valued by some valuing subject.

The crisp objective/subjective distinction in modern science, however, has been undermined by the Heisenberg Uncertainty Principle in quantum physics, as the observation of subatomic entities unavoidably affects their state of being. Therefore, the modern scientific worldview has become problematic. Seizing upon this circumstance, J. Baird Callicott (1989), among others, has broached a value theory for environmental ethics that is neither subjective nor objective. Just as experimental physicists actualize the potential of an electron to be at a particular place by observing it, so, Callicott suggests, the potential value of an entity, both instrumental and intrinsic, is actualized by a valuer appreciating it.

Although it may eventually give way to a postmodern scientific worldview, the modern scientific worldview continues to reign supreme. The "land ethic" sketched by Aldo Leopold (1949) has been the moral inspiration of the non-anthropocentric wing of the contemporary popular environmental movement, in part because Leopold respects the subjectivity of value required by the modern scientific world view without at the same time reducing nature to natural resources.

Callicott (1987) claims that Leopold's ecocentric environmental ethic may be traced to the eighteenth-century moral philosophy of David Hume and Adam Smith, who think that feelings lie at the foundations of value judgments. While feelings fall on the subjective side of the great subject/object divide, Hume and Smith also point out that our feelings may be altruistic or other-oriented as well as selfish. Hence we may value others for their own sakes, as ends-in-themselves. Further, Hume and Smith note that in addition to sympathy for others, respectively, we also experience a "public affection" and, accordingly, value the "interests of society even on their own account."

In *The Descent of Man,* Charles Darwin (1874) adopted the moral psychology of Hume and Smith and argued that the "moral sentiments" evolved among human beings in conjunction with the evolution of society, growing in compass and refinement along with the growth and refinement of human communities. He also developed the incipient holism of Hume and Smith, flatly stating that primeval ethical affections centered on the tribe not its individual members.

Leopold, building directly on Darwin's theory of the origin and evolution of ethics, points out that ecology represents human beings to be members not only of multiple human communities but also of the "biotic community." Hence, "the land ethic simply enlarges the boundaries of the community to include soils, waters, plants, and animals, or collectively: the land. . . . It implies respect for . . . fellow members and also respect for the community as such" (Leopold, 1949, p. 204).

Animal welfare ethicists and biocentrists claim that Leopold's ecocentrism is tantamount to "environmental fascism." Leopold wrote—and his exponents affirm—that "a thing is right when it tends to preserve the integrity, stability, and beauty of the biotic community [and] wrong when it tends otherwise (Leopold, 1949, pp. 224–225). If this is true, then not only would it be right deliberately to kill deer and burn bushes for the good of the biotic community, it would also be right to undertake draconian measures to reduce human overpopulation—the underlying cause, according to conventional environmental wisdom, of all environmental ills.

Providing for the possibility of moral consideration of wholes, however, does not necessarily disenfranchise individuals. The land ethic is holistic as well as (not instead of) individualistic, although in the case of the biotic community and its nonhuman members holistic concerns may eclipse individualistic ones. Nor does the land ethic replace or cancel previous socially generated human-oriented duties—to family and family members, to neighbors and neighborhood, to all human beings and humanity. Human social evolution consists of a series of additions rather than replacements. The moral sphere, growing in circumference with each stage of social development, does not expand like a balloon—leaving no trace of its previous boundaries. It adds, rather, new rings, new "accretions," as Leopold called each emergent social-ethical community. The discovery of the biotic community simply adds several new outer orbits of membership and attendant obligation. Our more intimate social bonds and their attendant obligations remain intact. Thus we may weigh and balance our more recently discovered duties to the biotic community and its members with our more venerable and insistent social obligations in ways that are entirely familiar, reasonable, and humane.

Ecofeminism

The term "ecofeminism" is a contraction of the phrase "ecological feminism," which may be understood as an analysis of environmental issues and concerns from a feminist point of view and, vice versa, as an enrichment and complication of feminism with insights drawn from ecology. Ecofeminism is both an approach to environmental ethics and an alternative feminism.

An axiom of ecofeminism is that, both historically and globally, men have dominated women and "man" has dominated nature. Further, many male-centered, culture-defining texts, such as the epics of Homer and Hesiod, the works of the ancient philosophers, and so forth, have associated women with nature and personified the Earth and nature generally as female (Griffin, 1978). The domination of women and nature appears to stem from a single source: patriarchy (literally, father-rule). Criticize and overcome patriarchy, the principal ideological force responsible for the domination of women, and one will at the same time have criticized and overcome the principal ideological force responsible for the degradation and destruction of nature. According to Marti Kheel, "for deep ecologists, it is the anthropocentric worldview that is foremost to blame. . . . Ecofeminists, on the other hand, argue that it is the androcentric worldview that deserves the primary blame" for the environmental crisis (Kheel, 1990, p. 129).

Some environmentalists suspect such an analysis to be a thinly disguised ploy to divert the energies of the environmental movement into the feminist movement. Deep ecologist Warwick Fox (1989), for example, argues that a feminist environmental ethic focused on abolishing patriarchy is too self-serving, simplistic, and facile to be taken seriously as a panacea for environmental ills. Other movements, he points out, can make, and have made, the same implausible claim: If we only abolish the ideology of racism, capitalism, imperialism, and so on, then we will usher in the millennium and all will be right with the world, natural as well as social.

Karen J. Warren (1990) does not follow Kheel and blame the domination and subordination of nature by "man" on the domination and subordination of women by men. Rather, she argues, both forms of "oppression" are "twin" expressions of hierarchically ordered "value dualisms" reinforced with a "logic of domination." Critiques of anthropocentrism and androcentrism are mutually illuminating and complementary. A person opposed to the one ought to be opposed to the other—because subordination, domination, and oppression are wrong, whether of women by men or of nature by "man." Environmentalists should also be feminists and feminists, environmentalists. Ecofeminism is the union of the two.

An ecofeminist approach seeks to correct an alleged "male bias" in environmental ethical theory—a selection of concepts and methodology that ignores, discounts, or denigrates women's issues, concerns, and experience. Alison M. Jagger has suggested that modern Western ethics, "Enlightenment moral theory," is thoroughly male-biased since it portrays moral agents as being "disembodied, asocial, autonomous, unified, rational, and essentially similar to all other" agents (Jagger, 1992, p. 367). In short, it abstracts, generalizes, universalizes. Intimately associated with this "Cartesian" moral psychology are such commonplaces of modern Western ethics as universal application of abstract principles and rules, impartiality, objectivity, rights, and the victory of synoptic and dispassionate reason over myopic and prejudicial feelings. Warren argues, accordingly, that "ecofeminism . . . involves a shift *from* a conception of ethics as primarily a matter of rights, rules, or principles predetermined and applied in specific cases to entities viewed as competitors in the contest of moral standing, *to* a conception of ethics as growing out of . . . defining relationships . . . and community" (Warren, 1990, pps. 141–142). She notes further that "ecofeminism makes a central place for [the more feminine, less male] values of care, friendship, trust, and appropriate reciprocity—values that presuppose that our relationships to others are central to our understanding of who we are" (Warren, 1990, p. 143).

It is surprising that ecofeminists have not warmly endorsed the Aldo Leopold land ethic, which grounds morality in such sentiments as love, sympathy, and fellow-feeling. The *locus classicus* for an environmental ethic growing out of "defining relationships" and "community" is found in Leopold's *A Sand County Almanac* (1949). Marti Kheel, however, castigates Leopold's land ethic, arguing that it epitomizes male bias. Leopold endorses hunting, historically a predominantly male activity, as a means not only of ecological management but also of experiencing our defining relationships with nature and cultivating a "love and respect" for "things natural, wild, and free."

Deep ecology

Just as there are Democrats (with a capital "D," members of one of the two major political parties in the United States) and democrats (with a lower-case "d," persons, irrespective of party affiliation, who agree with Winston Churchill that democracy is the worst form of government except for all the others), so there are Deep Ecologists (with a capital "D" and "E") and deep ecologists (with a lower-case "d" and "e"). The latter, such as Aldo Leopold, think that ecology has profound philosophical implications that it transforms our understanding of the world in which we live and what it means to be a human being. Deep Ecologists, on the other hand, endorse the eight-point "platform" of Deep Ecology that Arne Naess co-authored with George Sessions (Devall and Sessions, 1985). Moreover, they downplay the importance of environmental *ethics*, and advocate "Self-[with a capital 'S'] realization," instead. In short, deep ecology is a philosophical orientation; Deep Ecology is an ideology.

Ethics per se, Deep Ecologists allege, assumes "social atomism," a conception of each individual self as externally related to all other selves and to unselfconscious nature (Fox, 1990). Therefore, Deep Ecologists

suppose that an ethical act on the part of an atomic moral agent involves grudgingly considering the interests of other morally considerable beings equally and impartially with his or her own. But for people actually and consistently to behave ethically—as thus characterized—is as rare as it is noble. Therefore, even if environmental ethics could be broadly infused, environmental destruction and degradation would be little abated.

However, the metaphysical implications of ecology undermine the social atomism upon which ethics is supposedly premised. We human beings are internally, not externally, related to one another and to non-human natural entities and nature as a whole. "Others" cannot be cleanly and neatly distinguished from ourselves. Our relationships, natural as well as social, with "them" are mutually defining. We are embedded in communities, biotic as well as human. If we could only realize that the environing world is ultimately indistinguishable from ourselves, then we could enlist the powerful and reliable motive of self-interest in the effort to reverse environmental degradation and destruction (Naess, 1989).

The process of Deep Ecological Self-realization is experiential as well as intellectual. Through practice as well as study, we should cultivate a palpable sense of identification with the world. Nature-protecting behavior will flow from experiential identification with nature. Warwick Fox (1990) has suggested that Deep Ecology should actually be renamed "transpersonal ecology," since, as in transpersonal psychology, the goal of Self-(with a capital "S") realization involves self-(with a lower-case "s") transcendence.

Deep Ecology's suspicions about the efficacy of environmental ethics seems to be based upon a narrow characterization of ethics that excludes sentiment-based communitarian ethics like the Leopold land ethic and its ecofeminist correspondents. Ecofeminists have also sharply criticized Deep Ecology because it seems to "totalize" and "colonize" the "other" (Cheney 1987; Plumwood, 1993). With the important exception of Naess, Deep Ecologists either explicitly or implicitly claim that the integrated, systemic ecological world view is true and regard other ways of constructing nature and the relationship of people to nature to be false. A cornerstone of feminism is openness to the experience of women, experience that is quite varied. The experience of all or even of most women may not jibe well with Deep Ecological Self-realization. Hence the Deep Ecologists' often doctrinaire assertions about how the world is really and truly organized and how we *ought* to experience it are anathema to most ecofeminists.

Pluralism

The term "pluralism" in ethics characterizes two things equally well.

What we might call "social pluralism" is the view that diverse and often mutually inconsistent ethical outlooks should be respected and that there may not be any single moral principle or set of principles, however basic, that all moral agents must acknowledge. Human rights, for example, may be widely acknowledged in the West, but not in other parts of the world; hence, from a social pluralist's point of view, for Western governments to try to impose standards of human rights upon non-Western societies is inappropriate.

Personal pluralism, on the other hand, is the view that a single moral agent may endorse a variety of different moral principles, some of which may be mutually inconsistent, and employ one or another in different morally charged situations. For example, in resolving ethical questions about diet, a personal pluralist might apply Singer's principle that one should not cause sentient beings unnecessary suffering and therefore decide not to eat factory-farmed meat. In resolving ethical questions about abortion, he or she might apply Schweitzer's reverence-for-life principle and vote for an anti-abortion candidate for public office. And, in resolving ethical questions about species conservation, the same person might embrace Leopold's principle that one should preserve the integrity, stability, and beauty of the biotic community and help save an endemic plant species by shooting the feral goats or pigs threatening it.

Social pluralism appears attractive because it seems to imply inclusiveness and tolerance. In extremis, however, social pluralism is vulnerable to the same sort of criticism that ethical relativism, in extremis, has attracted. A social pluralist recognizes no universal ethical values or principles, he or she has no means of ethically challenging any one else's sincerely held moral beliefs. Further, if there are no universal ethical values or principles upon which to base agreement, then radical and intractable differences of moral outlook are irreconcilable. How then can they be resolved except by coercion?

Personal pluralism arose in environmental ethics because finding a single moral principle that could guide our actions in respect to other people, animals, plants, species, ecosystems, the atmosphere, the oceans, and the biosphere proved difficult (Stone, 1987). Moreover, our inherently rich and complicated moral lives may be distorted if reduced to a single master principle of action and we are frequently misled if we try rigorously to follow one (Brennan, 1992). According to Mary Midgley (1992), we may read the history of Western ethical theory, from Plato and Aristotle to Singer and Leopold, not as a series of formulations of and justifications for competing master principles of action, but as a series of illuminating insights into human ethical experience that can deepen our moral reflection and help us to make wise practical choices.

Proponents and critics alike of personal pluralism have noted some obvious problems. An agent who has a variety of principles and their theoretical justifications at the ready, with no faithful commitment to any of them required, may be tempted to choose the most convenient or self-serving. But all ethics, whether pluralistic or unitary, assume good will on the part of moral agents. A more difficult problem is how to select which principle to apply when more than one is relevant at some moment of decision, and when those that are relevant indicate different and incompatible courses of action. But to demand an algorithmic solution to this problem is to beg the question against personal pluralism.

Moral principles, however, do not exist in an intellectual vacuum (Callicott, 1990). They are often derived from and are always associated with a complex of supporting ideas—usually an ethical theory, which is in turn supported by a moral philosophy. In choosing to act upon a moral principle, a personal moral pluralist thus also endorses—whether consciously or not—the ethical theory and ultimately the moral philosophy supporting it. But the ethical theories and moral philosophies supporting such popular principles as the Christian golden rule, the Aristotelian golden mean, the Kantian categorical imperative, the utilitarian greatest-happiness principle, and so on, offer radically different visions of nature and human nature. Are we morally autonomous rational ends-in-ourselves for whom nature exists only as means, as Kant argues; or are we vessels of pleasure and pain, equal in this morally relevant respect to all other sentient animals, as Singer holds? How can we be both at once?

Communitarianism

A communitarian moral philosophy might provide a coherent sense of self and world without compromising the richness and complexity of our moral lives or attempting to derive all ethical actions from a single principle. Suppose that ethics, as Darwin argued, is correlative to society; that at this stage of human social evolution, we are simultaneously members of many communities or societies, including families, neighborhoods, towns or cities, nation-states, the global human community, the mixed human-domestic animal community, and the biotic community; and that a spectrum of different and not always compatible duties and obligations grow out of our various social relationships—for example, to provide our children with affection, to watch our neighbors' houses when they are away on vacation, to donate old clothes to the Salvation Army, to pay our taxes, to relieve world hunger, to boycott factory-farmed meat, and to help preserve biodiversity.

Right and wrong behavior in respect to family and family members, humanity and human beings, the biotic community and wild animals and plants, grows out of the very different kinds of communal relationships that we bear in these very different cases. Hence what is right in the context of one kind of community (feeding domestic animals, who are members of the "mixed community," for example) may be wrong in another (feeding wild animals, who are members of the biotic community). A multiplicity of community-generated principles guides our actions, but this multiplicity is united and coordinated by a single general understanding of how our various duties arise and to whom they apply. A coherent moral outlook like this certainly does not automatically determine the best course of action when one's multiple duties conflict. But one can at least hope rationally to decide, in circumstances of hard choice, which of several relevant but conflicting duties is the most pressing because they can all be expressed in comparable and commensurable terms.

J. BAIRD CALLICOTT

Directly related to this article are the other articles in this entry: DEEP ECOLOGY, LAND ETHIC, *and* ECOFEMINISM. *Also directly related are the entries* SUSTAINABLE DEVELOPMENT; ENVIRONMENTAL POLICY AND LAW; ENVIRONMENT AND RELIGION; ANIMAL WELFARE AND RIGHTS, *articles on* ETHICAL PERSPECTIVES ON THE TREATMENT AND STATUS OF ANIMALS, VEGETARIANISM, WILDLIFE CONSERVATION AND MANAGEMENT, *and* ANIMALS IN AGRICULTURE AND FACTORY FARMING; POPULATION ETHICS, *sections on* ELEMENTS OF POPULATIONS ETHICS, *and* NORMATIVE APPROACHES; ENVIRONMENTAL HEALTH; AGRICULTURE; FOOD POLICY; *and* HAZARDOUS WASTES AND TOXIC SUBSTANCES. *For a further discussion of ideas mentioned in this article, see the entries* BIOETHICS; FUTURE GENERATIONS, OBLIGATIONS TO; JUSTICE; NATURE; UTILITY; *and* VALUE AND VALUATION. *For a further discussion of topics mentioned in this article, see the entries* ANIMAL RESEARCH; GENETIC ENGINEERING, *article on* ANIMALS AND PLANTS; *and* TECHNOLOGY, *articles on* PHILOSOPHY OF TECHNOLOGY, *and* TECHNOLOGY ASSESSMENT. *Other relevant material may be found under the entries* INTERNATIONAL HEALTH; JAINISM; LAW AND BIOETHICS; NATIVE AMERICAN RELIGIONS; POPULATION ETHICS, *section on* RELIGIOUS TRADITIONS; POPULATION POLICIES; PUBLIC HEALTH, *article on* DETERMINANTS OF PUBLIC HEALTH; TAOISM; *and* VETERINARY ETHICS. *See also the* APPENDIX (CODES, OATHS, AND DIRECTIVES RELATED TO BIOETHICS), Section VI: ETHICAL DIRECTIVES PERTAINING TO THE ENVIRONMENT.

Bibliography

ATTFIELD, ROBIN. 1983. *The Ethics of Environmental Concern.* New York: Columbia University Press.

BRENNAN, ANDREW. 1992. "Moral Pluralism and the Environment." *Environmental Values* 1, no. 1:15–33.

CALLICOTT, J. BAIRD. 1987. *Companion to A Sand County Almanac: Interpretive and Critical Essays.* Madison: University of Wisconsin Press.

———. 1989. *In Defense of the Land Ethic: Essays in Environmental Philosophy.* Albany: State University of New York Press.

———. 1990. "The Case Against Moral Pluralism." *Environmental Ethics* 12, no. 2:99–124.

CHENEY, JIM. 1987. "Eco-Feminism and Deep Ecology." *Environmental Ethics* 9, no. 2:115–145.

DARWIN, CHARLES. 1874. *The Descent of Man and Selection in Relation to Sex.* London: John Murray.

DEVALL, BILL, and SESSIONS, GEORGE. 1985. *Deep Ecology: Living as if Nature Mattered.* Salt Lake City, Utah: G. M. Smith.

EHRENFELD, DAVID W. 1976. "The Conservation of Non-Resources." *American Scientist* 64, no. 6:648–656.

FEINBERG, JOEL. 1974. "The Rights of Animals and Unborn Generations." In *Philosophy and Environmental Crisis,* pp. 43–68. Edited by William T. Blackstone. Athens: University of Georgia Press.

FOX, WARWICK. 1989. "The Deep Ecology-Ecofeminism Debate and Its Parallels." *Environmental Ethics* 11, no. 1:5–25.

———. 1990. *Toward a Transpersonal Ecology: Developing New Foundations for Environmentalism.* Boston: Shambala.

———. 1993. "What Does the Recognition of Intrinsic Value Entail." *Trumpeter* 10, no. 3:101.

GOODPASTER, KENNETH E. 1978. "On Being Morally Considerable." *Journal of Philosophy* 75:308–325.

GRIFFIN, SUSAN. 1978. *Woman and Nature: The Roaring Inside Her.* New York: Harper & Row.

HARGROVE, EUGENE C. 1989. *Foundations of Environmental Ethics.* Englewood Cliffs, N.J.: Prentice Hall.

JAGGAR, ALISON M. 1992. "Feminist Ethics." In *Encyclopedia of Ethics,* pp. 361–370. Edited by Lawrence C. Becker and Charlotte B. Becker. New York: Garland Publishing.

JOHNSON, LAWRENCE E. 1991. *A Morally Deep World: An Essay on Moral Significance and Environmental Ethics.* Cambridge: At the University Press.

KHEEL, MARTI. 1990. "Ecofeminism and Deep Ecology: Reflections on Identity and Difference." In *Reweaving the World: The Emergence of Ecofeminism,* pp. 128–137. Edited by Irene Diamond and Gloria Feman Orenstein. San Francisco: Sierra Club Books.

LEOPOLD, ALDO. 1949. *A Sand County Almanac and Sketches Here and There.* New York: Oxford University Press.

LOVELOCK, JAMES. 1979. *Gaia: A New Look at Life on Earth.* Oxford: Oxford University Press.

MIDGLEY, MARY. 1992. "Beasts Versus the Biosphere." *Environmental Values* 1, no. 2:113–121.

NAESS, ARNE. 1989. *Ecology, Community and Lifestyle: Outline of an Ecosophy.* Translated by David Rothenberg. Cambridge: At the University Press.

NORTON, BRYAN G. 1987. *Why Preserve Natural Variety?* Princeton, N.J.: Princeton University Press.

———. 1991. *Toward Unity Among Environmentalists.* New York: Oxford University Press.

PASSMORE, JOHN. 1974. *Man's Responsibility for Nature: Ecological Problems and Western Traditions.* New York: Charles Scribner's Sons.

PLUMWOOD, VAL. 1993. *Feminism and the Mastery of Nature.* London: Routledge.

POTTER, VAN RENSSELAER. 1971. *Bioethics: Bridge to the Future.*

Prentice-Hall Biological Science Series. Edited by Carl P. Swanson. Englewood Cliffs, N.J.

REGAN, TOM. 1981. "The Nature and Possibility of an Environmental Ethic." *Environmental Ethics* 3, no. 1:19–34.

———. 1983. *The Case for Animal Rights*. Berkeley: University of California Press.

ROLSTON, HOLMES, III. 1988. *Environmental Ethics: Duties to and Values in the Natural World*. Philadelphia: Temple University Press.

SAGOFF, MARK. 1988. *The Economy of the Earth: Philosophy, Law, and the Environment*. Cambridge: At the University Press.

SCHWEITZER, ALBERT. 1969. [1966]. *Reverence for Life*. Translated by Reginald H. Fuller. New York: Harper & Row.

———. 1989. "The Ethic of Reverence for Life." Translated by John Naish. In *Animal Rights and Human Obligations*, 2d ed., pp. 32–37. Edited by Tom Regan and Peter Singer. Englewood Cliffs, N.J.: Prentice Hall.

SHRADER-FRECHETTE, KRISTEN S. 1981. *Environmental Ethics*. Pacific Grove, Calif.: Boxwood Press.

SINGER, PETER. 1975. *Animal Liberation: A New Ethics for Our Treatment of Animals*. New York: New York Review.

STONE, CHRISTOPHER D. 1987. *Earth and Other Ethics: The Case for Moral Pluralism*. New York: Harper & Row.

TAYLOR, PAUL W. 1986. *Respect for Nature: A Theory of Environmental Ethics*. Princeton, N.J.: Princeton University Press.

WARREN, KAREN J. 1990. "The Power and Promise of Ecofeminism." *Environmental Ethics* 12, no. 2:125–146.

WENZ, PETER S. 1988. *Environmental Justice*. Albany: State University of New York Press.

II. DEEP ECOLOGY

Deep ecology is a comprehensive worldview of humans in harmony with nature, an "ecosophy" ("ecowisdom") that responds to ecological crisis. It is also a movement to translate this worldview into radical societal reform. Supporters of the deep ecology movement contrast their position with "shallow" reform movements, holding that every living being has intrinsic or inherent value that gives it the right to flourish, independent of its usefulness for humans. All life is interrelated, and living things, humans included, depend on the support of others. For supporters of deep ecology, who tend to oppose the degradation of nature except to satisfy vital needs, the long-range integrity and health of the ecosystems of Earth are of fundamental ethical importance.

The ecological crisis has deep roots in misguided, anthropocentric attitudes about the dominion of humans on Earth. These exploitative, consumptive attitudes, according to the position of deep ecology, cannot be overcome without significant social changes, including changes in the lifestyles of those who live in the rich countries. Such changes can emerge only from a philosophical or religious basis that nurtures a sense of personal responsibility, not simply to persons living now but also to future human generations as well as fauna and flora. The current human population is already too large in many countries; further human population increases will lower the quality of life for both humans and nonhuman forms of life. A smaller human population is desirable and can be achieved by reduced birthrates over several centuries.

The position of the deep ecology movement can be illuminated by contrasting it with the position of so-called shallow ecology. The shallow position considers it unnecessary or even counterproductive to take up philosophical or religious questions to solve the ecological crisis. Its supporters argue that reforms of existing practices are needed, but reforms of basic principles are unnecessary. Those who advocate the shallow position do not find intrinsic value in nonhuman life forms, nor do they find the consumptive economic system problematic. Humans ought to exploit nature, though prudently. High standards of living are not objectionable, and can be raised even further by concentrating on investment in science and technology. Attempts should be made to bring less-developed nations up to this standard.

The deep ecology movement's historic forebears include Henry David Thoreau and John Muir. Aldo Leopold and Rachel Carson, also of the United States, are more recent pivotal figures. In 1962 Carson's book *Silent Spring* set off an ecological alarm. Starting with practical issues related to pesticides, Carson probed the philosophical assumptions underlying this attack on pests that stood in the way of human progress. In Europe such ecological concerns joined with the peace and social justice movements to create the first wave of the "green movement." Australians also became involved. In eastern Europe, ecologists were judged hostile to state-sponsored industrial development, and were banned. In the Third World, long-term ecological sustainability often had to take second place to short-term economic survival.

The deep ecology movement argues for ecological sustainability, human development that conserves the richness and diversity of life forms on Earth. This position, often said to be biocentric (centered on life) rather than anthropocentric (centered on human life only), includes what Leopold called "the land": the whole community of life on the landscape—rivers, mountains, canyons, forests, grasslands, and estuaries. Reforestation, for example, does not mean large tree plantations, producing timber and fiber for humans. Such plantations, which lack the biodiversity, complexity, health, and integrity of spontaneous natural ecosystems, are not genuine biological communities.

Those who advocate deep ecology and the more shallow reformers must learn to cooperate. Some strengths of each approach can be combined; some weakness of each, offset. The former sometimes become lost in utopian visions of a "green world"; the latter may be too absorbed in ad hoc, short-range solutions. The former can press for, and practice, more modest standards of living and support higher prices for nonvital products. Those who are less "deep" can be more pragmatic, willing to respond to what is currently politically realizable reform. Through such cooperation the supporters of both movements may help avoid crises likely to occur if ecologically responsible policies are forced too soon and too fast on populations that are not prepared for them. The deep premises of argumentation add to the utilitarian arguments, which are shallow in relation to philosophical and religious premises, needing more depth of analysis of the problem.

The discussions surrounding deep ecology have implications for the medical area of bioethics as well. "Rich life, simple means," an aphorism of the deep ecology movement, suggests for medical bioethics a strengthening of preventive medicine and a reduced reliance on technically advanced treatments, especially if they require large investments of resources and energy. Medical bioethics can learn from ecological bioethics the need for a moral vision that can reorder its priorities.

ARNE NAESS

Directly related to this article are the OVERVIEW *and other articles in this entry:* LAND ETHIC, *and* ECOFEMINISM. *Also directly related are the entries* ANIMAL WELFARE AND RIGHTS; ENDANGERED SPECIES AND BIODIVERSITY; FUTURE GENERATIONS, OBLIGATIONS TO; POPULATION ETHICS; POPULATION POLICIES; VALUE AND VALUATION; BIOETHICS; *and* RIGHTS, *article on* RIGHTS IN BIOETHICS. *For a discussion of related ideas, see the entries* ENVIRONMENT AND RELIGION; JAINISM; LIFE; NATIVE AMERICAN RELIGIONS; *and* NATURE. *Other relevant material may be found under the entries* ANIMAL RESEARCH; FOOD POLICY; HAZARDOUS WASTES AND TOXIC SUBSTANCES; VETERINARY ETHICS; *and* XENOGRAFTS.

Bibliography

DEVALL, BILL, and SESSIONS, GEORGE. 1985. *Deep Ecology.* Salt Lake City: Gibbs M. Smith.

FOX, WARWICK. 1990. *Towards a Transpersonal Ecology: Developing New Foundations.* Boston: Shambhala.

LEOPOLD, ALDO. 1949. *A Sand County Almanac: And Sketches Here and There.* New York: Oxford University Press.

NAESS, ARNE. 1989. *Ecology, Community and Lifestyle.* Translated and revised by David Rothenberg. Cambridge: At the University Press.

PEPPER, DAVID. 1984. *The Roots of Modern Environmentalism.* London: Croom Helm.

SNYDER, GARY. 1974. *Turtle Island.* New York: New Directions.

The Trumpeter: Canadian Journal of Ecosophy. P.O. Box 5853, Station B, Victoria, B.C., Canada V8R 6S8.

III. LAND ETHIC

After graduating from the Yale Forest School, Aldo Leopold (1887–1948) joined the U.S. Forest Service in 1909 and served for fifteen years. He resigned to pursue his interest in wildlife ecology and management; in 1933 he was named Professor of Game Management and inaugurated a doctoral program in the subject at the University of Wisconsin. Over the course of his multifaceted career, Leopold came to believe that human harmony with nature could be achieved only if, in addition to governmental management and regulation, private citizens (and property owners in particular) acquired a "land ethic." Such an ethic would make ecosystems and their parts direct beneficiaries of human morality: "A land ethic changes the role of Homo sapiens from conqueror of the land community to plain member and citizen of it. It implies respect for his fellow-members, and also respect for the community as such" (Leopold, 1949, p. 204).

Leopold is routinely called a modern American "prophet." *A Sand County Almanac,* his slender book of literary and philosophical essays, has become the "bible" of the contemporary environmental movement in the United States. And his land ethic is the environmental ethic of choice among most American environmentalists and conservationists, both amateur and professional. It rests upon secular scientific, not sectarian or supernatural religious, foundations. It is less rigidly doctrinaire than deep ecology's eight-point ethical "platform." Unlike ecofeminism, it focuses directly on the human–nature relationship, unrefracted by the alleged historical oppression of women by men. And, in sharp contrast to Western ethical paradigms, it has a holistic dimension that can ground environmental policy and law respecting endangered species and biodiversity.

In the foreword to *A Sand County Almanac,* Leopold (1949, pp. viii–ix) identifies the central eco-axiological theme: "That land is a community is the basic concept of ecology, but that land is to be loved and respected is an extension of ethics. That land yields a cultural harvest is a fact long known, but latterly often forgotten. These essays attempt to weld these three concepts." Its forty-odd essays document two decades of Leopold's reflective intimacy with the natural world; they span the North American continent from Mexico to Canada and from the Southwest to the Midwest; and they range in style from pastoral vignettes to didactic sermonettes. Part One introduces the basic ecological concept of a biotic community (or ecosystem) personally and experientially through artful seasonal sketches of Leopold's beloved 120 acres of Wisconsin River bottomland. The regional sketches of Part Two develop the community concept in ecology more intellectually, generally, and abstractly. The prescriptive essays of Part Three frankly and forcefully explore the ethical and aesthetic implications of the community concept in ecology. The final essay, "The Land Ethic," is the book's philosophical climax and consummation.

The biological paradigm

Though liberally educated, Leopold was primarily a student of biology, not of philosophy. Hence his thinking about ethics was influenced more by Charles Darwin than by Immanuel Kant and Jeremy Bentham, the fountainheads of the two major modern paradigms in ethics—deontology and utilitarianism, respectively—both of which proceed somewhat as follows: I demand that others dutifully respect my rights (in the deontological tradition) or take full account of how the consequences of their actions affect my interests (in the utilitarian). To defend that demand, I identify a characteristic I possess that arguably justifies my claim to moral rights or to consideration of my interests. According to Kant, it is rationality; according to Bentham, sentience. If I am to be consistent in my moral reasoning, then I must acknowledge that those who possess the same morally enfranchising property are entitled to the same regard from me as I demand of them. In short, the prevailing modern paradigms reach the moral standing of others starting from one's claim against others of one's own moral standing.

In sharp contrast, the biological paradigm, the paradigm in which Leopold works, starts with altruism, not egoism. Human beings are bonded to their fellows through sympathetic feelings and what David Hume and Adam Smith call the moral sentiments. The prehuman ancestors of *Homo sapiens*, whose survival and reproductive success greatly depended upon communal living, sympathy and the other moral sentiments, were strengthened by natural selection and ever more broadly cast through social expansion. With the evolution of the powers of speech and reflection, forms of behavior that accorded with altruistic and social sensibilities were articulated in codes of conduct. As clans merged into tribes, tribes into nations, and so on, such codes were extended to each emergent social whole and its members. Leopold (1949, p. 202) comments that "Ethics, so far studied only by philosophers, is actually a process in ecological evolution." And he alludes to natural selection when he defines an ethic from a biological point of view "as a limitation on freedom of action in the struggle for existence." That he built directly and self-consciously upon this scenario of ethics arising out of community membership, which Darwin had fully articulated in the *Descent of Man*, therefore, seems certain. To the evolutionary foundation laid by Darwin, Leopold adds crucial material from ecology—the "community concept," especially—in order to erect his land ethic.

In Leopold's (1949, p. 203) own words: "All ethics so far evolved rest upon a single premise: that the individual is a member of a community of interdependent parts." That is Darwin's account of the origin and development of ethics in a nutshell. Ecology "simply enlarges the boundaries of the community to include soils, waters, plants, and animals, or collectively: the land" (p. 204). When this novel ecological insight is added to Darwin's classic evolutionary account of ethics, Leopold believes that the land ethic follows. Therefore, he writes, "A thing is right when it tends to preserve the integrity, stability, and beauty of the biotic community. It is wrong when it tends otherwise" (pp. 224–225).

Most contemporary environmental philosophers follow another path to an environmental ethic. They work well within either deontology or utilitarianism, and proceed to extend ethical standing to nonhuman beings by lowering the qualifications for moral rights or for consideration of interests. "Animal liberation" follows from Bentham's first principles virtually without modification, if we acknowledge that most animals are sentient. And "animal rights" follows from Kant's first principles if we acknowledge that while few, if any, animals may be rational, many have sufficiently robust mental capacities to support claims of rights on their behalf. Of course, animal welfare ethics are not the same as environmental ethics. But, taking the next step along these parallel paths, other philosophers have variously argued that all things having interests, broadly construed, or goods of their own—that is, all living beings—deserve, if not rights, then either dutiful respect (according to the deontologists) or moral consideration (according to the utilitarians).

From facts to values

To most moral philosophers, the biological paradigm seems to be more a scientific theory about ethics than a normative theory of ethics. And Leopold's facile move from an ecological "is" (that *Homo sapiens* is a plain member and citizen of the biotic community) to an environmental "ought" (that *therefore* we ought to preserve the integrity, stability, and beauty of the biotic community) seems to commit the naturalistic fallacy—the fallacy (named by G. E. Moore, but attributed to David Hume) of deducing prescriptive statements about our moral obligations and ethical values exclusively from descriptive statements about the way things in fact are.

The two major modern philosophical paradigms, on the other hand, seem strained to the breaking point when one attempts to extend rights or entitlements to an entire species or to whole ecosystems, let alone "soils and waters." The Leopold land ethic, grounded in feeling and community, better accords with the holistic focus of contemporary environmental concerns. Environmentalists and conservationists are not too concerned about the well-being of individual grubs, bugs, and shrubs. They are concerned, rather, about what pollution is doing to Earth's atmosphere, fresh waters, and oceans; about what fragmentation is doing to ecosystems; about endangered species and biological diversity.

Contemporary environmental philosophers thus face a theoretical dilemma. Cling to the modern paradigm and remain out of phase with the more holistic character of genuine environmental concerns, or give up the intellectual security and familiarity of the modern paradigm, follow Leopold's application of the biological paradigm to environmental concerns, and work to solve the daunting problem of deriving environmental ethical values from facts about human moral psychology, evolutionary biology, and ecology.

Ironically, Hume himself may provide the key to bridging the lacuna between "is" and "ought," fact and value, and thus clear the way for environmental philosophers to embrace the biological paradigm of ethical theory that the land ethic extends. "Reason," our tool for determining facts, according to Hume (1960, p. 469), "in a strict and philosophical sense can have influence on conduct only after two ways: either when it excites a passion [such as the love and respect that Leopold identifies with ethics] by informing us of the existence of something which is a proper object of it; or when it discovers the connexion of causes and effects, so as to afford us means of exerting any passion." Dispassionate, descriptive evolutionary biology, a product of what Hume calls "reason," has discovered that human beings and other extant forms of life are descended from common ancestors. Evolutionary biology thus discloses a previously unknown fact: that we are literally kin to "our fellow-voyagers . . . in the odyssey of evolution," as Leopold (1949, p. 109) characterizes them. The discovery of the fact excites the passions—love and respect—we feel for our kin. Equally dispassionate and descriptive ecological biology has discovered the existence of the biotic community, of which we are no less members than of our various human communities. And the discovery of that fact excites the passions—loyalty and patriotism in this case—that we feel for the social wholes to which we belong. Thus may we move from facts to values, from "ises" to "oughts," in the land ethic, after a manner, according to Hume, that is so strict and philosophical.

J. BAIRD CALLICOTT

Directly related to this article are the OVERVIEW *and other articles in this entry:* DEEP ECOLOGY, *and* ECOFEMINISM. *Also directly related is the entry* ENDANGERED SPECIES AND BIODIVERSITY. *For a further discussion of topics mentioned in this article, see the entries* ANIMAL WELFARE AND RIGHTS; ENVIRONMENTAL HEALTH; ENVIRONMENTAL POLICY AND LAW; EVOLUTION; FEMINISM; LIFE; RIGHTS; UTILITY; *and* VIRTUE AND CHARACTER. *For a discussion of related ideas, see the entries* ANIMAL RESEARCH; AUTHORITY; BIOTECHNOLOGY; ENVIRONMENT AND RELIGION; EUGENICS; FAMILY; FETUS; FOOD POLICY; FUTURE GENERATIONS, OBLIGATIONS TO; GENETIC ENGINEERING, *article on* ANIMALS AND PLANTS; GENETICS AND ENVIRONMENT IN HUMAN HEALTH; HAZARDOUS WASTES AND TOXIC SUBSTANCES; NATIVE AMERICAN RELIGIONS; *and* SUSTAINABLE DEVELOPMENT.

Bibliography

CALLICOTT, J. BAIRD. 1987. *Companion to A Sand County Almanac: Interpretive and Critical Essays.* Madison: University of Wisconsin Press.

———. 1989. *In Defense of the Land Ethic: Essays in Environmental Philosophy.* Albany: State University of New York Press.

FLADER, SUSAN L. 1974. *Thinking like a Mountain: Aldo Leopold and the Evolution of an Ecological Attitude Toward Deer, Wolves, and Forests.* Columbia: University of Missouri Press.

HUME, DAVID. 1967. [1739]. *A Treatise of Human Nature.* Edited by L. A. Selby-Bigge. Oxford: At the Clarendon Press.

LEOPOLD, ALDO. 1933. *Game Management.* New York: Scribner's.

———. 1949. *A Sand County Almanac, and Sketches Here and There.* New York: Oxford University Press.

———. 1953. *Round River: From the Journals of Aldo Leopold.* Edited by Luna B. Leopold. New York: Oxford University Press.

———. 1991. *The River of the Mother of God and Other Essays by Aldo Leopold.* Edited by Susan L. Flader and J. Baird Callicott. Madison: University of Wisconsin Press.

MEINE, CURT. 1988. *Aldo Leopold: His Life and Work.* Madison: University of Wisconsin Press.

POTTER, VAN RENSSELAER. 1971. *Bioethics: Bridge to the Future.* Prentice-Hall Biological Science Series. Edited by Carl P. Swanson. Englewood Cliffs, N.J.: Prentice-Hall.

———. 1988. *Global Bioethics: Building on the Leopold Legacy.* East Lansing: Michigan State University Press.

IV. ECOFEMINISM

"Environmental ethics" refers to a wide range of normative positions, from traditional Western, utilitarian, rights- and justice-based ethics to nontraditional and non-Western ethics. Feminist concerns in environmental ethics span this broad range of positions. However, one feminist position is distinctive: ecological feminism.

"Ecofeminism" is expressly committed to making visible the nature and significance of connections between the treatment of women and the treatment of nonhuman nature, or "women–nature connections."

Ecofeminism claims that understanding women–nature connections is essential to any adequate feminism or environmental ethic.

Varieties of ecofeminism

Just as there is not one feminism, so there is not one ecofeminism. "Ecofeminism" is a term that refers collectively to various environmental perspectives with roots in different feminisms: liberal feminism, traditional Marxist feminism, radical feminism, socialist feminism, and Third World feminism. These roots give rise to different, sometimes competing, ecofeminist positions on the nature and resolution of contemporary environmental problems. What makes them ecofeminist is their explicit focus on "women–nature connections."

Consider the range of women–nature connections explored by ecofeminism (see Warren, 1993). Some ecofeminists discuss *historical* connections: for example, the role rationalism has played in Western philosophy and science in justifying the inferiorization of what is associated with female nature (Plumwood, 1991). They argue that to the extent that either the concept or the ascription of reason historically has been applied only to (some) human males, rationalism has been male-gender-biased. The male-gender bias arises from the mistaken assumption that women (and, typically, men of color) are incapable of the impartial, objective, abstract, universalizable reason by virtue of which rational men are both distinguished from and superior to nonrational "nature" (see Warren, 1989). These ecofeminists argue that philosophical conceptions of the human self, ethics, and culture that rely on Western historical conceptions of reason will thereby be male-gender biased (see Warren, 1989).

Some ecofeminists discuss *conceptual* women–nature connections: for example, the way women and nature have been conceived as inferior to male-identified reason and culture. Many ecofeminists claim that the twin dominations of women and nature grow out of and reflect oppressive ways of thinking. These are characterized at least minimally by value dualisms (mind/body, reason/emotion, man/woman, culture/nature), value hierarchies (assigning greater status, value, or prestige to what is "up" in "up–down" hierarchies), conceptions of power as power of "ups" over "downs," conceptions of privilege that systematically favor the "ups," and a logic of domination (the assumption that superiority justifies subordination) (Warren, 1990). On this view, oppressive patriarchal conceptual frameworks sanction behaviors that maintain the domination of women and nature.

Ecofeminists discuss *empirical* women–nature connections: for example, Third World women as managers of domestic households, primary gatherers of food and fuel (typically wood), and collectors and distributors of water (see Warren, 1992). These women must walk further for fuel and suffer greater exposure to contaminated water; in Western countries, poor women, men, and children of color face increased health risks associated with radioactive waste and hazardous waste incinerators (Warren, 1992; Commission for Racial Justice, 1987). Development policies and practices do not recognize the distinct gendered division of labor experienced by Third World women, or the gender, race, and class factors that contribute, even if unconsciously and unintentionally, to the subordination of women and people of color cross-culturally.

Ecofeminists also are interested in *epistemological* and *methodological* women–nature connections. At least 80 percent of the farmers in Africa are women, and women grow about 60 percent of the world's food (see Warren, 1992). A study in Sierra Leone showed that while local men could name an average of eight products of nearby bushes and trees, local women could identify thirty-one (see Warren, 1992). Such data suggest that women often have "indigenous technical knowledge" (ITK) or farming and forestry due to their gendered-role responsibilities in these areas (see Warren, 1992). Consequently, issues of epistemology and methodology in framing environmental ethics, policy, and decision making must ask not simply "What is known?" but "Who has the requisite knowledge and expertise?" According to ecofeminism, what women know as household managers of domestic economies, forests, and agriculture is important to the development of environmental ethics.

Symbolic associations between women and nature appear in art, literature, religion, and philosophy. This is especially evident in the sexist, naturist, and ageist language used to describe women and nonhuman nature. Women are characterized frequently as cows, sows, foxes, chicks, bitches, beavers, dogs, mares, dingbats, old bats, pussycats, birdbrains, harebrains, and serpents. They are pets, dolls, babes, childlike, whiny, "domesticated creatures." Nature is raped, mastered, mined, penetrated, domesticated, manipulated, conquered, and controlled by "the man of science." Virgin timber is felled, cut down; land that lies fallow is barren and useless (not "impotent" and "sterile"). (Similarly, men of color are disproportionately described in the subordinating language of the "downs" as animals, studs, dicks, weasels, wolves, unruly and dangerous "savages" driven by "animalistic instinct"; as docile, wimpy, sissy, childish, or childlike, and not fully rational; as childlike, simple [nonrational] "slaves" who need the guidance and protection of the paternalistic master, the "up.") In a patriarchal context, whatever is woman-, animal-, nature-, or even child-identified has historically been inferior ("down") to what is man-, male-, human-, adult-, or culture-identified. Thus language that feminizes animals and nature, animalizes and naturalizes women (and some men), or describes women, nature, and some men as domesticated pets or children, serves to reflect and reinforce their inferiorization.

What, then, about the allegedly positive connotations of "Mother Nature" or "Mother Earth"? Ecofeminists disagree about whether such female-gendered language truly liberates or merely reinforces harmful gender stereotypes (see Roach, 1991). However, all ecofeminists agree that within a patriarchal context, where gendered language has functioned historically to elevate that which is associated with men and male culture, its uncritical continued use in the prefeminist present is problematic.

Finally, there are *political* ("*praxis*") women–nature connections. The term "ecofeminism," coined by Françoise d'Eaubonne in 1974, has always referred to grass-roots activism by local women interested in bringing together feminist environmental concerns. Whether it is the Chipko women in India, who are attempting to save trees from commercial fiber producers by hugging the trees, or Native American women, who are protesting the dumping of uranium mining residue on their lands, or the thousands of women from various cultures who gathered to develop strategies for policy and community organizing to combat water pollution, soil erosion, deforestation, and desertification at planning sessions, conferences, and seminars in conjunction with the Earth Summit in Rio de Janeiro in 1992, ecofeminism has always been grounded in grass-roots, local community political organizing (see Lahar, 1991). Properly understood, then, ecofeminist ethics is largely a theoretical response to such grass-roots political concerns involving women's lives globally.

Contributions of ecofeminism

One might summarize ecofeminism's contributions to environmental ethics as threefold: First, ecofeminism challenges male-gender bias wherever and whenever it occurs. Second, ecofeminism offers a corrective lens to oppressive male-gender bias by self-consciously attempting to develop environmental analyses and positions that are not male-gender-biased. Third, ecofeminism offers a transformative perspective in environmental ethics, one that builds on but goes beyond both current feminisms that do not have an adequate environmental component and current environmental ethics that does not have a distinctly feminist component.

Ecofeminism does this by using a feminist lens to form different insights about women–nature connections; those environmental ethics that do not include (eco)feminist insights are viewed by ecofeminists as either antifeminist or nonfeminist. Nonfeminist environmental ethics, unlike antifeminist environmental ethics, is not ipso facto male-biased; its claims and con-

clusions might be quite compatible with and supportive of ecofeminist ethics. What an explicitly (eco)feminist environmental ethic does is overtly challenge androcentric (male-centered) bias in the way environmental ethics is conceived and practiced. For this reason, many ecofeminists criticize other environmental ethics (e.g., deep ecology, traditional Western ethics) for either their androcentric bias or their inattention (however inadvertent or unintentional) to important historical and empirical data about women–nature connections. Ecofeminists insist that within the intellectual traditions of the past few thousand years and at least of Western cultures, anthropocentrism (human-centeredness) has functioned historically as androcentrism (male-centeredness); failure to see this results in a gender blindness that is harmful to the framing of an environmental ethic or philosophy.

Similarly, ecofeminist conceptual concerns challenge the dominant notions of reason, knowledge, and objectivity, as well as the dominant notions of the human self that underlie them, that have been a mainstay of Western philosophical and environmental ethics. What ecofeminists seek is the development of different, nonoppressive notions of each that change or expand how the notions of reason, knowledge, objectivity, and the human self are conceived. In this vein, many ecofeminists challenge the extension of rights by animal-rights ethics to some nonhuman animals because those rights are based on historically intact, unrevised (and hence problematic) notions of the human self as moral agent (claimant, right holder, interest carrier) separate from and superior to lower plant and inorganic life.

Ecofeminist epistemological concerns raise related issues about the underrepresentation of women's voices in environmental ethics. Such concerns prompt ecofeminists to criticize, for example, land ethicists for their apparent lack of interest in gender issues. Ecofeminist concerns about gendered language and nature symbols (e.g., Mother Earth) challenge those environmental ethics (e.g., stewardship ethics) that uncritically adopt or perpetuate gender-exclusive or gender-problematic language and symbol systems (see Adams, 1993). Ecofeminist political concerns about unequal distributions of power and privilege in maintaining systems of domination (e.g., domination over women and nature) challenge any environmental ethic uncorrected by feminism to pay more attention to power and privilege in discussions of environmental ethics (see Warren, 1990).

Concluding remarks

In conclusion, ecofeminist ethics is a self-consciously feminist-biased ethics insofar as it consciously, intentionally, and explicitly adopts a feminist perspective as the organizing lens through which any environmental ethic is constructed. Despite their critics (see Biehl, 1991; Fox, 1989), ecofeminists argue that in contemporary patriarchal society, the label "feminist" *does* add something important to the nature and description of environmental ethics; in a nonpatriarchal context, "feminist" concerns may well be unnecessary and the label "feminist" may drop away (see Warren, 1990). But for now, ecofeminist ethics reminds us that in contemporary patriarchal culture, there are important ways in which the domination of nature and the domination of women are linked, and that failure to acknowledge such links perpetuates the mistaken view that feminism does not contribute anything significant to any environmental or biocentric ethics.

KAREN J. WARREN

Directly related to this article are the OVERVIEW *and other articles in this entry:* DEEP ECOLOGY, *and* LAND ETHIC. *Also directly related is the entry* FEMINISM. *For a further discussion of topics mentioned in this article, see the entries* ENDANGERED SPECIES AND BIODIVERSITY; ENVIRONMENTAL HEALTH; ENVIRONMENTAL POLICY AND LAW; ETHICS, *especially the article on* NORMATIVE ETHICAL THEORIES; HAZARDOUS WASTES AND TOXIC SUBSTANCES; RACE AND RACISM; SCIENCE, PHILOSOPHY OF; SEXISM; *and* SUSTAINABLE DEVELOPMENT. *For a discussion of related ideas, see the entries* AUTHORITY; ENVIRONMENT AND RELIGION; FOOD POLICY; FUTURE GENERATIONS, OBLIGATIONS TO; GENETICS AND ENVIRONMENT IN HUMAN HEALTH; HUMAN NATURE; *and* NATURE. *Other relevant material may be found under the entries* ABUSE, INTERPERSONAL, *article on* ABUSE BETWEEN DOMESTIC PARTNERS; ANIMAL WELFARE AND RIGHTS, *especially the articles on* ETHICAL PERSPECTIVES ON THE TREATMENT AND STATUS OF ANIMALS, *and* HUNTING; *and* CARE, *article on* CONTEMPORARY ETHICS OF CARE.

Bibliography

ADAMS, CAROL J., ed. 1993. *Ecofeminism and the Sacred.* New York: Continuum.

BIEHL, JANET. 1991. *Rethinking Ecofeminist Politics.* Boston: South End.

CALDECOTT, LEONIE, and LELAND, STEPHANIE, eds. 1983. *Reclaim the Earth: Women Speak out for Life on Earth.* London: Women's Press.

CHENEY, JIM. 1987. "Eco-Feminism and Deep Ecology." *Environmental Ethics* 9, no. 2:115–145.

D'EAUBONNE, FRANÇOISE. 1974. *Le feminisme ou la mort.* Paris: Pierre Horay.

DIAMOND, IRENE, and ORENSTEIN, GLORIA FEMAN, eds. 1990. *Reweaving the World: The Emergence of Ecofeminism.* San Francisco: Sierra Club.

FOX, WARWICK. 1989. "The Deep Ecology-Ecofeminism Debate and Its Parallels." *Environmental Ethics* 11, no. 1: 5–25.

GRAY, ELIZABETH DODSON. 1981. *Green Paradise Lost.* Wellesley, Mass.: Roundtable.

GRIFFIN, SUSAN. 1978. *Woman and Nature: The Roaring Inside Her.* New York: Harper & Row.

Heresies #13. 1981. H, no. 1. Special issue, "Feminism and Ecology."

KING, YNESTRA. 1981. "Feminism and the Revolt of Nature." *Heresies #13* 4, no. 1:12–16.

LAHAR, STEPHANIE. 1991. "Ecofeminist Theory and Grassroots Politics." *Hypatia* 6, no. 1:28–45.

MERCHANT, CAROLYN. 1980. *The Death of Nature: Women, Ecology, and the Scientific Revolution.* New York: Harper & Row.

———, ed. 1984. *Environmental Review* 8, no. 1. Special issue, "Women and Environmental History."

———. 1989. *Ecological Revolutions: Nature, Gender, and Science in New England.* Chapel Hill: University of North Carolina Press.

MURPHY, PATRICK, ed. 1988. *Studies in the Humanities* 15, no. 2. Special issue, "Feminism, Ecology, and the Future of the Humanities."

New Catalyst. 1987–1988. "Woman/Earth Speaking: Feminism and Ecology." No. 10.

ORTNER, SHERRY. 1974. "Is Female to Male as Nature is to Culture?" In *Woman, Culture, and Society,* pp. 67–87. Edited by Michelle Zimbalist Rosaldo. Stanford, Calif.: Stanford University Press.

PLANT, JUDITH, ed. 1989. *Healing the Wounds: The Promise of Ecofeminism.* Philadelphia: New Society.

PLUMWOOD, VAL. 1991. "Nature, Self, and Gender: Feminism, Environmental Philosophy, and the Critique of Rationalism." *Hypatia* 6, no. 1:3–27.

ROACH, CATHERINE. 1991. "Loving Your Mother: On the Woman-Nature Relationship." *Hypatia* 6, no. 1:46–59.

RUETHER, ROSEMARY RADFORD. 1975. *New Woman/New Earth: Sexist Ideologies and Human Liberation.* New York: Seabury.

SALLEH, ARIEL KAY. 1984. "Deeper Than Deep Ecology: The Eco-Feminist Connection." *Environmental Ethics* 6, no. 4:339–345.

SHIVA, VANDANA. 1988. *Staying Alive: Women, Ecology and Development.* London: Zed.

STURGEON, NOËL, ed. *Ecofeminist Newsletter.*

UNITED CHURCH OF CHRIST. COMMISSION FOR RACIAL JUSTICE. 1987. *Toxic Wastes and Race in the United States: A National Report on the Racial and Socio-Economic Characteristics of Communities with Hazardous Waste Sites.* New York: Author.

WARREN, KAREN J. 1987. "Feminism and Ecology: Making Connections." *Environmental Ethics* 9, no. 1:3–20.

———. 1989. "Male-Gender Bias and Western Conceptions of Reason and Rationality: A Literature Overview. *Newsletter on Philosophy and Feminism* 88, no. 2:48–53. Special Issue, "Gender, Reason, and Rationality."

———. 1990. "The Power and the Promise of Ecological Feminism." *Environmental Ethics* 12, no. 2:125–146.

———. 1992. "Taking Empirical Data Seriously: An Ecofeminist Philosophical Perspective." In *Human Values and the Environment: Conference Proceedings*, pp. 32–40. Madison: Wisconsin Academy of Sciences, Arts and Letters.

———. 1993. Introduction to ecofeminism section. In *Environmental Philosophy: From Animal Rights to Radical Ecology*. Edited by Michael E. Zimmerman, J. Baird Callicott, John Clark, George Sessions, and Karen J. Warren. Englewood Cliffs, N.J.: Prentice-Hall.

WARREN, KAREN J., ed. 1991. *Hypatia* 6, no. 1. Special issue, "Ecological Feminism."

woman of power: a magazine of feminism, spirituality, and politics. 1991. 9 (Spring). Special issue, "nature."

ENVIRONMENTAL HAZARDS

See ENVIRONMENTAL HEALTH; *and* HAZARDOUS WASTES AND TOXIC SUBSTANCES.

ENVIRONMENTAL HEALTH

Since the publication of *Silent Spring* (Carson, 1962), the world has been alerted to the mortal danger of exposing human beings, and other life forms, to many products and by-products of industrial civilization. Although the negative effects of environmental pollution on human health cannot be denied, the existence and magnitude of danger associated with particular processes and products often remain controversial.

One reason for controversy is that powerful interests typically have a stake in denying that their industries create health hazards. Nuclear industries, for example, deny that low-level radiation causes cancer. Cigarette manufacturers deny a causal link between passive smoking and cancer. Manufacturers of asbestos products take a similar stand about asbestos, as do manufacturers of agricultural pesticides about their products.

A second reason for continued controversy is that because causal connections in these matters are inherently difficult to establish, affected industries can hire competent scientists to dispute claims of environmental hazards to human health. In general, three types of evidence can be used to show that an environmental constituent is a health hazard. But none can establish connections beyond dispute (Luoma, 1988).

First, nonhuman animals can be exposed to a suspected health hazard and the effect observed. This cannot prove anything conclusively about human exposure, because human beings are biochemically different from nonhuman animals. Also, in order to establish a connection in short order and at minimal cost, nonhuman animals are often exposed to much larger doses than the expected exposure of human beings. The effect of a small dose on human beings cannot be established conclusively from evidence about the effects of much larger doses on nonhuman animals.

A second method of investigation is to expose human beings in controlled settings to mild doses, over short periods of time, to materials suspected of causing serious health problems when exposure in terms of amount or duration is considerably greater. The problem here is that some substances may be so toxic that it would violate human rights deliberately to expose people even to mild doses. Other substances, on the contrary, may have no deleterious effect at low levels of exposure but be toxic at higher levels of concentration or over longer periods of time. In such cases, public-health hazards may be underestimated or missed entirely.

Third, epidemiological studies test a substance by comparing the rate of disease in one population with that in another, attempting to correlate differences between the populations' rates of disease with differences in their rates of exposure. However, it is difficult to establish in this way a connection between a given suspected toxin and illness or death, because under normal conditions people are exposed all the time to many suspected toxins, of various strengths, for varying periods of time. It is difficult to isolate the effect of any one substance. Also, the effect of exposure, if there is any, is often a weak one. In a small population, for example, few additional cancers can be expected from exposure to low-level radiation. What is more, the cancer effect is long delayed and spread out in the population over a forty-year period, making it difficult to detect at any given time (Stewart, 1993). Finally, radiation exposure and cancer exist in the human population in any case, so it is impossible to know of any given cancer that it is caused by exposure to low-level radiation, or that the low-level radiation in question is related, for example, to a nuclear industry (Stewart, 1993).

Basically the same considerations apply where the issue is the effect of exposure to passive smoking, to asbestos, or to agricultural pesticides. Thus, controversies can be maintained for decades. Nevertheless, the weight of evidence supports the claim that the exposure of human beings to chemicals and other products and by-products of industrial civilization is often harmful to human health.

Evidence of environmental ill health

"Since the 1950s, age-standardized cancer incidence rates in the U.S. have increased by 43.5 percent" (Epstein, 1992, p. 233). Death from cancer has increased similarly. The best attempts to isolate the causes of cancer result in the conclusion that environmental factors account for between 60 and 90 percent of cancers. The rest are attributable to inherited tendencies or internal biochemical malfunctions (Epstein, 1987).

Studies have shown cancer effects from doses of radiation previously thought to be safe. In one study, a distinguishing fact about children who died of cancer before age ten, compared both with those who died of other causes and with those who survived to age ten, is that the cancer victims' mothers had, on average, twice as many X-rays while pregnant (Stewart, 1993). Another study showed a strong statistical association between a father's exposure to external radiation while working at a nuclear-waste reprocessing plant before the child was conceived, and the child's contracting leukemia (Gardner, 1991).

Radiation is not the only risk factor for cancer. Pesticides and other chemicals are implicated as well. A study showed that the mammary adipose tissue of women with breast cancer contained significantly more residues of chemicals associated with pesticides than did the tissue of women with nonmalignant tumors (Falck et al., 1992). Another study revealed that among white male scientists and engineers, those who were members of the American Chemical Society had significantly more deaths from leukemia and lymphatic cancer (Arnetz et al., 1991). A study of men from Iowa and Minnesota showed a link between elevated environmental chemical exposures, which resulted from living near a factory, and two types of cancer, non-Hodgkin's lymphoma and leukemia (Linos et al., 1991). Non-Hodgkin's lymphoma has been linked to the use of certain pesticides as well (Weber, 1992). Foundry workers in Denmark who were exposed to elevated levels of silica dust, metallic fumes, carbon monoxide, and several organic chemicals had markedly elevated rates of lung cancer (Sherson et al., 1991). Occupational exposure to asbestos is currently considered responsible for 8,000 to 12,000 deaths each year in the United States (Rauber, 1991).

Typically, years intervene between exposure to environmental contaminants and an associated cancer or death. But in some cases the connection between environmental pollution and human mortality is more direct. In Utah, for example, on days when air pollution (particulates and sulfur dioxide) was bad, almost 20 percent more people died than on days when air pollution was minimal; the increased deaths were mostly among those with respiratory and cardiovascular diseases (Pope et al., 1992). The "U.S. Office of Technology Assessment estimates that the current mix of sulphates and particulates in ambient air may cause 50,000 premature deaths in the United States each year—about 2 percent of annual mortality" (Postel, 1986, p. 34). Toxic chemicals released into the air in 1988 were estimated by the Environmental Protection Agency (EPA) to cause "up to 3,000 cases of fatal cancer yearly as well as birth de-

fects, lung disease, nervous system disorders, liver damage, and other health problems . . ." (U.S. General Accounting Office, 1991a, p. 8). When all types and sources of air pollution are considered, the American Lung Association puts the toll at 120,000 premature deaths per year (French, 1991).

There is increasing evidence that indoor air is often a health hazard. Radon in homes is believed to be a leading cause of cancer. The "sick building" syndrome is also a concern. It is the phenomenon of buildings inducing illnesses of various sorts in a large percentage of the people who spend considerable time in them. For example, chemicals in materials used to build and decorate the Dupage County Judicial and Office Facility in Wheaton, Illinois, were considered responsible for a variety of employee illnesses. As a result, a nearly new building was temporarily evacuated.

High levels of sulfur dioxide in the air, which, when combined with water, forms sulfuric acid, the main constituent of acid rain, can harm people when they drink water. Acidic water may dissolve lead and other metals. These metals enter the body when people drink the water. Late in 1992, the EPA estimated that 20 percent of the nation's municipal water supplies contained unacceptably high levels of lead due to the water's acidity. Lead has been linked to brain damage in children (Luoma, 1988).

Environmental racism

Risks of environmentally influenced diseases and deaths are not distributed evenly across the population. Geographically, the people at greatest risk are those who live near sources of industrial pollution, such as factories and certain types of mines, and those who live near deposits of toxic waste. For example, it seems that a geometrically increasing cancer rate for people in some communities on Cape Cod, Massachusetts, is due to toxic deposits from nearby Otis Air Force Base (Hallowell, 1991). By 1989, 14,401 sites of toxic contamination had been noted on 1,579 military installations around the United States (Renner, 1991). When cancer rates are plotted on a map of the United States, the areas showing the highest rates are areas of industrial production, such as Chicago, Detroit, northern New Jersey, and the lower Mississippi valley.

There is also a disparate impact on minority communities, referred to as "environmental racism." "Three out of every five African Americans and Hispanics live in a neighborhood with a hazardous waste site, and . . . race is the most significant variable in differentiating communities with such sites from the communities without them" (Steinhart, 1991, p. 18). "Probably the greatest concentration of hazardous-waste sites in the United States is on the predominantly black and Hispanic

South Side of Chicago" (Russell, 1989, p. 25). With 28 million pounds of toxics poured into the area annually, the EPA estimates the risk of cancer to be 100 to 1000 times normal (Lavelle, 1992). According to the federal Centers for Disease Control, "lead poisoning endangers the health of nearly 8 million inner-city, largely black and Hispanic children" all over the United States (Russell, 1989, p. 24). Rural minority groups suffer disproportionately as well: "2 million tons of radioactive uranium tailings have been dumped on Native American lands; reproductive organ cancer among Navajo teenagers is seventeen times the national average" (Russell, 1989, p. 24).

Environmental racism is international as well as domestic. Toxic waste from industrial countries has been deposited in Africa (Jacobson, 1989). Some corporations in industrial countries continue to manufacture pesticides considered too dangerous for use in their own countries. These are sold to farmers in the Third World, resulting in 10,000 to 40,000 poisonings a year (Postel, 1988). The Bhopal tragedy, in which 2,000 people were poisoned by a chemical that leaked from a factory in India, highlights the fact that environmental safeguards in the Third World are sometimes inadequate. The company that owns the factory is based in the United States, where it maintains higher standards of safety at its factories.

The legal structure

According to traditional Anglo-American jurisprudence, when one person injures another, the injured party can sue in court to recover damages. The legal rules governing such proceedings constitute the law of torts. This body of law is largely unhelpful, however, where injuries are due to most forms of environmental pollution. It is too difficult to prove that a harm—a case of cancer, for example—resulted from a particular emission of radioactivity or a certain dumping of toxic waste. Also, it would be inefficient for each injured party to sue individually, as was done traditionally, when the activity in question is alleged to affect many people, possibly thousands. Finally, tort actions can take place only after harm is done, and it is preferable to use the law to avoid harms where possible. So the major role of government in the area of environmental health is through the regulatory process.

In 1970, the National Environmental Policy Act was signed into law to "fulfill the responsibilities of each generation as trustee of the environment for succeeding generations." The EPA, established soon thereafter, required most federally funded projects to be accompanied by an Environmental Impact Statement so that any deleterious effects of such projects could be recognized and possibly ameliorated. Subsequent legislation has given the EPA authority, for example, to regulate processes that pollute the air and water (the Clean Air Act and the Clean Water Act); to locate, authorize, and fund the cleanup of hazardous wastes (the Resource Conservation and Recovery Act, which established the Superfund); and to control the use of pesticides (the Federal Insecticide, Fungicide, and Rodenticide Act). States now have their own EPAs that perform similar functions.

The federal EPA is not the only agency with responsibility to oversee activities that can affect environmental health. The Department of Energy (DOE), for example, oversees the disposal of nuclear waste; the Department of Agriculture (USDA) helps to determine consumer exposure to pesticide residues on food; and the Department of Labor protects the health of workers through the Occupational Safety and Health Administration (OSHA). In addition, most states have administrative agencies with similar responsibilities for intrastate activities.

Because Congress has authorized these agencies, and the many subagencies through which they operate, to protect the public, courts are reluctant to intervene, making private lawsuits particularly difficult. If an agency is operating within its congressional mandate, and is arguably doing its job in a reasonable fashion, the court will usually protect both the agency and those in compliance with its standards from private lawsuits seeking compensation for environmentally related illnesses. Thus, the protection of environmental health depends much more directly on the actions of these agencies than on the concerns of private citizens or their elected representatives.

Progress to date

It is sometimes claimed that the environment must be getting more healthful, since people are, on average, living longer (Simon, 1983). However, increased longevity may be due to such factors as more healthful lifestyles (less cigarette smoking and more exercise, for example), improved hygiene, more widespread prenatal care (in most industrial countries), and improved medical techniques (for example, in the treatment of heart disease). Increase longevity is not, by itself, evidence that the environment—the air that we breathe and the water that we drink—is more healthful.

There has been progress in air quality. The removal of lead from gasoline, begun in the early 1970s, resulted in a marked reduction of the general U.S. population's exposure to lead in the environment (Commoner, 1990). The problems of acid rain has been ameliorated somewhat. Owing largely to measures taken under the Clean Air Act, sulfur dioxide emission fell by 28 percent in the United States and particulates by 62 percent between 1970 and 1987 (French, 1991). As a result, the sulfur content of rain in the Northeast has decreased, and the rate at which lakes are acidifying has slowed, although much more improvement is needed for acidification to be reversed (Mohnen, 1988). The level of ozone, and thus of smog, in Los Angeles's air was less in 1991 than in any of the previous fifteen years ("Vital Signs," 1992).

Indoor air has improved as well. Smoking is increasingly restricted in indoor commercial environments or, as in the case of domestic airline flights in the United States, prohibited altogether. The overall rate of smoking is also down, although the rate among high school seniors remains 20 percent. As evidence mounts that passive smoking is a health hazard, exposure to it is declining.

Enforcement problems

As noted above, the protection of human health from environmental contamination is largely the responsibility of the EPA and other federal and state agencies. Unfortunately, the performance of these agencies is sometimes disappointing. The EPA's regulation of pesticides serves to exemplify the general problem. The EPA regulates pesticides under the Federal Insecticide, Fungicide, and Rodenticide Act. The general public is exposed to pesticides primarily through residues on food and through contamination of groundwater that serves as a major source of drinking water. The EPA recognized in 1988 that "forty-six pesticides . . . contaminate groundwater solely as a result of normal agricultural use" (Fultz, 1991, p. 3). But a registered chemical can remain in use for up to fifteen years after it is discovered in groundwater, before a decision is made about its continued use. An example is atrazine, a pesticide in widespread agricultural use (Fultz, 1991). What is more, for pesticides already found toxic, the EPA has not lowered acceptable exposure through residues on food in light of additional exposure through drinking water.

Worse yet, not all pesticides in widespread use are registered with the EPA, resulting in the continued exposure of the public through both food and water to pesticides not yet tested for their "potential to cause birth defects, cancer, and other chronic health effects" (Fultz, 1991, p. 5). Exemption from the registration requirement is given in so-called emergencies for one year at a time. But some exemptions have been granted for more than a decade, during which people are exposed to pesticides of unknown toxicity (Guerrero, 1991b). Also, the EPA continues to emphasize the control of point sources of water pollution, such as factories and municipal sewer systems, instead of nonpoint sources, such as agricultural runoff, despite evidence that the latter poses the greater water pollution problem (Guerrero, 1991b). This may be due to the fact that the USDA promotes the use of many pesticides to increase crop yields even though these chemicals constitute health hazards.

Unfortunately, the EPA's inadequate protection of public health from the dangers of pesticides is typical. Substantially similar stories can be told about surface-water pollution, hazardous waste management and cleanup, enforcement of the Clean Air Act, and DOE decisions about the disposal of nuclear waste. Consider the following: "The National Research Council estimated that only 2 percent of at least 60,000 chemicals that are used widely have been comprehensively studied for toxic effects" (Ziem and Davidoff, 1992, p. 88).

In addition to poor funding, a general reason for these inadequacies is that agencies tend to establish such close ties to the industries they are charged with regulating that they identify with industry perspectives and needs. The agency's capture by industry results partly from industry offers of future, high-paying employment to regulatory personnel who are "reasonable." Another factor may be pressure on the agency by legislators responsible for approving its budget. Such legislators may depend on the affected industry for campaign contributions (Sanjour, 1992). Conscientious federal employees who try to regulate effectively are relegated to tasks that have little impact. Those employees who blow the whistle on an agency's failure to do its job must go before the presidentially appointed Merit System Protection Board, which may be more interested in protecting the president and "the system" than the meritorious whistleblower (Sanjour, 1992).

Added to its other inadequacies is the appearance of racism in the EPA's enforcement efforts. "Penalties under hazardous waste laws at sites having the greatest white population were about 500 percent higher than penalties at sites with the greatest minority population" (Lavelle, 1992, p. S2). This disparity can be accounted for only by race, not by income. There is a similar disparity of 46 percent in penalties concerning nontoxic waste, air pollution, and water pollution. It takes 20 percent longer for toxic waste sites in minority areas to be placed on the priority list for cleanup, and the cleanup in minority areas is more likely than in white areas to be merely containment of the waste than treatment that removes its toxicity.

Environmental racism appears to affect government regulation of international trade. For example, pesticides banned in the United States due to their toxicity to human beings can be legally manufactured and then sold abroad. (Some return as residues on imported food.)

Future problems

Risks of cancer and cataracts will increase significantly as the result of a decrease in stratospheric ozone that will continue beyond the twentieth century. The human immune system may also be weakened by increased ultraviolet radiation, resulting in a variety of health problems (Stetson, 1992).

Genetically engineered microorganisms are being developed at an increasing rate. Their release into the environment to aid the cleanup of oil spills, for example, may at some time constitute a health hazard.

Trade agreements, such as the North American Free Trade Agreement (NAFTA), intended to lower barriers to free trade across national borders, may result in additional toxic pollution. NAFTA is likely to promote manufacturing and agriculture in Mexico, where pollution-control efforts appear to be less effective than in the United States. U.S. manufacturers and farmers may react to Mexican competition by obtaining lower standards of pollution control from the government. Many regulations that were supposed to be issued under the Clean Air Act of 1990 were delayed more than a year, and others were postponed indefinitely, owing to concerns in some quarters that industries complying with them would be less competitive economically.

Incineration of solid waste is increasingly popular in the United States. But "incinerators . . . pump into the air . . . dioxins and furans (extremely toxic substances suspected of causing cancer and genetic defects), and twenty-eight different types of heavy metals, including lead, cadmium, and mercury," which are also health hazards (Young, 1991, p. 9). The residues of incinerators are toxic wastes that threaten groundwater supplies when put into ordinary landfills.

Perhaps the greatest dangers to environmental health in the future will come from risks of exposure to nuclear radiation. The DOE is so interested in depositing high-level nuclear waste in Yucca Mountain, Nevada, that it has ceased its search for alternative sites. Yet the potential for long-term isolation of waste in Yucca Mountain is questionable. Volcanic activity occurred in the area only 20,000 years ago, rather than 270,000, as the DOE had previously contended. More generally, the National Research Council concluded in 1990 that studies during the preceding twenty years had increased uncertainties regarding long-term predictions in geology (Lenssen, 1992). This conclusion concerns all projects of long-term burial, including the burial of transuranic nuclear waste (radioactive elements heavier than uranium) in Carlsbad, New Mexico, and the burial of so-called low-level nuclear wastes in several states (Poole, 1992). The General Accounting Office has expressed concern that radioactive tritium buried at Hanford Nuclear Reservation in the state of Washington could explode, releasing considerable radiation into the atmosphere (U.S. General Accounting Office, 1990).

Other dangers from continued reliance on nuclear power around the world include massive shipments on the high seas of plutonium (from France to Japan during the 1990s) and the increasing use in Japan of breeder reactors, which many experts consider inherently unsafe. Such reactors produce plutonium by removing the moderator that slows down neutrons in conventional reactors. Additional heat is generated by increased neutron activity, requiring a special coolant, which is usually liquid sodium that can "catch fire on contact with air and explode on contact with water" (Mortimer, 1991, p. 130).

Decisional frameworks

How should decisions about environmental health be made? Advocates of free trade and free markets suggest that market mechanisms will protect public health adequately. But from the perspective of firms competing for customers, environmental protection seldom makes sense. A manufacturer's plastic toys, for example, seldom are more attractive to customers because water and air used in manufacturing processes were purified before being released into the environment. Similarly, catalytic converters on automobiles add to cost but do not improve cars in most customers' eyes. Without government mandates requiring all producers in an industry to protect the environment, the cost of such protection impairs competitiveness, or reduces profits, of conscientious firms that act alone. So the free market discourages the protection of environmental health in the absence of government-mandated regulations, such as those administered by OSHA and the EPA.

The EPA and other government agencies have been faulted for failure to oppose the market-driven activities of private enterprise with sufficient vigor. Three kinds of reforms may be ameliorative. First, agency personnel should be barred for five years from employment, directly or indirectly, by companies the agency regulates. This will encourage greater independence of agency personnel from the perspectives of regulated companies. Second, campaign finance reform could also help to diminish the influence of financial interests on the regulatory process. Finally, whistle-blowers should be given special job and financial protection (Sanjour, 1992).

What decisional framework should these agencies employ? Some libertarians, who stress the importance of individual rights, maintain that any environmental pollution that may harm anyone should be disallowed. The government should "enjoin anyone from injecting pollutants into the air, and thereby invading the rights of persons and property. Period" (Rothbard, 1970, p. 5). But this purist approach seems unrealistic, since it would disallow, for example, most manufacturing and almost all uses of fossil fuels, including that in automobiles. Polluting the environment in ways potentially harmful to human health is too ingrained in industrial ways of life to be eliminated entirely.

Pointing to benefits of industrialization—air-conditioning in summer, heating in winter, rapid transportation, sophisticated medical interventions—some people maintain that pollution should be allowed until risks to people outweigh benefits. According to this view, government agencies, such as the EPA, should use risk/benefit analysis to determine permissible kinds and levels of pollution (Ruckelshaus, 1983).

Critics maintain, however, that risk/benefit analysis favors continued pollution over health-related concerns. First, current levels of pollution are often assumed to be acceptable and are used as precedents for future decisions. Second, whereas benefits of current pollution practices are assumed, risks must be proven scientifically, a task already difficult. Finally, risk/benefit analysis depends largely on subjective judgments of "experts" whose opinions may reflect employers' interests (Winner, 1986).

Some suggest avoiding subjectivity by using cost–benefit analysis (CBA), in which all costs and benefits of proposed pollution-controlling regulations are put into monetary terms. The alternative with the highest net benefit should be chosen. Costly health hazards would thus be taken into account. The EPA usually allows environmental impact statements to employ CBA, and the Nuclear Regulatory Commission uses CBA regularly.

But there are many problems with CBA. Costs and benefits associated with the length and quality of human life, which are affected by environmental health, cannot reliably be translated into monetary terms. Second, subjectivism remains because there is great uncertainty in projections of health hazards (Shrader-Frechette, 1991). Third, by employing money as its standard, CBA takes into account views and desires only insofar as they are expressed in monetary terms. The opportunity for such expression is proportional to the money at people's disposal. Using CBA, then, agencies would give protection to people not equally but in proportion to their wealth or income. Where actions of government agencies are concerned, CBA denies equal protection of the laws. Finally, using normal economic techniques, CBA discounts the future, making a present cost or benefit larger than an otherwise equivalent, but future, cost or benefit. This biases public policy toward the short term. If the duty to avoid or minimize harming people is based on human rights, harming future generations is morally equivalent to harming contemporaries. CBA immorally discounts the lives and well-being of future generations (Wenz, 1988).

Instead of CBA, the following are suggested rules of thumb. First, the burden of proof should be reversed from that employed in risk/benefit analysis. Before a potentially harmful addition is made to the environment, its safety should be demonstrated. Currently, for example, potentially carcinogenic pesticides can be used widely for ten to fifteen years before investigations are completed. Products are withdrawn then only if demonstrated to harm public health. The burden to demonstrate its safety should be on those wanting to expose people to a new chemical.

Second, people at greatest risk should be given the greatest voice in decisions about creating or using potentially hazardous substances (Shrader-Frechette, 1991). For example, corporate officials and owners interested in manufacturing processes that create toxic wastes would legitimately retain a significant voice in regulatory decisions if they could, and would, store the wastes near themselves and their families.

Third, through subsidies the government should encourage sustainable agriculture, integrated pest management, mass transit, energy conservation, and other practices and products that reduce the introduction of health hazards into the environment.

Fourth, when indirect costs of a product can be calculated reliably, those costs should, over time, be added as a tax to the consumer price of the product. For example, the price of gasoline should reflect costs associated with the deleterious health effects of smog. Only then will consumers be guided by accurate information about how much a product actually costs them. Such information generally improves the results of relying on market mechanisms.

Finally, agencies should discourage practices that tend to hide the existence or severity of environmental health problems. Storage of nuclear wastes underground, so the continuing health hazard is not noticed, and the war on cancer, that lulls people into thinking a cure is near, lead the public to underestimate their jeopardy. This should be avoided in part because an informed public is central to addressing problems of pollution. Lacking any objective formula for balancing alleged benefits against alleged harms to determine the acceptability of pollution, an informed public must be the ultimate judge of government decisions related to environmental health.

PETER S. WENZ

Directly related to this entry are the entries HAZARDOUS WASTES AND TOXIC SUBSTANCES; *and* ENVIRONMENTAL POLICY AND LAW. *For a further discussion of topics mentioned in this article, see the entries* ENVIRONMENTAL ETHICS; FUTURE GENERATIONS, OBLIGATIONS TO; OCCUPATIONAL SAFETY AND HEALTH; *and* PUBLIC

HEALTH, *especially the article on* PUBLIC HEALTH METHODS: EPIDEMIOLOGY AND BIOSTATISTICS. *For a discussion of related ideas, see the entries* HARM; *and* RISK. *Other relevant material may be found under the entries* ANIMAL RESEARCH; ANIMAL WELFARE AND RIGHTS; ECONOMIC CONCEPTS IN HEALTH CARE; ENDANGERED SPECIES AND BIODIVERSITY; ENVIRONMENT AND RELIGION; GENETICS AND ENVIRONMENT IN HUMAN HEALTH; INTERNATIONAL HEALTH; RACE AND RACISM; *and* SUSTAINABLE DEVELOPMENT. *See also the* APPENDIX (CODES, OATHS, AND DIRECTIVES RELATED TO BIOETHICS), SECTION VI: ETHICAL DIRECTIVES PERTAINING TO THE ENVIRONMENT.

Bibliography

ARNETZ, BENGT B.; RAYMOND, LAWRENCE W.; NICOLICH, MARK J.; and VARGO, LISA. 1991. "Mortality Among Petrochemical Science and Engineering Employees." *Archives of Environmental Health* 46, no. 4:237–248.

CARSON, RACHEL. 1962. *Silent Spring*. Boston: Houghton Mifflin.

COMMONER, BARRY. 1990. "Ending the War Against Earth." *The Nation*, April 30, pp. 589–594.

EPSTEIN, SAMUEL S. 1987. "Losing the War Against Cancer." *Ecologist* 17, nos. 2–3:91–101.

———. 1992. "Profiting from Cancer: Vested Interests and the Cancer Epidemic." *Ecologist* 22, no. 5:233–240.

FALCK, FRANK, JR.; RICCI, ANDREW, JR.; WOLFF, MARY S.; GODBOLD, JAMES; and DECKERS, PETER. 1992. "Pesticides and Polychlorinated Biphenyl Residues in Human Breast Lipids and Their Relation to Breast Cancer." *Archives of Environmental Health* 47, no. 2:143–146.

FRENCH, HILARY F. 1991. "You Are What You Breathe." In *The World Watch Reader on Global Environmental Issues*, pp. 97–111. Edited by Lester R. Brown. New York: W. W. Norton.

FULTZ, KEITH O. 1991. *EPA Should Act Promptly to Minimize Contamination of Groundwater by Pesticides*. GAO/T-RCED-91-46. Washington, D.C.: U.S. General Accounting Office.

GARDNER, MARTIN J. 1991. "Father's Occupational Exposure to Radiation and the Raised Level of Childhood Leukemia near the Sellafield Nuclear Plant." *Environmental Health Perspectives* 94:5–7.

GUERRERO, PETER F. 1991a. *Greater EPA Leadership Needed to Reduce Nonpoint Source Pollution*. Testimony; GAO/T-RCED-91-34. Washington, D.C.: U.S. General Accounting Office.

———. 1991b. *Pesticides: EPA's Repeat Emergency Exemptions May Provide Potential for Abuse*. Testimony; GAO/T-RCED-91-83. Washington, D.C.: U.S. General Accounting Office.

HALLOWELL, CHRISTOPHER. 1991. "Water Crisis on the Cape." *Audubon*, July–August, pp. 65–74.

JACOBSON, JODI L. 1989. "Abandoning Homelands." In *State of the World, 1989: A Worldwatch Institute Report on Prog-*

ress Toward a Sustainable Society, pp. 59–76. Edited by Lester R. Brown. New York: W. W. Norton.

LAVELLE, MARIANNE. 1992. "Unequal Protection: The Racial Divide in Environmental Law." *National Law Journal*, September 21, pp. S1–S12.

LENSSEN, NICHOLAS. 1992. "Confronting Nuclear Waste." In *State of the World, 1992: A Worldwatch Institute Report on Progress Toward a Sustainable Society*, pp. 46–65. Edited by Lester R. Brown. London: Earthscan.

LINOS, ATHENA; BLAIR, AARON; GIBSON, ROBERT W.; EVERETT, GEORGE; VAN LIER, STEPHANIE; CANTOR, KENNETH P.; SCHUMAN, LEONARD; and BURMEISTER, LEON. 1991. "Leukemia and Non-Hodgkin's Lymphoma and Residential Proximity to Industrial Plants." *Archives of Environmental Health* 46, no. 2:70–74.

LUOMA, JON R. 1988. "The Human Cost of Acid Rain." *Audubon*, July, pp. 16–25.

MOHNEN, VOLKER A. 1988. "The Challenge of Acid Rain." *Scientific American* 259, no. 2:30–38.

MORTIMER, NIGEL. 1991. "Nuclear Power and Carbon Dioxide: The Fallacy of the Nuclear Industry's New Propaganda." *The Ecologist* 21, no. 3:129–132.

POOLE, WILLIAM. 1992. "Gambling with Tomorrow." *Sierra*, September–October, pp. 50–54, 89–92.

POPE, C. ARDEN; SCHWARTZ, JOEL; and RANSOM, MICHAEL R. 1992. "Daily Mortality and PM10 Pollution in Utah Valley." *Archives of Environmental Health* 47, no. 3:211–217.

POSTEL, SANDRA. 1986. *Altering the Earth's Chemistry: Assessing the Risks*. Worldwatch Paper 71. Washington, D.C.: Worldwatch Institute.

———. 1988. "Controlling Toxic Chemicals." In *State of the World, 1988: A Worldwatch Institute Report on Progress Toward a Sustainable Society*, pp. 118–136. Edited by Lester R. Brown. New York: W. W. Norton.

RAUBER, PAUL. 1991. "New Life for White Death." *Sierra*, September–October, pp. 62–65, 104–105, 110–111.

RENNER, MICHAEL. 1991. "Assessing the Military's War on the Environment." In *State of the World, 1991: A Worldwatch Institute Report on Progress Toward a Sustainable Society*, pp. 132–152. Edited by Lester R. Brown. New York: W. W. Norton.

ROTHBARD, MURRAY. 1970. "The Great Ecology Issue." *The Individualist* 2, no. 2:1–8.

RUCKELSHAUS, WILLIAM D. 1983. "Science, Risk, and Public Policy." *Science* 221, no. 4615:1026–1028.

RUSSELL, DICK. 1989. "Environmental Racism." *Amicus Journal* 11, no. 2:22–32.

SANJOUR, WILLIAM. 1992. "In Name Only." *Sierra*, September–October, pp. 74–77, 95–103.

SHERSON, DAVID; SVANE, OLE; and LYNGE, ELSEBETH. 1991. "Cancer Incidence Among Foundry Workers in Denmark." *Archives of Environmental Health* 46, no. 2:75–81.

SHRADER-FRECHETTE, KRISTIN S. 1991. *Risk and Rationality: Philosophical Foundations for Populist Reforms*. Berkeley: University of California Press.

SIMON, JULIAN L. 1983. "Life on Earth Is Getter Better, Not Worse." *Futurist* 17, no. 4:7–14.

STEINHART, PETER. 1991. "What Can We Do About Environmental Racism?" *Audubon*, May, pp. 18–21.

Stetson, Marnie. 1992. "Saving Nature's Sunscreen." *Worldwatch* 5, no. 2:34–36.

Stewart, Alice. 1993. "Low Level Radiation—The Effects on Human and Nonhuman Life." In *Poison Fire/Sacred Earth*, pp. 13–15. Edited by Sibylle Nahr and Uwe Peters. Munich: World Uranium Hearing.

U.S. General Accounting Office. 1990. *Nuclear Energy: Consequences of Explosion of Hanford's Single-Shell Tanks Are Understated: Report to the Chairman*. GAO/RCED–91–34. Washington, D.C.: Author.

———. 1991a. *Air Pollution: EPA's Strategy and Resources May be Inadequate to Control Air Toxics: Report to the Chairman*. GAO/RCED–91–143. Washington, D.C.: Author.

———. 1991b. *Pesticides: Food Consumption Data of Little Value to Estimate Some Exposures: Report to the Chairman*. GAO/RCED–91–125. Washington, D.C.: Author.

"Vital Signs." 1992. *Worldwatch* 5, no. 2:6.

Weber, Peter. 1992. "A Place for Pesticides?" *Worldwatch* 5, no. 3:18–25.

Wenz, Peter S. 1988. *Environmental Justice*. Albany: State University of New York Press.

Winner, Langdon. 1986. *The Whale and the Reactor: A Search for Limits in an Age of High Technology*. Chicago: University of Chicago Press.

Young, John E. 1991. "Burn Out." *Worldwatch* 4, no. 4:8–9.

Ziem, Grace E., and Davidoff, Linda L. 1992. "Illness from Chemical 'Odors': Is the Health Significance Understood?" *Archives of Environmental Health* 47, no. 1:88–91.

ENVIRONMENTAL POLICY AND LAW

Two legal traditions

Among the many purposes of environmental law, two stand out: the protection of property rights and the preservation of places. Laws controlling pollution serve primarily the first goal; they constrain the risks some people would impose on others. These laws typically treat pollution not as a social cost or "externality" but as a trespass or an invasion of personal and property rights. Statutes that pursue the second purpose seek to preserve national forests, landscapes, and landmarks; to protect historical districts; to maintain biodiversity; and to defend the integrity of ecological systems, such as rivers and wetlands.

These two sorts of statutes emerge from two foundational traditions in the political culture of the United States, the first of which draws on the values of individualism and autonomy; the second, on those of community and diversity. The first tradition, which we associate with libertarianism and individualism, insists that property rights are important; this tradition would protect the individual from imposed and unconsented-to risks associated with pollution.

The second tradition, which we associate with Madisonian republicanism, suggests that Americans may use the representative and participatory processes of democracy to ask and answer moral questions about the goals of a good society. Through the political process, Americans identify and pursue together conceptions of the common good that are not reducible to the good that individuals may pursue for themselves. Americans, most of whom are immigrants or descended from immigrants, discover in the natural environment a common heritage—a *res publica*—that unites them as a nation. Environmental laws, then, regard nature as having a cultural shape, form, or value we are responsible to maintain for its own sake and for the sake of future generations.

Laws that emerge from the second political tradition—that protect our natural heritage, the integrity of ecological systems, biodiversity, forests, and so on—like those that protect personal and property rights, often cannot be justified simply on economic grounds. Economic arguments concern preferences individuals satisfy to promote their own welfare as they see it. Environmental laws, in contrast, tend to engage deeply held human values that concern not only the welfare but also the dignity and autonomy of persons and the integrity of places.

Among nonwelfare-based values is the widely held conviction that a self-respecting nation as wealthy as the United States would not trade a magnificent natural birthright for bowls of consumer pottage. In this perspective, the protection of wetlands, estuaries, rivers, species, and old-growth forests may make sense less for economic than for ethical, aesthetic, and cultural reasons. Protective policies of this kind express a respect for nature, not a quest for wealth.

The Clean Air Act

The Clean Air Act seeks primarily to protect individuals from pollution and in that way to honor their personal and property rights. Yet it also seeks to protect air quality for cultural and aesthetic reasons, particularly when it affects national monuments and parks.

National ambient air quality standards (NAAQS). The law in 1970 required the then new Environmental Protection Agency (EPA) to set standards for a list of "criteria" pollutants in order to assure that air pollution would not endanger public health or welfare, or harm particularly sensitive individuals. In calling for "an adequate margin of safety," Congress suggested that safe thresholds existed for air pollutants and that standards could be set well under them. Yet Congress knew at the time that no such levels existed; nevertheless, it set the EPA the task of ratcheting pollution down to safe levels even at considerable costs.

To understand this, one might consider the case of *Boomer* v. *Atlantic Cement Co.* (1970), which came to trial in New York State as Congress worked on the Clean Air Act. There the plaintiff, a farmer, sought to enjoin a major cement manufacturer from spewing dust and fumes onto his land. New York State is a jurisdiction that usually grants injunctions in nuisance cases. In this instance, however, the trial court awarded the plaintiff compensatory damages instead, since Atlantic, an immense plant supporting the local economy, would have to cease operations in order to cease polluting. Thus, the court effectively gave the polluter the power of eminent domain—the power to coerce the plaintiff off his land at a price set not by the plaintiff but by the court.

What the court did was efficient from an economic point of view: It allocated resources according to market-based prices. This approach establishes economically "optimal" levels of pollution—levels at which those who benefit from polluting activities could still benefit even after compensating their victims. These levels, however, can be understood only in terms of a hypothetical market in which people discriminate among risks—and therefore demand countervailing "benefits" to accept them—wholly on the basis of the magnitude of those risks; in other words, the extent and probability of injury. In this context, the moral context or "meaning" of the risk (whether it is voluntary or imposed, for example) would not be relevant.

This is the reverse of what happens in an actual market in which people accept some risks and reject others, not necessarily because of the magnitude of those risks nor because of the benefits associated with them, but for moral reasons—for example, because they resent some risks more than others. Many Americans, like Mr. Boomer, seek just to live in peace. Ultimately, by forcing Boomer to accept compensatory damages, the court opted for "optimal" pollution but departed from the common-law defense of property rights.

Congress faced a similar dilemma. At one extreme, Congress might apply a cost–benefit or "compensation" test, permitting pollution to increase to levels it would reach in a hypothetical market in which people made "trade-offs" on the basis of the magnitude of risks, without regard to the moral context. This might vastly increase the amount of allowable pollution, in view of many risks people voluntarily accept (for example, by smoking). Thus, Congress could allow much more pollution if its goal were to bring to environmental risks the same cost–benefit ratios that people apparently accept in other areas of their lives.

At the other extreme, Congress could protect the right of individuals not to have risks imposed on them. To do this, however, Congress would have to force pollution down to levels at which no one would suffer any invasion of person or property. This could bring the economy to a halt.

The Clean Air Act, in setting NAAQS at "no-risk" levels, adopted the second extreme, and thus treated persons as ends-in-themselves and not as mere means to the efficiency of markets. Yet it also set up a goal so idealistic or aspirational that it had to be honored as much in the breach as in the observance. To make progress under the law, the EPA and state agencies generally "halved the difference" between the extremes by compelling polluters to develop and apply the best pollution-control technology. This may satisfy neither extreme because it may fail a cost–benefit test and also may fail to protect everyone's health.

Yet this approach sometimes pushed pollution control to the "knee of the curve"—the point at which the costs increase geometrically and further control could arguably exceed even what respect for persons and property reasonably demands. Thus, even if regulation does not take its cue from the efficiency of hypothetical markets, it can still be reasonable, as long as it does not force the protection of personal and property rights well beyond the point of rapidly diminishing returns.

Prevention of significant deterioration (PSD). This doctrine originated in a brief 1972 court order enjoining the EPA from approving state pollution-control plans that "permit the significant deterioration of existing air quality" where it exceeds NAAQS. After a series of judicial elaborations of PSD requirements, Congress in 1977 amended the Clean Air Act to forbid all but small increments of pollution in "clean" airsheds, such as "in national parks, national wilderness areas, national monuments, national seashores, and other areas of special . . . recreational, scenic, or historic value."

By prohibiting polluters from degrading pristine air quality in aesthetically and culturally sensitive areas, the act goes beyond the protection of the rights of individuals. It apparently respects the integrity of particular places and the interests of future generations in inheriting those places comparatively undisturbed. Because of these requirements, the Navaho Power Plant, for example, installed expensive scrubbers to prevent comparatively small losses of visibility in the Grand Canyon. This agreement is easier to justify on symbolic and aesthetic than on economic grounds.

Air-pollution law evolved, along with other forms of environmental protection, from an early preoccupation with health and safety issues to a larger concern with the sustainability of the economy within its ecological setting. A brief historical review will help us understand American environmental law.

The appeal to technology and administration: 1969–1979

Since the passage of the National Environmental Policy Act of 1969 (NEPA), American environmental law has undergone three distinct stages of development. During the first stage, the euphoria of the 1970s, Congress enacted, among other statutes, the Clean Air Act of 1970, the Occupational Safety and Health Act of 1970, the Clean Water Act of 1972, the Endangered Species Act of 1972, the Ocean Dumping Act of 1972, the Safe Drinking Water Act of 1974, the Toxic Substances Control Act of 1976, and the Resource Conservation and Recovery Act of 1976. These laws set aspirational (and, as it turned out, sometimes unrealistic) goals by calling, for example, for a workplace free of risks from toxic substances and for air quality standards well under "safe" thresholds.

Under the Clean Water Act, Congress did not contemplate setting standards for water quality, however, since outside of drinking water (covered by a different statute), the condition of the nation's aquatic ecosystems could not be valued simply in relation to human health and safety. Accordingly, the Clean Water Act called for new technologies to minimize water pollution and thus to attain a vague objective: the restoration and maintenance of the "chemical, physical, and biological integrity of the Nation's waters." Questions arose, however, concerning the precise goals of the law and the efficiency of government-mandated ("command-and-control") technical approaches to achieving them. Critics also questioned the expenditure of hundreds of billions of dollars to control pollution beyond what may be necessary to protect public health.

The rhetorical objectives of laws enacted during the 1970s, which are strong enough to warm the heart of the most ardent environmentalist, soon became fictions as deadlines passed, violations were not monitored or prosecuted, and the agencies fought uphill political and legal battles to make whatever gains they could, given their limited resources. On those rare occasions when the regulatory agencies threatened to enforce a statute to its full extent, Congress could be counted on to weaken it. In 1973, when a court ordered the EPA to bring California into compliance with the Clean Air Act, for example, EPA administrator William Ruckelshaus responded with gasoline rationing, since nothing less draconian would do the job. Congress intervened by extending the deadline, then by setting another and another; they, too, passed without action.

Other statutes display the same distance between the heaven of legislative rhetoric and the earthbound scaffolding of regulatory attempt and achievement. The Delaney clause of the Food, Drug and Cosmetic Act, which covers processed food, has for decades prohibited any trace of a pesticide that can be shown to induce cancer in animals at any dosage, but it has rarely been enforced. Only a handful of pesticides have been removed from the market since the 1970s, and pesticide use has doubled.

The Occupational Safety and Health Administration has regulated at a rate of about one hazardous substance a year. Administrations have avoided the effects of the Endangered Species Act by failing to list species as endangered and by approving inadequate plans to protect those that are listed. (Some biologists believe, for example, that Washington and Oregon would have to be depopulated to assure the survival of the grizzly bear.) And statutes protecting wetlands—Section 404 of the Clean Water Act, for example—depend on the ability and flexibility of officials to determine what and where a wetland is.

Laws enacted during the 1970s, even though they set goals so lofty as to become pious fictions, did slow environmental degradation and force the development of improved pollution-control technologies. This process had another advantage: American leadership in technical and regulatory know-how can be explained in part by what the nation learned from its own mistakes.

Retrospective liability and criminalization: 1980–1989

By 1981, environmental regulation had reached an impasse. Time and time again, Congress announced the good news of a risk-free, pollution-free environment and a nation with all its scenic wonders and biological integrity intact. The regulatory agencies then had to announce the bad news: what society would have to pay and who would have to pay it. Many of those who bore the costs then blamed the messenger; the EPA and other agencies came under enormous criticism for policies that required great outlays to achieve minor improvements. When President Ronald Reagan announced a program of regulatory rescission and appointed Anne Gorsuch at EPA and James Watt at the department of Interior to achieve it, it seemed that the goals of the 1970s would be abandoned if not reversed, especially in view of the ideological commitments and managerial styles of these appointees.

By 1981, however, the constituency of the environmental movement had dramatically changed. At first enlisting primarily upper-middle class, well-educated suburbanites, environmentalism had become a populism, including lower-middle-class Americans in the heartland who resented the effects of global markets on their communities. Social-science surveys showed overwhelming support among all economic and social groups for the strictest regulation, regardless of cost. Because of the strength of environmentalism among his own supporters, President Reagan found himself obliged to replace the head of the EPA and the secretary of the interior, and to accept a new barrage of environmental statutes. The new laws appealed to a populist rather than to a technocratic constituency.

Liability-based legislation.   During the 1970s, when regulatory agencies told industry what technologies to install, economists criticized this "command-and-control" approach as woefully inefficient, arguing that industry, given the right incentives, could control waste materials in more cost-effective ways. Congress acted on this criticism with a vengeance by passing laws that assigned strict liability to any corporation that might be involved in causing a pollution problem and by holding severe criminal penalties over the heads of corporate officials.

Laws enacted during the 1980s—including the Environmental Response, Compensation, and Liability Act of 1980, the Hazardous Waste Act of 1984, and the Superfund Amendments and Reauthorization Act of 1986—did not simply address present hazards but also dealt with remediation of past and prevention of future occurrences. Some of these statutes make polluters jointly and severally liable for the entire cost of cleanup, regardless of fault. Thus any company whose name appears on a manifest at a poorly operated waste dump might find itself legally liable to pay the entire cost of a gold-plated cleanup.

Laws of this kind take a moralistic or retributivist approach, associated with populist crusades, in regulating pollution. Instead of telling corporate polluters what they must do, these laws threaten to punish them for what they have done or might do. This contrasts with the approach of the 1970s, which allowed polluters to avoid blame by installing appropriate technologies. However fair or unfair the "retributivist" or "liability" approach may seem, it has been effective in chastening the behavior of polluters.

The executive versus the legislative branch. During the latter part of the 1980s, a pitched ideological and political battle arose between the White House and the Congress (controlled by different parties) concerning the enforcement or nonenforcement of environmental statutes. Starting with President Reagan's Executive Order 12291, issued in February 1981, the White House, operating through the Office of Management and Budget and then the Competitiveness Council, argued that environmental regulations should pass a cost–benefit test and not undermine the international competitiveness of American industry. Congressional committees replied that the executive branch has a duty to carry out the laws, not to amend them unilaterally to conform to a particular economic theory or ideology. Although the U.S. Supreme Court has found cost–benefit analysis irrelevant to health-and-safety-based legislation, the political standoff continued, putting agencies like the EPA in the tightening jaws of a vise formed by the legislative and executive branches of government.

In response to the resulting legislative "gridlock," many leaders in both the business and the environmental community reason that they have more to gain by working with each other—by negotiating their own compromises—than by supporting the combat of their partisans in the political process. Accordingly, environmental negotiation seems to many a much more promising road than political impasse. The move from opposition and litigation to negotiation requires leaders to adopt a pragmatic stance, however, rather than an ideological one. Both sides appear to have much to gain if they work together—and much to lose if they continue their ideological antagonism.

The Clinton administration.   When President Bill Clinton assumed office, studies showed that over the previous decade the regulatory agencies had met only a small fraction of the deadlines Congress set for the air to be clean, ocean dumping to cease, species habitats to be secure, and so on. The new administration promised to end the "gridlock" of divided government—a situation in the environmental area in which Congress pretended to make law and the executive branch pretended to enforce it.

The new administration soon found, however, that divided government was not the only problem. During the previous twenty years, Congress and the executive branch had engaged in what psychologists call "enabling behavior." Like an alcoholic and his or her spouse, Congress and the executive agencies may have quarreled, but at a deeper level they were in league with each other. By letting deadlines pass, accepting "reasonable progress" in lieu of compliance, substituting *de minimis* or "negligible risk" for statutory "zero risk" standards, and otherwise failing to enforce legislation, agencies such as the EPA spared Congress the unpleasantness of making hard choices and allowed it to parade itself as the defender of nature, personal rights, purity, and so on. Congress in turn gave the agencies autonomy—the ability to work the law as they liked, within the tolerance of the courts.

What is worse, both industry and environmental groups resisted attempts to reform the law to make its enforcement practicable. For example, when the Clinton administration proposed to replace the Delaney clause with an effective and enforceable health-based pesticide statute, the chemical industry opposed it because it threatened its profits. But environmental groups also opposed the Clinton administration proposal because it would allow some pesticide use, and thus would abandon the legislative fiction of the Delaney clause, which holds out the hope of a pesticide-free nation.

Thus, the Clinton administration had to take on an entrenched way of doing business in which all parties—environmentalists, industry groups, regulatory agencies, and congressional committees—played set roles in the expectation that other groups would follow their own assigned scripts. All of these players may feel they have more to gain by defending the entrenched system than by making the compromises necessary to enact statutes that are enforceable. Thus the Clinton administration requires a great deal of political genius to make progress. Having a "green" ideology will hardly be enough.

The road to sustainability: 1990–

In the 1970s, Americans confronted environmental problems that were primarily local in scale, recent in time, and near- or medium-term in their effects. Examples included belching smokestacks, persistent pesticides, automobile exhaust, burning rivers, groundwater contamination, and oil spills. Congress responded to these on a medium-by-medium basis as technical problems to be solved by improvements in science, technology, analysis, and regulation. These acute and obvious hazards often proved to be the cheapest to control; thus the EPA's initial efforts accomplished a great deal.

The problem of scale. The environmental problems of the 1990s, in contrast, tend to be global rather than local in scale, historical rather than recent in origin, and to concern the farther rather than the nearer future. These problems include global warming and climate change, deforestation, loss of genetic diversity, the ozone hole, and overpopulation. Environmental problems no longer seem to center on "spillovers" one activity may impose on another but on the aggregate and often synergistic and unpredictable effects of these activities on ecological and biospheric systems that sustain the economy as a whole.

Mainstream economists in the past tended to regard the environment as if it were a firm offering a flow of goods and services that, like those of any company, must be correctly priced in a market. If markets failed to attach the prices to those goods and services, then that task would fall to public officials guided by economic experts. Thus, the mainstream view regarded cost–benefit analysis and "shadow" pricing as the best ways to conserve resources over the long run. Many analysts today, in contrast, regard the environment (biospheric and ecological systems) as containing the economy, rather than the other way round. They understand environmental problems in terms of the scale effects of

economic activity as a whole on the global systems that sustain it.

In other words, the problem of the *scale* of the economy relative to the carrying capacity of the planet, rather than the problem of the *allocation* of resources within the economy, became a prominent issue of the 1990s. Many analysts questioned not so much the goals of economic development (employment, low inflation, prosperity) as the way we pursue these goals, that is, by continually increasing the amount of resources we take from nature and the amount of wastes we put back in (e.g., Daly, 1977). In the 1970s economic development threatened the environment. Today, the environment—rising sea levels, dying forests, eroding land, thinning stratospheric ozone, and the overexploitation of resources by burgeoning and impoverished populations—constrains economic development.

"Capping" emissions. The fundamental philosophy of domestic legislation has thus begun to change. By setting a "cap" or nationwide limit on the total allowable amount of sulfur dioxide emissions, for example, the 1990 Clean Air Act sought to control acid rain. By allowing polluters to sell to others the emission "allowances" or "permits" they do not use, the statute encourages industry to maximize productivity while minimizing wastes—and thus to find the cheapest ways of protecting the environment.

Analysts have suggested the use of "caps" to discipline virtually all of our relationships with the natural world—caps on carbon oxide production, road construction, deforestation, erosion, and so on. Biodiversity laws and treaties "cap" the extinction of species. Statutes that require recycling and resource recovery, specify fuel efficiency standards, call for renewable sources of energy and for conservation, and so forth, derive from macroeconomic thinking, consultation, and consensus-building to determine the aggregate levels of resource depletion and waste production that are compatible with a "sustainable" relationship with the environment. The point is not necessarily to allocate resources efficiently. It is to treat nature as a habitat for ourselves and other creatures—to establish between people and the environment they inhabit a viable relationship that makes ethical, cultural, and ecological as well as economic sense.

Yet the new "sustainability" approach has many hurdles to surmount. First, no one has found a way to measure the "scale" of economic activity that correlates with environmental deterioration. (Water vapor, for example, is a large-scale emission but causes little or no ecological damage.) Second, human ingenuity often finds ways to replace scarce natural resources with plentiful ones, so it is by no means clear that Earth is running out of resources. On the contrary, the real prices of many commodities, including agricultural products, have fallen for the last few decades and stand at historical lows, suggesting that they are becoming more and more plentiful, at least in relation to demand.

The international perspective. Debates over treaties initiated at the United Nations Conference on the Environment and Development in 1992 illustrate international concern with the sustainability of economic activity and the carrying capacity of the earth. To some extent the international community has dealt successfully with environmental threats; for example, the Montreal Protocol, an international accord signed in 1987, initiated controls on the production of chemicals that damage stratospheric ozone. And conventions aimed at preserving endangered species and controlling the harvest of resources held in common—whales, for example—have long exerted influence on the international community.

To an even larger extent, however, international environmental conventions and the institutions—called "regimes"—set up to implement them meet many of the same problems of enforcement that are familiar in domestic contexts. Many of the conventions—such as those that ban pollution in the North Sea—are hortatory or idealistic. Politicians enact these protocols under pressure from the "green" movement, but because of the very great costs involved, they make slow progress in enforcing them.

In eastern Europe and the former Soviet Union, central authority acting without accountability caused environmental devastation on an unprecedented scale. After the demise of communism and of Cold War ideology, people try to fill the moral vacuum with loyalty to local culture and tradition (hence the break-up of nations) and by making a greater commitment to landscape and place. This commitment, if accompanied by institutions that make people accountable for the consequences of their actions, may reverse a century-old pattern of environmental destruction. International financial assistance for environmental protection will provide the appropriate context for environmental as well as for economic renewal.

All sides appear to agree, however, that war poses the greatest threat to the environment and to human safety and health, especially given the proliferation of nuclear weapons. Environmental protocols, conventions, and regimes bring peoples closer together and teach nations to cooperate with and to trust each other. Insofar as environmental protection encourages a sustainable peace, it will lay the surest foundation for sustainable development.

MARK SAGOFF

Directly related to this entry are the entries ECONOMIC CONCEPTS IN HEALTH CARE; *and* SUSTAINABLE DEVELOP-

MENT. *For a further discussion of topics mentioned in this article, see the entries* ANIMAL WELFARE AND RIGHTS, *articles on* ETHICAL PERSPECTIVES ON THE TREATMENT AND STATUS OF ANIMALS, *and* WILDLIFE CONSERVATION AND MANAGEMENT; AUTONOMY; ENDANGERED SPECIES AND BIODIVERSITY; ENVIRONMENT AND RELIGION; ENVIRONMENTAL ETHICS; ENVIRONMENTAL HEALTH; FUTURE GENERATIONS, OBLIGATIONS TO; PATERNALISM; POPULATION ETHICS, *section on* ELEMENTS OF POPULATION ETHICS; POPULATION POLICIES; RIGHTS; RISK; *and* VALUE AND VALUATION. *For a discussion of related ideas, see the entries* INTERNATIONAL HEALTH; PUBLIC HEALTH, *article on* PHILOSOPHY OF PUBLIC HEALTH; PUBLIC HEALTH AND THE LAW; *and* WARFARE, *articles on* NUCLEAR WARFARE, CHEMICAL AND BIOLOGICAL WARFARE, *and* INTERNATIONAL WEAPONS TRADE. *Other relevant material may be found under the entries* ETHICS, *article on* TASK OF ETHICS; *and* HEALTH-CARE RESOURCES, ALLOCATION OF.

Bibliography

ACKERMAN, BRUCE A. 1974. *The Uncertain Search for Environmental Quality.* New York: Free Press.

ACKERMAN, BRUCE A., and HASSLER, WILLIAM T. 1981. *Clean Coal/Dirty Air: Or How the Clean Air Act Became a Multibillion-Dollar Bail-out for High-Sulfur Coal Producers and What Should Be Done About It.* New Haven, Conn.: Yale University Press.

Boomer v. Atlantic Cement Co. 1970. (N.Y.) 257 N.E.2d 870.

CONSTANZA, ROBERT, ed. 1991. *Ecological Economics: The Science and Management of Sustainability.* New York: Columbia University Press.

DALY, HERMAN E. 1977. *Steady-State Economics: The Economics of Biophysical Equilibrium and Moral Growth.* San Francisco: W. H. Freeman.

DALY, HERMAN E., and TOWNSEND, KENNETH N., eds. 1993. *Valuing the Earth: Economics, Ecology, Ethics.* Cambridge, Mass.: MIT Press.

FINDLEY, ROGER W., and FARBER, DANIEL A. 1992. *Environmental Law in a Nutshell.* 3d ed. St. Paul, Minn.: West.

GOODLAND ROBERT; DALY, HERMAN E.; and EL-SERAFY, SALAH, eds. 1992. *Population, Technology, and Lifestyle: The Transition to Sustainability.* Washington, D.C.: Island Press.

LESTER, JAMES P., ed. 1989. *Environmental Politics and Policy: Theories and Evidence.* Durham, N.C.: Duke University Press.

MELNICK, R. SHEP. 1983. *Regulation and the Courts: The Case of the Clean Air Act.* Washington, D.C.: Brookings Institution.

ROSENBAUM, WALTER A. 1991. *Environmental Politics and Policy.* 2d ed. Washington, D.C.: Congressional Quarterly Press.

SMITH, V. KERRY, ed. 1984. *Environmental Policy Under Reagan's Executive Order: The Role of Benefit-Cost Analysis.* Chapel Hill: University of North Carolina.

Vig, Norman J., and Kraft, Michael E., eds. 1994. *Environmental Policy in the 1990s: Toward a New Agenda*. 2d ed. Washington, D.C.: Congressional Quarterly Press.

World Bank. 1992. *World Development Report 1992*. New York: Oxford University Press.

ENVIRONMENT AND GENETICS

See Genetics and Environment in Human Health. *See also* Genetic Engineering.

ENVIRONMENT AND RELIGION

The closing decades of the twentieth century saw the appearance of a new field of religious interest, characterized by the conviction that religion and the environment stand in a profoundly reciprocal relationship. In the words of the philosopher of religion Steven C. Rockefeller, "The environmental crisis cannot be addressed without coming to terms with the spiritual dimension of the problem, and the spiritual problems of humanity cannot be worked out apart from a transformation of humanity's relations with nature" (Rockefeller and Elder, 1992, p. 141). The body of literature, community of scholarship, and network of institutional practices that have emerged are large and coherent enough to constitute a distinctive field of religious action and study.

The purpose of this entry is to provide, from a primarily Western, and chiefly U.S., standpoint, an introduction to this rapidly growing field by identifying its historical context, and the three principal stages in its development since the 1960s.

From one perspective, the new field of religious interest is simply another chapter in the history of religion, this one written under the stimulus of the global environmental crisis. Humanity's inability to live in harmony with the environment has always been an important subject for religion. It is typically conceived as a reflection of humanity's deep alienation from the true ground of its existence. This view is apparent, for example, in the biblical myth of the fall of Adam and Eve in the Garden of Eden. Adam and Eve disobey their Creator, and are expelled from the garden. Their descendants are doomed to everlasting enmity, among themselves and between themselves and the earth from which they must wrest their livelihood. This condition will not change until humanity is reconciled with its Creator.

Many of the world's religions also find in direct physical and spiritual encounter with nature a way to overcome alienation from the divine ground of their being. This conviction underlies the function of sacred places as places of religious renewal. It is present among a long line of Christian ascetics, from the desert fathers to Saint Francis of Assisi, to the New England Pilgrims, nerving their hope that by repeating the original pilgrimage of the Israelites into the wilderness and meeting the adversities encountered there, they would find a way to reenter paradise (Williams, 1962).

The transformation of modernity

Thus, one clear source of the contemporary interest in religion and the environment is the view that the world's religions bear in their myths and belief systems the wisdom required to address the environmental and spiritual crises of contemporary civilization. But this is not sufficient to understand why the contemporary interest in religion and the environment arose when and how it did. The new interest must be understood primarily as an effort to transform some of the most influential assumptions of the post-Enlightenment era, but to do so from a standpoint that is itself rooted in modes of thought and valuation that came to prominence with the Enlightenment. It is, in other words, an effort to place modernity upon a more authentic and sustainable spiritual foundation (Weiming, 1993).

From this perspective, the new concern for religion and the environment is the culmination of a cultural reaction against the mechanistic and anthropocentric modes of thought that achieved dominance in the post-Reformation era and that led to the desacralization of the natural world (Merchant, 1989). Martin Buber, Martin Heidegger, Alfred North Whitehead, Albert Schweitzer, and Paul Tillich, among others, carried this reaction into the twentieth century, and anticipated the contemporary religious interest in the environment. If there is greater moral outrage at the profanation of nature in the post–World War II period, it is because the modern environmental crisis has itself worsened.

The new field of religious interest is a distinctly modern endeavor in several respects. In the first place, it is global in focus and compass. Not only this holy place, or that holy mountain, but Earth itself is widely viewed as charged with religious significance. The modern process of globalization by which the world has become a single place, and the peoples of the world conscious of their shared dependence upon it, is perhaps the major context for contemporary concern for the sacred (Robertson, 1985). It is also a modern phenomenon that significant spokespersons should have arisen within virtually every religious tradition on the globe in defense of the environment, from the Dalai Lama, to Pope John Paul II and Leonardo Boff, to Chief Oren

Lyons, and that much of the activity generated on the subject should be ecumenical (e.g., the work of the World Council of Churches on the theme "Peace, Justice, and Integrity of Creation") and interfaith (e.g., the 1986 World Wide Fund for Nature celebration in Assisi, Italy). While these activities have been generated in most cases by small minorities within the world's religious and academic communities, they have often attracted wide public attention.

The new religious interest is also very much a creature of subversive democratic, aesthetic, and scientific movements, deriving much of its persuasive appeal from them. In place of the dominant ontology of autonomous and externally related individuals associated with the figures of René Descartes, John Locke, and Isaac Newton, these movements pursued an organic and relational vision of human and natural community (Albanese, 1990). The fundamental thrust of the eighteenth-century democratic revolutions on behalf of greater equality and opportunity of participation in social life is a primary motivation for the new field, undergirding practical efforts by religious communities to address the role of social injustice in environmental destruction, and serving as a wellspring of religiously resonant metaphors, such as Gary Snyder's praise for Native American religions, because they celebrate "a kind of ultimate democracy" (Nash, 1989, p. 114).

Associated with the democratic movement, especially in the nineteenth century, was a new aesthetic that perceived spirit immanent in ordinary human activities and throughout nature, an aesthetic manifest in new genres of nature poetry, nature essays, landscape painting, symphonic music, and landscape architecture. Equally important, the new scientific view of nature as an internally related, loosely integrated whole, a view based upon holistic tendencies in nineteenth-century evolutionary and ecological science, and twentieth-century developments in astronomical and atomic physics, was a powerful factor in reconceptualizing the relations of humanity, nature, and God.

Criticism of religious traditions

The new religious interest in religion and the environment also carries one step further the Enlightenment project of judging all received traditions from the standpoint of their consequences for practical life. It introduces a new pragmatic test for the adequacy of any particular religious symbol, attitude, or doctrine—its consequences for the environment.

Medieval historian Lynn White, Jr., crystallized this approach in 1967 in his widely read essay, "The Historical Roots of Our Ecological Crisis." Assuming that practical "human ecology is deeply conditioned by beliefs about our nature and destiny—that is, by religion,"

White argued that the primary source of the environmentally destructive practices of Western science and technology was to be found in an axiom peculiar to Latin Christianity: The world was created and planned by a transcendent God for the exclusive purpose of serving humanity (White, 1974). It followed that if the environmental behavior of Western civilization was to change, this axiom had to be replaced.

White set in motion a controversy that may be considered to mark the first stage in the new field of religion and the environment. The controversy was based upon three important arguments: first, that White's pragmatic approach was justified, even though he failed to discriminate the multiple causal factors involved in such an historical analysis; second, that he accurately identified a despotic strand in the Judeo-Christian tradition, especially as it had developed in the West; and third, that its continuing effects on the behavior of believers could be empirically verified (Eckberg, 1989). Theologian Gordon Kaufman (1972) argued that the inner logic of Western Christianity was anthropocentric because it used anthropomorphic moral categories to describe God. Other Christian theologians, such as Thomas Derr, generally agreed with White's analysis of Christianity, but disagreed with his conclusion, since in their view human history, not nature, is rightfully the primary locus of divine action in the world. Lutheran theologian H. Paul Santmire concluded that the tradition was "ambiguous," because two conflicting theological motifs—the one predicated on a vision of the human spirit rising above nature in order to commune with God, the other predicated on a vision of the human spirit celebrating God's presence in and with the biophysical order—contended with one another throughout the history of Western theology (Santmire, 1985).

The kind of critical evaluation that White made of Western Christianity was soon made of other faiths as well. The results were uniformly the same: All religious traditions (with the exception, perhaps, of the primal religions of indigenous peoples) have shortcomings when evaluated from the standpoint of their environmental practices and consequences.

Yi-Fu Tuan has argued, for example, that even in ancient China, whose religions taught that humanity was a part of nature, the environment suffered from overexploitation (Tuan, 1974). Tuan pointed out that in the Chinese case, as in other cases, there were not only conflicting teachings and unsuspected and unintentional consequences of particular beliefs, but an inevitable gap between ideal and practice. Other scholars have noted inherent liabilities in the belief structures of Asian salvation religions, comparable to the problem of anthropocentrism in Christianity. Classic Hinduism, for example, tends to be world-denying, and Buddhism and Taoism ethically passive. It is often difficult to reconcile the cosmologies of these faiths (e.g., the Taoist idea of *yin* and *yang*), or their beliefs concerning individual salvation and destiny (e.g., the Buddhist doctrine of karma) with contemporary scientific knowledge of evolutionary process, or with the need for science-based social interventions (Rolston, 1990). In the case of Native American environmental traditions, there is serious debate about whether they were, in truth, good conservationists. Criticism has centered on the authenticity of the documents by which their beliefs and practices are known, and on whether the lack of large-scale environmental disturbance was due to their religious beliefs or lack of technological development.

The recovery and reconstruction of religious traditions

White also gave momentum to a second and alternative train of inquiry, the deliberate construction of viable environmental faiths. He noted the environmentally positive natural theology of the Greek Orthodox tradition, in which nature was viewed as a symbolic system through which God speaks to humankind, and the figure of Saint Francis of Assisi, who saw all creatures glorifying their Creator (White, 1974). By the late 1970s, this more constructive attitude had replaced the attitude of suspicion. Scholars were setting about the selective reconstruction of the received religions with the double aim of recovering their authentic and positive environmental insights and making them important instruments for changing contemporary values and practices.

Five themes can be discerned within the immense body of work devoted to this reconstructive task: (1) the relation of God or the sacred to the world; (2) the religious significance of the land; (3) the value of other beings; (4) the nature of human being and moral responsibility; and (5) spirituality, or the immediate experience of the sacred in the world.

The Judaic and Christian traditions. Reconstructive work in the Judaic and Christian traditions has attempted, through a reinterpretation of scripture, theology, and cosmology, to articulate how God is both immanent within and transcendent of the world. Well before White's article, Lutheran theologian Joseph Sittler called, in 1954, for a theology for nature that would be responsive to the vitalities of Earth; in his prophetic 1961 address to the World Council of Churches in New Delhi, Sittler argued that to be true to the biblical witness, the doctrine of salvation must swing within the orbit of the doctrine of creation. Sittler sought to recover the authentic Christian vision of the world of nature as a "theater of grace" (Sittler, 1972).

The 1960s witnessed a shift of outlook in biblical studies that supported Sittler's call. Claus Westermann, among other biblical scholars, argued that the notion

that God acts only in history is a misreading of the Hebrew scriptures. Earth, as described in Genesis, is a "good creation" and the fruit of an original blessing. Yahweh, savior of Israel, is also the creator, sustainer, and savior of the world (Westermann, 1978). Biblical scholars also recovered the classical cosmological Christology of Paul as articulated in the hymn recorded in Colossians 1:15–20, wherein the divine Word or Logos through whom all things were made is the same as the Logos that became incarnate in Christ (Schillebeeckx, 1980). For Paul, "all creation is groaning in travail," awaiting its final redemption.

Building on these retrievals of the theology of nature in the Hebrew and Christian scriptures, as well as the long tradition of Christian natural theology, in which evidence for the existence of God is adduced from perceptions of design in nature, Christian theologians have sought to interpret the doctrine of God in relational terms. While God is not to be identified with the world, God and the world interpenetrate, or live within, one another. John Cobb took early leadership of efforts by theologians influenced by the process metaphysics of Alfred North Whitehead and Charles Hartshorne to replace the mechanistic model of evolution with an ecological and democratic model, in which subjective feeling and purpose are inherent in all entities. Cobb joined with Australian biologist Charles Birch to construct a naturalistic interpretation of God as the supreme and perfect exemplification of the ecological model of internal relations between organisms and their environment (Birch and Cobb, 1981). God is present to the feelings of every entity of the universe, luring it toward its maximal richness of experience and harmony with every other entity. By this means, Cobb and other process theologians seek to provide metaphysical warrant for their conviction that the caring and loving God of Jesus as portrayed in the Gospels is also the God of the cosmos.

James Gustafson, also drawing upon the contemporary sciences, believes that the task of a theocentric ethic of nature is to discern the parameters of responsible human action in the interdependent whole of creation, and to remind humans that God's will for creation is more comprehensive than an intention for the salvation and well-being of the human species alone (Gustafson, 1994). From a different doctrinal perspective, Jürgen Moltmann argues that a trinitarian notion of internal relations within the Godhead may be interpreted to mean that God and the world dwell within one another through the Spirit (Moltmann, 1985).

Perhaps the most radical reenvisaging of the relationship of God to the world has been given by feminist theologians, such as Sallie McFague and Rosemary Radford Ruether. In place of God as lord, king, and patriarch, with the world as his realm, McFague experiments with the models of God as mother, lover, and friend of the world, the world being conceived as God's body. As mother, God "bodies forth" creation and affirms all beings; as lover, God values creation, suffers with, and desires to heal it; as friend, God desires coworkers to extend fulfillment to all creation (McFague, 1987). Ruether presents the construct of the God/ess as the primal matrix of being and new being in order to combine both the masculine and feminine forms of the word for the divine, while preserving the Judeo-Christian affirmation that divinity is one (Ruether, 1992).

If, as the apostle Paul believed, all creation is an expression of God's creative activity, the object of God's self-giving love, and the medium of God's redemptive activity, then all living creatures and communities are worthy of respect and are coparticipants with human beings in the drama of liberation from oppression. It follows that the treatment of nature, on the one hand, and the ethical responsibility toward humans, on the other, may be distinguished but not separated. The primary ethical imperative before human beings is to conform to the will of God, which is to do justice to all creation, considered individually and in community. For this reason, it is claimed that the core ethic of the Semitic faiths is eco-justice, and it is true that this strong sense of the ethical interdependence of the welfare of human and nonhuman existence has been an important element in helping to heal divisions between advocates of social justice and environmentalists, restoring respect for the relevance of these faiths for contemporary social struggles.

Four competing models detail the moral responsibility of human beings within this total community of existence; each has scriptural basis, congruity with modern theories of environmental ethics, and advocates within particular historic strands of Jewish and Christian life.

1. The model of stewardship is based upon a rereading of the first account of the creation of human beings in Gen. 1:26–27 in light of the second and more explicitly ecological account of Gen. 2:15. In the first account, human beings are created in the image of God and given dominion over the rest of creation, but the second account places Adam in the Garden of Eden "to till it and keep it." According to the tradition of stewardship, "dominion" should be understood to mean acting as trustees for creation, as servants of its welfare. This is an eco-justice model in that the image of the good steward is one who manages Earth's natural systems in such a way that they are sustained for the future and that their resources are distributed equitably. Douglas John Hall has developed a relational interpretation of stewardship, interpreting the *imago Dei* as meaning that human beings are created to emulate God's care and love toward creation (Hall, 1986).

2. The second model lifts up two central symbols in the Judaic and Christian traditions: covenant and land. It depicts God entering into relationship with creation through the making of covenant—from the first covenant, "with day and night and the orders of heaven and earth" (Jer. 33:25), to the covenant with Noah and all living beings, to the covenant with Abraham that established the people of Israel and promised them a good land. Covenant is an inherently political–ethical concept denoting an unconditional agreement to be faithful to one another as members of one community enduring over space and time. Covenants also entail specific obligations. As Walter Brueggemann has pointed out, one of the primary responsibilities that human beings have in the covenant is to receive with gratitude the land as a gift and to assure its integrity while maintaining justice to all the people that dwell upon it. When human beings are unfaithful to the covenant, God expels them from the land (Brueggemann, 1977).

3. Whereas the first model provides a religious grounding for what is often referred to in secular ethics as resource conservation, and the second model provides a basis for Aldo Leopold's idea of human beings as citizens of the land community, the third model is closely associated with modern animal rights and animal-liberation ethics. In fact, Jews and Christians have a long record of concern for the welfare and suffering of domestic animals, an activity that draws upon biblical motifs, such as God as shepherd of all creatures. Andrew Linzey has developed a theory of animal rights which he calls "theos-rights," based on the notion that God has rights in the creation. That God has such rights is clear to him because of the fact of what he calls Spirit-filled creatures—sentient animals that stand, like human beings, in a subjective relationship to God. Human beings, the creatures most capable of spiritual communion, have a special responsibility to respect the theos-rights of other creatures in ways analogous to the respect for human rights (Linzey, 1987).

4. One of the most popular expressions of Christian environmental interest in the 1980s was the emergence of creation spirituality, associated with the writings of Matthew Fox. For Fox, authentic Christian spirituality is rooted in a vivid sense of the original goodness of creation, and he finds that sense most alive in the Christian mystical tradition running from Irenaeus to Hildegard of Bingen to Meister Eckhart. Creation spirituality holds up the vision of human beings performing a royal vocation, acting as cocreators with the cosmic Christ in bringing the cosmos to harmonious fulfillment. This model requires attending to the arts, liturgy, dance, and meditation, to awaken humanity's divine poetic powers (Fox, 1983). Other forms of Christian theology that emphasize an aesthetic, contemplative, and sacramental re-

lationship to the divine presence in nature include the Eastern Orthodox liturgical tradition, which views humanity as a priestly mediator between God and the world; the long tradition of Christian poetry—from Gerard Manley Hopkins to Denise Levertov; and feminist rituals of healing and focused attention on the body as a medium for the experience of grace.

Islam. For Islamic scholars, the environmental crisis affecting Islamic countries, as well as the rest of the world, stems from the modern Western value system, which divorces the natural and divine worlds. In Islam, no such clear demarcation is conceived to exist. Seyyed Hossein Nasr writes that one can claim that "God Himself *is* the ultimate environment which surrounds and encompasses humanity," a state of affairs that leads to such joyous celebrations of nature as that found within Sufi poetry (Rockefeller and Elder, 1992, p. 89). However, humanity is privileged. The Qur'an explicitly spells out human dominion over nature. In recent years, a number of articles available to an English-speaking audience probe the Qur'an and its body of interpretation to address the question of human responsibility in a universe where all creatures and resources are "subjected" to human beings. In general, the position taken is that the human relationship to nature should be that of stewardship rather than mastery. Mawil Y. Izzi Deen (Samarrai), drawing on the Qur'an, includes among the reasons for protecting the environment: because it is God's creation; because its component parts praise their Creator; because natural laws made by the Creator are based on the concept of the continuity of existence; because other creatures are "peoples" like humans and therefore worthy of respect; because Islamic ethics is based on justice and equity; because the universe is the gift of God to all ages; and because no other creature is able to perform the task (Deen, 1990).

Asian religions. Reappropriations of the Abrahamic faiths typically begin with an affirmation of faith in God's original intention for a "good creation" and the created nature of human beings as moral overseers of creation, and then ask what are the means by which humans may be enabled to exercise moral responsibility in the face of repeated evidence of their failure to do so. The Asian faiths begin at the opposite end, as it were, with the assumption that humans are alienated from their true existence, and that only by a path of spiritual enlightenment can they gain awareness of the world as it is and the kind of self-realization appropriate to it. Asian religions offer practical spiritual disciplines for liberation from the suffering and self-contradictions associated with the environmentally destructive individualism and materialism of modern civilization. The aim of these disciplines is to achieve an enlightened consciousness of existence as a seamless unity. It is no won-

der that these faiths have attracted the interest of environmentally sensitive Westerners for two centuries, and that as modern culture has increasingly transformed Asia itself, new efforts have arisen in the late twentieth century to renew and reinterpret these traditions in order to provide an indigenous cultural base for environmental ethics.

Significant differences among and within the several ancient Asian faiths are often lost to view when transferred to the West. Hinduism, for example, finds the source of earthly suffering in the illusion of the self's perception of itself as differentiated from other beings, and liberation in the meditative consciousness that one's true or transcendental self (*Atman*) is identical with the "undifferentiated fullness of being" (*Brahman*) within or behind all things (Callicott and Ames, 1989, p. 262). Sometimes the absolute reality of *Brahman* is conceived as a mystical monadic substance identical in each thing; at other times, as a one-in-many Divine Being called by many names and manifest in many gods, each one the Supreme Being; and at still other times, as the many incarnations of the Supreme Being in the forms of various species. However conceived, because all beings are victims of the same suffering as human beings and share the same divine essence as human beings, to be enlightened as to the true nature of reality is at one and the same time to practice *ahimsa*, or noninjury to all living creatures. The practice of *ahimsa*, to the point of sacrificing one's life for other creatures, led 363 members of the Bishnois sect of Hinduism to lay down their lives in defense of trees in the eighteenth century, an inspiration for the protest of the Chipko Andolan movement against deforestation by hugging trees two centuries later.

All schools of Buddhism originate in the discovery by Siddhartha Gautama, the Buddha, that desire is both the cause of human suffering and the only aspect of human nature over which individuals can exercise control. To extinguish desire, whether for pleasure, wisdom, or even salvation, is to realize peace with the world and the capacity to perceive the world as it is—a series of transient phenomena without ultimate cause or end. Thus, to achieve enlightenment, or *nirvana*, is to achieve a new consciousness, at once a new worldview and a new moral orientation to the world. Both of these—the Buddhist view of the world, and the Buddhist attitude of detachment from the world—are widely considered important religious bases for living in harmony with the environment.

Buddhist philosopher David Kalupahana points out that in Buddhism human beings are not the center of the universe, but like all other beings, dependently coarising parts of it (Callicott and Ames, 1989). Everything tends to become of equal value, since there is no human or divine point from which to grade the relative significance of everything. For philosophers such as Kalupahana, the Buddhist worldview is unsurprisingly congruent with the contemporary scientific ecological outlook in that it accepts the empirical givenness of the natural world as an ever-changing, interdependent unity in diversity.

Moreover, to be freed *from* the self-defeating desire to possess the world is to be freed *for* a life of enjoyment and appreciation of the world as it is, rather than as one wants it to be. The Buddhist attitude toward the world is one of disinterested contemplation rather than, as in the biblical view, active cocreation. But it is a misunderstanding to characterize this attitude as passive. The Buddha lived an active moral life of compassion born of the joy that he experienced with his release from the tyranny of personal craving, and the wish to share this joy with others. Contemporary Mahayana Buddhists stress that a Buddha-nature awaits realization in all humans and sentient beings, and its essence is a pure, disinterested love for all being. In Japanese Zen Buddhism, which has been especially influential with Western environmentalists, the emphasis shifts even further toward an ideal of active harmony between humanity and nature. Through arduous spiritual practices, the Zen initiate is led to a vivid aesthetic experience of nature, called *satori*, and to an active concern for harmonizing human dwelling with nature on the model of Japanese landscape architecture.

Contemporary environmental philosophers find Taoism to be an especially rich basis for environmental ethics. This is due to the fundamental notion of the Tao itself, the idea that there is an emergent harmony inherent in nature, and that to follow this unfolding evolutionary tendency, to "follow Nature," is to find peace and fulfillment. Of special import in this regard is the Taoist concept of *feng-shui*, or geomancy, which means adapting actions to the inherent ecological processes and tendencies of the environment, a promising basis for a new ethic of sustainable development.

Native American traditions.   Native Americans are widely perceived as having an ecologically sound religious attachment to Earth and its creatures. They are often viewed as spiritual environmentalists having something to teach other cultures about how to live in harmony with nature. This view is shared by Amerindians themselves. Vine Deloria, Jr., and N. Scott Momaday are prominent among Amerindian writers who contrast a rootless Christianity with native people's perception of themselves as dwellers within a sacred landscape. The following highlighting of environmentally significant beliefs glosses over the differences among tribes scattered over a vast continent and is true only to the general pattern of Amerindian thought and practice.

Aspects of Amerindian faith most often cited as environmentally viable include:

Belief in the familial relationship of all life.   Black Elk speaks of "us two-leggeds" who "with the four-leggeds and the wings of the air and of all green things . . . are children of one mother and their father is one Spirit" (Neihardt, 1961, p.1). This belief necessitates that one care for other creatures and natural phenomena as one would care for a family member. Frequently quoted is the ethical precept made by Smohalla, founder of the dreamer religion, "You ask me to plow the ground. Shall I take a knife and tear my mother's bosom?" (Vecsey and Venables, 1980, p. 26).

Belief in the in-dwelling spirit among all life forms. Missionary John Eliot listed first among the questions his would-be converts asked concerning Christian dogma, "Why have not beasts a soul as man hath, seeing they have love, anger, &c. as man hath?" (Albanese, 1990, p. 30). Not only plants and animals, but stones, wind, stars, and other natural phenomena are believed to be part of, to be alive with, the Great Spirit, and no opposition exists between spirit and nature. This belief necessitates that one respect and honor the spirits of animals and plants. Ojibwe stories convey an ethics of interspecies trade, animals who reveal themselves to the good hunter who does not overharvest them, who disposes of their bones properly, and makes as much use of the carcass as is possible. Killing as such is not a crime, but wanton slaughter is.

Religious attachment to specific places.   Rather than a vague, undifferentiated love of "nature," Amerindians have shown an attachment to specific places, sacred locales where power is concentrated, ancestors are buried, spirits reveal themselves. Continued relationship to these sacred spaces is thought to be essential for human survival.

Belief in the restorative power of ritual.   In disease, in hunting, in the life-sustaining activities of the tribe, Amerindians look to restoring harmony with nature, apologizing to the guardian spirit of an animal or plant when it is killed, seeking the cause of sickness or plant failure in relational disharmony with nature and attempting a ceremonial remedy.

Collective understanding of land tenure.   This aspect of Amerindian life is linked to a sense of mutuality and community and is in stark contrast to Euro-capitalist notions of private property.

Religious contributions to a global ethic

A third stage in the development of the field of religion and the environment began with the recognition in the 1980s that the religions of the world will need to play a major role in the elaboration and implementation of a global environmental ethic. Many religious, political, scientific, and environmental leaders share this recognition, which has been clearly articulated at international conferences, such as the 1992 Earth Summit in Rio de Janeiro, Brazil, and in international conservation strategies, such as *Caring for the Earth* (World Conservation Union, 1991). The challenge is multifaceted and will inevitably dominate discussions of religion and the environment into the twenty-first century.

There are three principal ways by which religious thinkers are responding to this challenge. First, they seek to integrate religious claims to truth with two important Enlightenment sources of a global environmental ethic—the traditions of moral democracy and universal human rights (Weiming, 1993), and the story of the universe as told by natural science (Swimme and Berry, 1992). Second, they seek to identify the distinctive contributions that each of the world's religious or wisdom traditions can make to a global environmental ethic. Charlene Spretnak, for example, argues that Buddhism offers a distinctive wisdom regarding how to transcend human greed and hatred; Native American spiritualities offer a distinctive wisdom regarding our intimate relationship with nature; the traditions of Goddess worship offer a distinctive wisdom regarding the wholeness of the body; and the Semitic religious traditions offer a distinctive wisdom regarding social justice and community (Spretnak, 1993). Third, they seek ways by which shared attention to the critical issues of the environmental crisis might help the religions of the world make peace with one another.

None of these endeavors will be successful unless there is a fundamental rapprochement between the universal humanism of modernity and the diverse, often conflicting, ethical claims of the historic religious traditions (Küng, 1991). Whether such a reconciliation is possible is an open question. Is it possible for each of the world's religions to understand the demand for dialogue—interfaith, cross-cultural and cross-disciplinary—as inherent in its unique revelation and tradition? Is it possible for branches of the world's religions to evolve into a reasoned world faith with the capacity to inspire and guide a religiously and culturally pluralistic world society?

J. RONALD ENGEL

Directly related to this entry are the entries ENVIRONMENTAL ETHICS; ETHICS, *article on* RELIGION AND MORALITY; *and* SUSTAINABLE DEVELOPMENT. *See also the entries* AFRICAN RELIGION; BUDDHISM; CONFUCIANISM; EASTERN ORTHODOX CHRISTIANITY; HINDUISM; ISLAM; JAINISM; JUDAISM; NATIVE AMERICAN RELIGIONS; ROMAN CATHOLICISM; SIKHISM; *and* TAOISM. *For a further discussion of topics mentioned in this article, see the entries* ANIMAL WELFARE AND RIGHTS; ENDANGERED SPECIES AND BIODIVERSITY; ENVIRONMENTAL HEALTH; ETHICS; EUGENICS; EUGENICS AND RELIGIOUS LAW; RESPONSIBILITY; *and* VALUE AND VALUATION. *Other relevant material may be found under the entries* COMPASSION; FAMILY; FEMINISM; HUMAN NATURE; JUSTICE; *and* METAPHOR AND ANALOGY.

Bibliography

ALBANESE, CATHERINE L. 1990. *Nature Religion in America: From the Algonkian Indians to the New Age.* Chicago: University of Chicago Press.

BIRCH, CHARLES, and COBB, JOHN B. 1981. *The Liberation of Life: From the Cell to the Community.* Cambridge: At the University Press.

BRAYBROOKE, MARCUS. 1992. *Stepping Stones to a Global Ethic.* London: SCM Press.

BRUEGGEMANN, WALTER. 1977. *The Land: Place as Gift, Promise and Challenge in Biblical Faith.* Philadelphia: Fortress Press.

CALLICOTT, J. BAIRD, and AMES, ROGER T., eds. 1989. *Nature in Asian Traditions of Thought: Essays in Environmental Philosophy.* Albany: State University of New York Press.

DEEN, MAWIL Y. IZZI (SAMARRAI). 1990. "Islamic Environmental Ethics, Law, and Society." In *Ethics of Environment and Development: Global Challenge, International Response,* pp. 189–198. Edited by J. Ronald Engel and Joan G. Engel. Tucson: University of Arizona Press.

ECKBERG, DOUGLAS LEE, and BLOCKER, T. JEAN. 1989. "Varieties of Religious Involvement and Environmental Concerns: Testing the Lynn White Thesis." *Journal of the Scientific Study of Religion* 28, no. 4:509–517.

ENGEL, J. RONALD. 1990. "Introduction: The Ethics of Sustainable Development." In *Ethics of Environment and Development: Global Challenge, International Response,* pp. 1–23. Edited by J. Ronald Engel and Joan G. Engel. Tucson: University of Arizona Press.

FOX, MATTHEW. 1983. *Original Blessing.* Santa Fe, N.M.: Bear.

GUSTAFSON, JAMES M. 1994. *A Sense of the Divine: The Natural Environment from a Theocentric Perspective.* Cleveland, Ohio: Pilgrim Press.

HALL, DOUGLAS JOHN. 1986. *Imaging God: Dominion as Stewardship.* Grand Rapids, Mich.: William B. Eerdmans Publishing.

KAUFMAN, GORDON D. 1972. "A Problem for Theology: The Concept of Nature." *Harvard Theological Review* 65, no. 3:337–366.

KÜNG, HANS. 1991. *Global Responsibility: In Search of a New World Ethic.* New York: Crossroad.

LINZEY, ANDREW. 1987. *Christianity and the Rights of Animals.* New York: Crossroad.

McFAGUE, SALLIE. 1987. *Models of God: Theology for an Ecological, Nuclear Age.* Philadelphia: Fortress Press.

MERCHANT, CAROLYN. 1989. *The Death of Nature: Women, Ecology and the Scientific Revolution.* New York: Harper & Row.

MOLTMANN, JÜRGEN. 1985. *God in Creation: A New Theology*

of Creation and the Spirit of God. Translated by Margaret Kohl. San Francisco: Harper & Row.

NASH, RODERICK FRAZIER. 1989. *The Rights of Nature: A History of Environmental Ethics.* Madison: University of Wisconsin Press.

NEIHARDT, JOHN G. 1961. *Black Elk Speaks, Being the Life Story of a Holy Man of the Oglala Sioux.* Lincoln: University of Nebraska Press.

ROBERTSON, ROLAND. 1985. "The Sacred and the World System." In *The Sacred in a Secular Age: Toward Revision in the Scientific Study of Religion,* pp. 347–358. Edited by Phillip E. Hammond. Berkeley: University of California Press.

ROCKEFELLER, STEVEN C., and ELDER, JOHN C. 1992. *Spirit and Nature: Why the Environment Is a Religious Issue: An Interfaith Dialogue.* Boston: Beacon Press.

ROLSTON, HOLMES, III. 1990. "Science-Based Versus Traditional Ethics." In *Ethics of Environment and Development: Global Challenge, International Response,* pp. 63–72. Edited by J. Ronald Engel and Joan G. Engel. Tucson: University of Arizona Press.

RUETHER, ROSEMARY RADFORD. 1992. *Gaia and God: An Ecofeminist Theology of Earth Healing.* San Francisco: HarperSan Francisco.

SANTMIRE, H. PAUL. 1985. *The Travail of Nature: The Ambiguous Ecological Promise of Christian Theology.* Philadelphia: Fortress Press.

SCHILLEBEECKX, EDWARD. 1980. "'All Is Grace.' Creation and Grace in the Old and New Testaments." In his *Christ: The Experience of Jesus as Lord,* pp. 515–530. New York: Seabury Press.

SITTLER, JOSEPH. 1972. *Essays on Nature and Grace.* Philadelphia: Fortress Press.

SPRETNAK, CHARLENE. 1993. *States of Grace: The Recovery of Meaning in the Postmodern Age.* San Francisco: HarperCollins.

SWIMME, BRIAN, and BERRY, THOMAS. 1992. *The Universe Story: From the Primordial Flaring Forth to the Ecozoic Era— A Celebration of the Unfolding of the Cosmos.* San Francisco: HarperSan Francisco.

TUAN, YI-FU. 1974. "Discrepancies Between Environmental Attitude and Behaviour: Examples from Europe and China." In *Ecology and Religion in History,* pp. 91–113. Edited by David Spring and Eileen Spring. New York: Harper & Row.

VECSEY, CHRISTOPHER, and VENABLES, ROBERT W., eds. 1980. *American Indian Environments: Ecological Issues in Native American History.* Syracuse, N.Y.: Syracuse University Press.

WEIMING, TU. 1993. "Toward the Possibility of a Global Community." In *Ethics, Religion and Biodiversity: Relations Between Conservation and Cultural Values,* pp. 65–74. Edited by Lawrence S. Hamilton and Helen F. Takevchi. Cambridge, Mass.: White Horse Press.

WESTERMANN, CLAUS. 1978. *Blessing in the Bible and the Life of the Church.* Translated by Keith Crim. Philadelphia: Fortress Press.

WHITE, LYNN, JR. 1974. "The Historical Roots of Our Ecologic Crisis." In *Ecology and Religion in History,* pp. 15–31.

Edited by David Spring and Eileen Spring. New York: Harper & Row.

WILLIAMS, GEORGE H. 1962. *Wilderness and Paradise in Christian Thought: The Biblical Experience of the Desert in the History of Christianity and the Paradise Theme in the Theological Idea of the University.* New York: Harper and Brothers.

World Conservation Union. 1991. *Caring for the Earth.* Gland, Switzerland: IUCN Publications.

EPIDEMICS

Epidemics may be defined as concentrated outbursts of infectious or noninfectious disease, often with unusually high mortality, affecting relatively large numbers of people within fairly narrow limits of time and space. They probably emerged in human populations with the "Neolithic Revolution," roughly eight to ten thousand years ago, as humans began to domesticate animals, practice agriculture, and settle into towns and villages, with a corresponding increase in the density of population. This article will cover the history of epidemics with particular reference to their implications for bioethics, beginning with a survey of ancient and medieval times, moving on to responses to epidemics before the nineteenth century, then examining in more detail the impact of cholera and the bacteriological revolution. It will conclude with a discussion of the epidemiological transition and its aftermath, the emergence of new epidemics in the late twentieth century, and the ethical implications of the data surveyed. The focus will be mainly but not exclusively on Europe and North America, where historical source material is richest, and scholarly and scientific studies are most numerous.

Ancient and medieval times

Hippocratic texts indicate the presence of tuberculosis, malaria, and influenza in the population of ancient Greece, and the historian Thucydides provides the first full description of a major plague, the precise nature of which remains uncertain, in Athens (430–429 B.C.E.), in his history of the Peloponnesian War. The increase in trade brought about by the growth of the Roman Empire facilitated the transmission of disease, and there were massive epidemics in the Mediterranean (165–180 C.E. and 211–266 C.E.). The "plague of Justinian" (542–547 C.E.), which was said to have killed ten thousand people a day in Constantinople, is the first recorded appearance of bubonic plague (McNeill, 1979). In Europe and Asia, diseases such as measles and smallpox gradually became endemic, affecting virtually all parts of the population on a regular basis, with occasional epidemic outbursts. Periodic epidemics of bubonic plague continued, most seriously in the fourteenth century, when perhaps as much as one-third of Europe's population perished.

When Europeans arrived in the Americas, from 1492 on, they brought many of these diseases to native American populations for the first time, with devastating effects. The importation of African slaves introduced malaria and yellow fever by the seventeenth century (Kiple, 1984). The merging of the disease pools of the Old and New Worlds was completed by what appeared to be the transmission of syphilis to Europe from the Americas at the end of the fifteenth century, though the subject remains disputed by historians, some arguing that it was a recurrence or mutation of a disease that already existed on the Continent (Crosby, 1972).

Responses to epidemics before the nineteenth century

The ancient Greeks and Romans commonly, though not universally, believed that epidemics were brought into human communities from outside. Thucydides, for example, described the plague that struck Athens during the Peloponnesian War as having arrived by sea. This belief was the basis of official reactions to epidemics in medieval Europe. Following the closure of the port at Venice to all shipping for thirty days as the plague threatened in 1346, regulations imposed in Marseilles in 1384, and in other ports thereafter, prescribed the biblical period of isolation for a "quarantine" (forty days) outside the harbor for any ship thought to have called previously at a place infected with the plague. In 1423 the Venetians set up a hospital where plague victims were isolated, and by 1485 the city had a sanitary authority armed with wide-ranging powers during epidemics. In some epidemics, as in the Great Plague of London in 1665, victims were compulsorily isolated in their own houses, which were marked with a red cross to warn the healthy not to enter. Compulsory screening was not an issue before the late nineteenth century, however, because diseases were recognized as such only after the onset of obvious symptoms, and the concept of the asymptomatic carrier did not exist. In addition to these measures, the authorities in many medieval towns, working on the theory that epidemics were spread through the contamination of the atmosphere, ordered the fumigation of the streets to try to clear the air. Doctors and priests were expected to attend to the sick; and those who fled, as many did, are strongly criticized in the chronicles of these events.

Popular reactions to epidemics included not only flight from infected areas and evasion of public health measures, but also attacks on already marginalized and stigmatized minorities. As bubonic plague spread in Europe in 1348–1349, for example, rumors that the Jews were poisoning water supplies led to widespread pogroms. Over nine hundred Jews were massacred in the German city of Erfurt alone (Vasold, 1991). Such actions reflected a general feeling, reinforced by the church, that plagues were visited upon humankind by a wrathful Deity angered by immorality, irreligion, and the toleration of infidels. A prominent part in these persecutions was played by the flagellants, lay religious orders whose self-flagellating processions were intended to divert divine retribution from the rest of the population. Jews were scapegoated because they were not part of the Christian community. Drawing upon a lengthy tradition of Christian anti-Semitism, which blamed the Jews for the killing of Christ, the people of medieval Europe regarded Jews at such times as little better than the agents of Satan (Delumeau, 1990).

State, popular, religious, and medical responses such as these remained essentially constant well into the nineteenth century. The medical understanding of plague continued throughout this period to draw heavily on humoral theories, so that therapy centered on bloodletting and similar treatments designed to restore the humoral balance in the patient's body. They were of limited effectiveness in combating bubonic plague, which was spread by flea-infested rats. The isolation and hospitalization of victims also therefore did little to prevent the spread of plague. Nevertheless, the disease gradually retreated from western Europe, for reasons that are still imperfectly understood. The introduction of more effective quarantines with the emergence of the strong state in the seventeenth and eighteenth centuries was almost certainly one of these reasons, however, and helped prevent the recurrence of epidemics in the seventeenth and eighteenth centuries (Vasold, 1991).

State intervention also played a role in reducing the impact of smallpox, the other major killer disease of the age after bubonic plague. Its spread was first reduced by inoculation, before compulsory programs of cowpox vaccination brought about a dramatic reduction in the impact of the disease in nineteenth-century Europe. Despite the imperfections of these new methods, which sometimes included accidentally spreading the disease, vaccination programs in particular may be regarded as the first major achievement of the "medical policing" favored by eighteenth-century absolutist monarchies such as Prussia. Police methods that paid scant attention to the liberties of the subjects were used to combat the spread of epidemics. They included the use of troops to seal off infected districts, quarantines by land and sea, and the compulsory isolation of individual victims. Most of these measures had little effect, however, either because of lack of medical knowledge or because poor communications and lack of police and military manpower prevented them from being applied comprehensively (Rosen, 1974).

The impact of cholera

These theories and practices were brought into question above all by the arrival in Europe and North America of Asiatic cholera. The growth of the British Empire, especially in India, improved communications and trade, and facilitated the spread of cholera from its base in the Ganges delta to other parts of Asia and to the Middle East. Reaching Europe by the end of the 1820s, the disease was spread further by unsanitary and overcrowded living conditions in the rapidly growing towns and cities of the new industrial era. At particular moments of political conflict, above all in the European revolutions of 1830 and 1848, the Austro-Prussian War of 1866, and the Franco-Prussian War of 1870–1871, it was carried rapidly across the continent by troop movements and the mass flight of affected civilian populations (Evans, 1988).

Cholera epidemics affected the United States in 1832, 1849, and 1866, on each occasion arriving from Europe in the aftermath of a major conflict. State, popular, and medical responses in 1830–1832 were unchanged from earlier reactions to epidemics. Quarantine regulations were imposed, military cordons established, victims isolated, hospitals prepared. In Prussia, the breaching of such regulations was made punishable by death. But the opposition that such measures aroused among increasingly powerful industrial and trading interests, and the feeling among many liberals that the policing of disease involved unwarranted interference with the liberty of the individual, forced the state to retreat from combating cholera by the time of the next epidemic, in the late 1840s. In addition, medical theories of contagion were brought into disrepute by the failure of quarantine and isolation to stop the spread of the disease in Europe. Until the 1880s, many doctors thought that cholera was caused by a "miasma" or vapor rising from the ground under certain climatic circumstances. It could be prevented by cleaning up the cities so as to prevent the source of infection from getting into the soil (Evans, 1987). This was a contributory factor in the spread of sanitary reform in Europe and the United States during this period. But its importance should not be overestimated. Boards of health established in American cities in the midst of the cholera epidemics of 1832 and 1849 were short-lived and of limited effectiveness, and even in 1866 the more determined official responses had less to do with the impact of cholera than with the changed political climate (Rosenberg, 1987).

The fact that cholera affected the poorest sectors of society most profoundly was the result above all of structural factors such as unsanitary and overcrowded living conditions, unhygienic water supplies, and ineffective methods of waste disposal. But state and public responses to epidemics in the nineteenth century, at least in the decades after the initial impact of cholera, were primarily voluntaristic. Religious and secular commentators blamed cholera on the alleged immorality, drunkenness, sexual excess, idleness, and lack of moral fiber of the victims. Fast days were held in eleven New England states in 1832, in the belief that piety would divert God's avenging hand. Once again, the socially marginal groups of industrial society, from vagrants and the unemployed to prostitutes and beggars—or, in the United States in 1866, the newly emancipated slaves and the newly arrived Irish immigrants—were blamed (Rosenberg, 1987).

The rise of the medical profession, with well-regulated training and a code of ethics, ensured that doctors were more consistently active in treating victims of epidemics in the nineteenth century than they had been in previous times. Partly as a result, there were popular attacks on the medical profession in Europe during the epidemic of 1830–1832. Angry crowds accused doctors of poisoning the poor in order to be able to reduce the burden of support they imposed on the state or, in Britain, in order to provide fresh bodies for the anatomy schools (Durey, 1979). As late as 1892, doctors and state officials were being killed in cholera riots in Russia (Frieden, 1977). There were also disturbances in the United States, where a hospital was burned down in Pittsburgh and a quarantine hospital on Staten Island, in New York City, was destroyed by rioters fearing the spread of yellow fever. However, in most of Europe, public disturbances caused by epidemics had largely ceased by the middle of the nineteenth century. Fear of disorder was another reason for the state's withdrawal from policing measures (Evans, 1988). In Europe, too, religious responses to epidemics had become less important by the end of the century as religious observance declined. In 1892, however, as cholera once more threatened America's shores, it fed nativist prejudice and led to the introduction of harsh new restrictions on immigration.

The bacteriological revolution

Cholera was only the most dramatic of a number of infectious diseases that took advantage of urbanization, poor hygiene, overcrowding, and improved communications in the nineteenth century (Bardet et al., 1988). Typhus, typhoid, diphtheria, yellow fever, tuberculosis, malaria, and syphilis continued to have a major impact, and even smallpox returned on a large scale during the Franco-Prussian War of 1870–1871. Treatment continued to be ineffective. But the rapid development of microscope technology in the last quarter of the century enabled medical science to discover the causative agents of many infectious diseases in humans and animals. Building on the achievements of Louis Pasteur, Robert Koch identified the tubercle bacillus in 1882 and the cholera bacillus in 1884. These discoveries marked the triumph of bacteriology and completed the swing of medical opinion back from belief in "miasmas" as causes of epidemics toward a contagionist point of view.

From the 1880s, states once more imposed quarantine and isolation, backed by preventive disinfection. The greater effectiveness of state controls, compared with the earlier part of the century, was combined with the more precise focus on eliminating bacterial organisms. Once the role of victims' excretions in contaminating water supplies with the cholera bacillus became known, it was possible to take preventive action by ensuring hygienic water supplies and safe waste disposal. By the outbreak of World War I in 1914, the role of the human body louse in spreading typhus, and that of the mosquito in transmitting malaria and yellow fever, had been identified. Mosquito control programs were launched by the U.S. Army in Cuba following the Spanish-American War of 1898, and subsequently in the Panama Canal Zone, in order to reduce the incidence of yellow fever cases to an acceptable level. Regular delousing reduced typhus among armies on the western front in Europe during World War I. The Japanese army prevented casualties from typhoid and smallpox by a campaign of systematic vaccination during the war with Russia in 1904–1905 (McNeill, 1979; Cartwright, 1972).

The bacteriological revolution thus inaugurated an age of sharply increased state controls over the spread of disease. Laws were introduced in many countries making the reporting of infectious diseases compulsory. The growth of a comprehensive, state-backed system of medical care, working through medical officers, medical insurance plans, and the like, made comprehensive reporting easier. Hospital building programs in the second half of the nineteenth century facilitated the isolation of victims in hygienic conditions where they could be prevented from spreading the disease. The greater prestige of the medical profession in most industrialized countries by the late nineteenth and early twentieth century ensured that doctors were no longer attacked, and that the necessity of compulsory reporting and isolation was widely accepted by the public. However, a bacteriological understanding of disease causation also involved a narrowing of focus, in which increased emphasis was placed on the compulsory reporting of cases, followed by their isolation, at the expense of broader measures of public health and environmental improvement (Porter, 1993).

The epidemiological transition

Lower death rates from diseases such as cholera, typhoid, and tuberculosis were only partially the consequence of bacteriologically inspired state preventive measures, and the disease burden from acute infectious disease began to decline rapidly. The provision of clean, properly filtered water supplies and effective sewage systems reflected growing municipal pride and the middle-class desire for cleanliness. It made epidemics such as the outbreak of cholera that killed over eight thousand people in Hamburg, Germany, in little over six weeks in the autumn of 1892 increasingly rare. Just as important were improvements in personal hygiene, which again reflected general social trends as well as the growing "medicalization" of society in western Europe and the United States. Such developments reinforced the stigmatization of poor and oppressed minorities as carriers of infection, since they were now blamed for ignoring official exhortations to maintain high standards of cleanliness, even though their living conditions and personal circumstances frequently made it difficult for them to do so. Particular attention was focused on working-class women, who were held responsible by official and medical opinion for any lack of hygiene in the home (Evans, 1987).

The development of tuberculin by Koch in 1890 made possible the compulsory screening of populations even for asymptomatic tuberculosis. This was increasingly implemented after 1900, in conjunction with the forcible removal of carriers to sanatoria, although this was more effective in isolating people than in curing them. Educational measures also helped reduce the spread of the disease. The development and compulsory administration in many countries of a preventive vaccine against tuberculosis from the 1920s aroused resistance among the medical community, not least because by creating a positive tuberculin reaction in noncarriers, it made it impossible to detect those who truly had the disease, except where symptoms were obvious. These measures had some effect in reducing the impact of the disease. However, although the precise causes of the retreat of tuberculosis remain a matter of controversy among historians, the long-term decline of the disease from the middle of the nineteenth century was probably more the result of improvements in housing, hygiene, environmental sanitation, and living standards than of direct medical intervention. The introduction of antibiotics such as streptomycin after World War II proved effective in reducing to insignificant levels mortality from a disease that had been the most frequent cause of death or disability among Americans aged fifteen to forty-five (Dubos and Dubos, 1987).

Similarly, official responses to syphilis centered, especially in Europe, on the forcible confinement of prostitutes to state-licensed brothels or locked hospital wards, where they were subjected to compulsory medical examination. Before World War I, New York, California, and other states had introduced compulsory reporting of cases of venereal disease, and official concern for the health of U.S. troops led to the jailing of prostitutes. Measures such as these had no discernible effect on infection rates, which rose sharply during the war. They also represented a serious restriction on the civil liberties of an already stigmatized group of women, while the men who were their customers, and equally active in the sexual transmission of disease, were regarded as irresponsible at worst, and were not subjected to similar measures. The development of Salvarsan (arsphenamine) by Paul Ehrlich in 1910 introduced the possibility of an effective treatment for syphilis. But here again there was resistance, both within the medical community and from outside, from those who considered that an increase in sexual promiscuity would be a result. This view became even more widespread following the use of penicillin on a large scale during World War II (Brandt, 1987).

Epidemics of the late twentieth century

In the West, epidemic infectious disease was regarded by the second half of the twentieth century as indicating an uncivilized state of mind, and was ascribed above all to nonwhite populations in parts of the world outside Europe and North America. This reflected structural inequalities in the world economy, as the great infections became increasingly concentrated in the poor countries of the Third World. By the middle of the twentieth century, however, rapidly increasing life expectancy was bringing rapid growth of noninfectious cardiac diseases, cancer, and other chronic conditions that posed new epidemic threats to an aging population in the affluent West. Under increasing pressure from the medical profession, the state responded not only with education initiatives but also with punitive measures directed toward habits, such as cigarette smoking, that were thought to make such conditions more likely. The arsenal of sanctions governments employed included punitive taxation on tobacco and the banning of smoking, under threat of fines and imprisonment, in a growing number of public places. Increasingly, institutions in the private sector also adopted these policies. They raised the question of how far state and nonstate institutions could go in forcing people to abandon pleasures that were demonstrably harmful to their own health. At the same time, they contrasted strongly with the reluctance

of many states and companies to admit responsibility for cancer epidemics caused by factors such as nuclear weapons testing, the proximity of nuclear power stations to human populations, or the lack of proper precautions in dealing with radioactivity in industrial production.

In the 1980s, the identification of a new epidemic, known as acquired immune deficiency syndrome (AIDS), once more raised the ethical problems faced by state and society, and by the medical profession, in the past. Lack of medical knowledge of the syndrome and the danger of infection from contact with blood or other body fluids, posed the question of whether the medical profession had a duty to treat AIDS sufferers in the absence of any cure. The evidence of the overwhelming majority of past epidemics, for which there was also no known cure, seems to be, however, that medical treatment, even in the Middle Ages, could alleviate suffering under some circumstances, and was therefore a duty of the practitioner. In a condition that could prove rapidly fatal, the ethics of prolonged tests of a drug such as AZT, in which control groups were given placebos, was contested by AIDS sufferers anxious to try anything that might possibly cure the condition, or at least slow its progress.

If this was a relatively novel ethical problem, then the question of compulsory public-health measures was a very old one. Like the sufferers in many previous epidemics, AIDS victims tended to come from already stigmatized social groups: gays, drug abusers and prostitutes, Haitians and Africans. The ability to screen these high-risk groups for the presence of the causative agent, the HIV retrovirus, even at the asymptomatic stage, raised the possibility of compulsory screening measures, quarantine, and isolation. On the other hand, individuals publicly identified as HIV-positive generally found it difficult or impossible to stay employed, to obtain life or health insurance, or to avoid eviction from their homes. In the absence of adequate supportive measures, public-health intervention reinforces existing discrimination against these groups, as in many past epidemics.

An alternative state response has consisted of neglect, on the assumption that AIDS is unlikely to affect the heterosexual, non-drug-abusing, nonpromiscuous majority of the voting public. It is noticeable that, generally, politicians have invested resources in public education and other preventive measures only when they have believed that the majority population is at risk. These problems have been raised again by the recent resurgence of tuberculosis in Western countries, among the HIV-positive but also among the poor and the homeless. Drug-resistant strains of the disease are now common, and the transient, jobless, and destitute have neither the means nor the stability of life-style to complete the lengthy course of drugs that is necessary to effect a cure. The compulsory isolation of victims and their forcible subjection to a course of treatment is not a satisfactory long-term solution to the problem, since reinfection is likely upon release, unless the social and personal circumstances of the affected groups undergo a dramatic improvement.

Conclusion: Ethical implications

The history of epidemics suggests that society's responses have usually included scapegoating marginal and already stigmatized groups and the restriction of their civil rights. From the Jews massacred during the Black Death in medieval Europe, through the beggars and vagrants blamed for the spread of cholera in the nineteenth century, to the prostitutes arrested for allegedly infecting troops with syphilis during World War I, and the minorities whose life-styles were widely regarded as responsible for the spread of AIDS in the 1980s and 1990s, such groups have frequently been subjected to social ostracism and official hostility in times of epidemic disease. Frequently, though not invariably, they have been the very people who have suffered most severely from the disease they were accused of spreading. Doctors have sometimes been reluctant to treat them; the state has often responded with punitive measures.

At no time have public-health measures to combat epidemics been politically uncontested. Nineteenth-century feminists, for example, campaigned vigorously against the state's restriction of the civil liberties of prostitutes in the name of disease control. The fact that their male customers were left free to spread sexually transmitted diseases unhampered by the attentions of the state implied an official endorsement of different standards of morality for men and for women, and it was this major structural element of the social value system that the feminists were seeking to change. Without such change, not only was medical intervention ethically indefensible, but there would never be any likelihood of effective control of sexually transmitted diseases. Similarly, many nineteenth-century epidemics, such as cholera or tuberculosis, were spread by poor nutrition, overcrowded housing, and inadequate sanitation. Social reformers therefore regarded major improvements in these areas as more important than direct medical intervention through measures such as compulsory hospitalization.

Epidemics are frequently caused by social and political upheavals. In the past, movements of large masses of troops and civilians across Europe, from the Crusades to the Crimean War, brought epidemics in their wake. In the early 1990s, a major cholera epidemic broke out in Peru as the result of the flight of thousands of peasants from their mountain settlements, driven out by the pitiless armed conflict between the army and the "Shining Path" guerrillas, to the narrow coastal strip, where they lived in makeshift shantytowns with no sanitation. Eco-

nomic crisis and the dismantling of welfare measures for the homeless, the mentally disturbed, and the destitute in many Western countries in the 1980s contributed to a massive increase in the transient population on the streets of the great cities. Discrimination against AIDS sufferers by landlords and employers has added to this problem. By the early 1990s there were an estimated ninety thousand homeless on the streets of New York City, half of whom were HIV-positive and several thousand of whom were suffering from tuberculosis. Any long-term solution to these epidemics must be more than merely medical, as must any explanation of their occurrence. Public-health measures are thus inevitably political in their implications, since they can be considered and administered only with reference to the wider social and cultural context within which the disease they seek to prevent or control has originated.

RICHARD J. EVANS

Directly related to this entry are the entries PUBLIC HEALTH AND THE LAW; PUBLIC HEALTH; HEALTH SCREENING AND TESTING IN THE PUBLIC HEALTH CONTEXT; *and* HEALTH PROMOTION AND HEALTH EDUCATION. *For a further discussion of topics mentioned in this article, see the entries* AIDS, *article on* PUBLIC HEALTH ISSUES; HEALTH POLICY, *article on* POLITICS AND HEALTH CARE; HOSPITAL; LIFESTYLES AND PUBLIC HEALTH; MEDICAL INFORMATION SYSTEMS; PATERNALISM; PROSTITUTION; *and* WARFARE, *articles on* PUBLIC HEALTH AND WAR, *and* NUCLEAR WARFARE. *For a discussion of related ideas, see the entries* HEALTH AND DISEASE, *article on* HISTORY OF THE CONCEPTS; *and* OCCUPATIONAL SAFETY AND HEALTH. *Other relevant ideas may be found under the entries* HEALTH OFFICIALS AND THEIR RESPONSIBILITIES; JUSTICE; RIGHTS; *and* VALUE AND VALUATION.

Bibliography

BARDET, JEAN-PIERRE; BOURDELAIS, PATRICE; GUILLAUME, PIERRE; LEBRUN, FRANÇOIS; and QUÉTEL, CLAUDE, eds. 1988. *Peurs et terreurs face à la contagion: Cholera, tuberculose, syphilis: XIXe-XXe siécles.* Paris: Fayard.

BRANDT, ALLAN M. 1987. *No Magic Bullet. A Social History of Venereal Disease in the United States Since 1880.* Rev. ed. New York: Oxford University Press.

CARTWRIGHT, FREDERICK F. 1972. *Disease and History.* London: Hart-Davis.

CROSBY, ALFRED W. 1972. *The Columbian Exchange: Biological and Cultural Consequences of 1492.* Westport, Conn.: Greenwood.

DELUMEAU, JEAN. 1990. *Sin and Fear: The Emergence of a Western Guilt Culture, 13th–18th Centuries.* New York: St. Martin's Press.

DUBOS, RENÉ, and DUBOS, JEAN. 1987. *The White Plague. Tuberculosis, Man and Society.* New Brunswick, N.J.: Rutgers University Press.

DUREY, MICHAEL. 1979. *The Return of the Plague: British Society and the Cholera*. Dublin: Gill & Macmillan.

EVANS, RICHARD J. 1987. *Death in Hamburg: Society and Politics in the Cholera Years 1830–1910*. Oxford: At the Clarendon Press.

———. 1988. "Epidemics and Revolutions: Cholera in Nineteenth-Century Europe." *Past and Present* No. 120: 123–146.

FRIEDEN, NANCY M. 1977. "The Russian Cholera Epidemic, 1892–93, and Medical Professionalization." *Journal of Social History* 10:538–559.

KIPLE, KENNETH F. 1984. *The Caribbean Slave: A Biological History*. Cambridge: At the University Press.

———. 1993. *The Cambridge World History and Geography of Human Disease*. Cambridge: At the University Press.

MCNEILL, WILLIAM H. 1979. *Plagues and Peoples*. Harmondsworth, U.K.: Penguin.

PORTER, DOROTHY. 1993. "Public Health." In *Companion Encyclopedia of the History of Medicine*. Edited by W. F. Bynum and Roy Porter. London: Routledge.

ROSEN, GEORGE, comp. 1974. *From Medical Police to Social Medicine: Essays on the History of Health Care*. New York: Social History Publications.

ROSENBERG, CHARLES E. 1987. *The Cholera Years: The United States in 1832, 1849, and 1866*. Rev. ed. Chicago: University of Chicago Press.

VASOLD, MANFRED. 1991. *Pest, Not und schwere Plagen: Seuchen und Epidemien von Mittelalter bis heute*. Munich: C. H. Beck.

EPIDEMIOLOGY AND BIOSTATISTICS

See PUBLIC HEALTH, *article on* PUBLIC-HEALTH METHODS: EPIDEMIOLOGY AND BIOSTATISTICS.

ETHICS

I. Task of Ethics
  Michael Slote
II. Moral Epistemology
  Michael J. Quirk
III. Normative Ethical Theories
  W. David Solomon
IV. Social and Political Theories
  Jean Bethke Elshtain
V. Religion and Morality
  Robin W. Lovin

I. TASK OF ETHICS

Ethics as a philosophical or theoretical discipline is concerned with tasks that concern ordinary, reflective individuals. Since its origins in classical and preclassical times, it has sought to understand how human beings should act and what kind of life is best for people. When Socrates and Plato dealt with such questions, they presupposed or at the very least hoped that they could be answered in "timeless" fashion, that is, with answers that were not dependent on the culture and circumstances of the answerer, but represented universally valid, rational conclusions.

In fact, however, the history of philosophical or theoretical ethics is intimately related to the ethical views and practices prevalent in various societies over the millennia. Although philosophers have usually sought to answer ethical questions without regard to (and sometimes in defiance of) some of the standards and traditions prevalent around them, the history of ethics as a philosophical discipline bears interesting connections to what has happened in given philosophers' societies and the world at large. Perhaps the clearest example of this lies in the influence of Christianity on the history of theoretical ethics.

Philosophical/theoretical ethics, of course, has had its own influence on Christianity, for example, Aristotle's influence on the philosophy of Thomas Aquinas and on the views and practices of the church. Nonetheless, to compare the character of the pre-Christian ethics of Socrates, Plato, Aristotle, the Stoics, the Epicureans, and other schools of ancient ethical thought with the kinds of ethics that have flourished in the academy since Christianity became a dominant social force is to recognize that larger social and historical currents play significant roles in the sphere of philosophical ethics.

Socrates, Plato, and Aristotle, for example, do not discuss kindness or compassion, moral guilt, or the virtue of self-denial, or selflessness. Christianity helped to bring these notions to the attention of philosophy and to make philosophers think that issues framed in terms of them were central to their task. By the same token, a late-twentieth-century revival of interest in ancient approaches to ethics may reflect the diminishing force and domination of Christian thinking in the contemporary world.

But if the concepts that ethics focuses on can change so profoundly, one may well wonder whether a single discipline of ethics can be said to persist across the ages, or even whether such a thing as "the task" of philosophical ethics can be said to endure. Socrates, and later Plato, were perhaps the first philosophers to make a self-conscious attempt to answer general ethical questions on the basis of reason and argument rather than convention and tradition. But was the task they accepted really the same as that of contemporary ethics? This issue needs to be addressed before the task of ethics can be described.

Despite the fact that the concepts and problems of physics have varied over the last few centuries, it is still possible to speak of the history of a single discipline called physics. Moreover, we might say that the task of physics has been and remains that of developing physical concepts for the explanation and description of physical phenomena. Something similar can be said about theoretical ethics. Over the millennia, thoughtful people and philosophers have asked what kind of life is best for the individual and how one ought to behave in regard to other individuals and society as a whole. Although different concepts have been proposed to assist in the task of answering these questions, the questions themselves have retained an identity substantial enough to allow one to speak of the task of philosophical ethics without doing an injustice to the history of ethics.

The history of ethical theories

There has been a good deal less variation in philosophical concepts between those Plato employed and those we employ than there has been in regard to physical concepts within the field of physics. Concepts in philosophical ethics are the instruments with which philosophers address perennial ethical questions, and the distinctive contribution of any given theoretical approach to ethics resides in how (and how well) it integrates such concepts into an overall ethical view.

The concepts of ethics fall into two main categories. The first category comprises notions having to do with morality, virtue, rationality, and other ideals or standards of conduct and motivation; the second, notions pertaining to human good or well-being and the "good life" generally. Notice that morality is only one part, albeit a major one, of the first category. Claims and ideals concerning how it is rational for us to behave are not necessarily "moral" within our rather narrow modern understanding of that notion. Prudence and far-sightedness, for example, are rational, but their absence is not usually regarded as any kind of moral fault; and since these traits are also usually regarded as virtues, it seems we have room for virtues that are not specifically moral virtues. In addition, questions about human well-being and about what kind of life is best to have are less clearly questions of morality, narrowly conceived, than of ethics regarded as an encompassing philosophical discipline. The two categories mentioned above basically divide the concepts of ethics understood in this broad sense, and all major, substantive ethical theories attempt to say something about how these two classes of concepts relate to one another. Since modern views employ concepts and ask specific questions that are more familiar to contemporary readers, these views will be discussed first.

Deontology.   Modern deontology treats moral obligations as requirements that bind us to act, in large measure, independent of the effects our actions may have on our own good or well-being, and to a substantial extent, even independent of the effects of our actions on the well-being of others. The categorical imperative of Immanuel Kant (1724–1804), in one of its main formulations, tells us that we may not use or mistreat other people as a means either to our own happiness or to that of other people, and various forms of moral intuitionism make similar claims (1964). Intuitionists typically differ from Kant in holding that there are several independent, fundamental moral requirements (e.g., to keep promises, not to harm others, to tell the truth). But they agree with Kant that moral obligation is not just a matter of good consequences for an individual agent or for sentient beings generally. Thus even though deontologists such as Kant and, in the twentieth century, W. D. Ross, have definite views about human well-being, they do not think of moral goodness and moral obligation as rooted in facts about human well-being (or the well-being of sentient beings generally); and here a comparison with Judeo-Christian religious thought seems not inappropriate.

The Ten Commandments are not a product of rational philosophy; they have their source in religious tradition and/or divine command. They do, however, represent a kind of answer to the question about how one should behave toward others; that is, they ask the question that philosophical ethics attempts to answer. Moreover, the way the Ten Commandments answer this question is somewhat analogous to the way moral principles are conceived by deontologists such as Kant and the intuitionists.

In religious thinking, the Ten Commandments are not morally binding through some connection to the well-being or happiness of individuals or even the larger community; they are binding because God has commanded them, and deontology seeks to substitute for the idea of a deity, the idea of requirements given by reason itself or of binding obligations perceivable by moral insight. The deontologist typically holds that one's own well-being and that of others are taken into account and given some weight by the set of binding moral requirements, but that these are not the only considerations that affect what we ought to do generally or on particular occasions. For deontologists, the end does not always justify the means, and certain kinds of actions—torture, betrayal, injustice—are wrong for reasons having little to do with good or desirable consequences.

Consequentialism.   The contrast here is with so-called consequentialists, for whom all moral obligation and virtue are to be understood in terms of good or desirable consequences. Typically, this has meant framing some conception of human or sentient good or well-being and claiming that all morality is derivative from or understandable in terms such as "good" or "well-being." Thus Jeremy Bentham, Henry Sidgwick (1981), and other utilitarian consequentialists regard pleasure or the satisfaction of desire as the sole, intrinsic human good, and pain or dissatisfaction as the sole, intrinsic evil or ill, and they conceive our moral obligations as grounded entirely in considerations of pleasure and pain. The idea that one should always act to secure the greatest good of the greatest number is simply a way of saying that whether an act is right or wrong depends solely on whether its overall and long-term consequences for human (or sentient) well-being are at least as good as those of any alternative act available to a given agent. And since classical utilitarianism conceives human good or well-being in terms of pleasure or satisfaction, it holds that the rightness of an action always depends on whether it produces, overall and in the long run, as great a net balance of pleasure over pain as could have been produced by performing any of its alternatives.

This utilitarian moral standard is rather demanding, because it says that anything less than the maximization of overall human good or pleasure is wrong, and that means that if I fail to sacrifice my own comfort or career when doing so would allow me to do more overall good for humanity, then I act wrongly. But apart from the fact of how much it demands—there is nothing, after all, in the Ten Commandments or in the obligations defended by deontologists that requires such extreme sacrifice—what is most distinctive about utilitarianism is its claim that moral right and wrong (and moral good and evil) are totally, not merely partially, concerned with producing desirable results. The end, indeed, does justify the means, according to utilitarianism, and thus one might even be justified in killing, say, one innocent person in order to preserve the lives of two others.

Most deontologists would regard this as the most implausible, vulnerable feature of utilitarian and other consequentialist moral conceptions. But the utilitarian can point out that if you do not make human or sentient happiness the touchstone of all morality, but rely instead on certain "given" intuitions about what morally must or must not be done, you have given yourself a formula for preserving all the moral prejudices that have come down to us from the past. We require, Bentham argued, some external standard by which not only the state of individuals and society, but also all our inherited moral beliefs and intuitions can be properly evaluated. Bentham claimed that judging everything in terms of pleasure and pain can enable us to accomplish this goal. Historically, utilitarianism was conceived and used as a reformist moral and political doctrine, and that is one of its main strengths. If overall human happiness is the measure of moral requirement and moral goodness, then aristocratic privilege and the political disenfranchisement of all but the landed and wealthy are clearly open to attack, and Bentham and his "radical" allied did, in

fact, make use of utilitarian ideas as a basis for making reforms in the British political and legal system.

But not all the reformist notions and energies lie on the side of consequentialism. The version of Kant's categorical imperative that speaks of never treating people merely as means, but always (also) as ends in themselves, was based on the idea of the fundamental dignity and worth of all human beings. Such a notion is clearly capable of being used—and, in fact, has been used—in reformist fashion to defend political and civil rights.

The debate between deontology and consequentialism has remained fundamentally important in philosophical ethics. Although there are other forms of consequentialism besides utilitarianism and other forms of deontology besides Kantian ethics, the main issue and choice has been widely regarded as lying between utilitarianism and Kant. This may be partly explained by the interest contemporary ethics has shown in understanding ethical and political issues as fundamentally interrelated; for both utilitarianism and Kantianism can claim to be "on the side of the angels" in regard to the large questions of social-political choice and reform that have exercised us in the modern period and may well continue to do so.

In the ancient world, the philosophical interest in ethics was also connected to larger political and social issues; both Plato (ca. 430–347 B.C.E.) and Aristotle sought to embed their ideas about personal morality within a larger picture of how society or the state should operate. Moreover, Plato was a radical and a reformer, though the *Republic* takes a direction precisely opposite to that of both utilitarianism and Kantianism. Plato was deeply distrustful of democratic politics and of the moral and political capacities of most human beings. His *Republic* (1974) advocates the rule of philosophers who have been specially trained to understand the nature of "the Good" over all those who have not attained such mystic/intellectual insight. Nor does Aristotle defend democracy. In somewhat milder form, he prefers the rule of virtuous individuals over those who lack—and lack the basic capacity for—virtue. If the ancient world contains any roots of democratic thinking, they lie in Stoicism, which emphasized the brotherhood of man (which seems to leave women out of account), but also spoke of the divine spark in every individual (including women). (Kant took the idea that all human beings have dignity, rather than mere price, from the Stoic Seneca [4 B.C.E.–C.E. 65].)

Virtue ethics.   All schools of ancient ethics defended one or another form of "virtue ethics." That is, they typically conceived what was admirable about individuals in terms of traits of character, rather than in terms of individual obedience to some set of moral or ethical rules or requirements. Ancient ethics was also predominantly eudaimonistic. *Eudaimonia* is the ancient Greek word for being fortunate or doing well in life, and eudaimonism is the view that our first concern in ethics is with the nature and conditions of human happiness/well-being and in particular our own happiness/well-being. This does not mean that all ancient ethics was egoistic, if by that term one refers to views according to which the moral or rational agent should always aim at his or her own (greatest) good or well-being. Aristotle is a clear example of an ethical thinker whose fundamental orientation is eudaimonistic, but who is far from advocating that people should always aim at their own self-interest.

For Aristotle, the question to begin with in ethics is the question of what is good for human beings. But Aristotle argues that human good or happiness largely consists in being actively virtuous, thus tying what is desirable in life to what is admirable in life in a rather distinctive way. For Aristotle, the virtuous individual will often aim at the good of others and/or at certain noble ideals, rather than seek to advance his or her own well-being, so egoism is no part of Aristotelianism.

But certainly most interpreters have regarded the Epicureans as having a basically egoistic doctrine. Epicureanism resembled utilitarianism in treating pleasure and the absence of pain as the sole conditions of human well-being. Rather than urge us to seek the greatest good of the greatest number, however, the Epicureans argued that virtue consisted in seeking one's own greatest pleasure/absence of pain. (Given certain pessimistic assumptions, the Epicureans thought this was best accomplished by minimizing one's desires and simplifying one's life.)

Although there are some notable modern egoists (e.g., Hobbes, Spinoza, and Nietzsche), most recent moral philosophers have assumed that there are fundamental, rational reasons for being concerned with something other than one's own well-being. Moreover, the eudaimonistic assumption that questions about individual happiness or well-being are the first concern of ethics has, in modern times, given way to a more basic emphasis on questions like, "How ought I to act?" and "What obligations have I?" The Jewish and Christian religious traditions seem to have made some difference here. In both traditions, God's commandments are supposed to have force for one independent of any question of one's own well-being (assuming that one is to obey because God has commanded, and not just because one fears divine punishment). For most Christians, moreover, Jesus sacrificing himself for our redemption places a totally non-egoistic motive at the pinnacle of the Christian vision of morality. So the notions that one should always be concerned with one's own well-being, and that ethics is chiefly about how one is to conceive and attain a good life, are both profoundly challenged by any moral philosophy that takes Judaism or Christianity, understood in the above fashion, seriously.

Recent developments

Twentieth-century philosophical ethics bears the imprint of much of the history of the discipline, and many of the more current, prominent approaches to the subject represent developments of historically important views. But earlier in the twentieth century, ethics, at least in Britain and in the United States, veered away from its past in the direction of what has come to be called metaethics. The move toward metaethics and away from traditional ethical theory resulted, in part, from the influence of a school of philosophy called logical positivism. The positivists held up experimentally verifiable science as the paradigm of cognitively meaningful discourse and claimed that any statement that was not empirically confirmable or mathematically demonstrable lacked real content. Since it is difficult to see how moral principles can be experimentally verified or mathematically proved, many positivist ethicists began to think of ethical claims as cognitively meaningless and refused to advance substantive moral views, turning instead to the analysis of ethical terms and ethical claims. Issues about the meaning of moral terms have a long history in philosophical ethics, but the idea that these metaethical tasks were the main task of philosophical ethics gained a prevalence in the early years of the twentieth century that it had never previously had.

In the latter half of the twentieth century, substantive or normative ethics (that is, ethics making real value judgments rather than simply analyzing such judgments) once again came to the fore and tended to displace metaethics as the center of interest in ethics. In particular, there was a resurgence of interest in Kantian ethics and utilitarianism, followed by a renewal of interest in the kind of virtue ethics that dominated the philosophical landscape of ancient philosophy.

The revival and further development of Kantian ethics received its principal impetus from John Rawls and younger philosophers influenced by him. Rawls's principal work, *A Theory of Justice* (1971) represents a sustained attack on utilitarianism and seeks to base its own positive conception of morality and social justice on an understanding of Kant's ethics that bypasses the controversial metaphysical assumptions Kant was thought to have made about absolute human freedom and rationality. Other Kantian ethicists (Christine Korsgaard, Onora O'Neill, and Barbara Herman), however, have sought to be somewhat truer to the historical Kant while developing Kant's doctrines in directions fruitful for contemporary ethical theorizing.

Meanwhile, the utilitarians responded to Rawls's critique with reinvigorated forms of their doctrine, and, in particular, Derek Parfit's *Reasons and Persons* (1984) seeks to advance the utilitarian tradition of ethical theory within a philosophical perspective that fully takes into account the insights of the Rawlsian approach.

Finally, virtue ethics has been undergoing a considerable revival. In a 1958 article, Elizabeth Anscombe argued that notions like moral obligation are bankrupt without the assumption of God (or someone else) as a lawgiver, whereas concepts of character excellence or virtue and of human flourishing can arise, without such assumptions, from within a properly conceived moral psychology. This challenge was taken up by philosophers interested in exploring the possibility that the notions of good character and motivation and of living well may be primary in ethics, with notions like right, wrong, and obligation taking a secondary or derivative place or perhaps even dropping out altogether. Such virtue ethics does not, however, abandon ethics' traditional task of telling us how to live, since, in fact, ideals of good character and motivation can naturally lead to views about how it is best to treat others and to promote our own character and happiness. Rather, the newer virtue ethics sought to learn from the virtue ethics of the ancient world, especially of Plato, Aristotle, and the Stoics, while making those lessons relevant to a climate of ethical theory that incorporates what has been learned in the long interval since ancient times.

More recently, however, a radical kind of virtue ethics without precedent in the ancient world has developed out of feminist thought and in the wake of Carol Gilligan's groundbreaking *In a Different Voice* (1982). Gilligan argued that men tend to conceive of morality in terms of rights, justice, and autonomy, whereas women more frequently think of morality in terms of caring, responsibility, and interrelation with others. And at about the same time as Gilligan wrote, Nel Noddings in *Caring: A Feminine Approach to Ethics and Moral Education* (1984) articulated and defended the idea of a feminine morality centered on caring.

The ideal of caring Noddings has in mind is particularistic: It is not the universally directed benevolence of the sort utilitarianism sometimes appeals to, but rather caring for certain particular people (e.g., one's friends and family) that she treats as the morally highest and best motivation. Actions then count as good or bad, better or worse, to the extent that they exhibit this kind of caring. Clearly, Nodding's view offers a potential answer to the traditional question of how one should live, but since the answer seems to be based on fundamental assumptions about what sorts of inner motivation are morally good or bad, it is a form of virtue ethics. Of course, her view can be stated in terms of the principle "Be caring and act caringly." But if we focus on conform-ing to the principle instead of on the needs of the individuals we care about, we risk falling short of what the principle itself recommends. It is the state or process of sensitive caring, rather than attention to principle, that generates what Noddings would take to be satisfying answers to moral questions and appropriate responses to particular situations.

Enriched by such feminine/feminist possibilities, ethical theory has been actively and fertilely involved with the perennial task(s) of ethics. But because few of the traditional questions have been answered to the satisfaction of all philosophers, one may well wonder whether philosophy will ever be able fully to answer those questions or even whether philosophers have, over the centuries, made real or sufficient progress in dealing with them. But it is also possible to attack the tradition(s) of philosophical ethics in a more radical fashion.

Modern challenges to philosophical ethics

Some modern intellectual and social traditions have questioned the notion that ethics can validly function as a distinct sphere of rational inquiry. One example of such questioning was the widespread view, earlier in the twentieth century, that ethics should confine itself to the metaethical analysis of concepts and epistemological issues (and possibly to the sociological description of the differing ethical mores of different times and places) rather than continue in its traditional role of advocating substantive ethical views. (Metaethics has undergone something of a revival, but largely in a form regarded as compatible with substantive ethical theorizing.)

Historically, various forms of religion and religious philosophy have also posed a challenge to the autonomy and validity of traditional ethics. The claims of faith and religious authority can readily be seen as overriding the kind of rational understanding that typifies traditional philosophical inquiry. Thus, Thomas Aquinas believed strongly in the importance of the ethical issues raised by Aristotle and in Aristotle's rational techniques of argument and analysis; but he also permitted his Christian faith to shape his response to Aristotle and did not fundamentally question the superiority of faith to reason. He believed, however, that reason and philosophy could accommodate and be accommodated to faith and religious authority.

Existentialism.   But more radical religionists have questioned the importance of reason and have even prided themselves in flying in the face of reason. Religious views that stress our dependent, finite, sinful creatureliness can lead one to view philosophical ethics as a rather limited and even perverse way to understand the problems of the human condition. In modern times this religion-inspired critique of ethics and the philosophical received a distinctive existentialist expression in the writings of Blaise Pascal (1966) and Søren Kierkegaard (1960, 1983).

It is very difficult to give a completely adequate characterization of existentialism as a philosophical movement or tendency of thought. It cuts across the distinction between theism and atheism, and some of the most prominent existentialists have, in fact, been atheists. But the earlier theistic existentialism that one finds in Pascal and, more fully developed, in Kierkegaard is principally concerned with attacking rationalistic Western philosophy and defending a more emotional and individualistic approach to life and thought. Plato and Aristotle, for example, sought rationally to circumscribe the human condition by treating "man" as by his very essence a "rational animal" and prescribing a way of life for human beings that acknowledged and totally incorporated the ideal of being rational. But for Pascal, the heart has reasons that reason cannot know, and Kierkegaard regarded certain kinds of rationally absurd religious faith and love as higher and more important than anything that could be circumscribed and understood in rational, ethical, or philosophical terms.

The atheistic Nietzsche (1844–1900) also attacked philosophical ethics and rational philosophy generally by attempting to deflate their pretensions to being rational. Nietzsche saw human life as characterized by a "will to power," that is, a desire for power over other individuals and for individual achievement, and in *The Genealogy of Morals* (1956) he argued that Judeo-Christian ethics, as well as philosophical views that reflect the influence of such ethics, are based in debilitating and poisonous emotions rather than having their source in rational thought or enlightened desire. What comes naturally to man is, he thought, an aristocratic morality that is comfortable with power and harsh in regard to failure, and the idea that the meek and self-sacrificing represents the highest form of human being he took to be the frustrated and angry response of those who have failed to attain power, but are unwilling to admit even to themselves how they really feel.

Nietzsche clearly expressed an antipathy to the whole tradition of philosophical ethics, and even if he did defend an iconoclastic ethics "of the superman," his writings point the way to an attitude like that of the more recent existentialist Jean-Paul Sartre (1905–1980). In his *Being and Nothingness* (1956), Sartre argued that all ethics is based in error and illusion, and he attempted instead to describe the human condition in nonjudgmental, nonmoral terms. Sartre argued that human beings are radically free in their choice of actions and values, and he claimed that all value judgments, because they purport to tell us what we really have to do, involve a misunderstanding, which he called "bad faith," of just how free we actually are. At the end of his book, Sartre proposed to write a future book on ethics,

but also set out, in compelling fashion, the reasons for thinking that any future ethics is likely to fall into error and illusion about the character of human freedom. Here, as in *Being and Time* of Martin Heidegger (1889–1976) which had a decisive influence on Sartre's existentialism, the existentialist philosopher is essentially critical of the role ethical thinking plays in philosophy and in life generally and says, in effect, that if we face the truth about our own radical freedom, we must stop doing ethics. Ethics may think of itself as a rational enterprise, but for Sartre, it was mainly a form of self-deception.

Marxism. Existentialism has had a great influence on Western culture, but Marxism has probably had a much greater influence, and Karl Marx's writings (*Capital* and *The German Ideology*), like those of some of the existentialists, attempt to accustom us to the idea of taking ethics less seriously than practitioners of philosophical ethics have tended to do. According to Marx (1818–1883) (and Friedrich Engels), philosophical ethics and philosophy generally are best understood as expressions of certain class interests, as ideological tools of class warfare, rather than as independently and timelessly valid methods of inquiry into questions that can be settled objectively and rationally.

For example, intellectual, philosophical defenses of property rights can be seen as expressing and asserting bourgeois class interests against a resentful and increasingly powerful proletariat. All philosophy, according to such a view, is merely the expression of underlying economic forces and struggles. A truly liberated view of human history requires us to stop moralizing and start understanding and harnessing the processes of history, using the tools of Marx's own "scientific socialism." While Marx believed that a "really human morality" might emerge under communism, philosophical ethics is seen more as a hindrance than as a means to enlightened understanding of human society.

Psychoanalysis. In addition, psychoanalysis, as a movement and style of thought, has often been taken to argue against traditional ethics as an objective discipline with a valid intellectual task of its own. The psychoanalytic account of moral conscience threatens to undercut traditional ethical views and traditional views of ethics by making our own ethical intuitions and feelings seem illusory. In a manner partly anticipated by Nietzsche, Sigmund Freud's original formulation of psychoanalytic theory (e.g. in *The Interpretation of Dreams* and *Introductory Lectures on Psychoanalysis*) treat conscience and guilt as forms of aggression directed by the individual against himself (Freud, 1989). (Freud [1856–1939] tended to focus on the development of conscience in males.) Rather than attack parental figures he feared, the individual psychologically incorporates the morality of these seemingly threatening figures. If conscience is a function of hatred against one or more parental figures, then its true nature is often obscured to those who have conscience. According to classic psychoanalysis, the very factors that make us redirect aggression in such a fashion also make it difficult consciously to acknowledge that conscience has such a source.

If moral thought has this dynamic, then much of moral life and moral philosophy is self-deluded. However, for some more recent psychoanalysts, not all forms of ethical thinking are illusory. Followers of the British psychoanalyst Melanie Klein (1975) have said that various ethical ideals can and do appeal to us and guide our behavior, once "persecutory guilt" of the kind based in aggression redirected against the self is dissolved through normal maturation or through psychotherapy. Moreover, the analyst Erik Erikson (1964) gave a developmental account of basic human virtues that has clear, ethical significance.

In the end, perhaps it should not be surprising that many attempts to undermine ethics eventually reintroduce something like familiar ethical notions and problems. We have to live with one another, and the problems of making life together possible and, if possible, beneficial are problems that will not and cannot go away. Even if a given society and generation has settled on a particular solution to the problems of living together, new historical developments can make these solutions come unstuck, or at least force people to reconsider their appropriateness. And even if different societies and cultures have different moral standards, it is possible to overestimate the differences. For example, however much aggression societies may allow toward outsiders and enemies, no society has a moral code that permits people, at will, to kill members of that society. Moreover, the very fact of moral differences among different societies indicates a need for cooperative and practical ethical thinking that will enable people either to resolve or live with the differences.

Applied ethics.   This is a point where the need for applied ethics most clearly comes into view. Whether it is in medicine, science, biotechnology, business, or the law, people have to come together to solve problems, and ethics or ethical thinking can play a role in generating cooperative solutions. If existentialism, religion, Marxism, and psychoanalysis all in varying degrees question the need for philosophical ethics, the practical problems of contemporary life seem to indicate some new ways and to highlight some old ways in which philosophical ethics has validity and value.

The explosive development of new knowledge and techniques in medicine and biology has made bioethics one of the central areas of practical, moral concern. And those seeking to solve moral problems in this area naturally appeal to philosophical ethics. To take just one controversial area, the question of euthanasia engages the ideas and energies of different ethical theories in different ways and often with differing results. Thus, the Kantian may focus on issues concerning the autonomy of the dying patient and the right to life, whereas utilitarians will stress issues about the quality of life and the effects of certain decisions on families and society as a whole, and defenders of an ethics of caring will perhaps see less significance in larger social consequences and focus on how a medical decision will affect those most intimately and immediately affected by it.

Applied ethics in our contemporary sense is not new: Socrates' discussion of the duty of obedience to unjust laws in the *Crito* and Henry David Thoreau's of civil disobedience are only two of countless historical instances of what we would call applied ethics. Today, we think, civilization is more complicated and our problems are more complex. Still, in facing those problems, bioethicists, business ethicists, and other applied ethicists typically look to philosophical ethics, to substantive theories like utilitarianism and virtue ethics and Kantianism, and to the criticisms each makes of the others, for some enlightenment on practical issues.

MICHAEL SLOTE

Directly related to this article are the other articles in this entry: MORAL EPISTEMOLOGY, NORMATIVE ETHICAL THEORIES, SOCIAL AND POLITICAL THEORIES, *and* RELIGION AND MORALITY. *For a further discussion of topics mentioned in this article, see the entries* AUTONOMY; CARE; EMOTIONS; FEMINISM; JUSTICE; LIFE; PSYCHOANALYSIS AND DYNAMIC THERAPIES; RIGHTS; UTILITY; *and* VIRTUE AND CHARACTER. *For a further discussion of related ideas, see the entries* JUDAISM; PROTESTANTISM; ROMAN CATHOLICISM; *and* VALUE AND VALUATION.

Bibliography

ANSCOMBE, G. E. M. 1958. "Modern Moral Philosophy." *Philosophy* 33:1–19.

ARISTOTLE. 1962. *Nicomachean Ethics.* Translated by Martin Ostwald. New York: Macmillan.

BENTHAM, JEREMY. 1982. *An Introduction to the Principles of Morals and Legislation.* New York: Methuen.

ERIKSON, ERIK H. 1964. *Insight and Responsibility.* New York: W. W. Norton.

FREUD, SIGMUND. 1989. *A General Selection from the Works of Sigmund Freud.* New York: Anchor.

GILLIGAN, CAROL. 1982. *In a Different Voice: Psychological Theory and Women's Development.* Cambridge, Mass.: Harvard University Press.

KANT, IMMANUEL. 1964. *Groundwork of the Metaphysic of Morals.* 3d ed. Translated by Herbert H. Paton. New York: Harper & Row.

KIERKEGAARD, SØREN. 1960. *Kierkegaard's Concluding Unscientific Postscript.* Translated by Walter Lowrie. Princeton, N.J.: Princeton University Press.

————. 1983. *Fear and Trembling: Repetition.* Translated by Howard V. Hong and Edna H. Hong. Princeton, N.J.: Princeton University Press.

KLEIN, MELANIE. 1975. *Love, Guilt, and Reparation and Other Works, 1921–1963.* New York: Delacorte Press.

LONG, A. A., and SEDLEY, D. N. eds. 1989. *The Hellenistic Philosophers.* 2 vols. New York: Cambridge University Press. See especially vol. 1, sections "Epicureanism" and "Stoicism."

MARX, KARL. 1977. *Selected Writings of Karl Marx.* Edited by David McLellan. Oxford: Oxford University Press.

NIETZSCHE, FRIEDRICH. 1956. *The Birth of Tragedy* and *The Genealogy of Morals.* Translated by Francis Gaffing. Garden City, N.Y.: Doubleday.

NODDINGS, NEL. 1984. *Caring: A Feminine Approach to Ethics and Moral Education.* Berkeley: University of California Press.

PARFIT, DEREK. 1984. *Reasons and Persons.* Oxford: At the Clarendon Press.

PASCAL, BLAISE. 1966. *Pensées.* Harmondsworth, U.K.: Penguin Books.

PLATO. 1974. *Republic.* Translated by G. M. A. Grube. Indianapolis, Ind.: Hackett Publishing.

RAWLS, JOHN. 1971. *A Theory of Justice.* Cambridge, Mass.: Harvard University Press.

ROSS, W. D. 1930. *The Right and the Good.* Oxford: At the Clarendon Press.

SARTRE, JEAN-PAUL. 1956. *Being and Nothingness: An Essay on Phenomenological Ontology.* Translated by Hazel E. Barnes. New York: Philosophical Library.

SIDGWICK, HENRY. 1981. [1907]. *The Methods of Ethics.* 7th ed. Indianapolis, Ind.: Hackett Publishing.

II. MORAL EPISTEMOLOGY

Moral epistemology is the systematic and critical study of morality as a body of knowledge. It is concerned with such issues as how or whether moral claims can be rationally justified, whether there are objective moral facts, whether moral statements strictly admit of truth or falsity, and whether moral claims are universally valid or relative to historically particular belief systems, conceptual schemes, social practices, or cultures.

The subdiscipline of moral epistemology is hardly a recent arrival on the philosophical scene. Plato's *Republic*, Aristotle's *Nicomachean Ethics*, Hume's *Treatise on Human Nature*, Kant's *Critique of Practical Reason*, and Hegel's *Phenomenology of Spirit* all grapple with moral-epistemological themes and issues. However, the lion's share of explicit, self-conscious reflection on moral-epistemological problems has taken place in the twentieth century, reflecting Western philosophy's more general preoccupation with the problem of knowledge since the time of Kant. This article describes and critically evaluates some of the major options in moral epistemology taken during that period.

Intuitionism

When one describes a person as "good," or when one says of an action that it is "the right thing to do" under the circumstances, is one pointing out an objective feature of the person or action, or is one expressing one's own subjective reaction? Is one stating something that could be either true or false? Is one making a claim that could be supported by reasons or evidence, and that would warrant the assent of any rational human being? Or is one merely giving voice to one's own attitudes or feelings? Much of the contemporary debate in moral epistemology turns on the answer to these questions.

Intuitionists, chief among whom were G. E. Moore and W. D. Ross, insist that moral terms such as "good" and "right" name objective properties, refer to real aspects of real things, events, activities, and persons, and claim that we have access to these properties by a form of direct insight or perception. Because of this, moral statements are genuine propositions capable of being assigned a truth value of "true" or "false." To use a technical, philosophical term, morality is "cognitive." Intuitionists, while drawing an analogy between sensory intuition and moral intuition, also generally insist that moral intuition is different in kind from sense perception. While sense perception acquaints us with objective facts, moral intuition acquaints us with equally objective values.

According to G. E. Moore's *Principia Ethica* (1903), "good" is a simple, unanalyzable concept. Like the property concept "yellow," "good" cannot be defined except by pointing out instances of the concept, which enables one to grasp its unitary meaning. Unlike "yellow," which denotes a property intuited by our ordinary sensory apparatus, "good" names a nonnatural property, which, despite the fact that it is not empirically given, is nonetheless just as objective and real as is the property "yellow." W. D. Ross, in *The Right and the Good*, expands Moore's table of simple, objective moral properties to include "duty," or "rightness," and the degrees of rightness that attach to conflicting prima facie duties in different circumstances (Ross, 1930).

Intuitionists like Moore do not deny that there is moral knowledge; in fact, they affirm it emphatically. But for both Moore and Ross, our knowledge of what is ultimately good or right is not inferred or deduced but immediately given; we do not need to define, rationalize, or justify it. Thus a physician, deciding to remove an irreversibly brain-dead patient from a respirator, might give reasons for her decision by citing the beneficial consequences (e.g., an end to the patient's fruitless suffering) that might be achieved, or by insisting that the duty to preserve life is trumped by the higher duty to preserve a patient's dignity. But as to why these consequences are good, or why these putative duties are duties, the intuitionist physician can rightfully appeal only to her perception of the basic quality of goodness or rightness in them. Look and you too shall see.

The very immediacy of moral knowledge poses a serious problem for the intuitionist, namely, how moral argument and moral disagreement are possible. According to Moore, one either "sees" that something is good or one doesn't, and if one doesn't, there's little to be done except to look again. But what if two or more competent moral agents persistently "see" different values in the same circumstances? Who is "seeing" what is really there, and who is "seeing" a moral illusion? The intuitionist faces the difficulty of accounting for genuine moral disagreement—disagreement not about the empirical, factual issues of how to bring about the greatest good or do one's duty, but the evaluative issue of what sorts of things are genuine, intrinsic goods or actual obligations. This faculty of moral intuition is therefore curious. It is supposed to yield insight into objective properties of things, outcomes, deeds, and institutions, yet it lacks any public criterion against which claims like "X is good" or "Y is the morally right thing to do" might be checked and rationally validated.

Emotivism

A number of thinkers influenced by logical positivism, most notably A. J. Ayer and Charles L. Stevenson, rejected intuitionism and with it the conviction that moral discourse was objective and cognitive. The resulting theory, emotivism, denied that "good" or "right" named any sort of objective, intuitable property. Rather, to say of something that it is "good" or "evil," "right" or "wrong," is to express a subjective attitude or emotional response toward it. For example, the proposition, "You ought not to have lied to that patient," asserts nothing more than "you lied to that patient"; the "ought" merely notes an attitude of disapproval on the part of the speaker. Emotivists emphasize the imperative quality of moral utterance. To say lying is wrong is, in effect, to issue the command, "Do not lie." To place ethical discourse in a recognizable context, the effort on the part of agents is to influence the behavior of others and to persuade them to adopt different beliefs. If emotivists like Ayer and Stevenson are right about the meaning of moral statements, the demand to account for "moral knowledge" is senseless, since all moral discourse is inherently noncognitive, nonrational, and subjective.

Perhaps this is an acceptable price to pay to make the phenomenon of moral disagreement intelligible. An intuitionist would be vexed by disagreements such as the following:

(1a) Active, involuntary euthanasia is morally acceptable under certain conditions,

versus

(1b) Active, involuntary euthanasia is always immoral, under any and all conditions.

Yet what for the intuitionist is an epistemological dilemma, for the emotivist is not a dilemma at all. The proponent of (1a) is "commending" the permissibility of involuntary, active euthanasia under certain conditions rather than asserting a true-or-false proposition; she is expressing a "pro-attitude" toward (1a), and trying to persuade others to do so as well. The proponent of (1b) is doing precisely the same thing, expressing an "anti-attitude." The disagreement is one of subjective attitude and feeling and does not concern anything objective; there is no deep, moral truth under dispute.

But perhaps it might be premature to claim that the ability to make sense of moral disagreement thereby vindicates emotivism. One serious difficulty with emotivism is that it narrows the human significance of moral discourse by flatly denying that whenever one makes a moral claim, one places oneself in the position of having to back up that claim by citing what one takes to be good reasons in its behalf.

Universal prescriptivism

Universal prescriptivism is a compromise between emotivism and the commonsense conviction that morality is a rational enterprise. Its chief exponent, R. M. Hare, argues in *The Language of Morals* (1952) that moral imperatives carry certain inexorable rational constraints. If I make the moral judgment, "Active, involuntary euthanasia is wrong," I am in effect declaring that one ought not to perform active, involuntary euthanasia on someone, and thus commanding, "Do not perform active, involuntary euthanasia," where the ought command is issued to anyone in the relevant situation, including me, the speaker. So while moral judgments have an imperative or prescriptive component—like Moore, Hare rejects naturalism—they exhibit a universality that binds the speaker's deeds to her claims, and enables the speaker to use reason to draw further moral conclusions on the basis of prescriptions that function as premises in deductive arguments.

In affirming the role of deductive reason in ethics, Hare's universal prescriptivism challenges the emotivist's assumption that only indicative premises are beyond suspicion in valid argumentation. For surely the following argument is a valid deduction:

(2a) I ought not to lie to my patients and thus intentionally mislead them.
(2b) My patient Bill asked me to tell him about his medical condition.
(2c) I ought not to lie to Bill about his condition.

All its premises are meaningful, and since the major premise is prescriptive, the taboo against deducing an "ought" from an "is" is not violated. Furthermore, (2a) itself could be justified by being a valid conclusion drawn from more general prescriptions:

(2d) I ought not to be unjust.
(2e) To lie to one's patients and thus intentionally mislead them is unjust.
(2f) I ought not to lie to my patients and thus intentionally mislead them.

However, there cannot be an infinite hierarchy of such deductions. For the prescriptivist, one's ultimate prescriptive or evaluative premises are chosen rather than deduced: One cannot ground one's moral convictions in premises more basic. The foundations for moral reasoning cannot themselves have a foundation; they reflect one's basic stance or attitude toward persons and things. No "ought" can be derived from an "is." One's moral first principles, being prescriptions, cannot be rooted in indicative soil.

This might lead one to wonder whether universal prescriptivism is more a refinement of emotivism than a genuine advance on it. It seems to push the point where ethical discourse is a matter of attitude and criterionless choice back to the most general evaluation the agent wishes to make. For example, substitute the following premise for (2a) above:

(2a¹) I ought not to lie to my patients and thus intentionally mislead them *unless* I have ample reason to judge that doing so will confer some psychological or medical benefit to them.

If a physician were to judge that some such benefit were to be obtained from intentional deception, then the conclusion that one may intentionally deceive a patient will follow, in direct contradiction to (2c) and (2f). Given the initial moral orientation, certain principles for action are validated, but the original moral orientation cannot itself be validated; it can only be accepted, endorsed, chosen. Since this nonrational, inaugural choice provides the basis for all subsequent moral reasoning, the content of an agent's morality appears to be ultimately arbitrary, even if it is not arbitrary in all its detail.

Hare disagrees. In *Freedom and Reason* (1963) he argues that universal prescriptivism sets limits on the kinds of fundamental moral choices an agent can make. Consider the following:

(3a) Certain people ought to be persecuted because, and only because, their skin is black.

If moral imperatives using "ought" are, as Hare claims, universal prescriptions, then the agent uttering these words is, or ought to be, committing himself to the proposition that if his skin were black he, too, ought to be persecuted. It is clear that few individuals who make such assertions, apart from those Hare dubs "fanatics," would assent to the latter claim. Yet it is entailed by the universal prescription (3a); hence, the morality of any agent who asserts (3a) and refuses to extend it to cover himself is, for that very reason, rationally inadequate.

Of course, there is no possibility of genuine argument with a genuine "fanatic": The fanatic's assertion of ultimate principles or fundamental commitments, however odious or bizarre they may be, can only be met with counterassertion and not counterreasoning. Hare seems willing to accept this lack of logical resources against fanaticism. Nevertheless it seems reasonable to ask universal prescriptivists such as Hare whether, by cutting off rational argument at fundamental principles, they are granting too much to fanatics by ruling out any way in which their convictions can be criticized, rather than their unpleasant characters. The fanatic may be vile and depraved, but by universal prescriptivist standards, he is not necessarily defective in reason.

Naturalism

Intuitionists, emotivists, and prescriptivists all agree that "facts" are distinct from "values"—that an "ought" cannot be deduced from an "is." G. E. Moore coined the term, "the naturalistic fallacy," to describe the frequent attempts on the part of philosophers to define "the good" by deducing it from some matter of fact about human beings and their desires. A number of philosophers have challenged this no-ought-from-an-is doctrine by providing counterexamples to it, in effect denying that the naturalistic fallacy is a fallacy.

Philippa Foot (1959), for example, has cited "rude" and "courageous" as concepts whose evaluative meaning cannot be pried from their descriptive meaning. The criteria for identifying someone as "rude" or "courageous" are factual. If someone fits a given description, one has warrant for saying that he or she is rude or courageous; thus, the proposition "She is rude/courageous" is cognitive. But to describe someone as rude is to evaluate that person negatively. Consider the absurdity of saying: "You're rude, cowardly, and abusive, but that isn't meant as a put-down." So, according to Foot, valid moral arguments can draw evaluative conclusions from factual premises.

Peter Geach (1956) makes an analogous point in his analyses of "good." To say that a thing is good is to say something concerning the kind of thing it is. "Good" does not mean precisely the same thing in the following sentences: "That car is good"; "that watch is a good watch"; and "Mohandas Gandhi was good." To say of each one of these that it is good is to employ criteria determined by the kind of thing being evaluated. But this is to say, again against the emotivist and the prescriptivist, that the criteria that fix the meaning of evaluative terms such as "good" are not ultimately matters of choice, but rather matters of fact. To know a good watch, one needs to know what a watch is and what it is for; to know a good person, one, likewise, must know what a human being is and those ends at which humans aim in their actions.

Finally, John Searle (1964) accuses noncognitivists of harboring an arbitrarily constricted notion of what constitutes a "fact." Human institutions are part of what is the case, and these "institutional facts" can appear in descriptive premises in valid deductive arguments that generate evaluative conclusions. For example, to acknowledge the institution of promising is to grant that under certain circumstances, when one utters the words, "I promise to do X," one places oneself under an obligation to do X, and therefore is obliged to do X, and therefore one ought to do X. Because institutional facts are determined by the rules guiding the aims and actions of participants, one can deduce values from them.

Naturalists sketch a picture of moral language in which moral concepts are understood by deriving them from nonmoral, "naturalistic" ones, upon which moral knowledge rests. A robust naturalism in bioethics, then, would show no qualms about defining "the good" or "the right" in a medical context by appealing to certain key facts about human beings (e.g., their pain, dignity, mortality, etc.) and about the social and institutional setting for these facts.

At this point, however, the prescriptivist can offer a rebuttal that is difficult to answer on the naturalist's own terms without begging an important question. The prescriptivist concedes that moral language necessarily has a factual or descriptive component, but insists that it also makes ineliminable reference to the agent's desires, aims, and wishes. These can be more or less rational depending on whether their satisfaction interferes with or complements other sets of desires, aims, and wishes, but no desire can be judged rational or irrational per se. These basic desires and attitudes might differ from person to person; there is no escaping the fundamental choice behind all evaluations and prescriptions. So when the naturalist claims to have deduced an "ought" from an "is," either the major premise harbors an implicit prescription (e.g., "One ought to honor institutions like promise-keeping") or the argument is not a strict deduction.

Naturalists might reply that the "natural" premises to which they appeal and that ground moral judgment and description are rooted not in the desires or aims of individuals but in general facts about human nature of which it is the philosopher's job to remind us. For example, Aristotle understood *eudaimonia*, or "human flourishing," to be the good for a human being, because it was a result of acting in accord with one's rational human nature; Thomas Aquinas defined the good in

terms of human creatures' reestablishing a right relation to God; and John Stuart Mill's psychological theories stand behind his definition of the good as pleasure seeking and pain avoidance. Aristotle, Thomas Aquinas, and Mill all pursued ethics in the context of what might be called "philosophical anthropology." Yet this simply elevates the naturalist's dispute with the prescriptivist to a higher level of abstraction. The prescriptivist could deny that there is any fact of the matter that might constrain the choice between philosophical anthropologies, while the naturalist could just as adamantly insist upon it. Thus naturalism might provide a coherent, consistent alternative to prescriptivism, but only by accepting philosophical stalemate at a higher level.

Rationalism

One possible avenue around the prescriptivist/naturalist impasse would be to repudiate the naturalistic fallacy, yet insist that moral principles are justified by examining the nature of rationality itself. This sort of moral epistemology owes much to Kant. A number of notable philosophers, inspired by Kant yet eager to avoid his dubious treatment of the self, have endeavored to ground moral knowledge in the reflective exercise of reason by actual human agents.

The most ambitious of these attempts is clearly that of Alan Gewirth, who in *Reason and Morality* tries to prove the fundamental principle of morality by analyzing the bare concept of rational agency. Every rational agent, Gewirth argues, must presuppose certain generic goods—namely, freedom and a degree of well-being—that make the exercise of his or her agency possible. If the agent must claim these generic goods as necessary, he or she must also claim them as rights. But since these goods flow from the generic features of agency, he or she must also concede that all other agents must claim them as rights, and that there is a corresponding obligation to acknowledge and respect them. Hence, the Principle of Generic Consistency (PGC)—"Act in accord with the generic rights of your recipients as well as yourself" (Gewirth, 1978, p. 135)—is the fundamental, categorical principle of morality, from which all other concrete moral norms and precepts can be derived, and which can be denied only on pain of logical self-contradiction.

Many of Gewirth's critics (e.g., Nielsen, 1984; MacIntyre, 1984; Arrington, 1989) have questioned a crucial move in his dialectical "proof" of the PGC: Acknowledging that there exist necessary goods of rational agency need not entail recognizing them as one's rights. If these critics are correct, Gewirth's foundational moral principle is not necessarily true. If it is only contingently true, Gewirth's claim to a proof of the one fundamental principle of morality has not been vindicated.

In contrast to Gewirth's "hard" rationalism, other moral rationalists adopt a "soft" rationalism that proceeds not from unassailable premises about rational agency, but from contingent truths about what all rational agents would, in fact, choose under ideal conditions. For example, John Rawls, in *A Theory of Justice* (1971), maintains that in a hypothetical "original position," where the specific identities, desires, and advantages of rational agents are deliberately obscured behind a perspective of impartiality—a "veil of ignorance"—rational agreement would be secured regarding two specific principles of justice, equal liberty and equal distribution of goods, except in those cases where an unequal distribution of goods would work to the benefit of the worst-off social group.

"Soft" rationalism proceeds from assumptions about the rational choices individuals would make in imagined, empirical situations; thus it lends itself well to concrete application in such fields as legal, business, and medical ethics. For example, Robert M. Veatch, in *A Theory of Medical Ethics* (1981), argues that the responsibilities of medical professionals are set in an implicit "triple contract" involving those professionals, their patients, and society at large; specifically, medical rights and obligations are fixed by determining what sorts of agreements would be rational for all three interested parties to agree upon.

There are serious difficulties with these "soft" forms of moral rationalism. Rawls's "original position" suggests that individuals could and should be able to abstract themselves from their specific, contingent identities when formulating and justifying the principles of justice. But, as Michael Sandel (1982) and Charles Taylor (1985) have argued, this project faces formidable epistemological difficulties. It presupposes that "the self" is prior to its ends, that one's identity as a pure, rational chooser is separable from and more basic than one's identity as, say, an American, a Christian, a physician, and so on—and that it can and must draw upon rational resources that are neutral with respect to the ends and desires connected with these identities. Yet it is questionable whether such an "unencumbered" self would have any rational resources upon which to draw or any concrete intentions upon which to act; whether, indeed, the contracting chooser in the "original position" could ever be more than a philosophical fiction. Thus it seems as if moral rationalism—if it is to remain on epistemologically solid ground—must compromise its purity by admitting that the contingencies of time, place, and personal identity do make at least some difference in determining which choices and which sets of moral beliefs will be accepted as rational.

Realism and antirealism

Another way to get around the prescriptivist/naturalist standoff would be to insist with the naturalist that there are objective moral truths, but to question whether such truths can be deduced from more basic facts concerning human nature or human institutions. On this "realist" account of moral knowledge (so called because it affirms objective moral realities independent of the knowing subject), moral discourse is less a matter of reason than of careful perception and insight, of developing the capacity to discriminate moral facts and to describe them accurately and adequately. To the extent that moral knowledge rests on "seeing" moral properties, moral realism suggests Moore's intuitionism. Yet, unlike Moore, moral realists claim no special faculty of moral intuition, insist that moral properties are observable in precisely the same way as are empirical properties, and hold that moral judgments and observations are fallible and revisable.

This renewed form of moral realism has been advanced by a number of British philosophers (Platts, 1979; McDowell, 1979; Lovibond, 1983) influenced by Donald Davidson's theory of meaning and Ludwig Wittgenstein's critique of reductionism in the philosophy of language. From Davidson they have borrowed the idea that to know what any sentence means is to be able to specify the conditions under which it is true. From Wittgenstein they have taken the conviction that there is no way to establish a ground for language that is independent of and cognitively superior to actual language in use. Taken together, these Davidsonian and Wittgensteinian commonplaces work to deflate all forms of noncognitivism.

The noncognitivist needs to rely on a contrast between two kinds of utterances—those that carry truth values and those that do not—and thus insists on two kinds of "meaning" and two kinds of discourse. One kind of discourse can accurately represent facts (usually assumed to be science), and the other does not represent facts, but expresses attitudes and imposes those attitudes on a world plastic enough to accept them (art, poetry, morality). But since determining the meaning of any linguistic statement is inseparable from determining whether that which it asserts is true or false, the noncognitivist cannot plausibly draw the required contrast between first-rate, fact-picturing discourse and second-rate, value-projecting discourse. To know what any expression means is to know what would make it true, and this ability neither demands nor supports any assumptions about the superior cognitive reliability of any one form of discourse (scientific) over any other (commonsense, literary, or moral).

The moral realist argues that there are moral facts just as there are scientific facts, and does not expect moral facts to be reducible to or deducible from any other kind of fact. Moral properties are "supervenient" upon nonmoral properties. One discerns a moral property by enumerating a number of nonmoral properties standing in relation to each other, from which the moral property "emerges" without being strictly entailed by them. "Supervenience" becomes clearer when one turns from examining "thin," abstract moral concepts ("good," "right," "duty") to "thick" moral concepts (concrete, specific concepts, like "courage," "loyalty," or "mercifulness"). To know, for example, that a physician's treatment of an end-stage cancer patient with larger than usual doses of painkillers was merciful involves knowing a great number of facts concerning cancer, pain, the special needs of the terminally ill in general and of this patient in particular, and so on. While one does not infer the moral property of being merciful from these nonmoral facts, the property is a function of them; one perceives the moral fact that this act is merciful in and through perceiving the aforementioned nonmoral facts.

"Seeing" the moral facts in the associated nonmoral facts is a complex skill, demanding discipline, practice, and attentiveness to matters of minute detail. For the moral realist, becoming a morally competent bioethicist is largely a matter of acquiring and honing a certain sensibility, akin to that of understanding a work of art or literature, whereby one comes to notice the moral goods and obligations in the context of medical practice, and to disclose and explicate them in descriptive speech.

A number of moral epistemologists (e.g., Mackie, 1977) have complained that the realists' account of supervenience is incoherent. If the supervenient moral properties of a person change (for example, if someone ceases to be courageous or just), it is necessary that other, nonmoral properties also have changed (fleeing from every danger; ceasing to give others their due). Yet if that person possesses all the nonmoral dispositions associated with a moral property (steadfastness in the face of danger; a consistent willingness to keep promises), it cannot be inferred that he or she necessarily possesses the associated moral properties (the person might not be courageous or just, "despite appearances"). Supervenience is supposedly a logical relation between properties, yet because it cannot be interpreted as a form of inference, it becomes an inexplicable fact.

John Mackie subscribes to a form of moral antirealism or "projectivism" that allows for cognitive expressions in moral discourse—that is, the truth or falsity of moral beliefs, the validity or invalidity of moral arguments—yet understands them in an equivocal sense, as a disguised, second-level reflection upon first-level moral judgments and attitudes. The moral idiom forces us to speak as if there were moral facts, but such "facts" are ultimately projections of our attitudes. To insist that moral judgments are more than expressions of attitude would be to reintroduce supervenience, with all its difficulties. Moral antirealists would not exactly deny, then, that moral knowledge is a result of coming to "see things" and describe them in a certain way; they would, however, deny that such descriptions bear more than an instrumental function. The physician who "sees" that a

particular act toward a patient is merciful is indeed "seeing" something, but that something is a function of the physician's subjective attitude projected outward toward the patient.

This may not be cause for genuine worry on the realist's part. He or she could, of course, stand firm and endorse the reality of objective moral facts—the instantiation of "thick," descriptive moral properties such as "courage," "patience," and "mercifulness"—in the face of the logically peculiar notion of supervenience. Perhaps supervenience is an inexplicable logical and epistemological fact. So what? Supervenience is a feature of ordinary moral discursive practice, one that morally competent speakers can handle without much trouble. The difficulties that antirealist moral epistemologists claim to have uncovered are more a matter of their a priori prejudices (perhaps their epistemological "scientism") than their discovery of a defect in moral language and moral practice.

The realist, like Wittgenstein, confidently affirms that ordinary moral language is in good working order as it is. The antirealist, of course, can reply that such "folk" moral philosophy is untidy, plagued with logical ambiguities and desperately in need of philosophical reinterpretation. Thus the clashes between moral realists and moral antirealists recapitulate the earlier standoff between prescriptivists and naturalists. What is at issue is not whether values can be derived from facts, but whether it even makes sense to speak of emergent "moral facts" alongside nonmoral ones.

Against epistemology

Virtually all the various schools of moral epistemology considered seem to employ an ahistorical approach to moral discourse, argument, and judgment. Both prescriptivists and naturalists confidently speak of "*the* language of morals," presupposing that "morality" has a singular essence lurking under all the various "moralities" of human history. Their dispute only concerns what this "essence" might be. Rationalists, realists, and antirealists also claim their particular moral epistemologies for morality per se, as opposed to the morality characteristic of a particular time, place, or community; these epistemologies are seen as perennial options for anyone who wishes to think about ethics.

The assumption that "epistemology" studies the invariant universal structures of human knowledge, entitling it to "legislate" over all knowledge claims, has been the target of sustained philosophical attack in the latter half of the twentieth century by Ludwig Wittgenstein, Martin Heidegger, and John Dewey, among others. Richard Rorty's landmark *Philosophy and the Mirror of Nature* (1979) was one of the first works to point out the affinities between the projects of Wittgenstein, Heidegger, and Dewey. Rorty showed that all three undermined the pretense of "epistemologically oriented philosophy" to have attained a timeless, ahistorical, necessary vantage point in its judgments about knowledge by pointing out, in different ways, how knowledge claims are situated and justified in shared practical and social contexts and are unintelligible apart from such contexts. From Rorty's perspective, the different approaches of moral epistemologists are less important than their common goal of discovering the foundations of moral reason and showing how these foundations might (or might not) be "justified" to any rational person. But Rorty insists that the epistemological assumptions undergirding their "common goals" are baseless. Among those assumptions are the idea that there are moral truths available to human rationality as such, or that "morality," like "knowledge" and "being," is a concept with a unique, stable core meaning. Rorty's Wittgensteinian, Heideggerian, and Deweyan case against foundationalist philosophy thus makes a new, antifoundationalist and self-consciously historical approach to moral knowledge all the more appealing.

Relativism and the feminist critique of objectivity

Antifoundationalism in moral philosophy has taken a number of different forms. One of them, relativism, has once again emerged as a serious option in moral epistemology. The doctrine associated with the ancient Sophists—that objectivity, truth, and knowledge are matters of adhering to sociocultural convention rather than of attaining insight into nature—has been revived and expressed in more sophisticated ways by Gilbert Harman (1975), Bernard Williams (1985), Joseph Margolis (1991), and David Wong (1984). Wong, for example, maintains that the concept of "an adequate moral system" is relative to particular places and times: There is no single, universally valid moral system available, even as an unattainable ideal. Within each extant system, there are resources available for evaluating and criticizing rival systems binding on all who share its standpoint. Wong is neither a subjectivist nor a noncognitivist. There is, however, no standpoint outside all such systems from which judgment could be passed upon each of them indifferently. For Wong, the collapse of epistemological foundationalism, and the acknowledgment that our "moral systems" are not the deliverances of pure, universal human reason but are products of historical contingencies, supports a form of relativism that is less concerned about specific judgments of right or wrong than with the assessment of moral systems or cultures on the widest scale.

Many critics of contemporary relativism have argued that it retains most of the self-referential inconsistencies that plagued its earlier incarnations. Can the relativist maintain that the relativistic thesis is "true" or "reasonable" without begging the question? (See Putnam, 1981.) Other critics argue that the historical contingency of moral beliefs and their lack of necessary epistemic foundations does not imply relativism, since it does not preclude the possibility of one moral system being more rationally adequate than its competitors (see Stout, 1989).

Yet this response elicits a further question: Whose conception of "rationality" is being employed when someone judges a moral system superior or inferior? Several important feminist philosophers have responded to this question by noting that, generally, the "rationality" employed and championed by moral philosophers has been "rationality" as understood and defined by men, who are ideologically biased by their place in a patriarchal social system and who tend to exclude the experiences and judgments of women (Tong, 1989; Code, 1991; Tuana, 1992). The idea that reason and objectivity could be "gendered" concepts has led some feminists to conclude that men and women evince different kinds of moral knowing, and to champion a feminine "ethic of care" as against a masculine "ethic of principles" (Gilligan, 1982), just as it has led others to reject those very "feminine virtues" as yet another aspect of women's oppression by men (Bartky, 1990; Puka, 1990). Whatever the ultimate outcome of these debates, contemporary feminism has done much to reinforce the antifoundationalist and historicist critique of "objectivity" and "rationality" as universal, unproblematic features of human thought and discourse. But does that critique undermine the idea of "moral knowledge" as such?

Historicism, virtue, and tradition

One systematic moral philosopher who disagrees with that sentiment, and who has used the insights of historicism and antifoundationalism in rethinking and recovering a workable notion of "moral knowledge," is Alasdair MacIntyre. *After Virtue* (1984) begins by noting both the interminable and arbitrary character of contemporary moral arguments and the vehemence with which they are conducted, and asks what might account for the powerlessness of contemporary moral philosophy to resolve moral conflict and secure agreement. MacIntyre attempts to answer this question by pursuing a historical inquiry into the succession of moral theories and the social contexts in which they arose. MacIntyre maintains that the intractability of moral disagreement is one aspect of the "emotivist culture" of late modernity that provides no solid basis for making shared, rational moral judgments and thus renders the idea of genuine moral knowledge unintelligible.

Most modern moral theory and practice has dispensed with the Aristotelian idea of a human *telos*, an "end" proper to human beings as such. Modern social and political orders have ceased to define their mission as that of articulating a shared vision of the good life and communally pursuing it, since it is assumed that there is no good-defining end to seek. Then what can moderns claim to "know" when they make ethical assertions, decisions, and judgments? MacIntyre dubs the standard modern response to this question "the Enlightenment project": the task of finding the universal rules or standards that guide conduct yet swing free from any substantive conception of a good life, and are justifiable by appealing to rationality.

All attempts to fulfill the ambitions of the Enlightenment project have failed, according to MacIntyre, by their own standards of success. Kantians, Utilitarians, Humeans, Intuitionists, and so on, all presuppose that there is something universally known or grasped (the Categorical Imperative, the principle of utility, the sentiment of benevolence, the self-validating property of goodness or rightness) that provides an adequate ground for moral judgment and action. Upon closer inspection, however, both the prescriptive force and the specific content of such moral foundations seem arbitrary and local rather than necessary and universal. If this is so, the epistemological universalism of the Enlightenment project functions as a mask, concealing the manipulative, will-driven ambitions of its disciples under guise of the objectivity of universal principle. Friedrich Nietzsche thus stands as both the fruition and the ruin of the Enlightenment project. His achievement is to have revealed that behind the rhetoric of objective, universal rational foundations, the morality of the modern West is yet another arbitrary upsurge of "will to power," and its impending collapse is testament to its own timid denial of this hard truth.

While MacIntyre insists that Nietzsche is certainly right about modern moral theory and practice, he has not thereby shown that all morality falls victim to the same disease. If the history of moral beliefs and moral theories can reveal the bankruptcy of the Enlightenment project and the moral nihilism of Nietzsche's "genealogical" critique of morality, it can also show how the moral philosophies they displaced can succeed where they themselves failed. MacIntyre contends that contemporary Aristotelians can draw upon epistemological resources that both Enlightenment rationalists and Nietzschean skeptics lack.

First, Aristotelians begin thinking about morality with a systematic conception of the virtues, a set of character traits that enable human agents to perfect their natures and thus realize, however imperfectly, their ultimate end. Duties and obligations—what one ought to do—begin to make sense only against the background of belief about what one ought to be. Since virtue is intrinsically connected to a conception of well-being or human flourishing shared by members of a moral community, one can establish a sound, rational motive for being moral, without reducing what one ought to prefer or desire, in light of one's true end, to what one empirically happens to prefer or desire.

Second, by understanding moral behavior as action that proceeds from a character perfected by these virtues, one eliminates the need for thinking of morality as exclusively, or even primarily, a matter of conscientious rule-following. Hence one evades the difficulty afflicting most forms of moral rationalism, that of specifying substantial moral principles, rather than empty generalities, to putatively compel the rational assent of anyone whosoever. For Aristotelians, as MacIntyre understands them, there is no moral knowledge apart from moral education and training, education not so much in assimilating precepts and norms, but in acquiring the skilled moral wisdom (*phronesis*) to express the proper responses and sentiments in the proper way at the proper times.

Finally, Aristotelianism, for MacIntyre, can make sense of the ways in which traditions of rational inquiry and communal practice can sustain a conception of the virtues while subjecting it to both internal scrutiny and external challenge. Most moral epistemologists make the false assumption that morality names a universal phenomenon rooted in universal human reason. If MacIntyre is right, there is no morality except as rooted in particular communities with their own particular traditions concerning the nature of the virtues and their role in promoting human well-being. This might seem to lend comfort to those moral and political conservatives who take reason and tradition to be polar opposites, and who denigrate the former and deify the latter. Yet only by participating in the common life and practices of a tradition can we come to recognize moral reasons as reasons. By dialectically examining and testing these reasons against those of rival traditions of thought and practice, we can confirm or deny their adequacy and provisionally justify our confidence in them. Traditions are the primary bearers of moral reasons; the internal evolution of traditions and the conflicts between alternative traditions indicates the way in which moral knowledge is embodied in time and history, and how moral knowers can yet transcend historical limitations.

Conclusion

The virtue-centered historicism exemplified by MacIntyre might seem, at first, to be yet another item on the menu of moral epistemologies, yet another intellectual position for ethicists to choose and then defend. But it would be a mistake to view it in this way. Moral epistemology, as a historicist like MacIntyre conceives of it, differs from moral epistemology as most moral epistemologists have conceived of it. MacIntyre denies the ability to transcend all traditional allegiances and to spell out the conditions for moral knowledge in general and as such. As MacIntyre suggests, the moral system it would be rational to adopt depends on who one is and how one understands oneself; there is no moral system that is rational without qualification (1988). This is certainly not to suggest a radical moral relativism, since one's initial loyalties, convictions, and self-understandings are precisely what are to be tested by inquiry and comparative criticism. One must begin inquiring somewhere, however, and the only available starting points are within the assumptions and ways of life of the specific traditions one happens to inhabit.

Thus, for historicists like MacIntyre, Rorty, Stanley Hauerwas, and Jeffrey Stout, moral epistemology can no more escape the gravitational pull of human practice and human history than can any other form of inquiry. Since they cannot be detached from the changing, finite traditions that give them rational legitimacy, it may be more accurate to speak of moral epistemologies in the plural rather than a singular moral epistemology.

The implications of historicism for bioethics are, if anything, even more profound. Since claims to moral knowledge are always made within specific traditions of thought and practice, the claims made by bioethicists about informed consent, active and passive euthanasia, paternalism and autonomy will inevitably reflect these particular traditions and will preclude appeal to any neutral ground transcending these traditions to bioethics as such. "Bioethics as such," like "rationality as such," is a post-Enlightenment fiction. Each moral tradition—whether Christian, Jewish, Islamic, or secular—will provide resources for bioethical reflection, but the individual bioethicist cannot escape reflecting and theorizing as a member of his or her tradition, as opposed to being a disengaged, impersonal spectator on "universal values." From the vantage point of historicism, bioethical inquiry and debate need to be reconfigured as conflict among and reconciliation between these traditions, which give moral thought and action their lease on life.

MICHAEL J. QUIRK

Directly related to this article are the other articles in this entry: TASK OF ETHICS, NORMATIVE ETHICAL THEORIES, SOCIAL AND POLITICAL THEORIES, *and* RELIGION AND MORALITY. *For a further discussion of topics mentioned in this article, see the entries* CARE; EMOTIONS; FEMINISM; HUMAN NATURE; UTILITY; VALUE AND VALUATION; *and* VIRTUE AND CHARACTER. *This article will find application in the entries* ABORTION; AUTONOMY; BENEFICENCE; BIOETHICS; DEATH AND DYING: EUTHANASIA AND SUSTAINING LIFE; INFORMED CONSENT; JUSTICE; *and* PATERNALISM. *For a discussion of related ideas, see* CASUISTRY; MEDICAL ETHICS, HISTORY OF, *section on* EUROPE; SCIENCE, PHILOSOPHY OF; *and* SEXISM.

Bibliography

ARRINGTON, ROBERT L. 1989. *Rationalism, Realism, and Relativism: Perspectives in Contemporary Moral Epistemology.* Ithaca, N.Y.: Cornell University Press.

AYER, A. J. 1946. *Language, Truth, and Logic.* New York: Dover.

BARTKY, SANDRA LEE. 1990. "Feeding Egos and Tending Wounds: Deference and Disaffection in Women's Emotional Labor." In her *Femininity and Domination: Studies in the Phenomenology of Oppression,* pp. 99–119. London: Routledge.

BERNSTEIN, RICHARD J. 1983. *Beyond Objectivism and Relativism: Science, Hermeneutics, and Praxis.* Philadelphia: University of Pennsylvania Press.

BLACKBURN, SIMON. 1971. "Moral Realism." In John Casey, ed., *Morality and Moral Reasoning.* London: Methuen.

CODE, LORRAINE. 1991. *What Can She Know? Feminist Theory and the Construction of Knowledge.* Ithaca, N.Y.: Cornell University Press.

DANCY, JONATHAN. 1991. "Intuitionism." In *A Companion to Ethics,* pp. 411–414. Edited by Peter Singer. Oxford: Basil Blackwell.

FOOT, PHILIPPA. 1959. "Moral Beliefs." *Proceedings of the Aristotelian Society* 59:83–104.

———. 1978. *Virtues and Vices: And Other Essays in Moral Philosophy.* Berkeley: University of California Press.

GEACH, PETER T. 1956. "Good and Evil." *Analysis* 17, no. 2:33–42.

GEWIRTH, ALAN. 1978. *Reason and Morality.* Chicago: University of Chicago Press.

———. 1982. *Human Rights: Essays on Justification and Applications.* Chicago: University of Chicago Press.

GILLIGAN, CAROL. 1982. *In a Different Voice: Psychological Theory and Women's Development.* Cambridge, Mass.: Harvard University Press.

GOLDMAN, ALAN H. 1988. *Moral Knowledge.* London: Routledge & Kegan Paul.

GRIMSHAW, JEAN. 1991. "The Idea of a Female Ethic." In *A Companion to Ethics,* pp. 491–499. Edited by Peter Singer. Oxford: Basil Blackwell.

HARE, R. M. 1952. *The Language of Morals.* Oxford: Oxford University Press.

———. 1957. "Geach: Good and Evil." *Analysis* 17, no. 5:103–11.

———. 1963. *Freedom and Reason.* Oxford: At the Clarendon Press.

———. 1964. "The Promising Game." *Revue Internationale de Philosophie* 70:398–412.

HARMAN, GILBERT. 1975. "Moral Relativism Defended." *Philosophical Review* 84, no. 1:3–22.

HAUERWAS, STANLEY. 1979. *The Peaceable Kingdom: A Primer in Christian Ethics.* Notre Dame, Ind.: University of Notre Dame Press.

———. 1986. *Suffering Presence: Theological Reflections on Medicine, the Mentally Handicapped, and the Church.* Notre Dame, Ind.: University of Notre Dame Press.

LOVIBOND, SABINA. 1983. *Realism and Imagination in Ethics.* Minneapolis, Minn.: University of Minnesota Press.

MacIntyre, Alasdair C. 1966. *A Short History of Ethics.* New York: Macmillan.

———. 1984. *After Virtue: A Study in Moral Theory.* 2d ed. Notre Dame, Ind.: University of Notre Dame Press.

———. 1988. *Whose Justice? Which Rationality?* Notre Dame, Ind.: University of Notre Dame Press.

———. 1990. *Three Rival Versions of Moral Enquiry: Encyclopaedia, Genealogy, and Tradition.* Notre Dame, Ind.: University of Notre Dame Press.

Mackie, John L. 1977. *Ethics: Inventing Right and Wrong.* New York: Penguin.

Margolis, Joseph. 1991. *The Truth About Relativism.* Oxford: Basil Blackwell.

McDowell, John. 1979. "Virtue and Reason." *Monist* 62, no. 3:331–50.

———. 1988. "Values and Secondary Qualities." In *Essays on Moral Realism.* Edited by Geoffrey Sayre-McCord. Ithaca, N.Y.: Cornell University Press.

McNaughton, David. 1988. *Moral Vision: An Introduction to Ethics.* Oxford: Basil Blackwell.

Moore, G. E. 1903. *Principia Ethica.* Cambridge: At the University Press.

Nielsen, Kai. 1984. "Against Ethical Rationalism." In *Gewirth's Ethical Rationalism: Critical Essays with a Reply by Alan Gewirth*, pp. 59–82. Edited by Edward Regis, Jr. Chicago: University of Chicago Press.

Platts, Mark de Bretton. 1979. *Ways of Meaning: An Introduction to a Philosophy of Language.* London: Routledge & Kegan Paul.

Pigden, Charles R. 1991. "Naturalism." In *A Companion to Ethics*, pp. 421–431. Edited by Peter Singer. Oxford: Basil Blackwell.

Puka, Bill. 1990. "The Liberation of Caring: A Different Voice for Gilligan's 'Different Voice.'" *Hypatia* 5, no. 1:58–82.

Putnam, Hilary. 1981. *Reason, Truth, and History.* Cambridge: At the University Press.

Rawls, John. 1971. *A Theory of Justice.* Cambridge, Mass.: Harvard University Press.

———. 1985. "Justice as Fairness: Political not Metaphysical." *Philosophy and Public Affairs* 14, no. 3:223–251.

Regis, Edward, Jr., ed. 1984. *Gewirth's Ethical Rationalism.* Chicago: University of Chicago Press.

Rorty, Richard. 1979. *Philosophy and the Mirror of Nature.* Princeton, N.J.: Princeton University Press.

Ross, W. D. 1930. *The Right and the Good.* Oxford: At the Clarendon Press.

Sandel, Michael. 1982. *Liberalism and the Limits of Justice.* Cambridge: At the University Press.

Sayre-McCord, Geoffrey, ed. 1988. *Essays on Moral Realism.* Ithaca, N.Y.: Cornell University Press.

Searle, John R. 1964. "How to Derive 'Ought' from 'Is.'" *Philosophical Review* 73, no. 1:43–58.

Stevenson, Charles L. 1944. *Ethics and Language.* New Haven, Conn.: Yale University Press.

———. 1963. *Facts and Values: Studies in Ethical Analysis.* New Haven, Conn.: Yale University Press.

Stout, Jeffrey. 1989. *Ethics After Babel: The Languages of Morals and Their Discontents.* Boston: Beacon Press.

Taylor, Charles. 1985. "The Nature and Scope of Distributive Justice." In *Philosophy and the Human Sciences.* Vol. 2 of his *Philosophical Papers.* Cambridge: At the University Press.

Tong, Rosemarie. 1989. *Feminist Thought: A Comprehensive Introduction.* Boulder, Colo.: Westview.

Tuana, Nancy. 1992. *Woman and the History of Philosophy.* New York: Paragon House.

Veatch, Robert M. 1981. *A Theory of Medical Ethics.* New York: Basic Books.

Williams, Bernard. 1985. *Ethics and the Limits of Philosophy.* Cambridge, Mass.: Harvard University Press.

Wong, David B. 1984. *Moral Relativity.* Berkeley: University of California Press.

———. 1991. "Relativism." In *A Companion to Ethics*, pp. 442–450. Edited by Peter Singer. Oxford: Basil Blackwell.

III. NORMATIVE ETHICAL THEORIES

The concept of normative ethics was invented early in the twentieth century to stand in contrast to the concept of metaethics. In ethical theories prior to the twentieth century, it is impossible to discern any sharp distinction between what have come to be called metaethics and normative ethics. In the first half of the twentieth century, however, this distinction began to structure ethics as an intellectual discipline and it continues to be influential at the end of the twentieth century even though crucial theoretical supports for it have disappeared.

Normative ethics was regarded as that branch of ethical inquiry that considered general ethical questions whose answers had some relatively direct bearing on practice. The answers had to be general rather than particular in order to distinguish normative ethics from casuistry; they had to have a bearing on practice in order to distinguish normative ethics from metaethics. Casuistry was understood in its classical sense as the study of particular cases, while metaethics was understood originally as the inquiry into the semantics of ethical language.

G. E. Moore's classic proposal for the structure of ethics distinguished three key questions: (1) What particular things are good? (2) What kinds of things are good? and (3) What is the meaning of "good"? (Moore, 1903). The first question is the central question of casuistry, while the second question falls within normative ethics, and the third, within metaethics (although Moore used neither the term "metaethics" or "normative ethics" in his early work). Normative ethics as a field of inquiry, then, is positioned somewhat precariously between the detail of casuistry and the abstractness of metaethics.

The character of normative ethics was also strongly influenced in the first half of the twentieth century by the almost universal acceptance of the principle of moral neutrality. This principle, accepted by virtually all mainstream Anglo-American moral philosophers from the 1930s to the 1960s, asserted that the results of metaethical investigations were logically independent of normative ethics. When coupled with the original understanding of metaethics as an account of the meaning of key ethical terms, it implied that such semantic investigations were logically irrelevant to inquiries about how to live. Under the influence of this principle, normative ethics was largely abandoned by Anglo-American moral philosophers in favor of a single-minded pursuit of metaethical inquiry. And since the metaethical views most in favor during this period were various forms of noncognitivism (e.g., emotivism and prescriptivism), it was regularly asserted that normative ethics should be relegated to preachers, novelists, and other nonphilosophers. The widely accepted noncognitivist views held that there was no cognitive content to normative ethical judgments since these judgments were primarily expressions of attitudes (as emotivists held) or primarily expressions of prescriptions (as prescriptivists held). But if normative judgments had no cognitive content—if, that is, they were primarily the expression of noncognitive attitudes or imperatives—then it was unclear why moral philosophers should be concerned with examining them. Normative ethics was regarded as largely a matter of exhortation and was removed from the standard repertoire of strictly philosophical concerns.

This sharp distinction between metaethical and normative inquiry, however, together with the relegation of normative ethics to nonphilosophical inquiry, was too unstable to last. Philosophers increasingly recognized that the principle of moral neutrality was not a theoretically neutral presupposition of ethical inquiry but rather drew a considerable amount of its support from the prevailing noncognitivist view. When these noncognitivist views were severely challenged in the late 1950s and 1960s (by, among others, Philippa Foot, Kurt Baier, Stephen Toulmin, and Alan Gewirth), the sharp distinction between metaethics and normative ethics was blunted; this opened the way to a resurgence of interest in normative ethics, expressed by new attempts to reformulate and to defend classical ethical views. Although a complete historical explanation of the remarkably sudden return of philosophers in the 1960s and 1970s to the classical questions of normative theory will no doubt be extremely complex, the decline of noncognitivism and the concomitant rejection of a sharp distinction between normative ethics and metaethics surely contributed to it. Classical Kantian theory was developed in a creative and persuasive manner by John Rawls and his student, Thomas Nagel, along with Alan Don-

agan, Alan Gewirth, and others. Utilitarianism received new attention from, among others, Richard Hare and his students Derek Parfit and Peter Singer. The classical Aristotelian/Thomist view was reformulated and defended by Elizabeth Anscombe, Peter Geach, Alasdair MacIntyre, and like-minded moral philosophers.

What was revived under the label "normative ethics," however, was not identical to what had previously been neglected by moral philosophers as normative ethics. The watershed in ethical theory in the 1960s changed not only the interests of moral philosophers but also changed their conception of their discipline. The task of metaethics was expanded from the narrow one of clarifying the semantics of ethical terms to a much broader investigation of the whole range of metaphysical, epistemological, and semantic questions associated with ethical inquiry. Metaethics came to be concerned not only with questions about the meaning of ethical terms and judgments, but also with metaphysical questions about the nature of ethical properties and epistemological questions about how claims to ethical knowledge are to be appraised. Normative ethics in turn came to be understood as that pole of ethical theory that stood closest to practice. Whereas previously the distinction that most clearly structured ethical inquiry was the distinction between metaethics and normative ethics, the crucial distinction increasingly came to be that between ethical theory and applied ethics.

Ethical theory was distinguished from applied ethics by being both more general and more abstract, and also by being less driven by a concern that its results would have some immediate consequences for action or policy. Within ethical theory, however, elements coexisted that, according to earlier views, would have been sharply distinguished as metaethical and normative. Ethical theory inquired into the epistemological and metaphysical features of ethics as well as into the most general truths about how we should live. Also, the new conception of ethical theory held that these two kinds of inquiry were continuous; it was not possible to pursue either kind without attending to its implications for the other. Ethical theory had become a seamless web with areas of greater or less practical relevance, roughly corresponding to those areas earlier distinguished as the normative and the metaethical.

One consequence of these complex historical developments is that it has become much more difficult to give a precise characterization of normative ethics than it would have been at an earlier time. Nevertheless, certain common assumptions about the nature of normative ethics, as well as a widely shared taxonomy of the varieties of normative theory, have persisted through these developments in the concept of normative ethics. The common assumptions include the claim that the central task of normative ethics is to define and to defend an adequate theory for guiding conduct. The received taxonomy divides normative theories into three basic types: virtue theories, deontological theories, and consequentialist theories. The following section will examine these three types of normative theory with the aim of exploring their distinctive features.

Types of normative theory

The basis for distinguishing the three types of normative theory lies in three universal features of human actions. This recourse to the features of actions should not be surprising, since the aim of normative theory is to guide action. Every human action involves (1) an agent who performs (2) some action that has (3) particular consequences. These three features may be set out as follows:

$$P \longrightarrow + + + + + + + + +$$
Agent   Action   Consequences

If Jones tells a lie to Smith that causes Smith to miss his train, then Jones is the agent, his telling a lie is the action, and Smith's missing the train is one of the consequences of the action. Difficulties arise, of course, in many cases in determining whether someone is an agent in a particular case (e.g., if Jones is insane when he shoots the president, is he really the agent of any action?); or the nature of the particular action performed (e.g., if Jones is cutting down a tree, believing reasonably that he is the only one in the forest, but Smith wanders by and the tree falls on him, causing his death, does a killing take place or merely a death?); or what the consequences of a particular action may be (e.g., if Jones tells Smith "Take the stuff," but Smith understands him to say "Take the snuff," with the consequence that he takes the snuff and due to a hitherto undiscovered allergy becomes ill, is his illness a consequence of Jones's action in saying "Take the stuff"?). These are difficult questions, of course, and they have been much discussed in contemporary action theory in philosophy. In the typical case of human action, however, agent, action, and consequences can be identified, and the typical case provides the basis for the widely shared taxonomy of normative theories.

Ethical or broadly evaluative judgments can also be classified using a taxonomy drawing on these features of human action. Some ethical judgments are primarily evaluations of agents, such as "Jones is a compassionate doctor" or "Smith is a conscientious nurse." In these cases the object evaluated is a particular person, and he or she is evaluated as a possible or actual agent of an action. Some other ethical judgments are primarily about actions in the narrow sense, such as "Jones has a duty to tell the patient the truth about the diagnosis" or "The direct killing of the innocent is always wrong." In

these cases, the primary object of ethical evaluation is an action—the thing done or to be done. This action may be characterized either as required ("X must be done") or as permitted ("X would be right to do) or as forbidden ("A would be wrong to do." More concrete characterizations of actions are also possible, such as "X was a vicious action" or "X was a heroic action." In all of the cases, however, the action is the primary object of evaluation.

A third class of ethical judgments is primarily about states of affairs or objects that are neither agents nor actions, such as "Health is more important than money" or "Human suffering is a terrible thing." Ethical judgments like these do not, directly at least, evaluate either agents or actions. However, the objects evaluated in them, may be, and frequently are, the possible consequences of actions. Thus, this last class of judgments can also be matched to one of the three basic features of human action.

Normative theories may have any of three basic structures, and the differences among these structures are determined by which of the three kinds of practical judgments is taken as basic by a particular theory. *Virtue* theories take judgments of agents or persons as most basic; *deontological* theories take judgments of actions as most basic; and *consequentialist* theories take judgments of the possible consequences of an action as more basic. The sense in which a theory takes a judgment of a certain kind as most basic will become clear in the discussion of each type of theory.

Virtue theories. Normative theories that regard judgments of agents or of character as most basic are called virtue theories because of the central role played in them by the notion of a virtue. In the context of these theories, a virtue is understood as a state of a thing "in virtue of which" it performs well or appropriately. In this broad understanding of virtue not only human beings possess virtues but also certain inanimate objects—a virtue of a knife, for example, will be a sharp blade. Indeed, anything that can be said to have a function or role attached to it because of the kind of thing it is may be said to possess virtues, at least potentially.

A virtue theory takes judgments of character or of agents as basic in that it regards the fundamental task of normative theory as depicting an ideal of human character. The ethical task of each person, correspondingly, is to become a person who has certain dispositions to respond in a characteristic way to situations in the world. Differences among persons may be of quite different kinds. Some people are shorter or fatter than others, some more or less intelligent, some better or worse at particular tasks, and some more courageous, just, or honest than others. These differences can be classified in various ways: physical versus mental differences, differences in ability versus differences in performance, and so on. Those features of human beings on which virtue theories concentrate in depicting the ideal human being are states of character. Such theories typically issue in a list of virtues for human beings. These virtues are states of character that human beings must possess if they are to be successful as human beings.

Typically, a virtue theory has three goals:

1. to develop and to defend some conception of the ideal person
2. to develop and to defend some list of virtues necessary for being a person of that type
3. to defend some view of how persons can come to possess the appropriate virtues.

Virtually all ancient moral philosophers developed normative ethical theories of this sort. The ethical theories of Plato and Aristotle, in particular, provide models of this kind of normative ethical theory. As a consequence, the particular disputes that occurred among ancient philosophers centered on questions that one would expect to arise within a virtue perspective. What are human virtues? How are they acquired? Are they essentially states of knowledge? Can one know that a certain trait of character is a virtue without possessing it? Is it possible to have one, or a few, of the virtues without possessing all of them? Are all human virtues of the same type or are there fundamentally different kinds? Are human virtues a matter of nature or of convention? And, most important of all, what is the correct list of moral virtues? Much of the discussion of ethics in ancient Greece centered on a particular short list of virtues—justice, temperance, courage, and wisdom—that came to be called the *cardinal virtues*. After the introduction of Christianity into Europe, these four virtues were joined by faith, hope, and charity—the so-called *Christian virtues*—to form the seven virtues; these, together with the seven deadly vices, dominated medieval thinking about ethics.

One can also see how questions of human character are basic according to virtue theories by seeing how questions about (1) which actions one ought to perform and (2) which consequences one ought to bring about are subordinated to questions of human character. For a virtue theory the question "Which actions ought one to perform?" receives the response "Those actions that would be performed by a perfectly virtuous agent." Similarly, those states of affairs one is required to bring about in the world as a consequence of one's actions are those states of affairs valued by a perfectly virtuous person. Of course, particular actions may also be required by one's particular virtues. For example, someone who possesses the virtue of honesty may be required by the virtue itself to tell the truth in certain cases. Or someone may be required to pursue certain consequences by certain virtues. For example, an agent who has the virtue of be-

nevolence may be required to pursue the happiness or well-being of others. But these requirements are derivative from the virtues, and the fundamental ethical question thus remains a question about the correct set of virtues for human beings.

Deontological theories.   Deontological normative theories take moral judgments of action as basic, and they regard the fundamental ethical task for persons as one of doing the right thing—or, perhaps more commonly, of avoiding doing the wrong thing. While virtue theories guide action by producing a picture of ideal human character and a list of virtues constitutive of that character, deontological theories characteristically guide action with a set of moral principles or moral rules. These rules may refer to particular circumstances and have the following form:

Actions of type T are never (always) to be performed in circumstance C.

Or, they may be absolute in that they forbid certain actions in all circumstances and have the following form:

Actions of type T′ are never to be performed.

The essential task of a deontological theory, then, is twofold:

1. to formulate and to defend a particular set of moral rules
2. to develop and to defend some method of determining what to do when the relevant moral rules come into conflict.

One must qualify, however, the claim that deontological theories make rules fundamental in ethics. What is fundamental, in fact, are actions themselves and their moral properties. This emphasis on actions can take either of two forms: A normative theory may guide action by requiring agents to perform certain kinds of action that can be specified by a rule or other general action guide. Alternatively, one might regard normative theories as requiring particular actions that in their "particularity" elude specification by a rule. This difference has led some moral philosophers to distinguish two forms of deontological normative theories: *rule deontological theories*, which guide action in the first manner, and *act deontological theories*, which guide action in the second. Virtually all influential deontological theories, however, have taken a rule form and, for this reason, this discussion will continue to emphasize the centrality of rules.

Just as a virtue theory subordinates judgments of actions and consequences in a characteristic way, a deontological theory subordinates judgments of character and consequence. The state of character ethically most important in a deontological view is *conscientiousness*— that state of character that disposes persons to follow rules punctiliously, whatever the temptations may be to make an exception in a particular case. Conscientiousness does not have value in itself, but it has value derivatively because it is the most important state of character for ensuring that persons follow rules and, hence, that they do what is right. In a similar way, the consequences of actions that deontologists are most concerned with are the consequences of particular rule-followings. Not all of an agent's practical life, however, need be reduced to rule-following. An agent may have certain personal ideals or particular projects that exist apart from moral rules. These personal ideals or personal projects may be pursued, according to the deontologist, but their pursuit is permitted only if it does not violate the moral rules. Moral rules define the limits of practical pursuits and projects. They are the moral framework within which nonmoral matters can go on. And this is the sense in which moral rules with their emphasis on judgments of actions are basic, according to the deontological view.

Just as virtue theory has its historical roots in the moral philosophy of ancient Greece, deontological theories have affinities with legalistic modes of thought characteristic of Judaic and later Roman thought. The Decalogue (Ten Commandments), although it functions in a religious context, provides a model of a set of rules of conduct that are basic in much the same way rules function in a deontological theory. One is required to follow the rules in the Decalogue because they are the commandments of God, and reasons can be given why it is appropriate to do what God tells one to do. When a deontological theory is deployed in a secular context, however, this reason for rule-following is necessarily absent. Nor can deontologists require that rules be followed because doing so is necessary to become persons of a certain sort or because doing so is necessary to bring about certain consequences. If they took the first route, their view would become a *virtue* theory; if they took the second route it would become a *consequentialist* theory. For a view to be genuinely deontological, it must claim that an agent's fundamental ethical task is to perform certain actions and that the value of this task cannot be dependent on the value of either virtues or consequences.

The most profound attempt to defend this view was anticipated in ancient moral philosophy by the Stoics and was developed in its most persuasive form by the modern German philosopher Immanuel Kant. The Stoics claimed that moral rules are expressions in the human realm of laws of nature and that rational creatures are required to follow these rules because, as creatures, they are parts of nature and, as such, obligated to bring their action in line with natural forces. Human beings differ from other objects of nature by possessing both freedom and reason. Since they are free, they may act against nature; since they have reason, however, they can understand natural laws and choose to bring their action in line with such forces. Kant's view agrees with the Stoic view in broad outline, but he develops the notions of freedom and reason far beyond the Stoic view. Kant's ultimate answer to questions about how we discover the correct set of moral rules is that only by following the dictates of reason can we be genuinely free.

Consequentialist theories.   Consequentialist normative theories take judgments of the value of the consequences of actions as most basic. According to these theories, one's crucial ethical task is to act so that one will bring about as much as possible of whatever the theory designates as most valuable. If a particular consequentialist theory designates, for example, that pleasure is the only thing valuable in itself, then one should act so as to bring about as much pleasure as possible. The goals of a consequentialist theory itself are threefold:

1. to specify and to defend some thing or list of things that are good in themselves
2. to provide some technique for measuring and comparing quantities of these intrinsically good things
3. to defend some practical policy for those cases where one is unable to determine which of a number of alternative actions will maximize the good thing or things

Like deontological theories, consequentialist theories can be divided into act and rule varieties. *Act consequentialism* requires agents to perform the particular action that in a particular situation is most likely to maximize good consequences. *Rule consequentialism* requires agents to follow those moral rules the observance of which will maximize good consequences. The difference between these two forms of consequentialism, however, is not as straightforward as it may at first seem. It is particularly difficult to precisely characterize rule consequentialism. Is the agent supposed to follow those rules that, if followed by everyone, would maximize good consequences, or rather those rules that will maximize goodness, regardless of how other agents act? There are a number of similar difficulties in characterizing rule consequentialism, and these difficulties have led some moral philosophers to deny that there is a genuine distinction here at all. They have argued, indeed, that when any form of rule consequentialism is rigorously characterized it will be found to degenerate into a form of act consequentialism.

For consequentialists, the distinction between *instrumentally* good things and *intrinsically* good things is also of special importance. Instrumentally good things are good only insofar as they play some role in bringing about intrinsically good things. If, in a particular case, some thing that is ordinarily instrumentally good does not stand in the appropriate relation to an intrinsically good object, then its goodness evaporates. Its goodness is merely dependent. Intrinsically good things, on the contrary, are good not because of any relation in which they may stand to other things. Their goodness is independent because it is constituted by the kind of thing the good thing is. Thus, a particular consequentialist theory may hold that only pleasure is intrinsically good, but that other things, including types of action and states of character, are instrumentally good. The virtue of honesty, for example, might be regarded as instrumentally good by such a theory since honesty is likely to contribute to maximizing human happiness. Even if honesty is typically instrumentally good, however, situations may arise in which one could maximize pleasure by acting deviously rather than honestly. In such cases, a consequentialist theory (complications about rule versions of the theory aside) would hold that one should perform the devious action. According to this view, there is nothing about honesty in itself that is good.

Consequentialist theories find their fullest expression in modern thought, especially in the thought of the British utilitarians Jeremy Bentham, John Stuart Mill, and Henry Sidgwick. Drawing on earlier work in the British empiricist tradition, the classic utilitarians claimed that the only intrinsically good thing is human happiness, which they understood as constituted by pleasure and the absence of pain. The utilitarian maxim, "Act always in such a way as to promote the greatest happiness to the greatest number," has been the paradigmatic consequentialist moral principle and has inspired many more recent consequentialists.

There was much disagreement among classical utilitarians, however, about the details of their view. Can pleasures be distinguished qualitatively as well as quantitatively? What role should rules and virtues play within the practical thought of a utilitarian? How can the flavor of the absolute prohibitions associated with justice and the inviolability of the person be preserved within a utilitarian framework? These questions, along with other similar ones, were answered differently by different utilitarians. They were at one, however, in aspiring to formulate and defend a particular version of consequentialism.

The distinction above between the instrumentally and intrinsically good makes it possible to specify more clearly what a consequentialist theory is and to overcome certain difficulties of definition that may creep in. If a consequentialist theory is characterized as one that specifies some object, state of affairs, or property that should be maximized, one might ask whether the object or state of affairs referred to in this definition might be either a state of character or the performance of certain

actions. If so, then the distinctions between a consequentialist theory, on the one hand, and a deontological theory or a virtue theory, on the other, seems to be in jeopardy. If the intrinsically valuable things specified by a consequentialist theory can include actions or states of character, then virtue theories and deontological theories would seem to be mere species of consequentialism, distinguished from other forms of consequentialism by the type of thing they specify as intrinsically valuable. Virtue theories would be consequentialist theories that specify states of character as intrinsically valuable; deontological theories would be consequentialist theories that specify the performance of certain actions as valuable. If deontological and virtue theories are merely varieties of consequentialism, however, there are not three basic structures but rather one basic structure with a number of varieties.

One might deal with this difficulty by defining a consequentialist theory as one that specifies what is intrinsically good but includes neither states of affairs nor actions, but this seems arbitrary. In addition, although this solution no longer allows that deontological theories and virtue theories are varieties of consequentialism, it does not make it possible to understand how these three types of theory exhibit different structures. One can see that there are different structures here, however, by looking more closely at the differences among these theories. Suppose that a particular consequentialist theory specifies certain virtues as the only intrinsically valuable things. Suppose, more specifically, that a particular consequentialist theory, C, specifies that the virtue of justice is the only intrinsically valuable thing. One can also suppose that a virtue theory, V, specifies the good for human beings such that it is constituted solely by the virtue of justice. Are these two theories practically equivalent? If virtue theories are a mere variety of consequentialism, they should be. If they are not, then virtue theories are not a mere variety of consequentialist theory.

One can see that these two theories are not practically equivalent by considering the practical requirements each imposes on an agent. C requires that an agent act in such a way that he or she will maximize the number of just persons. Since consequentialist theories require that agents maximize whatever is intrinsically valuable, and since the only intrinsically valuable thing according to C is the virtue of justice, agents are required by this theory to maximize justice. V, however, need not have this consequence. What V requires of an agent is that he or she develop those virtues that are constitutive of being a good human being. V requires, then, merely that an agent develop justice. There is nothing in V itself that requires an agent to try to bring about justness in others. A virtue theory more complicated than V may include a virtue—perhaps benevolence—that requires agents to promote the well-being of others as well as themselves. But this requirement to maximize the number of people who possess virtues is not a requirement derived from the nature of a virtue theory itself. It can be derived only from some particular virtue that may—or may not—be a component of a particular virtue theory.

One can arrive at this same point by considering an agent who finds herself in a situation where she can maximize the number of just persons only by becoming herself unjust. In order to make others just, she must become unjust. One example of such a case might be a politician who believes that the best way to make the citizens of her country just is to acquire political power and to exercise it in ways that only she can succeed in doing. Also, suppose she knows that only by renouncing justice herself, by being prepared to act unjustly, can she acquire political power. Thus it is only by becoming unjust that she can most efficiently make others just.

What do C and V have to say to this agent? It is clear that C would approve the renunciation of justice on her part if that would maximize the number of persons who possess justice. The loss of this particular agent's own justice to the sum of justice in the world is more than offset by the gain in the number of persons who are just. The sacrifice is worth it. But what would V require? It is equally clear that V does not require the agent to sacrifice her own justice. Virtue theories hold that an agent's own character plays a special role in his or her practical thinking that it does not play in a consequentialist theory. A virtue theory gives agents reasons to act because it is supposed that each person wants to be a flourishing and fulfilled human being. An agent's own life and character then will have a certain primacy according to a virtue theory. Virtues are not just intrinsically valuable things that should be inculcated in as many agents as possible. They are states of character that each agent must acquire in order to succeed as a human being. Thus, V will not necessarily require that this agent become unjust even if this would maximize the amount of justice in the world.

Similar conclusions follow with regard to a comparison between consequentialist theories and deontological theories. Consider a particular consequentialist teleological theory, C′, that specifies that the only intrinsically valuable things are acts of truth-telling, and a particular deontological theory, D, that specifies that the only moral rule is one that enjoins truth-telling in all cases. Are these two theories practically equivalent? Again it is useful to consider a case in which maximizing a particular good requires the renunciation of it by an agent. Suppose that an agent finds himself in a situation in which he can most efficiently produce the maximum

ratio of truth-tellings to lyings by himself telling a lie. Perhaps he has discovered that, by telling others that whenever they tell a lie their life is shortened by three weeks, he can most efficiently promote truth-telling. But he also knows that this is a lie. What should he do?

It seems clear that C′ would require him to act in whatever way will maximize the number of truth-tellings, and, if this requires him to lie, so be it. Although his lie may be intrinsically bad, its badness will be more than outweighed by the intrinsically good states of affairs it brings about. The person who accepts D, however, believes that there is a moral rule enjoining everyone always to tell the truth. This rule gives him a reason to act, because he is committed to doing the right thing. He is not committed primarily to bringing about as many right or dutiful actions as possible; rather, he is committed to doing the right thing. Just as a virtue theory holds that an agent stands in a more intimate relation to his own character than he does to the characters of other persons, a deontological theory holds that an agent stands in a more intimate relation to his own actions than he does to the actions of others. The action of an agent who follows a moral rule will have a different moral significance for a deontologist than the action of an agent who brings it about that someone else follows a moral rule. For a deontologist, it is not as important that there be rule-followings as that he or she follow moral rules. D need not then require, or even permit, that the agent tell a lie if this is necessary to maximize truth-telling, and hence C′ and D, like C and V, are not practically equivalent. If they are not practically equivalent, however, then deontological normative theories, like virtue theories, are not mere varieties of consequentialism.

Deeper differences among normative theories

This comparison of virtue, deontological, and consequentialist normative theories suggests that the differences among them are deeper than might at first appear. Indeed it suggests that while they certainly differ with regard to which of the three kinds of practical judgments they take as most basic, there are other, and more fundamental, differences among them. To accept one of these normative theories is to accept a particular attitude toward the relation of an agent to his or her character and actions. If one adopts a virtue theory, one's own character comes to have an especially important place in one's practical thinking. It is of the first importance that one become a person of a certain sort. This view need not imply, as it may seem to, that one is committed to an egoistic or selfish life. One may be guided by a virtue theory to pursue a life dominated by generosity and concern for others. One may, indeed, strive to become completely selfless in the sense of always putting the needs of others ahead of one's own needs. But even if this is one's goal, it is also true that one's own character forms the primary focus of one's practical life. The apparent combination here of concern for self and concern for others may appear paradoxical, but it is surely not incoherent. Some of the greatest moral heroes—for example, Gandhi, Jesus, and Albert Schweitzer—seem to have combined these two concerns in their lives.

In a similar way, if one adopts a deontological theory, one's own actions come to play an especially important role in one's practical thinking. It makes a difference to one that one's actions are wrong. It is more important practically to an agent that he or she has told a lie than that a lie has been told. In cases where one's telling a single lie will prevent three others from telling lies, one will not decide what to do by simple arithmetic. Of course, a deontologist will not expect that others will have the same concern for her lie as she will have for it. She may recognize that for someone else, his telling a lie will have a different practical significance for him than *her* telling a lie will have for him. And just as she may not be prepared to tell one lie to prevent him from telling two, she will not expect him to tell one lie to prevent her from telling two. Indeed, she will recognize that from his point of view, his telling one lie is worse in an important sense than her telling two, just as from her point of view her telling one lie is worse than his telling two.

The special significance given to one's actions by a deontological theory need not imply that a deontologist is egoistic or, in the ordinary sense of the term, self-centered. In this way the deontologist is in a situation similar to that of the virtue theorist. The particular moral rules that one is required to follow may give the needs and interests of others parity with one's own, or, more likely, they may require one to put others ahead of oneself. What they cannot require is that one take up a particular attitude toward the rules themselves. The rules cannot, as it were, define their own condition of application—nor can they specify how they relate to one's faculty of practical decision making at the deepest level.

To a consequentialist, giving this special significance to one's character or one's actions may seem confused and possibly morally corrupt. Of course, consequentialists may be concerned with questions of character, but character cannot be their central normative focus. According to consequentialism, what is of primary ethical importance is that the amount of the intrinsically valuable be maximized. Determining the most effective means for maximization involves straightforward questions of efficiency. These questions may be neither simple nor easily answered, but structurally they are straightforward: Which of the possible courses of action will most likely maximize the amount of goodness in the world? In canvassing the possible means to this end, the consequentialist requires an agent to throw his own character and actions into the same category with other possible means. The kind of character one should develop depends upon the kind of character that will contribute most to the relevant goal. The actions one should perform depend similarly on consequentialist goals. For a consequentialist, one must put a certain distance between oneself—considered as the agent who must make practical choices—and one's own character and actions. One's character and actions have the same role in one's practical thinking as would any other possible means—one's wealth, for example, or influence—that are in a more usual sense external. More important, one's own character and actions have no more special role in practical thinking than do the character and actions of others. All are regarded as possible means to maximize intrinsically good things, and one's own actions and character may have special significance only insofar as they may be more easily—because more directly—manipulated by oneself.

One might think, however, that one feature of the agent's character cannot be treated as a mere means, even by a consequentialist. For any consequentialist theory, it will surely be important that persons have those states of character that dispose them to pursue or to favor intrinsically good things. It might be argued that this state of character cannot be treated by the theory as a mere means. But this argument underestimates the resources within consequentialism for distancing an agent from his or her character. Suppose an agent holds a consequentialist normative theory, C'', according to which the only intrinsically good things are states of human pleasure. Suppose also that this agent has a character such that he is disposed always to act in ways he believes will maximize human pleasure. This argument suggests that this agent will not be prepared to sacrifice for the goal of maximal pleasure his own disposition to pursue this goal. But why should this be the case? One might think that a case could never arise in which an agent could contribute most to maximizing pleasure by changing his character to that of someone unconcerned with maximizing pleasure. But this view is surely wrong. Suppose the agent discovers an empirical law according to which human pleasure is maximized only if agents are disposed not to pursue human pleasure but to pursue knowledge. But if this is true—and it is surely possibly true—the agent should act to change as many persons' characters as possible from pleasure-seeking to knowledge-seeking characters. Nor is there any reason why, on consequentialist grounds, this agent should make an exception in his or her own case. So even those features of human character that lead an agent to pursue the maximization of intrinsically good things are not given a special place by consequentialists. Every feature of the character of an agent may be regarded as a possible means to the maximization of the relevant goal.

This feature of consequentialist theories was first emphasized by Henry Sidgwick, the greatest of modern utilitarians. Sidgwick was convinced that if the utilitarian goal of human happiness was to be maximized, then it was necessary that most persons *not* be utilitarians. Indeed, he thought that what was probably required was that most persons hold deontological views and have their character shaped in accordance with such views. He proposed then, for utilitarian reasons, that utilitarianism be propagated as an esoteric view, and that only a few of the most able and intelligent members of society have their characters shaped in accord with it (Sidgwick, 1972). These bearers of the esoteric view, in turn, would mold the characters of those less able and enlightened in accord with a deontological perspective. Had Sidgwick's enlightened few become convinced that maximal human happiness required that they, too, acquire "deontological characters," simple consistency would have required them to change their own characters appropriately. In this way, consequentialism might require that agents strive to bring about a world in which no one, not even oneself, has the kind of character that would dispose one to strive at the most basic practical level for consequentialist goods.

Justifying normative theories

The question of how, if at all, one can rationally choose among these three normative theories is a question taken up under the topic of moral epistemology. It is important to note here, however, that these normative theories emerge in Western thought as components in comprehensive philosophical theories developed by Plato, Aristotle, Aquinas, Kant, Mill, and other major philosophers. They are embedded in rich and complex worldviews in ways that make it difficult to discuss them in isolation from their theoretical and historical settings.

The tendency within contemporary ethical theory is to discuss the merits of these views in purely ethical terms and to ignore to a large extent their larger theoretical settings. Thus, consequentialism is frequently attacked because it is alleged to countenance the judicial punishment of the innocent if that is required for achieving some good end. In arguments like this one, the alleged ethical implications of a normative theory are appealed to in order to evaluate the theory. Similarly, deontologists may be criticized for holding that certain actions are morally forbidden even if performing them in a particular case might prevent an enormous tragedy. It is now a matter of record that these arguments

have been unsuccessful in producing agreement within normative ethics. Nevertheless, the same slightly tired arguments continue to be made.

The lesson from the history of these views would seem to be, however, that if any of them is to be adequately defended, or successfully criticized, its theoretical setting must be taken into account. Each of these theories has complex relations with particular philosophical accounts of rationality, explanation, nature, intention, the law, the passions, and other topics of central philosophical interest. A more adequate account of them, if possible here, would have to take these theoretical entanglements into account. Certainly any serious attempt to choose rationally among them would have to locate them in this larger theoretical setting.

Normative ethics and practice

The raison d'être for normative ethics, as we have seen, is to guide action, and the theories explored above have been developed with such guidance in mind. There is general disagreement, however, about exactly how these normative theories are to relate to the resolution of particular normative problems. It is not easy to demonstrate how the debate between consequentialists and deontologists is related to more concrete disagreements about physician-assisted suicide or recombinant DNA research. Part of the difficulty arises from the fact that each of the three normative theories embodies a particular conception of how it relates to concrete normative problems. There is no theory-independent criterion of how normative theories are to guide action, since each theory embodies a view about its own application. In this way normative theories double back on themselves with regard to their action-guiding function.

An illustration of this doubling-back phenomenon is found in current debates about the relation of virtue theories to practice. Virtue theories are frequently criticized because they do not yield concrete action guides in the way that consequentialist and deontological theories appear to do. The moral advice to "Be just" lacks the action-guiding bite of either a moral rule that requires an agent to perform certain actions or a consequentialist conception that specifies some good to be maximized. But this objection fails to take account of the distinctive way in which virtue theories purport to guide action. A central claim of virtue theories is that the action-guiding function of a normative theory is not to resolve concrete puzzles about action. Edmond Pincoffs, a leading contemporary virtue theorist, coined the useful term "quandary ethics" precisely to designate what virtue theories are against: a conception of normative ethics as guiding action by giving a particular solution to quandaries about action. If one supposes that the only way in which a normative theory can guide action is by resolving particular moral quandaries, then one is unlikely to take virtue theories seriously.

Virtue theories offer, however, an alternative account of the action-guiding function of normative theories. They claim that an adequate normative theory will prescribe something like a training program to make agents ethically "fit." This program may not specify exactly how one is to act in particular cases, because these decisions are best left to the prudential decisions of a "morally fit" agent in the concrete decison-making situation. Thus, virtue theories double back on themselves and specify how they are to relate to practice. Both deontological and consequentialist theories also contain such self-referential accounts of their own application.

An important implication of this doubling-back phenomenon is that one cannot assess the adequacy of normative theories by invoking a well-defined criterion for "successful" action-guiding without begging the question. To have such a well-defined criterion is already to have taken a position on some of the fundamental questions in normative ethics.

This difficulty is actually even more serious than this first point suggests. It is not just that each of the three normative theories embodies a well-defined criterion of how normative theory should relate to practice. Also, there are a number of different models of how general ethical thinking should relate to concrete practice. Some of these models have loose affinities with some of the normative theories, but there is not a fixed or necessary connection between them. Indeed, the conflicts among the normative theories cut across, in complex ways, the conflicts among these models for relating normative theory to practice. A representative collection of these models would include: (1) deductivism, (2) dialectical models, (3) principlism, (4) casuistical models, and (5) situation ethics. These models have been for the most part badly defined in the current literature, and the differences among them and their relations to traditional normative theories tend to be matters of dispute.

Deductivism. The deductivist model regards the action-guiding function of ethical theory to be the development of highly abstract and general first principles that, together with some factual description of a particular morally problematic situation, will entail concrete action guides. According to this model, moral principles developed and defended within normative ethical theory will play the role of premises in deductive arguments for ethical judgments about particular cases. This model of application is particularly attractive to some deontologists and consequentialists. It is related to more general accounts of justification in contemporary epistemology that suggest that all justification must come from some set of foundational claims in the area in question. It also makes large demands on the justificatory resources of a normative theory, since all of the justification for the

principles must come from the theory itself. There is no "bottom up" justification from particular moral beliefs to general principles, as will be found in some of the other models.

Dialectical models. Partly because of worries about the foundationalist character of deductivism, some moral theorists understand the relation between normative theory and practice in a dialectical way. Instead of supposing that justification is exclusively "top down," they suppose that there is dialectical interplay between the principles in a normative theory and particular moral judgments. Normative principles may be modified if they fail to fit our deeply held particular moral beliefs, just as our particular beliefs may be modified in order to fit principles. Whether agents modify principles or particular judgments will depend upon their degree of commitment to each and to the other beliefs they might hold. Just as the deductivist model has affinities with foundationalist theories in epistemology, the dialectical model is inspired by coherentist epistemological theories, which suggest that justification in general is to be understood as a function of how large sets of propositions "hang together" or cohere. The most influential form of the dialectical model is John Rawls's "method of reflective equilibrium," which he uses to support his deontological normative theory.

Principlism. Some philosophers have wanted to downplay the importance of normative theory for resolving concrete ethical problems. They emphasize, for example, that consequentialist and deontological normative theories in most cases mandate the same actions, and that it is only in exceptional cases that differences seem to emerge. And they add that the exceptional cases are likely to be so difficult to resolve that both consequentialists and deontologists disagree among themselves about what normative theory requires. They conclude that general ethical reflection should focus on what they call "middle-level" principles, that is, not the most general principles in any normative theory but those that are likely to be acceptable to adherents of different normative theories. They hope that agreement may be easier to achieve in practical matters if the premises for practical arguments are not sought at the deepest level of normative theory. This model has been especially influential in bioethics and has been developed and defended by Tom Beauchamp and James Childress (1989). The middle-level principles they propose are labeled autonomy, beneficence, nonmaleficence, and justice. Their claim is that these principles, when suitably refined, are likely to be acceptable to both rule consequentialists and deontologists.

Casuistical model. Some philosophers have understood genuinely practical and action-guiding thinking in a way that makes it even more remote from the disputes among the classical normative theories. They propose that the appropriate model for practical reflection is found in the case-based approach popular in late medieval and early modern moral thought. According to this approach, ethical reflection should focus on certain paradigm cases of morally good action or morally bad action. Arguments from these paradigm cases to more problematic cases may be made by exploring similarities and differences between the two. This approach rejects attempts to formulate the goodness or badness of paradigm cases in abstract and general principles, and emphasizes analogical as opposed to deductive reasoning. Albert Jonsen and Stephen Toulmin (1988) have been the leading advocates of this model in recent normative ethics.

Situation ethics.   Some might suggest that situation ethics is not so much a model for practical thinking as a rejection of any model. It claims that one should approach the resolution of particular moral problems by eschewing all general action guides in favor of concentrated attention to the details of the particular situation. In some of its versions it may look a bit like the casuistical model; but in its most radical formulations it would mandate that even paradigm cases should play no central role in particular reflection because they could deflect the agent's attention from the particular features of the case under consideration. Among contemporary thinkers, Joseph Fletcher has been the most prominent advocate of this view, although his early commitment to situation ethics developed later into a more general commitment to consequentialism. In his formulation of situation ethics, he suggests that reflection on particular cases should be guided by the general principle, "Do the loving thing!" However, he is insistent that this principle does not play the role of a premise in any deductive practical argument.

These five models represent different ways of thinking about how ethical reflection might be brought to bear on particular moral problems. They range from deductivism, in which successful ethical reflection requires premises drawn from an adequate normative theory, to situation ethics, which eschews any dependence on normative theory. The other three theories occupy the middle ground between these two extremes. In contemporary ethics there is no consensus on which of these models is most adequate. Each has its defenders and its critics, and there is a lively discussion in the contemporary literature about their respective merits.

When this disagreement about the correct approach to concrete ethical reflection is added to the disagreement among classical normative theories, it is easy to see why contemporary applied ethics involves conflicts of such depth and complexity. One is confronted not only with competing normative theories, but also with competing conceptions of how such theories would relate to concrete ethical problems. These two different

levels of disagreement indeed tend to reinforce one another, since particular disagreements at each level tend to be tied to particular disagreements at the other.

Normative theories and bioethics

The revival of normative ethics in the 1960s was associated with a general renewed interest, across Western culture, in applied ethics and especially in bioethics. Rational reflection on the difficult ethical issues associated with the expanded technological resources of the biological sciences demanded a theoretical structure of some richness, and the classical normative theories provided that structure.

The conflicts between deontological and consequentialist theories have been particularly salient in discussions within bioethics. Indeed, some general discussions of bioethics and many popular textbooks treat these two options as if they are the only possible theoretical perspectives. Part of the explanation for this is surely that so many of the ethical problems in medical practice, as well as in the biological sciences more generally, involve questions about whether actions that are generally regarded as morally problematic can be justified in cases where they appear to promise great benefits. Examples of this kind of conflict are plentiful in contemporary bioethics: Can information obtained by a physician in a doctor–patient encounter be revealed to a third party without the patient's consent, if doing so will prevent some great harm? Can physicians lie to their patients in cases where doing so will increase the effectiveness of therapy and decrease the chances of severe depression? Can physicians override the religious objections of patients to certain therapies when it is clear that these therapies will provide important benefits to the patients?

Moral difficulties like these have been at the center of contemporary discussions in bioethics from its inception. They lend themselves to an analysis that regards them as embodying a general conflict between the thought that some actions (e.g., revealing confidential information, lying, or paternalistic interference) are simply not to be done and the thought that one should be prepared to do whatever is necessary so that things go as well as they can. This conflict in turn seems very close to the fundamental issues at stake between the deontologist and the consequentialist.

Until recent years, virtue theories have been conspicuously absent from most discussions of bioethics. The renewed interest in these approaches is associated with their revival within moral philosophy generally. But there are also features of contemporary bioethics that explain the attention they receive. First, a kind of impasse has developed between consequentialist and deontological approaches to some bioethical problems, and bioethicists have turned to virtue theories with the hope that they can avoid this impasse. Second, there is a new interest in questions about the character of the various agents (e.g., physicians, nurses, researchers, and technicians) who work in settings where bioethical issues arise. This interest in character is partially a reflection of impatience with "quandary ethics." It also, however, grows out of the search for new models of moral education. Molding and shaping character has seemed to many a more attractive goal for moral education than the goal of inculcating rules. Shaping character indeed seems especially important in bioethics, where change is endemic and rules become outdated quickly.

Finally, virtue theories seem to be attracting more attention within bioethics because of the strong analogies between the notion of health and overall biological fitness, on the one hand, and, on the other, the more general notion of human flourishing that lies at the heart of virtue theories. For those who think that bioethical issues are best approached by getting clear on the goals of the biomedical sciences, this analogy is likely to lead them to take virtue theories seriously.

In spite of the recent revival of virtue ethics both within bioethics and within moral philosophy more generally, however, the dominant argumentative strategies in bioethics continue to be drawn from the deontological and consequentialist traditions. Nevertheless, each of the three traditions is now represented in the contemporary bioethical discussion by competent and enthusiastic advocates, and it seems certain that the central problems within bioethics will continue to be discussed in terms contributed by these normative traditions.

W. David Solomon

Directly related to this article are the other articles in this entry: TASK OF ETHICS, MORAL EPISTEMOLOGY, SOCIAL AND POLITICAL THEORIES, *and* RELIGION AND MORALITY. *For a further discussion of topics mentioned in this article, see the entries* ACTION; CARE; CASUISTRY; EMOTIONS; FIDELITY AND LOYALTY; FREEDOM AND COERCION; MEDICAL ETHICS, HISTORY OF, *section on* EUROPE, *subsection on* ANCIENT AND MEDIEVAL; OBLIGATION AND SUPEREROGATION; RIGHTS; UTILITY; *and* VIRTUE AND CHARACTER. *For a discussion of related ideas, see the entries* AUTONOMY; COMPASSION; DOUBLE EFFECT; *and* NATURAL LAW.

Bibliography

ANSCOMBE, G. E. M. 1958. "Modern Moral Philosophy." *Philosophy* 33:1–19. An influential attack on deontological and consequentialist normative theories and defense of a virtue approach to normative ethics.

BEAUCHAMP, TOM L., and CHILDRESS, JAMES F. 1989. *Principles of Biomedical Ethics.* 3d ed. New York: Oxford University Press. The most discussed contemporary defense of principlism.

BRANDT, RICHARD. 1979. *A Theory of the Good and the Right.* Oxford: At the Clarendon Press. A defense of ideal rule utilitarianism.

BROAD, CHARLIE D. 1930. *Five Types of Ethical Theory.* London: Routledge & Kegan Paul. An early attempt to develop a taxonomy of normative ethical theories.

DONAGAN, ALAN. 1977. *The Theory of Morality.* Chicago: University of Chicago Press. A defense of a comprehensive deontological normative theory.

FLETCHER, JOSEPH. 1966. *Situation Ethics: The New Morality.* Philadelphia: Westminster. The classic statement and defense of situation ethics.

FOOT, PHILIPPA. 1978. *Virtues and Vices; And Other Essays in Moral Philosophy.* Berkeley: University of California Press. A collection of influential articles defending a virtue approach to normative theory.

FRANKENA, WILLIAM K. 1973. *Ethics.* 2d ed. Englewood Cliffs, N.J.: Prentice-Hall. An influential discussion of the taxonomy of normative theories.

JONSEN, ALBERT R., and TOULMIN, STEPHEN E. 1988. *The Abuse of Casuistry: A History of Moral Reasoning.* Berkeley: University of California Press. The most important recent discussion of the casuistical model.

KITTAY, EVA FEDER, and MEYERS, DIANA T., eds. 1987. *Women and Moral Theory.* Totowa, N.J.: Rowman and Littlefield. A useful recent collection of articles developing the feminist critique of moral theory.

MACINTYRE, ALASDAIR C. 1981. *After Virtue: A Study in Moral Theory.* Notre Dame, Ind.: University of Notre Dame Press. The most important recent restatement and defense of an Aristotelian virtue theory.

MOORE, G. E. 1903. *Principia Ethica.* Cambridge: At the University Press.

NAGEL, THOMAS. 1970. *The Possibility of Altruism.* Oxford: At the Clarendon Press. An important defense of a deontological theory.

PARFIT, DEREK. 1984. *Reasons and Persons.* Oxford: At the Clarendon Press. The most sophisticated recent defense of utilitarianism.

RAWLS, JOHN. 1971. *A Theory of Justice.* Cambridge, Mass.: Harvard University Press. The most influential recent statement and defense of a Kantian deontological theory and a dialectical model for the justification of normative principles.

ROSS, W. D. 1930. *The Right and The Good.* Oxford: At the Clarendon Press. An enormously influential statement and defense of a deontological normative theory. It also contains important criticisms of consequentialism.

SCHEFFLER, SAMUEL, ed. 1988. *Consequentialism and Its Critics.* Oxford: Oxford University Press. A useful recent collection of articles exploring consequentialism.

SIDGWICK, HENRY. 1907. *The Methods of Ethics.* 7th ed. London: Macmillan.

SMART, JOHN JAMESON CARSWELL, and WILLIAMS, BERNARD A. 1973. *Utilitarianism: For and Against.* Cambridge: At the University Press. An important exchange between a prominent consequentialist and a critic of consequentialism.

WILLIAMS, BERNARD A. 1985. *Ethics and the Limits of Philosophy.* Cambridge, Mass.: Harvard University Press. A recent criticism of the very idea of a normative theory.

IV. SOCIAL AND POLITICAL THEORIES

Every social and political theory is entangled with ethics. The great political philosopher Jean-Jacques Rousseau proclaimed that the person who would separate politics from ethics will fail to understand both. Despite the efforts of practitioners of "value-free social science," the concepts and categories with which political theorists work—order, freedom, authority, legitimacy, justice—are part and parcel of competing ethical frameworks. It is very difficult to talk about justice without talking about fairness. What is fair is an ethical question that cannot be adjudicated without some reference to what is good for human beings or what kind of good human beings may strive to attain. Terms that circulate within ordinary discourse, such as "fairness" and "freedom," are also central themes within social and political thinking. The implication for bioethics is straightforward. No matter how strenuously the bioethicist may hope to isolate his or her perspective from metaphysical, ontological, epistemological, and civic imperatives, social and political theory frames and penetrates all bioethical considerations.

The human sciences cannot be value-free. In Charles Taylor's words, "they are moral sciences in a more radical sense than the eighteenth century understood" (Taylor, 1971, p. 51). There are, according to Taylor, inescapable epistemological arguments for what might be called an interpretive approach to the human sciences, for human beings are self-defining animals. These self-definitions, in turn, take place within a context that shapes our understanding of self and other as well as our appreciation of human possibilities and the need for constraint. We are caught in conceptual webs. It is the task of social and political theory to make more explicit the nature of the frameworks within which we think and act, and hence, the context within which bioethical imperatives make themselves felt, whether as advances in human freedom, triumphs of human control, or dangerous new forms of oppression. Based on an interpretive approach to political theory, this article will demonstrate why political theory must be normative and will go on to rehearse contemporary debates in social and political theory using the public/private distinction and the women's movement as illustrative examples.

Why social and political theory must be normative

Terms of ordinary discourse serve as a conceptual prism through which we view different human relationships, activities, and forms of life. Most of the time we take such terms for granted. We are all shaped by ways of life that are built upon basic notions and rules. Political theorists concern themselves with the ways in which a society's constitutive understandings either nourish or deplete human capacities for purposive activity. It is, therefore, one task of the political theorist to examine critically the resources of ordinary language, revealing latent meanings, nuances, and shades of interpretation others may have missed or ignored. When we examine our basic assumptions, we enhance our ability to sift out the most important issues (Elshtain, 1981).

Society's understanding of the terms "public" and "private," for example, are always defined and understood in relationship to each other. One version of private means "not open to the public," and public, by contrast, is "of or pertaining to the whole, done or made in behalf of the community as a whole." In part these contrasts derive from the Latin origin of "public," *pubes,* the age of maturity when signs of puberty begin to appear: Then and only then does the child enter, or become qualified for, public activity. Similarly, *publicus* is that which belongs to, or pertains to, "the public," the people. But there is another meaning: public as open to scrutiny; private as that not subjected to the persistent gaze of publicity. The protection of privacy is necessary, or so defenders of constitutional democracy have long insisted, in order to prevent government from becoming all-intrusive, as well as to preserve the possibility of different sorts of relationships—both mother and citizen, friend and official.

Our involvement in one of a number of competing ethical or normative perspectives is inescapable. It is influenced by what we take to be the appropriate relationship between public and private life, for this also defines our understanding of what politics should or should not attempt to define, regulate, or even control. There is widespread disagreement over the respective meaning of public and private within societies. Brian Fay sees the public and the private as part of a cluster of "basic notions" that serve to structure and give coherence to all known ways of life. The boundaries between the public and the private help to create a moral environment for individuals, singly and in groups; to dictate norms of appropriate or worthy action; and to establish barriers to action, particularly in areas such as the taking of human life, regulation of sexual relations, promulgation of familial duties and obligations, and the arena of political responsibility. Public and private are embedded within a dense web of meanings and intimations and are linked to other basic notions: nature and culture, male and female, and each society's "understanding of the meaning and role of work; its views of nature; . . . its concepts of agency; its ideas about authority, the community, the family; its notion of sex; its beliefs about God and death and so on" (Fay, 1975, p. 78). The content, meaning, and range of public and private vary within each society and turn on whether the virtues of political life or the values of private life are rich and vital or have been drained, singly or together, of their normative significance.

The social and political theorist recognizes that no idea or concept is an island unto itself. Basic notions comprise a society's intersubjectively shared realm. "Intersubjectivity" is a rather elusive term referring to shared ideas, symbols, and concepts that reverberate within a society and help to constitute a way of life. The philosopher Ludwig Wittgenstein claims that when we first "begin to believe anything, what we believe is not a single proposition, it is a whole system of propositions. (Light dawns gradually over the whole.)" (Wittgenstein, 1969, p. 21e). Similarly, when we use a concept, particularly one of the bedrock notions integral to a way of life, we do not do so as a discrete piece of "linguistic behavior" but with reference to other concepts, contrasts, and terms of comparison.

As with the concepts of public and private, there are no neatly defined and universally accepted limits on the boundaries of politics. Politics, too, is essentially contested. An essentially contested concept is internally complex or makes reference to several dimensions, which are, in turn, linked to other concepts. Such a concept is also open-textured, in that the rules of its application are relatively flexible, and it is appraisive or normative. For example, one political theorist might claim that a given social situation is unjust. Another might argue that to label the situation unjust only inflames matters, because he or she believes that certain underlying cherished social institutions and relations should not be tampered with or eliminated in the interest of attaining a political or ideological goal. In another example, the feminist political theorist who believes that being born female in and of itself constitutes an injustice on the "biological" level may want to eliminate all sex differences and a public/private distinction as well, for she will see in distinctions themselves a ploy to oppress women (Firestone, 1970). Other feminist thinkers may find this view reprehensible, as it deepens rather than challenges societal devaluation of female bodies and a woman's central role in reproduction. This latter group sees injustice in inequalities that are socially and politically, not biologically, constituted. The point is not to eliminate a public/private distinction but to push for parity in male and female participation in both realms.

Boundary shifts in our understanding of "the political" and hence, of what is public and what is private, have taken place throughout the history of Western life and thought. Minimally, a political perspective requires that some activity called politics be differentiated from other activities. If all conceptual boundaries are blurred and all distinctions between public and private are eliminated, no politics can, by definition, exist (Elshtain, 1981). The relatively open-textured quality of politics means that innovative and revolutionary thinkers are often those who declare politics to exist where politics was not thought to exist before. Should their reclassifications remain over time, the meaning of politics—indeed of human life itself—may be transformed. Altered social conditions may also provoke a reassessment of old, and a recognition of new, "political" realities. Sheldon Wolin observes, "The concepts and categories of a political philosophy may be likened to a net that is cast out to capture political phenomena, which are then drawn in and sorted in a way that seems meaningful and relevant to the particular thinker" (Wolin, 1960, p. 21). Thus each social and political theorist must be clear about what rules he or she is employing to sort the catch and to what ends and purposes.

Bioethical issues in the concepts of public and private

In the history of Western political thought, public and private imperatives, concepts, and symbols have been ordered in a number of ways, including the demand that the private world be integrated fully within the public arena; the insistence that the public realm be "privatized," with politics controlled by the standards, ideals, and purposes emerging from a particular vision of the private sphere; or, finally, a continued differentiation or bifurcation between the two spheres. Bioethics is deeply implicated in each of these broad, general theoretical tendencies that often touch on the private and the public, as in a case, for example, where a couple decides to conceive a child through artificial insemination by donor (AID). What happens to a society's view of the family and intergenerational ties if more couples resort to artificial insemination? What is the effect on the psychosocial development of donor children? What are the responsibilities, if any, of the donor father beyond the point of sperm donation for a fee? Do contractual agreements suffice to "cover" not just the legal but also the ethical implications of such agreements? Does society have a legitimate interest in such "private" choices, given the potential social consequences of private arrangements? Should such procedures be covered by health insurance, whether public or private?

Questions such as these pitch us into the world of social and political theory and the ways particular ideals are deeded to us. Thus, the social-contract liberal endorses a different cluster of human goods than the virtue theorist or the communitarian. Political and social theory yield ethical debates about these competing ideals of human existence. Moral rules—and whether they are to be endorsed or overridden—are inescapable in debating human existence and the human imperative to create meaning. "Public" and "private" and the relations of politics to each exist as loci of human activity, moral reflections, social and historic relations, the creation of meaning, and the construction of identity.

The ways in which our understanding of public, private, and politics plays itself out at present is dauntingly complex. Contemporary society is marked by moral conflicts. These conflicts have deep historical roots and are reflected in our institutions, practices, laws, norms, and values. For example, the continuing abortion debate in the United States taps strongly held, powerfully experienced moral and political imperatives. These imperatives are linked to concerns and images evoking what sort of people we are and what we aspire to be. The abortion debate will not "go away" because it is a debate about matters of life and death, freedom and obligation, and rights and duties.

Perhaps the intractability of many of the debates surrounding bioethics can best be understood as flowing from a central recognition that language itself has become a preoccupation for theorists and ethicists because of our growing concern for establishing norms, limits, and meanings in the absence of a shared ethical consensus. A persistent theme of contemporary social and political theory is that language helps to constitute social reality and frames available forms of action. We are all participants in a language community and hence share in a project of theoretical and moral self-understanding, definition, and redefinition. Our values, embedded in language, are not icing on the cake of social reasoning but are instead part of a densely articulated web of social, historical, and cultural meanings, traditions, rules, beliefs, norms, actions, and visions. A way of life, constituted in and through language, is a complex whole. One cannot separate attitudes toward surrogacy contracts, in vitro fertilization (IVF), use of fetal tissue for medical experimentation, sex selection as a basis for abortion, or genetic engineering to eliminate forms of genetically inherited "imperfection," from other features of a culture. These bioethical dilemmas do not take place in isolation but emerge from within a culture and thus engage in the wider contests over meaning that culture generates.

Contemporary debates in social and political theory

Current debate in social and political theory has focused on the question of whether to buttress or to challenge the liberal consensus that came to prevail in modern Western industrial societies. These broad, competing schools of thought are known as liberalism, civic republicanism, and communitarianism. A social movement informed by one or more of these traditions will exhibit conflicting tendencies and posit incompatible claims.

Liberalism comes in many different forms. Some liberal thinkers stress the individual and his or her rights, often downplaying notions of duty or obligation to a wider social whole. They assume, optimistically, that each individual's pursuit of self-interest will result in "good" for the society as a whole. Those whose analyses begin with the free-standing individual as the point of reference and the "good" of that individual as their normative ideal are often called individualists. In the nineteenth century, this standard of individualism was most cogently articulated by John Stuart Mill in his classic work, On Liberty (1859).

By contrast, communitarians begin not with the autonomous individual but with a social context out of which individuals emerge. They argue that the pursuit of individual self-interest is more likely to yield a fragmented society than a "good" and fair one. Communitarians insist that rights, while vital, are not the individual's alone. Instead, individual rights necessarily flow from rights recognized by others within a community of a particular sort in which responsibilities are also cherished, nourished, and required of individuals (Bellah et al., 1985).

Feminism.   The contemporary women's movement and the way in which it reflects, deepens, and extends features of these traditions illustrate the range of social and political debate. There is no single ethics or moral theory of feminism. Liberalism, with its vibrant individualist strand, has been attractive to feminist thinkers. The language of rights is a potent weapon against traditional obligations, particularly those of family duty or any social status declared "natural" on the basis of ascriptive characteristics. To be free and equal to men became a central aim of feminist reform. The political strategy that followed was one of inclusion. Since women, as well as men, are rational beings, it followed that women as well as men are bearers of inalienable rights. It followed further that there was no valid ground for discrimination against women as women. Leading proponents of women's suffrage in Britain and the United States undermined arguments that justified legal inequality on the basis of sex differences. Such feminists, including the leading American suffragists Susan B. Anthony and Elizabeth Cady Stanton, claimed that denying a group of persons basic rights on the grounds of difference could not be justified unless it could be shown that the difference was relevant to the distinction being made. Whatever differences might exist between the sexes, none, in this view, justified legal inequality and the denial of the rights and privileges of citizenship.

Few early feminists pushed this version of liberal individualist universalism to its most radical conclusion of arguing that there were no bases for exclusion of adult human beings from legal equality and citizenship. Nineteenth-century proponents of women's suffrage were also heirs to a civic-republican tradition that stressed the need for social order and shared values, emphasized civic education, and pressed the importance of having a propertied stake in society. Demands for the inclusion of women often did not extend to all women. Some women, and men, would be excluded by criteria of literacy, property ownership, disability or, in the United States, race. Thus liberal feminism often incorporated the civic-republican insistence on citizenship as a robust, civically demanding, and limited privilege rather than a legalistic and universalistic standing.

At times, feminist theory turned liberal egalitarianism on its head by arguing in favor of women's civic equality on grounds of difference, an argument that might be called neo-Aristotelianism. Ronald Beiner writes,

> The basic conception of neo-Aristotelianism is that moral reason consists not in a set of moral principles, apprehended and defined through procedures of detached rationality, but in the concrete embodiment of certain human capacities in a moral subject who knows those capacities to be constitutive of a consummately desirable life. (Beiner, 1990, p. 75)

Thus greater female political participation was promoted in terms of women's moral supremacy or characteristic forms of virtue. These appeals arose from and spoke to women's social location as mothers, using motherhood as a claim to citizenship, public identity, and civic virtue (Kraditor, 1971). To individualist, rights-based feminists, however, the emphasis on maternal virtue as a form of civic virtue was a trap, for they were, and are, convinced that only liberalism, with its more individualistic construal of the human subject, permits women's equality and standing.

The diverse history of feminism forms the basis for current feminist discourse and debate. These debates are rife with ethical imperatives and moral implications. Varieties of liberal, socialist, Marxist, and utopian feminism abound. Sexuality and sexual identity have become highly charged arenas of political redefinition. Some feminists see women as universal victims, some as a transhistorical sex class, others as oppressed "nature." A minority want separation from "male-dominated" society. Others want full integration into that society, hence its transformation toward liberal equality. Others insist that the feminist agenda will not be completed until "women's virtues," correctly understood, triumph. Feminism, too, is an essentially contested concept.

Divisions among feminists over such volatile matters as AIDS, IVF, surrogate embryo transfer, surrogate motherhood, sex selection—the entire menu of real or potential techniques for manipulating, controlling, and altering human reproduction—are strikingly manifest. One broad general tendency in feminist theory might be called noninterventionist. Noninterventionists see reproductive technologies as a strengthening of arrogant human control over nature and thus over women as part of the "nature" that is to be controlled. Alternatively, the prointerventionist stance foresees technological elimination of males and females themselves. Prointerventionists celebrate developments that promise control over nature.

The prointerventionists, who welcome and applaud any and all techniques that further sever biological reproduction from the social identity of maternity, are heavily indebted to a stance best called ultraliberalism. This theory is driven by a vision of the self that exists apart from any social order. This view of the self, in turn, is tied to one version of rights theory that considers human beings as self-sufficient, promoting a view of society that sees itself organized around contractual agreements between individuals.

The social-contract model.   The contract model has its historical roots in seventeenth-century social-contract theory, and it incorporates a view of society constituted by individuals for the fulfillment of individual ends, with social goods as aggregates of private goods. Critics claim that this vision of self and society ignores aspects of community life, such as reciprocal obligation and mutual interdependence, thereby eroding the bases of authority in family and polity alike.

The pervasiveness of the individualist position is further evident in the prointerventionist stance on bioethical innovations in the area of reproduction. In this view, new reproductive technologies present no problem as long as they can be wrested from male control (Donchin, 1986). Women, having been oppressed by "nature," can overthrow those shackles by seizing the "freedom" offered by technologies that promise deliverance from biological "tyranny." Strong prointerventionists go so far as to envisage forms of biological engineering that would make possible the following: "One woman could inseminate another, so that men and nonparturitive women could lactate and so that fertilized ova could be transplanted into women's or even into men's bodies" (Jaggar, 1983, p. 132). The standard of evaluation concerning these technologies is self-sufficiency and control, paving the way for invasive techniques that break women's links to biology, birth, and nurturance, the vestiges of our animal origins and patriarchal control.

The prointerventionist position owes a great deal to Simone de Beauvoir's feminist classic, *The Second Sex* (Beauvoir, 1968). Beauvoir argues that the woman's body does not "make sense" because women are "the victim of the species." The female, simply by being born female, suffers an alienation grounded in her biological capacity to bear a child. Women are invaded by the fetus, which Beauvoir describes as a "tenant" and a parasite upon the mother. Men, by contrast, are imbued with a sense of virile domination that extends to reproductive life. The life of the male is "transcended" in the sperm. Beauvoir's negative appraisal of the female body extends even to the claim that a woman's breasts are "mammary glands" that "play no role in woman's individual economy: they can be excised at any time of life" (Beauvoir, 1968, p. 24). If to this general repudiation of female embodiment one adds strong individualism, the prointerventionist stand becomes clearer.

Opposed to the radical prointerventionist stance is the noninterventionist voice associated with feminism in a less individualist, more communitarian frame. The noninterventionists ponder the nature of the many choices the new reproductive technology offers. They wonder whether amniocentesis is really a free choice or merely a coercive procedure with only one "correct" outcome: to abort if the fetus is defective. They speculate whether new reproductive technologies are an imposition upon women who see themselves as failures if they cannot become pregnant. Furthermore, noninterventionists reassess the values identified with mothering and encourage the growth and triumph of values they consider to be strongly, if not exclusively, female. They insist that technological progress is never neutral, stressing that "progress" requiring the invasion and manipulation of women's bodies must always be scrutinized critically and may need to be rejected.

Strong noninterventionists claim that women want nothing to do with new reproductive technologies. In the words of one, "The so-called new technology does not bring us and our children any kind of qualitative or quantitative improvement in our lives, it solves none of our basic problems, it will advance even more the exploitation and humiliation of women; therefore we do not need it" (Mies, 1985, p. 559). As with the prointerventionist posture, there are noninterventionists who maintain a critical stance but do not condemn all reproductive technologies outright. Moderate prointerventionists support some but not all of the technological possibilities presented by contemporary reproductive science.

These differences played themselves out in the quandaries confronted by feminists with the Baby M surrogacy-motherhood case, a situation in which biological motherhood and social parenting were severed—as feminists, especially strong individualist feminists, had long claimed they could or should be (*Baby M, in re*, 1988). It was also a case in which everyone presumably freely agreed to a contract. Baby M was born to Mary Beth Whitehead, who had contracted with a couple, the Sterns, to be artificially inseminated with Mr. Stern's sperm. She was to relinquish the baby on birth for $10,000. Ultimately, she could not give the baby up and refused the money. The Sterns sued on breach of contract grounds.

Although liberal feminism emphasizes contractarian imperatives, many liberal feminists, including such popular leaders of the women's movement as the liberal Betty Friedan, saw in the initial denial of any claim by Mary Beth Whitehead, the natural mother, to her child, "an utter denial of the personhood of women—the complete dehumanization of women. It is an important human rights case. To put it at the level of contract law is to dehumanize women and the human bond between mother and child" (Barron, 1987). Friedan implies an ethical limitation to freedom of choice and contract.

Clearly, feminist debates concerning reproductive technology and surrogacy inexorably lead feminists back into discussions of men, women, children, families, and the wider community. Once again we see that bioethical capabilities and possibilities cannot be severed from wider cultural and social surroundings, including our understanding of the human person and his or her private and public needs, identities, and commitments. One broad frame, the social contract, has been noted; it either assumes or promotes the image of the self-sufficient self and goods as the properties of individuals.

The social-compact model.   A second model of social theory, that of the social compact, or social covenant, offers a more rooted and historical picture of human beings than that of the social contract. Compact, or covenant, theory does not recognize primacy of rights and individual choice as the self-evident starting point. The compact self is a historical being who acknowledges that he or she has a "variety of debts, inheritance, rightful expectations, and obligations" and that these "constitute the given of my life, the moral starting point" (MacIntyre, 1981). Modern uprootedness is construed as a problem in the social compact. To be cut off from a wider community as well as from the past, as required by strong individualist modes, is to deform present relationships. The argument here is not that the compact self is totally defined by particular ties and identities, but that without a beginning that recognizes our essential sociality, there is no beginning at all.

The world endorsed in the social-compact model is in tension with the dominant individualist mindset. For this reason, individualists sometimes claim that communitarians, who endorse a social-compact idea, express little more than nostalgia for a simpler past. But the compact defenders argue, in turn, that the past presents itself as the living embodiment of vital traditional conflicts. The social compact makes room for rebellion against one's particular place as one way to forge an identity with reference to that place. But there is little space in the compact frame for social revolt to take a form that excises all social ties and relations if the individual "freely chooses" to do so, a possibility the contractarian must admit. It follows that the familial base of the social compact is opaque to the standpoint of contract theory, given its individualist foundation. This difference about the family, the social institution that first introduces the child into the world, is the focus of political theory debates that bear important implications for bioethics.

The family as a theoretical battleground

Given their individualist starting point, contractarians tend to devalue women's traditional roles and identities as mothers and familial beings. Proponents of the social-compact model, by contrast, understand women's contributions as wives, mothers, and social benefactors as vital to the creation and sustenance of life itself and, beyond that, of any possibility for a "good life." The compact theorist argues that community requires that an important segment or significant number of its members be devoted to the task of caring for the young, the vulnerable, and the elderly. Historically, the work of care has been seen by ethicists, political theorists, and political leaders, including many prominent women, as the mission of women. They worry that in a world of individualism, an ethic of care will be repudiated or replaced by modes of intervention less tied to concrete knowledge and concern of those being cared for (Ruddick, 1989; Tronto, 1993). They also advocate a reevaluation of families that gives conceptual weight to the "private realm" by showing that this sphere is central to social and political life. They insist that our understanding of justice must include a notion of what it means to be a caring society and to honor the work of care.

The compact theorist regrets the lack of a descriptive vocabulary that aptly and richly conveys what we mean when we talk about families and what makes caring commitments different from contractual agreements. The intergenerational family, for example, necessarily constitutes human beings in a particular web of relationships in a given time and place. Stanley Hauerwas, for example, claims that, "Set out in the world with no family, without a story of and for the self, we will simply be captured by the reigning ideologies of the day" (Hauerwas, 1981). We do not choose our relatives—they are given—and as a result, Hauerwas continues, we know what it means to have a history. Yet we continue to require a language to "help us articulate the experience of the family and the loyalty it represents. . . . Such a language must clearly denote our character as historical beings and how our moral lives are based in particular loyalties and relations. If we are to learn to care for others, we must first learn to care for those we find ourselves joined to by accident of birth" (Hauerwas, 1981).

Political theorists have grappled with the issue of the family's relationship to the larger society from the beginning: Where does the family fit in relation to the polity? In his work *Republic*, Plato eliminates the family for his ideal city. The ruler-philosophers he calls Guardians must take "the dispositions of human beings as though they were a tablet . . . which, in the first place, they would wipe clean" (Plato, 1986). Women must be held "in common." A powerful, all-encompassing bond between individuals and the state must be achieved such that all social and political conflict disappears, and the state comes to resemble a "single person," a fused, organic entity. All private loyalties and purposes must be eliminated.

Plato constructs a meritocracy that requires that all considerations of sex, race, age, class, family ties, tradition, and history be stripped away in order to fit people into their appropriate social slots, performing only that function to which each is suited. Children below the ruler class can be shunted upward or downward at the will of the Guardians, for they are so much raw material to be turned into instruments of social "good." A system of eugenics is devised for the Guardians. Children are removed from mothers at birth and placed in a child ghetto, tended to by those best suited for the job. No private loyalties of any kind are allowed to emerge: Homes and sexual attachments, devotion to friends, and dedication to individual or group aims militate against single-minded devotion to the city. Particular ties are a great evil. Only those that bind the individual to the state are good.

No doubt the modern reader finds this rather extreme. Many contemporary theorists contend that Plato constructed his utopia in an ironic mode. Whether Plato meant it or not, his vision is instructive, for it helps us to think about the relation of the family to wider civic loyalties and obligations. Plato aspired to "rational self-sufficiency." He would make the lives of human beings immune to the fragility of messy existence. The idea of self-sufficiency was one of mastery in which the male citizen was imbued with a "mythology of autochthony that persistently, and paradoxically, suppressed the biological role of the female and therefore the family in the continuity of the city" (Nussbaum, 1986).

Moral conflicts, for Plato, suggest irrationalism. If one cannot be loyal both to families and to the city, loyalty to one must be made to conform to the other. For Plato, then, "Our ordinary humanity is a source of confusion rather than of insight . . . [and] the philosopher alone judges the right criterion or from the appropriate standpoint" (Nussbaum, 1986). Hence the plan of *Republic*, which aims to purify and to control human relations and emotions. Later strong rationalists and individualists take a similar tack: They hold that all relationships that are not totally voluntary, rationalistic, and contractual are irrational and suspect. Because the family is the ultimate example of embedded particularity, ideal justice and order will be attained only when "the slate has been wiped clean" and human beings are no longer limited by familial obligations.

Yet a genuinely pluralist civic order would seem to require diversity on the level of families as well as other institutions which, in turn, promote and give rise to many stories and visions of virtue. This suggests the following questions for social and political theory: In what ways is the family issue also a civic issue with weighty public consequences? What is the relationship between democratic theory and practice and intergenerational family ties and commitments? Do we have a stake in sustaining some models of adults in relation to children compared to others? What do families, composed of parents and children, do that no other social institution can? How does current political rhetoric support family obligations and relations?

Equality among citizens was assumed from the beginning by liberals and democrats; indeed, the citizen was, by definition, equal to any other citizen. Not everyone, of course, could be a citizen. At different times and to different ends and purposes, women, slaves, and the propertyless were excluded. But these exclusions were slowly dropped. Whether the purview of some or all adults in a given society, liberal and democratic citizenship required the creation of persons with qualities of mind and spirit necessary for civic participation. This creation of citizens was seen as neither simple nor automatic by early liberal theorists, leading many to insist upon a structure of education in "the sentiments." This education should usher into a moral autonomy that stresses self-chosen obligations, thereby casting further suspicion upon all relations, practices, and loyalties deemed unchosen, involuntary, or natural.

Within such accounts of civic authority, the family emerged as a problem. For one does not enter a family through free consent; one is born into the world unwilled and unchosen by oneself, beginning life as a helpless and dependent infant. Before reaching "the age of consent," one is a child, not a citizen. This vexed liberal and democratic theorists, some of whom believed, at least abstractly, that the completion of the democratic ideal required bringing all of social life under the sway of a single democratic authority principle.

Communitarian versus individualist views of family: Mill and Tocqueville. In his tract *The Subjection of Women*, John Stuart Mill argued that his contemporaries, male and female alike, were tainted by the atavisms of family life with its illegitimate, or unchosen, male authority, and its illegitimate, or manipulative and irrational, female quests for private power (Mill, 1970). He believed that the family can become a school in the virtues of freedom only when parents live together without power on one side and obedience on the other.

Power, for Mill, is repugnant: True liberty must reign in all spheres. But what about the children? Mill's children emerge as blank slates on which parents must encode the lessons of obedience and the responsibilities of freedom. Stripped of undemocratic authority and privilege, the parental union serves as a model of democratic probity (Krouse, 1982).

Mill's paean to liberal individualism is an interesting contrast to Alexis de Tocqueville's observations of family life in nineteenth-century America, a society already showing the effects of the extension of democratic norms and the breakdown of patriarchal and Puritan norms and practices. Fathers in Tocqueville's America were at once stern and forgiving, strong and flexible. They listened to their children and humored them (Tocqueville, 1980). They educated as well as demanded obedience, promulgating a new ethic of child rearing. Like the new democratic father, the American political leader did not demand that citizens bow or stand transfixed in awe. The leader was owed respect and, if he urged a course of action upon his fellow citizens following proper consultation and procedural requirements, they had a patriotic duty to follow.

Tocqueville's discerning eye perceived changing public and private relationships in a liberal, democratic society. Although great care was taken "to trace two clearly distinct lines of action for the two sexes," women, in their domestic sphere, "nowhere occupied a loftier position of honor and importance," Tocqueville claimed. The mother's familial role was enhanced in her civic vocation as the chief inculcator of democratic values in her offspring. Commenting in a civic-republican vein, Tocqueville notes, "No free communities ever existed without morals and, as I observed . . . , morals are the work of women" (Tocqueville, 1945).

Clearly, Tocqueville rests in the social-covenant or communitarian camp; Mill, in the social-contract or individualist domain. In contrast to Mill, Tocqueville insisted that the father's authority in a liberal society was neither absolute nor arbitrary. In contrast to the patriarchal authoritarian family where the parent not only has a "natural right" but acquires a "political right" to command his children, in a democratic family the right and authority of parents is a natural right alone. This natural authority presents no problem for democratic practices as Tocqueville construed democracy, in contrast to Mill. Indeed, the fact that the "right to command" is natural, not political, signifies its special and temporary nature: Once the child is self-governing, the right dissolves. In this way, natural, legitimate paternal authority and maternal moral education reinforce a political order that values flexibility, freedom, and the absence of absolute rule, but requires order and stability as well.

Popular columnists and "child experts" in Tocqueville's America emphasized kindness and love as the preferred technique of child nurture. Obedience was still seen as necessary—to parents, elders, God, government, and the conscience. But the child was no longer construed as a depraved, sin-ridden, stiff-necked creature who needed harsh, unyielding instruction and reproof. A more benign view of the child's nature emerged as notions of infant depravity faded. The problem of discipline grew more, rather than less, complex. Parents were enjoined to get obedience without corporal punishment and rigid methods, using affection, issuing their commands in gentle but firm voices, insisting quietly on their authority lest contempt and chaos reign in the domestic sphere (Elshtain, 1990).

Family authority and the state.   In Tocqueville's image of the democratic family, children were seen both as ends and as means to a well-ordered family and polity. A widespread moral consensus reigned in the America of that era, a kind of Protestant civic religion. When this consensus began to erode under the force of rapid social change (and there are analogues to the American story in all modern democracies), certainties surrounding familial life and authority as a secure locus for the creation of democratic citizens were shaken as well. Tocqueville suggested that familial authority, though apparently at odds with the governing presumptions of democratic authority, is nonetheless part of the constitutive background required for the survival and flourishing of democracy.

Family relations, so this politico-ethical argument goes, could not exist without family authority. These relations and responsibilities, in turn, remain the best way to create human beings with a developed capacity to give ethical allegiance to the principles of democratic society. Because democratic citizenship relies on the self-limiting freedom of responsible adults, a mode of child rearing that builds on basic trust, loyalty, and a sense of commitment is necessary. Family authority structures the relationship between adult providers, nurturers, educators, and disciplinarians, and dependent children, who slowly acquire capacities for independence. Modern parental authority is shared by mother and father.

What makes family authority distinctive is its sense of stewardship: the recognition that parents undertake continuing obligations and responsibilities. Certainly in the modern West, given the long period of childhood and adolescence we honor and recognize, parenting is an ongoing task. The authority of the parent is special, limited, and particular. Parental authority, like any form of authority, may be abused, but unless it exists, the activity of parenting itself is impossible. The authority of parents is implicated in moral education required for the creation of a democratic political morality. The intense loyalties, obligations, and moral imperatives nurtured in families may clash with the requirements of public au-

thority, for example, when young men refuse to serve in a war they claim is unjust because war runs counter to the religious beliefs of their families. This, too, is vital for democracy. Keeping alive a potential locus for revolt, for particularity, for difference, sustains democracy in the long run. It is no coincidence, this argument concludes, that all twentieth-century totalitarian orders aimed to destroy the family as a locus of identity and meaning apart from the state. Totalitarian politics strives to require that individuals identify only with the state rather than with specific others, including family and friends.

Family authority within a democratic, pluralistic order, however, does not exist in a direct homologous relation to the principles of civil society. To establish an identity between public and private lives and purposes would weaken, not strengthen, democratic life overall. For children need particular, intense relations with specific adult others in order to learn to make choices as adults. The child confronted prematurely with the "right to choose" is likely to be less capable of choosing later on. To become a being capable of posing alternatives, one requires a sure and certain place from which to start. In Mary Midgley's words: "Children . . . have to live *now* in a particular culture; they must take some attitude to the nearest things right away" (Midgley, 1978). The social form best suited to provide children with a trusting, determinate sense of place and ultimately a "self" is a family in which parents provide ongoing care, protection, and concern.

The stance of the democratic political and social theorist toward family authority resists easy characterization. It involves a rejection of any ideal of political and familial life that absorbs all social relations under a single authority principle. Families are not democratic polities. The family helps to hold intact the respective goods and ends of exclusive relations and arrangements. Any further erosion of that ethical life embodied in the family bodes ill for democracy. For this reason, theorists representing the communitarian or social-covenant perspective are often among the most severe critics of contemporary consumerism, violence in streets and the media, the decline of public education, the rise in numbers of children being raised without fathers, and so on. They insist, against their critics, that a defense of the family—by which they mean a normative ideal of mothers and fathers in relation to children and to a wider community—can help to sustain a variety of ethical and social commitments, including providing a strong example of adults working together to create a home. Because democracy itself turns on a generalized notion of the fraternal bond between citizens (male and female), it is vital for children to have early experiences of trust and mutuality. The child who emerges from such a family is more likely to be capable of acting in the world as a complex moral being, one part of, yet somewhat detached from, the immediacy of his or her own concerns and desires.

Toward an ethical polity

All political and social theorists, whatever their particular philosophic frameworks and normative commitments, agree that social and political theories always embody some ideal of a preferred way of life. Although a handful of postmodern or deconstructive contemporary theorists disdain all normative standards, most social and political thinkers insist that no way of life can persist without a widely shared cluster of basic notions. Those who locate ethical concerns at the heart of their theories hope for a world in which private and public lives bearing their own intrinsic purpose are allowed to flourish. A richly complex private sphere requires freedom from some all-encompassing public imperative for survival. But in order for the private sphere to flourish, the public world itself must nurture and sustain a set of ethical imperatives, including a commitment to preserve, protect, and defend human beings in their capacities as private persons, and to allow men and women alike to partake in the good of the public sphere with participatory equality (Elshtain, 1981). Such an ideal seeks to keep alive rather than to eliminate tension between diverse spheres and competing ideals and purposes. There is always a danger that a too strong and overweening polity will overwhelm the individual, as well as a peril that life in a polity confronted with a continuing crisis of legitimacy may decivilize both those who oppose it and those who would defend it.

The prevailing image of the person in an ethical polity is that of a human being with a capacity for self-reflection. Such persons can tolerate the tension between public and private imperatives. They can distinguish between those conditions, events, or states of affairs that are part of a shared human condition—grief, loss through death, natural disasters, and decay of the flesh—and those humanly made injustices that can be remedied. Above all, human beings within the ethical polity never presume that ambivalence and conflict will one day end, for they have come to understand that ambivalence and conflict are the wellspring of a life lived reflectively. A clear notion of what ideals and obligations are required to animate an authentic public life, an ethical polity, must be adumbrated: authority, freedom, public law, civic virtue, the ideal of the citizen, all those beliefs, habits, and qualities that are integral to a political order.

Much of the richest theorizing of democratic civil society since 1980 has come from citizens of countries who were subjected for forty years or more to authoritarian, even totalitarian regimes. They pose alternatives both to collectivism and to individualism by urging that the associations of civil society be recognized as subjects in their own right. They call for a genuinely pluralist law to recognize and sustain this associative principle as a way to overcome excessive privatization, on the one hand, and overweening state control, on the other. Solidarity theorist Adam Michnik insists that democracy

> entails a vision of tolerance, and understanding of the importance of cultural traditions, and the realization that cherished human values can conflict with each other. . . . The essence of democracy as I understand it is freedom—the freedom which belongs to citizens endowed with a conscience. So understood, freedom implies pluralism, which is essential because conflict is a constant factor within a democratic social order. (Michnik, 1988, p. 198)

Michnik insists that the genuine democrat always struggles with his or her own tradition, eschewing the hopelessly heroic and individualist notion of going it alone. Michnik positions himself against contemporary tendencies to see any defense of tradition as necessarily "conservative"; indeed, he criticizes all rigidly ideological thinking that severs every political and ethical concern between right and left, proclaiming that "a world devoid of tradition would be nonsensical and anarchic. The human world should be constructed from a permanent conflict between conservatism and contestation; if either is absent from a society, pluralism is destroyed" (Michnik, 1988, p. 199).

A second vital political-ethical voice is that of Vaclav Havel, a playwright, dissident, political theorist, and, in the years following the "tender revolution" of 1989, the president of a then-united Czechoslovakia. In his essay, "Politics and Conscience," he writes:

> We must trust the voice of our conscience more than that of all abstract speculations and not invent other responsibilities than the one to which the voice calls us. We must not be ashamed that we are capable of love, friendship, solidarity, sympathy and tolerance, but just the opposite: we must see these fundamental dimensions of our humanity free from their "private" exile and accept them as the only genuine starting point of meaningful human community. (Havel, 1986, pp. 153–154)

To this end, he favors what he calls "anti-political politics," defined not as the technology of power and manipulation, of cybernetic rule over humans or as the art of the useful, but politics as one of the ways of seeking and achieving meaningful lives, of protecting them and serving them. "I favor politics as practical morality, as service to the truth, as essentially human and humanly measured care for our fellow humans. It is, I presume, an approach which, in this world, is extremely impractical and difficult to apply in daily life. Still, I know no better alternative" (Havel, 1986, p. 155). This is the voice of an ethical polity. Were this voice to prevail, the way in which our ethical dilemmas are adjudicated, including those emerging from bioethics, would be rich and complex enough to enable us to see the public and civic consequences of our private choices, even as it would guard against severe intrusion into intimate life from the outside.

Ethical dilemmas are inescapably political and political questions are unavoidably ethical. Bioethical matters can never be insulated from politics, nor should they be. But the way in which such matters are addressed will very much turn on the social or political theories to which the ethicist, the medical practitioner, the patient or consumer, and the wider, interested community are indebted.

JEAN BETHKE ELSHTAIN

Directly related to this article are the other articles in this entry: TASK OF ETHICS, MORAL EPISTEMOLOGY, NORMATIVE ETHICAL THEORIES, *and* RELIGION AND MORALITY. *For a further discussion of topics mentioned in this article, see the entries* ACTION; AUTHORITY; CARE; DEATH; FAMILY; FEMINISM; FREEDOM AND COERCION; HUMAN NATURE; INTERPRETATION; JUSTICE; LIFE; NATURE; RACE AND RACISM; REPRODUCTIVE TECHNOLOGIES; RIGHTS; SEXISM; VALUE AND VALUATION; VIRTUE AND CHARACTER; *and* WOMEN. *This article will find application in the entries* ABORTION; BIOETHICS; FIDELITY AND LOYALTY; PUBLIC POLICY IN BIOETHICS; RESPONSIBILITY; *and* TRUST. *For a discussion of related ideas, see the entries* ADOLESCENTS; CHILDREN; *and* CONSCIENCE.

Bibliography

Baby M, in re. 1988. 109 N.J. 396, 537 A.2d 1277.

BARRON, JAMES. 1987. "Views on Surrogacy Harden After Baby M Ruling." *New York Times* April 2, pp. A1, B2.

BEAUVOIR, SIMONE DE. 1968. *The Second Sex.* Translated by Howard Madison Parshley. New York: Bantam.

BEINER, RONALD. 1990. "The Liberal Regime." *Chicago-Kent Law Review* 66, no. 1:73–92.

BELLAH, ROBERT N.; SULLIVAN, WILLIAM; TIPTON, STEPHEN; MARSDEN, RICHARD; and SWIDLER, ANN. 1985. *Habits of the Heart. Individualism and Commitment in American Life.* Berkeley: University of California Press.

DONCHIN, ANNE. 1986. "The Future of Mothering: Reproductive Technology and Feminist Theory." *Hypatia* 1, no. 2:121–137.

ELSHTAIN, JEAN BETHKE. 1981. *Public Man, Private Woman: Women in Social and Political Thought.* Princeton, N.J.: Princeton University Press.

———. 1984. "Reflections on Abortion, Values, and the Family." In *Abortion: Understanding Differences,* 47–72. Edited by Sidney Callahan and Daniel Callahan. New York: Plenum.

———. 1990. *Power Trips and Other Journeys: Essays in Feminism as Civic Discourse.* Madison: University of Wisconsin Press.

———. ed. 1982. *The Family in Political Thought.* Amherst: University of Massachusetts Press.

FAY, BRIAN. 1975. *Social Theory and Political Practice.* London: Allen and Unwin.

FIELD, MARTHA A. 1988. *Surrogate Motherhood: The Legal and Human Issues.* Cambridge, Mass.: Harvard University Press.

FIRESTONE, SHULAMITH. 1970. *The Dialectic of Sex.* New York: Bantam Books.

HAUERWAS, STANLEY. 1981. "The Moral Value of the Family." In his *A Community of Character: Toward a Constructive Christian Social Ethic.* Notre Dame, Ind.: Notre Dame University Press.

HAVEL, VACLAV. 1986. *Living in Truth.* London: Faber and Faber.

JAGGAR, ALISON M. 1983. *Feminist Politics and Human Nature.* Totowa, N.J.: Rowman and Allanheld.

KRADITOR, AILEEN S. 1971. *The Ideas of the Woman Suffrage Movement 1890–1920.* Garden City, N.Y.: Doubleday.

KROUSE, RICHARD W. 1982. "Patriarchal Liberalism and Beyond: From John Stuart Mill to Harriet Taylor." In *The Family in Political Thought,* pp. 145–172. Edited by Jean Bethke Elshtain. Amherst: University of Massachusetts Press.

MACINTYRE, ALASDAIR C. 1981. *After Virtue: A Study in Moral Theory.* Notre Dame, Ind.: Notre Dame University Press.

MICHNIK, ADAM. Interviewed by Eric Blair. 1988. "Towards a Civil Society: Hopes for Polish Democracy." *Times Literary Supplement.* February 19–25, pp. 188, 198–199.

MIDGLEY, MARY. 1978. *Beast and Man: The Roots of Human Nature.* Ithaca, N.Y.: Cornell University Press.

MIES, MARK. 1985. " 'Why Do We Need All This?' A Call Against Genetic Engineering and Reproductive Technology." *Women's Studies International Forum* 8, no. 6:553–560.

MILL, JOHN STUART. 1970. [1869]. *The Subjection of Women.* Cambridge, Mass.: MIT Press.

———. 1989. [1859]. *On Liberty.* Edited by Alburey Castell. Arlington Heights, Ill.: H. Davidson.

NUSSBAUM, MARTHA C. 1986. *The Fragility of Goodness: Luck and Ethics in Greek Tragedy.* Cambridge: At the University Press.

PATEMAN, CAROLE. 1988. *The Sexual Contract.* Stanford, Calif.: Stanford University Press.

PLATO. 1986. *Republic.* Translated by Allan Bloom. New York: Basic Books.

ROTHMAN, BARBARA KATZ. 1989. *Recreating Motherhood: Ideology and Technology in Patriarchal Society.* New York: W. W. Norton.

RUDDICK, SARA. 1989. *Maternal Thinking: Toward a Politics of Peace.* Boston: Beacon Press.

SHANLEY, MARY LYNDON. 1989. *Feminism, Marriage, and the*

Law in Victorian England, 1850–1895. Princeton, N.J.: Princeton University Press.

TAYLOR, CHARLES. 1971. "Interpretation and the Sciences of Man." *Review of Metaphysics* 25, no. 1:3–51.

TOCQUEVILLE, ALEXIS DE. 1980. [1851]. *Democracy in America.* Edited by Phillips Bradley. New York: Knopf.

TRONTO, JOAN C. 1993. *Moral Boundaries: A Political Agreement for an Ethic of Care.* New York: Routledge.

WITTGENSTEIN, LUDWIG. 1969. *On Certainty.* Edited by G. E. C. Anscombe and G. H. von Wright. New York: Harper.

WOLIN, SHELDON S. 1960. *Politics and Vision: Continuity and Vision in Western Political Thought.* Boston: Little, Brown.

V. RELIGION AND MORALITY

In the minds of many people, religion and morality are closely connected. Even in secular discussions of ethics, law, and medicine, the presumption remains strong that religious beliefs are an important source of moral guidance, and that religious authorities have a significant influence in shaping attitudes toward biomedical research, new technologies, and medical interventions at the beginning and end of life. Both those who hold religious beliefs and those who do not expect that such beliefs will make a significant difference in the moral lives of their adherents.

When this commonplace assumption about the connection between religion and morality is subjected to examination, however, problems emerge. Although moral virtues and behaviors characteristic of Christian love or Buddhist compassion may be clearly associated with a specific religion, the human possibilities they describe are often familiar and admired, even among those who do not share the religious beliefs. Persons outside of a community of faith may display its characteristic virtues, and those who reject a particular religion may realize its moral ideals better than most of its adherents. For example, Christian writers often turn to Gandhi as the modern model of the love that Jesus preached, while Gandhi valued the life of Jesus as an example of the harmlessness he sought to encourage. This recognition of specific moral virtues in persons outside the community of belief in which those virtues are defined and taught is so common today as to be unremarkable, but it challenges the assumption that specific moral beliefs and practices can be tied to specific religious commitments.

The assumption that religion and morality are somehow related thus gives way to questions about exactly what forms this relationship may take and how it is understood. What claims are persons making when they relate a moral judgment to a religious belief, and how are we to understand the similar judgments that others make on nonreligious grounds? How will these different moral and religious orientations relate to the findings of the biomedical sciences? How should the providers of medical services relate to the diversity of these religious and moral orientations in a complex, pluralistic society?

Types of relationships

A first step toward answering these questions is to identify the variety of relationships between religion and morality that are found in the world's moral and religious traditions (Little and Twiss, 1978). In general, religion is an authoritative source of moral norms and a primary motivation for conformity to moral requirements. Significant variations on this general idea do, however, exist. Is religion the only source of the moral norms, or may those norms, or some of them, be discovered or created in other ways? Is the authoritative source the will of a divine lawgiver, or an intrinsic goodness in the nature of things themselves? Is the motive for moral action a religious love of the good for its own sake, or the hope for an ultimate compensation for the hardships that moral behavior sometimes requires?

Answers to these questions differ, both among different religious traditions and among different schools of thought within a single tradition. The major monotheistic traditions—Judaism, Christianity, and Islam—often represent key moral norms as direct commands of God. In the religions that originated in India—Hinduism, Jainism, and Buddhism—by contrast, the central concept is *karma*, a cosmic moral order that fixes inescapable consequences for any action (Green, 1978). Protestant Christianity has often stressed the word of God, the direct divine command that is independent of any human knowledge or wisdom, while Roman Catholic moral theology has relied more on the concept of "natural law," a moral order established by God, but knowable by human reason and apparent in the workings of the natural order (Gustafson, 1978).

While it would be possible to explore the relationships between religion and morality by surveying major religious traditions individually, that approach would quickly become a volume unto itself, and it would still do scant justice to the nuances and variety within each tradition. For present purposes, we must limit consideration to a typology of relationships that can be observed in a number of traditions, especially as these traditions come into contact with one another and with the forces of modern technological change. Examples of each type can be identified in a variety of religious traditions, but readers who seek a comprehensive understanding of morality in, for instance, Buddhism or Islam will need to consult other sources, some of which are identified in the bibliography for this article.

The wide variety of possible relationships between

religion and morality may be organized in three prominent types that have received most serious attention from modern scholars: (1) cosmic unity, in which moral obligations derive from a natural or metaphysical order that is understood in religious terms; (2) logical independence, in which moral norms, despite their historical connections to religion, do not depend directly on religion for their validity, and in which religious values must be sharply distinguished from judgments of moral worth; and (3) cultural interdependence, in which neither religion nor morality can be understood apart from the communities in which they have developed and in which their practices have become intertwined.

This typology is derived from modern Western scholarship and reflects particularly the development of religion in modern, secular societies. Each of the types, however, has roots in earlier developments in Western theology and philosophy, and most have parallels in other, non-Western religious and cultural communities. While the emphasis in what follows will be on the modern West, much will be relevant to modern and modernizing cultures in other parts of the world, and analogies to the relationship between religion and morality in other cultural settings may illuminate both those settings and the West's.

Cosmic unity. Many cultures have conceived moral and natural orders as an undifferentiated unity. The rewards and punishments associated with moral action are as much a part of reality as the forces of wind and water or the patterns of growth and development observed in plants and animals. To put the matter another way, both the observable patterns of nature and the system of moral requirements are part of a larger order that encompasses all reality, seen and unseen. This unity, expressed both in myths and poetry and in speculative metaphysics, comes into question as science and philosophy develop, but it remains a powerful influence, even in modern, secular societies.

Sometimes, the power that requires moral conduct is thought of in impersonal terms, as a force to be reckoned with by humans and by more powerful beings as well. Early Greek philosophers and poets understood justice (*diké*) in these terms. Justice keeps gods and humans from exceeding their limits, and those who ignore justice risk disaster for the whole community (Adkins, 1985). In ancient China, *tao* was a pervasive force that both regulated the order of natural events and set the standard for human conduct (Girardot, 1985). Similar concepts appear in other traditions.

In the Hebrew scriptures, the ultimate power is a personal God who is not subject to higher forces, but who addresses human beings in terms of moral commandments (Deut. 5:1–21). This God is also the creator of the natural forces with which humans must reckon.

A somewhat later strand of the tradition represents wisdom (*hokmah*) as the pervasive, unifying power by which God both shapes the material world and directs the conduct of good persons (Prov. 8:1–31).

These early conceptions of a moral order inherent in the order of things often gave way to an understanding of laws and obligations as purely human creations, having power only so far as they are enforced. The development of these skeptical ideas often coincided with the breakdown of traditional social patterns, or with the discovery of other peoples and cultures who lived by quite different rules. Both Greek and Roman philosophers, however, retained the notion that some requirements are not conventional, but natural. However much Greece and Persia otherwise may have differed, some moral requirements remained the same in both places (Aristotle, 1962).

This idea provided theologians with the basis for a concept of "natural law," through which God's commandments could be known by all rational persons. Thus, the same minimal requirements of morality apply to everyone, whether or not they share the same ideas about God. Both Judaism and Islam developed philosophical systems that transmitted the Hellenistic notion of natural law to the Christian West, and for a brief time in the Middle Ages, teachers in all three traditions could debate the relationship between God's will and the created order in a shared philosophical framework (Jacobs, 1978). In medieval Christian theology, natural law related all rational beings to God. Natural law was seen to be the way a finite, rational being participates in the eternal law by which God orders the universe.

The ever-present possibility of elevating a particular aspect of nature to the level of equality with God led, however, to widespread suspicion of natural law ideas among moral and religious reformers. The main line of development in Jewish ethics centered on observance of a code of law based on scripture and rabbinic interpretation, rather than on a rationalist moral philosophy (Lichtenstein, 1978). In Islam, the philosophical movement evolved in a more mystical direction, focused on the identity of the human spirit with the spiritual character of all reality, rather than on the moral requirements of a natural order (Rahman, 1979). In Western Christianity, the Protestant Reformation challenged all forms of religious legalism, including the precepts of natural law.

During the seventeenth century, however, a new group of legal and political theorists seized upon the concept of natural law as the key to understanding the relationships between nations as well as persons. While the religious significance of the natural law was not necessarily rejected, it was the universality of the obligation, not its divine origin, that attracted these jurists to the idea. In both legal and theological treatments of natural law, however, these highly articulated systems of moral thought share with the earliest myths of cosmic unity the notion that some moral requirements are inescapable because they are part of the structure of reality itself. Since World War II, renewed interest in theories of natural law as a starting point for an international recognition of basic human rights testifies to the continuing significance of this way of relating moral requirements to religious beliefs about the origin and end of the world in which the moral life is lived (Maritain, 1951).

The idea of a comprehensive order that encompasses both moral and religious requirements thus appears both in the most ancient religious traditions and in modern Western theories of natural law. Although reformers in many theistic traditions have sought to restore religious morality to a direct dependence on the will of God, the underlying idea that what God wills is also supported by the natural order that God has created never entirely disappears, even when the human ability to know God's will through the natural order is contested.

Logical independence. The fact that religion and morality are closely related in the history of Western thought does not, of itself, establish that their connection is important for contemporary moral decisions. The historical relationships might be viewed as accidental or contingent, subject to change without altering the basic requirements of morality. The links between religion and morality might even be points of confusion that obscure important features of both religious and moral truths. For some thinkers, then, it is important to establish the distinction between religious and moral evaluations, even though these may be commonly confused in practice, or integrally related in some more comprehensive system of ideas. Failure to make the distinction between religion and morality runs the risk of subordinating both to prevailing cultural practices, which may themselves be morally questionable.

By the eighteenth century, European philosophers had begun to advance theories about the historical development of religion that were not based on the history presented in the Bible. Religion could thus be given a "natural history," as opposed to the sacred history revealed in scripture. David Hume's "The Natural History of Religion," (Hume, 1927) postulated a primitive connection between fear of the awesome power of natural forces and dread of punishment for moral transgressions. Such fear may continue to serve as a useful inducement to moral conformity, but it leads only to confusion if the source of the moral imperatives is sought in a supernatural power. Against those who worried that a distinction between religion and morality would lead to a decline in moral standards, Hume argued that a sound logical con-

nection between moral requirements and the public good was the only secure basis for morality. A utilitarian calculation of the line of conduct that will produce the largest social benefits is the final source of moral norms, and respect for that public good is the only secure ground of moral motivation.

In addition to the possibility that the connection between religion and morality is simply a residue of primitive superstitions, philosophers noted another point that seemed not only to distinguish religion from morality, but also to give a logical priority to morality. Religious traditions frequently praise a divine center and origin of moral goodness, or point to the lives of exemplary religious figures as examples to be followed. To recognize that goodness seems, however, to require a moral judgment that precedes the religious assent. We can only praise God or emulate the saints for moral goodness if we have an idea of what is morally good, by which we measure even these supreme examples. "Even the Holy One of the gospel," wrote Immanuel Kant, "must first be compared with our ideal of moral perfection before we can recognize him as such" (Kant, 1964, p. 76).

Clearly, whether one begins with Hume's "natural history" of religion or Kant's rational foundation for moral judgments, morality and religion cannot be simply identical. The Christian natural law tradition used reason to discern God's will in the order of the created world. In Kant and Hume, reason formulates its requirements independently, on the basis of social utility or of logical necessity. The resulting standard of morality is then applied to religion, which may or may not measure up.

This separation of moral requirements from religious belief does not, however, imply that religion has no connection to morality. Many who accepted a rational morality, the requirements of which did not depend on faith, continued to value religion as a motive for the moral life. Love of a God who is perfect in goodness, and reverence for saints who have upheld the requirements of morality in the face of severe temptations, provide powerful motives for people to live up to moral expectations in more ordinary circumstances. Indeed, Kant argued that some conception of God is ultimately required to make sense of the sacrifices that all moral action requires of us. The logical independence of morality from religion does not require that religion be abandoned, but it does require that moral actions be undertaken precisely because we are convinced that they are morally right, and not because we believe that God commands us to do them.

These philosophical developments coincided with important historical changes in European religious life. By the end of the seventeenth century, the normative requirement of religious conformity was rapidly being replaced by practices of religious toleration and, eventually, by a civic commitment to religious freedom. The logical separation of religion from morality became a sociological necessity as well, if citizens who were no longer united in their religious beliefs were to acknowledge moral obligations to one another. In the United States, especially, the idea developed that a variety of quite different religious beliefs could support a common moral consensus (Frost, 1990). Because morality and religion are independent, diversity of religious beliefs need not lead to moral conflict, and moral order does not require religious agreement.

In other cases, where the break with traditional forms of religious and social life was sharper, or where the conflict between religious groups was more intense, public moral expectations were reformulated in nonreligious terms. Where cooperation between religion and government proved difficult, or where the moral consensus between different religious groups was obviously lacking, the concept of a "secular state" provided the necessary basis for social unity. A secular state not only refuses to privilege one or another religious perspective among its people, it resolutely excludes religious considerations from the formation of policy and regulations. Religion and religious morality become private considerations, subject to regulation for the public good.

This understanding first emerges clearly in the French Revolution, but the idea of a secular state has also provided hope for civil unity for many twentieth-century leaders in countries deeply divided by religious strife or torn by controversy over modernizations that undermine traditional forms of religious life. In the United States, where the prevailing model has been the religious consensus on moral expectations, elements of the secular state concept have nonetheless been invoked to curb sectarian religious practices that differ sharply from those of the majority, or to exclude religious arguments from controversial questions of policy. Judicial limitation of a parent's power to withhold medical care from children on religious grounds and political arguments that Roman Catholic opposition to abortion violates the constitutional separation of church and state are two instances in which the apparent lack of religious consensus has prompted arguments for policies of a secular state.

The logical separation of morality from religion, then, provides an important intellectual starting point for the ordering of societies divided by religious differences or seeking to modernize in the face of opposition by traditional religious groups. The distinction between religion and morality does not, by itself, prescribe a role for religion in public life. Religion may be one element in a powerful moral consensus that differs from the religious morality of a traditional society, or it may be vir-

tually excluded from influence by a secular state that defines public morality in terms of a utilitarian calculation of the public good.

Cultural interdependence.   Although the logical separation of morality from religion is a premise for much of Western European and North American thought in ethics, law, politics, and even theology, its relevance to other points in history and other parts of the world is less clear. The modern Western distinction between religion and morality is missing from many highly developed religious and cultural systems, which assign duties to persons on the basis of their position in society without obvious distinctions between what modern Westerners differentiate into moral requirements, common courtesy, religious obligations, and patriotic duties.

This is most clear in the traditional societies of India, China, and Japan. Hinduism recognizes few duties that correspond to the universal moral obligations of modern Western ethics. Specific persons owe duties to specific others, based on the place each occupies in a social, moral, and religious hierarchy, so that traditional Hinduism can hardly exist outside of the social system in which it originates. In China, a Confucian system of philosophical morality was tied to the details of the education and duties of an elite corps of governing intellectuals, while in Japan, the traditional religion of the people centered on the cults of specific ancestors and the spirits of specific places. Hinduism and, to a certain extent, Confucianism demonstrated in the nineteenth century that they could be reinterpreted in more universal philosophical terms, but the reconstruction of State Shintō in Japan during the same time period suggests that the unitary system of religion, state, and morals can also be adapted to the demands of modernizing societies (Hardacre, 1989).

While the interdependence of religion and culture is most clearly seen in these highly developed national traditions, the missionary religions that have moved across large parts of the world also illustrate this interdependence, precisely in their adaptability to very different cultural settings. Christianity presents very different appearances in Moscow and in Dallas. Buddhism in Tokyo is distinctively Japanese, as it is distinctively Thai in Bangkok. The same might be said for Islam in Cairo and in Kuala Lumpur. Nor are these variations simply the result of a constant teaching consciously applied to different situations. Religious traditions develop by interacting with the economic life and productive systems by which their adherents meet their material needs, as well as by the inner logic of their spiritual teachings. The modern sociological study of religion rests on this awareness of the nonreligious forces that operate on religious communities and the unintended consequences that religious beliefs have in the world of economic life (Weber, 1958).

Those who view religion from this perspective identify important changes that religions undergo in modern, technological societies. The institutions of religion no longer occupy the central positions of power and authority they once held. Wider knowledge of the world and more exposure to other cultures lead to an awareness of other religions beside one's own. These changes mark what sociologists call secularization, but the interactions of religion and culture are no less real in that context than they were when religion had a more dominant position.

Secularization may reduce the power of religions institutions and leaders, but it does not produce a neutral culture free of religious influences. A "secular" society is shaped in part by the historical interactions between the religion and culture that have shaped the particular place in which the society now exists. A modern economy influenced by a Confucian past differs significantly from one that has developed out of European Protestantism. The process of secularization, therefore, does not provide a neutral, universal standpoint from which to settle questions of morality and policy.

Since the 1970s, social scientists, philosophers, and theologians have widely accepted this contextualization of their work and have sought to explore its implications for their systematic thought (Stout, 1988). What was believed to be universal and rational is now widely seen to be particular. Notions of objectivity, tables of individual rights and duties—even, perhaps, the idea of rationality itself—are shaped by particular cultural starting points.

Where supposed neutrality and rational authority have been used to suppress religious conflict, the continuing influence of religion on culture sometimes results in violent rejection of the secular state and its institutions. Fundamentalist movements throughout the Islamic world and among Hindus in India reject modern secular culture as an alien Western imposition and reassert an identity of religion, morality, and culture. In the United States and elsewhere, renewed interest in the religions of indigenous peoples includes a rediscovery of their distinctive understandings of health and healing, which link religion, morality, and medicine in ways unfamiliar to modern medical science (Sullivan, 1988).

The implications of this reassertion of the cultural integrity of religion and morality are, however, variously construed by authors reflecting on modern pluralistic societies. One view suggests that the loss of community and the rise of social disorder is a direct result of the attempt to exclude from public discussion the religious values that are the only available foundation for morality. The social achievements that people in the United States most prize, including their individual rights and political freedoms, are simply the fruit of the Christian moral traditions that gave rise to them. If we hope to continue to enjoy them, we must restore those moral traditions in which they originate to a central role in shaping the life of society (Neuhaus, 1984).

Another point of view suggests, by contrast, that the public life of a pluralistic society can no longer provide a forum for genuine moral convictions, which always have a particular religious basis. If we seek to develop persons of moral character, we must do it within religious communities that have a distinctive identity. It may then be possible to translate some of these religious values into public policy through political action, but it will not be possible to offer a public argument for the values at stake. They can only be understood in a community where the way of life in which they originate is cherished and enacted (Hauerwas, 1981).

An understanding of the cultural interdependence of religion and morality thus calls into question both the cosmic order that sustains religion's requirements everywhere and the universal, rational morality that is characteristic of modern understandings of the independence of morality from religion. In this emphasis on cultural specificity that is sometimes called "postmodern," everything depends on the relationship between religion and morality in a particular place and time. Those who hold this view agree on the importance of the interaction of morality and religion. They differ over whether this interaction should take the form of cultural hegemony by a particular religious tradition, in order to provide the necessary foundation for public order, or should be practiced in small communities of shared faith, who venture into politics and public policy only for limited purposes and confine their virtues to their separated life.

Implications for bioethics

Perhaps the most striking result of this survey is the diversity of relationships between religion and morality that are held in different religious traditions and, indeed, within the same religious tradition, in different historical and cultural settings. In a pluralistic society, where researchers often work in global networks and medical-care providers deal with patients and families from many communities, many different understandings of morality and religion will impinge on their work, raising new issues in bioethics.

Questions of patient autonomy and appropriate respect for the human subjects of biomedical research become even more difficult when the parties have not only different religious beliefs about the nature of the human being, but also different understandings of how these beliefs appropriately relate to moral decisions that doctor and patient, researcher and subject, primary parties and review committees must make together. Conflicts may arise, for example, when medical personnel appeal for decisions on clinical or scientific grounds to patients and families whose beliefs do not admit nonreligious reasons for decisive personal choices. It is important in the first instance simply to be aware of this diversity of moral and religious perspectives and alert to their relevance to professional choices. Even specialists who are well trained in bioethics often uncritically accept the viewpoint that morality is logically independent of religion, because that is the position of the moral philosophy that has provided much of the theoretical framework for contemporary bioethics. Without awareness of the other possibilities this article has surveyed, significant moral issues may be overlooked until they become the subject of public controversy or undermine the relationship of trust between medical-care providers and patients.

Investigations of the cultural interdependence of religion and morality may make us aware of serious moral claims. What a patient believes about ritual purity or about the fate of the soul after death deserves more than just respectful interest. It may determine what it means to treat that patient as a free person with an inherent dignity. In any case, the cultural specificity of all moral and religious perspectives should also alert us to the limitations of the claims of biomedical science.

Cultural interdependence opens up possibilities for serious conflicts between cultural perspectives in medical and scientific institutions. Often, research and clinical personnel do not share the commitments of universities or hospitals that have religious sponsorship. An ethical commitment to scientific objectivity or clinical autonomy, which is easy to sustain when religion and morality are believed to be logically distinct, may come into conflict with the view that sustaining a distinctive religious culture within the institution is the only way to sustain it as a moral community. Alternatively, religious views that stress the importance of distinctive moral communities may withdraw from the more complex, pluralistic world of the medical center or research institute, thus eliminating a possibly important mediating influence between the narrowly focused aims of medical practice and the values of ordinary Jews, Catholics, Muslims, or Baptists who happen for the moment to be patients in a medical facility.

The increasing cultural complexity of biomedical science and its institutions prompts the search for a core of morality that would provide the basis for policy decisions, without requiring unanimity on the religious reasons for those moral requirements. Logical independence of this common morality from particular religious commitments seems to be required, whether the morality is to be founded on a universal moral logic or, less

ambitiously, on the necessary requirements of medical practice. Although the idea of a completely neutral, secular medical ethics may no longer be plausible, a standard of "secular arguments" for policy choices seems to some observers to solve the problem of moral and religious difference. By insisting that arguments for or against specific policy choices must be made for reasons accessible to all parties in the debate, we eliminate public choices based on specific religious convictions. Arguments for or against a program of acquired immunodeficiency syndrome (AIDS) education and prevention on ground of its effect on community health are acceptable. Arguments for or against it on grounds that it conforms to the requirements of a specific religious teaching are not.

While the standard of "secular arguments" or "publicly accessible reasons" is appealing, it presupposes a very large area of public moral consensus. Although some such consensus does exist, its scope is unclear, and there is no guarantee that it is actually broad enough to resolve the difficult bioethical issues that divide society today. In short, it may be that a strictly defined "secular argument" will be insufficient to yield a determinate solution to the problems, that some appeal to the religious convictions or other private views of the participants will be necessary if we are to settle the questions at all (Greenawalt, 1988).

Efforts to define an independent system of morality, in which bioethical issues could be resolved without reference to the diversity of religious moral positions, are thus subject to a variety of problems. The issues range from attacks on the supposed neutrality and objectivity of secular scientific inquiry, to the criticism that if it should achieve this neutrality, it would be unable to provide determinate solutions to policy questions that have been posed to medicine and science.

Another possibility, however, is to accept the unity of religious and moral discourse and ask whether biomedical science and clinical practice might participate in it. Physicians and other providers of medical services have ideas about human flourishing based on long experience with patients and clients. Scientific research may confirm or disprove widespread convictions about the best means to achieve and sustain a good life, and it may provide new evidence of causal links between choices and outcomes. Discussion of the human good typically takes quite different forms from the highly structured discourse of the biomedical sciences, but those sciences clearly do have a contribution to make to it.

Beliefs that hold that there is a cosmic unity of religion and morality, a single reality in which religious and moral truths make sense together, offer the clearest opportunities for biomedical participation. This openness is most apparent in contemporary formulations of natural law theory, which explicitly make use of biomedical knowledge as part of the determination of what is natural and what the conditions for human flourishing are. Even where religious traditions have not developed systematic statements, however, their narratives and rituals make implicit claims about the constraints that the world imposes on human life, and about what human beings must do to live well within those limits (Lovin and Reynolds, 1985).

Where these myths, narratives, hymns, and rites are taken to be rivals to a scientific account of reality, there will inevitably be conflicts between the biomedical sciences the religious ideas about morality. But religious discourse is never simply an objective account of the way things are. It is always also an orientation of human life within that world of facts, and the physician's or the medical researcher's account of those facts may have a place in that orientation. Such an understanding neither separates religion from morality, nor links them both to a specific cultural system, but regards morality as an orientation of human life within a reality that is susceptible both to scientific examination and to the imaginative and liberating comprehension that religion offers.

Those who seek to join a discussion of the human good in which both religious wisdom and scientific discovery have a place must acknowledge that there are other views, religious and scientific, that will reject that collaboration. A moral realism that links religion, science, and morality may provide the best framework for biomedical researchers and clinicians to explain the ethical implications of their work in terms that many religious traditions can accept.

ROBIN W. LOVIN

Directly related to this article are the other articles in this entry: TASK OF ETHICS, MORAL EPISTEMOLOGY, NORMATIVE ETHICAL THEORIES, *and* SOCIAL AND POLITICAL THEORIES. *For a further discussion of topics mentioned in this article, see the entries* AUTHORITY; AUTONOMY; BUDDHISM; CONFUCIANISM; HINDUISM; ISLAM; JAINISM; JUDAISM; JUSTICE; MEDICAL ETHICS, HISTORY OF, *sections on* EUROPE, *and* SOUTH AND EAST ASIA; NATURAL LAW; PROTESTANTISM; PUBLIC POLICY AND BIOETHICS; ROMAN CATHOLICISM; UTILITY; VALUE AND VALUATION; *and* VIRTUE AND CHARACTER. *This article will find application in the entries* ABORTION; *and* BIOETHICS. *For a discussion of related ideas, see the entries* ACADEMIC HEALTH CENTERS; ENVIRONMENT AND RELIGION; EUGENICS AND RELIGIOUS LAW; FRIENDSHIP; HEALING; INTERPRETATION; LAW AND MORALITY; LIFE; LOVE; NARRATIVE; SIKHISM; *and* TAOISM.

Bibliography

ADKINS, ARTHUR W. H. 1985. "Cosmogony and Order in Ancient Greece." In *Cosmogony and Ethical Order: New Essays in Comparative Ethics,* pp. 39–66. Edited by Robin W. Lovin and Frank E. Reynolds. Chicago: University of Chicago Press.

ARISTOTLE. 1962. *Nicomachean Ethics.* Translated by Martin Ostwald. Indianapolis, Ind.: Bobbs-Merrill.

FROST, J. WILLIAM. 1990. *A Perfect Freedom: Religious Liberty in Pennsylvania.* Cambridge: At the University Press.

GIRARDOT, NORMAN J. 1985. "Behaving Cosmogonically in Early Taoism." In *Cosmogony and Ethical Order: New Essays in Comparative Ethics,* pp. 67–97. Edited by Robin W. Lovin and Frank E. Reynolds. Chicago: University of Chicago Press.

GREEN, RONALD M. 1978. *Religious Reason: The Rational and Moral Basis of Religious Belief.* New York: Oxford University Press.

GREENAWALT, KENT. 1988. *Religious Convictions and Political Choice.* New York: Oxford University Press.

GUSTAFSON, JAMES M. 1978. *Protestant and Roman Catholic Ethics: Prospects for Rapprochement.* Chicago: University of Chicago Press.

HARDACRE, HELEN. 1989. *Shinto and the State, 1868–1988.* Princeton, N.J.: Princeton University Press.

HAUERWAS, STANLEY. 1981. *A Community of Character: Toward a Constructive Christian Social Ethic.* Notre Dame, Ind.: University of Notre Dame Press.

HUME, DAVID. 1927. "The Natural History of Religion." In *Hume: Selections,* pp. 253–283. Edited by Charles W. Hendel. New York: Scribner's.

JACOBS, LOUIS. 1978. "The Relationship Between Religion and Ethics in Jewish Thought." In *Contemporary Jewish Ethics,* pp. 41–58. Edited by Menachem Marc Kellner. New York: Sanhedrin Press.

KANT, IMMANUEL. 1964. *The Moral Law; or Kant's Groundwork of the Metaphysics of Morals.* Translated by Herbert J. Paton. New York: Harper & Row.

LICHTENSTEIN, AHARON. 1978. "Does Jewish Tradition Recognize an Ethic Independent of Halakha?" In *Contemporary Jewish Ethics,* pp. 102–123. Edited by Menachem Marc Kellner. New York: Sanhedrin Press.

LITTLE, DAVID, and TWISS, SUMNER B. 1978. *Comparative Religious Ethics: A New Method.* New York: Harper & Row.

LOVIN, ROBIN W., and REYNOLDS, FRANK E. 1985. "In the Beginning." In *Cosmogony and Ethical Order: New Essays in Comparative Ethics,* pp. 1–35. Edited by Robin W. Lovin and Frank E. Reynolds. Chicago: University of Chicago Press.

MARITAIN, JACQUES. 1951. *Man and the State.* Chicago: University of Chicago Press.

NEUHAUS, RICHARD J. 1984. *The Naked Public Square: Religion and Democracy in America.* Grand Rapids, Mich.: William B. Eerdmans.

RAHMAN, FAZLUR. 1979. *Islam.* 2d ed. Chicago: University of Chicago Press.

STOUT, JEFFREY. 1988. *Ethics after Babel: The Languages of Morals and Their Discontents.* Boston: Beacon Press.

SULLIVAN, LAWRENCE E. 1988. *Icanchu's Drum: An Orientation to Meaning in South American Religions*. New York: Macmillan.

WEBER, MAX. 1958. *The Protestant Ethic and the Spirit of Capitalism*. Translated by Talcott Parsons. New York: Scribner's.

ETHICS COMMITTEES

See CLINICAL ETHICS, *article on* INSTITUTIONAL ETHICS COMMITTEES; *and* RESEARCH ETHICS COMMITTEES. *See also* INFANTS, *article on* PUBLIC POLICY AND LEGAL ISSUES.

ETHICS CONSULTATION, CLINICAL

See CLINICAL ETHICS, *article on* CLINICAL ETHICS CONSULTATION.

EUGENICS

I. Historical Aspects
        Daniel J. Kevles
II. Ethical Issues
        Marc Lappé

I. HISTORICAL ASPECTS

The word "eugenics" was coined in 1883 by the English scientist Francis Galton, a cousin of Charles Darwin and a pioneer in the mathematical treatment of biological inheritance. Galton took the word from a Greek root meaning "good in birth" or "noble in heredity." He intended the term to denote the "science" of improving human stock by giving the "more suitable races or strains of blood a better chance of prevailing speedily over the less suitable" (Kevles, 1986, p. ix).

The idea of eugenics dated back at least to Plato, and discussion of actually achieving human biological melioration had been boosted by the Enlightenment. In Galton's day, the science of genetics had not yet emerged: Gregor Mendel's 1865 paper, the foundation of that discipline, was not only unappreciated but also generally unnoticed by the scientific community. Nevertheless, Darwin's theory of evolution taught that species did change as a result of natural selection, and it was well known that through artificial selection farmers and flower fanciers could obtain permanent breeds of animals and plants strong in particular characters. Galton thus supposed that the human race could be similarly improved—that through eugenics, human beings could take charge of their own evolution.

The idea of human biological improvement was slow to gather public support, but after the turn of the twentieth century, eugenics movements emerged in many countries. Eugenicists everywhere shared Galton's understanding that people might be improved in two complementary ways—to use Galton's language, by getting rid of the "undesirables" and by multiplying the "desirables" (Kevles, 1986, p. 3). They spoke of "positive" and "negative" eugenics. Positive eugenics aimed to foster greater representation in society of people whom eugenicists considered socially valuable. Negative eugenics sought to encourage the socially unworthy to breed less or, better yet, not at all.

How positive or negative ends were to be achieved depended heavily on which theory of human biology people brought to the eugenics movement. Many eugenicists, particularly in the United States, Britain, and Germany, believed that human beings were determined almost entirely by their germ plasm, which was passed from one generation to the next and overwhelmed environmental influences in shaping human development. Their belief was reinforced by the rediscovery, in 1900, of Mendel's theory that the biological makeup of organisms was determined by certain "factors," which were later identified with genes and were held to account for a wide array of human traits, both physical and behavioral, "good" as well as "bad."

In the first third of the twentieth century, eugenics drew the support of a number of leading biologists, not only in the United States and western Europe but also in the Soviet Union, Latin America, and elsewhere. Many of these biologists came to the creed from the practice of evolutionary biology, which they extrapolated to the Galtonian idea of taking charge of human evolution. One of the most influential was Charles B. Davenport, the head of the Station for Experimental Evolution, a part of the Carnegie Institution of Washington and located at Cold Spring Harbor, New York, where Davenport established the Eugenics Record Office. Other eugenic enthusiasts included, in the United States, the biologists Raymond Pearl, Herbert S. Jennings, Edwin Grant Conklin, William E. Castle, Edward M. East, and Herman Muller; in Britain, F. A. E. Crew, Ronald A. Fisher, and J. B. S. Haldane; and in Germany, Fritz Lenz, who held the chair of racial hygiene in Munich, and Otmar von Verschuer.

Some eugenicists, notably in France, assumed that biological organisms, including human beings, were formed primarily by their environments, physical as well as cultural. Like the early-nineteenth-century biologist Jean Baptiste Lamarck, they contended that environmental influences might even reconfigure hereditary material. Environmentalists were mainly interested in positive eugenics, contending that more attention to factors such as nutrition, medical care, education, and clean play would, by improving the young, better the human race. Some urged that the improvement should begin when children were in the womb, through sound prenatal care. The pregnant mother should avoid toxic substances, such as alcohol. She might even expose herself, for the sake of her fetus, to cultural enrichment, such as fine plays and concerts.

Individuals with good genes were assumed to be easily recognizable from their intelligence and character. Those with bad genes had to be ferreted out. For the purpose of identifying such genes, in the early twentieth century eugenics gave rise to the fist programs of research in human heredity, which were pursued in both state-supported and private laboratories established to develop eugenically useful knowledge. The Eugenics Record Office at Cold Spring Harbor was typical of these institutions; so were the Galton Laboratory for National Eugenics at University College (London), whose first director was the statistician and population biologist Karl Pearson, and the Kaiser Wilhelm Institute for Anthropology, Human Heredity, and Eugenics in Berlin, which was directed by the anthropologist Eugen Fischer. Staff at or affiliated with these laboratories gathered information bearing on human heredity by examining medical records or conducting extended family studies. Often they relied on field workers to construct trait pedigrees in selected populations—say, the residents of a rural community—on the basis of interviews and the examination of genealogical records. An important feature of German eugenic science was the study of twins.

However, social prejudices as well as dreams pervaded eugenic research, just as they did all of eugenics. Eugenic studies claimed to reveal that criminality, prostitution, and mental deficiency (which was commonly termed "feeblemindedness") were the products of bad genes. They concluded that socially desirable traits were associated with the "races" of northern Europe, especially the Nordic "race," and that undesirable ones were identified with those of eastern and southern Europe.

Eugenics entailed as many meanings as did terms such as "social adequacy" and "character." Indeed, eugenics mirrored a broad range of social attitudes, many of them centered on the role in society of women, since they were indispensable to the bearing of children. On the one hand, positive eugenicists of all stripes argued against the use of birth control or entrance into the work force of middle-class women, on grounds that any decline in their devotion to reproductive duties would lead to "race suicide." On the other hand, social radicals appealed to eugenics to justify the sexual emancipation of women. They contended that if contraception were freely available, women could pursue sexual pleasure with whomever they wished, without regard to whether a male partner was eugenically promising as a father. If and when a woman decided to become pregnant, then her choice of the father could focus on the production of a high-quality child. Sex for pleasure would thus be divorced from sex for eugenic reproduction.

In practice, little was done for positive eugenics, though eugenic claims did figure in the advent of family-allowance policies in Britain and Germany during the 1930s, and positive eugenic themes were certainly implied in the "Fitter Family" competitions that were a standard feature of eugenic programs held at state fairs in America during the 1920s. In the interest of negative eugenics, germ-plasm determinists insisted that "socially inadequate" people should be discouraged or prevented from reproducing themselves by urging or compelling them to undergo sterilization. They also argued for laws restricting marriage and immigration to their countries, in order to keep out genetically undesirable people.

In the United States, eugenicists helped obtain passage of the Immigration Act of 1924, which sharply reduced eastern and southern european immigration to the United States. By the late 1920s, some two dozen American states had enacted eugenic sterilization laws. The laws were declared constitutional in the 1927 U.S. Supreme Court decision of *Buck v. Bell,* in which Justice Oliver Wendell Holmes delivered the opinion that three generations of imbeciles are enough. The leading state in this endeavor was California, which as of 1933 had subjected more people to eugenic sterilization than had all other states of the union combined (Kevles, 1986).

At the time, a number of biologists, sociologists, anthropologists, and others increasingly criticized eugenic doctrines, contending that social deviancy is primarily the product of a disadvantageous social environment—notably, for example, of poverty and illiteracy—rather than of genes, and that apparent racial differences were not biological but cultural, the product of ethnicity rather than of germ plasm. In 1930, in the papal encyclical *Casti connubii,* the Roman Catholic church officially opposed eugenics, along with birth control. By the 1930s, a coalition of critics had helped bring a halt in most countries to the attempts of eugenicists to gain significant social and political influence. An exception to this tendency was Germany, where eugenics reached its apogee of power during the Nazi regime. Hundreds of thousands of people were sterilized for negative eugenic reasons and scientific authority joined with social hatred to send millions of the "racially unfit" to the gas chambers. Verschuer trained doctors for the SS in the intricacies of racial hygiene, and he analyzed data and specimens obtained in the concentration camps. In the years after World War II, eugenics became a dirty word.

In the 1930s, attempts to sanitize eugenics had been

made by various British and American biologists. They wanted to maintain Galton's idea of human biological improvement while rejecting the social prejudice that had pervaded the conception. They realized that a sound eugenics would have to rest on a solid science of human genetics, one that scrupulously rejected social bias and weighed the respective roles of biology and environment, of nature and nurture, in the making of the human animal. They succeeded in laying the foundation for such a science of human genetics, and that field made great strides in the following decades.

The advances in human genetics boosted the new field of genetic counseling, which provided prospective parents with advice about what their risk might be of bearing a child with a genetic disorder. In the 1950s, the early years of such counseling, some geneticists had sought to turn the practice to eugenic advantage—to reduce the incidence of genetic disease in the population, and by extension to reduce the frequency of deleterious genes in what population geneticists were coming to call the human gene pool. To that end, some claimed that it was the counselor's duty not simply to inform a couple about the possible genetic outcome of their union but also to instruct them whether to bear children at all. By the end of the 1950s, however, the informal standards of practice in genetic counseling were strongly against eugenically oriented advice—that is, advice aimed at the welfare of the gene pool rather than of the family. The standards had it that no counselor had the right to tell a couple not to have a child, even for the sake of the couple's welfare.

At first, genetic counseling could draw only on family histories and could tell parents nothing more than the odds that they might conceive a child with a recessive or dominant disease or abnormality. Since the 1960s, as the result of amniocentesis and advances in human biochemical and chromosomal genetics, genetic counseling has become coupled to technical analyses that can identify whether a prospective parent actually carries a deleterious gene and can determine prenatally whether a fetus truly suffers from a selection of genetic and chromosomal diseases or disorders. If the fetus is found to be at such a disadvantage, the parents have the option to abort—at least in countries where abortion is legal, which in 1993 included the United States, Great Britain, and France.

Reproductive selection on a genetic basis—by screening of parents, abortion of fetuses, or both—has found support among liberal religious groups, secular ethicists, and many feminists. They regard it as enlarging women's freedom to control their lives and as contributing to family well-being. However, reproductive selection has been contested by the Roman Catholic church and fundamentalist Protestants, mainly because of their opposition to abortion for any reason. Some feminists have interpreted such selection as yet another among several recent innovations in reproductive technology—for example, in vitro fertilization—that threaten to reduce women to mere reproductive machines in a patriarchal social order. Others have pointed to the heavy emotional and familial burdens placed upon women by prenatal diagnosis that reveals a fetus with a genetic disease or disorder. Genetic selection also has raised apprehensions among some members of minority groups and among disabled persons that it will lead to a revival of negative eugenics that may affect them disproportionately. Handicapped people and their advocates have attacked the attitude that a newly conceived child with a genetic affliction merits abortion, calling it a stigmatization of the living who have the ailment and the expression of a eugenics mentality (Stanworth, 1987; Rothman, 1986, 1989; Duster, 1989; Cowan, 1992).

The human genome project

These fears have been exacerbated by the Human Genome Project, the multinational effort, begun in the late 1980s, to obtain the sequence of all the DNA in the human genome. Once the complete sequence is obtained, it will in principle be easy to identify individuals with deleterious genes of a physical (or presumptively antisocial) type, and the state may intervene in reproductive behavior so as to discourage the transmission of these genes in the population. Such a policy could work special injury upon certain minority groups—for example, people of African origin, since the recessive gene for sickle-cell anemia occurs among them with comparatively high frequency. It could also threaten the disabled, since the only "therapy" currently available for most genetic or chromosomal diseases or disorders is abortion, and since identifying such fetuses as candidates for the procedure stigmatizes people who have been born with the handicap. In 1988, China's Gansu Province adopted a eugenic law that would—so the authorities said—improve population quality by banning the marriages of mentally retarded people unless they first submit to sterilization. Such laws have been adopted in other provinces and in 1991 were endorsed by Prime Minister Li Peng.

Negative eugenic intentions appeared to lie behind a July 1988 proposal from the European Commission for the creation of a human genome project in the European Community. Called a health measure, the proposal was entitled "Predictive Medicine: Human Genome Analysis." Its rationale rested on a simple syllogism—that many diseases result from interactions of genes and environment; that it would be impossible to remove all the environmental culprits from society; and that, hence, individuals could be better defended against disease by identifying their genetic predispositions to fall ill. According to the summary of the proposal: "Predictive Medicine seeks to protect individuals from the kinds of illnesses to which they are genetically most vulnerable and, where appropriate, to prevent the transmission of the genetic susceptibilities to the next generation." In the view of the European Commission, the genome proposal would make Europe more competitive—indirectly, by helping to slow the rate of increase in health expenditures; directly, by strengthening its scientific and technological base (Commission of the European Communities, 1988).

Economics may well prove to be a powerful incentive to a new negative eugenics. In the United States, the more that health care becomes a public responsibility, paid for through the tax system, and the more expensive this care becomes, the greater the possibility that taxpayers will rebel against paying for the care of those whose genetic makeup dooms them to severe disease or disability. Even in countries with national health systems, public officials might feel pressure to encourage, or even to compel, people not to bring genetically affected children into the world—not for the sake of the gene pool but in the interest of keeping public health costs down.

However, a number of factors are likely to offset a broad-based revival of negative eugenics. Eugenics profits from authoritarianism—indeed, almost requires it. The institutions of political democracy may not have been robust enough to resist altogether the violations of civil liberties characteristic of the early eugenics movement, but they did contest them effectively in many places. The British government refused to pass eugenic sterilization laws. So did many American states; and where they were enacted, they were often unenforced. Awareness of the barbarities and cruelties of state-sponsored eugenics in the past has tended to set most geneticists and the public at large against such programs. Moreover, persons with handicaps or diseases are politically empowered, as are minority groups, to a degree that they were not in the early twentieth century. They may not be sufficiently empowered to counter all quasi-eugenic threats to themselves, but they are politically positioned, with allies in the media, the medical profession, and elsewhere, including the Roman Catholic church, to block or at least to hinder eugenic proposals that might affect them.

The European Commission's proposal for a human genome project provoked the emergence of an antieugenic coalition in the European Parliament that was led by Benedikt Härlin, a member of the West German Green Party. The Greens had helped impose severe restrictions on biotechnology in West Germany and raised objections to human genome research on grounds that it might lead to a recrudescence of Nazi biological policies. Guided by Härlin, the European Parliament's

Committee on Energy, Research and Technology raised a red flag against the genome project as an enterprise in preventive medicine. It reminded the European Community that in the past, eugenic ideas had led to "horrific consequences" and declared that "clear pointers to eugenic tendencies and goals" inhered in the intention of protecting people from contracting and transmitting genetic diseases or conditions. The application of human genetic information for such purposes would almost always involve decisions—fundamentally eugenic ones—about what are "normal and abnormal, acceptable and unacceptable, viable and non-viable forms of the genetic make-up of individual human beings before and after birth." The Härlin Report also warned that the new biological and reproductive technologies could make for a "modern test tube eugenics," a eugenics all the more insidious because it could disguise more easily than its cruder ancestors "an even more radical and totalitarian form of 'biopolitics'" (European Parliament, Committee on Energy, Research, and Technology, 1988–1989, pp. 23–28).

The Härlin Report urged thirty-eight amendments to the European Commission's proposal, including the complete excision of the phrase "predictive medicine" from the text. As a result of the report, which won support not only from German Greens but also from conservatives on both sides of the English Channel, including German Catholics, the European Commission produced a modified proposal that accepted the thrust of the amendments and even the language of a number of them. The new proposal called for a three-year program of human genome analysis as such, without regard to predictive medicine, and committed the European Community in a variety of ways—most notably, by prohibiting human germ line research and genetic intervention with human embryos—to avoid eugenic practices, prevent ethical missteps, and protect individual rights and privacy. It also promised to keep the European Parliament and the public fully informed via annual reports on the moral and legal basis of human genome research. Formally adopted in June 1990, the European Community's human genome program will cost 15 million ECU (about $17 million) over three years, with some one million ECU devoted to ethical studies (Kevles and Hood, 1992).

In the United States, apprehensions of the ethical dangers in the Human Genome Project found expression in the Congress across the political spectrum—from liberals who had long been concerned about governmental intrusion into private genetic matters to conservatives who worried that the Human Genome Project might foster increased practice of prenatal diagnosis and abortion. Among the Americans most sensitive to the eugenic hazards and the ethical challenges inherent in the project were a number of its leading scientific enthusiasts, particularly James D. Watson, the first head of the National Center for Human Genome Research, who considered it both appropriate and imperative that the American genome program stimulate study and debate about its social, ethical, and legal implications. In 1988, Watson announced that such activities would be eligible for roughly 3 percent of the National Center's budget. He told a 1989 scientific conference on the genome: "We have to be aware of the really terrible past of eugenics, where incomplete knowledge was used in a very cavalier and rather awful way, both here in the United States and in Germany. We have to reassure people that their own DNA is private and that no one else can get at it" (Kevles and Hood, 1992, pp. 34–35).

Human genetics in a market economy

Despite the specter of eugenics that some see in the Human Genome Project, many observers hold that its near-term ethical challenges lie neither in private forays into human genetic improvement nor in some state-mandated program of eugenics. They lie in the grit of what the project will produce in abundance: genetic information. These challenges center on the control, diffusion, and use of that information within the context of a market economy.

The advance of human genetics and biotechnology has created the capacity for a kind of individual eugenics—families deciding what kinds of children they wish to have. At the moment, the kinds they can choose are those without certain disabilities or diseases, such as Down syndrome or Tay-Sachs disease. Although most parents would now probably prefer just a healthy baby, in the future they might be tempted by the opportunity—for example, via genetic analysis of embryos—to have improved babies, children who are likely to be more intelligent or more athletic or better-looking (whatever such terms might mean). People may well pursue such possibilities, given the interest that some parents have shown in choosing the sex of their child or that others have shown in the administration of growth hormone to offspring they think will grow up too short. In sum, a kind of private eugenics could arise from consumer demand.

Many commentators have noted that the torrent of new human genetic information will undoubtedly pose challenges to social fairness and equity. They have emphasized that employers may seek to deny jobs to applicants with a susceptibility—or an alleged susceptibility—to disorders such as manic depression or illnesses arising from features of the workplace. For example, around 1970, it came to be feared that people with sickle-cell trait—that is, who possess one of the recessive genes for the disease—might suffer the sickling of their red-blood cells in the reduced-oxygen environment of high altitudes. Such people were unjustly prohibited from entering the Air Force Academy, were restricted to ground jobs by several major commercial air carriers, and often were charged higher premiums by insurance companies. Life and medical insurance companies may well wish to know the genomic signatures of their clients, their profile of risk for disease and death. Even national health systems might choose to ration the provision of care on the basis of genetic propensity for disease, especially to families at risk for bearing diseased children (U.S. Congress, Office of Technology Assessment, 1990; Kevles, 1986).

In response to these threatening prospects, many analysts have contended that individual genomic information should be protected as strictly private. However, legal and insurance analysts have pointed out that insurance, and insurance premiums, depend on assessments of risk. If a client has a high genetic medical risk that is not reflected in the premium charged, then that person receives a high payout at low cost to himself or herself but at high cost to the company. The problem would be compounded if the person knows the risk—while the company does not—and purchases a large amount of insurance. In either case, the company would have to pass its increased costs to other policyholders, which is to say that high-risk policyholders would be taxing low-risk ones. Thus, insisting on a right to privacy in genetic information could well lead—at least under the largely private system of insurance that now prevails in the United States—to inequitable consequences.

American legislatures have already begun to focus on the genuine social, ethical, and policy issues that the Human Genome Project raises, particularly those concerning the use of private human genetic information. In the fall of 1991, a U.S. House of Representatives subcommittee held hearings on the challenge that such information posed to insurability. About the same time, the California state legislature passed a bill banning employers, health service agencies and disability insurers from withholding jobs or protection simply because a person is a carrier of a single gene associated with disability. Although California Governor Pete Wilson vetoed the bill, it was a harbinger of the type of public policy initiatives that the genome project no doubt will increasingly call forth. The Human Genome Project, like most of human and medical genetics, is less likely to foster a drive for a new eugenics than it is to pose vexing challenges to public policy and private practices for the control and use of human genetic information.

DANIEL J. KEVLES

Directly related to this article is the companion article in this entry: ETHICAL ISSUES. *Also directly related are the entries*

EUGENICS AND RELIGIOUS LAW; NATIONAL SOCIALISM; RACE AND RACISM; GENETIC ENGINEERING, *article on* HUMAN GENETIC ENGINEERING; *and* GENETICS AND RACIAL MINORITIES. *For a further discussion of topics mentioned in this article, see the entries* ABORTION; DEATH AND DYING: EUTHANASIA AND SUSTAINING LIFE, *article on* HISTORICAL ASPECTS; FERTILITY CONTROL; FUTURE GENERATIONS, OBLIGATIONS TO; GENE THERAPY; GENETIC COUNSELING; GENETIC TESTING AND SCREENING; GENETICS AND THE LAW; GENOME MAPPING AND SEQUENCING; HEALTH TESTING AND SCREENING IN THE PUBLIC-HEALTH CONTEXT; MEDICAL GENETICS; REPRODUCTIVE TECHNOLOGIES, *articles on* SEX SELECTION, *and* CRYOPRESERVATION OF SPERM, OVA, AND EMBRYOS; WARFARE, *article on* PUBLIC HEALTH AND WAR; *and* WOMEN; *articles on* HISTORICAL AND CROSS-CULTURAL PERSPECTIVES, *and* HEALTH-CARE ISSUES. *For a discussion of related ideas, see the entries* BIOLOGY, PHILOSOPHY OF; EVOLUTION; GENETICS AND HUMAN BEHAVIOR; GENETICS AND HUMAN SELF-UNDERSTANDING; *and* HEALTH AND DISEASE. *See also the* APPENDIX (CODES, OATHS, AND DIRECTIVES RELATED TO BIOETHICS), Section IV: ETHICAL DIRECTIVES FOR HUMAN RESEARCH.

Bibliography

ADAMS, MARK B., ed. 1990. *The Wellborn Science: Eugenics in Germany, France, Brazil, and Russia.* New York: Oxford University Press.

BERNARD, JEAN. 1990. *De la biologie à l'éthique: Nouveaux pouvoirs de la science, nouveaux devoirs de l'homme.* Paris: Éditions Buchet–Chastel.

COMMISSION OF THE EUROPEAN COMMUNITY. 1988. *Proposal for a Council Decision Adopting a Specific Research Programme in the Field of Health; Predictive Medicine: Human Genome Analysis (1989–1991).* COM (88) 424 final-SYN 146. Brussels: Author.

COWAN, RUTH SCHWARTZ. 1992. "Genetic Technology and Reproductive Choice: An Ethics for Autonomy." In *The Code of Codes: Scientific and Social Issues in the Human Genome Project,* pp. 244–263. Edited by Daniel J. Kevles and Leroy Hood. Cambridge, Mass.: Harvard University Press.

DAVIS, JOEL. 1990. *Mapping the Code: The Human Genome Project and the Choices of Modern Science.* New York: John Wiley.

DUSTER, TROY. 1990. *Backdoor to Eugenics.* New York: Routledge.

EUROPEAN PARLIAMENT, COMMITTEE ON ENERGY, RESEARCH AND TECHNOLOGY. 1988–1989. *Report Drawn up on Behalf of the Committee on Energy, Research and Technology on the Proposal from the Commission to the Council (COM/88/424-C2-119/88) for a Decision Adopting a Specific Research Programme in the Field of Health: Predictive Medicine: Human Genome Analysis (1989–1991).* Rapporteur European Parliament Session Documents, 1988–89, 30.01.1989, Series A, Doc. A2-0370/88 SYN 146. Benedikt Härlin, rapporteur. Brussels: Author.

FARRALL, LYNDSAY A. 1979. "The History of Eugenics: A Bibliographical Review." *Annals of Science* 36, no. 2: 111–123.

GERMAN BUNDESTAG. 1987. *Report of the Commission of Enquiry on Prospects and Risks of Genetic Engineering.* 10th Legislative Period, Paper 10/6775. Bonn: Author.

HOLTZMAN, NEIL A. 1989. *Proceed with Caution: Predicting Genetic Risks in the Recombinant DNA Era.* Baltimore: Johns Hopkins University Press.

KEVLES, DANIEL J. 1986. *In the Name of Eugenics: Genetics and the Uses of Human Heredity.* Berkeley: University of California Press.

KEVLES, DANIEL J., and HOOD, LEROY, eds. 1992. *The Code of Codes: Scientific and Social Issues in the Human Genome Project.* Cambridge, Mass.: Harvard University Press.

MÜLLER-HILL, BENNO. 1988. *Murderous Science: Elimination by Scientific Selection of Jews, Gypsies, and Others, Germany, 1933–1945.* Translated by George F. Fraser. New York: Oxford University Press.

PROCTOR, ROBERT. 1988. *Racial Hygiene: Medicine Under the Nazis.* Cambridge, Mass.: Harvard University Press.

ROTHMAN, BARBARA KATZ. 1986. *The Tentative Pregnancy: Prenatal Diagnosis and the Future of Motherhood.* New York: Viking.

———. 1989. *Recreating Motherhood: Ideology and Technology in a Patriarchal Society.* New York: W. W. Norton.

SCHNEIDER, WILLIAM H. 1990. *Quality and Quantity: The Quest for Biological Regeneration in Twentieth-Century France.* Cambridge: At the University Press.

STANWORTH, MICHELLE, ed. 1987. *Reproductive Technologies: Gender, Motherhood and Medicine.* Minneapolis: University of Minnesota Press.

U.S. CONGRESS. OFFICE OF TECHNOLOGY ASSESSMENT. 1990. *Genetic Monitoring and Screening in the Workplace.* Washington, D.C.: U.S. Government Printing Office.

WEINDLING, PAUL. 1989. *Health, Race and German Politics Between National Unification and Nazism, 1870–1945.* Cambridge: At the University Press.

WINGERSON, LOIS. 1990. *Mapping Our Genes: The Genome Project and the Future of Medicine.* New York: Dutton.

II. ETHICAL ISSUES

"Eugenics" (from the Greek for "wellborn") was coined in 1883 by Sir Francis Galton (1822–1911) to describe a form of applied heredity that could "improve the inborn qualities of a race" (Galton, 1869). The rationale for eugenic improvement came directly from the successes of animal breeders. Animal husbandmen who bred livestock and chickens discovered that they could increase the prevalence of desirable features (such as exceptional fatback thickness or egg production) by selectively mating specimens with the desired trait. These observations suggested to Galton and his cousin Charles Darwin the possibility of human "improvement" through genetic means (see Darwin, 1871).

Even in its earliest conception, eugenics raised ethical issues because it presupposed the acceptability of social institutions that would favor one group over another. Galton's vision was to encourage judicious mating practices, control of social institutions, and other policies that gave procreative advantage to persons with "superior" traits over those deemed less genetically worthy. What constitutes a superior genetic trait is but one of the many ethical issues raised by eugenics.

While such intuitive observations provided the rationale for eugenics, both moral and practical reasons limited the achievement of eugenic ends. The justification for eugenic programs in the United States (Kevles, 1985) and Europe (Ludmerer, 1972) during the 1920s and 1930s was at best quasi-scientific and based on the crudest of political theory. Political eugenics in the Third Reich reached a scientific nadir in programs like the *Lebensborn* ("Spring of Life") movement, in which SS (*Schutzstaffel*) officers were "selectively" mated to idealized Aryan young women without regard to morality or genotype, and "biologically valuable" infants were kidnapped and placed in orphanages. Later, the children were assigned to "suitable" Aryan families (Lifton, 1986). Such heinous acts, coupled with the attempt to extirpate whole peoples in the Holocaust, led to public revulsion and the precipitous decline of eugenics after World War II.

Scientific considerations

The likelihood that any given trait can be augmented through controlled mating is called the "opportunity for selection." This opportunity depends heavily on the extent of genetic diversity—the frequency and number of different genetic variants maintained in a population—and on the degree to which a given trait is determined by genetic factors. Extensive human genetic diversity affords ample opportunity for selection. Even among groups with long histories of common lineages, such as certain South American Indian tribes, sufficient genetic variation and evolutionary potential continue to exist to permit genetic change (Salzano and Callegari-Jacques, 1988). These observations suggest that some form of human eugenics remains theoretically possible, even in groups that have undergone evolutionary "bottlenecks" that in theory reduce their genetic variability.

In spite of genetic diversity, present patterns of human reproduction and demographics in most developed countries limit the opportunity for eugenics. Unlike the controlled breeding possible within domesticated animal populations or Nazi Germany, moral strictures on directed reproduction in most cultures make systematic control of reproduction infeasible. Where little variance exists in the numbers of children that families bear and low mortality across groups is the norm, genetic change

is largely stifled. Thus, little intrinsic opportunity exists in most developed countries for the enrichment of certain genotypes over others. This is particularly true in the United States and Scandinavian countries, where the population replacement rate barely exceeds or equals the death rate (zero population growth).

Even where population growth has slowed or stalled, microdemographic conditions can have subtle genetic impacts. Under such circumstances, if only a few families leave many offspring over several generations, their genetic contributions to society will increase disproportionately. For instance, in America some families with the Huntington's chorea gene were uncharacteristically large as a result of some as yet unknown "reproductive compensation" in those carrying the responsible gene(-s). Over several generations, these Huntington's family lineages have increased more rapidly than the surrounding population, thus increasing the frequency of Huntington's gene(-s). Since Huntington's chorea is caused by a single gene, giving such families the choice of not reproducing or selectively aborting Huntington's disease-positive fetuses could reduce the frequency of the Huntington's gene. Would this program be desirable?

It is important to note that the full "adaptive value or disvalue" of this and many other genes is incompletely understood. Moreover, the Huntington's mutation(-s), as well as those for hemophilia and other single-gene-determined conditions, are constantly reintroduced into the population at a relatively high rate through spontaneous mutation. In developed countries where the age of procreation is delayed and environmental mutagens are prevalent, high mutation "loads" in older sperm and eggs will tend to negate eugenic efforts. These factors increase the necessity for ethical analysis of various eugenic policies to include those designed to affect the occurrence of mutations as well as the transmission of genetic traits in populations.

Types of eugenics

Eugenic initiatives can be divided into two subcategories: *positive eugenics*, in which the frequency of presumptively desirable or beneficial genes is increased; and *negative eugenics*, in which deleterious genes are eliminated from the gene pool. Policies that reduce the frequency of desirable genetic combinations or increase those that are deleterious are said to be *dysgenic*. It is also useful to bifurcate eugenic policies into those that embrace whole populations or groups (*macro eugenics*) from those that affect only families or kinship groups (*micro eugenics*).

A program with a macroeugenic impact is one that gradually increases the frequency of presumptively beneficial genes over several generations. Positive macro eugenics occurs when whole cultural or ethnic groups with "desirable" genes are given incentives to adopt procreative methods that give them a selective advantage over other groups. Such a policy could result by default.

Simply discouraging certain forms of birth control or abortion in a targeted group, or providing tax advantages for procreation within certain social classes, offers a selective advantage to identified groups. While such policies do in fact occur, they are not at present linked to eugenic ends in any conscious way, largely because no "desirable" genotypes have been scientifically defined at a group level.

Similar macroeugenic impacts through negative eugenics are also possible: such ends were intended by the Nazi policies of forced sterilization and extermination of reproducing members of various ethnic groups, especially Jews. Today, no one would expect *intentionally genetic* macro policies to be countenanced in developed countries for both political and moral reasons; yet "ethnic cleansing" has occurred in regions of the former Yugoslavia, with little concerted opposition.

A program with a microeugenic impact is one in which an individual couple and their extended family are afforded access to greater genetic choice than is the norm. For instance, the early utilization of prenatal diagnosis was largely limited to certain high-income families (Lappe, 1981). Today, such a trend is evident in the selective availability and use of genetic tests by well-to-do couples during germ cell or zygote selection, in vitro fertilization, embryo transfer, and other forms of assisted fertility. These policies can in theory provide a microeugenic advantage to families that can afford these interventions by giving them some assurance of "genetic quality" in their offspring. This edge may be more imagined than real, depending on the actual ability of genetic testing to reduce the occurrence of abnormal or defective genes while not inadvertently introducing others. Because such policies are directed primarily at women, they raise special ethical issues discussed below.

Ethical perspectives

Proper ethical analysis of eugenic considerations is clouded by intrinsic uncertainties of the appropriate definition of the terms used in discussing eugenic initiatives. Each term carries poorly defined value connotations. Words like "normal," "deleterious," "desirable," "undesirable," and "improvement" are scientifically vague as they apply to the human genetic stock. A precise definition of a "deleterious genotype" remains unclear, in spite of our increased understanding of causation of genetic disease.

For instance, does a carrier of one or more recessive genes that in combination can cause genetic disease like sickle-cell anemia have a deleterious genotype? What about single genes, like those associated with colon cancer, that do not universally predict cancer occurrence

when present? Often, carrier status is associated with heightened resistance to disease (as appears to be the case for several genetic loci and malaria) rather than with the selective disadvantage implied by a "deleterious genotype." The acceptability of moving from the "is" of this sort of human genetic variation to the "ought" of using this variation to effect eugenic ends is a critical ethical issue in eugenics.

The overall moral acceptability of implementing any eugenic strategy turns on the definition, human cost, and justification for using genetics to effect human "improvement." A naturalistic view in ethics is that the place of humans in the order of nature makes it clear that evolution has a direction and, by inference, that improvement is an imperative because it is an extension of the natural order (Sperry, 1974). At least one prominent evolutionary biologist contests this view (Simpson, 1974) by noting that nothing in the evolutionary program would suggest an innate tendency toward "progress." Religious scholars have observed that no reason exists to interpret human destiny as indicative of a divine imperative toward species improvement (Ramsey, 1970).

The same argument may not apply to preventing harm to the gene pool and, by inference, to the species from dysgenic trends. While no duty may exist to effect improvement, assuring that no harm occurs generally carries a stronger moral imperative in medicine than does beneficence. Thus, some have argued for the critical importance of maintaining the integrity of the gene pool by protecting it from accumulation of excessive mutations (see Lappe, 1981). Reduction of environmental mutagens coupled with an emphasis on procreation at earlier ages might be such a combination.

Because eugenic methods have historically been offered by those who are "best off" in terms of political power (not necessarily genotype), eugenics raises issues of justice and fairness to those who, through no fault of their own, receive a poorer share of the genetic lottery. Historically, sterilization policies have been directed at the poor, in the mistaken belief that they were the embodiment of defective genes (Reilly, 1977).

Eugenics provides a lens through which to see this and other forms of reproductive coercion. Ethicists have long questioned the acceptability of using coercion through officially sanctioned policies or social suasion to influence the reproductive choices in certain groups. This can occur when welfare recipients are penalized for having children, or when genetic policies are directed at members of one sex and not the other.

Issues affecting women

Since many eugenic policies entail the tacit or conscripted cooperation of women, they can be highly discriminatory by posing disproportionate risks—both physical and psychosocial—to women. Examples include female-centered sterilization programs and protracted contraception policies (Depo-Provera), the use of prenatal diagnosis and abortion, and welfare payments linked to procreative status. Some states, notably California, have policies that mandate, with only a modicum of informed consent, that all women undergo prenatal serum tests (for alpha-fetoprotein) to detect pregnancies at risk for neural tube defects or Down syndrome. While amniocentesis previously was used primarily for identifying seriously affected fetuses (e.g., those with Tay-Sachs disease), serum alpha-fetoprotein testing of prospective mothers prior to amniocentesis has a high false-positive rate and provides test results that embrace a range of conditions. Some of the "affected" fetuses so detected include less severely impaired ones (e.g., those with Down syndrome or minor neural tube defects) and a small percentage of otherwise normal fetuses.

The nearly universal participation of women in serum alpha-fetoprotein programs and their high acceptance rate of the subsequent "indicated" abortions approximates a eugenic program. Such genetically "selective" abortion and prenatal diagnosis generally are said to place a high psychosocial burden on women (Rothman, 1992), and are deemed to reduce rather than enhance genetic diversity (Bonnicksen, 1992).

The expansion of the use of genetic diagnoses to embrace the testing of embryos during in vitro fertilization and embryo transfer also impacts directly on women's reproductive freedom. The advent of a large spectrum of testable genotypes through the Human Genome Program, coupled with gamete choice, pre-embryo genetic testing, and selective in vitro fertilization will likely place social and psychological pressure on women to opt for "quality" and not merely reproductive success.

Such programs raise the specter of a eugenics program in which women serve as passive receptacles of artificially selected embryos (Lippman, 1990). Were such programs to conscript poor women and deny them both free and fully informed consent, as many claim surrogate mother programs initially did, they would be especially objectionable. The venue for the choices involved in such genetic selection would most likely be a genetic counseling clinic.

Genetic counseling and eugenics

Eugenic considerations are not usually overtly identified in programs that might influence reproductive decision making. American and European genetic counselors openly disavow any eugenic objectives to their practice (Wertz and Fletcher, 1988). The American Society of Human Genetics does not have any policy statement that implies a eugenic ideal. It is neither the primary nor the secondary objective of any medical society in the United States to adopt policies that impact on future generations or their genetic composition. These policies are often the result of reaction against a eugenic taint, and not necessarily a rational conclusion. For this reason, stated and actual policies may be inconsistent.

For instance, most counselors recognize that many existing genetic programs, including prenatal diagnosis, newborn screening, and carrier screening may have subtle or profound eugenic or dysgenic impacts. A value-neutral stance, such as that taken by genetic counselors regarding the impact of their genetic information, may be dysgenic, eugenic, or neutral, depending on the circumstances.

Because of value neutrality, genetic counseling as presently practiced does not usually protect certain families or ethnic groups from passing on deleterious genes. Groups that intermarry among close relatives (like the Amish) have higher than normal coefficients of inbreeding and therefore may transmit more deleterious genes in a double-recessive state (i.e., both parents pass on the same gene) than will other populations who intermarry more randomly.

A closer examination of the counseling process and content reveals that eugenic ends may be subtly incorporated into the options and disease entities chosen for inclusion as "suitable" for selective abortion (see Lippman, 1990). An example would be sex chromosome abnormalities that usually are associated only with minor physical and mental abnormalities. Revealing to anxious parents the genetic status of a fetus with Turner's syndrome (where the absence of an X chromosome leads to short stature, webbed neck, and subtle neurological deficits in girls) is a case in point, since the child's ultimate well-being is only marginally impaired.

The value-neutral counseling ethic leads to a non-interventionism that may of necessity permit dysgenic outcomes. The process of aborting a fetus with a deleterious recessive disease and then compensating for the loss of the expected child by trying to have more children ultimately results in a subtle increase in frequency of the recessive gene over many generations. This is true because with reproductive compensation, two-thirds of all of the live children will be carriers of the recessive gene at issue, instead of the one-half normally expected without prenatal diagnosis. (Such a dysgenic trend will not be true for prenatal diagnosis of dominant disorders. For example, selective abortion directed against a fetus carrying the gene for a dominant condition like polycystic kidney disease will lead to a rapid decline in the gene frequency.)

For prenatal diagnosis programs directed against X-linked conditions, such as Duchenne's muscular dystrophy or hemophilia A, aborting male fetuses will lead to more births of girls, half of whom will be carriers of the gene. A "eugenic" policy that aborted female carrier *fetuses* is considered morally unacceptable. But with the ability to test *pre-embryos* for their carrier status, their destruction in order to find a noncarrier replacement may be seen as morally acceptable. With the advent of these pre-embryo and related germ cell selection technologies, counselors who espouse a "no eugenics" view may not convince couples eager to improve the genetic status of their offspring.

Justifying eugenic policies

The appropriateness of providing state-sponsored services to encourage reproductive choices (for example, the screening programs for alpha fetoprotein and neural tube defects) is a more subtle ethical issue than that of forced sterilization, mandatory genetic testing, or state-encouraged selective abortion. The major ethical questions posed by intentionally adopting (or ignoring) potential eugenic or dysgenic impacts of these or related reproductive choices turn on the following considerations, among others: our duties to present versus future generations; the obligation not to do harm versus the duty to benefit; and the obligation of health professionals to provide for the needs of individuals or families versus that of protecting the gene pool as a whole.

These problems arise in the context of consanguinity. Marriage between related individuals can be considered genetically disadvantageous to the extent it brings together otherwise rare, recessive genes. But for some cultures, "desirable" marriages may involve first- or second-cousin matings, while in others, interbreeding within ethnic or religious lineages is expressly proscribed by scripture or common law. When, if ever, should society intervene to discourage such marriages?

From a purely theoretical perspective, it is possible to entertain the idea of eugenics on the premise that there is nothing intrinsically wrong with considering ways to improve the human condition as long as societal values are reinforced and overt harms to vulnerable populations are avoided. It has been argued (in Singapore) that a state that is not unnecessarily burdened by individuals with "avoidable" genetic diseases will be one that can compete more efficiently in international markets. Such a simplistic assumption belies the ethical tensions that arise when societal benefits accrue only at the expense of restricting individual reproductive and social freedoms.

Eugenic programs may compromise persons in other ways. The well-being of extant individuals may suffer when social policy permits prenatal diagnosis and abortion of fetal individuals with the same condition. This conflict is exemplified by the alpha-fetoprotein screening program in California, which was opposed by persons with neural tube–related disabilities, out of concern that it would diminish social acceptance of their normalcy.

In theory, reproductive freedom is protected by affording an informed consent mechanism before embarking on any genetic testing or selective abortion. In practice, the fact that a certain policy is state-sanctioned can be taken to imply an ulterior motive to reduce the overall birth incidence of a costly disorder and to replace affected individuals with others more socially or medically acceptable. Some observers (Duster, 1990) regard genetic screening policies as tantamount to a back door to eugenics, since their existence reflects a de facto acceptance of a social policy of genetic exclusion.

Validating eugenic policies

Because genetic disease entails suffering, and minimization of suffering is a widely recognized and legitimate goal of medicine, all potentially eugenic policies that affect a whole population can be measured against this claim for legitimating genetic change. It is reasonable to ask if adopting a eugenic policy would materially reduce human suffering in the long run. Where and when does the current genetic status of a given group of extended family members warrant genetic intervention on this basis?

Eugenic interventions can be weighed against certain ethical tenets. While eugenic interventions are usually ethically suspect because they entail blunt and often coercive policies, there are special circumstances when such policies may be acceptable. Among the conditions that need to be met are at least the following:

1. The genetic condition of a particular group has been demonstrated to be sufficiently endangering to justify an intervention.
2. The persons who will be affected by the policy are given a voice in the decision making.
3. The ends sought are justified by the group's own standards and norms, at costs the group finds acceptable.
4. The means are necessary and ethically acceptable to the affected persons.
5. Policymakers can give reasonable assurances that both the risks and the benefits of the proposed policy will be equitably distributed.
6. Societal goals can be accomplished without infringing on other cultural or fundamental values.
7. The eugenic policy represents the least coercive option to attain the agreed upon objective.

To take the simplest example, an Indian population around Lake Maracaibo in Venezuela has one of the highest gene frequencies for Huntington's disease, a disorder that wreaks havoc in their indigenous cultural setting. This population also has an intrinsically high fertility rate, and hence could reduce or even eliminate most occurrences of the disease if restrictive reproductive policies were adopted for gene carriers. Would it be proper or acceptable to offer a populationwide program to identify and counsel persons with the Huntington's gene to not reproduce? Would such a policy be more acceptable than the present option of affording nondirective information through genetic counseling?

In the instance of the Maracaibo Indians, the conditions enumerated above could in theory be met, yet the question of respecting the cultural integrity of the group is not addressed. Eugenic questions almost always raise such political questions even after ethical issues are addressed.

Ethical/political interface

Constitutional and ethical arguments against eugenics turn on the primacy of privacy in reproductive decision making. Any moral justification for a postmodern eugenics must establish the legitimacy of the state's claim of a right to limit fundamental reproductive freedoms based on individual differences. The necessity for making political judgments about reproductive choice may intensify as the real or perceived impact of deleterious genes on social institutions and health-care costs becomes more evident. With the advent of expanded genetic testing the workplace-based health insurance, the reproductive decisions made by employees may become the province of the employer. A carrier of cystic fibrosis, while not himself at risk of serious illness, may produce a child who will carry great costs to the insurer if he is married to another carrier and wants to have progeny. Hence, the possibility that employers may discriminate based on genetic status can occur and may have unintended eugenic consequences must be considered (see Draper, 1992).

Although ostensibly "eugenic" changes in gene frequency can occur through chance events or crude public policies (for example, the use of tax incentives in Singapore to encourage the breeding of well-to-do individuals), ethical issues arise most graphically under circumstances in which the distribution of genetic material is controlled intentionally. This can occur when carriers of genetic disease–causing genes are subjected to screening programs with implied social objectives of limiting procreation. Such an event occurred in the early 1970s when African-Americans with sickle-cell trait, who were themselves largely unaffected by their genetic status, were excluded from certain jobs or military service, and were required in some states to take genetic tests (for sickle-cell trait) as a condition for a marriage license.

When policy decisions restrict the reproductive options of certain groups, they constitute a kind of back door to eugenics. Such policies can carry a social connotation that diminishes the perceived worth of groups with certain genotypes. Policies of reproductive screening and/or exclusion can be mistakenly associated with "solutions" to societal ills. Such events as testing of newborns for an extra Y chromosome, mistakenly believed to be associated with criminality, are freighted with moral weight. This is especially true when socially identified or targeted genes are localized in certain ethnic or cultural groups with a long tradition of social exclusion or discrimination. The roots of such genetic lineages will become more evident as data are generated by the initiative to map and sequence the human genome. Such data raise questions about the potential misuse of genetics in forensic and other societally sanctioned activities especially where incorporating ethnic differences may be crucial for accurate testing.

The human genome program

Because of the greatly expanded net of genes identified through the Human Genome Program as it proceeds to describe the full sequence of the three billion bases on the human chromosomes, the opportunity for eugenic applications in setting diagnostic policies will undoubtedly increase. This program will provide a data base for genetic screening and testing that could provide couples with greatly enhanced knowledge of the genetic consequences of their reproduction, and for the potential to select sperm and/or eggs with certain genotypes prior to fertilization. The availability of new "nondestructive" genetic tests (for example, the use of the discarded polar body to assess the genetic makeup of a recently fertilized zygote) provides a still more radical opportunity for microeugenic choices. Issues of intentional killing or elimination of embryos or fetuses with certain genotypes (a key argument against germline engineering) ostensibly would be obviated by the use of such techniques.

The Human Genome Program would also provide a means of identifying groups of persons whose load of putatively adverse genetic mutations is disproportionately high compared with that of the surrounding population. Such populations probably exist generally, and high concentrations may be found among offspring whose parents were exposed to highly mutagenic chemicals (e.g., ethylene oxide) or ionizing radiation.

Such an eventuality suggests that ethical considerations of the eugenic impact of reproductive choices have a component of distributive justice. Deciding what groups benefit by virtue of their good "gene quality" and who may be hurt by continued neglect of their "genetic burden" are ethical dilemmas of the next century. With a font of genetic knowledge, ignoring genetic differences is itself a policy that requires justification.

Applying ethical principles

The major ethical issues surrounding eugenics should focus on integrating existing ethical principles with the new science of defined human genetics. Among the principles that can be invoked are the following:

1. Intergenerational justice. It is desirable not to leave the next generation worse off than the present one.
2. Scientific responsibility. Before genetic tests are put into commerce, it is incumbent on scientists and clinicians to use moral imagination to project the consequences of applying them.
3. Not harming. The duty not to harm takes precedence over the duty to benefit, suggesting that negative eugenics, in which certain deleterious genes are kept from reentering the gene pool, has priority over positive eugenics.
4. Autonomy. Respecting autonomy requires a continuation of the present policies of allowing reproductive freedom and privacy in individual decision making (Lappé, 1986).
5. Justice. Any benefits or risks of new genetic programs should be equitably distributed, and new policies adjusted in favor of the least well-off (Rawls, 1971) should be given priority over those that appear to afford social benefit at the expense of the genetically "handicapped."

With these policies in place, small-scale eugenic programs could in theory be instituted, albeit not without much public dialogue and legal protections to assure that discrimination and coercion are minimized. Ultimately, however, eugenic programs will continue to be ethically suspect because to work, they must favor or penalize extant or unborn human beings by virtue of their genetic and not their intrinsic social worth.

MARC LAPPÉ

Directly related to this article is the companion article in this entry: HISTORICAL ASPECTS. *Also directly related are the entries* EUGENICS AND RELIGIOUS LAW; FUTURE GENERATIONS, OBLIGATIONS TO; GENE THERAPY; GENETIC COUNSELING; GENETIC ENGINEERING, *article on* HUMAN GENETIC ENGINEERING; GENETICS AND HUMAN SELF-UNDERSTANDING; GENETICS AND THE LAW; GENETICS AND RACIAL MINORITIES; GENETIC TESTING AND SCREENING; GENOME MAPPING AND SEQUENCING; HEALTH TESTING AND SCREENING IN THE PUBLIC HEALTH CONTEXT; MEDICAL GENETICS; NATIONAL SOCIALISM; RACE AND RACISM; *and* REPRODUCTIVE TECHNOLOGIES, *articles on* SEX SELECTION, *and* CRYOPRESERVATION OF SPERM, OVA, AND EMBRYOS. *For a further discussion of topics mentioned in this article, see the entries* ABORTION; CRYONICS; DEATH AND DYING: EUTHANASIA AND SUSTAINING LIFE, *article on* HISTORICAL ASPECTS; FERTILITY CONTROL; VALUE AND VALUATION; WARFARE, *article on* PUBLIC HEALTH AND WAR; *and* WOMEN, *articles on* HISTORICAL AND CROSS-CULTURAL PERSPECTIVES, *and* HEALTH-CARE ISSUES. *For a discussion of related ideas, see the entries* BIOLOGY, PHILOSOPHY OF; EVOLUTION; GENETICS AND HUMAN BEHAVIOR; *and* HEALTH AND DISEASE. *See also the* APPENDIX (CODES, OATHS, AND DIRECTIVES RELATED TO BIOETHICS), *Section* IV: ETHICAL DIRECTIVES FOR HUMAN RESEARCH.

Bibliography

BONNICKSEN, ANDREA. 1992. "Genetic Diagnosis of Human Embryos." *Hastings Center Report* 22, no. 4:S5–S11.

CLARKE, ANGUS. 1991. "Is Non-directive Genetic Counselling Possible?" *Lancet* 338, no. 8773:998–1001.

DARWIN, CHARLES. 1871. *The Descent of Man and Selection in Relation to Sex.* 2 vols. London: John Murray.

DRAPER, EILEEN. 1992. "Genetic Secrets: Social Issues of Medical Screening in a Genetic Age." *Hastings Center Report* 22, no. 4:S15–S18.

DUSTER, TROY. 1990. *Backdoor to Eugenics.* New York: Routledge.

GALTON, FRANCIS, SIR. 1869. *Hereditary Genius: An Inquiry into Its Laws and Consequences.* London: Macmillan. Repr. Gloucester, Mass.: Peter Smith, 1972.

HUBBARD, RUTH. 1986. "Eugenics and Prenatal Testing." *International Journal of Health Services* 16, no. 2:227–242.

KEVLES, DANIEL J. 1985. *In the Name of Eugenics: Genetics and the Uses of Human Heredity.* Berkeley: University of California Press.

LAPPÉ, MARC. 1975. "Can Eugenic Policy Be Just?" In *The Prevention of Genetic Disease and Mental Retardation,* pp. 456–475. Edited by Aubrey Milunsky. Philadelphia: W. B. Saunders.

———. 1981. "Justice and Prenatal Life." In *Justice and Health Care,* pp. 83–94. Edited by Earl E. Shelp. Dordrecht, Holland: D. Reidel.

———. 1986. *Broken Code: The Exploitation of DNA.* San Francisco: Sierra Club Books.

LIFTON, ROBERT J. 1986. *The Nazi Doctors: Medical Killing and the Psychology of Genocide.* New York: Basic Books.

LIPPMAN, ABBY. 1990. "Is Genome Mapping the Way to Improve Canadians' Health?" *Canadian Journal of Public Health* 81, no. 5:397–398.

———. 1991. "Prenatal Genetic Testing and Screening: Constructing Needs and Reinforcing Inequities." *American Journal of Law and Medicine* 17, no. 1–2:15–50.

LUDMERER, KENNETH M. 1972. *Genetics and American Society: A Historical Appraisal.* Baltimore: Johns Hopkins University Press.

PROCTOR, ROBERT. 1988. *Racial Hygiene: Medicine Under the Nazis.* Cambridge, Mass.: Harvard University Press.

RAMSEY, PAUL. 1970. *Fabricated Man: The Ethics of Genetic Control.* New Haven, Conn.: Yale University Press.

RAWLS, JOHN A. 1971. *A Theory of Justice.* Cambridge, Mass.: Harvard University Press/Belknap Press.

REILLY, PHILIP. 1977. *Genetics, Law and Social Policy.* Cambridge, Mass.: Harvard University Press.

ROTHMAN, BARBARA KATZ. 1992. "Not All That Glitters Is Gold." *Hastings Center Report* 22, no. 4:S11–S15.

SALZANO, FRANCISCO M., and CALLEGARI-JACQUES, SIDIA M. 1988. *South American Indians: A Case Study in Evolution.* New York: Oxford University Press.

SIMPSON, GEORGE GAYLORD. 1974. "The Concept of Progress in Organic Evolution." *Social Research* 41:28–51.

SPERRY, ROGER W. 1974. "Science and the Problem of Values." *Zygon* 9, no. 1:7–21.

TWISS, SUMNER B. 1976. "Ethical Issues in Priority-Setting for the Utilization of Genetic Technologies." In "Ethical and Scientific Issues Posed by the Human Uses of Molecular Genetics." Edited by Marc A. Lappé and Robert S. Morrison. *Annals of the New York Academy of Sciences* 265: 22–45.

WATSON, JAMES D., and COOK-DEEGAN, ROBERT MULLAN. 1990. "The Human Genome Project and International Health." *Journal of the American Medical Association* 263, no. 24:3322–3324.

WERTZ, DOROTHY, and FLETCHER, JOHN. 1988. "Attitudes of Genetic Counselors: A Multinational Survey." *American Journal of Human Genetics* 42, no. 4:592–600.

EUGENICS AND RELIGIOUS LAW

I. Judaism
>   *David Feldman*

II. Christianity
>   *William Bassett*

III. Islam
>   *Abdulaziz Sachedina*

IV. Hinduism and Buddhism
>   *Geoffrey P. Redmond*

I. JUDAISM

The laws against incest and consanguinity in the Old Testament would seem to have a rationale in eugenics, although this is never specified in the biblical text. The traditional commentators, too, advert only to the natural repugnance against incest. In the Talmudic discussion as well as in the legal codes, the subject is treated as a sexual offense, involving a breach of morality rather than a eugenic error. (The Talmud is the repository of rabbinic exposition of biblical law and teaching, spanning more than five centuries. The legal codes are based on the Talmud and on subsequent development of the law, such as in Responsa, formal opinions rendered by rabbinic authorities in response to new case-law inquiries.)

Even bastardy is a moral rather than a eugenic category. The *mamzer* (in Jewish law, the product of an adulterous or incestuous liaison, not of a relationship between two persons who are not married to one another) is not legally ill-born; his or her status is compromised only legally and socially, rendered so in punitive or deterrent judgment against parents not free to have entered the relationship. But no difference obtains between the *mamzer* born of adultery—even a technical adultery, such as when the document of divorce for the mother's previous marriage was impugned—and the *mamzer* born of incest. Hence, no eugenic motive can be assigned here.

A man "maimed in his privy parts" bears the same legal disabilities as the *mamzer.* Thus, a man of "crushed testicles or severed member" is excluded from "the congregation of the Lord" (Deut. 23:2). This verse is interpreted to mean only that he may not enter into conjugal union with an Israelite woman. Thus, the castrated male is under the ban because the act of castration is forbidden. But one "maimed in his privy parts" as a result of a birth defect or disease, as opposed to one castrated by his own or another's deliberate assault, is free of this disability. The legal situations were thus analogized: "Just as the *mamzer* is the result of human misdeeds, so only the castrated one who is such as a result of human misdeeds is to be banned." Since that distinction is made in both cases, and since the banned *mamzer* and the castrated are permitted to marry, for example, another *mamzer* or a proselyte, it must be concluded that moral outrage and punitive judgment rather than eugenic considerations are operative.

Eugenics, in the sense of choosing a marriage partner with the well-being of progeny in mind, is more clearly present in Talmudic counsel and legislation. A man is counseled to choose a wife prudently, and guidance is offered in doing so in accordance with the intellectual and moral virtues of the prospective bride. And since, we are told, a son, for example, normally takes after his mother's brothers, a man should regard the maternal uncles in making his decision (Bava Batra, 110a). A hidden physical blemish in a spouse is grounds for invalidating a marriage, unless the other spouse can be presumed to have known of it in advance.

Heredity as a eugenic principle takes its legal model from rulings with respect to circumcision. A male infant whose two brothers died possibly as a result of this operation may not be circumcised. He is deemed to have inherited the illness (probably hemophilia) that proved fatal to his two brothers. The Talmud goes on to say that an infant whose two maternal cousins showed that weakness may not be circumcised either. That is, statistical evidence yielded by two sons from the same mother can also be reflected in two sisters of that mother (Yevamot, 64b). Coming from Talmudic times (before 500

C.E.), this is a remarkably early recognition that hemophilia is transmitted through maternal lineage—in itself a significant eugenic discovery.

The statistical evidence or the presumption of adverse hereditary factors in a third family member, when those factors are seen to exist in two others, thus becomes the basis of Talmudic laws of eugenics. With modern laboratory means to determine the presence of these factors, the principle of course operates even sooner, without waiting for statistical evidence in two members. The Talmud rules that one may not marry into a family of epileptics or lepers (Yevamot, 64b) or—by extension—a family in which tuberculosis or any similar disease appears in multiple members. This may be the first eugenic edict in any social or religious system.

The pure "heredity" underlying this recommendation is not unanimously agreed upon. While one view in the Talmud attributes the transmission of characteristics in the pre-Mendelian age to heredity, another view sees it as "bad luck." In a Responsum where the questioner considered abortion because the mother was epileptic, the rabbi responded that the latter of the two views stated above may be the right one, and that fear of bad luck is an inadequate warrant for abortion (Feldman, 1968).

In an earlier context, the Mishnah (the foundation layer of the Talmud) speaks of the faculties that a father bequeaths to his son: "looks, strength, riches, and length of years" (Eduyot, II, 9). Here, too, the commentaries align themselves on both sides: one sees the bequeathing of faculties as a natural hereditary process, the other sees them as divine reward for the father's virtues.

Two other Talmudic ideas with eugenic motifs are reflected in current practice. In the interests of fulfilling the injunction to "love one's wife as much as himself and honor her more than himself," a man is advised to seek his sister's daughter as a bride; his care for her will be the more tender due to his affection for his own sister. Yet in the thirteenth century, Rabbi Judah the Pious left a testamentary charge to his children and grandchildren that became a source of guidance to others on the level of precedent for subsequent Jewish law. In this famous testament, he advises against marriage with a niece because it may have adverse genetic results. Modern rabbinic authorities dismiss such fears as unjustified unless they are medically warranted.

A second point is a Talmudic notion that eugenic factors operate in intercourse during pregnancy. Conjugal relations, we are told, should be avoided during the first trimester as "injurious to the embryo"; but they are encouraged during the final trimester as desirable for both mother and fetus, for then the child is born "well-formed and of strong vitality" (Niddah, 31a). A medieval Jewish authority makes the matter a point of pride in comparative culture: the Talmud recommends coitus during the final trimester, whereas the Greek and Arab scholars say it is harmful. Do not listen to them, he says (Responsa Bar Sheshet, no. 447). Nonetheless, the Talmud prohibits the marriage of a pregnant or nursing widow or divorcee. In the case of a pregnant woman, the second husband, it is suggested, may be less considerate of a fetus fathered by another man and may inadvertently damage it through abdominal pressure during intercourse (Yevamot, 36a). In the nursing situation, the new father may fail to take the necessary steps to supplement the diet of his stepchild (it is assumed that a pregnancy diminishes the mother's milk). And a pregnant woman who feels an urgent physical or psychological need for food during the Yom Kippur fast is to be fed for the sake of her fetus's welfare as well as her own (Yoma, 82a).

More a matter of preaching than of law is the notion that defective children can be the result of immoral or inconsiderate modes of intercourse—an idea expounded but ultimately rejected by the Talmud (Nedarim, 20a). Yet in more modern times, the Hasidim (pietistic Jewish groups with a mystical orientation) maintain that spiritual consequences of the act are indeed possible; that if a man has pure and lofty thoughts during or preparatory to cohabitation, he can succeed in transmitting to the child of either sex an especially lofty soul. Hence dynastic succession of leadership, presuming the inheritance of that loftier soul, as opposed to democratic selection, obtains among Hasidic groups.

A study of biblical and Talmudic sources written by Max Grunwald in 1930, cited by Immanuel Jakobovits, discerns a broad eugenic motif. Grunwald writes that Judaism

> quite consciously strives for the promotion of the quantity of progeny by the compulsion of matrimony, the insistence on early marriage, the sexual purity of the marital partners and the harmony of their ages and characters, the dissolubility of unhappy unions, the regulation of conjugal intercourse, the high esteem of maternity, the stress on parental responsibility, the protection of the embryo, etc. To be sure, there can be no question here of a compulsory public control over the health conditions of the marriage candidates, but that would positively be in line with the principles of Jewish eugenics: the pursuit after the most numerous and physically, mentally, and morally sound natural increase of the people, without thinking of an exclusive race protection. (Jakobovits, 1975, p. 154)

Although abortion is warranted primarily for maternal rather than fetal indications, screening of would-be parents for actual or potential defective genes, such as in Tay-Sachs disease, would, like premarital blood tests, be much in keeping with the Jewish traditional eugenic concern. Such genetic screening is, in fact, facilitated by a unique computerized system under the auspices of the New York–based Dor Yesharim (Generation of Upright [Descendants], from Psalms 112:2). Young men and women diagnosed as Tay-Sachs carriers are identified by code number. When marriage is contemplated, the couple is alerted to the fact that both are carriers, with one chance in four of a homozygous fetus, so that marriage plans may be reconsidered. Besides Tay-Sachs, which is fatal to the child by about age five, nonfatal disabilities have been added to Dor Yesharim's data base.

Although surrogate parenting and artificial insemination create social and family problems, the conceptional procedures that make them possible are in and of themselves acceptable when natural means are ineffective. In vitro fertilization, to assist in a conception that might otherwise be thwarted by blocked fallopian tubes or by sperm inadequacy, has been accorded full moral and legal sanction. Genetic engineering that alters the germ line has been ruled out by Jewish ethicists, but gene therapy, removing or correcting defective genes, would be a proper extension of the mandate to heal. The newly announced technology for cloning embryos has been greeted with more caution than hope—hope for improved procreational prospects for couples otherwise limited to one or no progeny, but caution against creating multiple embryos deprived of their distinctiveness as individuals. Safeguards are called for against the dangers of genetic mutation, or of political or profit-motive "baby farming" that could result from abuse of broader eugenic techniques.

DAVID M. FELDMAN

Directly related to this article are the other articles in this entry: CHRISTIANITY, ISLAM, *and* HINDUISM AND BUDDHISM. *Also directly related are the entries* ETHICS, *article on* RELIGION AND MORALITY; EUGENICS, *articles on* HISTORICAL ASPECTS, *and* ETHICAL ISSUES; GENETIC ENGINEERING, *article on* HUMAN GENETIC ENGINEERING; *and* INFANTS, *article on* HISTORY OF INFANTICIDE. *For a further discussion of Jewish religious tradition, see the entries* ABORTION, *section on* RELIGIOUS TRADITIONS, *article on* JEWISH PERSPECTIVES; DEATH, *article on* WESTERN RELIGIOUS THOUGHT; JUDAISM; MEDICAL ETHICS, HISTORY OF, *section on* NEAR AND MIDDLE EAST, *articles on* ANCIENT NEAR EAST, *and* ISRAEL; *and* POPULATION ETHICS, *section on* RELIGIOUS TRADITIONS, *article on* JEWISH PERSPECTIVES. *Other relevant material may be found under the entries* FERTILITY CONTROL, *article on* ETHICAL ISSUES; GENETICS AND HUMAN BEHAVIOR; GENETICS AND HUMAN SELF-UNDERSTANDING; GENETICS AND RACIAL MINORITIES; MEDICAL GENETICS; *and* REPRODUCTIVE TECHNOLOGIES, *article on* ETHICAL ISSUES.

Bibliography

FELDMAN, DAVID M. 1968. *Birth Control in Jewish Law: Marital Relations, Contraception, and Abortion as Set Forth in the Classical Texts of Jewish Law.* New York: New York University Press.

———. 1991. "The Case of Baby M." In *Jewish Values in Health and Medicine,* pp. 163–169. Edited by Levi Meier. Lanham, Md.: University Press of America.

JACOBS, LOUIS. 1974. "Heredity." In *What Does Judaism Say About . . . ?,* pp. 165–166. New York: Quadrangle/New York Times.

JAKOBOVITS, IMMANUEL. 1975. *Jewish Medical Ethics: A Comparative and Historical Study of the Jewish Religious Attitude to Medicine and Its Practice.* New ed. New York: Bloch Publishing Company.

KOLATA, GINA. 1994. "Reproductive Revolution Is Jolting Old Views." *New York Times,* January 11, pp. A1, C12.

ROSNER, FRED. 1986. *Modern Medicine and Jewish Ethics.* Hoboken, N.J.: Ktav Publishing House.

ZEVIN, SHELOMOH YOSEF. 1957. *Le'Or Ha-Halakhah: Be-ayot u-verurim,* pp. 147–158. 2d ed. Tel Aviv: Abraham Zioni.

II. CHRISTIANITY

The following is a revision and update of the first-edition article "Eugenics and Religious Law: Christian Religious Laws" by the same author. Portions of the first-edition article appear in the revised version.

Christian religious laws historically comprehend a large spectrum of rules to guide individual conduct and social relationships among the baptized. The laws most likely to have eugenic significance are the canons prohibiting the marriage of relatives. These regulations also form the basis for the modern civil law prohibitions against the marriage of relatives in both the Continental legal systems and the Anglo-Saxon statutory scheme. Though the principal justification given for such prohibitions in Christian law has been ethical and social, there is substantial evidence that they also may reflect considerations classified as eugenic in contemporary scientific research.

The ecclesiastical regulations that forbid marriage between persons closely related by consanguinity are among the most ancient canons of the Christian tradition. Penalties attached to the violation of religious exogamic laws have varied historically in their severity, as, indeed, have the ways of measuring the degrees of kinship and defining within which degrees the crime of incest shall be punished. But the core of the tradition of canon law remains constant and reflects an extreme reluctance to accept the marriages of close relatives as humanly or religiously feasible.

For Roman Catholics all marriages within the direct line of blood relationship, that is, between an ancestor and a descendant by parentage, and within the collateral line to the fourth degree, that is, to third cousins, are forbidden (*Code of Canon Law*, 1983, canon 1091). The definition of marriages within four degrees of relationship as incestuous dates to the Fourth Lateran Council in 1215 (c. 50). In the Greek Orthodox tradition, marriage in the direct line and in the collateral line to the sixth or seventh degree by the Roman method of computation is prohibited in canon 54 of the Synod in Trullo, 691/692 (Hefele, 1896). All Oriental Christians forbid marriages in the direct line; Armenians, Jacobites, and Copts prohibit it in the collateral line to the fourth degree, Melkites to the sixth degree, Serbs and Chaldeans to the third degree, and Ethiopians without distinction. Among Protestant reformers the restrictions of the medieval canon law were accepted by some, such as Phillip Melanchthon and Martin Chemnitz (Kemnitz); only the Old Testament regulations of Leviticus 18:6-18 by others, such as Martin Bucer and, perhaps, Martin Luther; and only the closest ties of direct parental relationship by still others, such as John Wycliffe. In the Anglican community, The Book of Common Prayer contains a table drawn up by Archbishop Matthew Parker based on Leviticus in naming relatives incapable of marriage (Wheatly). Most Protestant churches today follow the prohibitions of civil law regarding incest and kinship marriage (Acte for Kynges Succession; Acte for Succession of Imperyall Crowne; Concerning Precontracte and Degrees).

The sources of and commentaries upon the Christian laws record debate about the extent of the prohibition, the possibility of dispensation within certain close degrees of kinship, and the related question of the divine or natural law origin of the laws (e.g., Burchard of Worms, *Decretum*, bk. 7, "De Incesto"; Burchard of Worms, *Collection in 74 titulis* 65.281-284). They reveal, however, only the most sketchy discussion of the foundations of the regulations themselves.

The classical reasons given for the prohibition of consanguineous marriages are ethical and social. The first reason was called the *respectus parentelae*, namely, that such marriages would undermine the respect due to parents and consequently to all those who are closely related (Aquinas, Thomas 1948, *Summa theologiae* II-II, 154, 9). Second, they constitute a moral danger to family life arising from the possibility of early moral corruption of the young dwelling within the same household in which marriage could be allowed (ibid.; Sánchez 1605, 7.52.12, 7.53). Third, the prohibition of consanguineous marriages prevents the disruption of the family by sexual competition and forces the multiplication of friendships and the spread of charity (Augustine). These three reasons seem to have been sufficient to justify the laws, so that most scholars did not go beyond them to seek a further justification. Adhémar Esmein, for example, said the laws arose out of an instinctive repulsion for incest and were not reflective of any known adverse physical consequences. Some modern authors speculate that the reason for strict enforcement of prohibitions against incestuous marriages was to force the breakup of landed family estates (Duby, 1983).

It is only in comparatively modern times that an explicitly eugenic reason for the prohibition has received scientific attention. Writing in 1673, Samuel Dugard noted: "There is a *judgment* which is said often to accompany these Marriages, and that is *Want of Children* and a *Barrennesse*" (p. 53). "The Children are weak, it may be; grow crooked, or, what is worse, do not prove well; presently, Sir, it shall be said what better could be expected? an unlawfull Wedlock must have an unprosperous successe" (p. 51). Ambrosius J. Stapf's *Theologia moralis* in 1827 alluded to this possibility (p. 359). A fuller treatment is found in Dominic Le Noir's 1873 edition of St. Alphonsus's *Theologia moralis*. Edward Westermarck in 1889 and Eduard Laurent in 1895 spoke at length of a physiological justification of the canons to prevent indiscriminate inbreeding and the risk of a high incidence of deleterious genetic effects. Franz Wernz, in 1928 (n. 352 [70]), writing from a comprehensive knowledge of the canonical tradition, said the ancient writers also knew of the undesirable effects of excessive inbreeding. He noted reasons derived from contemporary medical science in the writings of Gratian (early twelfth century) (C.xx "Anglis permittitur, ut in quarta vel in quinta generatione cognibitur," c. 20, c. 35, q. 2), Pope Innocent III (1161–1216) (Schroeder, 1937), and Thomas Aquinas (*Commentum in libros IV Sententiarum*, dist. 40 and 41, q. 1, art. 4). Since the late nineteenth century nearly all commentators on the canonical rules speak of eugenic objections to marriages of blood relatives.

It is possible to find in the ancient ecclesiastical commentators an awareness of a eugenic foundation to the prohibition expressed in primitive and undifferentiated modes of speech. For example, a persistent belief was kept alive among theologians and canonists that children of incestuous relationships will die or will be greatly debilitated, or that the familial line will be cursed with sterility. Benedict the Levite (850?) wrote of these marriages: "From these are usually born the blind, the deaf, hunchbacks, the mentally defective, and others afflicted with loathsome infirmities" (*Capitularum collectio*). Furthermore, in the explanations of the name of the impediment (i.e., the impediment of consanguinity), if one traces their origins through medieval glossography to the *Etymologies* of Isidore of Seville (560?–636), there appears an awareness of a physiological factor in the blood bond of close relatives that must be weakened before marriage can be contracted safely.

The antecedents of the Christian canons in the Mosaic law (Lev. 18:6–18) and the Roman law (Burge) were taken as expressions of natural law by the canonists and were continued in the barbarian codes (*Pactum legis salicae* 13.11; *Leges visigothae* 4.1.1–7; *Codex Euriciani* 2). In his *Ecclesiastical History* (I, 27), where the Venerable Bede (673–735) notes these laws, he records a quotation from a letter of Pope Gregory I to Augustine of Canterbury, written in 601 (*Responsa Gregorii*). The reason given by Gregory for forbidding marriages of close relatives is, "We have learned from experience that from such a marriage offspring cannot grow up." This letter and this reason not only are later picked up and cited by Gratian ("Anglis permittatur," c. 2, c. 35, q. 5) and Thomas Aquinas (*Summa theologiae suppl.* 54, 3), but may be found in virtually all the canonical collections of the early Middle Ages. Though comment on this passage is rare, comment was, perhaps, unnecessary. The passage from Gregory seems clearly to say that experience teaches that children from forbidden consanguineous marriages are affected or unable to grow up. There is thought to be a physiological consequence to incest. In the light of this it seems probable that the labored argumentation over the question of how close the relationship must be for marriage to be forbidden by natural law must have been conducted in some awareness of a popular belief in the biological consequences of such unions. The fear of genetic anomalies or biological debilitation from indiscriminate inbreeding may not be perfectly articulated. It is difficult to imagine, however, that warning of some physiological dangers to offspring may not have been intended in the frequent citation of Pope Gregory to sustain the severity of the prohibition.

Tomás Sánchez (1605), who wrote the greatest of the canonical commentaries on marriage, says that the most suasive ground for forbidding incestuous unions is that there is a sharing of the blood among close relatives and that the physical image of a progenitor (*imago, complexio, effigies, mores, virtus paterna*) passes to offspring, so that the blood must be weakened through successive generations before marriage should be contracted (7.50; 7.51.1–2). Thus, preventing marriages of close relatives to protect the offspring by allowing several generations to pass before procreation can be called a measure of eugenic foresight, however simple the scientific awareness to support it may have been.

In summary, a eugenic foundation to Christian religious laws forbidding the marriage of close relatives is clearly articulated and commented upon by modern scholars from the late eighteenth and nineteenth centuries. Evidence of this kind of awareness may be discovered earlier in the canonical sources, however, going back at least to the seventh century. It would seem consistent with the eugenic connotation of those laws rooted in antiquity, together with a Christian sense of

responsibility for offspring that partly motivated them, to consider further eugenic restrictions on marriage in Christian communities today, in light of contemporary knowledge of genetics.

WILLIAM W. BASSETT

Directly related to this article are the other articles in this entry: JUDAISM, ISLAM, *and* HINDUISM AND BUDDHISM. *Also directly related are the entries* ROMAN CATHOLICISM; PROTESTANTISM; EASTERN ORTHODOX CHRISTIANITY; *and* EUGENICS. *For a further discussion of topics mentioned in this article, see the entries* CHILDREN, *especially the article on* HISTORY OF CHILDHOOD; FAMILY; MARRIAGE AND OTHER DOMESTIC PARTNERSHIPS; *and* SEXUAL ETHICS. *For a discussion of related ideas, see the entry* GENETIC TESTING AND SCREENING.

Bibliography

An Acte for the Establishement of the Kynges Succession. 1533–1534. 25 Hen. VIII, c. 22. *The Statutes of the Realm*, vol. 3, pp. 471–474, esp. 472–473.

An Acte for the Establisshement of the Succession of the Imperyall Crowne of This Realme. 1536. 28 Hen. VIII, c. 7. *The Statutes of the Realm*, vol. 3, pp. 655–662, esp. pp. 658–659.

AQUINAS, THOMAS. 1878. *Commentum in libros IV sententiarum*, dists. 40 and 41, ques. 1, art 4, pp. 770–771. Vol. 30 of *Opera omnia*. Edited by Stanislai Eduardi Frette. Paris: Ludovicum Vivès.

———. 1948. "Utrum consanguinitas de iure naturali impediat matrimonium," ques. 54, art. 3. In vol. 4 of *Summa theologiae*, pp. 838–840, esp. "Sed contra," p. 839. Rome: Marietti. Translated by the Fathers of the English Dominican Province under the title "Whether Consanguinity Is an Impediment to Marriage by Virtue of Natural Law." In vol. 3 of *Summa Theologica: First Complete American Edition*, pp. 2758–2760, esp. "On the Contrary," p. 2759. New York: Benziger Brothers.

———. 1948. "Utrum incestus sit species determinata luxuriae," ques. 154, art 9. In vol. 3 of *Summa theologiae*, pp. 722–723. Rome: Marietti. Translated by the Fathers of the English Dominican Province under the title "Whether Incest Is a Determinate Species of Lust?" In vol. 2 of *Summa Theologica: First Complete American Edition*, pp. 1823–1824. New York: Benziger Brothers.

AUGUSTINE. 1844–1891. "De jure conjugiorum, quod dissimile a subsequentibus matrimoniis habuerint prima connubia." In *Patrologiae cursus completus: Series Latina*, vol. 41, cols. 457–460. Compiled by Jacques-Paul Migne. Paris: Garnier Fratres.

———. 1950. "Of Marriage Between Blood-Relations, in Regard to Which the Present Law Could Not Bind the Men of Earliest Ages." *The City of God*, bk. 15, ch. 16, pp. 500–502. Translated by Marcus Dods. New York: Modern Library.

BEDE (VENERABLE BEDE). 1969. *Bede's Ecclesiastical History of the English People*, bk. 1, ch. 27, pp. 78–102, esp. p. 85. Edited by Bertram Colgrave and R. A. B. Mynors. Oxford: At the Clarendon Press. Facing Latin and English texts.

BENEDICT THE LEVITE (BENEDICTUS DIACONI). 1844–1891. "Captularum collectio: Pertz monitum." In *Patrologiae cursus completus: Series Latina*, vol. 97, bk. 3, sec. 179, col. 820. Compiled by Jacques-Paul Migne. Paris: Garnier Fratres.

BOUCHARD, CONSTANCE B. 1981. "Consanguinity and Noble Marriage in the Tenth and Eleventh Centuries." *Speculum* 56, no. 2: 268–287.

BRUNDAGE, JAMES A. 1987. *Law, Sex, and Christian Society in Medieval Europe*. Chicago: University of Chicago Press.

BURCHARD OF WORMS. 1965. [1915]. *Collectio in 74 titulis*. In *Anselmi episcopi Lucensis collectio una cum collectione minore*. Aalen: Scientia Verlage. Translated by John Gilchrist under the title *The Collection in Seventy-four Titles: A Canon Law Manual of the Gregorian Reform*. Toronto: Pontifical Institute of Medieval Studies, 1980.

BURGE, WILLIAM. 1910. *The Comparative Law of Marriage and Divorce*. Edited by Alexander W. Renton and George G. Phillimore. London: Sweet and Maxwell.

Code of Canon Law: A Text and Commentary. 1976. Canon 1976, secs. 1 and 2, pp. 487–489. Edited by Timothy Lincoln Bouscaren and Adam C. Ellis. Milwaukee: Bruce. English text with commentary.

Code of Canon Law: Latin-English Edition. 1983. Washington, D.C.: Canon Law Society of America.

Concerning Precontracte and Degrees of Consanguinite. 1540. 32 Hen. VIII, c. 38. *The Statutes of the Realm*, vol. 3, p. 792.

COUSSA, ACACIO. 1948. *Epitome praelectionem de iure ecclesiastico orientali*, vol. 3, *De matrimonio*. Rome: Typis Monasterii Exarchici Cryptoferratensis.

DAUVILLIER, JEAN-DECLERCQ CHARLES. 1936. *Le mariage en droit canonique oriental*. Paris: Recueil Sirey.

DUBY, GEORGES. 1983. *The Knight, the Lady, and the Priest: The Making of Modern Marriage in Medieval France*. New York: Pantheon.

DUGARD, SAMUEL. 1673. *The Marriages of Cousins German, Vindicated from the Censures of Unlawfullnesse, and Inexpediency, Being a Letter Written to His Much Honour'd T.D.* Oxford: Printed by Hen. Hall for Thomas Bowman. Attributed to Dugard although it is taken largely from Jeremy Taylor's *Ductor dubitantium*. Attributed to Simon Dugard in the British Museum Catalog.

ESMEIN, ADHÉMAR. 1929. *Le mariage en droit canonique*. 2 vols. 2d ed. Paris: Recueil Sirey.

FLEURY, JACQUES. 1933. *Recherches historiques sur les empêchements de parenté dans le mariage canonique dès origines aux fausses décrétales*. Paris: Recueil Sirey.

GOODY, JACK. 1983. *The Development of the Family and Marriage in Europe*. Cambridge: Cambridge University Press.

GRATIAN (GRATIANUS, THE CANONIST). 1554. *Decretum divi Gratiani, universi iuris canonici pontificias constitutiones & canonicas brevi compendio complectens*, pt. 2, causa 35, ques. 2, canon 20, p. 1217; ques. 5, canon 2, pp. 1218–1221. Lyons: I. Pideoius.

GREGORY I. 1957. "Gregorius Augustino Episcopo." *Registrum epistolarum*, vol. 2, pp. 332–343, esp. pp. 335–336. 2d ed. Edited by Paulus Ewald and Ludovicus M. Hartman. Monumenta Germaniae Historica, vols. 1 and 2. Berlin: Weidmannos.

HEFELE, KARL JOSEPH VON. 1896. "The Quinsext or Trullan Synod, A.D. 692." In *A History of the Councils of the Church: From the Original Documents*, vol. 5, sec. 327, pp. 221–239, esp. canon 54, p. 231. 2d ed., rev. Edited and translated by William R. Clark. Edinburgh: T. & T. Clark, 1896.

HERLIHY, DAVID. 1985. *Medieval Households*. Cambridge, Mass.: Harvard University Press.

ISIDORE OF SEVILLE. 1911. "De adfinitatibus et gradibus," "De agnatis et cognatis," "De conivgiis." *Etymologiarum sive originum, libri XX*, vol. 1, bk. 9, chs. 5–7. Edited by Wallace Martin Lindsay. Oxford: At the Clarendon Press. See also *Patro-logia cursus completus: Series Latina*, vol. 82, cols. 353–368.

LAURENT, EMILE. 1895. *Mariages consanguins et dégénérescences*. Paris: A. Maloine.

LIGUORI, ALFONSO MARIA DE' (ALFONSUS LIGUORI). 1872–1874. "De matrimonio." *Theologia moralis*, vol. 3, bk. 5, tract. 6, pp. 661–858, esp. pp. 783–784. Edited by Dominic Le Noir. 4 vols. Paris: Ludovicum Vivès.

MEYVAERT, PAUL. 1971. "Bede's Text of the *Libellus Responsionem* of Gregory the Great to Augustine of Canterbury." In *England Before the Conquest: Studies in Primary Sources Presented to Dorothy Whitelock*, pp. 15–33. Edited by Peter Clemoes and Kathleen Hughes. Cambridge: Cambridge University Press.

Patrologiae cursus completus. Series latina [*Patrologia latina*]. 1851–1894. 221 vols. Paris: Garnier Fratres *Supplementum*. Paris: Editions Garnier Frères.

SÁNCHEZ, TOMÁS. 1605. "De impedimentis." In his *Disputationum de sancto matrimonio sacramento*, vol. 3, bk. 7, dis. 50, pp. 332–336; dis. 51, pars. 1–2, pp. 336–337; dis. 52, par. 12, p. 352; dis. 53, pp. 352–354. 3 vols. in 4. Vols. 1 and 2, Genoa: Iosephum Pavonem, 1602. Vols. 3 and 4, Madrid: Ludouici Sanchez.

SCHROEDER, HENRY JOSEPH. 1937. [1215]. "The Twelfth General Council: Fourth Lateran Council." *Disciplinary Decrees of the General Councils: Text, Translation, and Commentary*, pp. 236–296, esp. canon 50, pp. 279–280. St. Louis: B. Herder. Latin text: "Canones Concilii Lateranensis IV (Oecumen XII): Anno 1215 habiti." *Disciplinary Decrees*, pp. 560–584, esp. canon 50, p. 578.

STAPF, AMBROSIUS JOSEPH. 1827. *Theologiae moralis*, vol. 2, sec. 312, p. 359. Innsbruck: Typis and Sumtibus Wagnerianis.

The Statutes of the Realm, Printed by Command of His Majesty King George the Third, in Pursuance of an Address of the House of Commons of Great Britain, from the Original Records and Authentic Manuscripts. 1963. Repr. 11 vols. in 12. London: Dawsons of Pall Mall.

WAHL, FRANCIS X. 1934. *The Matrimonial Impediments of Consanguinity and Affinity: An Historical Synopsis and Commentary*. Washington, D.C.: Catholic University of America Press.

WERNZ, FRANZ XAVIER. 1928. *Ius decretalium*, vol. 4. Rev. ed. Florence: Libraria Gaichetti.

WESTERMARCK, EDWARD A. 1921. *The History of Human Mar-

riage. 3 vols. 5th ed., rev. London: Macmillan; New York: Allerton, 1922. Repr. New York: Johnson Reprint Corp., 1971.

WHEATLY, CHARLES. 1759. [1710]. "Of the Preface and Charge and the Several Impediments to Matrimony." In his *A Rational Illustration of the Book of Common Prayer of the Church of England,* ch. 10, sec. 3, pp. 376–383. 8th ed. London: C. Hitch et al. A commentary.

III. ISLAM

The idea of eugenics is not well developed in the Islamic world. Both Islamic law and tradition generally condemn abortion, which is permitted only if the mother's life is endangered, so there is no genetic counseling that would lead to abortion. Both religious law and tradition do include references to a man's choosing an appropriate wife, but these concerns have been interpreted as moral and social, rather than eugenic.

Islamic religious-moral law, the Shari'a, deals with questions concerning laws of incest and consanguinity from the perspective of moral and social relationships rather than eugenic concerns. The general counsel of the Qur'an and the Prophetic traditions regarding marriage is promulgated in the laws that require a Muslim to marry within the community of believers. A Muslim is better than a non-Muslim as a spouse. "A woman may be married for four reasons: for her property, her status, her beauty, and her religion; so try to get one who is religious" (Muslim, 1956, tradition 3457). There is no law to suggest choosing a marriage partner with the intention of improving the progeny through the control of hereditary factors. With slight variations among the Sunni and Shiite schools, the law specifies that a woman may not marry a man who is not equal to her. The earliest ruling to require equality in matters of piety and freedom from physical defects detrimental to marriage is found among the Malikis (see al-Juzayri, 1969, for variations among the four schools of Sunni law).

In the Qur'an the main source for marriage law is book 4, verse 23. This prohibits marriage between persons closely related by blood, but this ban reflects ethical and social, rather than eugenic, considerations. Thus in Muslim jurisprudence a man and a woman may be forbidden to marry either because of blood relationship (e.g., a man may not marry his mother or either of his grandmothers, etc.) or relationships established through marriage (e.g., he may not marry the mother or grandmothers of his wife, etc.). Moreover, there are women whom a man may marry singly, but not be married to at the same time (e.g., two sisters, a woman and the sister of her mother or father). This latter prohibition seems to be more for psychological than for eugenic reasons.

Evidence that the Qur'an (or Shari'a) considers nurture, or the environment, to have impact on a child perhaps comparable to that of nature, or genetic inheritance, comes from the Book of Marriage, which prohibits marriage not only between a man and the woman who gave birth to him but also between a man and the foster mother who breastfed him at least a certain number of times.

The ruling seems to indicate similar consequences for foster relations established through suckling: "What is unlawful because of blood relations, is also unlawful because of corresponding foster suckling relations" (al-Bukhari, 1986, tradition 46; al-E'Amili, 7/281, tradition 2). In establishing unmarriageability, a foster mother who suckles an infant is regarded exactly as the infant's real mother.

There is further evidence of the Islamic tradition's lack of interest in eugenics. Islam abolished one of the four types of marriages among Arabs, the one described in Arab tradition in terms that may reflect eugenic concerns. The tradition says:

> The second type [of marriage] was that a man would say to his wife after she had become clean from her period, "Send for so-and-so [whose nobility is well established] and have sexual relations with him." Her husband would then keep away from her and would not touch her at all till her pregnancy became evident from that man with whom she was sleeping. After the pregnancy was established her husband would sleep with her if he wished. However, he allowed his wife to sleep with that person being desirous of the nobility of the child (*naja-bat al-walad*). Such marriage was called "marriage seeking advancement" (*nikah al-istibda'*). (al-Bukhari, 1986, sec. 37)

Islam, which insisted that faith in God was the main source of all human nobility, was uninterested in this practice, traditional in the Arab tribal culture, for the improvement of the human race through the control of hereditary factors.

Other traditions counsel the believers to choose a partner for breeding (*al-nutaf*) "bravery among the people of Khurasan" [in Iran], sexual potency among the Berber [in North Africa], and "generosity and envy among the Arabs" (al-'Amili, 1965, 7/29, tradition #6). The Islamic traditions (hadith literature) do reflect explicit knowledge of eugenics in choosing a marriage partner. The source of these eugenic considerations seems to be the Irano–Semitic culture, in which such interests were commonplace. Although these traditions were never used as authoritative precedents for legislation in the Shari'a, they express the popular piety connected with marital relations. For example, the Prophet is quoted saying, "Anyone wishing to follow my tradition should know that among my traditions is marriage. Seek children [through it]. . . . Protect your children from the milk of the prostitute and the insane among women, because milk makes inroads [in the character of a child]" (al-'Amili, 1969, 7/4, tradition 6). Moreover, in the case of a person drinking wine, the Prophet regarded it permissible to annul the marriage contract, especially, if the person was alcoholic (literally, "sick" with alcohol) (al-'Amili, 1969). There also existed a warning against marrying fatuous individuals because their offspring would be a loss. However, it was acceptable to marry them for sexual reasons, as long as one did not seek children through such a union. These traditions reveal the concern about hereditary factors in the progeny.

Other traditions encourage marriages within one's own collateral line, to first cousins. The Prophet, who belonged to the Hashimite clan, at one time looked at the children of 'Ali and Ja'far, two brothers and his paternal cousins by relation, and said, "Our daughters for our sons, and our sons for our daughters" (al-'Amili, 1969, 7/49, tradition 7). This encouragement is contradicted by other traditions that recommend exogamous marriage and even intermarriage between Arab and non-Arab, and between a free person and a slave. There does not seem to be any awareness in these early traditions of deleterious genetic effects from excessive inbreeding. However, since 1970 there has been a growing debate among traditional Muslim jurists over the authenticity of the tradition that encourages endogamy indiscriminately. Certain injurious hereditary conditions have been detected in the fourth and fifth generations of some tribes in Muslim societies where endogamy is the norm.

Muslim traditions also speak about the negative impact on the fetus of "improper" modes of intercourse rejected by the Qur'an. Yet it was believed that special prayer when one intends to have intercourse with his wife keeps the devil away from what God has ordained to be created. The pure state of the parents' minds and bodies can be transmitted to the child through the invocation of the Divine Name before intercourse. In light of belief in the divine purpose and decree in the creation of offspring ("It is God who brought you forth from your mothers' wombs," Qur'an 16:78), either born with birth defects or normal, there does not seem to be any indication to support genetic diagnosis or screening that would justify abortion, which Islam permits primarily to safeguard the mother's health.

ABDULAZIZ SACHEDINA

Directly related to this article are the other articles in this entry: JUDAISM, CHRISTIANITY, *and* HINDUISM AND BUDDHISM. *Also directly related are the entries* EUGENICS; *and* ISLAM. *For a further discussion of topics mentioned in this article, see the entry* ABORTION, *section on* RELIGIOUS TRADITIONS, *article on* ISLAMIC PERSPECTIVES. *Other relevant material may be found under the entries* ETHICS, *article on* RELIGION AND MORALITY; MARRIAGE AND OTHER DOMESTIC RELATIONSHIPS; *and* POPULATION ETHICS, *section on* RELIGIOUS TRADITIONS, *article on* ISLAMIC PERSPECTIVES.

Bibliography

Sunni views

AL-BUKHARI, MUHAMMAD IBN ISMA'IL. 1986. *Kitab al-nikah.* Vol. 4. In *Sahih al-Bukhari.* Beirut: 'Alam al-Kutub.
AL-JUZAYRI, 'ABD AL-RAHMAN. 1969. *al-Fiqh 'ala al-madhahib al-arba'a.* Vol. 4. Cairo: Dar al-Fikr al-'Arabi.
MUSLIM IBN AL-HAJJAJ AL-QUSHAYRI. 1956. *Kitab al-nikah.* In *Sahih al-Muslim.* Beirut: Dar Ihya' al-Turath al-'Arabi.

Shiite views

AL-'AMILI, AL-SHAHID AL-THANI. 1969. *Al-Rawdat al-bahiyya fi sharh al-lum'at al-dimashqiyya.* Vol. 5. An-Najaf, Iraq: Matba'a al-Adab.
AL-HURR, AL-'AMILI, MUHAMMAD IBN AL-HASAN. 1968. *Wasa'il al-shi'a.* Vol. 14. In *Kitab al-nikah.* Beirut: Dar Ihya' al-Turath al-'Arabi.

IV. HINDUISM AND BUDDHISM

Because reproduction is one of the most important concerns of human life, most religions concern themselves with the regulation of sexual activity, marriage, and production of children. Hinduism and Buddhism also guide their followers in these matters, but in ways very different both from each other and from Western religions.

Eugenics might be defined as controlling human reproduction to modify or benefit the species. Prior to the present innovation of genetic engineering, eugenics meant restrictions on who could reproduce and with which partner. The recent development of methods of altering the human genome has opened a new area of ethical discussion: the propriety of voluntarily altering the human genome. Eugenics has also been used to excuse genocide, but this aspect will not be discussed here since nothing in Hinduism or Buddhism allows rationalization of genocide.

Although Hinduism and Buddhism have highly developed ethical philosophies, neither religion produces set positions on such contemporary matters as eugenics, nor is it likely that they will, given the nature and organization of the two religions. In both religions, ethics are developed by the individual or the social community; there is no official body that produces ethical statements. Hence there are no official Hindu or Buddhist positions on issues that were not envisioned when their scriptures were composed over 2,000 years ago. However, both religions have ethical ideas or methods that can be applied to modern problems.

Hinduism has its beginnings in the two millennia before the Common Era; the historical Buddha, Shakyamuni, died about 500 B.C.E. In those remote times there were no concepts akin to those of modern genetics and hence there could be no ethical discussions of genetic manipulation. Rather than a single scripture analogous to the Judeo-Christian Bible or the Koran, Hinduism and Buddhism have vast collections of diverse canonical texts that have appeared over millennia. Hinduism does have several authoritative legal texts, the most important of which, *The Laws of Manu,* was composed from about 200 B.C.E. to 200 C.E. These texts codify religious law (*dharma*) but are not regarded as the only legal or ethical authority. Buddhist texts are concerned with spiritual development and give only very general precepts for regulation of lay life. However, it is possible to develop Hindu or Buddhist positions on eugenics.

Hinduism and Buddhism both arose in India and share many common beliefs, such as the doctrine of *karma* (discussed below), yet the differences between the two religions must not be underestimated. Generally speaking, Hinduism is a legalistic religion and pays great attention to regulating life in the world. Buddhism sees worldly life as secondary in importance; attainment of release from suffering in this or subsequent existences is its central concern.

Reproduction in Hindu religious law

Although Hinduism recognizes a final stage of life in which the individual is released from domestic and social obligations in order to be able to pursue enlightenment (*moksha*), in the earlier, householder stage, detailed rules define acceptable behavior. Among the most important are those that regulate reproduction. The intent of these rules is to maintain the hereditary caste distinctions. Here Hinduism's outlook is very similar to that of nineteenth- and early twentieth-century Western eugenics, which proposed controlling reproduction to prevent what were considered undesirable unions. Although the specific rules for regulating marriage and reproduction were different from those proposed by Western eugenics, the spirit is the same: to protect the human species from degeneration due to unsuitable matches. Hinduism does not define suitability for marriage according to scientific understanding of genetics, but by caste membership, which is hereditary, and by physical traits, which are correlated with astrology. Traditionally, prospective brides were inspected undressed and an elaborate system of body divination existed for interpreting body markings, particularly on erogenous areas. Manu states, "A man should not marry a girl who is a redhead or has an extra limb or is sickly or has not body hair or . . . is too sallow . . . He should marry a woman who does not lack any part of her body . . . whose body hair and hair on the head is fine . . ." (Manu, p. 44). There are also rules for selecting the sex

of children (males are conceived on even-numbered nights) and in all cases, the social class of husband and wife must match.

These procedures amount to methods of selecting marriage partners according to biological suitability, although the biological traits selected for concern may not seem very appropriate today. Marriage is discouraged if partners are not biologically and astrologically suited. In India, marriages have been and still are arranged by parents on the basis of social, economic, and reproductive suitability. Romantic interest is at best a very secondary consideration. The entire basis of marriage in Hinduism is eugenic, but the factors felt to predispose favorably to suitable offspring are quite different from modern Western ones. Marriage in Hinduism exists to ensure offspring and perpetuate family distinction and caste separation. These laws were intended to regulate reproduction rather than sexuality. Sexual liaison outside of marriage and across caste, though not approved of, was not considered wrong so long as no offspring resulted.

Hinduism does not contemplate elimination of inferior castes, but simply limitation of physical contact between them and higher ones. The higher castes must preserve their purity, but all castes are necessary and have their place in the cosmos (Danielou, 1993). This contrasts with the extreme, modern racism, in which one group, which considers itself superior, aims at the elimination of others. There is no idea of altering the genetic or social situation of humanity as a whole. On the contrary, marriage rules attempt to maintain the status quo. Their rationale is not to improve the human species but to prevent its degeneration.

In general, Hinduism has not been opposed to attempts to control reproduction. Female infanticide has been extensively practiced in India. An innovation is the use of ultrasound machines by entrepreneurs; at village marketplaces a pregnant woman can find out whether she is carrying a boy or girl, with abortion elected in the instance of the latter. A similar practice exists in China. Although the practice of female infanticide can be explained in economic terms (a girl's parents must provide a dowry if she is to be married), it represents a practice of controlling reproductive outcome for family or social goals. Infanticide has not been viewed with the same opprobrium as in the West, although it is certainly not fair to imply that the Hindu religion condones such acts.

The Indian concept of karma, which is fundamental to all its philosophical and religious systems, has some similarities to modern genetics. It is a law of moral cause and effect. The literal meaning of karma is action, and the theory holds that one's present state is the result of personal and collective actions in this and previous lives. Actions, like genes, have effects that persist across lifetimes. Much of each individual's present circumstances are the result of previous actions carried across generations. Karma and scientific genetics seek to account for the human experience that the past tends to repeat itself in the present. Both offer an explanation of how an individual comes to have certain traits.

Buddhism and human reproduction

Buddhism, which abolishes the caste system, has no concern with the suitability of marriages. Indeed, its monastic nature has made Buddhism generally uninterested in family life and reproduction. Throughout Buddhist history, clergy were forbidden to solemnize marriages; this was seen as inappropriate involvement in worldly affairs. (Wedding ceremonies officiated by Buddhist monks are a recent innovation.) Nor does Buddhism have an elaborate ethical code for regulation of lay behavior. Throughout most of its 2,500-year history, Buddhism has been monastic; lay life was not considered conducive for progress toward enlightenment. However, the sangha, the order of monks and nuns, did try to inculcate simple moral understanding in the laity.

In the Theravada form of Buddhism, which most closely resembles early Buddhism, the laity is taught the Five Precepts, which call on the Buddhist to avoid (1) unnecessary killing, (2) taking what is not given, (3) sexual misconduct, (4) harmful speech, and (5) use of intoxicants. Although Buddhist teachers will offer their particular interpretations of these principles, detailed rules are not given in any canonical text. Sexual misconduct, for example, is rarely defined and there is no position on contraception. Nor are there specific rules on suitability of marriage or sexual partners. The first precept might be interpreted as discouraging abortion; however, termination of pregnancy is not absolutely forbidden, though it is considered highly undesirable. Buddhism would see the ideal situation as one in which the partners are mindful of the consequences of their actions and avoid a situation in which abortion is a consideration. If carried out, abortion should use a method that minimizes any suffering. (For Buddhist analyses of the abortion issue see Taniguchi, 1987, and Redmond, 1991.) In Japan, where abortion is used as a method of family planning, Buddhist monks are involved in practices that women use to atone for abortion.

In contrast to the religious law of Judaism, Christianity, and Islam, the Buddhist precepts are very general, expressing morality in spirit rather than letter. Nothing in the five lay precepts can be construed to oppose genetic manipulation, provided that it is not harmful. Buddhism does not try to regulate lay behavior by detailed codes of laws, but rather by teaching sati, "mindfulness" and ahimsa, "harmlessness." The ultimate value in Buddhism is not living in accordance with a code of religious laws but being aware of the effects of one's actions so as to minimize harm. In general, a Buddhist would be concerned that genetic knowledge not be used in a way that causes suffering, but would not be opposed in principle to the acquisition or application of such knowledge. Buddhism places its highest value on knowledge, which it sees as the sole vehicle for enlightenment and release from suffering. Ignorance, not sin or disobedience, is the case of a human's unhappy state. Hence, Buddhism may be seen as favoring the acquisition and use of genetic knowledge, provided that it is applied in ways that help, rather than harm, living beings. Changing the genetic code so as to eliminate a disease in the offspring would be quite acceptable so long as it was carried out skillfully, that is, not harmfully. Partner selection for genetic or ethnic reasons is not supported by Buddhism, which abolished the Hindu caste system. However, such selection would not be ethically improper if it did not cause suffering to those involved.

Cosmology and eugenics

There are two commonly held contemporary Western positions about eugenics that Hinduism and Buddhism see rather differently from most Western ethicists. One position is that since the world and everything in it, including human beings, are held to be created by God according to a divine plan, then altering the human genome is altering the very basis of God's creation, which is impermissible. Thus the Vatican's statement on reproductive technology holds that "no biologist or doctor can reasonably claim, by virtue of his scientific competence, to be able to decide on people's origin or destiny" (Vatican, Congregation for the Doctrine of the Faith, 1992, p. 84). A similar but secular argument holds that we should not alter nature. Although altering nature may not be inherently wrong, pragmatically such alterations are much more likely to do harm than good. The only safe course is stringently to restrict novel technologies such as genetic engineering.

Neither Hinduism nor Buddhism conceives of a creator God whose divine plan might be altered by genetic manipulation. (Although Brahma is considered the creator in Hinduism, the metaphysics of creation are quite different. Creation occurs from moment to moment and not according to a perfect plan.) Far from seeing the world as divine or perfect, both religions regard the world as inevitably a place of suffering. The fundamental virtue in both Hinduism and Buddhism is practicing ahimsa, or harmlessness, which means to avoid making living beings suffer. For example, the environment should not be harmed because living creatures are dependent on it. Since the universe was not created by divine plan, altering it is not considered a repudiation of God. In this context genetic manipulation is perfectly acceptable.

As to the second argument, that humans cannot handle their power over the genome, neither Hinduism nor Buddhism can be held to have a clear position on this. Evil is the result, respectively, of delusion, *moha,* or ignorance, *avidya.* Ethical ignorance is simply an aspect of more general spiritual ignorance, which clouds perception of the true nature of existence. However, Buddhism and Hinduism conceive of ethical ignorance somewhat differently. In Hinduism, it is necessary to be aware of the complex laws, or *dharma,* regulating human behavior. In Buddhism, ignorance is lack of awareness of the law of cause and effect, for example, of knowing how one's actions will affect oneself and others (Taniguchi, 1994). Mindfulness shows that an action harmful to another will cause suffering just as it would if done to oneself. A unique moral insight of Buddhism is that ethical behavior requires factual knowledge (Redmond, 1989)—for example, what effects behavior will have on others—as well as knowledge of ethical precepts. The way to this knowledge is through self-cultivation such as meditation, study of religious texts, and, especially, the influence of a teacher. Ethical behavior results from personal moral development rather than detailed moral legislation.

Karma and eugenics

The concept of karma can be interpreted, or sometimes misinterpreted, so that it appears to oppose eugenics. Karma holds that misfortunes in this life are due to harmful actions in a former life (although there are also social sources of unfavorable karma). By this interpretation, if a child is born with a genetic disorder, then the misfortune is due to previous voluntary actions that harmed others and hence is deserved. Furthermore, this karma must be worked off; the suffering must be endured to expiate the previous wrongdoing. If the suffering is prevented, it will simply occur later. Thus, if a fetus with Down syndrome is aborted, the same individual will simply be reincarnated later with a similar affliction.

The idea that suffering should not be relieved, because karmically deserved, is widespread in India and Buddhist countries and is sometimes articulated by Buddhist teachers in the West. It is a misunderstanding of the Buddha's teaching, which was concerned to explain the way of release from suffering. Although Buddhism teaches compassion, some Buddhists, in common with some followers of other religions, find interpretations that rationalize evasion of the ethical obligation to be kind to others. It is not consistent with Buddhist teachings on compassion to refrain from relieving another's suffering on the grounds that it is due to the operation of karma.

Buddhism, although not opposed to eugenics if it is skillfully applied, does not require it. In contrast to Hinduism, it does not establish rules regarding reproductive behavior. Some contemporary Buddhists believe that each individual has his or her tasks in life and that, although these might be different for someone with a birth defect, others should not assume that such a life is therefore less worthy. This has affinities with the idea that we should not interfere with nature because we may not fully understand the effects of what we do.

Hinduism, then, requires a form of eugenics, and Buddhism is essentially neutral on eugenics as such, but would be greatly concerned to ensure that eugenic practice decreased suffering rather than increasing it. Neither religion sees eugenics as in itself improper, but both concern themselves with how it is carried out. However, Hinduism and Buddhism produce no set positions, and individual Hindus and Buddhists may have views different from those summarized here.

GEOFFREY P. REDMOND

Directly related to this article are the other articles in this entry: JUDAISM; CHRISTIANITY; *and* ISLAM. *Also directly related to this article are the entries* HINDUISM; BUDDHISM; ETHICS, *article on* RELIGION AND MORALITY; EUGENICS; GENETIC ENGINEERING, *article on* HUMAN GENETIC ENGINEERING; *and* INFANTS, *article on* HISTORY OF INFANTICIDE. *For a further discussion of Hinduism and/or Buddhism, see the entries* DEATH, *article on* EASTERN THOUGHT; MEDICAL ETHICS, HISTORY OF, *section on* SOUTH AND EAST ASIA, *articles on* INDIA, *and* SOUTHEAST ASIAN COUNTRIES, *and subsections on* CHINA, *and* JAPAN; *and* POPULATION ETHICS, *section on* RELIGIOUS TRADITIONS, *articles on* HINDU PERSPECTIVES, *and* BUDDHIST PERSPECTIVES. *Other relevant material may be found under the entries* CONFUCIANISM; FERTILITY CONTROL, *article on* ETHICAL ISSUES; GENETICS AND HUMAN BEHAVIOR; GENETICS AND HUMAN SELF-UNDERSTANDING; GENETICS AND RACIAL MINORITIES; JAINISM; MEDICAL GENETICS; REPRODUCTIVE TECHNOLOGIES, *article on* ETHICAL ISSUES; SIKHISM; *and* TAOISM.

Bibliography

DANIELOU, ALAIN. 1993. *Virtue, Success, Pleasure, and Liberation: The Four Aims of Life in the Tradition of Ancient India.* Rochester, Vt.: Inner Traditions International.

MANU. 1991. *The Laws of Manu.* Translated and with an introduction and notes by Wendy Doniger, with Brian K. Smith. London: Penguin.

REDMOND, GEOFFREY P. 1989. "Application of the Buddhist Anatma Doctrine to the Problems of Biomedical Ethics." *Ninth Conference of the International Association of Buddhist Studies Abstracts.* Taipei, Taiwan: Institute for Sino-Indian Buddhist Studies.

———. 1991. "Buddhism and Abortion." *Newsletter on International Buddhist Women's Activities,* no. 26 (January–March), pp. 7–11.

TANIGUCHI, SHOYO. 1987. "Biomedical Ethics from a Buddhist Perspective." *The Pacific World.* New Series no. 3, pp. 75–83.

———. 1994. "Methodology of Buddhist Biomedical Ethics." *Religious Methods and Resources in Bioethics,* pp. 31–65. Edited by Paul F. Camenisch. Dordrecht, Netherlands: Kluwer Academic Publishers.

VATICAN. CONGREGATION FOR THE DOCTRINE OF THE FAITH. 1992. "Instruction of Respect for Human Life in Its Origin and on the Dignity of Procreation." In *The Ethics of Reproductive Technology,* pp. 83–97. Edited by Kenneth D. Alpern. New York: Oxford University Press.

EUTHANASIA, ACTIVE AND PASSIVE

See DEATH AND DYING: EUTHANASIA AND SUSTAINING LIFE; *and* INFANTS, *articles on* HISTORY OF INFANTICIDE, *and* ETHICAL ISSUES.

EVOLUTION

Evolution is the central scientific concept in biology that describes the mode of origin of biological diversity. The idea is simple and may be defined as a process of descent with change. More explicitly, it states that all animals and plants existing on the earth today are the changed descendants of animals and plants that existed on the earth in the past. "Changed" refers to permanent modifications of structure and function encoded in the genetic material deoxyribonucleic acid (DNA), a substance that is present in the cells of all organisms and is the link between generations.

In biology, the twentieth century has been the age of genetics. The influence of the science of molecular coding has reached into every corner of the life sciences. Nowhere is its influence greater than in the understanding of the manner in which life evolves. This article deals with the living state, and is not concerned with the evolution of either the universe or the heavenly bodies.

Evolution versus the origin of life

The question of the ultimate origin of life is distinct from the consideration of descent with change. There are good scientific reasons for separating these matters. Life is not now arising spontaneously; all living organisms can be traced through their DNA to preexisting parental forms. The elementary conditions that existed when the planet was young and life arose from nonliving materials may be absent or difficult to identify or duplicate at present. One can perhaps surmise what those conditions were and attempt to investigate them now, but this approach has not been successful. The point of separating "origin" from "evolution" is to emphasize that the evolutionist works on the assumption that, given the basic properties of the living state (metabolism, irritability, mutability, and self-reproduction), descent with change in DNA codes can explain the diversity of life as now observed.

Evolution: Fact, course, and cause

Consideration of three separate questions can illuminate the concept of evolution:

1. *Is evolution a fact?* In deciding whether a concept has the status of fact, the scientist must consider all the evidence for and against the proposal and its alternatives. Biological diversity has only two possible explanations: Either each animal or plant existing on the earth today is the changed descendant of life existing in the past or each form of life was created or arose spontaneously in essentially its present form.

Evidence for the first alternative comes from such diverse areas of biological science as comparative anatomy and embryology, comparative biochemistry and molecular biology of proteins and nucleic acids, cell and chromosome structure and function, the record of fossils in the earth's crust, and the present and past geography and ecology of species. This evidence overwhelmingly supports evolution as a fact (see reviews in Futuyma and in Strickberger). Conversely, biological evidence does not support the theory of a special, separate origin or creation of the species on the planet. To the professional biologist, the evidence for the fact of evolution is so strong as to establish evolution as the central law of life on earth. As the title of Dobzhansky's article states: "Nothing in biology makes sense except in the light of evolution" (Dobzhansky, 1973, p. 125).

Evolution versus creation is thus not a serious scientific controversy. Rather, it is a clash between two incommensurate views of the living world that confront each other across a perpetual chasm (Eve and Harrold, 1991).

Answers to the next two questions about evolution assume at least a provisional acceptance of evolution as a fact. Even those who deny the fact will find it useful to consider these additional questions as part of a process of clarification, particularly since, unlike the first question, they concern areas wherein scientists differ from each other in their interpretations of data.

2. *What has been the* course *of evolution?* What can be determined about the pathways of descent from ancestral forms? Paleontology, a biological science based on the fossil remains of past animals and plants, is the main branch of biology that produces information on the course that evolution has followed leading to present

conditions. In many cases, the tracing of ancestry through a series of forms is supported by extensive evidence.

For some organisms, however, fossil remains are inadequate. Nevertheless, recent biochemical studies of the DNA and the proteins it encodes have led to a realization that these molecules themselves embody information that amounts to a detailed historical record that can supplement or even replace phylogenies (family trees) built on the fossil record or on morphology of existing forms. This discovery has spawned a modern science of biological history based on code similarities and differences. Scientists seeking patterns of descent using morphology of living forms or fossils and those who work on protein or genetic codes sometimes differ in their interpretations.

3. What is the *cause* of evolution? Why do animals and plants change with time? Why have they not remained the same from generation to generation? Why are there so many different forms of life recognizable as species, and why are there so many structures, functions, and behaviors that closely fit their carriers to differing environments? Until the middle of the nineteenth century, the idea of descent with change had been considered but lacked a plausible causal-analytical explanation. Charles Darwin (1859) proposed natural selection as a process that could explain continual, directed change in populations (Table 1). Although this outline of natural selection theory has been confirmed in modern biology, some disagree about the details and where the emphasis should be placed. Such disagreements among scientists over the factors that cause evolutionary change by no means indicate that these scientists disagree with one another about the fact of evolution.

Some modern analysts have recast some of the Darwinian emphases. There is a widespread view, for example, that "survival of the fittest" is not a good synonym for "natural selection." From the evolutionary point of view, it is not enough to simply survive: The individual organism must leave more progeny than other members of its population in order to be "fitter" in the Darwinian sense. Individuals having genes and gene combinations that lead to early death or relatively sparse reproduction are eliminated by natural selection, since those individuals make little or no contribution to the next generation and their descendants are sooner or later lost entirely. A second, and strongly positive, aspect of natural selection is that it progressively facilitates fitness by multiplying genetic variations that serve to increase relative reproductive efficiency.

Species and evolution in populations

Living organisms are naturally organized into distinct groups called species. A common genetic definition of a species emphasizes that it is an interbreeding group of closely related individuals that are reproductively isolated from other such groups. Using the criterion of absolute reproductive isolation between closely related species, especially in plants, is often difficult and has led to a contentious debate over the best way to define the species.

Disagreements among scientists over the definition of the species, however, do not affect studies of the dynamics of genetic change in populations. Most organisms naturally exist in geographically local interbreeding populations. No matter what their precise boundaries are, such populations constitute the site where natural selection is especially powerful because of the large size of the field of genetic variability. Sewall Wright calculated the size of an example of such a field of variability: "With 10 allelomorphs in each of 1000 loci, the number of possible combinations is 10^{1000} which is a very large number. It has been estimated that the total number of electrons and protons in the whole visible universe is much less than 10^{100}" (Wright, 1932, p. 356).

Since such estimates were first made, the specific genetic content of samples of populations of individuals facing the process of natural selection in a changing environment has been examined. The results are clear:

TABLE 1 Darwin's Theory of Natural Selection

Facts	*Observed Consequences*
1. There is a tendency to overpopulation, yet total numbers are stationary.	Struggle for existence
2. The struggle for existence occurs along with hereditary variation.	Natural selection ("survival of the fittest")
3. Natural selection occurs in a changing environment.	Incorporation of modifications leading to the origin of new adaptations or species

Each such population is indeed made up of a variable field of individual organisms that carry slightly differing genetic codes. The variability arises from novel mutations and from various combinations of existing genes that are formed at the time of reproduction. New gene combinations are produced in each succeeding generation. The process of natural selection ensures that those gene combinations that have survived best out-reproduce less fortunate individuals in the population. As this is repeated generation after generation, the population changes genetically in a manner that reflects adaptation to the environment. As the environment changes, the population is able to change with it; natural selection performs a genetic tracking of the changing environment.

Evolution of this sort has been repeatedly observed in living populations. For example, when DDT was first used to kill many different species of insects in the 1940s, a relatively small concentration was sufficient to achieve satisfactory pest control. In a few years, however, the earlier concentrations became ineffective. Tests revealed that this was due to genetic changes in the heredity of the insects themselves; through natural selection, they had acquired gene combinations that conferred varying degrees of physiological resistance to the poison. In the original population, such variants were very rare. Selection has naturally multiplied these combinations so that they have come to characterize the majority of the population.

The experiments of Crow (1954) mimicked these natural evolutionary changes. DDT-sensitive but genetically variable populations of fruit flies were allowed to live and reproduce in cages which had DDT applied to the inside surface. A large proportion of the adult flies died, but after a few weeks, the numbers were back up to the previous level. When this happened, a higher concentration of DDT was added; this process was repeated over a three-year period. Tests showed that the flies from the DDT cages had become about 2,000 times more resistant to the chemical than specimens reared in the absence of DDT. Genetic tests showed that the difference was inherited. The rapidity of such selective change depends partly on the time it takes for one generation to succeed the next. For the fruit flies in these population cages, this time was about one month, so that changes of this sort were incorporated into the population quite rapidly. Presented with many generations, many individuals, recombination of genes at reproduction and novel mutations, the process of natural selection effectively screens out inferior combinations and multiplies those that serve their carriers best in the environment that the species inhabits. The process not only continuously monitors the species and keeps it closely adapted to its present environment but also permits change if the population comes to face a novel environmental challenge.

Selection among groups of species, or among smaller groups within species, is theoretically possible under some conditions, but the field of variability on which natural selection may operate is very small compared with that between genetically variable individuals within a single interbreeding population.

The formation of species.   Just as all individuals arise from preexisting individuals, all species arise from preexisting species. Species formation appears to be most commonly accomplished by a demographic process that splits off a "daughter" population from the population of the ancestral species. Factors that promote this isolation are primarily environmental ones, such as geography and/or selection for novel modes of reproduction or habitat preferences. If spatially isolated from the parent species, the new population accumulates genetic differences that may ultimately result in reproductive isolation from the parent species. The circumstances under which this biologically based isolation arises have been the subject of much empirical and theoretical work in evolutionary biology. Throughout the process, however, the local interbreeding population continues to be the site of gradual genetic change.

Small-scale evolution.   Modern genetic work on populations has established that evolution is continuous—that is, increments of minor change occur with each succeeding generation. The animal or plant breeder produces a changed population over each successive generation by selecting some individuals for breeding stock and removing others by culling. Artificial selection thus mimics natural selection very closely. As Darwin aptly pointed out, the breeder who uses artificial selection can properly be viewed as a biological engineer who is applying the basic principles of evolution for human-directed purposeful ends. In nature, however, it is the contingency of the ecological moment that rules. Only the modern human's complex brain injects "purpose" or "direction" into the evolutionary system by trying to see the observed changes as progress toward a predetermined goal. As Stephen Jay Gould puts it: "Continents fragment and disperse; oceanic circulation changes; rivers alter their course; mountains rise; estuaries dry up. If life works more by tracking environment than by climbing up a ladder of progress, then contingency should reign" (Gould, 1989, p. 300).

Large-scale evolution.   To what degree do the slight changes that occur in each generation add up to produce the major evolutionary differences that are seen when different species are compared? Most geneticists believe that if selection continues to operate in a certain direction over many generations, the result may ultimately add up to quite large and conspicuous characters.

For example, a forelimb adapted for swimming might slowly be converted, by selection for certain gene mutations and combinations, to one adapted for walking on land. This is an area where evolutionists tend to disagree, since some contend that special single mutations of large effect, or special population conditions, must ensue before such large changes can become established. This argument states that, over geological time, evolution typically proceeds in spurts (punctuations) separated by periods of little or no change (equilibrium).

Evolution of the human species

From a geological perspective, the human species has evolved very recently. There is no evidence in the genetic or fossil history that the population structure or genetic variability of *Homo sapiens* is basically different from that of other large vertebrates, such as the great apes to which *Homo sapiens* is closely related. The human basic body structure, however, shows few specialized adaptive features. To the evolutionary biologist, it is clear that the overriding biological success of humans in the few hundred thousand years since the species originated is due to a pervasive mental capacity that is universal in all subdivisions of the modern species. The human brain apparently evolved at an early time in the history of the species. The brain provides an adaptability that substitutes conscious behavioral alteration for specific, codified somatic adaptation.

All humans belong to a single species, distinguishable by the large brain and distinctive capacity for cultural evolution. *Homo sapiens* arose in Africa and spread rapidly to all parts of the globe. Coincidentally, populations of previous hominids disappeared. Human migrations were accompanied by the formation of many relatively small, isolated, culturally distinct local populations on all the continents and most of the islands. Population groups remained small and local until about 12,000 years ago, when the population of the world was still only about 10 million. Agricultural development led to local population increases that were followed by spreading from these centers into areas already occupied, leading to the partial or complete breakdown of most of the old local populations. Exponential population growth, reaching about five billion, has continued to the present day.

All modern humans show striking genetic similarity that is somewhat hidden by conspicuous but biologically minor differences in stature, pigmentation, and physiognomy that evolved during the early phase of population spread. Variability also exists in biochemical properties and notably in brain function. Just as no two individuals are genetically identical, it is clear that each individual is born with a genetically unique brain. Some individuals in a population, for example, may show a genetically determined mental retardation or impairment relative to the mean, whereas other individuals may have brains that are especially adept at assimilating and processing information. Retarded, average, or enhanced mental abilities are found within all subdivisions of modern man (nuclear families, clans, local populations, geographic races, ethnic groups, and nations) and significant variability exists in differing individuals within the group rather than between groups.

Evolution: Supporters and opponents

To this point, the article has described the main outlines of the scientific concept of evolution and Darwin's theory of natural selection. The remainder of the article discusses major philosophical and religious controversies that have been provoked by a Darwinian view of evolution. These controversies go to the premises of bioethics and to considerations of what constitutes adequate teaching of biology and the implications of that instruction for bioethics.

Charles Darwin's studies and travels as a naturalist and his reading in 1838 of Thomas Malthus on population and the struggle for existence shaped his development of the concept of natural selection. He prepared several written accounts of his theory but did not publish them. In 1858, he received a paper to read from a biologist, Alfred R. Wallace, who, also stimulated by the work of Malthus, had described independently the elements in the theory that Darwin assumed was his alone. Charles Lyell, a geologist and Darwin's friend, persuaded him that the two men's accounts should be published simultaneously, even though Wallace had no thought of publication when he sent Darwin the paper. Darwin reluctantly agreed, and an "Abstract" of his major work, *The Origin of Species,* appeared in 1859.

Why did Darwin wait twenty years to publish his major discovery (Gould, 1977)? Presumably, he wanted to assemble all known data to support his theory. However, his notebooks (1987) also show that Darwin, familiar with prevailing views in philosophy and theology, was hesitant and even fearful of reactions to a materialistic explanation for human existence, the mind, ethics, and even religion itself. The idea of evolution was not new. Eighteenth-century naturalists like Georges de Buffon and Carolus Linnaeus had discussed it, as had Jean-Baptiste Lamarck and Lyell in the nineteenth. While other naturalists who explained evolution drew upon concepts like "vital forces, directed history, organic striving, and the essential irreducibility of mind," however, Darwin spoke "only of random variation and natural selection" (Gould, 1977, pp. 24–25).

The theological doctrine of creation teaches that the primary cause of the universe and all within it is an act *ex nihilo* ("from nothing") of a transcendent, beneficent Creator. Post-Darwinian reinterpretations of this doctrine explained evolution as guided by an intelligible purpose or design within nature. Darwin's theory rested on a premise that mental, moral, or spiritual phenomena are by-products of underlying physical and material causes. His position negated the plausibility of an intelligent design. Further, the idea of a God who had been continuously creating since the ultimate beginning of things—which one could now argue occurred *through* evolution—was unnecessary in view of Darwin's materialistic premise, which excluded all explanations for evolution beyond random variation and natural selection. Darwin chose to be skeptical about the likelihood that God continued to create through evolution; He simply saw no plausible reason to believe that all variations in nature were intentionally guided by an omniscient Creator.

Darwin was painfully aware that his position provided substantial reasons to doubt the inherited forms of and arguments for theism. He desired to avoid debate on religious topics and doubted that "direct arguments" had an effect on the public. It was possible to explain evolution in terms of variation and natural selection and still hold to a view, as the eighteenth-century deists had argued, that God was the ultimate and primary cause of creation but was now divorced from the ongoing process of evolution. But in the face of this possibility, Darwin thought it best to "admit one's ignorance and remain silent" (Rachels, 1990, p. 126). In short, the doctrine of God the Creator, acting in history and continuously creating out of boundless love, was logically incompatible with Darwin's explanation of evolution. A large part of the intellectual history of late-nineteenth- and early-twentieth-century religious thought and its relation to science can be understood as challenges to and compromises with Darwin's writings and the interpretations of them by scientists and theologians (Gilkey, 1965).

For opponents of Darwinism, a main point of contention concerned the origin of human beings and their moral standing in the world. The traditional religious view was that human beings, having been created "in the image" of God (Genesis 1:26), had special status and dominion over other animals. Darwin's earliest readers, as well as his latest, saw that an evolutionary view threatened to undermine one of the main premises of the traditional core of Western ethics, the origin of humans in a divine act of creation (Rachels, 1990). A second premise, that the special status of human beings resided in their rationality and distinctiveness when compared with animals, was also threatened by Darwin's position. Darwin himself was aware of this threat when he wrote in his notebook in 1838: "Man in his arrogance thinks himself a great work worthy of the interposition of a deity. More humble and I think truer to consider him created from animals" (1987, p. 300).

Darwin's friends as well as his enemies were troubled by the implications of the theory. Lyell, who was gradually persuaded of Darwin's central thesis, wrote:

> You may well believe that it cost me a struggle to renounce my old creed. One of Darwin's reviewers put the alternative strongly by asking "whether we are to believe that man is modified mud or modified monkey." The mud is a great comedown from the "archangel ruined." (1881, vol. 2, p. 376)

Darwin, described by Gould and others as a "gentle revolutionary" anxious to avoid paining his wife, friends, and a public that held tightly to their religious views, desired to leave the philosophical defense of his theory from attacks by opponents to supporters like Thomas H. Huxley and Joseph Hooker or to his belief in the "gradual enlightening of human understanding which follows the progress of science" (Gould, 1977, pp. 26, 27). Only a year after the publication of *Origin,* a famous confrontation occurred in a debate at Oxford University between Huxley and Hooker and the Anglican bishop Samuel Wilberforce. The accounts of this debate vary widely, but it was widely regarded as a prelude to many self-defeating attempts by religious leaders to challenge the scientific merits of Darwin's theory. The story is often retold in the chronicles of conflicts between science and religion. Gould's (1992) historical research into this legendary and ambiguously reported debate is probably the most accurate.

Evolution versus fundamentalism and "creation science"

In the United States, sharp public conflicts over evolution resulted from fundamentalist and evangelical Christian churches' efforts to influence legislatures to ban the teaching of evolution in public schools. Decisions on the curricula in public schools clearly have an ethical dimension involving respect for academic freedom and resolving conflicts between society's interests in education and challenges by groups interested in preserving cultural and religious identity. Fundamentalist and conservative churches hold that the Bible is verbally inerrant and has complete authority over belief and morals. In the early twentieth century, viewing the state of society as evidence of a breakdown in traditional morality, fundamentalist leaders attacked Darwinism and the growth of biblical criticism, terming them both "modernism." The modernist-fundamentalist controversy dominated U.S. Protestant church history in that period.

In the 1920s, aided by William Jennings Bryan, a populist who had been the Democratic nominee for

President in 1896, fundamentalists attacked evolution theory and lobbied for laws against teaching it in public schools. In 1925 Tennessee passed a law declaring it unlawful to teach any doctrine denying the divine creation of man as taught by the Bible. That law was challenged in the courts by the American Civil Liberties Union. John T. Scopes, a science teacher in Dayton, Tennessee, volunteered to serve as defendant against the charge of having taught evolution. Bryan assisted the prosecution, and Clarence Darrow, a nationally known criminal defense counsel, represented Scopes.

The ensuing "monkey trial" gained world attention. The judge did not permit a test of the state law's constitutionality or argument on the validity of the concept of evolution; according to him, the trial turned on the question of whether Scopes had taught evolution. Scopes admitted that he had; he was convicted and fined $100. On appeal, the Tennessee Supreme Court upheld the constitutionality of the 1925 law but acquitted Scopes on the technicality that he had been fined excessively. This decision blocked a planned appeal to the U.S. Supreme Court. In 1929, Arkansas passed a law forbidding the teaching of evolution in public schools; this law was struck down by the U.S. Supreme Court in 1968 (*Epperson v. Arkansas*). The Tennessee law was repealed by the state legislature in 1967.

In the 1930s, opposition to the teaching of evolution prevailed. Mention of evolution or Darwin was largely omitted from science textbooks (Nelkin, 1982). In the aftermath of the Soviet Union's successful launch of the Sputnik satellite in 1957, the National Science Foundation supported efforts to improve science teaching in the nation's schools. The Biological Sciences Curriculum Study (BSCS), a nonprofit organization, then issued a series of biology texts, used in many states, that described the concept of evolution as central to biology.

In the 1960s and 1970s, a reawakening of fundamentalism was accompanied by stronger, more thoughtful opposition to evolution, provoked in part by the widespread use of the BSCS curriculum. A few scientists with fundamentalist commitments organized to produce writings and debate with mainstream biologists. They named their movement "creation science" and argued that the Genesis creation account was supported by scientific data (Morris, 1977). The major claims of creation science are that the universe, energy, and life were created suddenly, from nothing; that mutations and natural selection were insufficient to bring about the development of living species and that change had occurred within fixed limits from original species; that humans and apes have separate ancestries; that geology is explained by catastrophism, including the occurrence of a worldwide flood (Whitcomb and Morris, 1961); and, finally, that the age of the earth was far less than the billions of years claimed by paleontologists.

Creation scientists and their advocates designed a model state law requiring that if evolution were taught, creation science would have to be given equal teaching time. They argued that respect for academic freedom should permit the teaching of both theories. Accordingly, in 1981 the Arkansas legislature enacted a law requiring "balanced treatment of creation science and evolution science" in public schools. The law stressed that academic freedom should permit the teaching of both approaches. A coalition of opponents—including religious leaders, educational groups, and parents—brought suit the same year in Federal court. They sought, among other things, to void the law as a violation of the First Amendment's prohibition against the establishment of religion. The diverse makeup of the coalition demonstrated how deeply evolution had been embraced by some contemporary religious thought.

Theologians and scientists testified for the plaintiffs (Gilkey, 1985; Gould, 1983). Judge William R. Overton found in favor of the plaintiffs, ruling that creation science appealed not to the criteria of the scientific method but to belief in a supernatural Creator whose acts were described in the book of Genesis and, further, that creation science was a particular religious view of origins with a history of its own in American fundamentalism (*McLean et al. v. Arkansas Board of Education*, 1983). The ruling struck down the Arkansas law, holding that a state requirement that biology instructors teach creation science was a clear violation of the establishment clause of the First Amendment.

In 1987 the U.S. Supreme Court heard an appeal of a Louisiana case that contested the constitutionality of a similar "balanced treatment" law enacted by the state legislature. Justice William Brennan wrote the majority opinion finding the law unconstitutional because it served no identified secular purpose and promoted a particular religious belief (*Edwards v. Aguillard*). Justice Antonin Scalia's dissent for the minority found the Louisiana legislature's position defensible in terms of protecting "students' freedom from indoctrination," and maintaining that students should receive "all of the evidence." That the justices held differing views on the status of evolution as a scientific fact portends continuing controversy. However, since the Arkansas and Louisiana cases, advocates of creation science have made no further attempt to use state legislation to achieve "equal treatment."

Evolution and ethics

The philosopher in Darwin's era who most vigorously discussed the implications of evolution for ethics was Herbert Spencer, who coined the term "survival of the fittest." Spencer based his treatise on ethics (1879) on a view that a "higher," or "more evolved," stage of human conduct was more fitting and conducive to peaceful, co-operative communities than older, or "lower," stages. He saw Darwin's theory of natural selection as providing a scientific basis for rules of conduct, family life, and reproduction. Popularization of Spencer's philosophy was an important factor in the eugenics movement in the early twentieth century. This movement oversimplified genetic and evolutionary explanations for social conditions of poverty and behavior that included alcoholism and criminality.

Spencer's arguments, and all naturalistic approaches to ethics, were soundly criticized by G. E. Moore in *Principia Ethica* in 1903. Moore argued that Spencer had committed the "naturalistic fallacy": The right and the good (the "ought" that is the aim of ethics) could not be identified with or derived from "natural" properties, with facts about what "is" the case. Moore's critique, when added to Spencer's misunderstandings of Darwin, who never argued for "higher" or "lower" stages or levels of evolution, abruptly ended a period in which Spencer and his views on social evolution were widely praised, especially in the United States.

Darwin and evolutionary biology strongly influenced the thought of the American pragmatist John Dewey, who stated that Darwin had introduced a "mode of thinking that in the end was bound to transform the logic of knowledge . . . [in] morals, politics, and religion" (1910, p. 2). In this spirit, Dewey adopted an experimentalist approach to ethical problems. In his view of reality, nature, as understood in scientific and ordinary experience, is the ultimate reality. Human beings are best understood as intelligent products of nature who find meaning and goals in life here and now. Dewey's influence on educational philosophy and practices has been profound.

Henri Bergson's *Creative Evolution* (1911) drew on Darwin's formulation but countered his materialistic theory with an explanation of how evolution toward complexity takes place using a principle he called *élan vital*, or "life force." Bergson could not accept that the complexities in human consciousness and the capacity to be moral could be explained by Darwin's materialist theory.

In the 1970s, a long debate about the genetic contributions to human social and ethical behavior culminated in Edward O. Wilson's *Sociobiology: The New Synthesis* (1975). Wilson argued that sociobiology would replace moral philosophy, since the former explained ethics "at all depths" as a product of the hypothalamus and the limbic system. Wilson did not attempt this explanation. His accomplishment was to explain the evolutionary significance of altruism, which had been a puzzle for Darwin and other evolutionists. At first view, altruism—helping others at the helper's expense—should be reproductively counterproductive and gradually eliminated by natural selection. Building on the earlier work of William Hamilton (1964), Wilson clarified the role of "kin altruism": Acting to increase the chances of a genetically similar individual's survival is a way of ensuring that one's own genes are transmitted, even in the cases of cousins. Kin altruism provides the basis for a significant biological contribution to moral behavior, which is favored by natural selection. The place of kin and reciprocal altruism for ethics was later developed in moral philosophy by Peter Singer (1981) and figures in the work of James Rachels (1990). Wilson's reductionistic claims for sociobiology were persuasively refuted by Mary Midgley (1978) and Michael Ruse (1979), followed by Singer and Rachels. They argued that ethics, a field of inquiry with its own internal standards of argument and justification, cannot be "taken over" by biological neurology any more than any other field, such as mathematics, could be so subsumed. Singer demonstrates clearly that although sociobiology can offer a scientific explanation of the development of ethics, it cannot be the source of ethical guidance, which can come only from choices of the ultimate premises of ethics.

Ruse (1989), Midgley, Singer, and Rachels are the contemporary philosophers who have most thoroughly discussed the significance of Darwin's discovery and evolution for human ethics. Gilkey (1965, 1985), more than any other theologian of the liberal tradition, has explicated ways that evolution can enrich understandings of religion. In religious ethics, the work of Charles Birch and John Cobb (1981) and other thinkers of the "process" school of thought following Alfred North Whitehead (1978) built upon the richness of evolutionary understandings of biology and culture to create a perspective to meet the challenges of the Darwinian view.

Conclusion

Reconciliation of the scientific and religious views of the human individual and species has continued to be a source of difficulty for contemporary society. Before Darwin, philosophers of the Enlightenment (e.g., David Hume, François-Marie Voltaire) challenged the credibility of received religious views of the existence of a special deity and the ethical implications of living without such beliefs. Before Darwin's work, however, there was no serious challenge to prevailing religious views of the creation of species, including human beings and, by extension, modern humans. Beginning with Darwin and continuing into the twentieth century, developments in modern paleontology, molecular genetics, and population biology have amassed an immense amount of data that illuminate evolution as a process that has been ongoing for hundreds of millions of years. The course that evolution has followed in reaching the present state has been delineated and clarified for many species, including *Homo sapiens*. Data produced by analytical studies of the cause of evolution strongly support Darwin's theory of natural selection as the leading directive agent of adaptive change in populations. These discoveries have yielded the fundamental conclusion that evolution, defined as descent with genetic change, is indeed a fact—a major law of life on Earth, from microorganism to modern man.

The enormous increase in population size of the human species has been accompanied by widespread internecine struggle, dangerously severe environmental degradation, and the global pandemic of AIDS. Dashing the hopes of Enlightenment thinkers, the social, political, and biological sciences have been unable to provide the grounds for a compelling vision of ethics and normative guidance. Those devoted to religious and philosophical inquiry into the meaning of human life thus find themselves facing a new challenge of unprecedented proportions. What is needed is leadership emphasizing the development of normative ethics and codes of behavior based on a genuine understanding of the human species as part of the natural world rather than as somehow separate from it.

The evidence of the unity and diversity of all species in the context of evolution is there for all to examine. The problems facing all cultures should be sufficiently compelling to unify all who care for the future of the earth and its communities. Yet it remains to be seen whether accounts of normative ethics, especially those conceived in philosophy and religion, will seriously consider the implications of biological evolution for ethical guidance.

HAMPTON L. CARSON
JOHN C. FLETCHER

For a further discussion of topics mentioned in this entry, see the entries BIOLOGY, PHILOSOPHY OF; GENETICS AND ENVIRONMENT IN HUMAN HEALTH; GENETICS AND HUMAN BEHAVIOR, *article on* SCIENTIFIC AND RESEARCH ISSUES; GENETICS AND HUMAN SELF-UNDERSTANDING; HUMAN NATURE; JUDAISM; LIFE; PROTESTANTISM; *and* ROMAN CATHOLICISM. *For a discussion of related ideas, see the entries* INTERPRETATION; *and* VALUE AND VALUATION. *Other relevant material may be found under the entries* ANIMAL WELFARE AND RIGHTS; ENVIRONMENTAL ETHICS; NATURAL LAW; *and* SCIENCE, PHILOSOPHY OF.

Bibliography

BERGSON, HENRI. 1944. [1911]. *Creative Evolution.* Translated by Arthur Mitchell. New York: Modern Library.

BIRCH, CHARLES, and COBB, JOHN B., JR. 1981. *The Liberation of Life.* Cambridge: At the University Press.

CROW, J. F. 1954. "Analysis of a DDT-Resistant Strain of Drosophila." *Journal of Economic Entomology* 47:393–398.

DARWIN, CHARLES. 1859. *On the Origin of Species by Means of Natural Selection or the Preservation of Favoured Races in the Struggle for Life.* London: John Murray.

———. 1987. *Charles Darwin's Notebooks, 1836–1844: Geology, Transmutation of Species, Metaphysical Inquiries.* Transcribed and edited by Paul H. Barrett et al. Ithaca, N.Y.: Cornell University Press.

DEWEY, JOHN. 1910. "The Influence of Darwin on Philosophy." In his *The Influence of Darwin on Philosophy, and Other Essays in Contemporary Thought,* pp. 1–19. New York: Henry Holt.

DOBZHANSKY, THEODOSIUS. 1973. "Nothing in Biology Makes Sense Except in the Light of Evolution." *American Biology Teacher* 35:125–29.

Edwards v. Aguillard. 1987. 482 U.S. 578.

Epperson v. Arkansas. 1968. 393 U.S. 97.

EVE, RAYMOND, A., and HARROLD, FRANCIS B. 1991. *The Creationist Movement in Modern America.* Boston: G. K. Hall.

FUTUYMA, DOUGLAS J. 1986. *Evolutionary Biology.* 2d ed. Sunderland, Mass.: Sinauer.

GILKEY, LANGDON. 1965. *Maker of Heaven and Earth: A Study of the Christian Doctrine of Creation.* New York: Anchor.

———. 1985. *Creationism on Trial.* Minneapolis: Winston Press.

GOULD, STEPHEN JAY. 1977. *Ever Since Darwin: Reflections in Natural History.* New York: Norton.

———. 1983. *Hen's Teeth and Horse's Shoes: Further Reflections in Natural History.* New York: Norton.

———. 1989. *Wonderful Life: The Burgess Shale and the Nature of History.* New York: Norton.

———. 1991. *Bully for Brontosaurus: Reflections in Natural History.* New York: Norton.

HAMILTON, WILLIAM D. 1964a. "The Genetical Evolution of Social Behavior I." *Journal of a Theoretical Biology* 7, no. 1:1–16.

———. 1964b. "The Genetical Evolution of Social Behavior II." *Journal of Theoretical Biology* 7, no. 1:17–52.

LYELL, KATHERINE MURRAY, ed. 1881. *Life, Letters and Journals of Sir Charles Lyell.* 2 vols. London: John Murray.

McLean v. Arkansas Board of Education. 1983. 529 F. Supp. 1255 (E.D. Ark. 1982).

MIDGLEY, MARY. 1978. *Beast and Man. The Roots of Human Nature.* Ithaca, N.Y.: Cornell University Press.

MOORE, G. E. 1993. [1903]. *Principia Ethica.* Revised ed. Cambridge: At the University Press.

MORRIS, HENRY M. 1977. *The Scientific Case for Creation.* San Diego, Calif.: Creation-Life.

NELKIN, DOROTHY. 1982. *The Creation Controversy: Science or Scripture in the Schools.* New York: W. W. Norton.

RACHELS, JAMES. 1990. *Created from Animals: The Moral Implications of Darwinism.* New York: Oxford University Press.

RUSE, MICHAEL. 1979. *Sociobiology: Sense or Nonsense?* Dordrecht, The Netherlands: D. Reidel.

———. 1989. *The Darwinian Paradigm: Essays on Its History, Philosophy, and Religious Implications.* London: Routledge & Kegan Paul.

SINGER, PETER. 1981. *The Expanding Circle: Ethics and Sociobiology.* New York: Farrar, Straus and Giroux.

SPENCER, HERBERT. 1879. *The Data of Ethics.* New York: Thomas Y. Crowell.

STRICKBERGER, MONROE W. 1990. *Evolution*. Boston: Jones and Bartlett.

WHITCOMB, JOHN C., JR. and MORRIS, HENRY M. 1961. *The Genesis Flood: The Biblical Record and Its Scientific Implications*. Philadelphia, Pa.: Presbyterian and Reformed Publishing Company.

WHITEHEAD, ALFRED N. 1978. [1929]. *Process and Reality: An Essay in Cosmology*. Corrected ed. New York: Free Press.

WILSON, EDWARD O. 1975. *Sociobiology: The New Synthesis*. Cambridge, Mass.: Harvard University Press.

WRIGHT, SEWALL. 1932. "The Roles of Mutation, Inbreeding, Crossbreeding and Selection in Evolution." *Proceedings of the Sixth International Congress of Genetics* 1:356–66.

EXPERIMENTATION, ANIMAL

See ANIMAL RESEARCH. *See also* ANIMAL WELFARE AND RIGHTS, *article on* ETHICAL PERSPECTIVES ON THE TREATMENT AND STATUS OF ANIMALS.

EXPERIMENTATION WITH HUMAN SUBJECTS

See INFORMED CONSENT, *article on* CONSENT ISSUES IN HUMAN RESEARCH; RESEARCH, HUMAN: HISTORICAL ASPECTS; RESEARCH, UNETHICAL; RESEARCH BIAS; RESEARCH METHODOLOGY; *and* RESEARCH POLICY. *For discussion of various research subjects, see the entries* ADOLESCENTS; AGING AND THE AGED, *article on* HEALTH CARE AND RESEARCH ISSUES; AUTOEXPERIMENTATION; CHILDREN, *article on* HEALTH CARE AND RESEARCH ISSUES; FETUS, *article on* FETAL RESEARCH; INFANTS, *article on* ETHICAL ISSUES; MILITARY PERSONNEL AS RESEARCH SUBJECTS; MINORITIES AS RESEARCH SUBJECTS; MULTINATIONAL RESEARCH; PRISONERS, *article on* RESEARCH ISSUES; STUDENTS AS RESEARCH SUBJECTS; SEX THERAPY AND SEX RESEARCH; *and* WOMEN, *article on* RESEARCH ISSUES.

EXPERT TESTIMONY

Courts frequently look to the testimony of expert medical witnesses to assist them in the search for legal truth. In addition to Egyptian and Biblical references to forensic medicine, physicians in Greece and Rome functioned as expert witnesses. A physician testifying at the inquest into Julius Caesar's death stated that he found twenty-three stab wounds on the corpse but only one wound, a wound in the throat, that could have caused death. The Institutes of Justinian (529–533 C.E.) and the codices of Charles V, the Lex Bambergensis (1507), also made provisions for expert medical testimony (Landé, 1936; Clements and Ciccone, 1984). Today in

the United States, physicians are called on to testify as expert witnesses in a variety of civil and criminal matters. The civil issues range from workers' compensation to child custody, from physical and emotional damages to malpractice. The issues in criminal cases range from cause of death to competence to stand trial, from deoxyribonucleic acid (DNA) typing to the insanity defense. This entry traces how a physician becomes involved as a medical expert witness, what the requirements of the role are, and the ethical issues that may arise.

Courts of law distinguish between fact witnesses and expert witnesses. Fact witnesses may be required to testify if they have some direct knowledge about the issue before the court, but may not express opinions. Expert witnesses have knowledge that goes beyond that of the ordinary citizen and agree to undertake the role of expert witness and are permitted to express opinions.

The difference between a "fact" and an "opinion" is the degree of concreteness of the description, or the difference in the "nearness or remoteness of inference" (McCormick, 1986, p. 26). The courts and the public receive expert testimony with both admiration and suspicion. There is appreciation for the clarity provided, but fear that experts may control the legal outcome. This fear may be accentuated in a democratic society that mistrusts those with special knowledge. In 1986, the American Medical Association (AMA) took the position that "as a citizen and as a professional with special training and experience, the physician has an ethical obligation to assist in the administration of justice" (Council on Ethical and Judicial Affairs of the AMA, 1994, p. 138). The participation of the medical expert may be justified on the basis that a meaningful concept of justice requires empirical data on the function of the human organism in health and disease—data that the medical expert can provide (Ciccone and Clements, 1987).

The expert-witness role

Expert-witness testimony in an adversarial legal system may lead to a battle of the experts, a battle that may be avoided if the court appoints an expert approved by both sides of a legal action. There are different models for the expert-witness role. In the first model, the court-appointed or "impartial expert" witness model, the expert witness is still subjected to cross-examination, yet has the implied endorsement of the court—the court would not hire an unqualified expert. However, the view that such an expert witness is neutral is a fallacy (American Academy of Orthopedic Surgeons, 1992) because the expert is necessarily an advocate for his or her opinion. In the second, the objective "expert-model," the expert is hired by or appointed to one party, but the expert's role is limited to a comprehensive examination of the evidence and formulation of an opinion, if possible. In the third, the "consultant" model, the expert functions as a consultant to the attorney. The expert provides an accurate statement of the examination conducted, the findings of the examination, and the opinion and reasoning used to arrive at the opinion, and provides assistance with trial strategy and cross-examination (Appelbaum, 1987). The ethical hazard of this model is that the expert may identify with the attorney's position and become an advocate.

In each model, the medical expert is expected to provide a clinical evaluation and a review of the applicable data in light of the legal question posed and in the spirit of honesty and striving for objectivity—the expert's ethical and professional obligation. This includes a thorough, fair, and impartial review and should not exclude any relevant information in order to create a view favoring either the plaintiff or the defendant (American Academy of Psychiatry and the Law, 1987). The treating physician, whom the court may compel to testify as a fact witness regarding contact with a patient, is frequently sought to provide expert-witness testimony. The legal system assumes that the treating doctor is more credible than a nontreating doctor. The treating physician has a specific therapeutic focus—the patient's health—that may not allow service as an expert witness. The treating physician may encounter a conflict of interest (e.g., maintaining the patient's confidentiality versus providing the court with information).

When taking on the functions and obligations of the expert-medical-witness role, the treating physician may, out of loyalty to the patient's best interests, act as an advocate for the patient. This distorts the obligation of the expert witness. On the other hand, if the treating doctor's expert testimony does not have the effect of adequately supporting the patient's position, the doctor–patient relationship may deteriorate as a result. Hence, the role of physician as advocate for the patient may be inconsistent with the role of physician as expert witness and pose the ethical issue of conflict of role obligation. This conflict should be avoided. When this is not possible, self-awareness of the possible conflict and awareness by the court of the conflict may minimize its effects.

The ethics of being a medical expert witness

Medical professionals who undertake the role of expert witness are generally expected to have an unrestricted license to practice medicine, to be knowledgeable and experienced in the area in which they are functioning as a medical expert, and to have knowledge of the legal system. At the initial contact by the court or an attorney, the expert clarifies the question being asked and explores the relevant information about the case. The discussion of the question also permits the expert to be explicit about limitations of the evaluation he or she can offer. The expert witness must know the law that is relevant to the forensic question in the jurisdiction in which the expert may testify. The court or the attorney can provide the applicable statutes. Professional values require such obligations. In addition, legal consequences involving criminal and civil verdicts with ensuing penalties require this standard of obligation.

Medical experts can expect cooperation from the court or attorney in obtaining all the relevant legal, social, and medical documents. Medical experts should obtain consultations from others when there are important areas outside of the expert's knowledge. The medical expert must also be aware that the attorney may have a hidden agenda—understanding the hidden agenda may influence the expert's decision to accept or refuse the case. For example, when the evidence is not strong, is the prosecuting attorney's raising the question of competence to stand trial (CST) a way to keep the individual from being released? Is the defense attorney's request for an evaluation of CST a way to prolong the legal process so that prosecution witnesses may become difficult to locate, thereby weakening the district attorney's case? These are ethical questions the legal system must address, but medical experts who work with the legal system have a clinical obligation to avoid abuse of their role.

The individual who agrees to function as an expert witness is entitled to an expert witness fee, the terms of which should be clear and explicit at the time that the work is started. It is unethical for expert witnesses to make their fees contingent on the outcome of trials. In fact, there are advantages to the expert working with a retainer fee, against which the work of the forensic expert may be charged: (1) it diminishes whatever influence the examiner's concern for payment has on the quality of the work, and (2) if asked on cross-examination if the experts are being paid for their opinions, the experts are able to respond that in fact they were paid on a retainer basis for their time. Such arrangements avoid the ethical problem of experts being seen as "hired guns."

The informed consent of the individual to undergo a forensic medical evaluation should be obtained whenever possible. This includes a description of the purpose of the evaluation, the limits to confidentiality that may exist, and to whom a report will be made. The doctor–patient relationship includes, as one of its ethical requirements, the qualified obligation that the physician maintain confidentiality. The examinations conducted by the medical expert witness are usually outside the scope of the doctor–patient relationship; however, the bioethical obligations remain, and the physician must be aware of the bioethical obligation not to harm the individual unnecessarily by gratuitous disclosure of information. The disclosure of information must conform with the requirements of the law and the explanation made to the individual examined. In a legal context, the medical expert is bound not by rules of medical confidentiality, but by the rules of confidentiality that the legal circumstances require. It is expected that the medical expert witness will be aware of and abide by the specific rules of confidentiality applicable to work with the legal system. Informing the examinee may not be sufficient protection because the physician can create a relationship in which the examinee forgets the warning (Diamond, 1959). There are circumstances in medical–legal evaluations where consent is not required. The individual is then informed that the evaluation is legally required. However, if the individual chooses not to participate, the refusal will be included in any report or testimony.

Admission of expert testimony

The role of the expert witness is based on education, training, and experience that gives the expert knowledge in a particular discipline. The United States Supreme Court in *Daubert v. Merrell Dow Pharmaceuticals* (1993) described the limits of expert scientific testimony and endorsed the *Federal Rules of Evidence* (United States, 1975) that had broadened the admissibility of scientific testimony to include theories that were not widely held. The *Daubert* decision rejected the restrictive standard that permitted the judge to exclude expert testimony that the judge found was not "sufficiently established to have gained general acceptance in the particular field to which it belongs" (*Frye v. United States*, 1923). However, the U.S. Supreme Court also put limits on "the admissibility of purportedly scientific evidence" by requiring the trial judge to determine whether the reasoning or methodology underlying the testimony is scientifically valid and whether that reasoning or methodology properly can be applied to the facts in issue (*Daubert v. Merrell Dow Pharmaceuticals*, 1993, p. 2796). This gatekeeping function of the judge on expert scientific testimony may lead to judges who appoint their own experts to examine the experts put forward by opposing parties in the litigation.

Ethics and medical expert testimony

The medical expert may be required to testify in perhaps one of ten cases that the expert is called upon to evaluate. It is this public role that causes the most discomfort and is the most sensationalized of all the expert's functions. The medical expert witness usually engages in this work as a part of a larger clinical practice. While some experts have given up clinical work, this is rare. Medical experts who have not actively engaged in their discipline or who have given it up may find their credibility questioned in court. Medical experts have the ethical obligation to inform the court or attorney hiring them of the status of their clinical practice. Prior to entering the courtroom, experts assist the attorney as well as they can "but only within the requirement of medical ethics" (Stone, 1981, p. 27). Each of the three models carries the ethical obligation that the expert be honest and, even when assisting an attorney, not become an advocate. The medical expert who is called to testify should require full and complete preparation from the attorney. Preparation for testimony, which almost always includes at least one pretrial conference between attorney and expert, is essential to adequate work in the courtroom.

In court, medical expert witnesses are not advocates for either side in the litigation, but may advocate their opinion. The most effective role of the expert witness is that of teacher—that is, one who elucidates the nature of the evaluations and the reasoning used to arrive at his or her opinions. The expert should present credentials without exaggeration. The expert should be prepared to present specific perspectives or bias and identify value components that are always present in interpretations of the data. If the issue before the court presents an ethical dilemma for the expert, whether as a result of personal belief or from concerns about societal harm that his or her opinion may cause, the expert has the obligation to avoid involvement in such cases. The requirement of truthfulness on the part of the medical expert witness requires that relevant information not be kept secret (Rappeport, 1981). In addition, there are limitations that occur in medical examinations, and these limitations of reviewed materials (e.g., completeness of the examination or knowledge of that area of medicine) may require the expert to qualify an opinion or, at times, to decline to provide an opinion to a particular question.

The attorney who retained the medical expert will call and question the expert with direct examination. This usually begins with eliciting the expert's credentials; the questions present the expert's education, training, experience, and other information that chronicle the achievements of the expert to the court. Using the *Daubert* directives, the judge may rule to exclude the expert. Medical-expert witnesses are expected to present their testimony—avoiding jargon—with sufficient clarity so that those lacking expertise can understand the findings and follow the reasoning. The attorney who has retained the expert can be expected to emphasize his or her ability and the brilliance of the conclusions. The cross-examining attorney, both in speech and gesture, will often attempt to convey to the court that the expert witness lacks credibility and that his or her conclusions are worthless.

The expert may be presented a hypothetical question, which is a conflation of assumptions and proven facts into an organized account of a situation. The hypothetical question calls for expert witnesses to assume the information in the question to be fact. Then experts are asked if they have an opinion derived from those facts and, if they do, to state that opinion. The hypothetical question is used because there is a dispute about the facts, and the hypothetical question allows the court to hear the expert's opinion without deciding if the facts in evidence are true.

The expert witness has rights in the courtroom and may ask the judge to clarify when material that is asked for is privileged. The expert witness may ask for clarification of a question or refuse to answer questions the expert does not understand. Experts may and should say that they do not have a response to the question, if in fact they do not have one. Experts, when asked a yes or no question, can ask the judge whether the answer can be qualified. If on cross-examination this is not permitted, on subsequent redirect examination the attorney who retained the expert may ask for further clarification. The expert has a right to complete an answer and should protest if interrupted. Expert witnesses, as contrasted with fact witnesses, may refresh their recollections using written notes and records.

The courtroom, the most visible portion of the adversarial system with its "battle of the experts," is viewed by some critics as a three-ring circus. Even when expert witnesses agree substantially, small differences may be exaggerated by an attorney and held up as proof that the entire discipline has nothing to offer the courts. If expert witnesses are expected to provide absolute certainty, the witnesses will inevitably be clowns in the courtroom. However, the opinion of the expert witness, as with a medical diagnosis, is a probability statement and as such, is the best conclusion given the analysis of the data. This conclusion may certainly be open to question. Although the credibility of the expert witness is important, the courtroom belongs to the attorneys. The weight given to the testimony of the expert is markedly influenced by the courtroom skill of the attorneys involved. Do the faults of the legal system outweigh its benefits and is there an alternative, superior system for arriving at legal verdicts? This is a question better considered in an analysis of the adversarial system.

At a trial, the ultimate issue is the question about which the jury or judge must arrive at a verdict (e.g., did the defendant's negligence cause the injury to the plaintiff?). It has been suggested that the medical expert respond only to questions about the medical condition and avoid responding to the ultimate issue, which some have called either a leap in logic (American Psychiatric Association [APA] Statement on the Insanity Defense, 1983) or the application of medical reality to a legal procedure. It is contended that the ultimate issue is an issue of social and moral policy and, therefore, is beyond the province of scientific inquiry. While there are circumstances when the information does not permit the medical expert to arrive at an opinion, the fact that the question has been framed in a legal context may make it appropriate for the expert to express an opinion. This opinion need not usurp the role of the trier of fact.

Conclusion

Much of society's ambivalence toward expert witnesses is derived from society's unrealistic hopes and fears of expert witnesses. The hope that the expert will have secret skills, which provide special access to absolute truth, imbues the expert role with unrealistic authority and certainty. This expectation of expert witnesses is not consistent with the reality of scientific expertise that allows for probable conclusions. The fear that the expert will take over the legal process and subvert justice is also exaggerated. The legal system has rules of procedure that limit the influence of the expert witness. Functioning within the boundaries of science and governed by ethical guidelines, experts are not oracles whose conclusions are not open to question, but witnesses who can provide the legal system with useful information.

J. RICHARD CICCONE

For a further discussion of topics mentioned in this article, see the entries AUTHORITY; CONFIDENTIALITY; CONFLICT OF INTEREST; DNA TYPING; *and* MEDICAL MALPRACTICE. *Other relevant material may be found under the entries* LAW AND BIOETHICS; *and* LAW AND MORALITY.

Bibliography

AMERICAN ACADEMY OF ORTHOPEDIC SURGEONS. 1992. "Orthopaedic Medical Testimony." In *Guide to the Ethical Practice of Orthopaedic Surgery.* Rosement, IL.: American Academy of Orthopaedic Surgeons.

AMERICAN ACADEMY OF PSYCHIATRY AND THE LAW. 1987. "Ethical Guidelines for the Practice of Forensic Psychiatry." *Newsletter* 12(1):16–17.

AMERICAN PSYCHIATRIC ASSOCIATION. 1983. "American Psychiatric Association Statement on the Insanity Defense." *American Journal of Psychiatry* 140, no. 6:681–688.

APPELBAUM, PAUL S. 1987. "In the Wake of Ake: The Ethics of Expert Testimony in an Advocate's Word." *Bulletin of the American Academy of Psychiatry and the Law* 15, no. 1:15–25.

CICCONE, J. RICHARD, and CLEMENTS, COLLEEN D. 1987. "The Insanity Defense: Asking and Answering the Ultimate Question." *Bulletin of the American Academy of Psychiatry and the Law* 15, no. 4:329–338.

CLEARY, EDWARD W., ed. 1986. *McCormick on Evidence.* St. Paul, Minn.: West Publishing.

CLEMENTS, COLLEEN D., and CICCONE, J. RICHARD. 1984. "Ethics and Expert Witnesses: The Troubled Role of Psychiatrists in Court." *Bulletin of the American Academy of Psychiatry and the Law* 12, no. 2:127–136.

COUNCIL ON ETHICAL AND JUDICIAL AFFAIRS OF THE AMERICAN MEDICAL ASSOCIATION. 1994. *Code of Medical Ethics: Current Opinions with Annotations.* Chicago: Author.

Daubert v. Merrell Dow Pharmaceuticals, Inc. 1993. 113 S.Ct. 2786. U.S.L.W. #4805.

DIAMOND, BERNARD L. 1959. "The Fallacy of the Impartial Expert." *Archives of Criminal Psychodynamics* 3:221–236.

FEDERAL RULES OF EVIDENCE. 1994. 702, 28 U.S.C.A. St. Paul, Minn.: West Publishing.

Frye v. United States. 1923. 293 Fed. 1013 (D.C. Cir.).

HALLECK, SEYMOUR L.; APPELBAUM, PAUL S.; RAPPEPORT, JONAS; and DIX, G. 1984. "Psychiatry in the Sentencing Process. A Report of the Task Force on the Role of Psychiatry in the Sentencing Process." In *Issues in Forensic Psychiatry: Insanity Defense, Hospitalization of Adults, Model Civil Commitment Law, Sentencing Process, Child Custody Consultation.* Washington, D.C.: American Psychiatric Press.

LANDÉ, KURT E. 1936. "Forensic Medicine in Europe—Legal Medicine in America." *New England Journal of Medicine* 215, no. 18:826–834.

McCORMICK, CHARLES T. 1986. *Handbook of the Law of Evidence.* St. Paul, Minn.: West Publishing.

MENNINGER, KARL. 1969. *The Crime of Punishment.* New York: The Viking Press.

RAPPEPORT, JONAS. 1981. "Ethics and Forensic Psychiatry." In *Psychiatric Ethics* pp. 285–276. Edited by Sidney Block and Paul Chodoff. Oxford: Oxford University Press.

STONE, ALAN A. 1981. "The Ethical Boundaries of Forensic Psychiatry: A View from the Ivory Tower." *Bulletin of the American Academy of Psychiatry and the Law* 12, no. 3:209–227.

UNITED STATES. 1975. Federal Rules of Evidence, Annotated. New York: M. Berder.

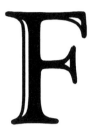

FAITH HEALING

See ALTERNATIVE THERAPIES; HEALING; *and* HEALTH AND DISEASE.

FALSIFICATION OF RESEARCH DATA

See FRAUD, THEFT, AND PLAGIARISM.

FAMILY

Families have played a most important role in the history of medicine, tending the sick when doctors were unavailable or unavailing. These two ancient, and in some respects rival, systems of care for the very vulnerable—medicine and the family—are each in part shaped by the other and rely upon the other for certain kinds of help. When illness or injury exhausts a family's capacity for care, it looks to professional medicine for the necessary facilities and expertise; in turn, technological advances in medicine have driven the health-care system to depend on families for what can be enormous sacrifices of time, money, caring labor, and even spare body parts on behalf of its patients. Recent developments in medicine have not only expanded the options for forming families—for example, through in vitro fertilization and contract pregnancy—but they have also had an impact on familial demographics: artificial means of birth control have helped reduce family size, while improve-

ments in health care have extended longevity, though they have not eradicated the ills of old age.

By and large, bioethics has had little to say about the moral significance of the family within the context of medicine. The explicit discussion of the family in the third edition of Tom Beauchamp and James Childress's *Principles of Biomedical Ethics* is confined to one paragraph stating that the burden on the family must not be determinative in decisions to refuse treatment (Beauchamp and Childress, 1989). The U.S. President's Commission for the Study of Ethical Problems in Medicine and Biomedical and Behavioral Research devotes no more than ten lines of text in 545 pages of *Deciding to Forego Life-Sustaining Treatment* to the family's role in medical decision making at the end of life (U.S. President's Commission, 1983). The Hastings Center's *Guidelines on the Termination of Life-Sustaining Treatment and the Care of the Dying* mentions families only in passing, in their role as surrogate decision makers or people who have feelings for the patient (Hastings Center, 1987). Allen E. Buchanan and Dan W. Brock's *Deciding for Others* views families as aggregates of competing individual interests and devotes much of its brief discussion of the family to the possibility of selfishness and disagreement among family members (Buchanan and Brock, 1989). We note also that the first edition of this Encyclopedia contained no "Family" entry.

The nature of the family

This neglect admits of several different explanations. For some bioethicists, the family is such a commonplace moral entity that its significance is left tacit in their analyses; unargued assumptions about family form a strong subtext, for example, in many discussions of decision making for incompetent patients. For others, the dramatic shifts in the demographics of American families over the last several decades renders families deeply suspect: they have become so fragile and their configurations so arbitrary, compared with what they once were, that we do better to exclude them altogether from our bioethical accounts.

The first view obscures the moral character of families; as we will attempt to show, they are complex and puzzling entities. But the second view is problematic as well, substituting myth for history. American families have always been somewhat fragile and subject to rapid reconfigurations. Families in the Chesapeake colonies of Virginia and Maryland, to take only one instance, were so vulnerable to malaria and other fatal illnesses that it was not at all unusual for an adult, whether slave or free, to bury three or even four spouses, or for half-orphaned children to be reared by relatives other than the surviving parent. In the matrilineal Iroquois societies of that same period, divorce was quite common. It is true that middle-class families gained a certain solidity when they underwent a shift around 1800 to a sentimental, child-centered model of domestic life, but this was achieved through an arguably unjust gendered division of labor, in which the father was increasingly absent from home and the mother's work was narrowed principally to unpaid domestic concerns. For many poor young nineteenth-century mothers—whether black, Latina, Irish, or east European—this arrangement was not an option, and the long hours spent working outside the home left the care of their children a somewhat haphazard business. Death in childbed and other premature deaths once threatened the family's integrity as much as the divorce rate, which has risen by a steady 3 percent in every decade since the Civil War, does now. In short, there is good reason to think that stress, turmoil, and identity crises have long been a feature of American families (Mintz and Kellogg, 1988).

A measure both of the importance of families to our lives and of our ambivalence about them is that any discussion of the topic quickly elicits a demand for an explicit statement of what is meant by "family." The most useful such account is perhaps a normative one, which identifies features of special moral significance in the clear paradigm cases. These features can then be used to determine what counts as a family in the less clear cases. Ludwig Wittgenstein's notion of family resemblances serves us here: any social configuration that incorporates at least most of the morally significant features of, say, marital and parent–child relationships can be thought of as a family for present purposes. These features include long-standing, committed relationships; blood ties; emotional intimacy; shared histories; shared projects that produce solidarity among family members. Other crucial features identify functions: families forge the selves of their youngest members and help maintain the selves of adults. Further, familial relationships go beyond the contractual and the voluntary; in them we incur responsibilities not of our own choosing.

Relationships within families will take on greater or lesser bioethical significance, depending on the familial question under consideration. If treatment decisions for a badly damaged neonate are at issue, "family" means the mother and father; if the issue at hand is pedigree testing for a genetic disorder, "family" means blood kinship; if the issue is determining the appropriate caregiver for a person with progressive dementia, "family" may mean spouse or child.

Family and the law

Discussions in family law echo the question of how we are to define families. While there was for many years no basis in common law for family members to make treatment decisions for incompetent adults, for example, a number of court decisions in the 1980s and recent legislative action now give families decisional authority in some twenty states (Areen, 1987, 1991). This makes it all the more necessary to know just who is entitled to count as family. A strictly biological definition does not capture what seems socially significant about single parenting, stepparenting, and contract pregnancy. The legal notion of marriage skips over "kith"—long-standing committed relationships resembling kinship that might give, say, a neighbor or housemate moral authority to speak on behalf of a patient who is too ill to make treatment decisions; the law also fails to recognize gay and lesbian relationships, which may be more significant than blood ties to a person with AIDS or a brain-injured person caught in a custody dispute between lover and parents. On the other hand, functionalist definitions of families require courts to determine whether a particular relationship closely enough approximates an accepted norm of "family" to count as one. This involves inquiry into such areas as sexual activity, management of finances, and degree of exclusivity and commitment—a profound intrusion into personal privacy.

When one compares the body of family law against the body of law dealing with, for example, commercial transactions, family law seems distinctly underdeveloped and lacking in detail. The reason for this, Lee Teitelbaum argues, is that families, incorporating "diffuse, particularistic, and collective values and relations," tend to reflect a wide-ranging set of circumstances and goals, while law is better suited to consider individuals as abstracted from these particulars, in public settings that can be assimilated into a formal, rational scheme (Teitelbaum, 1992, p. 789). There is a further problem. As

Carl Schneider points out, in the last few decades family law has increasingly eschewed moral discourse. The temptation is understandable: the problems within families are complex and often "reduce to unresolvable disputes over unverifiable beliefs." But by avoiding the language of morality, family law has stripped itself of conceptual notions that might help resolve such bioethical perplexities as contract pregnancy and the family's role in decision making for incapacitated patients (Schneider, 1992, p. 822).

Challenges to an ethics of strangers

Bioethics, however, need not lie down with law. Because it can achieve a high degree of particularity, it is better suited than the law to use a working definition of families that identifies morally relevant features and notes family resemblances—so to speak—among various small-scale human groups that include some such features. While bioethics has been slow to take families seriously, there are signs that the period of neglect is over. Roughly speaking, two approaches have been used to incorporate into bioethics what is morally valuable about families.

The first approach assumes the moral framework characteristic of the Enlightenment, with its stress on the impartial and the universalizable. Within this tradition, Nancy Rhoden has criticized the suspicion of the motives and interests of family members that has opened to court review their decisions concerning nontreatment of incapacitated relatives. Arguing that because family members "are in the best position to reproduce the preferences of an incompetent patient," Rhoden concludes that the burden of proof should be on the physician rather than the family (as is currently the case) to convince a court of law that an unwise decision has been made (Rhoden, 1988). In a more radical departure from current practice, John Hardwig has attacked the exclusionary bias of the doctor–patient relationship, insisting that the interests of all those with a stake in a medical decision, not just the patient's, be honored impartially (Hardwig, 1990).

At the same time, the so-called personal turn in ethics explored by Bernard Williams, Lawrence Blum, Jeffrey Blustein, Margaret Urban Walker, and others has challenged the orthodox assumption that ethics has primarily to do with right conduct among strangers—an ethics that favors no one and has dictates that are universalizable. The personal turn might be said to have begun with Williams's (1981) germinal observation that impartialist dictates, if followed scrupulously, leave insufficient room for moral agents to pursue their own individual interests, desires, and projects—all the substance, in fact, that gives life its meaning, though such meaning is what motivates one to go on. The task of

Williams and others has been to construct moral accounts that honor the particular and the personal but do so in a nonarbitrary way. Feminist ethical theory has devoted much attention to this task (Kittay and Meyers, 1987; Card, 1991).

In bioethics one can see the direct impact of the personal turn in the writings of Ferdinand Schoeman. He has argued that a Kantian ethics for strangers, which insists that medical decisions for an incompetent person can be made only in accordance with what is in that person's best interests, provides an inadequate basis for understanding the parent–child relationship. That relationship, because it is intimate, permits parents to compromise the child's interests to promote the family's goals and purposes. Parents could, for example, permit a child to donate bone marrow to save a sibling's life, even though donating the marrow is not in the child's medical interests. In Schoeman's view, then, the family is seen as an entity with an integrity of its own that is greater than the sum total of the interests of its members (Schoeman, 1985).

Rhoden's attempt to vindicate the decisional authority of families and Hardwig's challenge to the patient-centered focus of conventional bioethics use the relatively straightforward strategy of applying impartialist standards to a context—the doctor–patient relationship—where they have not been applied before. Both writers are concerned with decision making, and more particularly with the locus of the decision. The personal turn in bioethics, which is concerned with a more fine-grained understanding of the structures of interpersonal relationships and their importance for human action, is less developed. But attention to the personal suggests certain moral features of family life that might be used to construct an ethics of the family.

Some elements of an ethics of the family

Social critics from Plato through Shulamith Firestone have argued that the distinctive features of the family constitute moral liabilities, and that families ought to be altered or abolished. In *A Theory of Justice*, John Rawls notes quite explicitly that the family is always a problem for egalitarian social theory (Rawls, 1971). A more sympathetic approach would portray those features as morally valuable, but whatever one's basic stance toward families, they do possess features that require moral attention and analysis.

One rather marked characteristic of families is their tendency to favor members over nonintimates. A central question is whether this sort of bias can be adequately understood inside a universalizable, impersonal framework. For example, can the favoritism parents show their children be justified insofar, and only insofar, as it increases the overall utility? James Rachels has argued for a position he calls "partial bias," which allows the expression of particular regard for children (and presumably for one's intimates in general) in those cases where their needs are in conflict with similarly serious needs of others, but not otherwise; this approach, he suggests, allows the special goods of intimacy to flourish within the context of appropriate regard for the needs of all, impartially considered (Rachels, 1989). It is, however, questionable whether a truly disinterested regard for the needs of others, in a world where resources are so massively maldistributed as ours, would leave any appreciable room for special regard for the needs of our own, particularly for those of us living in affluence. But even if some measure of special attention to loved ones could be made consistent with general impartialist norms, unless family members favor their own to at least a slightly greater degree than impartialist considerations mandate, it would seem they express only an ersatz partiality, not true loyalty, love, or commitment. To feel the force of this point, consider our intuitive response to a father who, when his only daughter thanks him affectionately for taking her to a baseball game, tells her, "Oh, I would have had to do the same for any child of mine." Rather than attempt, as Rachels does, to assimilate personal loyalty into an impartialist framework, a promising strategy might be to put less emphasis on individual integrity and the separateness of individuals, and attend a little more to the connections among individuals. A careful attention to these interconnections offers a basis for just dealings with others that takes account of the difference between strangers and intimates.

A second notable feature of families is that not all of its relationships fit comfortably under what has come to be modern ethics' most favored image of relationship: the contract. Children notoriously "didn't ask to be born," and none of us has chosen our blood relations. This fact has important implications for any theory that bases duties solely on consent; indeed, families are perhaps the most plausible counterexample to such theories. It is sometimes claimed that parental duties toward children arise from the parents' having tacitly consented to the child's existence, first, by agreeing to have sexual intercourse and second, by choosing not to abort the fetus. But this analysis entails that where intercourse was forced or good-faith efforts at contraception failed, and where abortion is for ethical or economic reasons not an option, the parents are off the moral hook; many will be reluctant to pay this dearly to retain the contract as the model of obligation. Ordinarily, responsibilities can arise from causal as well as contractual relationships; a proximate causal role in putting another in danger, for example, obligates one to stand ready to provide aid. This suggests that parental responsibility may stem from the fact that parents caused the child's existence, and not because they contracted for the child (Nelson and Nelson, 1989). In fact it can be maintained that inti-

mate living as such creates expectations and other vulnerabilities, which, as Robert E. Goodin has argued, carry with them certain prima facie noncontractual duties. Such an analysis would embrace family members other than parents in a web of moral but nonconsensual relationship.

A third feature of the ethos that typifies families is a less individualistic image of persons than is customary in impersonal ethics. Actions are often assessed in terms of their impact on the family overall, and there is a certain amount of collective responsibility for family members' well-being. A family of immigrants might, for example, devote its resources to settling other relatives in the new country, an enterprise that requires individual family members to subsume their own projects and goals to the familial one. While the communitarian feature of family ethics has often lent itself to abuse as repeated sacrifices are demanded of certain family members (particularly women) to carry out a family agenda set by its dominant members, it is also true that a family cannot function if its members are altogether unwilling to pull in common. An ethics of the family, in contrast to the broad ethical theories, will concern itself with interests that are essentially held in common, as well as with individual interests.

A fourth distinguishing feature of what might emerge as an ethics of the family is that it is particularistic. *Pace* Tolstoy, all happy families are not like one another; there are myriad differences among and within them—as there are, for that matter, among unhappy ones. Because familial relationships are not only intimate but also of long standing, family members can come to know each other in rich, particular detail and from a highly specific standpoint. This means that the principles governing their behavior toward one another can be fine-tuned to a pitch of precision that is impossible, say, in law, where individual differences are perforce flattened out. What Iris Murdoch (1970) has called loving attention, and Martha Nussbaum (1990) calls fine awareness, would likely play an important role in any ethics of intimacy, whether among friends or within families. Attention to the particulars is what allows people involved in intimate relationships to focus on who they are together. This self-awareness, guided by general moral ideas such as justice, permits intimates to arrive at ethical decisions that are highly sensitive to circumstances and persons; the ethical work can be done "close up." Further, as these ethical deliberations become a part of the history of the relationship, their results can be used to guide future decisions that will be just as sensitive to the particulars (Walker, 1987).

Implications for medicine

Medical decision making.   When a patient is incompetent to decide about his or her own medical treatment, or when competence is intermittent, physicians turn to the family for help, since families are presumed to know best what the patient would want, and also to care about the patient's interests. Families are instructed to make their decision on the basis of what the patient would want—the "substituted judgment" standard established in the *Quinlan* case (1976)—or, if the patient was never competent, on the basis of what is best for the patient—the "best interests" standard. Tightly focused on the patient, either standard is open to challenge.

Linda L. Emanuel and Ezekiel J. Emanuel (1992) observe that the "substituted judgment" standard has been objected to on both theoretical and empirical grounds. An important theoretical objection is that reconstructing what a patient would want in highly specific circumstances from a general knowledge of the person's values requires a tremendous imaginative effort that may be beyond most people, while the empirical objections are that patients do not in fact discuss their preferences with family members, that family members are not good at assessing a patient's quality of life, and that proxies' selection is not much better than random chance in predicting patients' preferences for life-sustaining interventions. As Patricia White (1992) points out, people often do not know what they themselves would want if seriously ill.

The "best interests" standard is open to the objection that it cannot be seen as a patient's exercise (by proxy) of his or her right to refuse or consent to treatment, but instead gives the family power to exercise its own authority over the incompetent patient—something our society is reluctant to do because of the fear of abuse. While there are certainly instances of familial abuse of patients, one might question whether we ought to base social policy on the assumption that abuse is the possibility most to be feared. Yet if this objection to the "best interests" standard is unpersuasive, there is another that may be less so: the standard is not suitable to families because they are not simply a group of people each seeking to maximize his or her own self-interest. There is a collective character to family life that is not easily accommodated by the notion of individual best interests, and so the "best interests" standard is a code of conscience that from the family's point of view is distinctly second best. In fact, the standard is invoked primarily in adversarial situations where the family's solidarity has broken down, as in child-custody disputes.

An ethics of the family might suggest that what family members owe each other is not the best, understood abstractly. If it were, each of us would have a duty to find better parents for our children than we are ourselves. Rather, what is owed is the good that inheres in this particular set of relationships. If this is right, then at the sickbed it is less important that a brother, lover, or daughter-in-law will correctly decide what is best for an incompetent patient than that the decision be made by this particular person, the person who stands as close to the patient as possible and so serves the patient as an extended self. Here, as well as where the patient is competent, decision making that recognizes morally salient features of family life might set the needs and desires of the patient into careful balance against the family's resources for care, bringing a nuanced understanding of all the relevant particulars to bear on the decision.

The elderly and the end of life.   What, if anything, do adult children owe their frail elderly parents? Theories affirming a duty of reciprocity argue that our parents gave us life and cared for us when we needed care; in return, we owe them care when they are in need. The difficulty with such theories (held by Aristotle and Aquinas, and more recently by William Blackstone [1856]) is that they do not seem to recognize that parents owe their children a decent minimum of goods and services. If parents are merely paying what they owe, it is hard to see why the child need respond with anything more than a thank-you. Following this line of reasoning, Jane English (1979) and Norman Daniels (1988) cannot defend a duty of adult children to care for their parents: the child, not having contracted for the parental sacrifices made on his or her behalf, has no duty to reciprocate, since sacrifices that have not been requested require no return. A third view, shared by Joel Feinberg (1966) and Jeffrey Blustein (1982), distinguishes between duties of indebtedness and duties of gratitude, and concludes that duties of gratitude are owed even for those actions that are included in the parents' moral duties; children must help their parents when help is needed. And a fourth theory bases a duty to parents in the parents' own moral duties, for the parental duty consists in part in encumbering the child with a loving relationship that in the child's maturity will be mutual, and that cannot then legitimately be broken without cause (Nelson and Nelson, 1992).

Whatever the source of duties to frail elderly parents, the content of those duties is not easy to ascertain. If postindustrial societies do not set limits on the amount of increasingly costly medical care they offer the old as they leave this life, they may impoverish the young. Within a family, this dilemma might be played out in terms of nursing-home care for a grandparent (now costing upward of $35,000 a year) versus a child's college fund. Margaret Urban Walker (1987) has described such a decision as an opportunity for defining oneself morally, ratifying or breaking from a past course of action as one sets the course of one's future. Families, too, might be capable of strong moral self-definition of this kind.

Reproductive issues.   Medical solutions to infertility are genetic solutions; there is an attempt to establish a genetic tie between the child and at least one parent. In "traditional" contract pregnancy (in which the birth mother's egg is used to produce a child for people who have paid her to have the baby on their behalf) the importance of the maternal genes is played down, but the paternal genes—those of the contracting father—are considered crucial. In the far less common arrangement whereby the birth mother is hired to carry to term an embryo formed in vitro by the contracting couple's egg and sperm (this is called gestational contract pregnancy), the maternal genes regain their standard social meaning, designating the woman who will rear the child. In artificial insemination by donor, the paternal genes are seen to carry no social responsibility for the child. The model for all this is one of consumer choice, in which the infertile parties are at liberty to decide for themselves what weight to give genetic ties.

This model raises important questions about the moral significance of being a parent. If those who contribute genetically to a child can be said to cause that particular child to exist, and if an ethics of the family adopts a causal rather than a contractual model of responsibility, then the child's genetic parents would seem to have a prima facie obligation to remain in the child's life in an ongoing way; even if they delegate much of their responsibility for rearing the child, it does not follow that they may put themselves totally out of power to keep the child from harm. Thus lesbian or gay couples might have a duty to foster a loving bond between the child and the biological parent of the opposite gender.

Medicine invites a consumer-choice approach not only in the matter of genetic ties but also in the matter of genetic screening. While it is reasonable to protect one's family by trying to avoid giving birth to a child with a serious genetic defect, the choices made possible by genetic screening can be a burden as well as a benefit. An important mechanism for drawing new members into the family—the pregnant woman's continual process of making friends with her fetus—is distorted and interrupted by amniocentesis, endoscopy, chorionic villus sampling, ultrasound, alpha-fetoprotein assays. Such screening, along with the new possibility of fetal surgery, prompts the question, contrary to when the fetus becomes a human individual, of how and when the fetus joins the family. As Stanley Hauerwas and William Ruddick ask (Hauerwas, 1981; Ruddick, 1988), when is a fetus a child? At what point in the process of family creation ought the pregnant woman to make specific sacrifices on the fetus/child's behalf, and to what extent should these sacrifices be socially imposed?

Allocation of health-care resources.   A major function of the family is the care of its sick and vulnerable members. Because the United States has not acknowledged a basic responsibility to provide a minimum of health care for all its citizens, the burden of providing that care has fallen disproportionately on families—and within families, on adult women. The difficulty in achieving gender justice with respect to health care is not conceptual but political: how can we reconfigure our

society—and our families—to eliminate the bias that sees unpaid care as a natural task for women?

A further allocation issue concerns the range of the family's care. To whom is it owed, and when is it discretionary? What about adult siblings? Cousins? Grandparents? A lesbian daughter's partner? Need and the person's role in the family's history are both relevant considerations, as are the family's resources: If, after all, familial caregiving is exhausted, no further care will be forthcoming. What limits may the family set on the care it owes to its own? What limits may the family set on individual members' sacrifices? More particularly, in light of the fact that women assume a greatly disproportionate amount of the burden of care (Okin, 1989; Brody, 1990), what steps should be taken both within families and in the larger society to achieve gender justice? An ethics of the family might offer guidance in the notion of familial integrity: the particular way in which a given family strives to sustain a fruitful tension between intimacy and autonomy, and the way it engages in its characteristic projects and activities. Family integrity cannot, perhaps, be preserved at any price, but it is important to recognize that families as well as individuals can be destroyed unless justice forbids it.

Implementing an ethics of the family

Just as medical care is ethically inadequate when the focus is on the organ to be treated rather than on the person in whom the organ resides, so it is likely to be inadequate when no notice is taken of the families in which patients reside. An ethics that treats people as if they were unconnected and self-centered is not up to the task of promoting either justice or human flourishing. Primary-care physicians—not only practitioners of family medicine but also pediatricians and internists—are often adept at seeing beyond the patient to the nest of relationships within which that patient lives. They, like nurses and social workers, although hampered by institutional pressures that push families into the background, tend to be attuned to these relationships even when they cannot give a formal moral account of them. That account has been slow in coming; the values of families remain much more diffuse and implicit than the well-articulated values of medicine. But the relationship between the two systems of care is beginning to receive systematic exploration.

As we continue to discuss what that relationship should be in the twenty-first century, we may discover that taking families seriously requires major institutional changes. Hospitals might need to be restructured so that patients are not so estranged from their families; hospital ethics committees might have to take on a mediator's role for disputes among family members concerning patient care; the moral significance of families might have to be better reflected in case law; the conditions under which care is delivered will certainly have to be more hospitable to an ongoing relationship between patients and those who care for them; there will have to be a greater acknowledgment that families—the true source of primary care—are as essential a source of health care as medicine is. The practical difficulties in implementing an ethics of the family as it relates to health care, while daunting, are surely counterbalanced by the importance of the enterprise to the larger task of bioethics: thinking well and carefully about the concrete human realities—our differences, our similarities, our particularities, our intimacies—that have a direct bearing on health, whether within a medical or a familial setting.

HILDE LINDEMANN NELSON
JAMES LINDEMANN NELSON

For a further discussion of topics mentioned in this entry, see the entries CARE; CHILDREN; FEMINISM; GENETIC COUNSELING; GENETIC TESTING AND SCREENING; HOMOSEXUALITY; LOVE; MARRIAGE AND OTHER DOMESTIC PARTNERSHIPS; MATERNAL–FETAL RELATIONSHIP, *article on* ETHICAL ISSUES; REPRODUCTIVE TECHNOLOGIES; SEXISM; *and* WOMEN, *article on* HISTORICAL AND CROSS-CULTURAL PERSPECTIVES. *For a discussion of related ideas, see the entries* ABORTION, *section on* CONTEMPORARY ETHICAL AND LEGAL ASPECTS; ABUSE, INTERPERSONAL; ADOLESCENTS; ADOPTION; AGING AND THE AGED, *articles on* HEALTH-CARE AND RESEARCH ISSUES, *and* OLD AGE; FERTILITY CONTROL; FUTURE GENERATIONS, OBLIGATIONS TO; FETUS, *article on* HUMAN DEVELOPMENT FROM FERTILIZATION TO BIRTH; INFANTS; INFORMED CONSENT, *article on* LEGAL AND ETHICAL ISSUES OF CONSENT IN HEALTH CARE (*with its* POSTSCRIPT); LAW AND BIOETHICS; PERSON; TECHNOLOGY; *and* UTILITY. *Other relevant material may be found under the entries* ANIMAL WELFARE AND RIGHTS, *article on* PET AND COMPANION ANIMALS; AUTHORITY; LIFE; *and* PRIVACY IN HEALTH CARE.

Bibliography

AREEN, JUDITH. 1987. "The Legal Status of Consent Obtained from Families of Adult Patients to Withhold or Withdraw Treatment." *Journal of the American Medical Association* 258, no. 2:229–235.

———. 1991. "Advance Directives Under State Law and Judicial Decisions." *Law, Medicine and Health Care* 19, nos. 1–2:91–100.

BEAUCHAMP, TOM L., and CHILDRESS, JAMES F. 1989. *Principles of Biomedical Ethics.* 3d ed. New York: Oxford University Press.

BLACKSTONE, WILLIAM. 1856. Vol. 1 of *Commentaries on the Laws of England.* Philadelphia: J. B. Lippincott.

BLUM, LAWRENCE A. 1980. *Friendship, Altruism, and Morality.* New York: Routledge & Kegan Paul.

BLUSTEIN, JEFFREY. 1982. *Parents and Children: The Ethics of the Family.* New York: Oxford University Press.

———. 1993. "The Family in Medical Decisionmaking." *Hastings Center Report* 23, no. 3:6–13.

BRODY, ELAINE M. 1990. *Women in the Middle: Their Parent-Care Years.* New York: Springer.

BUCHANAN, ALLEN E., and BROCK, DAN W. 1989. *Deciding for Others: The Ethics of Surrogate Decisionmaking.* Cambridge: At the University Press.

CARD, CLAUDIA, ed. 1991. *Feminist Ethics.* Lawrence: University Press of Kansas.

DANIELS, NORMAN. 1988. *Am I My Parents' Keeper? An Essay on Justice Between the Young and the Old.* New York: Oxford University Press.

EMANUEL, EZEKIEL J., and EMANUEL, LINDA L. 1992. "Proxy Decision Making for Incompetent Patients: An Ethical and Empirical Analysis." *Journal of the American Medical Association* 267, no. 15:2067–2071.

ENGLISH, JANE. 1979. "What Do Grown Children Owe Their Parents?" In *Having Children: Philosophical and Legal Reflections on Parenthood,* pp. 351–356. Edited by Onoro O'Neill and William Ruddick. New York: Oxford University Press.

FEINBERG, JOEL. 1966. "Duties, Rights, and Claims." *American Philosophical Quarterly* 3, no. 2:139–144.

GOODIN, ROBERT E. 1985. *Protecting the Vulnerable: A Reanalysis of Our Social Responsibilities.* Chicago: University of Chicago Press.

HANEN, MARSHA, and NIELSEN, KAI, eds. 1987. *Science, Morality and Feminist Theory.* Calgary: University of Calgary Press.

HARDWIG, JOHN. 1990. "What About the Family?" *Hastings Center Report* 20, no. 2:5–10.

HASTINGS CENTER. 1987. *Guidelines on the Termination of Life-Sustaining Treatment and the Care of the Dying.* Briarcliff Manor, N.Y.: Author.

HAUERWAS, STANLEY. 1981. "Abortion: Why the Arguments Fail." In his *A Community of Character: Toward a Constructive Christian Social Ethic.* Notre Dame, Ind.: University of Notre Dame Press.

KITTAY, EVA FEDER, and MEYERS, DIANA T., eds. 1987. *Women and Moral Theory.* Totowa, N.J.: Rowman & Littlefield.

"Looking for a Family Resemblance: The Limits of the Functional Approach to the Legal Definition of Family." 1991. *Harvard Law Review* 104, no. 7:1640–1659.

MAHOWALD, MARY B. 1993. *Women and Children in Health Care: An Unequal Majority.* New York: Oxford University Press.

MINTZ, STEVEN, and KELLOGG, SUSAN. 1988. *Domestic Revolutions: A Social History of American Family Life.* New York: Free Press.

MURDOCH, IRIS. 1970. *The Sovereignty of Good.* London: Routledge & Kegan Paul.

NELSON, HILDE LINDEMANN, and NELSON, JAMES LINDEMANN. 1989. "Cutting Motherhood in Two: Some Suspicions Concerning Surrogacy." *Hypatia* 4, no. 3:85–94.

———. 1992. "Frail Parents, Robust Duties." *Utah Law Review* 1992, no. 3:747–763.

NELSON, JAMES LINDEMANN. 1990. "Partialism and Parenthood." *Journal of Social Philosophy* 21, no. 1:107–118.

———. 1992. "Taking Families Seriously." *Hastings Center Report* 22, no. 4:6–12.

Nussbaum, Martha C. 1990. *Love's Knowledge: Essays on Philosophy and Literature.* New York: Oxford University Press.

Okin, Susan Moller. 1989. *Justice, Gender, and the Family.* New York: Basic Books.

O'Neill, Onora, and Ruddick, William, eds. 1979. *Having Children: Philosophical and Legal Reflections on Parenthood.* New York: Oxford University Press.

Quinlan, In re. 1976. 70 N.J. 10–55, 355 A.2d 647-672, certiorari denied, 429 U.S. 922.

Rachels, James. 1989. "Morality, Parents and Children." In *Person to Person,* pp. 46–62. Edited by George Graham and Hugh LaFollette. Philadelphia: Temple University Press.

Rawls, John. 1971. *A Theory of Justice.* Cambridge, Mass.: Harvard University Press.

Rhoden, Nancy K. 1988. "Litigating Life and Death." *Harvard Law Review* 102, no. 2:375–446.

Rothman, Barbara Katz. 1986. *The Tentative Pregnancy: Prenatal Diagnosis and the Future of Motherhood.* New York: Viking.

Ruddick, Sara. 1989. *Maternal Thinking: Toward a Politics of Peace.* Boston: Beacon Press.

Ruddick, William. 1988. "Are Fetuses Becoming Children?" In *Biomedical Ethics and Fetal Therapy,* pp. 107–119. Edited by Carl Nimrod and Glenn Griener. Waterloo, Ont.: Wilfrid Laurier University Press.

———. 1989. "When Does Childhood Begin?" In *Children, Parents, and Politics,* pp. 25–35. Edited by Geoffrey Scarre. Cambridge: At the University Press.

Schneider, Carl E. 1992. "Bioethics and the Family: The Cautionary View from Family Law." *Utah Law Review* 1992, no. 3:819–847.

Schoeman, Ferdinand. 1980. "Rights of Children, Rights of Parents, and the Moral Basis of the Family." *Ethics* 91, no. 1:6–19.

———. 1985. "Parental Discretion and Children's Rights: Background and Implications for Medical Decision-Making." *Journal of Medicine and Philosophy* 10, no. 1:45–61.

Teitelbaum, Lee. 1992. "Intergenerational Responsibility and Family Obligation: On Sharing." *Utah Law Review* 1992, no. 3:765–802.

U.S. President's Commission for the Study of Ethical Problems in Medicine and Biomedical and Behavioral Research. 1983. *Deciding to Forego Life-Sustaining Treatment: A Report on the Ethical, Medical, and Legal Issues in Treatment Decisions.* Washington, D.C.: U.S. Government Printing Office.

Walker, Margaret Urban. 1987. "Moral Particularity." *Metaphilosophy* 18, nos. 3–4:171–185.

White, Patricia. 1992. "Appointing a Proxy Under the Best of Circumstances." *Utah Law Review* 1992, no. 3:849–860.

Williams, Bernard A. O. 1981. *Moral Luck: Philosophical Papers, 1973–1980.* Cambridge: At the University Press.

FEMALE CIRCUMCISION

See Circumcision, *article on* female circumcision.

FEMINISM

"One is not born, but rather becomes, a woman." These ringing words from *The Second Sex* (Beauvoir, 1988, p. 295) signal both the renaissance of feminism in the twentieth century and also one of its central themes: the social construction of women's reality. Feminists agree that what has historically been taken as "women's lot" and often understood as women's biologically determined destiny is rather a construction of patriarchal cultures. Feminism involves both the task of "deconstructing" those cultures, unmasking the theories, methods and structures that contribute to the oppression of women, and also the task of "reconstructing" alternative cultures, finding new ways of thinking, new methods and theories, new perspectives and meanings. "Feminism . . . stands as the mark of desire for a new way to conduct human affairs, to think about the human being as an entity, as well as being the expression of a political will to achieve justice for women" (Braidotti, 1986, p. 60).

All feminists agree that women are oppressed and that this oppression is wrong. Thus, at root, "feminism is a struggle to end sexist oppression" (hooks, 1984, p. 24). However, feminists characterize the oppression differently and hence stress different approaches to overcoming it (Sherwin, 1992; Dreifus, 1978; Douglas, 1990). Liberal feminists affirm individual choice and urge equal rights for women and reform of systems to include women. Socialist feminists utilize Marxist analysis to focus primarily on the role of economic oppression in women's lives; in this framework, reform is not enough. Radical feminists argue that women's oppression cannot be explained in economic terms alone and that gender oppression is the crucial variable. Focusing on gender oppression has also resulted in fundamental challenges to the concepts and frameworks of traditional philosophical and scientific theory. Hence, for example, traditional rights language of liberal theory is not taken as adequate to frame the discussion of justice for women.

Iris Marion Young (1990) identifies five "faces" of oppression: exploitation, marginalization, powerlessness, cultural imperialism, and violence. Historically, feminists have challenged all of these oppressions, some focusing on ending economic exploitation, others on moving women from the margins into the mainstream, others on eradicating violence toward women, others on gaining power for women, and yet others on challenging the cultural imperialism imposed on women by dominant "malestream" thought.

History

The term "feminism" was coined in France and came into wide usage in the late nineteenth century (Pateman, 1986). Although the roots of modern feminism may be traced back centuries (Lerner, 1993), its immediate beginnings lie in the eighteenth and nineteenth centuries. From Mary Wollstonecraft's early *Vindication of the Rights of Woman* (1891) to Margaret Sanger's campaign for birth control, feminists of the eighteenth and nineteenth centuries advocated women's rights to vote, to hold property, to receive an education, and to be in control of their own destinies and values, including their reproductive processes. They railed against the unjust treatment of women in the economic arena, against the intellectual and social inferiority ascribed to women, against the rights given to husbands over their wives, and against what George Sand called the "social nullity" of women—their marginalization (signified, for example, by being called "Mrs.") (Sand, 1972, p. 30).

Early feminists engaged in various forms of social action and civil disobedience: refusing to pay taxes, going on strike, keeping their own names after marriage or even refusing to marry at all. They argued vociferously against the ideologies of the day that rendered women second-class citizens. Lucretia Mott, Elizabeth Cady Stanton, Sojourner Truth, Lucy Stone, Harriet Taylor, Sarah and Angelina Grimke, Susan B. Anthony, Charlotte Perkins Gilman—these are but a few of the early feminists who laid the groundwork for both social action on behalf of women and for women's theorizing. Most of them accepted at least some of the tenets of liberalism, such as the rights of individuals and the necessity of the family, but within this acceptance they pushed for what one commentator calls the "envaluing" of women's activities (Thornton, 1986).

Betty Friedan and Simone de Beauvoir opened the modern era of feminism—the "second wave"—by naming femininity a "mystique" and challenging whether women's destiny was biological or socially imposed. They exposed social practices in which women are excluded, degraded, and socialized into the role of "other." They invited women to imagine a different social order in which they might be truly free. Significantly, Friedan (1965) talked *to* women about their lived experiences instead of talking *about* them in categories determined by the male-dominated social establishment; thus, voices of women began to enter the public arena and shape theory.

During the formational period of modern feminism (ca. 1950–1980), numerous theoretical developments took place. Kate Millett (1990; Lerner, 1986) described male power over women as a blatant political system: patriarchy. She raised fundamental challenges to the notion that women would "choose" their subordinate roles. Shulamith Firestone (1983) saw no solution until women could free themselves from their biological role as reproducers of the species; she therefore welcomed new reproductive technologies. Jill Johnston (1973) argued that women could not be free until they were free

of men politically and socially; she urged a "lesbian nation." Sarah Hoagland (1988) gives a contemporary and more nuanced voice to the ethical position that urges separation from dominant culture as a legitimate option; Rosi Braidotti (1986) challenges such separatist alternatives.

Feminists in this second wave also attended to symbols, myths, and psychic realities. Mary Daly (1973, 1990) gave voice to the power of language and the naming of reality by redefining words and challenging her readers to unmask linguistic attacks on women. Germaine Greer (1971) urged women to speak out and be outrageous (Daly did precisely that), refusing to accept men's power and asserting their own. Women, Greer believed, could claim the power that had been taken away from them by refusing to comply with the male system. While Millett and others focused on the political structures of oppression, Greer focused on women's internal revolution (Steinem, 1992).

Robin Morgan (1984) linked the two: Women's personal pains are symptomatic of and point to political and social structures and ideologies that support them. The slogan "the personal is political" thus became a common rallying point for feminist theory and ethics. Indeed, modern feminism grew in grass-roots "consciousness raising" sessions where women came together to share their plight and find a common language. As Nancy Hartsock suggests, "The practice of small-group consciousness raising, with its stress on examining and understanding experience and on connecting personal experience to the structures that define our lives, is the clearest example of the method basic to feminism" (Hartsock, quoted in Douglas, 1990, p. 19). Although contemporary feminism has also developed sophisticated and significant theory, theory has generally followed practices of women working for their rights, for a living wage, and for liberation from the myriad forms of oppression that they face.

These struggles gave rise to searing critiques of rape (Brownmiller, 1986), pornography (Dworkin, 1981), motherhood (Rich, 1976), racism (Moraga and Anzaldua, 1983; hooks, 1984), clitoridectomy (Daly, 1990), and other practices seen as oppressive to women. This period saw the emergence of the National Organization for Women, the Equal Rights Amendment, the development of sexual harassment theory, and arguments for affirmative action and preferential treatment. Women rallied around child-care and maternity leave issues, but also addressed broad social questions such as war (Elshtain, 1987). As was true in the first wave, there was no single approach to feminism and no single agenda among feminists. A variety of theories and actions were espoused in order to name and eradicate women's oppression.

Since women's reality is socially constructed, it can be deconstructed—the ideologies and injustices it perpetuates can be exposed. Political, social, historical, and economic tools of analysis are crucial to the task of unmasking ideology and injustice. Though they raised some challenges to traditional methods and theories, feminists of this period generally used those methods and theories. Some feminists drew on Buddhist, Jewish, Christian, and other theological traditions to ground their feminist claims, while others rejected traditional religions as contributing to the oppression of women and used primarily philosophical, political, or economic analysis. Women became focal points of investigation and were conceptualized as men's equals, and there was tremendous emphasis on "women's issues" such as childbearing and personal safety, but there was little challenge to fundamental assumptions of ontological, epistemological, or political frameworks (Gross, 1986).

Since 1980, the focus in feminism has shifted to a more profound criticism not merely of social structures and practices and their impact on women's oppression, but to a criticism of method and theory itself. Patriarchal discourse and its presuppositions have come under attack (Gross, 1986). Intensified concern has been addressed to the ways in which rationality itself reflects patriarchal assumptions and thus to the development of new modes of thinking and new definitions of theory and method. "Resistance to the tyranny of monolithic discourse has been the underlying issue in feminist theory in the 1980's" (Donovan, 1992, p. 187).

Feminism has therefore begun to take seriously the question of difference. Feminists of the previous century tended to stress women's equality with men. Women were then viewed only for their generalized "human" characteristics, those things that they shared with men. This left feminism unable to address the importance of women's distinctiveness. Feminists during the formational period of modern feminism tended to stress "sisterhood," focusing on those things that women were presumed to share with each other. This allowed the development of theories to account for specific skills of women, but it ignored differences between groups of women.

African-American women criticized feminism, charging white feminists with "ghettoizing" women of color (hooks, 1984). While white feminists railed against limited depictions of women as objects of beauty, for example, black women pointed out that they themselves were not depicted as beautiful at all, but as evil or sinful. An adequate feminist analysis, many argued, must attend not only to sex, but also to race and class and to the intersection of all three. It must abolish not only patriarchy but also capitalism and imperialism (Moraga and Anzaldua, 1983; Hull et al., 1982; Spelman, 1988). Some have coined the term "womanist" to describe a position in which concerns for race, sex, and class are never separated.

Thus, second-wave feminism was seen as blind to its own presuppositions and limitations, and as itself culturally conditioned and bounded. Women from Third World countries see feminism as too Western, focusing on those liberations that are of particular concern to white middle-class women rather than to poor women of color or women from exploited lands and subjugated countries. First World feminists were accused of developing analyses that "abound" in racism by defining as "women's" experience what is actually middle-class white Western women's experience (hooks, 1984; cf. Fox-Genovese, 1991).

In the "postmodern" phase of feminism, therefore, feminists are more attentive to differences—sexual, racial, class, and ethnic—and attempt to present analyses that are more contextual and recognize the influence of social location on theory and practice. Still, critics charge that contemporary feminism, at least in the United States, fails to shake the shackles of liberalism and remains "hostage to the history as well as the contemporary reality of our advanced capitalist society" (Fox-Genovese, 1991, p. 17). U.S. feminists are also accused of not taking seriously enough the theories that inform French feminism and other feminisms from around the world. Finally, the postmodern tendency to eschew theory has led some critics to charge that feminism is in danger of having no grounds for social criticism and therefore of leaving power in the hands of patriarchy (Donovan, 1992). Feminism must challenge its own presuppositions, including its metatheory.

Feminist ethics

During the postmodern phase characterized by criticism of method and theory, the assertion that women think differently than men do has been particularly important for the field of ethics. This assertion has come from two directions.

Drawing on Nancy Chodorow's (1978) crucial work on object relations theory, Carol Gilligan (1982) proposed that there is a "different voice" in ethics, largely associated with women. This voice reasons not in the language of rights and justice but in the language of relationship and caring.

Numerous feminists have used Gilligan's work to argue for an "ethic of care." Mary Field Belenky and her associates (1986) argued that women use an empathetic form of reasoning. Using motherhood as prototypical caring, Nel Noddings (1984) argued for a "feminine" mode of ethical reflection that was responsive to the needs of others, care-oriented, and based in prerational affections. While Noddings assumed a universal phenomenology of mothering, Sara Ruddick (1989) recognized the influence of culture on any definition of mothering. She nonetheless argued for a nearly universal mode of "maternal thinking" which she called "attentive love." She proposed that maternal thinking is always open to the new and therefore does not depend on repeatable knowledge, as does Western science. Other feminists have used nursing rather than mothering as the basis for an ethic of care (Fry, 1992).

Although neither Gilligan nor other "care" theorists would limit such modes of thinking exclusively to women, there is nonetheless a strong presumption that women have a "different" way of moral reasoning than men do. This way of reasoning is generally called an ethic of caring, and is contrasted with an ethic of justice. The ethic of caring is said to be relational, contextual, and empathic, as opposed to abstract, universalized, and principled approach of an ethic of justice.

Criticisms of this claim for difference abound, and developments on the theory have become a virtual industry (see Larrabbee, 1993; Kittay and Meyers, 1987; Cole and Coultrap-McQuin, 1992). Urging women to "care" for others can become a "compassion trap" that keeps women in traditional roles (Adams, 1971). Caring is a vague notion, not yet well defined (Nelson, 1992; Boyer and Nelson, 1992). Susan Sherwin (1992) has proposed that caring may constitute a "feminine" ethic based on attending to women's actual care-giving experiences, but that it is not sufficient for a "feminist" ethic. For a feminist ethic, a political perspective is needed: "[feminist ethics] derives from an explicitly political perspective of feminism, wherein the oppression of women is seen to be morally and politically unacceptable" (Sherwin, 1992, p. 49). Thus, for Sherwin, feminist ethics has at least one general principle: a principle of nonexploitation or nonoppression.

In particular, critics of the ethic of caring point out that what women do or how women think in a sexist culture will reflect the structures and practices embedded in the culture (see especially Romain, 1992). Others argue that the "caring" approach is ethnocentric and generalizes about the experiences of women rather than developing attention to context (see especially Benhabib, 1987).

Still others have argued that justice and care are not antithetical but mutually supportive, or that justice is needed in addition to care in order to have a viable ethic for the social order (see especially Held, 1987; Meyers, 1987). For example, the characterization of the "justice" approach to ethics is drawn from liberal philosophical tradition. But this is only one understanding of justice. Drawing partly on liberation theology, which urges human liberation as the primary commandment of God, some feminists have urged a concept of justice that is partial, impassioned, contextual, and requires positive supports for living (Lebacqz, 1991; Harrison, 1983; Heyward, 1984). Such a concept of justice comes close to feminists' characterization of "caring."

Indeed, although some feminists appear ready to urge caring as a priority over justice, others are less sanguine. The concern for women's oppression and liberation that has grounded feminism over the centuries implies that a concern for justice is central to feminism and should not be too sharply divided from a concern for caring. Women are often the caregivers for elderly relatives. But this means that caring itself must of necessity raise issues of justice such as the failure of current medical systems to provide long-term care (Muller, 1990).

While many feminists have stressed caring, therefore, others stress justice. Susan Okin (1989) argues that liberal theory on justice ignores women's care-giving roles, and that any adequate theory of justice must attend to the structures of the family. Karen Lebacqz (1987) argues that justice may not require the same thing from the oppressed as from the oppressor. Iris Marion Young (1990) suggests that justice needs to attend to the realities of group identity. These feminist theories push beyond the liberal notion that justice is giving to each (individual) what is due. Hence, justice may not be as opposed to caring as some feminists have argued, and an adequate feminist ethic must include attention to both caring and justice.

An alternative approach to difference in moral theory comes not from psychoanalytic roots but from Marxist analysis. If women's experiences are socially conditioned, then that conditioning itself can suggest that women have a particular "standpoint" from which society can be judged (Hartsock, 1983). The claim need not be made that sex alone yields a different perspective, but only that material and historical conditions have placed women in a particular social location from which they view the world, and that this social location is morally relevant and yields ethical insight. Much feminist liberation theology takes a similar stance, arguing for the "epistemological privilege" of the oppressed.

However, this perspective, too, raises difficulties. Not all women's experience is the same, nor would it yield a unified "standpoint" from which social structures, practices, and theories can be judged. Not all women are feminists. Feminists who claim to speak from women's standpoint, therefore, appear to be claiming a special privilege (Donovan, 1992).

The care-versus-justice debate and the question of whether there is a distinctive "standpoint" for women's theorizing are not the only important moments in contemporary feminist ethics. Some feminists have begun working with notions of communitarian ethics, drawing on the work of Alasdair MacIntyre and others. Others, such as French feminists, have begun to recapture existentialist traditions or to utilize the theories of power and sexuality developed by Michel Foucault (Cole and Coultrap-McQuin, 1992). Ecofeminism is emerging as a unified theory that connects women's concerns with concerns for nature more broadly.

What feminists agree upon in the field of ethics can be generally summarized into the following tenets (Scaltsas, 1992; Walker, 1992; Gross, 1986).

1. A critique of abstract theory, including its claims for objectivity and rationality, and a view of moral life not in terms of an overarching theory or central principle but rather as a tissue of understandings;
2. A concomitant focus on the concrete and contextual, emphasizing the knowing subject as embodied and socially situated, so that knowledge is not universal but mediated;
3. A new concept of reason as including feelings and emotions, stressing empathy and caring as distinctive modes of reasoning and ethical response;
4. A critique of choice as central to morality, and a recognition of the demands of relationships and situations and the necessity for attention to discern those demands;
5. A call for new modes of discourse and openness to development of additional forms of analysis and theory;
6. A recognition that equality of women with men is not sufficient, and that the goal is genuine liberation for all, including liberation from oppression in all its forms.

The focus on liberation from oppression provides a constant in feminist theory. Further, the focus includes both social structures and practices, and ideologies and forms of thinking. Both of these have been important in the growing feminist literature on bioethics.

Feminist bioethics

Feminist bioethics has followed the trends of modern feminism. The formational period of the second wave of feminism saw the development of significant social criticism of the medical profession and how it affects women's reality. In 1972, Phyllis Chesler's *Women and Madness* accused the mental-health-care system of failure to recognize women's oppression. Passivity, low self-esteem, and other characteristics that would be considered ill health for a man were considered "normal" and acceptable for a woman. Psychiatry had become a tool for the oppression of women, reinforcing their limited social roles (Ritchie, 1989).

What Chesler did for mental health, Barbara Ehrenreich and Dierdre English did for the health-care system in general. They argued that medicine functions as a legitimizing agent, providing "scientific" justification for particular social roles and dividing men from women. Normal female functions such as menstruation and menopause become "illnesses" to be defined and addressed by the medical profession. Women no longer birth babies; rather, they must be "delivered" by doctors (Ehrenreich and English, 1973). Scathing critiques of obstetrical and gynecological practices followed (Daly, 1990; Rich, 1976; Haire, 1972).

The medical system is seen by many feminists as strategic for women's oppression. Standing between biology and social policy, medical practices often serve as sources of powerful sexist ideology, defining normalcy for women and men. For example, Jo Ann Ashley (1976) showed that the development of nursing as a "woman's" profession was fraught with sexism and oppression of women. Janice Raymond (1979) argued that transsexual surgery was a medical "empire" designed to obscure legitimate questions that might be raised about women's roles in society. Mary Daly (1990) argued that gynecology was a "mind-binding" institution intent on imposing order on women under the guise of medical care—for example, by shaping women's medical "needs." Both moderate and more strident feminists were united in their opposition to ways in which the medical profession, wittingly or unwittingly, reinforces social discrimination against women (Muller, 1990).

Some feminists therefore circumvented or redefined the medical profession. The Boston Women's Health Collective's *Our Bodies, Ourselves* (1973) urged women to claim their own bodies. Women established self-help clinics, teaching each other diagnostic and contraceptive techniques. They founded organizations to enable women to obtain abortions ("Jane," in Fried, 1990).

Such alternative practices in health care have implications for bioethics: The activist thrust that undergirded the women's movement during this time implies an impatience with abstract modes of ethical argument that are traditional in bioethics.

Indeed, recent feminist work in bioethics have argued precisely against such abstract and principled approaches to bioethics as tend to dominate the field (Beauchamp and Childress, 1989). Following the general trend in feminist ethics of eschewing principles and their application, Helen B. Holmes, an editor of one recent volume of feminist bioethics, claims that "all our authors would agree that no single theory or no single strategy is adequate for settling every kind of ethical question" (Holmes, 1992).

Yet feminists are united in trying to unmask the ways in which the medical profession has contributed to the oppression of women. From specific critiques of the profession and its practices, contemporary feminism has moved to criticisms of medical ethics or bioethics as a discipline. The field of bioethics itself has come under attack for simply accepting the practices of medicine and for providing little political or institutional analysis and criticism.

For example, feminists have offered scathing critiques of new reproductive technologies such as in vitro fertilization (IVF) and concomitant arrangements such as surrogate motherhood. At first glance, this opposition seems surprising. In light of the strong feminist support for women's reproductive freedom (and remembering Shulamith Firestone's early call [1983] for new reproductive technologies), one might expect that feminists would affirm any technologies or arrangements that appear to enhance women's reproductive options. Both IVF and surrogacy appear to do just that. Yet feminists have generally denounced both.

The reasons are complicated and varied. They include the charge that the claims for success of IVF are inflated and therefore women's consent to such procedures is not genuinely "informed," and the charge that programs reinforce cultural stereotypes of women by requiring them to be married in order to be candidates for IVF. There are also concerns that allowing children or women's bodies to be "sold" contributes to "commodifying" human life and bodies; that IVF may be exploiting women to compensate for men's infertility; and that women's desire for children is itself socially conditioned and thus practices such as IVF simply reinforce women's oppression (Baruch et al., 1988; Corea, 1985; Holmes et al., 1980). But above all, feminists argue that IVF and surrogacy will take power away from women and put men in control of reproductive processes: "The new reproductive technologies are being developed and marketed primarily by men and for the profit of men. . . . These technologies are part of the historical process by which men have gradually extended their control of human reproduction" (Warren, 1985, p. 143).

Thus, an underlying issue is the balance and distribution of power in society. Taking a Marxist perspective, some feminists argue that surrogate contracts would not exist at all if the parties had equal power at the outset: women are "forced" into surrogate arrangements because of lack of economic means (Oliver, 1992). Others reject this argument, but point out that surrogacy allows someone to "own" another's body in a way that treats that person—the woman—as an object (Ketchum, 1992). Still others object to the entire notion of surrogate contracts on grounds that such contracts assume an individualistic, contract orientation that denies basic feminist claims about the relational nature of human life (Nelson and Nelson, 1992). Contracts are themselves embedded in and cannot be understood apart from noncontractual relationships (Hirschmann, 1992). Whether the ethical framework is Marxist, Kantian, or radical, the practice of IVF is seen by many feminists as undermining women's moral agency and their effective power in society.

These analyses of IVF and surrogacy highlight several aspects of feminist ethical analysis in the field of bioethics. First, it is practices and systems that are ex-

amined, not individual actions. Second, the concern is for the impact of those practices and systems on the oppression or liberation of women. Third, the impact on oppression or liberation must consider fundamental issues of whether women's moral agency is supported or denied, and this question includes but goes beyond the simple question of "informed consent." A full assessment of the impact on women's moral agency also considers how a practice contributes to views of women and to the breaking or perpetuating of stereotypes. Finally, the assessment will include both issues of relationship and care, and also issues of basic justice, seen in overcoming the five types of oppression identified by Iris Marion Young (1990).

This same cluster of concerns helps to explain why almost all feminists support women's access to safe, legal abortion. Although feminists use the language of a woman's "right" to abortion (Harrison, 1983; Fried, 1990), the argument for abortion is not generally a simple matter of asserting rights in a liberal framework.

An early and influential proponent of women's right to abortion did operate out of a liberal framework. Judith Jarvis Thomson argued (1986) that the right to life of the fetus did not give it a right to use another person's body. Hence, the woman has a right to remove her body from the fetus. Thomson picked up a feminist theme: the woman's right to her own body. However, her argument was still framed within liberal philosophical assumptions regarding freedom of choice; these assumptions are rejected by many contemporary feminists, who refuse to see the abortion debate as a question of pitting the "right to life" of a fetus against the "right to choose" of a woman.

Some feminists argue that the fetus is not fully human (Harrison, 1983; Sherwin, 1992). Because personhood is socially constructed, and because the fetus cannot exist independently of the woman, she is crucial to determining its status. There is no "personhood" for the fetus apart from its relationship to the woman.

But the moral legitimacy of abortion for most feminists does not hinge on the question of the status of the fetus. Contemporary feminists argue that no discussion of abortion is valid unless it attends to the general social and political climate of oppression of women. Opposition to abortion must be understood in part as opposition to women's freedom from male control (Harrison, 1983). Crucial to the abortion debate, therefore, is the question of honoring women's full moral agency and freeing women from male control.

A society that denies women freedom of reproductive choice is using women as a means to some end and therefore is making women less than fully human. If women are to be accorded full status as moral agents, then the decision about abortion must be left to them. Without this, women are denied their intrinsic value as persons. There can be no good society that denies the intrinsic value of persons. The "right to choose," therefore, is not a narrow individual right framed within liberal assumptions, but is an expression of concern for the fabric of social relationships and the moral status of women.

Furthermore, feminists point out that women often do not have genuine "choice" regarding pregnancy or abortion. In a culture that oppresses women, the power of sexual politics is such that women are often not free to resist male sexual advances or to control the circumstances of sexual contact. Pregnancy may not be "freely" chosen. Similarly, in cultures where women are economically oppressed and little support is provided for raising children, it is questionable whether women are truly "free" to choose to bear a child. The abortion question cannot be settled without attention to economic and sociopolitical agendas.

The status of the fetus is therefore not the only relevant moral question in the abortion debate; justice for women is equally important. Access to abortion or a "right to choose" is not a simple matter of freedom from interference by others; it is a larger matter of recognizing and rectifying women's oppression in society.

Still other feminists have raised questions about particular practices of abortion because of their potential impact on women's overall freedom and self-determination. Barbara Katz Rothman (1987) charges that prenatal diagnosis and selective abortion changes the experience of pregnancy for women, forcing them to distance themselves from the fetus so as to be able to abort it if necessary. Prenatal diagnosis begins to "commodify" pregnancy, turning it into a search for the perfect product. Selective abortion can also be used as a tool for sex selection, which has the potential—perhaps especially in so-called Third World countries—for reinforcing cultural stereotypes and discrimination against women (Warren, 1985; Wertz and Fletcher, 1992).

These arguments illustrate several aspects of feminist moral argument (cf. Lebacqz, 1987, 1991). First, feminist moral argument takes women's experience seriously. Second, it operates on a "hermeneutic of suspicion" about the prevailing social order and how that order affects women. Third, it is historical, exposing cultural myths—for example, showing that past prohibitions of abortion were not based on a consistent societal affirmation of the value of the fetus, but on a desire to keep control of women's bodies. Fourth, it focuses on the meaning of practices, not of individual acts alone. Fifth, it takes a global perspective, asking what the implications of practices will be for women around the world. Sixth, it utilizes rights language, but within a larger concern for what makes an acceptable or life-giving society. Seventh, it takes women's survival, women's

well-being, and women's power as central criteria. Only those practices that are life-giving and justice-making for women as defined by women will be considered morally acceptable.

Conclusion

Feminist approaches to bioethics have historically attempted to expose the ways in which medical practices contribute to the oppression of women. Contemporary feminist bioethics raises questions about bioethics itself, challenging the paradigms in which bioethics proceeds. For example, the rejection of liberal assumptions about autonomous individuals highlights the central claim of contemporary feminism that humans are at root relational, and that this relational nature of human life is morally significant in ways that are not easily comprehended by the dominant Western ethical paradigm.

Nonetheless, tensions emerge in feminist bioethics. Freedom of access to abortion can imply encouragement for the development of technologies such as prenatal diagnosis and selective abortion. Yet selective abortion raises justice questions for women, particularly when its global implications for sex selection are considered. Although feminists generally reject IVF and surrogacy on justice grounds, it is difficult to reconcile this rejection with their strong emphasis on woman's control of their own bodies and freedom of reproductive choice. Freedom and justice are not always easily reconciled.

Similarly, caring and justice are not always easily reconciled. Home health care in the United States is often provided by poor women of color from other countries who do not receive health benefits. In "caring" for others, their own health may be jeopardized, while at the same time they lack the resources to gain access to health care. Under those circumstances, caring and justice may conflict: justice for the home health worker might require that she give less care to others.

The three strong values of freedom, caring, and justice that have emerged within the field of feminist bioethics stand therefore in possible tension. Much normative work remains to be done.

Feminists draw on a long history to affirm a core of shared assumptions. These include the one voiced so powerfully by Simone de Beauvoir (1988): Reality is socially constructed, not biologically determined. Being female is not the same as being "feminine" or "woman." These are social constructions. Because they are social constructions, they can be deconstructed and reconstructed. Much effort has gone into the deconstructive task, exposing the oppressions that characterize women's lives. Here, contemporary feminists agree on the central role of power and on the interlocking effects of racist, classist, and sexist ideologies with political, economic, and social structures. Oppression is carried by language and symbol systems; hence, the deconstruction of patriarchy requires attention to the nature of rationality itself and to religious ritual and cultural myth as well as to concrete social issues.

The task of reconstruction continues. Central to it is claiming women's own experience as "different" and finding new ways to think about that difference. Feminists agree that women have been and still are oppressed because of their sex. They further agree that this oppression is wrong. Yet as feminism is diverse, so will feminist arguments in bioethics be diverse. Feminism is what Mary Daly once called "ludic cerebration": "the free play of intuition in our own space, giving rise to thinking that is vigorous, informed, multi-dimensional, independent, tough, creative" (1990, p. 23). Feminists will not agree on all social issues, though they show remarkable agreement on some. But what they will agree about is the necessity for new forms of cerebration—for ethical thinking that is contextual, informed by social analysis, in touch with women's real lived experiences, focused on the impact of practices on the poor and oppressed, justice-making, and life-giving.

KAREN LEBACQZ

Directly related to this entry are the entries SEXISM; *and* WOMEN. *For a further discussion of topics mentioned in this article, see the entries* ABORTION; ABUSE, INTERPERSONAL, *article on* ABUSE BETWEEN DOMESTIC PARTNERS; AUTHORITY; CARE; COMPASSION; ENVIRONMENTAL ETHICS, *article on* ECOFEMINISM; FERTILITY CONTROL; FETUS, *articles on* HUMAN DEVELOPMENT FROM FERTILIZATION TO BIRTH, *and* FETAL RESEARCH; GENDER IDENTITY AND GENDER IDENTITY DISORDERS; MENTAL ILLNESS, *articles on* CONCEPTIONS OF MENTAL ILLNESS, *and* ISSUES IN DIAGNOSIS; NURSING, THEORIES AND PHILOSOPHY OF; PSYCHIATRY, ABUSES OF; RACE AND RACISM; REPRODUCTIVE TECHNOLOGIES; RIGHTS; SEXUAL IDENTITY; *and* VALUE AND VALUATION. *For a discussion of related ideas, see the entries* AUTONOMY; BIOETHICS EDUCATION, *article on* NURSING; BIOLOGY, PHILOSOPHY OF; BODY, *article on* EMBODIMENT: THE PHENOMENOLOGICAL TRADITION; CHILDREN, *articles on* HISTORY OF CHILDHOOD, *and* RIGHTS OF CHILDREN; CIRCUMCISION, *article on* FEMALE CIRCUMCISION; FAMILY; FREEDOM AND COERCION; GENETIC TESTING AND SCREENING; INTERPRETATION; LONG-TERM CARE; MARRIAGE AND OTHER DOMESTIC PARTNERSHIPS; MATERNAL–FETAL RELATIONSHIP; PROSTITUTION; SEXUAL ETHICS AND PROFESSIONAL STANDARDS; SEXUALITY IN SOCIETY; *and* WARFARE. *Other relevant material may be found under the entries* ADOPTION; EMOTIONS; EVOLUTION; HARM; INFORMED CONSENT; LIFE; MEDICAL EDUCATION; *and* PERSON.

Bibliography

ADAMS, MARGARET. 1971. "The Compassion Trap." In *Woman in Sexist Society: Studies in Power and Powerlessness*, pp. 401–416. Edited by Vivian Gornick and Barbara K. Moran. New York: New American Library.

ANDOLSEN, BARBARA HILKERT; GUDORF, CHRISTINE E.; and PELLAUER, MARY D. 1985. *Women's Consciousness, Women's Conscience: A Reader in Feminist Ethics.* New York: Harper & Row.

ARDITTI, RITA; KLEIN, RENATE DUELLI; and MINDEN, SHELLEY, eds. 1984. *Test-Tube Women: What Future for Motherhood?* London: Pandora.

ASHLEY, JO ANN. 1976. *Hospitals, Paternalism, and the Role of the Nurse.* New York: Teachers College Press.

Atlantis: A Women's Studies Journal. 1975–. Toronto, Ont.: Micromedia.

BAIER, ANNETTE. 1985. *Postures of the Mind: Essays on Mind and Morals.* Minneapolis: University of Minnesota Press.

BARUCH, ELAINE HOFFMAN; D'AMAO, AMADEO F.; and SEAGER, JONI, eds. 1988. *Embryos, Ethics and Women's Rights: Exploring the New Reproductive Technologies.* New York: Harrington Park Press.

BEAUCHAMP, TOM L., and CHILDRESS, JAMES F. 1989. *Principles of Biomedical Ethics.* 3d ed. New York: Oxford University Press.

BEAUVOIR, SIMONE DE. 1988. *The Second Sex.* Translated by Howard Madison Parshley. London: David Campbell.

BELENKY, MARY FIELD; CLINCHY, BLYTHE McVICKER; GOLDBERGER, NANCY RULE; and TARULE, JILL MATTUCK. 1986. *Women's Ways of Knowing: The Development of Self, Voice, and Mind.* New York: Basic Books.

BENHABIB, SEYLA. 1987. "The Generalized and the Concrete Other: The Kohlberg-Gilligan Controversy and Moral Theory." In *Women and Moral Theory*, pp. 154–177. Edited by Eva Feder Kittay and Diana T. Meyers. Totowa, N.J.: Rowman & Littlefield.

BENHABIB, SEYLA, and CORNELL, DRUCILLA, eds. 1987. *Feminism as Critique: On the Politics of Gender.* Minneapolis: University of Minnesota Press.

BOSTON WOMEN'S HEALTH BOOK COLLECTIVE. 1973. *Our Bodies, Ourselves: A Book by and for Women.* New York: Simon & Schuster.

———. 1984. *The New Our Bodies, Ourselves: A Book by and for Women.* New York: Simon & Schuster.

BOYER, JEANNINE ROSS, and NELSON, JAMES LINDEMANN. 1992. "A Comment on Fry's 'The Role of Caring in a Theory of Nursing.'" In *Feminist Perspectives in Medical Ethics*, pp. 107–112. Edited by Helen B. Holmes and Laura M. Purdy. Bloomington: Indiana University Press.

BRAIDOTTI, ROSI. 1986. "Ethics Revisited: Women and/in Philosophy." In *Feminist Challenges: Social and Political Theory*, pp. 44–60. Edited by Carole Pateman and Elizabeth Gross. Boston: Northeastern University Press.

BROWNMILLER, SUSAN. 1986. *Against Our Will: Men, Women, and Rape.* New York: Bantam.

CARSE, ALISA L. 1991. "The 'Voice of Care': Implications for Bioethical Education." *Journal of Medicine and Philosophy* 16, no. 1:5–28.

CHESLER, PHYLLIS. 1972. *Women and Madness.* New York: Harcourt Brace Jovanovich.

CHODOROW, NANCY. 1978. *The Reproduction of Mothering: Psychoanalysis and the Sociology of Gender.* Berkeley: University of California Press.

CODE, LORRAINE; MULLETT, SHEILA; and OVERALL, CHRISTINE, eds. 1988. *Feminist Perspectives: Philosophical Essays on Method and Morals.* Toronto: Toronto University Press.

COHEN, SHERRILL, and TAUB, NADINE, eds. 1989. *Reproductive Laws for the 1990s.* Clifton, N.J.: Humana.

COLE, EVA BROWNING, and COULTRAP-MCQUIN, SUSAN, eds. 1992. *Explorations in Feminist Ethics: Theory and Practice.* Bloomington: Indiana University Press.

COLLINS, PATRICIA HILL. 1990. *Black Feminist Thought: Knowledge, Consciousness, and the Politics of Empowerment.* New York: Routledge.

COREA, GENA. 1985. *The Mother Machine: Reproductive Technologies from Artificial Insemination to Artificial Wombs.* New York: Harper & Row.

CRYSDALE, CYNTHIA S. W. 1994. "Gilligan and the Ethics of Care: An Update." *Religious Studies Review* 20, no. 1:21–28.

DALY, MARY. 1973. *Beyond God the Father: Toward a Philosophy of Women's Liberation.* Boston: Beacon Press.

———. 1990. *Gyn/Ecology: The Metaethics of Radical Feminism.* Boston: Beacon Press.

DONOVAN, JOSEPHINE. 1992. *Feminist Theory: The Intellectual Traditions of American Feminism.* New ed. New York: Continuum.

DOUGLAS, CAROL ANNE. 1990. *Love and Politics: Radical Feminist and Lesbian Theories.* San Francisco: ISM Press.

DREIFUS, CLAUDIA. 1978. *Seizing Our Bodies: The Politics of Women's Health.* New York: Vintage.

DWORKIN, ANDREA. 1981. *Pornography: Men Possessing Women.* New York: E. P. Dutton.

EHRENREICH, BARBARA, and ENGLISH, DIERDRE. 1973. *Complaints and Disorders: The Sexual Politics of Sickness.* Old Westbury, N.Y.: Feminist Press.

———. 1973. *Witches, Midwives, and Nurses: A History of Women Healers.* 2d ed. Old Westbury, N.Y.: Feminist Press.

ELSHTAIN, JEAN BETHKE. 1987. *Women and War.* New York: Basic Books.

FARLEY, MARGARET A. 1985. "Feminist Theology and Bioethics." In *Women's Consciousness, Women's Conscience: A Reader in Feminist Ethics,* pp. 285–305. Edited by Barbara Hilkert Andolsen, Christine E. Gudorf, and Mary Pellauer. New York: Harper & Row.

"Feminist Classics of This Wave." 1992. *Ms.,* July–August, pp. 64–65.

Feminist Issues. 1980–. New Brunswick, N.J.: Transaction Periodicals Consortium.

Feminist Review. 1979–. London: Feminist Review.

Feminist Studies. 1972–. College Park, Md.: Feminist Studies.

FIRESTONE, SHULAMITH. 1983. *The Dialectic of Sex: The Case for Feminist Revolution.* London: Women's Press.

FOX-GENOVESE, ELIZABETH. 1991. *Feminism Without Illusions: A Critique of Individualism.* Chapel Hill: University of North Carolina Press.

FRAZER, ELIZABETH; HORNSBY, JENNIFER; and LOVIBOND, SABINA, eds. 1992. *Ethics: A Feminist Reader.* London: Basil Blackwell.

FRIED, MARLENE GERBER, ed. 1990. *From Abortion to Reproductive Freedom: Transforming a Movement.* Boston: South End Press.

FRIEDAN, BETTY. 1965. *The Feminine Mystique.* New York: Penguin.

FRY, SARA T. 1992. "The Role of Caring in a Theory of Nursing Ethics." In *Feminist Perspectives in Medical Ethics,* pp. 93–106. Edited by Helen B. Holmes and Laura M. Purdy. Bloomington: Indiana University Press.

GILLIGAN, CAROL. 1982. *In a Different Voice: Psychological Theory and Women's Development.* Cambridge, Mass.: Harvard University Press.

GREER, GERMAINE. 1971. *The Female Eunuch.* New York: McGraw-Hill.

GROSS, ELIZABETH. 1986a. "Conclusion: What Is Feminism?" In *Feminist Challenges: Social and Political Theory,* pp. 190–204. Edited by Carole Pateman and Elizabeth Gross. Boston: Northeastern University Press.

———. 1986b. "Philosophy, Subjectivity, and the Body: Kristera and Irigaray. In *Feminist Challenges: Social and Political Theory,* pp. 125–143. Edited by Carole Pateman and Elizabeth Gross. Boston: Northeastern University Press.

HAIRE, DORIS. 1972. *The Cultural Warping of Childbirth: A Special Report.* Hillside, N.J.: International Childbirth Education Association.

HARRISON, BEVERLY WILDUNG. 1983. *Our Right to Choose: Toward a New Ethic of Abortion.* Boston: Beacon Press.

HARTSOCK, NANCY C. M. 1983. *Money, Sex and Power: Toward a Feminist Historical Materialism.* Boston: Northeastern University Press.

HELD, VIRGINIA. 1987. "Feminism and Moral Theory." In *Women and Moral Theory,* pp. 111–128. Edited by Eva Feder Kittay and Diana T. Meyers. Totowa, N.J.: Rowman & Littlefield.

HEYWARD, CARTER. 1984. *Our Passion for Justice: Images of Power, Sexuality and Liberation.* New York: Pilgrim.

HIRSCHMANN, NANCY J. 1992. *Rethinking Obligation: A Feminist Method for Political Theory.* Ithaca, N.Y.: Cornell University Press.

HOAGLAND, SARAH LUCIA. 1988. *Lesbian Ethics: Toward New Value.* Palo Alto, Calif.: Institute of Lesbian Studies.

HOLMES, HELEN B. 1992. "A Call to Heal Medicine." In *Feminist Perspectives in Medical Ethics,* pp. 1–8. Edited by Helen B. Holmes and Laura M. Purdy. Bloomington: Indiana University Press.

HOLMES, HELEN B.; HOSKINS, BETTY B.; AND GROSS, MICHAEL, eds. 1980. *Birth Control and Controlling Birth: Women-Centered Perspectives.* Clifton, N.J.: Humana.

———, eds. 1981. *The Custom-Made Child? Women-Centered Perspectives.* Clifton, N.J.: Humana.

HOLMES, HELEN B., and PURDY, LAURA M., eds. 1992. *Feminist Perspectives in Medical Ethics.* Bloomington: Indiana University Press.

HOOKS, BELL. 1984. *Feminist Theory: From Margin to Center.* Boston: South End Press.

HORTON, JACQUELINE A., ed. 1992. *The Women's Health Data Book: A Profile of Women's Health in the United States.* New York: Elsevier.

HULL, GLORIA T.; BELL-SCOTT, PATRICIA; and SMITH, BARBARA, eds. 1982. *All the Women Are White, All the Blacks Are Men, But Some of Us Are Brave.* New York: Feminist Press.

Hypatia: A Journal of Feminist Philosophy. 1983–. Oxford: Pergamon.

JARDINE, ALICE, and SMITH, PAUL. 1989. *Men in Feminism.* New York: Routledge.

JOHNSTON, JILL. 1973. *Lesbian Nation: The Feminist Solution.* New York: Simon & Schuster.

KETCHUM, SARA ANN. 1992. "Selling Babies and Selling Bodies." In *Feminist Perspectives in Medical Ethics,* pp. 284–294. Edited by Helen B. Holmes and Laura M. Purdy. Bloomington: Indiana University Press.

KITTAY, EVA FEDER, and MEYERS, DIANA T., eds. 1987. *Women and Moral Theory.* Totowa, N.J.: Rowman & Littlefield.

LARRABEE, MARY JEANNE, ed. 1993. *An Ethic of Care: Feminist and Interdisciplinary Perspectives.* New York: Routledge.

LEBACQZ, KAREN. 1987. *Justice in An Unjust World: Foundations for a Christian Approach to Justice.* Minneapolis, Minn.: Augsburg.

———. 1991. "Feminism and Bioethics: An Overview." *Second Opinion* 17 (October):11–25.

LERNER, GERDA. 1986. *The Creation of Patriarchy.* New York: Oxford University Press.

———. 1993. *The Creation of Feminist Consciousness: From the Middle Ages to Eighteen-Seventy.* New York: Oxford University Press.

MEYERS, DIANA T. 1987. "The Socialized Individual and Individual Autonomy: An Intersection Between Philosophy and Psychology." In *Women and Moral Theory,* pp. 139–153. Edited by Eva Feder Kittay and Diana T. Meyers. Totowa, N.J.: Rowman & Littlefield.

MILLETT, KATE. 1990. *Sexual Politics.* New York: Simon & Schuster.

MORAGA, CHERRIE, and ANZALDUA, GLORIA, eds. 1983. *This Bridge Called My Back: Writings of Radical Women of Color.* New York: Kitchen Table, Women of Color Press.

MORGAN, ROBIN, ed. 1984. *Sisterhood Is Global: The International Women's Movement Anthology.* New York: Anchor.

MORRISON, TONI, ed. 1992. *Race-ing Justice, En-Gendering Power: Essays on Anita Hill, Clarence Thomas, and the Construction of Social Reality.* New York: Pantheon.

MULLER, CHARLOTTE F. 1990. *Health Care and Gender.* New York: Russell Sage Foundation.

NELSON, HILDE LINDEMANN. 1992. "Against Caring." *Journal of Clinical Ethics* 3, no. 1:8–15.

NELSON, HILDE LINDEMANN, and NELSON, JAMES LINDEMANN. 1992. "Cutting Motherhood in Two: Some Suspicions Concerning Surgery." In *Feminist Perspectives in Medical Ethics,* pp. 257–265. Edited by Helen B. Holmes and Laura M. Purdy. Bloomington: Indiana University Press.

NODDINGS, NEL. 1984. *Caring: A Feminine Approach to Ethics and Moral Education.* Berkeley: University of California Press.

OKIN, SUSAN MOLLER. 1989. *Justice, Gender, and the Family.* New York: Basic Books.

OLIVER, KELLY. 1992. "Marxism and Surrogacy." In *Feminist Perspectives in Medical Ethics,* pp. 266–283. Edited by Helen B. Holmes and Laura M. Purdy. Bloomington: Indiana University Press.

PATEMAN, CAROLE. 1983. "Introduction: The Theoretical Subversiveness of Feminism." In *Feminist Challenges: Social and Political Theory,* pp. 1–10. Edited by Carole Pateman and Elizabeth Gross. Boston: Northeastern University Press.

PATEMAN, CAROLE, and GROSS, ELIZABETH, eds. 1986. *Feminist Challenges: Social and Political Theory.* Boston: Northeastern University Press.

PERALES, CESAR A., and YOUNG, LAUREN S., eds. 1988. *Too Little, Too Late: Dealing with the Health Needs of Women in Poverty.* New York: Harrington Park Press.

RAYMOND, JANICE G. 1979. *The Transsexual Empire: The Making of the She-Male.* Boston: Beacon Press.

RHODE, DEBORA L. 1989. *Justice and Gender: Sex Discrimination and the Law.* Cambridge, Mass.: Harvard University Press.

RICH, ADRIENNE C. 1976. *Of Woman Born: Motherhood as Experience and Institution.* New York: W. W. Norton.

RITCHIE, KAREN. 1989. "The Little Woman Meets Son of DSM-III." *Journal of Medicine and Philosophy* 14, no. 6:695–708.

ROMAIN, DIANNE. 1992. "Care and Confusion." In *Explorations in Feminist Ethics: Theory and Practice,* pp. 27–37. Edited by Eva Browning Cole and Susan Coultrap-McQuin. Bloomington: Indiana University Press.

ROTHMAN, BARBARA KATZ. 1987. *The Tentative Pregnancy: Prenatal Diagnosis and the Future of Motherhood.* New York: Penguin.

RUDDICK, SARA. 1989. *Maternal Thinking: Toward a Politics of Peace.* New York: Ballantine.

RUSSELL, LETTY M.; KWOK, PUI-LAN; ISASI-DIAZ, ADA MARIE; and CANNON, KATIE GENEVA, eds. 1988. *Inheriting Our Mothers' Gardens: Feminist Theology in Third World Perspective.* Philadelphia: Westminster.

SAND, GEORGE. 1972. "Indiana; Letters of George Sand; and The Intimate Journal of George Sand." In *Feminism: The Essential Historical Writings,* pp. 25–34. Edited by Miriam Schneir. New York: Random House.

SCALTSAS, PATRICIA WARD. 1992. "Do Feminist Ethics Counter Feminist Aims?" In *Explorations in Feminist Ethics: Theory and Practice,* pp. 15–26. Edited by Eva Browning Cole and Susan Coultrap-McQuin. Bloomington: Indiana University Press.

SCHNEIR, MIRIAM, ed. 1972. *Feminism: The Essential Historical Writings.* New York: Random House.

SHERWIN, SUSAN. 1992. *No Longer Patient: Feminist Ethics and Health Care.* Philadelphia: Temple University Press.

Signs: A Journal of Women in Culture and Society. 1975–. Chicago: University of Chicago Press.

SNITOW, ANN BARR; STANSELL, CHRISTINE; and THOMPSON, SHARON, eds. 1983. *Powers of Desire: The Politics of Sexuality.* New York: Monthly Review Press.

SPELMAN, ELIZABETH V. 1988. *Inessential Woman: Problems of Exclusion in Feminist Thought*. Boston: Beacon Press.

SPENDER, DALE. 1983. *Feminist Theorists: Three Centuries of Key Women Thinkers*. New York: Pantheon.

———. 1985. *For the Record: The Making and Meaning of Feminist Knowledge*. London: Women's Press.

STEINEM, GLORIA. 1983. *Outrageous Acts and Everyday Rebellions*. New York: New American Library.

———. 1992. *Revolution from Within: A Book of Self-Esteem*. Boston: Little, Brown.

THOMSON, JUDITH JARVIS. 1986. "A Defense of Abortion." In *Women and Values: Readings in Recent Feminist Philosophy*. New York: Wadsworth.

THORNTON, MERLE. 1986. "Sex Equality Is Not Enough for Feminism." In *Feminist Challenges: Social and Political Theory*, pp. 77–98. Edited by Carole Pateman and Elizabeth Gross. Boston: Northeastern University Press.

WALKER, MARGARET URBAN. 1992. "Moral Understandings: Alternative 'Epistemology' for a Feminist Ethics." In *Explorations in Feminist Ethics: Theory and Practice*, pp. 165–175. Edited by Eva Browning Cole and Susan Coultrap-McQuin. Bloomington: Indiana University Press.

WARREN, MARY ANNE. 1985. *Gendercide: The Implications of Sex Selection*. New York: Rowman & Allanheld.

WERTZ, DOROTHY C., and FLETCHER, JOHN C. 1992. "Sex Selection Through Prenatal Diagnosis: A Feminist Critique." In *Feminist Perspectives in Medical Ethics*, pp. 240–253. Edited by Helen B. Holmes and Laura M. Purdy. Bloomington: Indiana University Press.

WERTZ, RICHARD W., and WERTZ, DOROTHY C. 1977. *Lying-In: A History of Childbirth in America*. New York: Free Press.

WHITBECK, CAROLYN, ed. 1982. "Women and Medicine." *Journal of Medicine and Philosophy* 7, no. 2.

WILLIS, DAVID P., ed. 1989. *Health Policies and Black Americans*. New Brunswick, N.J.: Transaction.

WOLLSTONECRAFT, MARY. 1891. *Vindication of the Rights of Woman*. London: W. Scott.

YOUNG, IRIS MARION. 1990. *Justice and the Politics of Difference*. Princeton, N.J.: Princeton University Press.

FERTILITY CONTROL

I. MEDICAL ASPECTS

The ability of individuals to regulate their own childbearing represents one of the great medical advances of the twentieth century. As a result of demographic trends, which indicate an earlier onset of sexual activity and smaller family size, a woman may spend as long as thirty-five years purposefully avoiding pregnancy. An array of contraceptive methods is necessary to provide individuals with options that are most appropriate to their lifestyle, motivation, desire for effectiveness and convenience, and acceptance of medical risk. Two fundamental trends have affected contraceptive practice since 1960: the development of safe, continuous, and highly effective hormonal contraception, and more recently, an increased awareness of the role of barrier contraceptives for the dual purposes of pregnancy prevention and protection against sexually transmitted infections.

Currently available contraceptive methods include permanent methods that cause sterility—such as vasectomy in men and tubal occlusion in women—and reversible methods. Reversible methods include oral contraceptives (OCs); subdermal implants (Norplant®); progestin injections (depot-medroxyprogesterone acetate; DMPA; Depo-Provera®); intrauterine devices (IUDs); barrier methods (male and female condoms, diaphragm, cervical cap, and spermicidal products); and "natural" methods such as celibacy, periodic abstinence (natural family-planning and fertility-awareness methods), and withdrawal.

General considerations

It is unreasonable to assume that there is an ideal contraceptive method for each couple; more commonly, couples alternate among various methods over time. A number of general considerations can help to guide an individual (or couple) in the selection of an appropriate contraceptive method.

Frequency of sexual intercourse. Couples who have frequent intercourse (arbitrarily defined as more than two to three episodes of intercourse per week) should consider the more continuous, non-coitus-related methods of contraception: OCs, IUDs, implants, injectables, or if childbearing is completed, permanent sterilization. For less sexually active couples (those who have intercourse less than once per week), an episodic method, such as a barrier contraceptive, would provide protection without exposure to method-related risks at other times.

Number of sexual partners. Individuals who have multiple sexual partners, or whose partners have other partners, should be advised to consider one or more barrier methods, with the dual purposes of protection against sexually transmitted infections (STIs) and prevention of pregnancy. For couples who desire an optimal degree of pregnancy prevention, a combined approach of a barrier method plus a highly effective contraceptive will compensate for the relatively high pregnancy rate associated with barrier methods. Additionally, women in this category should not wear an IUD, as the risk of pelvic inflammatory disease (PID) and tubal infertility in IUD wearers is increased significantly in women with multiple sexual partners. For couples who are involved in a mutually monogamous relationship, no method of reversible contraception, including the IUD, increases the risk of PID or tubal infertility.

User acceptability. Personal attitudes regarding the acceptability of certain methods may influence the success of use. These include religious beliefs, which may preclude the use of "mechanical" and hormonal contraceptives; tolerance of "nuisance" side effects, such as breast changes and vaginal bleeding; willingness to touch the genitals (of self or partner); and aesthetic concerns, such as tolerance of the "messiness" of spermicidal creams and jellies.

Motivation and self-discipline. The degree of motivation to avoid pregnancy has a strong impact upon the successful use of contraceptives. Women who contracept to "delay" pregnancy have a higher failure rate than those who are intent on pregnancy prevention. Self-discipline also must be assessed, as women who are highly motivated may do well with intercourse-related (barrier) methods, while individuals who are poorly motivated should choose continuous non-intercourse-related methods such as OCs, IUDs, implantable or injectable methods, or sterilization.

Access to medical care. Because of the risk of medical complications, certain methods should be used only on the condition of reasonable access to medical care. This concern centers mainly on IUDs and to a lesser extent, hormonal methods. Users of barrier methods, natural methods, and those who have been successfully surgically sterilized have a negligible risk of life-threatening method-related complications.

Effectiveness. Desire for high effectiveness versus willingness to accept a degree of risk of failure is a primary concern for many contraceptors. Those who insist upon a high degree of efficacy are best advised to use a combination OC (discussed below), an IUD, an implantable or injectable method, or sterilization. Alternatively, for individuals who will accept a higher method failure rate, coupled with an understanding that such failures will result in a choice between delivery and abortion, less effective methods, including barriers and natural methods, may be used.

Safety. Medical safety is a major concern for most contraceptors, and concerns regarding health risks are a major reason for discontinuation of use. Paradoxically, adolescents are more likely to avoid or prematurely discontinue contraceptives for fear of adverse health effects, yet they comprise the age group least likely to experience them. The risks associated with contraceptive use are dependent on the following four variables, with an example of each:

1. *Age.* The risk of arterial complications (adverse effect on the heart and blood vessels, e.g., heart attack) of OCs is age-related; this risk is greatly compounded by cigarette smoking.
2. *Underlying medical conditions.* Women with underlying cardiovascular risk factors (e.g., hypertension, glucose intolerance, hyperlipidemia, cigarette use) are more likely to experience myocardial infarction (heart attack) while using OCs.
3. *Sexual behaviors.* A pattern of multiple sexual partners increases the risk of STIs. In particular, IUD wearers would have a greater risk of PID resulting in primary tubal infertility (fallopian tubes blocked by scar tissue).
4. *Method-specific risk.* Complications are intrinsic to the method, regardless of age, health, and sexual behaviors. Examples include the risk of hepatic adenomas (liver tumors that are noncancerous but that may hemorrhage) in OC users; and pelvic actinomycosis (infection) in long-term IUD users.

A key component of contraceptive efficacy and safety resides in the quality and clarity of instruction and counseling given to the user. Initial instruction should include a description of the methods of contraception currently available, their relative effectiveness, the advantages and disadvantages of each method, and, if appropriate, a comparison of short- and long-term costs. Once a method has been chosen, instruction should center on method-specific advice, such as information regarding method use and danger signals that should be reported to the provider. If the individual will be learning the use of a relatively complex method, or one with an increased likelihood of side effects, it is prudent to provide a simple backup contraceptive method, such as condoms, should the user decide to abandon the initial method. Method-specific counseling should be supplemented with a written fact sheet or other instructional material at a reading and comprehension level appropriate to the individual. Finally, the user should be encouraged to telephone or visit the office of the provider, as necessary, for further advice or modification of contraceptive use.

Oral contraceptives

The oral contraceptive (OC) is the method of reversible contraception used most widely in the United States. Two types are available: "combination" OCs, which contain fixed (monophasic) or variable (multiphasic) doses of synthetic estrogen and progestin, and progestin-only pills (POPs, mini pills). OCs primarily prevent pregnancy by preventing ovulation (release of an egg from the ovary). The estrogen and progestin in the pill exert negative feedback on the hypothalamus (the part of the brain that controls hormone production by the pituitary gland) to suppress the release of the hormone GnRH, which in turn decreases secretion of the pituitary hormones LH and FSH, preventing ovulation. OCs also thicken cervical mucus, which promotes an environment hostile to sperm and alters the endometrium (the lining of the uterus), so that implantation of an embryo is unlikely to occur even if an egg "breaks through" (is released) and is then fertilized. The failure rate of combined oral contraceptives when used correctly and consistently is 0.1 pregnancies per one hundred women per year. In typical use, the failure rate is three pregnancies per one hundred women per year.

Beneficial effects of OCs. *Prevention of pregnancy:* When used correctly, OCs are highly effective in preventing pregnancy. This includes ectopic pregnancies (those that implant outside the uterus), thus preventing an important cause of maternal morbidity and mortality. There is no increase in the rate of spontaneous abortion or fetal anomalies in former users of OCs, and no long-term reduction in fertility has been demonstrated.

Prevention of acute salpingitis (also called pelvic inflammatory disease, or PID): Even when controlled for sexual behavior and for the coincident use of barrier contraceptives, studies have shown that OC users have a decreased risk of acute salpingitis. It also appears that cases of salpingitis are less severe in OC users overall when compared to controls. Paradoxically, OC users seem to have a higher rate of chlamydial endocervicitis (an STI, with inflammation of the cervix, which may or may not progress to PID).

Prevention of genital tract cancers: Data from the Centers for Disease Control and Prevention's (CDCP) Cancer and Steroid Hormone (CASH) study show a 50 percent reduction in risk for the development of both endometrial and ovarian cancer. Past use of OCs appears to bestow this protective effect for as long as fifteen years after the user has discontinued OC use. The relationship of OCs and cervical dysplasia (abnormal cells of the cervix that, if not monitored, sometimes progress to cancer) and carcinoma is somewhat more complex because of confounding biases, but overall, OC use neither causes nor protects against cervical neoplasia (abnormal tissue formation).

Relief of menstrual symptoms: OCs provide excellent therapy for primary dysmenorrhea ("normal" painful or difficult menstruation that is not related to a disease) because they suppress the endometrium (the lining of the uterus). Consequently, the endometrium does not produce as much prostaglandin, the substance that produces cramping of the uterus. There is a more variable effect on premenstrual syndrome, in that while many women have a decrease in symptoms, others have no change, and a small percentage have worsening symptoms. Because of shorter and lighter menses, the incidence of iron deficiency anemia is reduced by 65 percent. There is also a reduced risk of toxic shock syndrome.

Reduced risk of benign breast disease: OC users have a significant reduction in the incidence of benign (noncancerous) breast conditions, including fibroadenoma and fibrocystic change.

Prevention and treatment of functional ovarian cysts: As a result of the pharmacologic suppression of GnRH release and consequent blunting of pituitary gonadotrophin release, women who use OCs are less likely to develop functional ovarian cysts than women who do not use hormonal contraception. This effect appears to be dose-related, and users of low-dose OC products have less protection than those using stronger formulations. If OCs are given in an attempt to suppress an existing ovarian cyst, it is necessary to utilize a relatively strong product (e.g., Ovral) in order to achieve an effective degree of hypothalamic/pituitary suppression.

Other beneficial effects: For reasons that are unclear, OC users also have a lower incidence of rheumatoid arthritis and peptic ulcer disease.

Adverse effects of OCs. The most common OC-related side effects are relatively minor. However, the patient may perceive them as major, and this may result in OC discontinuation and subsequent pregnancy. Effective management of minor or "nuisance" OC side effects consists mainly of patient education, and occasionally, medical intervention. Side effects include nausea, weight gain, spotting or breakthrough bleeding between menstrual periods, failure to have a menstrual period during the seven days off OCs, new onset or exacerbation of headaches, and chloasma (darkening of facial skin). Complications, while rare on low-dose combined oral contraceptives, can be serious.

Vascular complications: While initial studies indicated a direct relationship between estrogen dose and an increased risk of deep vein thrombosis (clotting) and pulmonary thromboembolism, more recent studies with low-estrogen-dose products have demonstrated only a minimally elevated attributable risk of these complications. For this reason, OC products containing thirty-five mcg of estrogen or less should be used routinely. In early studies of unselected women using relatively high-dose products, OC users also demonstrated an increased risk of myocardial infarction and stroke in comparison to controls. As a result of exclusion of women with major cardiovascular risk factors and a progressive trend toward the use of lower-dose products, OC users as a group no longer have an elevated attributable risk of OC-induced morbidity or mortality from arterial disease.

Hypertension: The estrogen and progestin components of OCs act in concert to occasionally cause the development of blood-pressure elevation in a small number of OC users. Hypertension is reversible with discontinuation of OCs.

Carbohydrate intolerance: The progestin component of OCs is known to cause peripheral glucose resistance and consequent elevation of insulin levels. In most cases, these effects are minor and are not clinically significant. If a diabetic woman is started on OCs, frequent blood glucose monitoring is necessary initially, as insulin requirements may change. OCs should not be given to diabetics who have clinically manifested vascular or kidney disease or to those with such cardiovascular risk factors as smoking, hypertension, hyperlipidemia (elevated fatty substances in the blood), or age over forty.

Breast cancer: The relationship between OC use and breast cancer has been studied extensively since the mid-1970s. In aggregate, the studies show that the relative risk of breast cancer in a present or former OC user is 1.0, implying neither protection nor increased risk. This relationship was present with a number of subgroups, including women who had initiated OCs at an early age, those who used OCs for longer than ten years, women with a history of benign breast disease, and those with a positive family history. However, a number of studies performed in the early 1980s demonstrated a possible association between OC use and breast cancer in other subgroups. The only thread of consistency in these studies was to show a small increase in the risk of breast cancer for recent OC users who developed breast cancer at an age younger than thirty-five. In that there seems to be a small reduction in breast cancers in past OC users older than thirty-five, it has been hypothesized that OCs, like pregnancy and exposure to other hormonal contraceptives, may be a weak breast cancer promoter, and that OCs may hasten the growth of a tumor already in existence.

DMPA

On October 29, 1992, the U.S. Food and Drug Administration (FDA) approved contraceptive labeling for depot-medroxyprogesterone (DMPA); commonly known by its trade name, Depo-Provera. This culminated a twenty-year effort to make a long-acting injectable contraceptive available to American women. Based upon the findings of extensive clinical research done outside the United States over a decade, the FDA determined that while some concerns remained, DMPA was considered to be as safe as other hormonal contraceptives already on the market.

DMPA's mechanism of action is quite similar to that of all other hormonal methods of contraception: inhibition of ovulation; thickening of cervical mucus, which makes sperm penetration through the cervical mucus more difficult; and induction of endometrial atrophy, which prevents implantation in the highly unlikely event of fertilization. The chemical structure of DMPA is much closer to that of natural progesterone than that of the 19-nortestosterone progestins used in oral contraceptives and Norplant. This may account for the fact that DMPA users have little, if any, change in a number of metabolic parameters over time. In particular, there is no change in clotting factors, globulin levels, or glucose metabolism in DMPA users when compared to pretreatment levels. The slight decrease in total cholesterol levels seen in DMPA users is the result of a minor drop in high-density lipoprotein, the "good" cholesterol, although neither change is clinically significant. Interestingly, DMPA positively affects the central nervous system, causing the seizure threshold to increase, thus making seizures less likely in women with seizure disorders (e.g., epilepsy). Estrogen levels in DMPA users remain at early follicular phase levels, and while other menopausal symptoms do not occur, there is a possibility that some DMPA users may lose a small amount of bone mass over time.

With DMPA there are 0.3 failures per one hundred women during the first year of typical use. This high efficacy is due both to DMPA's efficiency in inhibiting ovulation and the fact that it is a relatively "user friendly" method of contraception. The long interval between injections, a two-week grace period for injections given beyond twelve weeks, and the absence of need for any user or partner intervention at intercourse all contribute to DMPA's high effectiveness.

DMPA is given as a deep intramuscular injection into the deltoid (upper arm) or buttocks every twelve weeks. Since administration most optimally is provided with a 1½″ needle, most DMPA users, particularly thin women, will prefer the buttocks site. The initial injection of 150 mg of DMPA must be given within the first five days after the onset of menses, unless the woman has effectively been using the pill or has an IUD, in which case the first injection can be given any time during the month. Subsequent 150-mg injections are given at twelve-week intervals, although pregnancy is highly unlikely during the following two-week grace period. If fourteen weeks or more have elapsed since the last DMPA injection, a negative highly sensitive urine pregnancy test must be documented before the next injection is given.

The ideal candidate for DMPA is a woman who is seeking continuous contraception; wants long-term birth spacing; desires a method that is neither coitus-dependent nor requires daily motivation; or who cannot use, or chooses not to use, a barrier method, an IUD, or an estrogen-containing method. It may be particularly appropriate for women who cannot use OCs because of a history of thrombophlebitis, hypertension, heavy smoking, or other cardiovascular risk factors.

Women with sickle-cell anemia or seizure disorders actually may experience an improvement in their medical condition. DMPA is an excellent method for postpartum and post-abortal women and can be initiated immediately after completion of the pregnancy. Postpartum women who are lactating (nursing) should not be given DMPA until lactation has been established, usually one to two weeks after delivery. Women who desire a high degree of confidentiality in contraceptive use are attracted to DMPA because it does not require the personal possession of medications or devices, nor does it leave marks of administration or current use.

DMPA has few contraindications: active thrombophlebitis; undiagnosed abnormal genital bleeding; known or suspected pregnancy; active liver disease; a history of benign or malignant liver tumors; known or suspected carcinoma of the breast; and sensitivity (allergy) to the medication. Special conditions requiring more detailed medical evaluation and follow-up include a history of heart attack or stroke; diabetes mellitus; current migraine headaches; a history of severe endogenous depression; and chronic hypertension.

Menstrual changes are universal in women using DMPA and include episodes of irregular bleeding and spotting (lasting seven days or more during the first months of use) and amenorrhea (no menses). Sixty percent of women using DMPA for one year report amenorrhea, and the percentage increases with progressively longer use. Menstrual changes are the most frequent cause for dissatisfaction and discontinuation among women using DMPA, and appropriate patient education and selection and supportive follow-up measures can markedly reduce patient discontent. Medical intervention for irregular or heavy bleeding rarely is necessary, and anemia is uncommon. While counseling and reassurance are initial measures, medical therapy consisting of low-dose oral estrogen for one to three weeks may give temporary respite from bleeding. Women persistently dissatisfied may be better served by discontinuing this method and seeking alternative types of contraception rather than by repetitive medical or surgical intervention. In cases of heavy vaginal bleeding, gynecologic evaluation to rule out such unrelated conditions as vaginitis, cervicitis, or cervical lesions should be performed.

Another group of side effects that occur fairly frequently among DMPA users are pregnancy symptoms such as nausea, breast tenderness, abdominal bloating, and tiredness. While these symptoms are prevalent in the first few months of DMPA use, persistence is uncommon and they rarely are cause for discontinuation.

Weight gain occurs in two-thirds of DMPA users owing to the drug's anabolic effect and its resultant impact on appetite. On average, DMPA users gain four pounds per year for each of the first two years of use. Women concerned or dissatisfied with weight gain should be counseled that it may be controlled with adequate exercise and moderate dietary restriction. Many women notice weight stabilization or improvement with time. If these measures fail and weight gain becomes problematic, DMPA discontinuation may become necessary.

Headache is a relatively common complaint in DMPA users, although not all headaches are necessarily related to the hormone in the drug. If the headaches are mild and without neurologic changes, treatment may be attempted with oral analgesics.

After a 150-mg injection of DMPA, the mean interval until return of ovulation is four to six months. Conception usually is delayed in former DMPA users when compared with women discontinuing oral contraceptives or IUDs. The median time to pregnancy following the last injection is nine to ten months, and studies have shown that almost 70 percent of former DMPA users conceive within the first twelve months following discontinuation, and over 90 percent conceive by twenty-four months, a rate comparable to that of oral contraceptive users. Nulliparous women (those who have never given birth to a child) and those using DMPA for many years experience the same return of fertility as other women studied.

Recent medical studies have addressed other safety issues regarding DMPA use. A large study conducted by the World Health Organization (WHO) showed that in aggregate, there is no overall increased risk of breast, cervical, or ovarian cancers in users of DMPA. DMPA users have a reduction in endometrial cancer for as long as ten years after discontinuation of the method. While there was evidence of a weak association between DMPA use and breast cancer in the subgroup of women under thirty-five who had used the drug within the previous four years, most experts feel that this represents a very weak promoter effect at a level similar to OC use. A single study showed a 7 percent reduction in bone density in premenopausal DMPA users compared to controls, but it is not clear whether this is a true biologic effect caused by low estrogen levels or due to selection bias. Until more work is done in this area, some believe that it is prudent to screen potential DMPA users for osteoporosis risk factors and to provide additional counseling or evaluation for those with multiple risk factors.

Norplant

Norplant is a sustained-release contraceptive system that acts continuously for five years. It consists of six silicone rubber capsules, each the length and diameter of a matchstick, which are surgically implanted under the skin of the upper arm. The synthetic progestin Levonorgestrel, a hormone found in many oral contraceptives, is slowly released into the bloodstream, resulting in a constant hormone level. The contraceptive effect of Norplant is due primarily to inhibition of ovulation, although secondary mechanisms include thickening of cervical mucus, and formation of an atrophic endometrium. Although 20 percent of Norplant users ovulate in year one and up to 50 percent ovulate by year five of use, studies suggest that when ovulation does occur, it is defective and the ovum is not subject to fertilization. The cumulative pregnancy rate of Norplant users is 3.8 pregnancies per one hundred women over five years; the first-year failure rate is only 0.09 per hundred women per year. Ectopic (tubal) pregnancies are reduced by two-thirds in comparison to noncontracepting women, although should Norplant fail, there is a greater conditional probability (proportionate risk) that the pregnancy will be located in the fallopian tube rather than in the uterus.

Studies that have evaluated the metabolic effects of Norplant have found minimal impact. There is no effect on cholesterol or lipoprotein metabolism, glucose metabolism, or propensity to blood clotting. Norplant is an appropriate method of contraception for women who desire long-term contraception, who have completed childbearing but do not desire permanent sterilization and have had problems with other methods of contraception (including combined OCs), and for postpartum women, whether nursing or not.

The technique of insertion of Norplant involves anesthetizing the skin with local anesthetic and creation of a four-millimeter incision, followed by placement of a twelve-gauge trochar to insert the capsules in a fan-shaped pattern. The procedure takes less than ten minutes and is well tolerated by most women. The method should be inserted within five days of the onset of the menses and provides a contraceptive effect within twenty-four hours. More problematic is Norplant removal, which requires substantially more skill and takes between fifteen and forty minutes. The ease of removal is related to a number of factors, including the correctness of the initial Norplant insertion, the amount of fibrous tissue that has developed around the capsules, and the skill of the clinician.

The most prevalent adverse effect of Norplant is the unpredictability and irregularity of menstrual cycles, especially in the first year of use. Cycles may be shorter or longer than usual and associated with more or less bleeding; there may be bleeding between cycles, or no bleeding at all. Although there is no "cure" for irregular bleeding patterns, short-term palliation of the problem can be achieved by the use of low-dose oral estrogen therapy (e.g., ethinyl estradiol 20 mcg orally per day for two to three weeks). Other side effects include mild weight gain, headaches, hair loss, and new onset or exacerbation of depression.

Intrauterine devices (IUDs)

Although the IUD is used by only 1 to 2 percent of contracepting women in the United States, it is one of the most widely used methods worldwide. A popular method in the United States in the 1970s, IUD use dropped precipitously as a result of the high rate of pelvic infection and consequent tubal infertility experienced by women who used the Dalkon Shield IUD, which was removed from the market for this reason. Mainly because of business concerns related to the risk of product liability suits, manufacturers of most other IUDs voluntarily withdrew their devices over the next decade. The two IUDs currently available in the U.S. include a progesterone-releasing T-shaped IUD (Progestasert®), which must be exchanged yearly, and a copper-bearing T-shaped device called the Cu-T-380-A (ParaGard®), which exerts its contraceptive effect for eight years.

The IUD's mechanism of action is still a matter of conjecture. In copper IUDs, it is likely that copper ions released by the device have a toxic effect on sperm, rendering them incapable of fertilizing an ovum. Progesterone-releasing IUDs probably exert their contraceptive effect by converting the endometrium to a chronically atrophic state, preventing implantation of the zygote (fertilized egg). IUDs are known to be a relatively effective contraceptive, with failure rates in the range of 0.6 to 2.0 pregnancies per one hundred women per year. While many clinicians assume that the IUD increases a woman's risk of experiencing an ectopic (tubal) pregnancy, studies clearly show that users of progesterone-bearing IUDs have no increased risk of ectopic pregnancy when compared to nonusers of contraception, while users of copper IUDs experience profound protection.

Women best suited for the use of an intrauterine device are those who desire continuous contraception; who want long-term birth spacing or have completed their families but do not want to be sterilized; who require very high contraceptive efficacy; who desire a method that neither is coitus-dependent nor requires daily motivation; and who cannot use or choose not to use a barrier method or a hormonal method of contraception. IUD insertion and removal are simple office procedures that may result in temporary uterine cramping, but rarely require the use of local anesthesia or analgesia.

IUD use may result in relatively minor side effects such as heavy menstrual periods or cramping (less so with the progesterone-releasing type) and increased vaginal discharge. The relationship between IUD use and pelvic infection and consequent infertility has been studied in great detail. Early studies demonstrated that the major risk associations were recent insertion (within twenty days) and the type of IUD used (the Dalkon Shield bestowing the greatest risk). More recent studies have suggested that an IUD wearer's sexual behavior is the single most relevant risk factor for pelvic infection; a woman in a mutually monogamous sexual relationship has no increased risk of pelvic infection or tubal infertility ("blocked" or scarred tubes from PID) compared to the sexually active woman who uses no method. Conversely, women who have multiple concurrent sexual partners, or those who themselves are monogamous, but whose male partner has other sexual partners, appear to be at increased risk of IUD-associated pelvic infection.

In light of these considerations, contraindications to IUD use include the following:

- pelvic inflammatory disease within the past twelve months or recurrent PID (more than one episode in the past two years);
- post-abortal or postpartum endometritis or septic abortion in the past three months;
- known or suspected untreated endocervical gonorrhea, chlamydia, or mucopurulent cervicitis;
- undiagnosed abnormal vaginal bleeding;
- pregnancy or suspicion of pregnancy;
- history of impaired fertility in a woman who desires future pregnancy;
- known or suspected uterine or cervical malignancy;
- small uterine cavity;
- history of pelvic actinomycosis infection (not asymptomatic presence of the organism);
- known or suspected allergy to copper or, for copper IUD only, a history of Wilson's Disease (an inability to metabolize copper).

While young age may be associated with certain risky sexual behaviors, young age alone is not an absolute contraindication to IUD use. Correspondingly, a history of previous childbearing should not be an absolute prerequisite for IUD use. If a young woman is involved in a long-term mutually monogamous relationship and has no other risk factors, she may be considered a candidate for an IUD.

Barrier methods

Barrier methods include mechanical barriers such as male and female condoms, the female diaphragm and cervical cap, and chemical barriers such as spermicidal products. Nonprescription barrier contraceptives are an important contraceptive option because of their wide availability, relative ease of use, and acceptably high efficacy when used correctly and consistently. While the contraceptive efficacies of the various barrier methods when used alone are comparable to each other (typically about twenty pregnancies per one hundred women per year), their use in combination adds significantly to their effectiveness. In addition, male latex condoms and female vaginal sheaths, when used consistently and correctly, provide a high degree of protection against both the acquisition and the transmission of a number of sexually transmitted pathogens, including gonorrhea, chlamydia, syphilis, and some viral pathogens, including hepatitis B virus and HIV (human immunodeficiency virus), the virus that causes AIDS (acquired immunodeficiency syndrome). Spermicidal products, in addition to their contraceptive effect, have in vitro microbicidal properties and appear to provide some protection against gonorrhea and chlamydia. Nonprescription barrier contraceptives include male latex and animal membrane condoms; female polyurethane vaginal sheaths; the contraceptive sponge; and spermicidal films, foams, jellies, creams, and suppositories. Contraindications include allergy to latex rubber (in the case of male condoms, diaphragm, or cervical cap), a history of significant skin irritation with acute or chronic exposure to spermicides, and inability to understand instructions for use.

The contraceptive diaphragm is a dome-shaped latex device that serves as a mechanical barrier against the cervix and also holds a spermicidal preparation in place within the vagina. The diaphragm is one of the oldest barrier methods of the modern era, and has retained its popularity because of its nonhormonal nature, ease of use, and reasonable efficacy. It may be an appropriate method of contraception for women who prefer an intercourse-related nonhormonal method of contraception; desire a barrier method that can provide continuous protection over twenty-four hours; and feel that the diaphragm is less noticeable during intercourse than other barrier methods. The diaphragm should fit comfortably with the anterior (front) rim tucked behind the pubic bone in front and the posterior (back) rim seated deep in the vagina and behind the cervix, so that the cervix is covered by the dome of the diaphragm. The largest, most comfortable diaphragm that fits well should be chosen. Use of a backup method of contraception until the return visit, or until the patient is sure that the diaphragm is staying in place during intercourse, should be advised.

No attempt should be made to use the diaphragm if the woman cannot be fitted with the device due to physical characteristics of the vagina, cervix, or uterus that interfere with proper placement, or if the proper size diaphragm is not available. Other contraindications include a recent history of frequent lower urinary tract infections (e.g., cystitis), especially if associated with prior diaphragm use; less than three months since cervical surgery; less than two weeks since mid-trimester abortion or less than six weeks postpartum (after delivery of a child); allergy to rubber or to all spermicides; inability to understand instructions for use; and inability to insert, remove, and care for the device correctly.

The cervical cap is a thimble-shaped latex device that fits over the cervix and stays in place by mild suction. When used with a spermicide, it is a reliable barrier method of contraception that can be used continuously for up to forty-eight hours. In use in European countries since the 1930s, it was approved by the FDA for contraceptive use in the United States in 1988. The efficacy of the cervical cap in preventing pregnancy is similar to that of the diaphragm in nulliparous women, although the failure rate of the cap is greater in parous women.

The Prentif Cavity Rim Cervical Cap® is the only cap currently approved by the FDA. It is available in four sizes: 22-, 25-, 28-, and 31-mm internal diameter. Because cervix size may vary considerably, these sizes fit approximately 70–75 percent of women. The cap may be an appropriate choice for women who have experienced frequent urinary tract infections, especially if they occurred in association with the contraceptive diaphragm. Because there is less pressure on the urethra and bladder, the cap may be more comfortable than a diaphragm and less likely to predispose the user to a lower urinary tract infection.

Natural Methods

The most effective methods of fertility control are those in which sexual intercourse is avoided entirely. Abstinence is defined as a limited period of time in which intercourse is avoided, while celibacy refers to a lifestyle decision in which an individual chooses to avoid intercourse for a longer time interval, which may be lifelong in some cases.

Fertility awareness methods are those in which sexually active individuals avoid unprotected intercourse during the "fertile period," which is defined as the time in each cycle that ovulation is estimated to occur. Since the ovum survives for about 48 hours after ovulation and sperm can survive in the fallopian tubes for up to five days, the length of the fertile period is about seven days in most women. Couples who practice the fertility awareness method use a barrier method of contraception with intercourse during the fertile period and no method for the remainder of the cycle. In the "natural family planning" technique, a variant of fertility awareness, intercourse is avoided entirely during the fertile period and mechanical contraceptive methods are not used at any time in the cycle. The latter approach generally is endorsed by religious groups who object to the use of other birth-control methods, which they consider to be "artificial" in nature.

Four techniques, which can be used alone or in combination, are used to estimate the fertile period.

- The "calendar" method, in which previous menstrual cycling patterns are charted and from which future ovulatory patterns may be predicted. This method is comparatively inaccurate, as factors such as stress or illness can affect the time of ovulation and thereby shorten or lengthen a given cycle. In addition, many women have such variable cycle lengths that the estimated duration of the fertile period can be as long as two weeks.

- The "basal body charting" or "temperature" method, which is based upon the fact that a woman's basal temperature will increase by 0.5° to 1.0°F twelve to twenty-four hours after ovulation and will remain elevated until the next menstrual period. Women using this method are expected to check their temperature each morning upon arising until the temperature rise has been confirmed. Once two days have passed after the temperature rise, the fertile period is considered to be completed, and unprotected intercourse can resume until the next menstrual period.

- The "cervical mucus" method, also called the "Billings" or "ovulation" method, which relies upon the fact that a woman's cervical mucus becomes copious and watery in the few days before ovulation. The presence of characteristic mucus at the vaginal opening is a sign of impending ovulation and, hence, defines the existence of the fertile period.

- The "sympto-thermal" method uses a combination of two or more of the above techniques. The use of the cervical mucus to signal the beginning of the fertile period and the basal body temperature rise to predict its completion is the most accurate of the fertility awareness methods.

The effectiveness of the fertility awareness methods depends upon the couple's consistency of use and ability to avoid unprotected intercourse during the fertile period. When practiced correctly and consistently, the symptothermal method has a failure rate as low as two failures per one hundred women per year, while for the typical use failure rate for all methods of periodic abstinence is twenty pregnancies per one hundred women per year.

Sterilization

Voluntary surgical sterilization (VSS) is the most prevalent form of contraception in the United States; 60 percent of those surgically sterilized are women who have had tubal ligation, and 40 percent are men with vasectomies. Most couples who choose surgical sterilization have completed their families, although for some individuals this choice is prompted by an inability or unwillingness to use reversible methods of birth control. Criteria once used to determine the appropriateness of sterilization based on age and parity (number of children born) are no longer appropriate, and a woman's considered, informed decision should be respected by the provider, regardless of her age, parity, and social circumstances.

Tubal ligation. The most important point to be made in counseling a woman regarding tubal ligation is that the procedure must be considered permanent and should be performed only when she is sure that she desires no further children. Alternative (reversible) methods of birth control should be discussed to ensure that these methods have not been rejected on the basis of misunderstanding or other biases. Other important aspects of counseling include a description of the surgical risks of tubal ligation, failure rates, and a comparison to the various methods of sterilization available, including vasectomy for the woman's partner. If consent cannot be obtained from a severely mentally disabled woman, a legal guardian may provide consent in some cases.

Both the federal government and individual states have regulations regarding minimum age requirements and waiting periods from the time of written consent until the date that the operation may be performed if federal or state funding is to be used. For this reason, women who plan to undergo postpartum tubal ligation should receive counseling and consent before thirty-four weeks gestation.

The surgical approach to tubal ligation is primarily dependent upon whether the procedure is performed in the postpartum period, or longer than six weeks after delivery, in which case it is considered to be an interval tubal ligation. In a postpartum tubal ligation, a minilaparotomy performed within four to twenty-four hours of delivery is the preferred approach subsequent to a vaginal delivery. After receiving a regional or general anesthetic, a three-centimeter curvilinear or vertical incision is made immediately under the umbilicus. Once the peritoneal cavity has been entered, either the operator's finger can be used to sweep each tube into the incision or each tube can be grasped under direct vision. In either case, positive identification of the tube can be made by visualizing the fringelike portion at the abdominal end of each tube and by demonstrating that the nearby round ligament is uninvolved. After completion of the tubal occlusion, each excised tubal fragment must be sent for histological confirmation. In a woman delivered by cesarean section, any of the three techniques described below can be performed after repair of the uterine incision has been completed.

A number of techniques are available when there is direct access to the fallopian tubes via minilaparotomy or cesarean section. They include the following methods:

- modified Pomeroy method, in which two ligatures (sutures, "ties") are placed in the mid-portion of each of the tubes and then the pieces of tube between the ligatures are removed. The closed ends retract, leaving a gap between the closed-off tubal segments.
- Irving method, whereby the tubal stump nearest the uterus is tucked into a tunnel made in the myometrium (muscular structure) of the large upper part of the uterus.

- Uchida method, which involves excision of a five-centimeter segment of tube, followed by burying the tubal stump farthest from the uterus within the mesosalpinx (the free margin of the upper part of the broad ligament).

While the failure rates of the Irving and Uchida techniques are exceedingly low (less than 1/1,000) in comparison to the Pomeroy method (1/250), the former take longer to perform and therefore are relegated to special cases.

Interval tubal ligation may be performed with a laparoscope (a narrow lighted tube) via a low minilaparotomy incision (a small horizontal incision, 2–5 cm long, just above the pubic hairline), the former being much more prevalent in the United States. Laparoscopic approaches ("band-aid" surgery) include either open or closed laparoscopy, and both one- and two-puncture instruments (laparoscopes) are available. While a large majority of laparoscopic tubal ligations are performed under general anesthesia, there is a growing trend to perform these procedures under local anesthesia, thereby reducing cost and avoiding the risk of general anesthetic complications, which is the most common cause of tubal ligation deaths. If local anesthesia is used, the tubes must be bathed in a long-acting local anesthetic, then banded or clipped, rather than electrocoagulated (coagulation or clotting of tissue using a high-frequency electric current).

Minilaparotomy for interval tubal ligation is performed via a three-centimeter low horizontal incision. Because of the difficulty entailed in working through a small incision, the procedure is facilitated by using a uterine elevator, an instrument placed in the vagina to lift the uterus. The procedure may be performed with general, regional, or local anesthesia. Minilaparotomy is contraindicated when the patient is obese, has an enlarged or immobile uterus, or when adnexal disease (in the areas adjacent to the uterus, e.g., ovaries and tubes) such as endometriosis is suspected. Nonetheless, minilaparotomy can be a safer, simpler, and less expensive procedure than laparoscopy, which requires more technical equipment and endoscopy experience.

If minilaparotomy is chosen, any of the occlusion techniques outlined above for postpartum tubal ligation may be used. In addition, spring-loaded tubal clips are available that can be easily applied through a minilaparotomy incision. With the laparoscopic approach, three methods of tubal occlusion are available:

- Electrocautery, with a coagulation or "blend" current, used at two or three sites along the mid-fallopian tube. Either unipolar or bipolar cautery may be used; while bipolar cautery is safer (since it is less prone to cause bowel burns), it takes longer and has a higher failure rate. Unipolar electrocautery is faster and more effective, but there is a risk of sparking between the electrode and the bowel, resulting in an unrecognized injury. Fallopian tubes occluded by electrocautery may be quite difficult to reanastomose (reconnect, in the event the woman changes her mind and wants to try to achieve pregnancy) because of extensive scarring.

• Silastic (silicone rubber) rings may be applied with a forceps-type applicator to a loop of mid-portion fallopian tube. This approach avoids the risk of electrical injury to the bowel and preserves much larger segments of healthy ends of the severed fallopian tube should later reversal be considered.

• Spring-loaded clips may be placed at a single site in the middle of the tube and can be used with double-puncture laparoscopy or at minilaparotomy.

The provider must explain that with tubal interruption alone, no organ is removed; tubal sterilization merely prevents conception. The operation is not "desexing" and will not reduce libido, vary the woman's menses, or alter her appearance. There is usually no adverse change in sexual function following tubal sterilization; on the contrary, many women who feared pregnancy before the operation report increased satisfaction in sexual intercourse and are pleased with the operative result. However, 2 to 5 percent report less frequent orgasm and a similar percentage have delayed regret that the procedure was performed.

Only hypophysectomy (excision of the pituitary gland), bilateral oophorectomy (removal of both ovaries), and ovarian damage by radiation are certain methods of sterilization. Abdominal and tubal pregnancies have occurred (rarely) even after total hysterectomy (removal of the uterus). Oophorectomy and sterilization by radiation are usually followed within four weeks by vasomotor reactions (symptoms associated with menopause such as "hot flashes") and a gradual diminution in libido or sexual satisfaction during the next six months.

Vasectomy.   Sterilization of the man by vasectomy is both less dangerous and less expensive than tubal ligation, as it is routinely performed as an office procedure under local anesthesia. Through one or two small incisions in the scrotum, the vas deferens (the tube or duct that carries sperm) is isolated and occluded and usually a small segment of each vas is removed. Neither physiologic impotence nor changes in libido result from the procedure. Sterility cannot be assumed until postoperative ejaculates are found to be completely free of sperm. Failure of the vasectomy, as manifested by pregnancy in a partner, occurs in 0.1 percent of patients. Medical risks of vasectomy include hematoma (blood clot or bruise) formation, epididymitis (congestion or inflammation of the epididymis, the coiled tubular structure where sperm cells mature), spontaneous recanalization of the vas (reconnection of the ends with restored patency) (incidence of less than 1 percent), and the development of a spermatocele (cystic nodule containing sperm). Atrophy of the testes very rarely results from ligation of excessive vasculature (blood supply). Vasectomy often is reversible—up to 90 percent in some reports—but requires expensive microsurgery and special skill with no guarantee of success. Pregnancy results in only about 60 percent of cases after reversal; factors that influence success include (but are not limited to) the surgeon's skill, the type of procedure used, and time interval since vasectomy.

MICHAEL POLICAR

Directly related to this article are the other articles in this entry: SOCIAL ISSUES, ETHICAL ISSUES, *and* LEGAL AND REGULATORY ISSUES. *Also directly related are the entries* POPULATION POLICIES; POPULATION ETHICS, *especially the article on* NORMATIVE APPROACHES; *and* WOMEN, *article on* HEALTH-CARE ISSUES. *Other relevant material may be found under the entries* ABORTION, *article on* MEDICAL PERSPECTIVES; EUGENICS, *article on* ETHICAL ISSUES; FETUS, *article on* HUMAN DEVELOPMENT FROM FERTILIZATION TO BIRTH; FEMINISM; FREEDOM AND COERCION; INTERNATIONAL HEALTH; REPRODUCTIVE TECHNOLOGIES; *and* SEXISM.

Bibliography

BERMAN, S. M. 1991. "Fertility Control and HIV Infection." *Archives of AIDS Research* 5, nos. 1–2:25–28.

CHICA, M. D., and BARRANCO, E. 1994. "Fertility Control by Natural Methods: Analysis of 218 Cycles." *Advances in Contraception* 10, no. 1:33–36.

HATCHER, ROBERT A., ed. 1994. *Contraceptive Technology.* 16th rev. ed. New York: Irvington.

JUDKINS, DAVID R. 1991. *National Survey of Family Growth: Design, Estimation, and Inference.* Hyattsville, Md.: U.S. Department of Health and Human Services, Public Health Service, National Center for Health Statistics.

KUBBA, ALI. 1991. "New Thinking in Contraception." *Practitioner* 235, no. 1508:878–882.

ROBERTSON, WILLIAM H. 1990. *An Illustrated History of Contraception: A Concise Account of the Quest for Fertility Control.* Park Ridge, N.J.: Parthenon.

SLAWSON, DAVID C., and SHAUGHNESSY, ALLEN F. 1994. "Norplant vs. Oral Contraceptives." *Journal of Family Practice.* 38, no. 6:631–632.

STEDMAN, THOMAS LATHROP. 1990. *Stedman's Medical Dictionary.* 25th ed. Baltimore, Md.: Williams and Wilkins.

WEBB, ANNE. 1994. Long-Term Contraception: Assessing the Alternatives—Norplant and IUDs." *British Journal of Sexual Medicine* 21, no. 2:12–14.

II. SOCIAL ISSUES

The status of birth-control, sterilization, and abortion services in the United States has always been linked to the various social movements that have been engaged with issues of reproduction and sexuality. Since the nineteenth century, different groups have advocated for and against family planning (used here to refer to both birth control and abortion) for different reasons, and with differing levels of success.

While issues pertaining to reproductive control have always caused some degree of social conflict, this has been especially true since the mid-1970s, when the polarization over the abortion issue became intense and spread to other reproductive health services (e.g., contraception and sex education). The emergence of AIDS and rising rates of sexually transmitted diseases (STDs) have also contributed to the controversy surrounding family planning in the United States in the late twentieth century. This article discusses various groups that claim a stake to "ownership" (Gusfield, 1981) of family-planning issues, indicates some of the specialized populations that require family-planning services, and speculates briefly about the uncertain future of birth-control and abortion services in the United States. Finally, the article touches on debates on family planning that are taking place in the developing world.

Interest groups and family planning

Providers of family-planning services. Family-planning services in the United States are offered by both private and public agencies. Public providers of family-planning services at the local level include public-health clinics in hospitals or neighborhood health centers, which often provide birth-control services along with other primary health services, and hospital-based clinics, which often specialize in family-planning delivery. At the county, state, regional, and national levels, various arms of government are involved with the setting of policy for these publicly supported clinics and in devising formulas to disburse funding. The major conduit for public funding of family-planning services is Title X of the Public Health Act of 1970. Title X has never allowed funding for abortion services.

In the private sector, abortion and birth-control services are offered both by for-profit and not-for-profit clinics, and by private physicians. The not-for-profit Planned Parenthood Federation of America, Inc., with some 170 affiliates across the country in the 1990s, has been the most important provider of family-planning services in the private sector.

In theory, the public and private components of the family-planning delivery system share similar goals: the dissemination of contraceptive services and education under a public-health model, with the prevention of AIDS and sexually transmitted diseases a more recent addition to the previous agenda of fertility control. Yet the relationship between the private and the public components is quite complicated for two reasons. First, family-planning services, like other publicly provided social services in the United States, are typically delivered through a system that relies at least partly on private agencies, or "subcontractors," rather than directly by the government itself.

Second, the intense politicization of family-planning issues since the 1980 election of President Ronald Reagan has meant that often the agendas of public and private providers of family-planning services have been very much at odds. Title X—the major federal program for the provision of family-planning services—illustrates these contradictions. A significant proportion of Title X-funded services in many communities across the country is provided by Planned Parenthood, which is also a prime target of those who can be called "sexual conservatives" (see "Pro-Family Movement" below), because of the organization's visibility as an abortion provider. Political appointees within the U.S. Department of Health and Human Services, which oversees Title X and related services, have, at times, been aligned with political groups committed to the defunding of this program, because of some conservatives' opposition to birth-control programs. Between 1980 and 1990, the number of publicly funded family-planning clinics across the country declined 20 percent, from 5,000 to 4,000 clinics (Ettinger, 1992; Scott, 1991); this decline reflects the bitter ideological wrangling over the concept of publicly funded family planning.

The women's movement. Since the reemergence of a visible women's movement in the United States in the late 1960s—the "second wave" of feminism—various groups associated with the movement have been forceful advocates for family-planning services, and particularly for abortion services. (Indeed, a significant difference between first- and second-wave feminists was the willingness of the latter to engage in issues of reproduction rights and sexuality [Joffe, 1986]). For example, the campaign to make abortion legal and accessible was a major focus of the feminist movement at the time of its reemergence in the late 1960s. During the 1980s, when legal abortion became threatened, women's organizations such as the National Organization for Women (NOW) played a highly visible role in pro-choice activities, and worked closely with such organizations as Planned Parenthood and the National Abortion Rights Action League (NARAL). Similarly, the National Women's Health Network and the Federation of Feminist Health Centers represent specialized interest groups within the larger women's movement that have focused on reproductive issues.

With respect to other reproductive issues, however, the relation of sectors of the women's movement to its abortion allies has been more complex. At times, the responses of some feminist health activists to prevailing contraceptive practices and new contraceptive innovations have conflicted with sometime allies, such as Planned Parenthood. These activists, for example, raised doubts early on about the safety of oral contraception ("birth-control" pills); objected to testing new contraceptive technologies on women in developing nations (Seaman, 1969; Gordon, 1976); and more recently, voiced reservations about the likely social abuses of Norplant, a contraceptive implant.

The pro-family movement. Beginning in the 1970s, a movement of sexual conservatism—the "pro-family" movement—became a significant presence in family-planning politics (Petchesky, 1990; McKeegan, 1992). In broadest terms, this movement's main concern has been the breakdown of sexual morality in contemporary society, as evidenced by high rates of abortion, teenage pregnancy, out-of-wedlock births, and STDs. For sexual conservatives, widely available family-planning services—especially those supported by public funds—represent a temptation to break with traditional morality (Marshner, 1982). Though the pro-family movement is most visible in antiabortion activity, its interests and interventions extend to a broad range of reproductive and sexual matters—contraceptive services, sex education, teenage pregnancy prevention efforts, AIDS prevention services, and so forth (Joffe, 1986; Nathanson, 1991). Among the specific organizations affiliated with the pro-family movement that have engaged politically with family-planning issues are the Family Research Council, the Eagle Forum, the Moral Majority, the Concerned Women of America, and the Religious Roundtable. Some antiabortion groups, such as the American Life League, have recorded strong opposition to publicly funded birth-control programs.

Family-planning services for teenagers have been a major focal point of pro-family activity (Joffe, 1993). Conservative activists have persuaded legislators in a number of states to adopt parental notification and consent rules for teenagers seeking abortions, and have sought regulations that would include parental notification policies for federally funded clinics providing contraceptive services. Perhaps the key achievement of the pro-family movement has been the promotion of sexual abstinence as a major public-policy response to teenage pregnancy. One of the earliest and most controversial policy initiatives of pro-family political appointees was the establishment of so-called chastity centers. These centers, aimed at teenage females, focused exclusively on abstinence, and were forbidden by statute from mentioning abortion as an option in an unwanted pregnancy (Nathanson, 1991). Similarly, the Sex Respect curriculum, a sex-education program widely promoted by pro-family forces, contained no mention of birth control or abortion, focusing instead on abstinence.

The "gag-rule" controversy, which spanned the presidencies of Ronald Reagan and George Bush, is further illustration of the efforts of conservatives to link attacks on abortion and birth-control issues. Originally written as an administrative guideline during the Reagan administration, the gag rule forbade employees in Title X family-planning clinics to provide counseling about abortion options, even when clients asked. For many within the health-care community and the public at large, this ruling raised concerns about free speech for health professionals. In the space of several years, the gag rule was upheld by the Supreme Court and overturned by congressional legislation, which was promptly vetoed by then-President Bush, under intense pressure from conservatives. In one of his first acts after taking office in 1993, President Bill Clinton abolished the gag rule, under similar pressure from the pro-choice and family-planning communities.

Welfare conservatives. An interesting split within conservatism became increasingly evident in the early 1990s, with potentially profound implications for reproductive politics. "Welfare conservatives" differ from conservatives in the pro-family movement in arguing economic issues, especially issues of public spending (Nathanson, 1991). In contrast to the pro-family movement, whose defining issue is the breakdown of sexual morality, welfare conservatives are concerned about the rising welfare costs resulting from teenage pregnancies, out-of-wedlock births, and failure of fathers to make child-support payments. Welfare conservatives have made a number of policy proposals that either mandate use of contraception as a condition of receiving welfare or offer financial incentives for such contraceptive use, that penalize recipients financially for having additional children, and that forbid teenage mothers from receiving welfare assistance directly, providing instead that the grant go to their parents or guardians (Peirce, 1992).

The contraceptive implant, Norplant, introduced into the United States in late 1990, quickly became implicated in a number of policies advocated by welfare conservatives. Once inserted, the implant prevents pregnancy for up to five years. Both the insertion and the removal must be done by a health-care professional. After the patient has submitted to the insertion, no further "user compliance" is required, making this contraception far more effective than other birth-control methods. Within eighteen months of the introduction into the United States of this new method, virtually all states approved the public funding of Norplant insertion for welfare recipients. The potential for coercion is evident. Already, there have been instances where judges have required Norplant use as a condition of probation or child custody for women convicted on drug-related charges or of child abuse (Forrest and Kaeser, 1993).

Minority communities.   Minority communities in the United States—most notably, African-Americans and Hispanics—have long had a wary relationship with family-planning services. The historical links between the first generation of "birth controllers," such as Margaret Sanger, and those in the eugenics movement with an avowedly racist ideology (Chesler, 1992; Gordon, 1976) created for many minorities a lasting sense of distrust as to the intentions of some within the family-planning movement (Gordon, 1976). Such distrust reached a height in the late 1960s and early 1970s when many of the new government-funded clinics appeared to be targeted specifically at African-Americans, leading some African-American leaders to accuse family planners of "genocidal" intentions (Littlewood, 1977). More recently, some leaders—most notably, clergy—within minority communities have joined forces with the pro-family movement, arguing against such measures as condom distribution in inner-city high schools.

At the same time, the rates of premarital sexual activity, STDs, teenage pregnancy, and abortion have been disproportionately higher for African-Americans and Hispanics than for others. Thus, a number of minority organizations argue forcefully for the retention and expansion of family-planning and abortion services in their communities. Perhaps the most prominent example of such minority advocacy for family planning has been the teenage pregnancy initiative of the Children's Defense Fund. Other relevant minority groups in this regard include the National Black Women's Health Project and Latinas for Choice.

Services to specialized populations

Teenagers.   In the early 1990s, teenagers were entitled to receive low-cost or free confidential contraceptive services at Title X sites. Teenagers as a class did not receive any public funds for abortion.

The rising rates of sexual activity among teenagers (Alan Guttmacher Institute, 1991), particularly among younger teens, increased concern within the family-planning community about teenage pregnancy and this group's vulnerability to AIDS and STDs. Starting in the 1980s, a major response to both these issues was the establishment of school-based clinics (Kirby et al., 1991), on the theory that while few teens would make their way to a free-standing clinic, clinics located within the school would reach a much larger public. Predictably, such school-based clinics were controversial from the start, strongly opposed by conservatives, and just as strongly advocated by health professionals who feared an epidemic of STDs among teenagers if such preventive measures were not taken. The movement to establish school-based clinics proceeded very slowly.

A number of school districts, particularly those in large urban areas, began distributing condoms to students in response to the AIDS crisis. Here, too, there has been massive controversy, with many parent and church groups opposing such efforts. Generally speaking, however, AIDS-related interventions in schools seemed more acceptable to the public and to educators than specific efforts for pregnancy prevention. A national study of sex education in U.S. schools in the late 1980s found far more attention paid to AIDS and STDs than to contraceptive education (Forrest and Silverman, 1989).

Services to the disabled.   Case law in the United States generally recognizes that developmentally disabled individuals have the same fundamental rights regarding procreative choice as nondisabled individuals. There are, however, difficulties in implementing family-planning services for disabled persons. The issue of informed consent—to birth control, abortion, or sterilization, for example—is particularly relevant. Is the individual in question capable of giving informed consent, and if not, who is the appropriate surrogate empowered to make such decisions (Stavis, 1991)?

In spite of legal decisions supporting provision of such services, relatively few disabled persons are served in Title X clinics (Moore and Lieber, 1988). Few clinic staffs have received the specialized training necessary to work effectively with this population. In addition, many caretakers, especially parents, seem reluctant to ensure that these individuals receive such services. Finally, would-be recipients and caretakers alike are typically not aware of the entitlement of the disabled to family planning, which implies a need for more outreach services to this population.

The future of fertility control

The future of family-planning services in the United States is unclear. The presidential election of Bill Clinton in 1992, in certain significant respects, muted the influence of conservatives in public-policy debates about family-planning issues. Clinton's appointments to key health-policy positions of individuals strongly committed to family planning, especially in the area of teenage pregnancy prevention, sharply reversed the trends of the Reagan-Bush era. Ideological battles may be temporarily muted, but they will not disappear entirely because of a change in presidential administration. At the state and local levels, many of the bitter struggles over the public provision of reproductive health services will continue. And given the salience of sexuality-related issues in U.S. political culture, future Republican presidential victories very likely will imply a return to some of the policies that characterized the Reagan-Bush era.

The major—and, at the time of this writing, unknown—factor in the status of these services in the near future will be the ultimate character of health-reform efforts initiated by the Clinton administration. Early drafts of this proposed reform speak of coverage of "pregnancy-related services," but it is not clear what precisely will be made available under this plan. The abortion issue, of course, is among the most politically explosive items in this category, and many observers feel that disagreements about the inclusion of abortion have the potential to jeopardize the entire health-care-reform effort.

Beyond abortion, however, there are other important, as yet unanswered, questions. The Norplant insert, for example, when introduced in 1991, cost patients over $500, thus making this method accessible only to high-income women or those women whose incomes were low enough to qualify for Medicaid (Forrest and Kaeser, 1993). Thus it is not clear that all American women will have access to all contraceptive methods or to the more expensive fertility treatments, such as in vitro fertilization, under the new health measure. Generally speaking, however, we can assume that health-care reform will bring greater access to a broad range of family-planning services.

International issues

The highly politicized nature of family planning in the United States has had implications for the developing world. The Reagan-Bush era gave legitimacy to previously discredited theories of the relationship between population growth and economic growth, which argued the two were not incompatible. In response to pressures by conservatives, the emphasis of U.S. population programs abroad shifted heavily to programs promoting "natural family planning," rather than the more medically reliable methods of birth control, such as oral contraception. Most notably, the "Mexico City policy" adopted by the Reagan administration in 1984 stipulated that no U.S. aid would go to any international organizations that supported abortion, even if the U.S. funds were separated and used only for nonabortion purposes (McKeegan, 1992). The Mexico City policy was overturned in the early days of the Clinton administration in 1993, thus renewing a commitment on the part of the United States to international family-planning efforts, after a period of marked decline.

Family-planning issues appear increasingly to be a high priority for many developing nations. Concerns about the ability to feed fast-growing populations, the dramatic spread of AIDS in the Third World, especially in parts of Africa, and the estimated 200,000 to 250,000 deaths that occur each year from illegal abortions (United Nations, 1991) create constituencies for family-planning services within these countries—notwithstanding significant religious and cultural objections.

Finally, the rise of indigenous women's movements within the developing world has served as a particularly important stimulus for both additional family-planning services and the demand that such services be offered in a culturally appropriate manner (Bruce, 1987; Dixon-Mueller, 1993). The International Women's Health Coalition has been one of the most successful international population groups in terms of its ability to work closely with local, grass roots women's organizations in the design and delivery of family-planning programs.

CAROLE JOFFE

Directly related to this article are the other articles in this entry: MEDICAL ASPECTS, ETHICAL ISSUES, *and* LEGAL AND REGULATORY ISSUES. *Also directly related are the entries* ABORTION, *section on* CONTEMPORARY ETHICAL AND LEGAL ASPECTS; *and* POPULATION POLICIES. *For further discussion of topics mentioned in this article, see the entries* ADOLESCENTS; AIDS, *article on* PUBLIC-HEALTH ISSUES; ECONOMIC CONCEPTS IN HEALTH CARE; EUGENICS; FEMINISM; FREEDOM AND COERCION; HEALTH POLICY, *article on* POLITICS AND HEALTH CARE; INFORMED CONSENT, *article on* LEGAL AND ETHICAL ISSUES OF CONSENT IN HEALTH CARE (*with its* POSTSCRIPT); PUBLIC POLICY AND BIOETHICS; SEXUAL ETHICS; SEXUALITY IN SOCIETY; *and* WOMEN, *article on* HEALTH-CARE ISSUES. *Other relevant material may be found under the entries* HEALTH PROMOTION AND HEALTH EDUCATION; LIFESTYLES AND PUBLIC HEALTH; MARRIAGE AND OTHER DOMESTIC PARTNERSHIPS; PATERNALISM; PRIVACY IN HEALTH CARE; PUBLIC HEALTH, *article on* PHILOSOPHY OF PUBLIC HEALTH; *and* VALUE AND VALUATION.

Bibliography

ALAN GUTTMACHER INSTITUTE. 1991. *Facts in Brief: Teenage Sexual and Reproductive Behavior in the United States.* New York: Author.

BRUCE, JUDITH. 1987. "Users' Perspectives on Contraceptive Technology and Delivery Systems: Highlighting Some Feminist Issues." *Technology and Society* 9, nos. 3–4: 359–383.

CHESLER, ELLEN. 1992. *Woman of Valor: Margaret Sanger and the Birth Control Movement in America.* New York: Simon and Schuster.

DIXON-MUELLER, RUTH. 1993. *Population Policy and Women's Rights: Transforming Reproductive Choice.* Westport, Conn.: Praeger.

FORREST, JACQUELINE D., and KAESER, LISA. 1993. "Questions of Balance: Issues Emerging from the Introduction of the Hormonal Implant." *Family Planning Perspectives* 25, no. 3:127–132.

FORREST, JACQUELINE D., and SILVERMAN, JANE. 1989. "What Public School Teachers Teach About Preventing Pregnancy, AIDS, and Sexually Transmitted Diseases." *Family Planning Perspectives* 21, no. 2:65–72.

GORDON, LINDA. 1976. *Women's Body, Women's Right: A Social History of Birth Control in America.* New York: Grossman.

GUSFIELD, JOSEPH R. 1981. *The Culture of Public Problems: Drinking–Driving and the Symbolic Order.* Chicago: University of Chicago Press.

JOFFE, CAROLE E. 1986. *The Regulation of Sexuality: Experiences of Family Planning Workers.* Philadelphia: Temple University Press.

————. 1993. "Sexual Politics and the Teenage Pregnancy Prevention Worker in the United States." In *The Politics of Pregnancy,* pp. 289–300. Edited by Annette Lawson and Deborah L. Rhode. New Haven, Conn.: Yale University Press.

KIRBY, DOUGLAS; WASZAK, CYNTHIA; and ZIEGLER, JULIE. 1991. "Six School-Based Clinics: Their Reproductive Health Services and Impact on Sexual Behavior." *Family Planning Perspectives* 23, no. 1:6–16.

LITTLEWOOD, THOMAS B. 1977. *The Politics of Population Control.* Notre Dame, Ind.: University of Notre Dame Press.

MARSHNER, CONNAUGHT C. 1982. *The New Traditional Woman.* Washington, D.C.: Free Congress Research and Education Foundation.

MCKEEGAN, MICHELE. 1992. *Abortion Politics: Mutiny in the Ranks of the Right.* New York: Free Press.

MOORE, MELINDA, and LIEBER, CAROLYN. 1988. *Assessing Reproductive Health-Care Services: An Assessment of Service Availability to Learning and Developmentally Disabled Individuals Through Title X-Funded Clinics.* Washington, D.C.: Polaris Research and Development.

NATHANSON, CONSTANCE A. 1991. *Dangerous Passage: The Social Control of Sexuality in Women's Adolescence.* Philadelphia: Temple University Press.

NATIONAL ABORTION FEDERATION. 1990. *Who Will Provide Abortions? Report of a National Symposium.* Washington, D.C.: Author.

PEIRCE, NEAL. 1992. "Cold Approaches to a Hot-Button Issue." *National Journal* 24, no. 15:890.

PETCHESKY, ROSALIND P. 1990. *Abortion and Woman's Choice: The State, Sexuality, and Reproductive Freedom.* Rev. ed. Boston: Northeastern University Press.

SCOTT, JENNY. 1991. "Public Funding for Family Planning Drops." *Los Angeles Times,* September 27, p. A33.

SEAMAN, BARBARA. 1969. *The Doctor's Case Against the Pill.* New York: Avon.

STAVIS, PAUL F. 1991. "Harmonizing the Right to Sexual Expression and the Right to Protection from Harm for Persons with Mental Disability." *Sexuality and Disability* 9, no. 2:131–141.

UNITED NATIONS. 1991. *The World's Women, 1970–1990: Trends and Statistics.* New York: Author.

III. ETHICAL ISSUES

Fertility control gives people the power and the means to limit and prevent the procreative aspects of human sexuality. Terminology prior to the mid-twentieth century often referred to birth control and family planning to describe the same basic reality. This article deals with the three means of fertility control most often used—contraception, sterilization, and abortion. Technological developments and contemporary theories blur the absolute distinction among these three means, but ethical perspectives both in the past and in the present recognize important differences among them.

Contraception

Contraception, in the strict sense, interferes with the sexual act in order to prevent conception. In the broad sense, contraception includes all the means that can be used to prevent conception, including sterilization, which interferes with the sexual faculty or power. A close, logical connection exists between the ethical evaluation of contraception and of contraceptive sterilization. Judgments about the morality of contraception have traditionally distinguished between contraception within marriage and contraception outside marriage, based on the moral principle, often challenged today, that condemns sexual relations outside marriage.

Contraception within marriage. Most people today, along with philosophical ethicists, religious ethicists, and religious bodies, generally accept the morality of contraception within marriage, often appealing to the need for family planning. Most recognize a relationship between marital sexuality and procreation, but marital sexuality also has other significant purposes such as expressing and enhancing the love union of the partners and thereby the good of the marriage. Unlimited procreation, or at times any procreation, could be harmful to one of the spouses, the marriage relationship itself, the good of already existing children, or the needs of the broader society. No perfect contraception exists, but most ethical reasoning sees no significant moral differences among the various means, provided they are not harmful to the individuals who use them or to others. Logically, one could justify contraception on the basis of an absolute autonomy, giving the individual control over his or her body and the right to make all decisions concerning it; but most justifications of family planning, which by definition concerns more than the individual, avoid such a radical individual autonomy. The official teaching of the Roman Catholic church constitutes the strongest and the primary contemporary moral opposition to the use of contraception for spouses.

The widespread moral acceptance of contraception has taken place well within the twentieth century. Individuals do not make moral judgments in the abstract but in the concrete situation. A number of very significant social factors have influenced the near-unanimous acceptance of contraceptive practices within marriage: the increased life expectancy of all human beings; the massive improvements in infant and child health care; the realities of an increasingly urban and industrialized society; the changing role and function of women in society; the wider and more accurate understanding of the physiology of human reproduction; the recognition of the population explosion and the need to limit population; and the development, ready availability, and active promotion of newer, more effective forms of contraception.

The Christian religion played a most significant role in the ethical approach to contraception in the West. John T. Noonan's writings (1978, 1986, 1987) constitute the best source for the historical development of moral approaches to contraception in Catholicism, in Christianity in general, and in the West.

The ancient world of both East and West knew the reality of contraception either by avoiding insemination of the female or by using potions or magic. In the Greco-Roman world, some philosophers (e.g., Plato, Aristotle) and some gynecologists (e.g., Soranos of Ephesus) apparently accepted contraception. The Roman Empire, however, tended to encourage childbearing. The influential Stoic philosophers insisted that procreation constituted the only purpose of sexual intercourse, and thus logically condemned contraception.

The Hebrew scriptures contain no law condemning contraception, but the concentration on Israel as God's people, the descendants of Abraham and Sarah, emphasized the need for procreation and fertility. Thus the scriptures were generally negative toward contraception. Onan merited God's punishment by spilling his seed and by failing to provide his brother's widow with offspring (Gen. 38:10). Onan's wrongdoing did not involve contraception as such but the refusal of family responsibilities, although some later Jewish writings used Onan's punishment to vindicate the wrongness of coitus interruptus. Some Jewish authorities came to recognize limits on procreation and in certain cases even approved a woman's using root potions as a contraceptive (Noonan, 1986).

The Christian approach to contraception developed in this milieu and also in the context in which contraception was associated with prostitution and extramarital sexuality, which Christians strongly opposed. In addition, the potions used for contraception could not clearly be differentiated from abortifacients. The Christian condemnation of contraception followed from its understanding of human sexuality. Clement of Alexandria (d. 215? c.e.), and the Christian tradition following him, adopted the Stoic rule that marriage and sexuality existed for the purpose of procreation—proposed as a middle position between the Gnostic right (opposing all sexual contact, in imitation of Jesus) and the Gnostic left (celebrating the freedom to use sexuality in any manner). The influential Saint Augustine of Hippo (d. 430 c.e.), in opposition to his earlier acceptance of Manicheanism, which excluded procreation but accepted sexual intercourse and contraception, strongly asserted the procreative rule condemning contraception. Augustine's negative view of sexuality (common to many in the early church and perhaps even stronger in others such as Jerome) strengthened his support of the Stoic procreative rule. According to Augustine, sexual intercourse transmits original sin, since concupiscence as the disordered inclination to sexual pleasure always accompanies sexual relations.

Medieval theologians (e.g., Thomas Aquinas) and their successors maintained that procreation did not constitute the exclusive lawful purpose for marital sexuality. The church, for example, accepted the marital sexuality of the sterile and those no longer able to procreate. The procreation of offspring also included responsibility for the well-being and education of the children. However, the condemnation of contraception remained, with emphasis on its violation of the order of nature calling for the depositing of male seed in the vagina of the female. This nature-based rationale also served as the basis for the condemnation of sodomy, oral and anal intercourse, and masturbation. The split between eastern and western Christianity in the eleventh century and the Protestant Reformation in the sixteenth century did not change the universal Christian condemnation of contraception within marriage. This teaching continued well into the twentieth century.

The impetus for change came not from religious bodies or philosophical ethicists in general, but from popular morality and especially from people committed to improving the human condition. In France, for example, the use of contraception brought about a precipitous drop in the birthrate between 1750 and 1800. At the end of the eighteenth century, Thomas Malthus, in *An Essay on the Principle of Population* (1993), recognized the problems caused by overpopulation and called for restraints on procreation but not contraception. Francis Place in England in 1820 first advocated birth control as a solution to economic and family problems. In the United States, Robert Dale Owens in 1830 advocated the use of contraception. A Malthusian League came into existence in England in 1878, proposing contraception as a solution to the problems connected with large families; similar groups were established in many other parts of the Western world (Noonan, 1986).

Early proponents of contraception and family planning ran into strong popular opposition. In the United States, Anthony Comstock (d. 1915), a Protestant moral reformer and crusader, succeeded in influencing Congress to pass the law bearing his name, prohibiting the use of the mails for obscene materials, including contraceptives. Many states passed even more restrictive laws, and the Comstock-inspired legislation had some effect in the United States until 1965. Early proponents of family planning included many urban radicals and anarchists. Margaret Sanger, who truly merits the title of mother and founder of the family-planning movement, came from such a background but soon made common cause with the medical profession and middle-class women. Sanger publicized family planning and set up clinics to educate and provide contraceptive help for the community at large, especially poorer women. The movement gained considerably from the amalgamation of rival factions into the American Birth Control Federation in 1939, which changed its name in 1942 to the Planned Parenthood Federation. Some charitable foundations (e.g., Rockefeller and Ford) became more interested in family planning and population problems. By 1970, family planning had become a successful popular movement enjoying widespread public support. People in general wholeheartedly accepted the morality of family planning and contraception (Back, 1989).

Although some Protestant laypersons were involved in the early birth-control movements in the Anglo-Saxon countries, the Christian churches remained firm in their condemnation of artificial contraception, as distinguished from abstinence, well into the twentieth century. The Church of England became the first Christian church to accept officially the morality of artificial contraception for spouses. Although the Lambeth Conferences of 1908 and 1920 (official meetings of the bishops of the Anglican Church) condemned birth control, some Anglican statements supportive of birth control appeared in the 1920s. In 1930, the Lambeth Conference, by a vote of 193 to 67, adopted a resolution recognizing a moral obligation to limit or avoid parenthood and proposing complete abstinence as the primary and most obvious way while also accepting other methods (Fagley, 1960).

The Committee on Marriage and Home of the United States Federal Council of Churches in March 1931 issued an influential statement in which the majority of its members accepted the careful and restrained use of contraception by spouses. However, the Federal Council of Churches did not act upon this report. Subsequently, the major Protestant churches and the most significant Protestant theological ethicists (e.g., Karl Barth, Reinhold Niebuhr) accepted contraception as a way to ensure responsible parenthood. The social, cultural, and historical conditions mentioned earlier obviously influenced this massive change in church teaching, but the proponents of change also pointed to aspects in the Christian tradition supporting such a move. Christians had gradually come to recognize the loving or unitive aspect of marital sexuality in addition to the procreative aspect. The procreative aspect itself included not only the procreation but also the education of offspring. The very possibility of procreation and education called for the good health of the parents. In this light, Protestantism in general justified the use of contraception as a way for spouses to realize responsible parenthood (Fagley, 1960).

Roman Catholic official teachings steadfastly opposed artificial contraception within marriage. In 1930, Pope Pius XI in his encyclical *Casti connubii*, in obvious reaction to the Church of England's moral stand, strongly reiterated the condemnation of artificial contraception. Some Catholic theologians even before that time had been advocating the use of the infertile period, or the so-called rhythm method. In a 1951 address to the Italian Catholic Union of Midwives, Pope Pius XII taught that serious medical, eugenic, economic, and social indications justified the use of the sterile periods even on a permanent basis.

The renewal of Roman Catholicism at the Second Vatican Council (1962–1965) created great ferment and introduced many changes in the church. Pope John XXIII established, and Pope Paul VI continued and enlarged, a commission to study the question of the church's teaching. The majority of the commission favored changing the teaching to allow for artificial contraception, but in July 1968, Pope Paul VI issued his encyclical *Humanae vitae*, reiterating the condemnation of artificial contraception (Kaiser, 1985); Pope John Paul II continued the same teaching.

Humanae vitae sets forth the rationale for the condemnation of artificial contraception. Paragraph 11 states that the natural law "teaches that each and every marriage act must remain open to the transmission of life." In the next paragraph the pope refers to "the inseparable connection, willed by God and unable to be broken by man on his own initiative, between the two meanings of the conjugal act: the unitive and the procreative meaning" (Paul VI, 1968).

According to official, hierarchical Roman Catholic teaching, couples can and, at times, should limit their family in the name of responsible parenthood. *Humanae vitae* implies that, although artificial contraception is morally wrong, in practice—because of all the pressures couples experience—the use of artificial contraception might not always involve grave sin (Paul VI, 1968). Rhythm (or natural family planning) is acceptable because it does not interfere with the natural act. Supporters of the Billings method—that is, rhythm based on observation of changes in the vaginal mucus—point out other advantages of their approach, especially the necessary cooperation of husband and wife and the fact that the method does not subject the wife to medical risks (Billings and Westmore, 1980).

Humanae vitae set off a lively discussion within Roman Catholicism. Many theologians disagreed with the natural-law rationale proposed for the condemnation of artificial contraception and often argued that a loyal Roman Catholic could, in theory and in practice, legitimately dissent from such fallible teaching. Some theologians and ethicists continue to defend the hierarchical teaching (magisterium) and a few even claim that the teaching is infallible and no dissent is possible. The hierarchical teaching office, which continues to assert its position strenuously, has not claimed officially that the teaching is infallible but has sometimes taken actions against some theologians who dissent. In practice, the vast majority of Catholic spouses use contraception (Curran, 1979).

Other religious bodies today generally support artificial contraception in the context of responsible parenthood. The Eastern Orthodox church accepts responsible contraception while condemning abortion and infanticide. The multiple purposes of marriage, the lack of any definitive statement against contraception by the church, a synergistic cooperation between God and humans, and the need for responsible parenthood serve as the basis for the responsible use of contraception in marriage (Harakas, 1991; Zaphiris, 1974).

Orthodox Judaism gives a limited acceptance to some forms of contraception, based on the early Talmudic acceptance of the woman's using root potions. Jewish law puts the duty of procreation on the male, and this obligation militates against the use of condoms or coitus interruptus. In this view, the most acceptable contraception is that which interferes the least with the natural sexual act (Rosner, 1979). Conservative and Reform Judaism fully accept and endorse contraception provided it is not harmful to the parties involved.

Islam accepts contraception if it does not entail the radical separation of procreation from marriage. All forms of contraception are acceptable provided they are not harmful and do not involve abortion. Justification for contraception in Islam rests on reports that the Prophet Muhammad did not forbid the contraceptive practices of some of his companions (Hathout, 1991).

Ancient Hindu medicine and Hindu tradition did not contemplate contraception, but did sanction means to enhance conception. In time, medical texts such as the sixteenth-century *Bhavaprakasha* took the step toward contraception by advising a few oral preparations to prevent conception. When India embarked on a national family-planning program after its independence in 1947, the discussions accepted the morality of contraception but centered on the relative population sizes of the higher and lower castes (Desai, 1991).

Western philosophers today generally do not discuss in great detail the morality of contraception within marriage primarily because the basic issue is not controversial. Ethicists generally recognize that spouses have at times an obligation not to procreate, but they would not agree on the reasons for such an obligation.

Concerns of feminists have greatly influenced the contemporary discussion about fertility control in general and contraception in particular. The growing equality and full participation of women in marriage in the global context has definitely given impetus to a wider use of contraception. Feminist ethics starts from the experience of the oppression of women and seeks to unmask and do away with the patriarchal structures of society. Feminists see an important connection between the personal and the political. The practice of medicine involves patriarchal structures and practices that have oppressed women in general and especially in the matter of reproduction, which ordinarily takes place within the woman's own body. Feminists stress the need for women to control their own fertility and reproduction and to have the requisite freedom and autonomy to do so (Overall, 1987; Sherwin, 1992).

Contemporary popular morality—the behavior and values of ordinary people—as well as contemporary philosophy, theological ethics, and religious bodies (with the major exception of Roman Catholicism), accept the morality of contraception for spouses in practicing responsible parenthood. General agreement exists that on the microlevel of the family, the decision about contraception should be made by the spouses themselves in the light of their own health, the good of their marriage, the education and formation of their children, and population and environmental needs, both local and global (Curran, 1979). Population ethics deals with the ethical question of what steps individual governments can and should take in educating, persuading, encouraging, and perhaps even coercing citizens in the light of the population situation of the particular country.

Efficient and effective contraception has been a boon to human existence by giving spouses the means to control their procreation. Like any human good, contraception can be abused, but such abuse does not cancel out the great good that it has provided for humankind.

Contraception as a means of power, however, can be used by the strong against the weak. Population ethics deals with how contraceptive power has been used against the poor, the lower classes, and people of color, both within and across national boundaries. Feminists and others recognize the victimization of women by contraceptive power. Society has often forced women to bear the burden of contraception and especially to live with the medical risks of contraception. The contraceptive pill and the intrauterine device (IUD) definitely involve medical risks for women.

Contraception outside marriage. Judgments about the ethical use of contraception outside marriage depend on one's understanding of the morality of extramarital sexual activity. As a matter of fact many unmarried people are sexually active. Truly there has been a sexual revolution. The majority of adolescents in the United States have had sexual intercourse by the time they are nineteen years old; the problem of teenage pregnancies continues to grow (Demetriou and Kaplan, 1989).

Many feminists with their emphasis on reproductive rights, freedom, control of one's body, and autonomy emphasize the right of individuals to make contraceptive decisions in all cases (Harrison, 1985). Although society at large in the United States no longer condemns all extramarital sexuality as immoral and irresponsible, the mainstream churches and religions still generally maintain the immorality of sexual relations outside marriage (Lebacqz, 1989). The use of condoms enters into the discussion of extramarital sexuality not only because of the desire to prevent procreation, but also because condoms can help to prevent the spread of AIDS and sexually transmitted diseases (STDs). If one believes that extramarital sexual relations are morally responsible, then the use of contraception to prevent unwanted procreation is morally acceptable.

Problems arise when one believes that extramarital sexual relations, especially among adolescents, are morally wrong. Two different positions exist. One position maintains that readily available contraception itself facilitates such morally wrong behavior, and that encouraging the use of such contraception contributes to this immorality. A second position holds that people are going to have sexual relations regardless, so it is better to make sure they do not conceive and do not transmit diseases. Many ethicists who hold this position have accepted the general precept of counseling the lesser of two evils when someone is determined to do the wrong in the first place. It is a lesser evil to have sexual relations in a way that prevents procreation and/or avoids the transmission of harmful diseases (Keenan, 1989).

The provision of contraception to adolescents involves other moral issues, especially parental consent. Parents have responsibility for their children and the right and the obligation to teach their children morality. Some people maintain that the rights and obligations of parents mean that no contraception should be dispensed to adolescents without the permission of the parents. Others maintain that contraception can be provided without parental consent and propose a variety of reasons: Some children do not and cannot communicate with their parents about sexuality; some are going to be sexually active anyway, and it is better for them to use contraception than not to use it; and some are mature enough to make their own decisions in this area.

The Committee on Adolescence of the American Academy of Pediatrics (1990) issued a statement that tries to balance the different ethical responsibilities. According to the statement, pediatricians should actively work to relieve the negative consequences of adolescent sexual activity. Preventive measures involve counseling on responsible sexual decision making—including the counseling of abstinence—and providing contraceptive services for sexually active patients. A general policy guaranteeing confidentiality to the adolescent patient should be clearly stated to the patient and the parent at the time of the initiation of the professional relationship. The goal is to enhance conversation between the adolescent and the parent and to enlist parental support for the adolescent's responsible sexual behavior, including contraceptive use, whenever possible.

Sterilization

Sterilization in the narrow sense is the procedure that takes away one's capacity to procreate. In this sense, sterilization differs from contraception, which interferes with the sexual act and not with the sexual capacity or faculty. According to this understanding, which was standard in Roman Catholic medical ethics and accepted by others, sterilization can be either temporary or permanent. The anovulant pill technically constitutes a temporary sterilization because the pill temporarily suppresses ovulation. This entry employs the broader description of sterilization as the permanent (or somewhat permanent because of some possibility of reversal) removal of procreative capacity. Older forms of sterilization include hysterectomy and castration, but tubal ligation and vasectomy, procedures that are less than a century old, have become comparatively simple and fairly common. The primary ethical distinction concerns voluntary and nonvoluntary sterilization.

Voluntary sterilization.   Religions and religious ethicists generally recognize that individual human beings have stewardship over their bodies and that they should make the medical decisions that affect their lives and health. Philosophers usually recognize the primacy of the person as the decision maker in matters affecting his or her human good. Voluntary consent, in general, has become a primary canon in medical ethics. Some feminists and others insist on an individual's total autonomy with regard to decisions involving reproductive capacity. Religious approaches, in general, and most philosophers as well as medical codes recognize that the individual makes the decision, but that justifying reasons are required to make the decision for sterilization a good and morally acceptable one. Sterilization is proposed for either contraceptive or therapeutic reasons.

Contraceptive sterilization has become increasingly common both in the United States and throughout the world. As the very name indicates, contraceptive sterilization logically follows the same moral judgments as contraception. The one significant difference concerns the somewhat permanent nature of the procedure because of which many ethicists require a more serious and permanent reason to justify it. A basic maxim of medical ethics insists that one should never do more than is necessary to overcome the problem. With a similar consistency, the official teaching of the Roman Catholic church strongly opposes contraceptive sterilization (O'Rourke and Boyle, 1989). Again, many Catholics dissent in theory and in practice from this position.

Therapeutic sterilization is done for the good of the individual and not for contraceptive reasons. The general literature does not frequently discuss therapeutic sterilization as such, because the same standards govern therapeutic sterilization as govern other therapeutic interventions—the procedure must ultimately be for the good of the person and the evil or loss involved must be proportionately less than the good attained. Official Roman Catholic teaching and ethics have treated therapeutic sterilization at length and have developed an elaborate casuistry—or method of resolution through discussion of cases—in distinguishing the morally accepted therapeutic sterilization from the morally condemned contraceptive sterilization. Since sterilization has two different effects—sterilization of the procreative power and protection of the health of the individual—Roman Catholic medical ethics traditionally has applied the principle of double effect, according to which direct sterilization is always wrong but indirect sterilization may be justified for a proportionate reason. Direct sterilization is that which aims at making procreation impossible either as a means or as an end. Therapeutic or indirect sterilization aims directly at the health or good of the individual. Thus, a cancerous uterus can be removed, but hysterectomy to prevent harm to the woman from a pregnancy involves a direct and morally wrong sterilization (Boyle, 1977).

The issue of informed consent, a basic principle in contemporary bioethics, arises in different circumstances. Feminist literature, with its emphasis on reproductive rights and women's control over their bodies and because of many potential and actual abuses, strongly insists on informed consent. Until recently, women have borne the burden of sterilization much more than have men, even though female sterilization is a more difficult and risky procedure than male sterilization. Some poor women have been sterilized immediately after childbirth, having been "informed" about the sterilization and "given consent" just before the delivery of their children (Sherwin, 1992). Most people would also object to employers demanding that people, especially women, be sterilized as a precondition for certain types of employment.

Many writings deal with the sterilization of the mentally retarded who are somewhat incapacitated or even totally incapable of giving informed consent (Macklin and Gaylin, 1981). The Committee on Ethics of the American College of Obstetricians and Gynecologists (1988) issued a statement on "Sterilization of Women Who Are Mentally Handicapped," which urges all possible attempts to communicate with the person involved on whatever level is possible. In case the individual is mentally incompetent, the decision should be made by an appropriate surrogate or proxy, based on the best interests of the patient after considering alternative methods of dealing with the situation.

Nonvoluntary sterilization. Can some other purpose or goal ever override the important value of free consent? Population ethics considers the role of government, which can go from merely providing information to advocacy, providing incentives, or coercing with regard to sterilization. There has been some discussion of the ethics of eugenic and punitive sterilization.

Proposals (e.g., the Human Betterment Foundation) and even legislation for mandatory sterilization (thirty states in the United States passed such laws between 1907 and 1931) appeared in the early part of the twentieth century. Since mental disease and defects that are passed on by heredity create a menace for society and the state, advocates argued the good of the group can override the freedom of the individual. The Nazi eugenic laws and practices of this time have become notorious (Trombley, 1988).

In the second half of the twentieth century, only a few advocates have proposed some eugenic sterilization (e.g., Fletcher, 1960). The horrors occasioned by Nazi practice, the erroneous scientific foundation of the eugenic movement in the early part of the twentieth century, the fear of errors, the hubris of making eugenic decisions for others, the overly intrusive role of the state, and the continuing and growing emphasis on the freedom and rights of all, have contributed to the general consensus against eugenic sterilization. Some proposals have been made to cut off welfare funds to poor women who have children and refuse to undergo sterilization, but such proposals have not received much support (Lebacqz, 1978).

The fact that there is little or no discussion of punitive sterilization in the more recent literature hints at a consensus against the practice. However, Francis Hürth, a conservative Roman Catholic theologian in the 1930s, proposed limited cases in which punitive sterilization might be justified. Pope Pius XI went out of his way not to condemn punitive sterilization in his 1931 encyclical *Casti connubii*. Proponents maintain that if the state can inflict capital punishment for certain crimes, it can also inflict the lesser punishment of sterilization in limited, appropriate cases. Critics reply that punitive sterilization does not achieve the purposes of punishment and does not even inhibit future sex crimes (McCarthy, 1960). Punitive sterilization appears to be virtually unsupported (Mason, 1990).

Abortion

Abortion, or the termination of pregnancy, also constitutes a means of fertility control. This section briefly explains the logical application of moral positions on abortion to judgments about abortion as a means of fertility control.

All those who oppose abortion as a general principle also oppose abortion as a means of fertility control. Those who hold that from the first moment of conception the zygote should be treated as an individual human being, or who attribute a high value to the early conceptus, oppose forms of contraception that work as abortifacients. Here again technological developments blur the clear distinction between contraception and abortion. Doubts about how the IUD actually works led some people to condemn it as an abortifacient because of the theory that the IUD prevents the implantation of the early conceptus in the endometrium of the uterus (McCormick, 1981). Those who hold this view of the early conceptus strongly oppose the RU-486 pill, which definitely works as an abortifacient. On the other hand, those who do not attribute any value or great value to the early conceptus have no moral qualms about the RU-486.

Many (e.g., Harrison, 1985) who advocate the morality of abortion in general recognize significant moral differences between abortion and contraception. Some attribute more value and worth to the fetus as it develops in the maternal womb. Consequently, abortion (at least after the first few weeks) should not be used as the regular and ordinary method of fertility control for a number of reasons—the danger of some risk to the mother, the problems caused by multiple abortions, and the value that is attributed to the fetus. However, many believe that abortion may still be used in the case of contraceptive failure.

Fertility control has always been significant for humankind, but contemporary scientific, social, philosophical, theological, and feminist developments have focused even more attention on this issue.

CHARLES E. CURRAN

Directly related to this article are the other articles in this entry: MEDICAL ASPECTS, SOCIAL ISSUES, *and* LEGAL AND REGULATORY ISSUES. *Also directly related are the entries* SEXUAL ETHICS; SEXUALITY IN SOCIETY; POPULATION POLICIES; *and* ABORTION. *For a further discussion of topics mentioned in this article, see the entries* ADOLESCENTS; AUTONOMY; DOUBLE EFFECT; FEMINISM; FREEDOM AND COERCION; INFORMED CONSENT; JUDAISM; MARRIAGE AND OTHER DOMESTIC PARTNERSHIPS; NATURAL LAW; *and* ROMAN CATHOLICISM. *For a discussion of related ideas, see the entries* MULTINATIONAL RESEARCH; POPULATION ETHICS; *and* REPRODUCTIVE TECHNOLOGIES,

article on ETHICAL ISSUES. *Other relevant material may be found under the entries* BIOLOGY, PHILOSOPHY OF; BODY, *article on* CULTURAL AND RELIGIOUS PERSPECTIVES; EUGENICS; EUGENICS AND RELIGIOUS LAW; LIFE; *and* VALUE AND VALUATION.

Bibliography

AMERICAN ACADEMY OF PEDIATRICS. COMMITTEE ON ADOLESCENCE. 1990. "Contraception and Adolescents." *Pediatrics* 86, no. 1:134–138.

AMERICAN COLLEGE OF OBSTETRICIANS AND GYNECOLOGISTS. COMMITTEE ON ETHICS. 1988. "Sterilization of Women Who Are Mentally Handicapped." Committee Opinion 63. Washington, D.C.: Author.

BACK, KURT W. 1989. *Family Planning and Population Control: The Challenges of a Successful Movement.* Boston: Twayne

BILLINGS, EVELYN, and WESTMORE, ANN. 1980. *The Billings Method: Controlling Fertility Without Drugs or Devices.* Richmond, Victoria, Australia: Anne O'Donovan.

BOYLE, JOHN P. 1977. *The Sterilization Controversy: A New Crisis for the Catholic Hospital?* New York: Paulist Press.

CURRAN, CHARLES E. 1979. *Transition and Tradition in Moral Theology.* Notre Dame, Ind.: University of Notre Dame Press.

DEMETRIOU, EFSTRATIOS, and KAPLAN, DAVID W. 1989. "Adolescent Contraceptive Use and Parental Notification." *American Journal of Diseases of Children* 143, no. 10:1166–1172.

DESAI, PRAKASH N. 1991. "Hinduism and Bioethics in India: A Tradition in Transition." In *Theological Developments in Bioethics: 1988–1990,* pp. 41–60. Edited by Baruch A. Brody, B. Andrew Lustig, H. Tristram Engelhardt, Jr., and Laurence McCullough. Bioethics Yearbook, vol. 1. Dordrecht, Netherlands: Kluwer.

FAGLEY, RICHARD M. 1960. *The Population Explosion and Christian Responsibility.* New York: Oxford University Press.

FLETCHER, JOSEPH F. 1960. *Morals and Medicine: The Moral Problems of: The Patient's Right to Know the Truth, Contraception, Artificial Insemination, and Sterilization.* Boston: Beacon Press.

HARAKAS, STANLEY SAMUEL. 1991. "Eastern Orthodox Bioethics." In *Theological Developments in Bioethics, 1988–1990,* pp. 85–101. Edited by Baruch A. Brody, B. Andrew Lustig, H. Tristram Engelhardt, Jr., and Laurence McCullough. Bioethics Yearbook, vol. 1. Dordrecht, Netherlands: Kluwer.

HARRISON, BEVERLY WILDUNG. 1985. *Making the Connections: Essays in Feminist Social Ethics.* Edited by Carol S. Robb. Boston: Beacon Press.

HATHOUT, HASSAN. 1991. "Islamic Concepts and Bioethics." In *Theological Developments in Bioethics: 1988–1990,* pp. 103–117. Edited by Baruch A. Brody, B. Andrew Lustig, H. Tristram Engelhardt, Jr., and Laurence McCullough. Bioethics Yearbook, vol. 1. Dordrecht, Netherlands: Kluwer.

HOYT, ROBERT G., ed. 1968. *The Birth Control Debate.* Kansas City, Mo.: National Catholic Reporter.

INTERNATIONAL ISLAMIC CONFERENCE. 1974. *Islam and Family*

Planning. 2 vols. Beirut: International Planned Parenthood Federation, Middle East and North Africa Region. A faithful translation of the Arabic edition of the proceedings of the International Islamic Conference held in Rabat [Morocco], December 1971.

KAISER, ROBERT BLAIR. 1985. *The Politics of Sex and Religion: A Case History in the Development of Doctrine, 1962–1984.* Kansas City, Mo.: Leaven.

KEENAN, JAMES F. 1989. "Prophylactics, Toleration, and Co-operation: Contemporary Problems and Traditional Principles." *International Philosophical Quarterly* 29, no. 2: 205–220.

LEBACQZ, KAREN. 1978. "Sterilization: Ethical Aspects." In vol. 4 of *Encyclopedia of Bioethics,* pp. 1609–1613. Edited by Warren T. Reich. New York: Macmillan.

———. 1989. "Appropriate Vulnerability: A Sexual Ethic for Singles." In *Sexual Ethics and the Church: After the Revolution: A Christian Century Symposium,* pp. 18–23. Edited by John J. McNeill and James B. Nelson. Chicago: Christian Century Foundation.

MACKLIN, RUTH, and GAYLIN, WILLARD, eds. 1981. *Mental Retardation and Sterilization: A Problem of Competency and Paternalism.* New York: Plenum.

MALTHUS, THOMAS R. 1993. *An Essay on the Principle of Population.* New York: Oxford University Press. The original 1798 volume went through many editions.

MASON, JOHN KENYON. 1990. *Medico-Legal Aspects of Reproduction and Parenthood.* Brookfield, Vt.: Dartmouth.

MCCARTHY, JOHN. 1960. *The Commandments.* Vol. 2 of his *Problems in Theology.* Westminster, Md.: Newman.

MCCORMICK, RICHARD A. 1981. *Notes on Moral Theology, 1965 through 1980.* Washington, D.C.: University Press of America.

NOONAN, JOHN T., JR. 1978. "Contraception." In vol. 1 of *Encyclopedia of Bioethics,* pp. 204–216. Edited by Warren T. Reich. New York: Macmillan.

———. 1986. *Contraception: A History of Its Treatment by the Catholic Theologians and Canonists.* Enl. ed. Cambridge, Mass.: Harvard University Press.

———. 1987. "The History of Contraception: Seven Choices." In *The Contraceptive Ethos: Reproductive Rights and Responsibilities,* pp. 3–14. Edited by Stuart F. Spicker, William B. Bondeson, and H. Tristram Engelhardt, Jr. Philosophy and Medicine, vol. 27. Dordrecht, Netherlands: D. Reidel.

O'ROURKE, KEVIN D., and BOYLE, PHILIP. 1989. *Medical Ethics: Sources of Catholic Teaching.* St. Louis: Catholic Health Association of the United States.

OVERALL, CHRISTINE. 1987. *Ethics and Human Reproduction: A Feminist Analysis.* Boston: Allen and Unwin.

PAUL VI. 1968. "Humanae vitae." *Acta Apostolicae Sedis* 60:481–503. Translated under the title "Humanae Vitae (Human Life)." *Catholic Mind* 66 (September 30, 1968): 35–48.

ROSNER, FRED. 1979. "Contraception in Jewish Law." In *Jewish Bioethics,* pp. 86–96. Edited by Fred Rosner and J. David Bleich. New York: Sanhedrin.

SHERWIN, SUSAN. 1992. *No Longer Patient: Feminist Ethics and Health Care.* Philadelphia: Temple University Press.

TROMBLEY, STEPHEN. 1988. *The Right to Reproduce: A History of Coercive Sterilization.* London: Weidenfeld and Nicolson.

ZAPHIRIS, CHRYSOSTOM. 1974. "The Morality of Contraception: An Eastern Orthodox Opinion." *Journal of Ecumenical Studies* 11, no. 4:661–675.

IV. LEGAL AND REGULATORY ISSUES

A person's ability to control his or her fertility depends on available technology, moral and religious acceptability, and legal permissibility or the threat of sanction. A man or a woman's ability to prevent pregnancy when exercised knowingly and voluntarily enhances autonomy and liberty. Coercive control of fertility by the state or its agents poses a threat to dignity and reproductive freedom. The major fertility-control mechanisms are contraception and sterilization and, when neither is used or the chosen method fails, abortion. The mechanical and physiological characteristics of each method determine the ease and comfort of individual use, the likelihood of success, and the potential for coercion.

In many cultures men view children as proof of virility and power. They see attempts by women to limit or terminate pregnancy as an attack on male authority and reproductive potential, which in many societies equals wealth. For many women a desire to limit pregnancy must often be pursued furtively, with fear of violence and retaliation. Biology and the threat to a woman's independence, health status, and well-being make the control of fertility primarily a woman's concern. A woman's ability to limit and control her fertility may be a necessary precondition for equality and personal economic status. Control of fertility is central to modern notions of emancipated or liberated womanhood.

Because they affect relationships between the sexes, population growth, and a woman's status, contraception, sterilization, and abortion are and have been problematic for many societies. Secular societies committed to individual rights and liberties are less likely to intervene in reproductive decisions. But all societies have tried in the past and still attempt, to some degree, to influence individual reproductive choices—especially the choices of the less powerful, a status often identified with women of color.

History of contraception use and control

General. Various societies have for centuries interceded in the free use of contraception, largely for moral and/or religious reasons. Classical Islam permitted the use of birth control and even early abortion (Fathalla et al., 1990). Biblical Judaism, based on interpretations of the story of Onan in Gen. 38:8–10, condemned coitus interruptus and the use of male condoms. Christianity gradually evolved a doctrine, based on biblical references, interpretations of natural law, and the writings of Saint Augustine, that prohibited use of all contraceptive devices (St. John-Stevas, 1971). Widespread, class-linked knowledge of contraceptive practices was effectively withheld from most of the population following the condemnation of birth control by Thomas Aquinas in the mid-thirteenth century (Fathalla et al., 1990). As religion formed part of the basis for modern secular law, control of fertility became a subject of legal attention and regulation.

Abortion, as a method of fertility control, has always been especially controversial. Despite its morally and legally complex past and its tendentious present, there is evidence today that abortion remains a favored method of birth control for many women, both as a preferred method of fertility control and as a backup to failed contraception. Fifty million abortions are performed worldwide each year. In 1991, Romania, with little access to and inaccurate information about contraceptives, had the highest abortion ratio: three abortions for every one live birth, totalling 884,000 in 1991 (Stephen, 1992). In the United States 1.5 million abortions are performed per year, 25.9 per 1,000 women aged fifteen to forty-four; in China, ten million, one for every two live births (Preston, 1992).

While contraception and abortion address the prevention or termination of any specific pregnancy, sterilization terminates individual fecundity. With the development of modern, comparatively safe and effective means of sterilization (vasectomy, or surgical excision of the duct carrying sperm from the testicles; and salpingectomy, or surgical removal of one or both fallopian tubes), individuals can choose, by means of one medical intervention, to detach sexual intercourse from reproductive consequences. If chosen by individuals, these simple and almost always irreversible interventions extend autonomy; if imposed by the state, they can become instruments of repression.

Whether contraception, sterilization, and abortion should be permitted, prohibited, or coerced by government has generated intense controversy in countries as different as the United States, Romania, India, Ireland, and China. In each country, legislators, judges, individuals, and special-interest lobbies have struggled to affect how citizens will think about their options for controlling fertility, how the individual decision-making process will be informed and supervised, how access to contraception, abortion, and sterilization will be ensured or precluded, and whether coercion will be encouraged, permitted, or prohibited (Weston, 1990; Thomas, 1990).

Both female and male condoms have been available for centuries. Roman women attempted to use goat bladders (Fathalla et al., 1990), and some African women hollowed out okra pods (Robertson, 1990). A picture of a penile sheath is recorded as early as 1350 B.C.E., although male condoms did not come into general use in Europe until 1671 and became reliable only with the vulcanization of rubber in 1843 (Robertson, 1990). Monitoring and prohibiting use of birth-control devices such as condoms are difficult because of the inherently private nature of their use. Manufacture, distribution, sale, and advertising are more easily regulated and prohibited.

Despite the long history and the private nature of fertility control, various legal and theological systems have attempted prohibition. The early Christian (Roman Catholic and Protestant) argument against contraception, influential as the model for legal regulation, holds that God's purpose for sex is conservation of the species, which is frustrated when people have intercourse for nonprocreative purposes (St. John-Stevas, 1971). The Catholic church first proscribed contraception in canon law in 1140 (St. John-Stevas, 1971). While not all religions have been as resistant to the idea of contraception as the Catholic church, contraceptive use has traditionally been considered an appropriate area for moral guidance and proscription and not until the beginning of the twentieth century did significant numbers of Protestant theologians provide moral approval (Larson, 1991).

Religious regulation has been selective. Some forms of birth control were interdicted, while others were and have remained relatively unnoticed. In addition, prolonged lactation, postpartum abstinence, delayed marriage, celibacy, and to some extent infanticide, are all techniques of fertility management that have been and continue to be used.

United States history. Puritan theology dominated the early American colonists. The Puritans considered sex-related matters part of the devil's province, to be shunned and ignored, and they tolerated little open discussion (Robertson, 1990). In the 1830s some popular literature on contraception, such as Robert Dale Owen's *Moral Physiology*, began to be generally available (Robertson, 1990; Reed, 1978). Not until 1873 did law begin regulating distribution of contraceptives in the United States. The Comstock Act ("An Act for the Suppression of Trade in, and Circulation of, Obscene Literature and Articles of Immoral Use") equated contraception with obscenity and made it a federal offense to use the postal service for transporting obscene materials, defined to include contraceptive and abortion information and equipment. The act also banned importation and interstate transportation of such items (Sloan, 1988). After the act's passage, many states adopted their own regulations on the sale, advertising, and display of contraceptive devices.

Margaret Sanger, a nurse affected by her work in poor communities where morbidity (the incidence of disease) and mortality from abortion was high, was a vociferous advocate for birth control (Reed, 1978; Peo-

ple v. *Sanger,* 1918). She founded a monthly magazine, *The Woman Rebel,* for which she was arrested and indicted under the Comstock Act. She fled to Europe and returned in 1916 to establish the first American birth-control clinic in Brooklyn, a borough of New York City (Chessler, 1992). In 1918, she was convicted and sentenced to thirty days in the workhouse under New York State's Comstock law. Years later, a physician in one of Margaret Sanger's clinics who had ordered a package of contraceptives through the mail was charged with violating the Tariff Act of 1930, a statute based on the Comstock Act that prohibited importation of "any article whatever for the prevention of conception or for causing unlawful abortion" (Tariff Act, 1930). On appeal, the federal circuit court for the second circuit held that the act did not apply when the article imported was not intended for an immoral purpose. Judge Augustus Hand declared that the Tariff Act was part of a "continuous scheme to suppress immoral articles and obscene literature," and refused to find proper medical use of a contraceptive by a licensed physician to be immoral or obscene (*U.S. vs. One Package . . . , 1936,* p. 739). Though the court did not invalidate the statute, its interpretation limited the sweeping definition of morality and obscenity that had previously held sway.

Statutes modeled after the Comstock Act continued to exist, however, until 1965, when the U.S. Supreme Court in the case of *Griswold* v. *Connecticut* invalidated a Connecticut statute prohibiting the use of contraceptives. The Court held, citing prior cases that had created a zone of privacy protecting certain personal behaviors, that these penumbral rights of "privacy and repose," based on several fundamental constitutional guarantees, protected the use of contraceptives by married persons (*Griswold* v. *Connecticut,* 1965, p. 481). *Griswold* was followed by *Eisenstadt* v. *Baird* (1972), extending this reasoning to nonmarried individuals. The statute that was invalidated in *Eisenstadt* prohibited single persons from obtaining contraceptives to prevent pregnancy, and permitted contraceptives only on a physician's prescription for the purpose of disease prevention. The statute was held to violate the equal protection clause of the Fourteenth Amendment:

> [W]hatever the rights of the individual to access to contraceptives may be, the rights must be the same for the unmarried and the married alike. . . . If the right of privacy means anything, it is the right of the individual, married or single, to be free from unwarranted governmental intrusion into matters so fundamentally affecting a person as the decision whether to bear or beget a child. (*Eisenstadt* v. *Baird,* 1965, pp. 452–453)

Minors gradually attained access to contraceptive advice and devices. In 1977, in the case of *Carey* v. *Population Services International,* the U.S. Supreme Court invalidated a New York State statute that had banned the sale or distribution of contraceptives to persons below the age of sixteen and had prohibited the advertising or display of contraceptives by any person, including a pharmacist. In 1983, the Supreme Court struck down a federal statute prohibiting unsolicited advertisements of contraceptives (*Bolger* v. *Young Drug Products Corp.,* 1983). In addition, under Title X of the Public Health Services Act and Title XIX of the Social Security Act, receipt of federal funds prohibits a requirement of parental consent for services and requires confidentiality. Efforts to require parental notification under these acts have been held unconstitutional (*Jane Does 1 through 4* v. *State of Utah Dept. of Health,* 1985; *Planned Parenthood Association of Utah* v. *Dandoy,* 1987).

In 1988 the government attempted to impose a "gag" rule preventing providers at federally funded family-planning clinics from mentioning abortion as a possible solution to an unwanted pregnancy. The rule was reversed early in 1993, permitting federally funded clinics to provide a full range of advice and service for fertility control for men and women whether married, unmarried, or minors.

New contraceptive technologies

A revolution in birth control techniques has created new possibilities for individual choice and new dangers of coercive action by legislatures, bureaucrats, and judges. Additional dangers arise from inadequate new-product testing and from lack of information or misinformation about risks and benefits of use. Female condoms, Norplant, and Depo-Provera are increasingly available to women for contraception.

The female condom or vaginal pouch was approved by the U.S. Food and Drug Administration (FDA) in 1993. The device, developed and marketed by Wisconsin Pharmaceuticals, consists of a polyurethane sheath secured inside the vagina by a small metal ring and outside by a large metal ring. It is the only barrier contraceptive that is under the control of a woman, an increasingly important factor for women seeking to protect themselves from sexually transmitted diseases and human immunodeficiency virus (HIV) infection when their partners refuse or neglect to use condoms. The device was approved by the FDA despite concerns that it was not proved as effective as the male condom for prevention of pregnancy or prevention of transmission of infection.

Norplant (levonorgestrel), approved by the FDA in 1990, is a long-term implantable contraceptive comprised of six capsules that gradually release progestin, thereby providing effective contraception for five years. A two-capsule version provides protection for three years. Norplant, like other contraceptive devices, is morally neutral; it may enhance the range of individual choice or, because of its long-acting nature, lend itself to coercive action by others. It permits a woman to protect herself without conscious attention to contraception but makes her dependent on medical intervention for removal, a dependency many women resent.

Norplant suppresses ovulation, and changes the female physiology to discourage pregnancy. For women who choose this contraceptive technique, it offers 100 percent compliance and effectiveness without the need to attend to individual acts of intercourse or to daily medications. There are some side effects and contraindications for use, including the possibilities of weight gain, headaches, and a general feeling of malaise. A major problem in the United States is the cost, up to $700 to insert and remove (Board of Trustees, American Medical Association [AMA], 1992).

The only way to stop the contraceptive effect of the device is to have it surgically removed. Removal is more complicated than insertion and more than one session may be required to remove all the capsules; removal may also be painful. Norplant provides either long-acting contraception or time-limited sterilization (Mertus and Heller, 1992; Arthur, 1992).

Norplant presents an easy potential for coercive use by judges and legislatures. Problematic uses include requiring Norplant as a condition of parole following a conviction for child abuse, and paying women on welfare for consenting to initial and continued placement of the contraceptive. The first is clearly coercive. The second is potentially coercive depending on the context of a woman's poverty. Various state legislatures have considered statutes that would pay women receiving welfare to use Norplant or mandate its use by women convicted of child neglect and drug use, or both (Mertus and Heller, 1992; Board of Trustees, AMA, 1992).

Judicial or legislative imposition of Norplant may violate a woman's constitutionally protected rights to choose how to manage reproduction and to choose whether or not to consent to or refuse medical care (*Cruzan*, 1990). The U.S. Supreme Court has not yet ruled on this matter. Any long-acting male contraceptive would implicate these same rights. In addition, because long-acting contraception amounts to temporary sterilization, it raises the specter of eugenics—policies that are often directed at people of color, the poor, the retarded, the mentally ill, and other persons designated by those in power as undesirable. Norplant offers effective contraception when chosen voluntarily by a woman informed of the risks and benefits, and a potential for tyranny when imposed by judges or legislatures.

Regulation of contraceptive technologies

In addition to enhancing individual choice and restricting abuse, regulation of new technologies must ensure access and quality control. The development of new technologies is regulated formally by the approval process of the FDA, and informally by compensation awards under tort law for harm caused by defective products.

The FDA regulates the development of new drugs and contraceptive devices under the Federal Food, Drug and Cosmetic Act of 1938. Under this law, a company interested in marketing new contraceptive drugs or devices must submit data, including results from various tests for safety, effectiveness, and dosage, as part of an extensive approval process. In addition to approving new drugs and devices, the FDA reviews labeling and assesses data in a postmarketing surveillance program. The FDA approval process has been criticized as expensive, time consuming, and a barrier to new techniques. It has also been praised for protecting consumers from the harm of untested substances.

The FDA approval process is not the sole factor dictating whether a reproductive technology reaches U.S. consumers, however. The American tort system is designed to compensate those injured, deter the marketing of dangerous and defective products, and resolve disputes between the injured person and the manufacturer.

A person may recover damages for dangerous or defective products, including contraceptive devices, if either negligence or a strict liability is established. Negligence requires proof that the manufacturer was at fault. However, sometimes the fault of a large company is difficult to establish, and therefore the interests of justice dictate that a victim should be allowed to recover damages without proving specific fault. According to the strict products-liability principle, if a product is sold in a defective condition, and is unreasonably dangerous to the consumer, there is liability regardless of the care taken, that is, regardless of negligence in any individual case. Strict liability may make manufacturers apprehensive about putting new contraceptive products on the market.

This is the case especially since the litigation experience of the A. H. Robins Company, developer and marketer of the Dalkon Shield, an intrauterine contraceptive device. In a series of court cases in the early 1980s, this device was proved to cause pelvic inflammatory disease, infertility, birth defects, perforated uterus, and spontaneous abortion. In a series of jury verdicts throughout the United States, A. H. Robins was forced to pay compensatory damages and punitive damages because plaintiffs proved that the company had understood the dangers of the device, withheld this knowledge from prospective users, and misrepresented the nature and safety of the device (Mintz, 1985). Despite this experience, cases brought by women seeking recovery for harm from contraceptive devices have usually found the manufacturer liable only under theories of negligence—for example, negligent failure to comply with the duty of care, negligent failure to warn of risks, or fraudulent misrepresentation (*Hilliard* v. *A. H. Robins Co.*, 1984; *Tetuan* v. *A. H. Robins Co.*, 1987). In fact, even those courts purporting to apply strict liability seem to be applying a theory of negligent failure to warn under the rhetoric of strict liability (Henderson and Twerski, 1990; Fox and Traynor, 1990). Some case law holds manufacturers liable for failure to warn of risks that were unknown; this more closely resembles strict liability, but few states have applied such a standard (Fox and Traynor, 1990).

How tort law is interpreted is in a state of flux. Some judges and juries appear to view manufacturers as "deep pockets" (Reilly, 1989) and to see tort law as a vehicle for providing social insurance for injury victims. Many critics of large jury awards argue that the size of jury awards often bears no relationship to actual economic loss or to pain and suffering, and that awards of punitive damages are arbitrary and unfair. Supporters of the present pattern of trial awards argue that claims of a law crisis in this area are exaggerated because of manufacturers' dislike for how the law determines their liability (Fox and Traynor, 1990). However, as long as manufacturers fear they will have to pay large financial penalties to women who suffer the consequences of their new products, many may be reluctant to market new products, a trend that may limit women's access to new contraceptive technologies.

Postcontraception, the "morning-after" pill, is widely dispensed on college campuses after unprotected intercourse and in emergency rooms for rape victims; it promises to be another barrier to unwanted pregnancy. The process generally entails two treatments of oral contraceptives within seventy-two hours of intercourse and is thought to prevent pregnancy either by blocking fertilization or by blocking implantation of the fertilized egg. An antihormone product called RU-486, discussed in the following section, has also shown promise as a "morning-after" pill.

Despite the convenience and desirability of postcontraceptive options, manufacturers of oral contraceptives have not sought FDA approval for use of drugs for this purpose. Their reluctance may be motivated by fear of liability, fear of anti-abortion publicity, or by the cost of financing the complex studies that are required for FDA approval.

Abortion

This article will not survey the legal history and the current status of abortion law and regulation. This discussion will be limited to RU-486 (mifepristone) which, while functioning as an abortion inducer, is thought of by many users as similar to oral contraceptives.

RU-486 is a steroid analogue that, when used with prostaglandin (PG), is able to induce menses within eight weeks of the last menstrual period. It has been called a "menstrual regulator" in an attempt to distinguish it from contraceptives and abortion inducers, al-

though to theologians the physiological function is clearly that of an abortion inducer. It was approved for use in France in 1988. Limited trials in the United States began in 1994. Shortly after its introduction in France, the manufacturer, Roussel Uclaf, attempted to halt distribution for fear of anti-abortion protests. The French government, a one-third owner of the company, ordered continued manufacture and distribution (Banwell and Paxman, 1992).

Whether RU-486/PG will become readily available will depend on each nation's interpretation of relevant abortion laws and regulations. If abortion "is defined to include techniques that operate before implantation is complete, RU-486/PG will be regulated by abortion law. If not, RU-486/PG might be considered similar to a contraceptive and could be made more widely available. This distinction is particularly important because abortion legislation generally imposes criminal penalties" (Banwell and Paxman, 1992, p. 1400).

While France considers RU-486/PG an abortion inducer, Germany, New Zealand, and Liberia use a definition of pregnancy in their abortion statutes providing that pregnancy begins only after complete implantation. In these countries, RU-486/PG and any other menses-inducing technique is regulated as a form of contraception. In countries with strict abortion laws in which pregnancy is defined as beginning with fertilization, even early use of RU-486/PG might be barred (Banwell and Paxman, 1992).

Many countries in Latin America and Africa have restrictive abortion statutes that require proof of pregnancy. Statutes that require proof of pregnancy will be difficult to use as a barrier to RU-486/PG. Other national statutes criminalize the intent to abort whether or not the woman is pregnant. In these countries, many of which are former French colonies, the widespread use of RU-486/PG is effectively precluded. In societies governed by Islamic law, where pregnancy may be terminated until quickening—when fetal movement is felt—RU-486/PG would likely be acceptable (Banwell and Paxman, 1992).

Sterilization

Sterilization is a particularly useful technique for men and women who are certain that they have fulfilled their reproductive agenda. For these individuals sterilization provides an uncomplicated and generally certain method of limiting fertility. Whereas sterilization done competently is 100 percent effective, cases have claimed damages for children conceived as the result of incomplete sterilizations.

The key legal issues in sterilization involve the need to ensure that the choice is made by a competent adult who has chosen voluntarily; the need to decide for some persons, almost always women, who are clearly incapable of deciding for themselves; and the need to prevent notions of eugenics from dictating sterilization policy and practice. Sterilization, because it requires only one medical intervention, has been particularly susceptible to government abuse.

Women or men who choose sterilization must be counseled about the risks and benefits of the intervention itself and about the very slim chances for reversal if permanent infertility is no longer desired. Some localities have regulations requiring a waiting period between a request for sterilization and the actual procedure. Others preclude caregivers from soliciting consent for sterilization from women during the birthing process. Both restrictions offer protection against coercion, especially for low-income women and women of color who have been historically at risk for nonconsensual sterilization.

Sterilization has been used by physicians and by state and federal governments since the turn of the century (Mertus and Heller, 1992), in order to limit the reproduction of low-income women and women of color. It has also been used as a method of eugenics "to weed out traits or characteristics that are held to be undesirable. Further, sterilization was simultaneously discouraged among affluent white women" (Mertus and Heller, 1992, p. 377).

The history of involuntary sterilization of incompetent and developmentally disabled individuals in the first half of the twentieth century is a history of "wholesale violations of constitutional rights carried out with the approval of the highest judicial tribunals." Eugenic sterilization—the attempt to rid the collective gene pool of hereditary mental and physical defects—was the result of the "enthusiastic application of Mendelian genetics" to population policy (*Conservatorship of Valerie N.*, 1985, p. 148).

In the early twentieth century, thousands of young women and men were sterilized as the result of decisions by the directors of mental institutions or prisons in which they were housed, or by decisions of their conservators or guardians. The impulse to control the reproductive capacity of these people was fueled by the dual fears that children would perpetuate their parents' mental or physical "deformity" and would be a drain on state coffers. But there is another basis, never articulated as such in legislation or by the courts, and that is a general revulsion at the concept of mentally "defective" persons acting sexually. Indeed, a 1913 California statute granted authority to "asexualize" committed mental patients and developmentally disabled persons prior to their release from state institutions (*Conservatorship of Valerie N.*, 1985). Sexuality, as well as reproductive capacity, was at issue.

By the second decade of the twentieth century, twenty-two states had eugenic sterilization statutes. Between 1907 and 1921, 3,233 sterilizations were performed, of which California was responsible for 2,558. By 1927, California had performed over 5,000 sterilizations, four times as many as had been performed by any national government worldwide. By 1960, approximately 60,000 persons had been subjected to compulsory sterilization in the United States, with nearly 20,000 in California (Mertus and Heller, 1992).

In 1927, the U.S. Supreme Court upheld a Virginia statute permitting the sterilization of the "mental defectives" (*Buck v. Bell*, 1927). The Court based its decision on two lines of reasoning: that if rendered unable to procreate, the person might more easily become self-supporting; and that society can choose to protect itself from further dissemination of defective genes. Justice Oliver Wendell Holmes wrote, "The principle that sustains compulsory vaccination is broad enough to cover cutting the Fallopian tubes. . . . Three generations of imbeciles are enough" (*Buck v. Bell*, 1927, p. 207).

Buck v. Bell, though never overruled, has been severely limited by later decisions. In 1942, the U.S. Supreme Court invalidated the Oklahoma Habitual Criminal Sterilization Act, which ordered the sterilization of anyone convicted of three crimes involving "moral turpitude"; however, the contested law excepted certain white-collar crimes. In *Skinner* v. *Oklahoma* (1942), declaring the Sterilization Act unconstitutional on equal-protection grounds, the Court ruled that procreation is a basic civil right that can be abridged only by showing compelling state interest. The Court referred to the right to marriage and procreation as a basic liberty and as one of the basic civil rights. The Court's reluctance to approve the Oklahoma statute appears to reflect apprehension that sterilization could be used oppressively (*Skinner* v. *Oklahoma*, 1942).

The second half of the twentieth century has witnessed a revulsion against nonconsensual sterilization, based on the revelations of Nazi abuses and the emergence of various rights movements in the United States—civil, women's, welfare, mentally ill, the disabled, and prisoners. Sociological and medical research regarding the nature of mental illness and developmental disability also enlightened the public regarding the ability of developmentally disabled and mentally ill persons to lead constructive, competent, loving lives as partners and parents.

Beginning in the 1950s, numerous states repealed legislation permitting eugenic sterilization for institutionalized persons or limited the powers of conservators and guardians to procure individual sterilization. Yet in many states these statutes are still law. This has led to the ironic position, in many states, that no one can consent for the incapable, thus denying them access to sterilization even when sterilization is the only or arguably the best contraceptive solution—and even when it is required to protect health or life itself.

Arguments regarding sterilization for incompetent persons pit advocates of reproductive choice for the disabled against those who argue that the right to "bear or beget" a child includes the right to choose reproduction, contraception, or sterilization. Federal (*Hathaway v. Worcester City Hospital*, 1973; *Ruby v. Massey*, 1978) and state courts (*Moe*, 1982; *Grady*, 1981; *A.W.*, 1981) have generally held that developmentally disabled persons have fundamental privacy and liberty interests in making decisions about procreation and that these interests require sterilization to be an option for fertility control. Some state courts, however, have refused to authorize sterilization of an incompetent person unless the state legislature has specifically authorized the decision and specified a process (*Hudson v. Hudson*, 1979; *Eberhardy*, 1980). The U.S. Supreme Court has yet to examine the issue, but prior cases would seem to support a right of access to sterilization for incompetent persons.

Cases claiming rights of protection from sterilization most often involve consent for severely disabled young women for whom menstruation and pregnancy would be painful, provoking, upsetting, or possibly life-threatening (for example, one woman for whom the sight of her own blood caused a pattern of severe self-mutilation [*P.S.*, 1983]). In most states, courts appoint an independent guardian to protect the interests of the person and then base their decision on the standard of "best interest" (*P.S.*, 1983; *Hayes*, 1980) or substituted judgment (*Moe*, 1982; *Grady*, 1981).

The dangers of forced sterilizations are apparent outside the realm of prisoners, developmentally disabled, and incompetent individuals, largely where issues of race and class are present. The indigent, who are often persons of color, have been particularly subject to sterilization abuses by public officials and collaborating physicians. Numerous cases have been documented of coerced sterilization of Native Americans (Kelly, 1977), Latinos (particularly those who spoke little or no English), and African-Americans (*Relf v. Weinberger*, 1977). In response to one egregious incident (*Relf v. Weinberger*, 1977), the district court examined the practice of physicians at federally funded clinics who were using sterilization to limit the reproduction of African-American teenagers. The court invalidated federal regulations that permitted involuntary, coerced sterilization, including sterilization of minors or persons incapable of providing consent. The court further held that such sterilizations could not be funded under the Social Security Act or the Public Health Service Act. The court found that minors and other incompetents had undergone federally funded sterilization and that an indefinite number of poor people had been improperly coerced into accepting sterilization operations under the threat that various federally supported welfare benefits would be withdrawn unless they submitted.

Local statutes and federal regulations have further limited the use of sterilization. In New York City, for example, statutes passed in 1985 require completion of a complicated informed-consent process and a thirty-day waiting period before sterilization is permitted (*New York City, N.Y., Charter and Administrative Code* §17-401 *et seq.*). Federal regulations also prescribe special informed consent procedures and waiting periods for federally funded sterilizations ("Sterilization of Persons," 1993; "Sterilizations," 1993).

Much current law attempts to protect vulnerable women and limit potential abuse by emphasizing voluntary, informed consent and limiting sterilizations to which individual, capable consent is not given. Even where there is no specific legislation to that effect, compulsory sterilization has become rare; those states that have retained compulsory sterilization statutes on the books have, for the most part, let them slip into disuse (Haavik and Menninger, 1981).

Discussion of eugenics as appropriate public policy for the protection of future generations has largely been discredited because of the Nazis' horrendous abuse of the concept, because of scientific and societal disaffection with eugenic theories, and because of increasing respect for those with developmental and other disabilities. Nonetheless, eugenics is not yet dead. Increasing knowledge about genetics and new reproductive technologies such as in vitro fertilization, artificial insemination, and surrogate motherhood, may allow people to selectively create babies of "higher quality," and may renew the specter of eugenics, albeit in a new light (Neuhaus, 1988).

An ethical policy controlling reproduction must offer a range of contraceptive services to women and men and simultaneously protect adults with reproductive potential from state coercion. New technologies offer increased protection from unwanted pregnancy and increased potential for overriding individual preferences.

NANCY NEVELOFF DUBLER
AMANDA WHITE

Directly related to this article are the other articles in this entry: MEDICAL ASPECTS, SOCIAL ISSUES, *and* ETHICAL ISSUES. *For a further discussion of topics mentioned in this article, see the entries* ABORTION; ABUSE, INTERPERSONAL, *article on* ABUSE BETWEEN DOMESTIC PARTNERS; ADOLESCENTS; AIDS; AUTONOMY; EASTERN ORTHODOX CHRISTIANITY; ETHICS, *articles on* SOCIAL AND POLITICAL THEORIES, *and* RELIGION AND MORALITY; EUGENICS; FAMILY; FREEDOM AND COERCION; INFANTS, *article on* HISTORY OF INFANTICIDE; INFORMED CONSENT; ISLAM; JUDAISM; JUSTICE; LAW AND BIOETHICS; LAW AND MORALITY; MARRIAGE AND OTHER DOMESTIC PARTNERSHIPS; MENTALLY DISABLED AND MENTALLY

ILL PERSONS; NATIONAL SOCIALISM; NATURAL LAW; PAIN AND SUFFERING; POPULATION ETHICS; POPULATION POLICIES, *especially the section on* STRATEGIES OF FERTILITY CONTROL; PRISONERS; PROTESTANTISM; RACE AND RACISM; REPRODUCTIVE TECHNOLOGIES; RIGHTS; RISK; ROMAN CATHOLICISM; SEXISM; SEXUAL ETHICS; SEXUALITY IN SOCIETY; *and* WOMEN, *especially the article on* HISTORICAL AND CROSS-CULTURAL PERSPECTIVES. *For a discussion of related ideas, see the entries* AUTHORITY; BEHAVIOR CONTROL; COMPETENCE; EUGENICS AND RELIGIOUS LAW; GENETIC COUNSELING; GENETICS AND THE LAW; GENETIC TESTING AND SCREENING; LIFE; PERSON; PHARMACEUTICS; PROSTITUTION; PUBLIC POLICY AND BIOETHICS; *and* TECHNOLOGY.

Bibliography

ARTHUR, STACEY L. 1992. "The Norplant Prescription: Birth Control, Woman Control, or Crime Control?" *UCLA Law Review* 40, no. 1:1–101.

A.W., In re. 1981. 637 P.2d 366 (Colo.).

BANWELL, SUZANNA S., and PAXMAN, JOHN M. 1992. "The Search for Meaning: RU 486 and the Law of Abortion." *American Journal of Public Health* 82, no. 10:1399–1406.

"Birth Control, Pregnancy, Child Placement, and Abortion." 1993. 28 C.F.R. 551.23.

BOARD OF TRUSTEES. AMERICAN MEDICAL ASSOCIATION. 1992. "Requirements or Incentives by Government for the Use of Long-Acting Contraceptives." *Journal of the American Medical Association* 267, no. 13:1818–1821.

Bolger vs. Young Drug Products Corp. 1983. 463 U.S. 60.

Buck v. Bell. 1927. 274 U.S. 200.

Carey v. Population Services International. 1977. 431 U.S. 678.

CHESSLER, ELLEN. 1992. *Women of Valor: Margaret Sanger and the Birth Control Movement in America.* New York: Simon & Schuster.

Conservatorship of Valerie N., In re. 1985. 707 P.2d 760 (Cal.).

Cruzan v. Director, Missouri Department of Health. 1990. 497 U.S. 261.

Eberhardy, In re. 1980. 294 N.W.2d 540, 97 Wis.2d 654 (Wis.Ct.App.).

Eisenstadt v. Baird. 1972. 405 U.S. 438.

FATHALLA, MAHMOUD; ROSENFIELD, ALLAN; and INDRISO, CYNTHIA. 1990. "Family Planning." In *Family Planning.* Edited by Mahmoud Fathalla and Allan Rosenfield. Vol. 2 of *The FIGO Manual of Human Reproduction.* Park Ridge, N.J.: Parthenon.

Federal Food, Drug, and Cosmetic Act. 1938. 21 U.S.C. §301 *et seq.*

FOX, ELEANOR M., and TRAYNOR, MICHAEL. 1990. "Biotechnology and Products Liability." *ALI-ABA Continuing Course of Study: Biotechnology Law.* American Law Institute: Nov. 8.

FRANCOME, COLIN. 1984. *Abortion Freedom: A Worldwide Movement.* Boston: Allen & Unwin.

Grady, In re. 1981. 85 N.J. 235, 426 A.2d 467.

Griswold v. Connecticut. 1965. 381 U.S. 479.

HAAVIK, SARAH F., and MENNINGER, KARL A. 1981. *Sexuality, Law, and the Developmentally Disabled Person: Legal and Clinical Aspects of Marriage, Parenthood, and Sterilization.* Baltimore: Paul H. Brookes.

Hathaway v. Worcester City Hospital. 1973. 475 F.2d 701 (1st Cir.).

Hayes, In re. 1980. 93 Wash.2d 228, 608 P.2d 635.

HENDERSON, JAMES A., JR., and TWERSKI, AARON D. 1990. "Doctrinal Collapse in Products Liability: The Empty Shell of Failure to Warn." *New York University Law Review* 65, no. 2:265–327.

Hilliard v. A. H. Robins Co. 1984. 196 Cal.Rptr. 117, 148 Cal.App.3d 374 (2nd Dist.).

Hudson v. Hudson. 1979. 373 So.2d 310 (Ala.).

Jane Does 1 Through 4 v. State of Utah Department of Health. 1985. 776 F.2d 253 (10th Cir.).

KELLY, JOAN. 1977. "Sterilization and Civil Rights." *Rights* 23, no. 5:9–11.

LARSON, DAVID R. 1991. "Contraception and Coercion: Theological Reflections, Update." *Loma Linda University Center for Christian Bioethics* 7, no. 2 (June):4–5.

LEEBRON, DAVID W. 1990. "An Introduction to Products Liability: Origins, Issues and Trends." *Annual Survey of American Law* 1990, bk. 2:395–458.

MASTROIANNI, LUIGI; DONALDSON, PETER J.; and KANE, THOMAS T., eds. 1990. *Developing New Contraceptives: Obstacles and Opportunities.* Washington, D.C.: National Academy Press.

MEANS, CYRIL C., JR. 1971. "The Phoenix of Abortional Freedom: Is a Penumbral or Ninth-Amendment Right About to Arise from the Nineteenth-Century Legislative Ashes of a Fourteenth-Century Common-Law Liberty?" *New York Law Forum* 22, no. 2:335–410.

MERTUS, JULIE, and HELLER, SIMON. 1992. "Norplant Meets the New Eugenicists: The Impermissibility of Coerced Contraception." *Saint Louis University Public Law Review,* 11, no. 2:359–383.

MINTZ, MORTON. 1985. *At Any Cost: Corporate Greed, Women and the Dalkon Shield.* New York: Pantheon.

Moe, In re. 1982. 432 N.E. 2d 712, 385 Mass, 555 (Sup.Ct. Mass.).

MOHR, JAMES C. 1978. *Abortion in America: The Origins and Evolutions of National Policy, 1800–1900.* New York: Oxford University Press.

NEUHAUS, JOHN. 1988. "The Return of Eugenics." *Commentary* 15:26.

People v. Sanger. 1918. 222 N.E. 192, 118 N.E. 637; 251 U.S. 536 (1919).

PETCHESKY, ROSALIND P. 1990. *Abortion and Women's Choice: The State, Sexuality, and Reproductive Freedom.* Rev. ed. Boston: Northeastern University Press.

Planned Parenthood Association of Utah v. Dandoy. 1987. 810 F.2d 984 (10th Cir).

Planned Parenthood of Central Missouri v. Danforth. 1976. 428 U.S. 52.

PRESTON, YVONNE. 1992. "China's Shadow Population." *Straits Times,* June 21, pp. 1–2.

P.S., In re. 1983. 452 N.E.2d 969 (Sup.Ct.Ind.).

REED, JAMES. 1978. *From Private Vice to Public Virtue: The Birth Control Movement and American Society Since 1830.* New York: Basic Books.

REILLY, JOHN P. 1989. "The Erosion of Comment K." *University of Dayton Law Review* 14, no. 2:255–278.

Relf v. Weinberger. 1977. 372 F.Supp. 1196 (Dist. D.C.); motion denied, *sub nom. Relf* v. *Matthews*, 403 F.Supp. 1235 (Dist. D.C. 1975): order vacated, *Relf* v. *Weinberger,* 565 F.2d 722, 184 U.S.App.D.C. 147 (1977).

ROBERTSON, WILLIAM. 1990. *An Illustrated History of Contraception: A Concise Account of the Quest for Fertility Control.* Park Ridge, N.J.: Parthenon.

Roe v. Wade. 1973. 410 U.S. 113.

Ruby v. Massey. 1978. 452 R.Supp. 361 (Dist. Conn.).

Rust v. Sullivan. 1991. 111 S.Ct. 1759.

Skinner v. Oklahoma ex-rel. Williamson. 1942. 62 S.Ct. 1110.

SLOAN, IRVING J. 1988. *The Law Governing Abortion, Contraception and Sterilization.* New York: Oceana.

STEPHEN, CHRIS. "Romania: Abortions Skyrocket, Contraception Yet to Take Hold." International Press Service release, August 19.

"Sterilization of Persons in Federally Assisted Programs of the Public Health Service." 1993. 42 C.F.R. 50,201 *et seq.*

"Sterilizations." 1993. 42 C.F.R. 441.250 *et seq.*

ST. JOHN-STEVAS, NORMAN. 1971. *Agonizing Choice: Birth Control, Religion, and the Law.* Bloomington: Indiana University Press.

Tariff Act. 1930. 19 U.S.C.A. §305(a).

Tetuan v. A. H. Robins Co. 1987. 241 Kan. 441, 738 P.2d 1210.

THOMAS, CHRISTOPHER. 1990. "A Society Defeats Its Own Rules." *Times* (London), January 6.

U.S. v. One Package Containing 120, More or Less, Rubber Pessaries to Prevent Conception. 1936. 86 F.2d 737.

WESTON, MARK. 1990. "Where the World's Major Religions Disagree." *Washington Post,* January 23, p. Z12.

FETAL–MATERNAL RELATIONSHIP

See MATERNAL–FETAL RELATIONSHIP.

FETAL RESEARCH AND THERAPY

See FETUS.

FETAL TISSUE TRANSPLANTS

See ORGAN AND TISSUE PROCUREMENT, *article on* ETHICAL AND LEGAL ISSUES REGARDING CADAVERS; *and* FETUS.

FETUS

The first of the following three articles describes human development from the initial meeting of ovum and sperm until birth; the second article presents and comments on the philosophical, ethical, and legal issues dealing with the human conceptus; and the third article deals in a special way with research utilizing the human fetus. The title of the entire entry is "Fetus" because that is the term most commonly consulted when information on ethical debates pertaining to prenatal stages of human development is being sought. A variety of accepted usages of the term "fetus" is found in the following articles.

I. Human Development from Fertilization to Birth
> *Clifford Grobstein*
II. Philosophical and Ethical Issues
> *Mary B. Mahowald*
III. Fetal Research
> *LeRoy Walters*

I. HUMAN DEVELOPMENT FROM FERTILIZATION TO BIRTH

The overall developmental process that gives rise to a new human being is initiated by fertilization, the union of two specialized cells or gametes—egg and sperm—produced by two adult individuals of one species but opposite gender. The product of this union is the zygote (or fusion cell), which combines genetic information received from two hereditarily different parental lineages of the human species.

The word "zygote" is often used loosely. It is derived from the Greek *zygotos* (yoked together). In the strict sense, it should be applied to the one-cell fertilizing egg only after commingling of the genetic material from the mother and father, that is, after the dissolution of the membranes that surround and separate the two genetic messages—the two pronuclei. Prior to dissolution of the pronuclear membranes, the one-cell fertilizing egg is often called a prezygote. With the first cell division, the zygote gives way to the pre-embryo. The pre-embryo comes into existence with the first cell division and lasts until the appearance of a single primitive streak, which is the first sign of organ differentiation. This occurs at about fourteen days of development, after which the word "embryo" can be properly applied. The pre-embryonic interval can be further subdivided, depending upon the developmental state of the conceptus, as will be noted. For the purpose of this article, unless a technical meaning as just described is required, the generic word "conceptus" will be used. "Conceptus" can be used to describe any stage of development from fertilization to birth.

While these minutiae of definition are of interest mainly to the biologist, the details of the fertilizing process (which takes about twenty-four hours) and the pre-embryonic span (which lasts about fourteen days) have acquired moral significance. From a biological viewpoint, fertilization is a process, not an event; it is not possible to identify a biological moment of fertilization. The pre-embryonic span is marked by a biological instability, such as the possibility of tumor formation or twinning, so that biological individuation is not guaranteed until embryonic differentiation begins, marked by the appearance of the primitive streak. The complex interaction of these processes will be described below.

The cellular union takes place soon after the egg has been discharged (ovulated) from a mature ovarian follicle, usually into or near the funnel-shaped upper end of the oviduct (fallopian tube). The resulting conceptus is then propelled along the oviduct toward the uterus by ciliary action of the tubal lining.

During tubal transit the conceptus undergoes cleavage, a series of cell divisions that occur without significant intervening cellular growth. The cleavage process thus converts the single-celled zygote into a spherical cluster of smaller cells (blastomeres) making up the morula. Subsequently, a central cavity forms within the morula, converting it into the fluid-filled blastocyst. Still later a cluster of blastomeres at one pole of the blastocyst projects into the central cavity, or blastocoele. The cell aggregate thus produced from the blastocyst is referred to as the inner cell mass. It is the precursor to the entire later embryo.

The blastocyst and its immediately preceding and succeeding stages take place within the pre-embryo period. At this time the developing entity displays significant organization above the level of individual cells but has not yet begun formation of the recognizable organ rudiments characteristic of a typical embryo. In fact, the outer cellular layer of the pre-embryonic blastocyst never becomes part of the later embryo. Instead, it specializes as the peripheral trophoblast (feeding layer) of the developing entity. It is this outer trophoblast that makes first contact—on arrival of the blastocyst in the uterus—with the uterine lining, becoming incorporated into it in the process of implantation. Thus, none of the outer trophoblast cells participate in the embryo itself; rather, derivatives of these cells contribute to the later placenta, which is discarded as part of the afterbirth.

While these events are occurring, the inner cell mass organizes as the direct precursor of the entire new organism-to-be, first as the pre-embryo, then sequentially as the embryo, the fetus, and eventually the neonate. It is to be especially noted that the preliminary steps toward embryo formation are closely associated in

time with implantation, thereby constituting the first stages of actual pregnancy in the mother. In this process, what in the earlier pre-embryonic stage was a helter-skelter "inner cell mass" begins to aggregate into two distinct and coherent cell layers, one within the other. The outer of these, in relation to the embryo-to-be, is referred to as the ectoderm; the inner one, as the endoderm.

A little later there can be observed in the transforming pre-embryo a linear "primitive streak" that is significant in several important ways. First, the streak corresponds in its location and orientation to the major head-to-tail axis of the embryo-to-be—which will arise directly in front of and in line with the streak. This new axis provides the foundation of the embryo as a *single* multicellular individual. Second, the primitive streak turns out to be a thickening marked by inturning of surface cells into a new middle layer (the mesoderm), expanding as a third cellular sheet between the established ectoderm and endoderm. Third, later close interactions between the mesoderm and either the ectoderm or the endoderm are essential to subsequent embryogenesis, both of the embryo as a whole and in initiation and formation (morphogenesis) of individual embryonic organ rudiments.

Through these processes and events the pre-embryo transforms to a higher level of organization manifested as the embryo proper. The orientation (axiation) and development of organs (organogenesis) that mark the period of the embryo are regarded as terminating at about eight weeks after fertilization, when human bodily form and most major organs can be recognized as at least rudimentary precursors. Among the organs thus emerging are the heart and its major circulation, the tubular and elongating central nervous system, the segmented major skeletal axis and associated muscle groups, and the paired limbs. It should come as no surprise, therefore, that near the end of the embryonic period, limited bodily movements are detectable and visualized by ultrasonography. Indeed, it seems reasonable to interpret such bodily movements as indicators of the transition from embryo to fetus, where the latter exhibits increasing structural organization and functional maturation.

However, there are important caveats to be noted with regard to such simplifying generalizations. Primitive movement, such as the first turning of the head, observed six to eight weeks after fertilization, is certainly an indicator of deeper neuromuscular maturation. But such movements do not require or demonstrate higher-order cognitive function—such as later-appearing sensation, pain, or intention. The latter require and are manifestations of significant brain function. But at eight weeks the brain is anatomically only a rudiment, without the differentiated cellular neurons essential to neural function. Movements at this stage, therefore, are important indicators of developing neuromuscular connection but offer no evidence of such cognitive activities as are known to be associated with the more mature and functional brain.

The lesson provided by this cautionary note can be generalized to other differences between embryonic and fetal properties and capabilities. In fact, the embryo can be regarded as occupied largely with generating new structures and their relationships—what embryologists call morphogenesis and construction workers speak of as "roughing out" a planned construction. The fetus, on the other hand, is largely involved with establishment and maturation of functional activity patterns—processes that will continue into and even beyond the newborn.

Thus, to say that by eight weeks the embryo has become a fetus is a legitimate broad generalization of an overall course. It does not, however, deny that a beating heart and early circulation of primitive blood were established considerably before eight weeks. Nor, on the other hand, does it convey the clear fact that fetal kidneys and lungs are still inadequate for effective extrauterine function even at twenty weeks.

Thus, the terms "embryo" and "fetus" are valid in distinguishing broadly different overall periods in a complex developmental continuum. The two periods are very different in their dominant developmental nature, particularly if one focuses on their initial states and their terminations. But the overall difference does not precisely apply to each and every time and aspect throughout the complex developmental course. The initiation of bodily movements, as now revealed by ultrasonography in the sixth and seventh weeks, is as good a marker as any other in defining the embryo–fetal transition.

Developmental stages and moral status

Why should the limits of particular developmental periods become the subject of vigorous and even contentious debate? Because such limits offer possibilities for dealing with a deeply divisive issue—the assignment of status and rights to human offspring during the course of their development. The problem is epitomized in the activist claim that the human conceptus has a right to life. To generalize the question thus posed: At what points in the course of development does human offspring acquire increasing value and entitlement rights as a person? Should such status be assigned at sharply delineated developmental times, technically defined and specified once and for all? Or should status arise—as realization itself proceeds in most gradual becomings—over extended periods that include and are influenced by changing circumstances? Should the defined circumstances be subject to judgments by evaluators who may take into account wider contexts, including ethical and

religious teachings? And if such broader approaches seem reasonable or necessary, what are the critical developmental transitions that must be evaluated with respect to so central and complex a matter as personhood? And what contextual factors are to be taken into account in making such judgments?

Certainly a first step in any such difficult process is to establish which developmental transitions impinge critically upon the concepts of a person held by various informed parties. For example, fertilization restores an ovum to the diploid chromosomal state, in the process combining in a single cell what are the essentially equal but nonidentical genetic contributions from the two parental lineages. Few knowledgeable observers would doubt that when fertilization is completed, it has established the significant genetic foundation for the resulting person-to-be. On this basis, many argue that fertilization is, in fact, the definitive event in the process of human neogenesis.

But even this group would not seriously propose that zygotes should be counted as persons by the Census Bureau, or should be enfranchised to vote, or should be drafted into military service—all of these being reasonably applicable to the term "person" as it is variously defined in the law. Moreover, reestablishment of multicellularity in the course of cleavage of the zygote certainly makes a major contribution to essential aspects of a person—in this instance the unity of one individual despite a multiplicity of cellular components. In experiments on mice and other mammals, separation of blastomeres during the first several cleavages allows each blastomere to become a complete individual of the same genotype; that is, it produces identical twins. Identical human twins sometimes arise spontaneously, presumably by similar mechanisms. These observations suggest that multicellular singleness depends upon significant interactions among the early blastomeres, interactions that are, then, certainly prerequisite to the origin of a person.

Moreover, such interactive cellular processes also occur in the later developmental course. In both the embryo and the fetus, genetic defects or exposure to toxic substances in the environment can disrupt normal development, leading to severe abnormality and even premature death. Thus development must be regarded as a series of sequelae to hereditary intergenerational messages played out in particular environments and circumstances, which can also influence the developmental course.

Indeed, in carefully tracing such developmental courses we become aware of a stepwise progression through which the realized, most significant properties of a human person evolve—until it is generally acknowledged as fully human and endowed with the rights and privileges respected and guaranteed by the entire company of persons. And is such a definition and its resultant not a shared goal of advocates of both the opposing positions in the abortion wars?

Can persuasive examples of such steps and processes be brought forward? Certainly fertilization involves some of the required characteristics and is regarded by some as having all that are necessary. During fertilization, hereditary entities (chromosomes) contributed by two previously unrelated individuals are combined in one new entity that has a unique hereditary constitution with characteristics traceable back to both parents. Such a unique individual stemming from human parentage certainly, it is argued, makes a strong claim to recognition as possessing moral status as a human person.

However, to others the case seems insufficient and far from fully convincing. Such a conceptus may be acknowledged as a step in the right direction, but the step is by no means fully determinative. For example, a person is a *single* individual, whereas a human pre-embryo is still potentially at least a pair of identical twins, that is, at least two individual persons. Indeed, in armadillos, the early conceptus regularly produces four individuals following regular separation of the first four blastomeres.

Therefore, the claim that fertilization immediately results in a single person in the full moral sense is unconvincing to those who defend a woman's right to choose what happens to her own body. Nonetheless, even this group has to acknowledge that significant steps toward a person occur during the course of fertilization, in particular formation of a new genetic entity—a zygote both developmentally activated and possessing established kinship with the two parental lineages that contributed to it. And the latter heritage includes not only the direct parental donors of the chromosomes but also the ancestral lineage network that contributed to each parent.

In consequence, it would seem, the zygote and its derivative pre-embryo should have a moral and legal status that acknowledges its complex biological genesis as well as its resulting developmental potential. Accordingly, the significance and value of pre-embryos should be recognized as more than that of individual gametes but less than that of fully developed, existential persons.

Following initiation by fertilization, a next major event requiring consideration for significant moral status is implantation and its associated complications. During implantation the pre-embryo—previously floating free and therefore at least physically independent—enters into intimately interactive coexistence with its female parent. Thanks to the erosive effects of its peripheral trophoblast on the uterine lining, the pre-embryo penetrates the underlying, highly vascular endometrium of the uterine wall.

Implantation, like fertilization, is a process, not an event. The pre-embryo attaches to the endometrial surface at about the fifth day after fertilization but is not completely within the endometrium; it is not completely implanted until about the twelfth day after fertilization. While this implantation process is under way or soon after completion, the conceptus is undergoing the other developmental events described here, such as the appearance of the primitive streak. Thus, the continuum of development and the changes in nomenclature from pre-embryo to embryo take place during or immediately after the implantation process.

Important support for this implantation process is provided by the maternal ovary, within which the ruptured follicle has transformed into the corpus luteum (yellow body). The luteal cells produce the pregnancy-fostering hormone progesterone. This hormone, on reaching the endometrium via the maternal circulation, stabilizes its highly vascular state; if progesterone is withdrawn or blocked in its action, the endometrium sloughs and bleeding occurs, as in monthly menstruation. Therefore, premature termination of the action of progesterone is contragestational, blocking implantation or terminating it (abortion) if it has already begun.

In a stable pregnancy, however, as noted, transformation of the pre-embryo into an embryo continues—as does expansion of the area of interaction between the trophoblast and the maternal endometrium. Thus, both embryonic organization and maternal adaptation to the presence and needs of the offspring significantly increase as implantation proceeds. In the case of the pre-embryo, it has now become established as a single individual in continuing development. In the case of the mother, she is now pregnant in the full sense. Her uterine lining has been invaded, and her hormonal status has been profoundly altered. Therefore, both mother and offspring have passed the point of high risk of biological error, and the reproductive process is fully under way.

These changes call for careful reconsideration of the status of the conceptus, now entering early embryonic stages (as evidenced by the soon recognizable primitive streak). Such conceptuses, unlike earlier stages, have become developmentally single—that is, so far as is known, they do not, and presumably cannot, undergo twinning. Their definitive singleness clearly constitutes an important step toward what we commonly think of as a single human individual. Achievement of this stage establishes a claim that the early embryo is entitled to some measure of personhood even if pre-embryonic stages are not.

However, also to be noted is the fact that developmental singleness is not characteristic only of the human species, nor even of mammalian lineages. Therefore, something further must be added before a developing *human* entity is clearly to be regarded as a person. This additional requirement is among the most difficult to define precisely. It clearly involves the behavioral realm but is more than the simple occurrence of behavior. It involves activities of the brain but not just any brain activity. Certain parts of the brain and their activities are especially relevant. Moreover, the necessary activities are among those that are regarded as most uniquely human—even though details of the activities are still an enigma. Stated synoptically, to be a person requires particular activities of the brain, activities at least on the way toward a self-image with some capacity to generate behavior on its own behalf.

This sketch of a concept and possible genesis of a person is hardly a satisfying or definitive answer to the question of when a human person comes into being, that is, becomes a human being, in the course of its development. But it suggests a process that is gradual and stepwise rather than a sudden transformation. It places special emphasis on maturation of the brain. In these terms, fertilization, implantation, embryonic morphogenesis, and fetal maturation all play roles in establishing the foundations of personhood. But the definitive realization of the moral status of a person would seem to await appropriate maturation of the brain, which is achieved only marginally even in the newborn. Thus, in this view, the immediate major substrate of what is diagnostic of a person lies in the brain and is not fully developed even in the newborn. Better understanding of this substrate requires greater knowledge of brain function and its maturation.

Conclusion

The genesis of a person begins at fertilization and proceeds stepwise throughout gestation. The generative process is not completed and terminated even at birth. An understanding of the moral significance of the various stages of prenatal human development requires further investigation and reflection. Meanwhile, practical policy governing the status and treatment of developing persons might recognize such subcategories as nonpersons, prepersons, protopersons, quasi persons, and neopersons—each meriting specification within the individual life history of human personhood.

CLIFFORD GROBSTEIN

Directly related to this article are the other articles in this entry: PHILOSOPHICAL AND ETHICAL ISSUES, *and* FETAL RESEARCH. *Also directly related are the entries* PERSON; *and* LIFE. *This article will find application in the entries* ABORTION, *article on* MEDICAL PERSPECTIVES, *and section on* CONTEMPORARY ETHICAL AND LEGAL ASPECTS; FERTILITY CONTROL, *article on* MEDICAL ASPECTS; MATERNAL–FETAL RELATIONSHIP, *article on* MEDICAL ASPECTS; *and* REPRODUCTIVE TECHNOLOGIES. *For a discussion of related ideas, see the entry* BIOLOGY, PHILOSOPHY OF.

Bibliography

ETHICS COMMITTEE OF THE AMERICAN FERTILITY SOCIETY. 1988. "Ethical Considerations of the New Reproductive Technologies." *Fertility and Sterility* 49, no. 6 (Suppl. 1).
———. 1990. "Ethical Considerations of the New Reproductive Technologies." *Fertility and Sterility* 53, no. 6 (Suppl. 2).
GROBSTEIN, CLIFFORD. 1988. *Science and the Unborn: Choosing Human Futures.* New York: Basic Books.
MCCORMICK, RICHARD A. 1991. "Who or What Is the Preembryo?" *Kennedy Institute of Ethics Journal* 1, no. 1:1–15.
MORGAN, DEREK, and LEE, ROBERT G. 1991. *Blackstone's Guide to the Human Fertilization and Embryology Act, 1990: Abortion and Embryo Research, the New Law.* Arlington, Texas: Blackstone Press.
ROBERTSON, JOHN A. 1991. "What We May Do with the Preembryos: A Response to Richard A. McCormick." *Kennedy Institute of Ethics Journal* 1, no. 4:293–302.

II. PHILOSOPHICAL AND ETHICAL ISSUES

Fetuses are generally defined as "the unborn young of a viviparous animal" (*Stedman's Medical Dictionary,* 1990, p. 573). Although the focus of this article is human fetuses, some morally relevant considerations, such as the ability to experience pain, apply to nonhuman fetuses as well.

The "viviparous [live-bearing] animal" in which the human fetus develops is female. Once removed or delivered from the body of a pregnant woman, it is no longer a fetus but an abortus or a newborn. Thus, the meaning and existence of human fetuses cannot be adequately understood apart from their crucial relationship to pregnant women.

While the end of fetal development is clearly marked by termination of pregnancy through birth or abortion, the origin of fetal development is more difficult to specify. In ordinary language, the term "fetus" is sometimes used to describe the developing organism from fertilization until birth. For opponents of elective abortion, for example, a "fetal right to life" is generally attributed to embryos as well as fetuses. If this usage were followed with regard to organisms whose development is initiated in the laboratory, it would be appropriate to speak of fetuses as existing apart from women's bodies.

Development of the embryo precedes that of the fetus, and the term "pre-embryo" has been used to characterize the developing organism from fertilization until implantation. Although the term "conceptus" is sometimes used for the developing organism from fertilization until birth, this term also applies to other products of conception, including the placenta and embryonic or fetal membranes. Some authors prefer the term "preimplantation embryo" for the period immediately following fertilization (Michaeli et al., 1990, p. 341).

In what follows, the term "embryo" refers to the developing organism from fertilization until fetal stage, regardless of whether development occurs in vivo or in vitro. The term "preimplantation embryo" identifies the organism prior to implantation, when pregnancy is established. The term "fetus" is used for organisms that have developed beyond the embryonic period but have not yet been born or aborted. Where developmental stage is not pertinent to the discussion, the term "fetus" refers to the organism at any stage of its development, including the embryonic and preimplantation stages.

What kind of beings are fetuses?

The principal philosophical question to be addressed regarding fetuses is "What kind of beings are they?" Answers to this question determine the legal and moral status of the fetus, which is essential to resolution of a variety of ethical issues. At least four factors must be considered in answering the question: (1) its immaturity; (2) its presence in, and dependence (if its potential is to be realized) on, a biologically mature female; (3) its species membership; (4) its property of or potential for personhood.

A mature human adult is capable of reproducing its own kind. Children as well as fetuses are immature by this standard, but most fetuses are also immature by a standard that measures maturity as ability to survive outside a woman's body, that is, viability. Prenatal tests for fetal maturity, for example, measure the ability of the fetus to breathe on its own. Fetuses are more mature or less immature by either standard than embryos, including preimplantation embryos, despite the ability of the latter to survive briefly in vitro. Some fetuses are more mature than some preterm or premature infants because the latter have not completed the duration of gestation that generally precedes birth.

The more immature the organism, the greater degree of maturation it is capable of achieving during its life span. At the same time, the probability of maturation is increased during the course of early development. It is estimated that up to 75 percent of all human conceptions and 15–25 percent of all physiologically recognized pregnancies are aborted spontaneously (Knight and Callahan, 1989). If a fetus is viable, its probability of survival approaches that of a newborn. Viability is morally significant because it reduces the dependence of the fetus on the pregnant woman. If the pregnancy is then interrupted, others may determine the fate of the newborn.

Neither embryonic nor fetal development is possible apart from a woman's body. Even preimplantation embryos can be sustained for only about two days in vitro. At that point they must be frozen or placed within a woman's body in order to survive. The woman who gestates the embryo or fetus need not be genetically related to the offspring to whom she gives birth. Freezing results in 25 to 50 percent loss of embryos; the process arrests development, which can recommence only if the embryo is thawed and placed within a woman's body (Bonnicksen, 1988).

Although some believe that the entire duration of embryonic and fetal development may someday take place in vitro, it is not clear that this is biologically possible. If such development were possible, the dependence on women that has characterized the developing organism from the origin of humankind would no longer hold. Pregnancy would no longer be necessary. Even if the definition of a fetus were expanded to accommodate that state of affairs, a morally relevant distinction would still obtain between fetuses that develop in vitro and those that develop in vivo. If the fetus could be brought to term in vitro, the claim of women's right to determine the fate of the fetus would be considerably weakened.

While the in vitro status of the developing organism may seem to equalize the claims of men and women regarding the fate of externalized "fetuses," two factors argue against this: the fact that women experience both risk and discomfort in providing gametes, while men do not, and the fact that women are much more likely than men to be the principal caregivers of their offspring. It may further be argued that an externalized "fetus" capable of full development in vitro is comparable with a newborn, having rights of its own that supersede those of either genetic parent.

Because an embryo or fetus develops from human gametes, it is human. However, this does not imply that the human fetus is a person or has rights. It may be argued that even if human fetuses are not persons, we are obliged to avoid killing or inflicting pain on them. The concepts of humanness, sentience (the ability to feel pain or pleasure), and personhood are thus separable in their application to human fetuses. Although humanness is a matter of fact and the onset of sentience is a matter of uncertainty, both concepts are empirically grounded and definable. Because personhood is not necessarily empirically grounded, its definition is more difficult and controversial.

While the question of whether human fetuses are persons is debated by philosophers and theologians, their potential for personhood is accepted even by those who deny that they are persons. The potential for personhood also distinguishes human fetuses from other human tissue and organs. R. M. Hare maintains that human gametes are potential human beings, thus attributing the potential to separate cells (ova and sperm) existing in different bodies (Hare, 1975). Unlike separate gametes, however, the human zygote is a single cell that will naturally develop toward birth and unquestionable personhood unless impeded by spontaneous or elective means.

The legal status of human fetuses

Throughout the world, the legal status of fetuses is generally subordinated to that of pregnant women, but the degree to which women's interests or preferences are given priority varies from country to country, depending on the circumstances. Laws regulating abortion are generally indicative of the range of views. In countries such as Ireland and Honduras, for example, abortion is legal only if the woman's life is threatened by the pregnancy; the rationale for this position is that "the right to life [of the fetus] is inviolable" (Cook and Dickens, 1988, p. 1305). In countries such as Hungary, Norway, Taiwan, and Barbados, socioeconomic reasons are sufficient to override a fetal "right to life." In most countries, the legal status of the fetus is strengthened as gestation progresses. However, laws restricting or permitting abortion do not address the legal status of in vivo preimplantation embryos whose implantation may be prevented through use of contraceptive measures such as intrauterine devices. Neither do abortion laws address the legal status of in vitro preimplantation embryos.

In 1973, the *Roe* v. *Wade* decision of the U.S. Supreme Court maintained that "the word 'person,' as used in the Fourteenth Amendment, does not include the unborn" (*Roe* v. *Wade*, 1972, p. 158). Nonetheless, the Supreme Court affirmed that the states may prohibit abortion subsequent to fetal viability unless the pregnant woman's health is threatened by continuation of the pregnancy. Thus, although the fetus is not legally a person at any stage of its development, viability signifies a change in its legal status. Accordingly, some judicial rulings have compelled women to undergo surgery for the sake of a viable or possibly viable fetus (Kolder et al., 1987).

With the liberalization of abortion legislation in the United States in 1973, some feared that greater availability of abortuses might lead to widespread abuse involving fetal experimentation. The following year, a congressional moratorium was imposed upon federal funding of fetal research until the National Commission for the Protection of Human Subjects of Biomedical and Behavioral Research developed guidelines for such research. A fundamental principle of the commission was that fetuses to be aborted should not be subject to research procedures that were not also applicable to fetuses to be carried to term. Because fetuses in either category

were to be treated in accordance with the same standard, this was called "the equality principle" (Fletcher and Ryan, 1987, p. 127). The commission's recommendations were partially codified in 1975 as federal regulations.

The regulations governing fetal research in the United States refer to the abortus as a "fetus ex utero" (Baron, 1985, p. 13). Requirements vary, depending on whether the experimental procedure is therapeutic to the pregnant woman or to the fetus, whether the procedure is performed in utero or ex utero, whether the fetus is living or dead, and if living, whether it is viable, nonviable, or possibly viable. Research involving pregnant women must have a therapeutic goal for the woman, or risks to the fetus must be minimal. Research with fetuses must be therapeutic or involve minimal risk for the fetus, and must be intended to provide significant knowledge that is inaccessible by other means. The last requirement is also applicable to research with nonviable and possibly viable abortuses. Additionally, research with nonviable living abortuses must avoid artificial maintenance of vital functions or deliberate termination of the abortus's heartbeat or respiration. Research with possibly viable abortuses must have a therapeutic goal and must avoid added risk for the abortus. Research with "viable abortuses" is subject to the same standard as research with newborns. Since abortion is clinically defined as termination of a pregnancy before viability, the term "viable abortus" is problematic. By that definition, a living human organism capable of surviving ex utero is not an abortus.

Research with dead fetuses in the United States is covered by the Uniform Anatomical Gift Act, which specifies that the "decedents" to which it applies include any "stillborn infant or a fetus" (Baron, 1985, p. 13). The act permits the gift of "all or part of the . . . body" of a dead fetus to be used for research or therapeutic purposes, so long as consent is obtained from "either parent" (Baron, 1985, p. 13). This act has been adopted in some form by all fifty states and the District of Columbia. Jurisdictions vary in their requirements for research with human fetuses, both living and dead. Some, for example, distinguish between the use of fetal tissue obtained from elective abortions and tissue obtained from spontaneous abortions: the latter is permitted, while the former is not.

Federal regulations governing fetal research in the United States virtually preclude research with preimplantation embryos developed through in vitro technology. In contrast, the United Kingdom, following the recommendations of the Warnock Commission, enacted legislation that permits fetal experimentation until about fourteen days after fertilization. This point coincides with the formation of "the primitive streak" and the end of the possibility of twinning or recombination of the developing embryo (Glover, 1989, p. 100).

The moral status of human fetuses

Views about the moral status of human fetuses are even more far-ranging than views about their legal status. Because fetuses develop within women's bodies, some have characterized them as extraneous and sometimes unwanted tissue that women are as morally free to dispose of as they are free to dispose of growths or tumors. Because of the dependence of the fetus on the pregnant woman, some authors have characterized it as parasitic. On either of these accounts, the fetus has no moral status of its own.

At the opposite end of the spectrum is the view that the fetus has an independent moral status, despite the fact that it can exist only within the body of a pregnant woman. John Noonan, for example, maintains that the genetic humanity of the embryo, initiated at fertilization, gives it a right to life equal to that of any adult human being, including the pregnant woman (Noonan, 1970). Between these opposing views are positions that attribute to the fetus some moral status, but a status that is always subordinate to that of those who are unquestionably persons. As with its legal status, the moral status of the fetus is more likely to be supported late in its gestation. Carson Strong and Garland Anderson, for example, argue that the viable fetus has rights comparable with those of the newborn, while the nonviable fetus lacks those rights (Strong and Anderson, 1989). In contrast, Mary Anne Warren maintains that "the moral significance of birth" is such that the moral status of a developmentally younger newborn supersedes that of an older viable fetus. Her defense of this position is that "it is impossible to treat fetuses in utero as if they were persons without treating women as if they were something less than persons" (Warren, 1989, p. 59). Other authors place the point for affirming a fetal right to life earlier in gestation, some arguing that this occurs when individuation (the potential for separate existence) is established, others arguing that the onset of brain activity is the crucial threshold (Ford, 1988; Sass, 1989).

Another variable in views about the moral status of the fetus is an alleged distinction between those destined to be brought to term and those destined to be aborted. The argument here is that once a woman has declined the option of abortion, she is morally bound to make subsequent decisions that are protective of her developing fetus (Mattingly, 1992). Obviously, this distinction is at odds with the equality principle mentioned above, because obligations to fetuses destined to be born are more stringent than those toward fetuses destined to be aborted. It is also at odds with the principle of respect for autonomy, so long as that principle entails recognition of the fact that autonomous persons (including pregnant women) sometimes change their minds. The distinction is generally based on moral obligations to the potential child rather than to the fetus. On such an account we do not necessarily have responsibilities to fetuses as such.

It is not surprising that much of the debate about the moral status of the fetus focuses on the relevance of its potential for full or unquestionable personhood. Brian Johnstone supports the position that potential for personhood is morally compelling by distinguishing among three uses of the term "potential": a weak sense, in which one thing can be transformed into another by any kind of cause; a strong sense, in which something has the capacity for transformation within itself; and a statistical sense, which simply means that there is "high probability" that one thing will be transformed into another (Walters and Singer, 1982, pp. 49–50). Johnstone attributes all three of these senses to the human embryo, contrasting these with the absence of the strong or statistical sense of potential in human gametes. The implication is that human embryos, in virtue of their greater potential for personhood, have a moral status that lies somewhere between that of gametes and mature (born) human beings.

Like Hare, Helga Kuhse and Peter Singer argue that the potentiality argument is inadequate because all that can be said about the potential of embryos can also be said about the potential of ova and sperm (Walters and Singer, 1982). Consider, they suggest, a situation in which excess ova and sperm obtained for in vitro fertilization are disposed of by being flushed separately down the sink. No one, they believe, would find this action morally problematic. But suppose that after the ova and sperm are disposed of separately, a blockage in the sink occurs, and this causes them to remain lodged together, allowing fertilization to occur. According to Kuhse and Singer, "Those who believe that the embryo has a special moral status which makes it wrong to destroy it must now believe that it would be wrong to clear the blockage; instead the egg must now be rescued from the sink, checked to see if fertilization has occurred, and if it has, efforts should presumably be made to keep it alive" (Walters and Singer, 1982, p. 59). Assuming that reasonable people would not attempt such a rescue, they conclude that there is no sharp distinction between the moral status of human embryos and that of human gametes.

Specific issues

The preceding considerations are applicable to a broad range of ethical issues that involve human fetuses. These include abortion, coercive treatment during pregnancy, fetal therapy, custody disputes regarding extra embryos, fetal reduction, and fetal tissue transplantation. In what follows, each of these issues is considered with particular reference to the characteristics and status of the fetus.

Abortion may have three different meanings with regard to fetuses. First, it may mean termination of pregnancy, that is, the severance of the tie between the pregnant woman and her fetus. In some cases, severance of the tie has not resulted in fetal death, and the U.S. courts have held that the right to terminate the pregnancy does not imply the right to terminate fetal life in such circumstances. Second, abortion may mean termination of fetal life, which implies the intention of killing the fetus. In second-trimester gestations, different methods of abortion are more or less likely to accomplish that intent. Third, abortion may be defined as applicable not only to fetuses in utero but also to in vitro embryos. In this definition, the disposal of affected embryos after positive preimplantation genetic testing constitutes abortion. The second and third definitions are morally equivalent to feticide or embryocide.

Regardless of the definition and intention of abortion, the possibility of fetal sentience presents a moral consideration relevant to the selection of a method of abortion. Among techniques used in second-trimester terminations, for example, dilatation and evacuation (removal of fetal parts through the vagina) is more directly damaging to the fetus than other methods. Hysterotomy, the surgical removal of the fetus from the uterus, is least damaging to the fetus but most invasive for the woman. As already mentioned, the equality principle argues for providing comparable consideration to fetuses destined to be aborted and those destined to come to term. In the United States, this principle is not legally applicable to conflicts between the health of pregnant women and their fetuses because abortions are always permissible if the woman's health is endangered by the pregnancy.

Although most pregnant women willingly accept the inconveniences and discomforts of pregnancy, and some risk their own health in order to optimize fetal outcome, occasionally women refuse treatment recommended for the sake of the fetus. Pregnant women's refusal of hospitalization, intrauterine transfusion, or surgical delivery have been challenged on grounds of an obligation to the fetus or to the potential child (Kolder et al., 1987). Suits have also been brought against pregnant women for lifestyle decisions that endanger the fetus, such as drug and alcohol abuse. Most of these legal challenges have been unsuccessful because they are based on child abuse laws. Fetuses, even when viable, do not have equal legal standing with children. However, to the extent that human beings are responsible for others whose lives or welfare depend on them, a woman who has opted to continue her pregnancy may be morally responsible for avoiding behaviors that endanger the fetus.

When women accept treatment that jeopardizes their own health for the sake of their fetuses, their behavior may be considered virtuous rather than obligatory. However, their voluntariness in such situations may be compromised by social pressures that influence their decision making. George Annas suggests the possibility of such pressures when he compares the refusal of cesarean section recommended for treatment of fetal distress with a parent's refusal to donate an organ for his or her child (Annas, 1982). In both cases, parents may feel obliged to take risks in behalf of their offspring. Despite the fact that the personhood of the child is clearly established, while that of the fetus is controversial, judges have mandated that surgery be performed in the latter case but not the former (Annas, 1982). This implies that organ donation to one's child is superogatory, whereas cesarean section to benefit the fetus is obligatory.

Arguments in favor of overriding the pregnant woman's autonomy in behalf of the fetus have been made on grounds that harms to the developing organism are harms to the future child. Awards made to parents whose children were injured in utero are made on this basis. If a woman miscarries because of an accident or injury, an award may be made for the loss of the fetus, but this is not legally equivalent to the loss of a child. The duration of gestation and the possibility of viability are morally and legally relevant in such cases.

Advances in medical and surgical techniques for treatment of fetuses provide the prospect of women undergoing even more experimental and invasive procedures than they have accepted in the past. For example, it is possible to remove a nonviable fetus from a woman's uterus, surgically repair problems such as a hernia in its diaphragm, and return the fetus to the uterus to continue gestation (Ohlendorf-Moffat, 1991). Such procedures are morally different from those that a newborn might undergo because they necessarily involve risk to the pregnant woman, for which her consent is morally and legally indispensable.

Custody disputes regarding embryos have arisen because of their in vitro status. So long as embryos remain within the woman's body, others' claims regarding their disposition are unlikely to be upheld. When embryos have developed and have been preserved in vitro, however, disputes about their fate have involved potential heirs, gamete providers, and institutions in which the embryos were developed or preserved. Claims by institutions have been rejected by the U.S. courts in favor of the gamete providers. A complicating possibility arises from the fact that the only claimant capable of both genetic and gestational relationship to the embryo is the woman who provided the ova. If she is unwilling to gestate one or more embryos, and her decision regarding its disposition is contested, the embryo can develop further only through involvement of a third party, that is, through contract motherhood or surrogate gestation. An offspring that develops from such an arrangement has in fact three biologically related parents. The development of the fetus is dependent on only one of these, the gestational parent. In situations where each of the biological parents desires, and is competent to raise, the offspring, their disparate risks and involvement with the fetus suggest an ordering by which to determine whose wishes have priority: first, the gestational parent; second, the ovum provider; third, the sperm provider (Mahowald, 1993). Some authors consider the genetic tie more compelling than the gestational relationship, and some give equal weight to claims of ovum and sperm provider. In the trial court decision regarding the case of "Baby M," Judge Harvey R. Sorkow gave greater weight to the sperm provider than to the woman who was both genetically and gestationally related to the offspring (Sorkow, 1988).

Advances in treatment of infertility have led to an increased incidence of multiple gestations. At times, the expectation of live birth is reduced or even negated because so many fetuses are not likely to survive in utero for the entirety of gestation. Fetal reduction, which is also called "selective termination," "selective abortion," "selective birth," and "selective feticide," may be performed in order to facilitate the birth of one or more healthy infants (Evans et al., 1988, p. 293). When the mortality and morbidity of a multiple gestation are high, the intention of the procedure is not to terminate the pregnancy but to promote the healthy live birth of one or more infants. Ordinarily, an attempt is made to reduce the pregnancy to twins rather than a single fetus. Whether to provide the procedure for triplet gestations is more controversial than for gestations of a greater number of fetuses, in part because the procedure carries a risk to the remaining fetuses. The recommended criterion for determining which fetuses to terminate is one of efficiency: those that can technically be most easily reached and effectively terminated. Unlike most abortion procedures, fetal reduction involves direct termination of fetal life. Although only a few centers in the United States perform this procedure, the number is growing.

The issue of fetal tissue transplantation exemplifies the apparently inevitable linkage between fetuses and concerns about abortion. Although fetal tissue has long been used in treatment of some diseases (such as DiGeorge's syndrome), its use for treatment of severe neurological conditions such as Parkinson's disease is new and experimental. The symptoms of patients suffering from Parkinson's disease have apparently improved through grafts of fetal tissue obtained through routine suction abortions at six to eight weeks' gestation (Widner et al., 1992). Fetal tissue can be transplanted with greater success than adult tissue because it is less immunologically reactive, reducing the incidence of rejection. It also has a greater capacity to develop than adult tissue. Most ethicists support the use of fetal tissue for transplantation as an issue separate from that of abortion. This view has been challenged by some on empirical as well as ethical grounds (Mahowald, 1991). Those who oppose the use of fetal tissue for transplantation claim that it unavoidably involves complicity in, and legitimation of, abortion.

To some, just as a parent's abuse of a child provides grounds for others to decide about the child's fate, so a pregnant woman's choice of abortion compromises her right to consent to transplantation of fetal tissue. To others, the fetus is the pregnant woman's property, and this gives her the right to dispose of it as she wishes, even when it is no longer within her body. As with custody disputes concerning frozen embryos, others in addition to the woman who is genetically related to the fetus may claim ownership of the abortus. Institutions, for example, may argue that the abortus is discarded tissue, which they are legally entitled to dispose of as such; the sperm or ova providers may argue that they own the tissue generated by fertilization of their gametes. Conflicts are also possible between ova providers and gestational parents. The in vitro status of the abortus is critical to support of claims by those who are not gestationally related to it. Once the fetus is aborted or delivered, the pregnant woman's right to determine its fate is clearly less compelling.

In sum, human fetuses raise unique philosophical, legal, and ethical issues that are inseparable from their immature but human status, their relationship to pregnant women, and their potential for unquestioned personhood. All of these factors are relevant to issues that involve pregnant women: abortion, coercive treatment during pregnancy, possibilities for fetal therapy, custody disputes regarding embryos, fetal reduction, fetal research, and fetal tissue transplantation. Just as fetuses as such are inseparable from pregnant women, so the issues themselves inevitably overlap and are particularly likely to intersect with the controversial issue of elective abortion. So long as there are relievable threats to fetuses, and fetuses develop within women's bodies, this will continue to be the case.

MARY B. MAHOWALD

Directly related to this article are the other articles in this entry: HUMAN DEVELOPMENT FROM FERTILIZATION TO BIRTH, *and* FETAL RESEARCH. *Also directly related are the entries* PERSON; *and* LIFE. *For a further discussion of topics mentioned in this article, see the entries* AUTONOMY; *and* FREEDOM AND COERCION. *This article will find application in the entries* ABORTION, *sections on* CONTEMPORARY

ETHICAL AND LEGAL ASPECTS, *and* RELIGIOUS TRADITIONS; GENETIC TESTING AND SCREENING, *articles on* PRE-IMPLANTATION EMBRYO DIAGNOSIS, *and* PRENATAL DIAGNOSIS; MATERNAL–FETAL RELATIONSHIP, *articles on* ETHICAL ISSUES, *and* LEGAL AND REGULATORY ISSUES; *and* REPRODUCTIVE TECHNOLOGIES. *Other relevant material may be found under* BIOLOGY, PHILOSOPHY OF.

Bibliography

ANNAS, GEORGE J. 1982. "Forced Cesareans: The Most Unkindest Cut of All." *Hastings Center Report* 12, no. 3:16, 17, 45.

BARON, CHARLES H. 1985. "Fetal Research: The Question in the States." *Hastings Center Report* 15, no. 2: 12–16.

BONNICKSEN, ANDREA L. 1988. "Embryo Freezing: Ethical Issues in the Clinical Setting." *Hastings Center Report* 18, no. 6:26–30.

COOK, REBECCA J., and DICKENS, BERNARD M. 1988. "International Developments in Abortion Laws: 1977–88." *American Journal of Public Health* 78, no. 10:1305–1311.

EVANS, MARK I.; FLETCHER, JOHN C.; ZADOR, IVAN E.; NEWTON, BURRITT W.; QUIGG, MARY HELEN; and STRUYK, CURTIS D. 1988. "Selective First-Trimester Termination in Octuplet and Quadruplet Pregnancies: Clinical and Ethical Issues." *Obstetrics and Gynecology* 71, no. 3, pt. 1: 289–296.

FLETCHER, JOHN C., and RYAN, KENNETH J. 1987. "Federal Regulations for Fetal Research: A Case for Reform." *Law, Medicine and Health Care* 15, no. 3:126–138.

FORD, NORMAN M. 1988. *When Did I Begin? Conception of the Human Individual in History, Philosophy, and Science.* Cambridge: At the University Press.

GLOVER, JONATHAN. 1989. *Ethics of New Reproductive Technologies: The Glover Report to the European Commission.* De Kalb: Northern Illinois University Press.

GROBSTEIN, CLIFFORD. 1988. *Science and the Unborn: Choosing Human Futures.* New York: Basic Books.

HARE, R. M. 1975. "Abortion and the Golden Rule." *Philosophy and Public Affairs* 4, no. 3:201–222.

KNIGHT, JAMES W., and CALLAHAN, JOAN C. 1989. *Preventing Birth: Contemporary Methods and Related Moral Controversies.* Salt Lake City: University of Utah Press.

KOLDER, VERONIKA E. B.; GALLAGHER, JANET; and PARSONS, MICHAEL T. 1987. "Court-Ordered Obstetrical Interventions." *New England Journal of Medicine* 316, no. 19: 1192–1196.

KUHSE, HELGA, and SINGER, PETER. 1982. "The Moral Status of the Embryo: Two Viewpoints." In *Test-Tube Babies: A Guide to Moral Questions, Present Techniques and Future Possibilities,* pp. 57–63. Edited by William Walters and Peter Singer. New York: Oxford University Press.

LANDWIRTH, JULIUS. 1987. "Fetal Abuse and Neglect: An Emerging Controversy." *Pediatrics* 79, no. 4:508–514.

MAHOWALD, MARY B. 1991. "Fetal Tissue Transplantation: An Update." In *Bioethics and the Fetus: Medical, Moral and Legal Issues,* pp. 103–121. Edited by James M. Humber and Robert F. Almeder. Biomedical Ethics Reviews. Totowa, N.J.: Humana Press.

———. 1993. *Women and Children in Health Care: An Unequal Majority.* New York: Oxford University Press.

MATTINGLY, SUSAN S. 1992. "The Maternal-Fetal Dyad: Exploring the Two-Patient Obstetric Model." *Hastings Center Report* 22, no. 1:13–18.

MICHAELI, GALIA; FEJGIN, MOSHE; GHETLER, YEHUDIT; BEN NUN, ISAAC; BEYTHE, YORAN; and AMIEL ALIZA. 1990. "Chromosomal Analysis of Unfertilized Oocytes and Morphologically Abnormal Preimplantation Embryos from an *in Vitro* Fertilization Program. *Journal of in Vitro Fertilization and Embryo Transfer* 7, no. 6:341–346.

NOONAN, JOHN T., JR., ed. 1970. *The Morality of Abortion: Legal and Historical Perspectives.* Cambridge, Mass.: Harvard University Press.

OHLENDORF-MOFFAT, PAT. 1991. "Surgery Before Birth." *Discover,* February, pp. 59–65.

Roe v. Wade. 1972. No. 70-18. U.S. District Court 410. Syllabus, pp. 113–178.

SASS, HANS-MARTIN. 1989. "Brain Life and Brain Death: A Proposal for a Normative Agreement." *Journal of Medicine and Philosophy* 14, no. 1:45–59.

SORKOW, HARVEY R. 1988. "Ruling on Baby M." In *Intervention and Reflection: Basic Issues in Medical Ethics,* 3d ed., pp. 438–440. Edited by Ronald Munson. Belmont, Calif.: Wadsworth.

Stedman's Medical Dictionary. 1990. Baltimore: Williams and Wilkins.

STRONG, CARSON, and ANDERSON, GARLAND. 1989. "The Moral Status of the Near-Term Fetus." *Journal of Medical Ethics* 15, no. 1:25–27.

WALTERS, WILLIAM, and SINGER, PETER. 1982. *Test-Tube Babies: A Guide to Moral Questions, Present Techniques and Future Possibilities.* New York: Oxford University Press.

WARREN, MARY ANNE. 1989. "The Moral Significance of Birth." *Hypatia* 4, no. 3:46–65.

WIDNER, HÅKAN; TETRUD, JAMES; REHNCRONA, STIG; SNOW, BARRY; BRUNDIN, PATRICK; GUSTAVII, BJÖRN; BJÖRKLUND, ANDERS; LINDVALL, OLLE; and LANGSTON, J. WILLIAM. 1992. "Bilateral Fetal Mesencephalic Grafting in Two Patients with Parkinsonism Induced by 1-Methyl-a4-Phenyl-1,2,3,6-Tetrahydropyridine (MPT)." *New England Journal of Medicine* 327, no. 22:1556–1563.

III. FETAL RESEARCH

The following is an update of the first-edition article "Fetal Research" by the late André E. Hellegers.

All of the research discussed in this article involves women and men, as well as human embryos and fetuses. When implantation is a necessary condition for the research, as in the case of most fetal research, the fetus is implanted in the uterus of a woman. For all of the research considered in the article, the oocytes (eggs) of at least one woman are required; in cases involving in vitro fertilization, the oocyte retrieval process can be onerous for the woman involved. In addition, sperm from at least one man are required for fertilization. For reasons of brevity, this essay focuses primary attention on the developing human embryo and fetus, referring only incidentally to the woman and man who provide the gametes that give rise to the embryo and fetus or to the woman in whom gestation occurs.

Four major types of research will be analyzed in this article: (1) research on preimplantation embryos; (2) research on unimplanted embryos and fetuses beyond the fourteenth day of development; (3) research on implanted embryos and fetuses; and (4) research on aborted, live embryos and fetuses. The topic of research on living tissue derived from fetal remains is discussed in a separate article.

Preimplantation embryo research

The human preimplantation embryo can be defined as the developing organism from the time of fertilization to approximately the fourteenth day after fertilization, assuming a normal rate of development. The major preimplantation stages in human and other mammalian embryos are usually distinguished by such names as zygote, morula, and blastocyst. By the end of fourteen days the early human embryo has, except in rare cases, lost the capacity to divide into two individuals; it has also begun to exhibit a longitudinal axis that forms the template for the spinal column, an axis called the primitive streak (McLaren, 1986; Dawson, 1990a).

Preimplantation embryo research generally requires the associated procedure of in vitro fertilization (although it would in principle be possible to retrieve an early embryo by flushing it from the uterus of a woman following in vivo fertilization of an ovum). Thus, the question of research on preimplantation embryos did not arise until in vitro fertilization techniques had been developed and validated, first in laboratory animals, then in humans. M. C. Chang of the Worcester Foundation in Massachusetts was the first scientist to demonstrate unambiguously the fertilization of nonhuman mammalian oocytes in vitro (Chang, 1959). Chang's success was followed in 1969 by the first confirmed report of in vitro fertilization with human gametes by three British researchers (Edwards et al., 1969). Only nine years later the first human birth after in vitro fertilization—the infant's name was Louise Brown—was reported by members of the same British research team (Steptoe and Edwards, 1978).

There are two major contexts for research on preimplantation embryos. The first is one in which the transfer of the embryo into the uterus of a woman (or perhaps, in the future, into a device that can support full-term fetal development) is planned. In the second context, no embryo transfer is envisioned and, accordingly, the death of the embryo or later fetus at a stage before viability is intended. These two research contexts raise somewhat different ethical issues.

Research followed by embryo transfer.   In the years preceding the birth of Louise Brown in 1978, researchers devoted substantial attention to improving the prospects for successful in vitro fertilization and embryo transfer. This research focused on methods for maturing oocytes, facilitating fertilization, and culturing or cryopreserving early embryos (Biggers, 1979). During the 1990s, researchers continued this type of research. New methods for assisting fertilization have been devised, including the drilling of a small hole in the outer shell of an oocyte or the injection of a sperm directly into an oocyte (Van Steirteghem, 1993). Similarly, researchers have developed methods for removing one or two cells from an eight- or sixteen-cell embryo in order to perform preimplantation diagnosis of genetic or chromosomal abnormalities (Edwards, 1993). In the twenty-first century, one can anticipate research that attempts to prevent the later development of a genetic disease (for example, cystic fibrosis) by treating an individual at the embryonic stage of life. If successful, this kind of disease prevention by means of gene modification would be likely to affect all of the cells of the person, including his or her reproductive cells (Wivel and Walters, 1993).

The ethical issues that arise with preimplantation embryo research when embryo transfer is planned are at least analogous to those that arise with fetal research in anticipation of birth, with research on infants, and with research on children. That is, one attempts to perform a careful analysis of the probable benefits and harms of the research to the individual and to others; one seeks an appropriate decision maker, usually a genetic parent or a guardian, who can represent the best interests of the potential research subject; and one looks for a disinterested mechanism for prior ethical review of the proposed research. This kind of embryo research, in which the research procedures are often designated "therapeutic" or "beneficial," is generally approved by commentators on the ethics of such research, even if they diverge widely in their attitudes toward in vitro fertilization, the moral status of preimplantation embryos, and abortion (see, e.g., Ramsey, 1970; Catholic Church, 1987; Singer et al., 1990).

Research not followed by embryo transfer. Research in this context may be proposed for a variety of reasons. The goal of the research may be to assess the safety and efficacy of clinical practices, for example, in vitro fertilization or the use of contraceptive vaccines. Alternatively, the goal may be epidemiological, for example, to estimate the frequency of chromosomal abnormalities in early human embryos. In other cases the research has little reference to clinical medicine or human pathology. That is, research with preimplantation embryos may be much more basic, seeking to compare early development in various species of mammals or to explore the limits of embryo fusion or hybrid creation among different species.

Two distinct ethical questions have received primary attention in the international bioethics debate about preimplantation embryo research without embryo transfer. The first question is, Is research on such embryos morally permissible if it has no intention of benefiting the embryos themselves? If the answer to the first question is negative, the second question is irrelevant. However, if the answer to the first question is affirmative, there remains a second question: Is it morally permissible to fertilize human oocytes for the sole purpose of performing research on the resulting embryos and in the absence of any intention to transfer the embryos for further development?

In their responses to the first question, proponents of nonbeneficial (to the embryos) research procedures adduce several arguments. First, the research may produce benefits, either for clinical practice or in terms of basic knowledge, that are not attainable by any other means (U.S. Department of Health, Education and Welfare, 1979; Warnock, 1984; Ethics Committee, 1990; Robertson, 1994). One variant of this argument asserts that it is morally irresponsible to introduce new techniques (for example, cryopreservation of embryos) into clinical practice without first performing extensive laboratory studies of the technique.

Second, proponents of preimplantation embryo research note that the biological individuality of the embryo is not firmly established until approximately fourteen (or perhaps twenty-one) days after fertilization. Before that time twinning can occur, or two embryos can fuse into a single new embryo called a chimera (Hellegers, 1970; Dawson, 1987; Grobstein, 1988). If developmental individuality does not occur until after the preimplantation stage, research proponents argue, the preimplantation embryo is not protectable as a unique human being.

Third, proponents of research cite the apparently high embryo loss rate that occurs in natural human reproduction. The most reliable estimates are that approximately 50 percent of the human eggs that are fertilized either fail to develop or die within two weeks after fertilization occurs (Chard, 1991). To this factual evidence is added the metaphysical assertion that entities with such a high rate of natural death within two weeks of coming into being cannot be morally significant at this early stage of their existence. Proponents of embryo research may acknowledge that adult persons have some moral obligations toward early embryos, but these obligations are viewed as relatively weak and are thought to be outweighed by, for example, substantial clinical benefits to many future patients.

Opponents of preimplantation embryo research have replies to these arguments and adduce other arguments of their own. In response to the first argument of proponents, the opponents assert that the end of desirable clinical consequences does not justify the means of performing research that seriously damages or destroys the embryo. To the consequential argument of proponents, conservatives may counterpose a consequential argument of their own, namely, that negative consequences will result from research on early embryos. For example, researchers may become desensitized to the value of human life, or bizarre human–nonhuman hybrids may be produced in the laboratory (Catholic Church, 1987; Dawson, 1990b).

The second and third arguments of the proponents are viewed as mere descriptions of natural phenomena that carry no particular moral weight. Twinning, recombination, and embryo loss, if they occur naturally and are beyond human control, are in this view no more morally relevant than other natural evils like earthquakes or volcanic eruptions. For their part, opponents put forward two additional arguments. First, the genotype of a new individual is firmly established at the time when the pronuclei from the sperm cell and the ovum fuse. This fusion, sometimes called syngamy, occurs at the conclusion of fertilization. Thus, from a genetic standpoint, a new individual exists from syngamy forward. Second, opponents of preimplantation embryo research often adduce the potentiality argument: that the early embryo contains within itself all of the genetic instructions necessary for the development of a fetus, an infant, and an adult, provided only that the embryo is placed in an environment that will nurture its further development. Therefore, the person that the early embryo may one day become should be respected in an anticipatory way even at the early stages of development, when it lacks many of the characteristics of persons in the full sense.

Proponents of research do not deny that a new genotype is established at the time of fertilization. They simply point to other factual considerations that are in their view more relevant to moral judgments about the acceptability of embryo research. In response to the potentiality argument, research proponents note that a single sperm cell and a single oocyte have the potential to become an embryo, yet opponents of embryo research do not accord special moral status to reproductive cells. Further, only a few cells of the preimplantation embryo develop into the embryo proper; the rest become the placenta, the amniotic sac, and the chorionic villi (McLaren, 1986). In other words, potentiality is a continuous notion, or a matter of degree, not an all-or-nothing concept (Singer and Dawson, 1988).

Among proponents of research on preimplantation embryos there is a division of opinion on the second question noted above—whether the creation of human embryos specifically for research purposes is morally permissible. Proponents of the conservative answer to this question argue that only embryos left over from the clinical practice of in vitro fertilization and embryo transfer should be used in research (Steinbock, 1992). Such embryos might include those selected out when the number of embryos available for transfer exceeds a number that is considered safe for the woman (for example, more than four embryos). Leftover or surplus embryos might also become available in the context of cryopreservation, if a couple completes its desired family size or if both genetic parents die in an accident while some embryos remain in frozen storage.

The principal argument of conservatives on the deliberate-creation question is a Kantian argument against using early human embryos merely as means. In the opinion of conservatives, creating embryos with the prior intent of destroying them at an early stage of development is incompatible with the respect that should be accorded to human embryos. Conservatives can accept the use of leftover embryos for research because there was at least at one time an intention to transfer the preimplantation embryos to the uterus of a woman, where they could develop into viable fetuses. In their view, the research use of such "spare" embryos is a morally acceptable alternative to donation or discard (Steinbock, 1992). The primary argument of those who do not object to creating embryos for research is a composite. Proponents of this view argue, first, that our moral obligations to early human embryos are relatively weak. Further, proponents of the liberal view note that good research design may require either a larger number of embryos than the clinical context can provide or unselected embryos rather than those that have been rejected for embryo transfer, perhaps because they are malformed or slow in developing (Ethics Committee, 1990).

Practice vs. ethics.   In the 1990s international practice and ethical opinion regarding human embryo research diverged sharply. One polar position in practice was that of the United Kingdom, where research on preimplantation embryos was conducted in numerous laboratories under the supervision of voluntary and (later) statutory licensing authorities (United Kingdom, 1992). At the other pole was Germany, which prohibited the fertilization of ova for the practice of research, as well as any research that was likely to destroy or damage the embryo.

Ethics advisory bodies of the 1970s and 1980s were far from unanimous in their evaluations of research involving preimplantation embryos. The earliest report on this topic, produced by the Ethics Advisory Board for the U.S. Department of Health, Education, and Welfare (1979), judged embryo research to be ethically acceptable if it was designed primarily to "assess the safety and efficacy of embryo transfer" (p. 106). During the 1980s there emerged three general positions among such advisory bodies. Several Australian committees rejected the idea of any human embryo research. A few Australian committees and most of the committees based in continental Europe approved embryo research but rejected

the deliberate creation of embryos for research purposes. In the Netherlands, the United Kingdom, Canada, and the United States, advisory committees tended to approve both human embryo research and the creation of embryos for research (Walters, 1987). The 1989 recommendation of the Parliamentary Assembly of the Council of Europe adopted the intermediate position, requiring as well the prior approval of the "appropriate public health or scientific authority" or "the relevant national multidisciplinary committee" (Council of Europe, 1989).

Research on unimplanted embryos and fetuses beyond the fourteenth day of development

The developing human organism is technically called an embryo during the first eight weeks following fertilization. It is called a fetus for the remainder of its development. In this section, prolonged in vitro culture of embryos and fetuses will be evaluated.

Prolonged embryo culture has been undertaken in several species of nonhuman mammals, especially rats and mice. In the early years of research, embryos at various stages of development were removed (or "explanted") from the uteri of pregnant females and sustained in various kinds of laboratory devices that delivered oxygen and nutrients (New, 1973). More recently, unimplanted mouse and cattle embryos have been sustained in culture to developmental stages more complex than those attained by preimplantation human embryos (Chen and Hsu, 1982; Thomas and Seidel, 1993).

At present, no researchers are proposing to perform studies of either of these types with human embryos. The explantation mode of research will probably not be undertaken in humans because of the risks to the pregnant woman and because the need is questionable. However, sustained culture of human embryos after in vitro fertilization would in principle be possible. It is not clear whether the current lack of proposals to culture embryos in vitro beyond fourteen days is based on technical or ethical considerations. The longest well-documented periods for human embryo culture are eight days and thirteen days (Fishel et al., 1984). Possible rationales for extending embryo culture beyond fourteen days could include studying differentiation, the anatomy and physiology of the embryo, the implantation process, or the effect of drugs or radiation on the developing embryo (Karp, 1976; Edwards, 1989; Sass, 1989).

There has been relatively little ethical discussion of embryo research beyond fourteen days. Most advisory committees have simply accepted the fourteen-day limit without extensive discussion. In the case of the Warnock Committee report from the United Kingdom, this limit was said to be appropriate because it correlates with the appearance of the primitive streak in the embryo

(Warnock, 1984). The primitive streak is the first indication of the embryo's body axis. Several commentators have suggested that the justification for the fourteen-day limit is relatively weak and have proposed extending the limit for in vitro human embryo research to approximately twenty-eight days (Dawson, 1987; Edwards, 1989; Kuhse and Singer, 1990).

If embryo culture methods improve sufficiently, it may one day be possible to sustain either a nonhuman or a human embryo and fetus in vitro for an extended period, or even through an entire gestation. The technological support system that sustains such development will probably be called an artificial placenta. If prolonged embryo culture is employed with human embryos and fetuses, decisions will be required about whether to sustain development to the point of viability. At some point a transition will undoubtedly be made from laboratory research designed to test the technical feasibility of long-term culture to an actual attempt to produce a human child by means of ectogenesis (extrauterine development) (Kass, 1972; Fletcher, 1974; Karp, 1976; Walters, 1979).

Research on implanted embryos and fetuses

The ethical questions that surround research on implanted embryos and on implanted fetuses are virtually identical, except for the different stages of development involved. This continuity in biological development and similarity in ethical analysis is so striking that both the American National Commission for the Protection of Human Subjects and the British Polkinghorne Committee employed the term "fetus" to refer to the developing entity from the time of implantation through the whole of gestation (U.S. National Commission, 1975; Polkinghorne, 1989). In the following discussion the word "fetus" and its derivatives will be employed to refer to the embryo or fetus from the time of implantation in the uterus of a woman through the point at which physical separation from the woman occurs.

As in the case of preimplantation embryo research, one can distinguish two major contexts for fetal research. The first is one in which further development and delivery of an infant are anticipated. The second context is one in which induced abortion is either planned or in progress.

Fetal research in anticipation of birth. The ethical issues involved in fetal research conducted at any stage of gestation in anticipation of birth closely parallel the ethical issues in research on newborns. The main reason for the close parallel is that the further development of the fetus or newborn into an adult person is planned. No research procedure that is likely to threaten the life or damage the health of a future person would be either proposed or carried out by responsible scientists. For this reason, research not intended to benefit a particular fetus (in anticipation of birth) or a particular newborn is generally constrained by the no-risk or minimal-risk rule (U.S. National Commission, 1975; Polkinghorne, 1989). That is, the research must be judged to pose either no risk at all (as in certain observational studies) or only minimal risk to the potential subject. For research intended to benefit a particular fetus or newborn, a careful weighing and balancing of likely benefits and harms to the subject is required (Polkinghorne, 1989).

The major difference between neonatal research and fetal research in anticipation of birth is that the fetus is contained within the pregnant woman's body, and any research intervention will require physical contact with, or at least physical proximity to, the pregnant woman. Thus, fetal research inevitably and simultaneously affects a pregnant woman. For this reason it requires a careful weighing and balancing of the risks to her, as well as her informed consent.

Many clinical procedures that are now routinely employed in obstetrical practice were first tested on pregnant women and fetuses in anticipation of birth. One early therapy was the use of exchange transfusions to overcome Rh incompatibility between a pregnant woman and her fetus. In the 1980s experimental types of fetal surgery were undertaken to correct problems like urinary-tract obstructions. The worldwide epidemic of HIV infection and AIDS provided the context for important fetal research in the 1990s. In one randomized clinical trial, the antiviral drug AZT (azidothymidine) was administered to HIV-infected pregnant women in an effort to delay the progression of disease in them, as well as to prevent the transmission of infection to their fetuses.

Fetal research in anticipation of or during induced abortion. Fetal research conducted before or during induced abortion could have various aims. One possible goal would be to develop better techniques for prenatal diagnosis, for example, by means of fetoscopy or chorionic villi sampling. Another possible goal would be to study whether drugs, viruses, vaccines, or radioisotopes cross the placental barrier between pregnant woman and fetus. A third aim of such studies could be to develop techniques for induced abortion that are safer for pregnant women or more humane in the termination of fetal life. Fourth, during abortion by hysterotomy (a seldom-used procedure similar to a cesarean section), fetal physiology can be studied after the fetus has been removed from the uterus of the pregnant woman and before the umbilical cord has been severed (Walters, 1975).

Commentators on the ethics of fetal research in anticipation of induced abortion have always been aware that a pregnant woman who intends to terminate her pregnancy can change her decision about abortion even after a research procedure has been performed. In addition, in rare cases an attempt at induced abortion results in a live birth. Thus, except in the case of research procedures performed during the abortion procedure itself, the distinction between a fetus-to-be-aborted and a fetus-to-be-born is statistical rather than metaphysical. One study performed for the U.S. National Commission in the 1970s estimated the change-of-decision rate between a visit to an abortion facility and the scheduled time of termination to be in the range of 1–2 percent (Bracken, 1975).

The possibility that a pregnant woman may change her decision to undergo induced abortion after a research intervention sets an outer limit on the types of interventions that prudent researchers would be willing to perform. For example, it would be useful to know at what stages of pregnancy alcohol, drugs, or viral infections are most likely to produce malformations in human fetuses; however, in the view of most commentators on the ethics of fetal research, such studies ought not to be performed in humans. In the words of the Peel Committee report, "In our view it is unethical for a medical practitioner to administer drugs or carry out any procedures on the mother with the deliberate intent of ascertaining the harm that these might do to the fetus, notwithstanding that arrangements may have been made to terminate the pregnancy and even if the mother is willing to give her consent to such an experiment" (United Kingdom, 1972, p. 6).

Even if research likely to cause serious damage to the fetus is ethically proscribed, there are at least two different ethical standards that can be adopted with respect to fetal research in anticipation of or during induced abortion. The first standard asks for equal treatment of the fetus-to-be-born and the fetus-to-be aborted. In brief, this standard requires either that one should perform research procedures on fetuses-to-be-born concurrently with performing the same procedures on fetuses-to-be-aborted, or at least that one should be *willing to* perform the same procedure on both groups of fetuses. In practice, this standard would be virtually equivalent to the no-risk or minimal-risk rule discussed in connection with fetal research in anticipation of birth (McCormick, 1975; Walters, 1975; Ramsey, 1975; Polkinghorne, 1989).

An alternative standard would reject the equal-treatment requirement. What is proposed instead is a kind of case-by-case approach to fetal research (U.S. National Commission, 1975; Fletcher and Ryan, 1987). For example, if the primary risk of a research procedure like chorionic villi sampling is that it will cause abortion in a small percentage of pregnant women, then it can be argued that research on this diagnostic procedure should be performed on women who plan to undergo induced abortion. If the research procedure itself is unlikely to injure the fetus, then the major remaining risk is that the abortion that the pregnant woman planned to have

induced in the future would instead occur spontaneously. The major ethical questions remaining in a case of this kind have to do with the timing of abortion: Is a later rather than an earlier induced abortion less respectful of the developing fetus? Does a later abortion entail greater risks to the physical and mental health of the pregnant woman?

An important dimension of the fetal research discussion is the possibility that research procedures will cause pain to the fetus (Steinbock, 1992). One of the difficulties in coming to terms with this issue is that the word "pain" probably has different meanings at different developmental stages. The anatomical basis for simple spinal reflexes seems to be present in human embryos at about 7.5 weeks post fertilization. Between the ninth and twelfth weeks of development, the fetal brain stem begins to function as a rudimentary information processor. However, only at twenty-two–twenty-three weeks of gestation is the cerebral neocortex connected to the other parts of the brain (Flower, 1985). Presumably the fetal capacity to perceive pain would differ at each of these three steps, but it is difficult to know precisely to what extent painful stimuli would be felt or remembered.

Research on aborted, live embryos and fetuses

There are major conceptual difficulties involved in describing a previously implanted entity that is expelled or removed alive from a pregnant woman's body (or removed alive from attachment to an artificial placenta). One candidate term is "abortus"; another is "fetus ex utero" or "embryo or fetus outside the uterus." Adjectives applied to such entities include "previable" or "nonviable" and "viable." A "viable fetus outside the uterus" is in fact a newborn infant, albeit one that may be seriously premature. In addition, the notion of viability is elastic, sometimes seeming to mean the gestational age, weight, or length at which the smallest known infant has survived, at other times seeming to mean the stage at which a stipulated percentage of infants survive, given the assistance of technological means of life support.

Three circumstances can be envisioned in which the question of research on formerly implanted, living embryos or fetuses could arise. First, the surgical removal of an ectopic pregnancy could provide a still-living embryo or fetus. Second, a spontaneous miscarriage could result in the delivery of a live embryo or fetus. Third, an already implanted embryo or fetus could be aborted by means that make it either possible or likely that an intact, living embryo or fetus will result from the abortion procedure.

There is no clear consensus on the ethical justifiability of research on living human embryos or fetuses outside the uterus. In the United Kingdom, two official reports reflect a clear trend in a more conservative direction. In 1972, the Peel Committee affirmed the scientific value of research on clearly previable fetuses outside the uterus and permitted many kinds of research on such fetuses (United Kingdom, 1972). However, the Polkinghorne Committee report of 1989 expressly rejected the position of the Peel Committee, arguing that the only morally relevant distinction was between living and dead fetuses, not the distinction between previable and viable fetuses (Polkinghorne, 1989). In the United States, the National Commission for the Protection of Human Subjects allowed no significant procedural changes in the abortion procedure solely for research purposes and restricted what could be done with the live, delivered embryo or fetus to intrusions that would not alter the duration of its life (U.S. National Commission, 1975). Recommendation 1100 by the Parliamentary Assembly of the Council of Europe (1989) also discussed "the use of human embryos and fetuses in scientific research." Its recommendation clearly reflected the ambivalence of ethical opinion on research involving live embryos or fetuses outside the uterus. After stating that "Experiments on living embryos or foetuses, whether viable or not, shall be prohibited," the recommendation continued as follows: "None the less, where a state authorises certain experiments on non-viable foetuses or embryos only, these experiments may be undertaken in accordance with the terms of this recommendation and subject to prior authorisation from the health or scientific authorities or, where applicable, the national multidisciplinary body" (Council of Europe, 1989, p. 6).

Conclusion

Since André Hellegers's 1978 essay, the ethical discussion of research involving implanted fetuses and live, aborted fetuses has matured, but it has proceeded largely along the lines established in the 1970s. In contrast, the success of clinical in vitro fertilization has given new impetus to the ethical debate about research on preimplantation embryos. In the future it is at least possible that new methods for sustained embryo and fetal culture in vitro will give rise to additional ethical challenges.

LeRoy Walters

Directly related to this article are the other articles in this entry: human development from fertilization to birth, *and* philosophical and ethical issues. *Also directly related are the entries* Life; Person; Genetic Testing and Screening, *articles on* pre-implantation embryo diagnosis, prenatal diagnosis, legal issues, *and* ethical issues; Justice; *and* Utility. *For a further discussion of topics mentioned in this article, see the entries* Children, *article on* health-care and research issues; Informed Consent, *article on* consent issues in human research; Research Ethics Committees; *and* Research Policy. *The topics in this article will find application in the entry* Organ and Tissue Procurement, *article on* ethical and legal issues regarding cadavers. *For a discussion of related ideas, see the entries* Abortion, *sections on* contemporary ethical and legal aspects, *and* religious traditions; Gene Therapy; *and* Reproductive Technologies.

Bibliography

Biggers, John D. 1979. "*In Vitro* Fertilization, Embryo Culture and Embryo Transfer in the Human." Appendix, *HEW Support of Research Involving Human in Vitro Fertilization and Embryo Transfer,* chap. 8. Department of Health, Education and Welfare, Ethics Advisory Board. Washington, D.C.: Author.

Bracken, Michael B. 1975. "The Stability of the Decision to Seek Induced Abortion." In *Research on the Fetus, Appendix,* pp. 16-1 to 16-23. U.S. National Commission for the Protection of Human Subjects of Biomedical and Behavioral Research. Washington, D.C.: U.S. Department of Health, Education, and Welfare.

Catholic Church. Congregation for the Doctrine of the Faith. 1987. *Instruction on Respect for Human Life in Its Origin and on the Dignity of Procreation.* Vatican City: Author.

Chang, M. C. 1959. "Fertilization of Rabbit Ova *in Vitro.*" *Nature* 184, no. 4684:466–467.

Chard, T. 1991. "Frequency of Implantation and Early Pregnancy Loss in Natural Cycles." *Baillière's Clinical Obstetrics and Gynaecology* 5, no. 1:179–189.

Chen, L. T., and Hsu, Y. C. 1982. "Development of Mouse Embryos in Vitro: Preimplantation to the Limb Bud Stage." *Science* 218, no. 4567:66–68.

Council of Europe. Parliamentary Assembly. 1989. *Recommendation 1100: On the Use of Human Embryos and Fetuses in Scientific Research.* Strasbourg: Author.

Dawson, Karen. 1990a. "Introduction: An Outline of Scientific Aspects of Human Embryo Research." In *Embryo Experimentation,* pp. 3–13. Edited by Peter Singer, Helga Kuhse, Stephen Buckle, Karen Dawson, and Pascal Kasimba. New York: Cambridge University Press.

———. 1990b. "A Scientific Examination of Some Speculations About Continuing Human Pre-Embryo Research." In *Embryo Experimentation,* pp. 26–34. Edited by Peter Singer et al. New York: Cambridge University Press.

Edwards, Robert G. 1989. *Life Before Birth: Reflections on the Embryo Debate.* New York: Basic Books.

———, ed. 1993. *Preconception and Preimplantation Diagnosis of Human Genetic Disease.* Cambridge: At the University Press.

Edwards, Robert G.; Bavister, Barry D.; and Steptoe, Patrick C. 1969. "Early Stages of Fertilization *in Vitro* of Human Oocytes Matured *in Vitro.*" *Nature* 221, no. 5181:632–635.

Ethics Committee. American Fertility Society. 1990. "Ethical Considerations of the New Reproductive Technologies." *Fertility and Sterility* 53, no. 6 (supp. 2):1S–104S.

FISHEL, S. B.; EDWARDS, ROBERT G.; and EVANS, C. J. 1980. "Human Chorionic Gonadotropin Secreted by Pre-Implantation Embryos Cultured *in Vitro.*" *Science* 223, no. 4638:816–818.

FLETCHER, JOHN C.; and RYAN, KENNETH J. 1987. "Federal Regulations for Fetal Research: A Case for Reform." *Law, Medicine and Health Care* 15, no. 3:126–138.

FLETCHER, JOSEPH F. 1974. *The Ethics of Genetic Control: Ending Reproductive Roulette.* Garden City, N.Y.: Anchor.

FLOWER, MICHAEL J. 1985. "Neuromaturation of the Human Fetus." *Journal of Medicine and Philosophy* 10, no. 7:237–251.

GROBSTEIN, CLIFFORD. 1988. *Science and the Unborn: Choosing Human Futures.* New York: Basic Books.

HELLEGERS, ANDRÉ E. 1970. "Fetal Development." *Theological Studies* 31, no. 1:3–9.

KARP, LAURENCE E. 1976. *Genetic Engineering: Threat or Promise?* Chicago: Nelson-Hall.

KASS, LEON R. 1972. "Making Babies—the New Biology and the 'Old' Morality." *Public Interest* 26:18–56.

KUHSE, HELGA, and SINGER, PETER. 1990. "Individuals, Humans and Persons: The Issue of Moral Status." In *Embryo Experimentation,* pp. 65–75. Edited by Peter Singer, Helga Kuhse, Stephen Buckle, Karen Dawson, and Pascal Kasimba. New York: Cambridge University Press.

MCCORMICK, RICHARD A. 1975. "Experimentation on the Fetus: Policy Proposals." In *Research on the Fetus, Appendix,* pp. 5-1 to 5-11. U.S. National Commission for the Protection of Human Subjects of Biomedical and Behavioral Research. Washington, D.C.: U.S. Department of Health, Education and Welfare.

MCLAREN, ANNE. 1986. "Prelude to Embryogenesis." In *Human Embryo Research: Yes or No?,* pp. 5–23. Edited by Gregory Bock and Maeve O'Connor. London: Tavistock.

NEW, D. A. T. 1973. "Studies on Mammalian Fetuses *in Vitro* During the Period of Organogenesis." In *The Mammalian Fetus in Vitro,* pp. 15–65. Edited by C. R. Austin. London: Chapman & Hall.

POLKINGHORNE, J. C. 1989. *Review of the Guidance on the Research Use of Fetuses and Fetal Material.* London: Her Majesty's Stationery Office.

RAMSEY, PAUL. 1970. "Moral and Religious Implications of Genetic Control." In his *Fabricated Man: The Ethics of Genetic Control,* pp. 1–59. New Haven, Conn.: Yale University Press.

———. 1975. *The Ethics of Fetal Research.* New Haven, Conn.: Yale University Press.

ROBERTSON, JOHN A. 1994. *Children of Choice: Freedom and the New Reproductive Technologies.* Princeton, N.J.: Princeton University Press.

SASS, HANS-MARTIN. 1989. "Brain Life and Brain Death: A Proposal for a Normative Agreement." *Journal of Medicine and Philosophy* 14, no. 1:45–59.

SINGER, PETER, and DAWSON, KAREN. 1988. "IVF Technology and the Argument from Potential." *Philosophy and Public Affairs* 17, no. 2:87–104.

SINGER, PETER; KUHSE, HELGA; BUCKLE, STEPHEN; DAWSON, KAREN, and KASIMBA, PASCAL, eds. 1990. *Embryo Experimentation.* New York: Cambridge University Press.

STEINBOCK, BONNIE. 1992. *Life Before Birth: The Moral and Legal Status of Embryos and Fetuses.* New York: Oxford University Press.

STEPTOE, PATRICK C., and EDWARDS, ROBERT G. 1978. "Birth After the Reimplantation of a Human Embryo." *Lancet* 2, no. 8085:366.

THOMAS, WENDELL K., and SEIDEL, GEORGE E., JR. 1993. "Effects of Cumulus Cells on Culture of Bovine Embryos Derived from Oocytes Matured and Fertilized in Vitro." *Journal of Animal Science* 71, no. 9:2506–2510.

UNITED KINGDOM. DEPARTMENT OF HEALTH AND SOCIAL SECURITY ADVISORY GROUP. 1972. *The Use of Fetuses and Fetal Material for Research: Report.* London: Her Majesty's Stationery Office.

———. HUMAN FERTILISATION AND EMBRYOLOGY AUTHORITY. 1992. *Annual Report: 1992.* London: Author.

U.S. DEPARTMENT OF HEALTH, EDUCATION AND WELFARE. ETHICS ADVISORY BOARD. 1979. *HEW Support of Research Involving in Vitro Fertilization and Embryo Transfer: Report and Conclusions.* Washington, D.C.: Author.

U.S. NATIONAL COMMISSION FOR THE PROTECTION OF HUMAN SUBJECTS OF BIOMEDICAL AND BEHAVIORAL RESEARCH. 1975. *Research on the Fetus: Report and Recommendations.* Washington, D.C.: U.S. Department of Health, Education and Welfare.

VAN STEIRTEGHEM, ANDRÉ C. 1993. "High Fertilization and Implantation Rates After Intracytoplasmic Sperm Injection." *Human Reproduction* 8, no. 7:1061–1066.

WALTERS, LEROY. 1975. "Ethical and Public Policy Issues in Fetal Research." In *Research on the Fetus: Appendix,* pp. 8-1 to 8-18. U.S. National Commission for the Protection of Human Subjects of Biomedical and Behavioral Research. Washington, D.C.: U.S. Department of Health, Education and Welfare.

———. 1979. "Ethical Issues in Human *in Vitro* Fertilization and Research Involving Early Human Embryos." In *HEW Support of Research Involving Human in Vitro Fertilization and Embryo Transfer: Appendix,* chap. 1. U.S. Department of Health, Education and Welfare, Ethics Advisory Board. Washington, D.C.: U.S. Department of Health, Education and Welfare.

———. 1987. "Ethics and New Reproductive Technologies: An International Review of Committee Statements." *Hastings Center Report* 17 (spec. suppl., June):3–9.

WARNOCK, HENRY. 1984. *Report of the Committee of Inquiry into Human Fertilisation and Embryology.* London: Her Majesty's Stationery Office.

WIVEL, NELSON A., and WALTERS, LEROY. 1993. "Germ-Line Gene Modification and Disease Prevention: Some Medical and Ethical Perspectives." *Science* 262, no. 5133:533–538.

FIDELITY AND LOYALTY

Fidelity stems from the Latin word *fidelitas*; it can denote truth, and its common English connotation is conjugal. Etymologically, loyalty relates to the French word *loi,* or "law"; it may be said to have its natural context in the political community. The medical ethics literature since 1965 makes no systematic distinctions between the terms, and none will be attempted here.

In law, fidelity is associated with "fiduciary" relationships in which "there is special confidence reposed in one who in equity and good conscience is bound to act in good faith and with due regard to interests of one reposing the confidence" (Black, 1979, p. 564). The context may be domestic, commercial, or professional. Although this entry will focus on moral rather than legal issues and perspectives, the themes of trust, altruism, and commitment are reflected in the medical ethics literature under consideration. (For a general discussion of loyalty, and loyalty in the law, see the references to George Fletcher [1993] and Charles Fried [1976].)

However, consistent with legal usage, the first reference to fidelity in medical ethics is to the relationship between professionals, especially physicians, and patients. Thus, the term naturally relates to discussions of special obligations in those relationships, such as duties of telling the truth, preserving confidentiality, or securing the patient's consent before undertaking a treatment. Fidelity may offer a justification for such duties or a rationale for exceptions to them. An interesting question concerns the reciprocity of duties of fidelity. To what extent do patients owe fidelity to their physicians or other caregivers? The fact "that honesty with doctors is viewed as relative and contingent by many patients" calls into question the idea that physicians can count on real partnership with the persons they are trying to help (Vanderpool and Weiss, 1984, p. 368). Perhaps there are minimal demands of fidelity on those who expect it.

Fidelity-based theories

The focus on loyalty as a basic moral concept may have roots in social psychology or philosophy, as well as in law. However, in medical ethics the term appears most often in the work of religiously self-conscious writers. The most powerful source is the idea of covenantal loyalty that goes back to the Hebrew Bible, and the idea is central in Jewish ethics (Fletcher, 1993). In medical ethics it has been most thoroughly developed by Christian theologians. For Paul Ramsey and William F. May, fidelity or loyalty is the key term in a theory of medical ethics. In his preface to *The Patient as Person* (1970) Ramsey identified the fundamental norm to which he would appeal as "covenant loyalty," or "fidelity to covenant." This norm had clear religious roots, he thought, but it was not exclusive or esoteric; it was a norm that persons could understand regardless of their religious tradition, if any.

The term "loyalty" carried important connotations for Ramsey. The concept was pivotal in the work of his teacher, the theological moralist H. Richard Niebuhr (1960, 1963), and attention had been focused on the concept by Josiah Royce (1897, 1908), an American philosopher whose influence on Niebuhr—and Ramsey—was substantial. Royce had argued that the struggle of the moral life is the search for an adequate cause to which to be loyal. The self finds fulfillment in identification with something beyond itself. In the good life, an adequate cause is found. For Niebuhr, the right object of loyalty was the transcendent God of Western monotheism, but only a blasphemous imagination would say that loyalty would lead to identification with God; rather, loyalty required faithful response to God. For both Royce and Niebuhr, the self is moved away from the center of the moral universe. Persons do not live for themselves; they find themselves in loyalty to God or to a cause.

Ramsey developed these themes in his earlier work, notably *Basic Christian Ethics* (1950), where he argued that the central moral norm of the New Testament is agape, or love, which denoted, he thought, commitment to meeting the needs of individual other persons. He claimed that Christian ethics was an ethics of radical altruism; care for the self was justifiable only on instrumental grounds—when self-preservation or nurture was necessary for others. In the argument of that book, fidelity or faith refers to the Christian's responsive relationship to God, whereas agape or love refers to duties to other persons. Fidelity to God requires love for neighbor. Thus, for Ramsey, Christian ethics had to be a matter of faithful service to other persons, and fidelity was the most basic principle of the moral life, not merely one of several competing considerations to be weighed and balanced against other goods, rules, or principles.

Fifteen years later, it was natural for Ramsey to conflate terms and refer to the duties human beings owe each other in medical care as duties of covenant loyalty. His work in medical ethics in the 1970s and 1980s consisted of attempts to specify what those duties might be. In *The Patient as Person*, his overriding concern was with social and psychological forces that led to abuses of persons, in particular the fear of death and a thoughtless commitment to medical progress. Research subjects needed protection against caregivers who succumbed to these pressures; persons needed to be allowed to die rather than be kept alive in torment or loneliness.

The momentum of the argument in *The Patient as Person* was so overwhelming that Ramsey did not immediately confront an important question central to an ethic of fidelity: "Am I to be faithful to what the 'neighbors' say they need—or to what they really need?" In fact, throughout his career Ramsey was willing to stipulate only a very few basic human needs, for example, protection from physical attack. In the medical context, however, the issue became unavoidable. "To what in the other am I to be faithful?" Does fidelity look to the "best interests" of the patient or to the patient's autonomous choices? In *Ethics at the Edges of Life* (1978), Ramsey clearly opted for best interests or a "medical indications policy" in decisions about care for the dying. There is no doubt that this view is paternalistic from the perspective of an ethic in which autonomy and patients' rights count for more (Childress, 1982). The harder issues are: (1) the theological and moral adequacy of the alternatives, and (2) whether any ethic of fidelity must be paternalistic in a bad sense.

William F. May (1975, 1983) has developed the fidelity idea in a somewhat different direction. His basic strategy has been to characterize alternative models, metaphors, or images for the relationship between healer and patient. The assumption is that reality is shaped by perception. May has identified a set of images of the healing relationship: physicians as "fighters," "philanthropists," or artistic virtuosi. Because physicians see themselves in these ways, and are so seen by patients, interactions between physicians and patients tend to take on the characteristics of wars, generous acts of assistance, or skilled performance. Something is left out. That something is found when the relationship between physician and patient is seen primarily as one of fidelity. If one starts with covenant fidelity between selves, the other ways of imagining self and other are brought into perspective.

May wrote his doctoral thesis about responses to death in the works of Albert Camus and Martin Heidegger; his views on fidelity show the influence of Gabriel Marcel. May argues that fidelity is made possible by a realization that the power of death has been defeated. Without that realization, people can act only from motives of anxiety, and their behavior amounts to anxious searching for security and self-protection. Fidelity requires "nonchalance" and the courage to establish ties to the perishing world around one. The belief that the power of death is broken is the core idea of Christian theology; for May, as for Paul Ramsey, fidelity is clearly a theological concept.

May has traced out at least three other implications of the notion of fidelity as a norm in medical ethics. First, he has explicitly contrasted it with contract—unlike Robert M. Veatch and others, who have tended to see the terms as synonymous, differing only in connotation (Veatch, 1981). May sees contract as a term drawn from liberal economics and politics, one suggesting a bargain struck by equally informed and powerful actors. Contracts clearly specify what is to be done by whom; contracts may be canceled. Against this conception, May claims that covenantal relationships arise in contexts of inequality; they are not the result of rational bargains; they make demands beyond their explicit terms; and they alter the selves of the covenant part-

ners. Contract language is the language of the sovereign self; covenant language, of the responsive self.

Second, consistent with this understanding, May has insisted that the appropriate manifestation of fidelity in a physician–patient relationship is the fact that the faithful one serves as a teacher. Fidelity to a patient should not mean simply imposing one's will on the patient or guiltlessly accepting a patient's destructive choice. It means working with the patient to try to help the patient make a sound choice. I am faithful to you when I am willing to take the risk of trying to teach you. The stress on the pedagogical nature of the relationship between healer and patient softens the paternalism of Ramsey's formulation.

Third, May clearly acknowledges the communal and social aspects of faithful care. He argues for rethinking the way health care is provided, suggesting an increased role for nurses and a reorganization of health-care delivery. It is a first step in the direction of adopting the fidelity norm in an institutional, not merely an interpersonal, context.

Fidelity as part of a theory. Although Ramsey and May have been the most influential and distinctive users of the fidelity idea in twentieth-century medical ethics, they are not alone. Several other important approaches should be mentioned.

One significant application appears in the complex feminist literature on ethics. While some feminists have stressed autonomy and independence, others have attempted to develop a distinctive ethic of care. These contrasting concerns in normative ethics are related to the relationship between gender and moral intuitions, perceptions, judgments, and theories. (See, for example, Gilligan, 1982; Bebeau and Brabeck, 1989.) An ethic of care, with its concern for relationships, clearly addresses issues paralleling those raised by writers for whom fidelity is the basic norm. That overlap is increased insofar as feminist theory entails a view of the self as engaged and encumbered, skepticism about the possibility of a completely neutral moral perspective, and attention to "housekeeping"—that is, ongoing, chronic—issues rather than those of crisis or critical care (Warren, 1989).

The medical ethics literature offers many explorations of the relationship between physician and patient that have an obvious affinity with the discussion of fidelity to be found in Ramsey or May. For example, Pedro Láin Entralgo (1969) describes the normative core of the patient–physician relationship as "medical philia"; John C. Fletcher (1982) has suggested that clergy could function as "faithful companions" to patients and physicians at times of stress; and Eric Cassell (1991) has written at length about the healing power of the role of the physician. Clear, substantive overlap is evident between these works and writers who use "fidelity" in a more self-conscious and perhaps systematic way. The preoccupation with a healing relationship is constant, but separating terminological from substantive differences is no easy task.

Finally, the principle of fidelity plays an important, if subordinate, role in the ethic of principles developed by Tom L. Beauchamp and James F. Childress (1989). For them, fidelity is a form of promise-keeping, a duty justified in terms of basic principles of utility and autonomy. Fidelity is not the basic principle of morality, nor is it the controlling metaphor for the healing relationship. But it comes into play when people make agreements, and the duties associated with fidelity are a function of the nature of relationships and the expectations brought to them. While Beauchamp and Childress place fidelity in a very different theoretical context than Ramsey or May, it is not entirely clear how great a difference that will make in recommendations for the resolution of difficult cases.

Issues

Conflicts of loyalty.   Common in health care, conflicts of loyalty may include conflicts between a provider's duty to the person employing the provider and to the patient (e.g., over insurance or conditions of work); conflicts among various roles a provider may play (e.g., as caregiver, teacher, or researcher); and conflicting duties to various members of a family, perhaps complicated if more than one of them is the provider's patient. Conflicting loyalties among members of the health-care team (physicians, nurses, physical and occupational therapists, allied health personnel) and between caregivers and management are everyday issues in health care. Somehow, providers must balance professional and other personal loyalties and engagements.

In attempting to sort out these moral conflicts, at least two variables must be borne in mind. One concerns *to whom* a duty is owed: patient, employer, patient's family member, colleague. The other bears on *what* loyalty requires, the *substance or magnitude* of the duty: to protect a life, keep a confidence, or provide personal support. It is relatively easy in the abstract to assert that major duties to patients trump all other considerations, for example, that life-threatening, professionally incompetent care must be stopped. But even in that case, less pressing but significant loyalties to others may rightly determine how, where, and when action is taken. Complex balancing may be required to reconcile conflicting loyalties.

There may turn out to be a close connection between commitment to loyalty, as a fundamental principle, and use of casuistry as a method of analysis. It is possible that general rules of priority among loyalties can be formulated, for example: "Always stand by the choices a patient made when competent." But beginning with the loyalties, rather than the principles, forces one to acknowledge complexity and ambiguity at the core of the moral life, because there is always more than one loyalty and more than one requirement of a given loyalty. So the rule gets complicated: Which "rational" self is the true one? What of the feelings and needs of family? The complexities must be worked out carefully using imagination and precedent.

Creating fidelity bonds.   Views of human selfhood or human nature are often at stake in the disagreements over the role of loyalty in medical ethics, or in the moral life generally. Many pluralist theories in which fidelity is one of several basic but derivative principles tend to be concerned with the dangers of imposing one person's values on another. These theories are especially sensitive to the dangers of well-intentioned but disrespectful beneficence, and they want to speak of fidelity bonds—the generators of beneficence—as the product of freely entered agreements.

In contrast, fidelity-centered theories suggest that fidelity bonds may be created in other ways: through dependence as between children and parents, through membership such as citizenship, or simply through proximity. Josiah Royce (1897) suggested that bonding was associated with a sense of suffering together, and David Smith (1987) has argued that fidelity entails identification with the suffering of another, suggesting a notion of interdependent selfhood that is also to be found in Christian theology. For these writers, the greatest evil to be avoided is indifference, and they are clearly working with a different view of self and social relations than many pluralists.

Other considerations.   Fidelity theories must work out several other issues of consistency and adequacy. Some of these points have already been mentioned: Why is fidelity important? What is the relationship between fidelity and self-fulfillment? What moral principles, rules, or other considerations, if any, can justify disloyalty or breaking a fiduciary relationship? If loyalty means more than honoring another's choices, what more? Are universal demands of fidelity required, whatever the consequences?

Conclusion

However these issues may be resolved, some things are clear. The notion of fidelity or loyalty informed some of the most important work in medical ethics in the 1970s and 1980s. It is a suggestive notion that often carries theological connotations, and it stands as an alternative to theories that focus on the self and its basic autonomy. Newborns, children, the retarded and demented are not capable of autonomy as that term is often used in the medical ethics literature, but they can be loyal; others can be loyal to them, and they can be treated with dignity—or indignity. Nor is it clear that our "best" selves are our most competent or autonomous selves.

A loyalty-based ethic coheres with our experience of ourselves and illness; it meshes with clinical reality in which bonding between professional and patient, as well as among professionals—and within the family—is fundamental to therapy. Selves are not understood if those bonds, and their pathologies, are misunderstood. Although focusing on loyalties does not guarantee an accurate moral diagnosis or prescription, it does provide a helpful starting point for sorting out moral matters, a starting point that ensures the patient will be seen in his or her social context, and that the social self of the caregiver is taken into account.

DAVID H. SMITH

Directly related to this entry is the entry DIVIDED LOYALTIES IN MENTAL-HEALTH CARE. *For a further discussion of topics mentioned in this article, see the entries* CARE; CASUISTRY; ETHICS; FEMINISM; FRIENDSHIP; HUMAN NATURE; LOVE; METAPHOR AND ANALOGY; PATIENTS' RESPONSIBILITIES; PERSON; PROFESSIONAL–PATIENT RELATIONSHIP; *and* RIGHTS, *article on* RIGHTS IN BIOETHICS. *This article will find application in the entries* FAMILY; FRAUD, THEFT, AND PLAGIARISM; MARRIAGE AND OTHER DOMESTIC PARTNERSHIPS; PROFESSION AND PROFESSIONAL ETHICS; PSYCHIATRY, ABUSES OF; TEAMS, HEALTH-CARE; *and* WHISTLEBLOWING. *For a discussion of related ideas, see the entries* AUTONOMY; CONFIDENTIALITY; INFORMATION DISCLOSURE; INFORMED CONSENT; TRUST; UTILITY; VALUE AND VALUATION; *and* VIRTUE AND CHARACTER.

Bibliography

BEAUCHAMP, TOM L., and CHILDRESS, JAMES F. 1989. *Principles of Biomedical Ethics.* 3d ed. New York: Oxford University Press.

BEBEAU, MURIEL J., and BRABECK, MARY M. 1989. "Ethical Sensitivity and Moral Reasoning Among Men and Women in the Professions." In *Who Cares? Theory, Research, and Educational Implications of the Ethic of Care,* pp. 144–163. Edited by Mary M. Brabeck. New York: Praeger.

BLACK, HENRY CAMPBELL. 1979. *Black's Law Dictionary.* 5th ed. St. Paul: West Publishing.

CASSELL, ERIC J. 1991. *The Nature of Suffering: And the Goals of Medicine.* New York: Oxford University Press.

CHILDRESS, JAMES F. 1982. *Who Should Decide? Paternalism in Health Care.* New York: Oxford University Press.

FLETCHER, GEORGE P. 1993. *Loyalty: An Essay on the Morality of Relationships.* New York: Oxford University Press.

FLETCHER, JOHN C. 1982. *Coping with Genetic Disorders.* New York: Harper & Row.

FRIED, CHARLES. 1976. "The Lawyer as Friend: The Moral Foundations of the Lawyer–Client Relationship." *Yale Law Journal* 85, no. 7:1060–1089.

GILLIGAN, CAROL. 1982. *In a Different Voice: Psychological Theory and Women's Development.* Cambridge, Mass.: Harvard University Press.

LAÍN ENTRALGO, PEDRO. 1969. *Doctor and Patient.* New York: McGraw-Hill.

MAY, WILLIAM F. 1975. "Code, Covenant, Contract or Philanthropy." *Hastings Center Report* 5:29–38.

———. 1983. *The Physician's Covenant: Images of the Healer in Medical Ethics.* Philadelphia: Westminster.

McGILL, ARTHUR C. 1967. *Suffering: A Test of Theological Method.* Philadelphia: Geneva.

MURRAY, THOMAS H. 1986. "Divided Loyalties for Physicians: Social Context and Moral Problems." *Social Science and Medicine* 23, no. 8:827–832.

NIEBUHR, H. RICHARD. 1960. *Radical Monotheism and Western Culture.* New York: Harper & Row.

———. 1963. *The Responsible Self.* New York: Harper & Row.

RAMSEY, PAUL. 1950. *Basic Christian Ethics.* New York: Scribner.

———. 1970. *The Patient as Person: Explorations in Medical Ethics.* New Haven, Conn.: Yale University Press.

———. 1978. *Ethics at the Edges of Life: Medical and Legal Intersections.* New Haven, Conn.: Yale University Press.

ROYCE, JOSIAH. 1969. [1897]. "The Problem of Job." In vol. 2 of *The Basic Writings of Josiah Royce,* pp. 833–854. Edited by John J. McDermott. Chicago: University of Chicago Press. On suffering and theodicy.

———. 1969. [1908]. *The Philosophy of Loyalty.* In vol. 2 of *The Basic Writings of Josiah Royce,* pp. 855–1013. Edited by John J. McDermott. Chicago: University of Chicago Press.

SMITH, DAVID H. 1985. "Medical Loyalty: Dimensions and Problems of a Rich Idea." In *Theology and Bioethics: Exploring the Foundations and Frontiers,* pp. 267–282. Edited by Earl L. Shelp. Dordrecht, Netherlands: D. Reidel.

———. 1987. "Suffering, Medicine and Christian Theology." In *On Moral Medicine: Theological Perspectives in Medical Ethics.* Edited by Stephen E. Lammers and Allen Verhey. Grand Rapids, Mich.: William B. Eerdmans.

TOULMIN, STEPHEN. 1986. "Divided Loyalties and Ambiguous Relationships." *Social Science and Medicine* 23, no. 8:783–787.

VANDERPOOL, HAROLD Y., and WEISS, GARY B. 1984. "Patient Truthfulness: A Test of Models of the Physician–Patient Relationship." *Journal of Medicine and Philosophy* 9, no. 4:353–372.

VEATCH, ROBERT M. 1981. *A Theory of Medical Ethics.* New York: Basic Books.

WARREN, VIRGINIA L. 1989. "Feminist Directions in Medical Ethics." *Hypatia* 4, no. 2:73–87. This is part of a special issue of *Hypatia,* edited by Helen Bequaert Holmes, entitled "Feminist Ethics and Medicine."

FINLAND

See MEDICAL ETHICS, HISTORY OF, *section on* EUROPE, *subsection on* CONTEMPORARY PERIOD, *article on* NORDIC COUNTRIES.

FOOD POLICY

Widespread hunger and malnutrition are not new in the history of humankind. What is new is a deepening conviction that famine and starvation are by no means inevitable. The technical ability to feed a growing human family exists even if the political and economic structures and the political will for that purpose are inadequate or absent. To create that political will is the central ethical issue in planning and implementing a food policy that meets the needs of the post–Cold War world. The basic ethical concern focuses not only on hunger events, such as famine, that afflict particular populations at particular times, but even more on the chronic, debilitating hunger from which more than 10 percent of the human race suffers constantly.

This entry presents an overview of the world food situation; an examination of the policy framework situating and informing hunger; an exploration of policy responses; and a survey of the ethical questions involved in alleviating hunger on a world scale.

The condition of world hunger

Most authorities agree that the world produces enough food to feed every person on earth, and this production is expected to continue. Yet, nearly 800 million people are malnourished and face a daily struggle to find enough food to survive. Food security—access, through either production or purchase, to a diet adequate for normal human activity—eludes them. The international system of producers, processors, suppliers, marketers, regulators, and consumers that produces and distributes the world's food is not moving a fair share of it to these people. Military activity, moreover, by disrupting production and distribution and by displacing people, adds another set of obstacles.

The persistence of widespread hunger and malnutrition underscores the weaknesses of past efforts to improve the international food system, efforts focused mainly on increasing production rather than on addressing the underlying social, political, and economic forces that keep people hungry. If every person on earth received the two pounds of grain per capita that the world produces every day, everybody would have at least a minimum adequate diet. Increased production of food is surely an important goal, but distribution is at least equally salient, given existing imbalances between supply and need. Because peasant producers and agricultural laborers are most at risk of hunger, it is important to increase their food production and earnings. This requires priority support for small-scale and labor-intensive agriculture in order to meet supply, distribution, demand, and need simultaneously. The key is to raise the rural poor above subsistence.

Convened to deal with this problem, the U.N. World Food Conference of November 1974 concluded, "Every man, woman, and child has the inalienable right to be free from hunger and malnutrition in order to develop fully and maintain his physical and mental faculties" (U.N. World Food Conference, pp. 5–16). The 1974 World Food Conference was followed by the 1979 World Conference on Agrarian Reform and Rural Development (WCARRD), as well as several reports related to the same subject, including the report of the U.S. Presidential Commission on World Hunger (1980), the Brandt Commission reports, the U.S. Council on Environmental Quality's *Global 2000 Report to the President,* the 1980 Brundtland Commission report (World Commission, 1987) that led to the U.N. Conference on Environment and Development (UNCED) and its report known as Agenda-21 (U.N. Conference, 1992). All these events and reports stressed the need for increased food production by small farmers in food-deficit countries, better allocation of available food, fairer distribution of income through land reform and other measures, and efforts to sustain hungry people until they can achieve the food security to which the United Nations (U.N. World Food Conference, 1974) and most observers believe they have a right.

Despite some progress in a few developing countries, the world continues to face the same chronic, subtle, and dangerous food crisis that has persisted for many decades. According to the 1993 U.N. Food and Agriculture Organization (FAO) report, the worldwide total of malnourished people grows each year. The hunger these people suffer is not a dramatic famine that commands public attention but a daily struggle for survival that receives little coverage in the media, precisely because it is not dramatic. The FAO report indicates that most malnourished people live in the villages of developing countries.

While some countries are struggling to correct past neglect of the food sector and to increase investment in agriculture, in many cases their populations continue to grow faster than their own production of needed food. Despite the fact that food production has increased more rapidly in many developing countries than in the industrialized world, per capita food production in the former has barely kept pace with population growth. In some sub-Saharan African countries, where the outlook is especially bleak, the ratio has actually declined; and the additional food requirements of millions of refugees fleeing drought and violence (e.g., in Somalia and Rwanda) have greatly increased the region's already acute food needs.

Cereal grains account for about 85 percent of worldwide human food consumption. Nearly 90 percent of the grain is consumed in the countries in which it is grown, either directly as cereal food (mainly in poor countries) or indirectly as the products of animal consumers of grain, for example, meat, milk, and eggs (mainly in rich countries). A major part of the other 10 percent moves from the so-called North American breadbasket to the developing countries of Africa, Asia, and Latin America. Production and consumption of cereals have maintained a fragile equilibrium over the years; some years see production decreases, and others show increases.

Aggregate figures from the United Nations and the World Bank (1986) suggest that production will continue to match consumption, even with population growth; but the numbers do not reflect the differential food intake and, consequently, the endemic, chronic hunger, that results from income disparities among and within countries. Most people in the industrialized world, as well as the minorities associated with the modern economic sector in the developing countries, consume nearly four times as much grain per capita as poor people in developing countries. Moreover, as noted above, about 85 percent of the grain is consumed indirectly in industrialized countries and among the relatively affluent in the developing countries in the form of dairy products and the meat of grain-fed animals. Other people—mainly poor people in poor countries—consume their grain directly (e.g., as bowls of rice); thus not only do they get less food less reliably, but the food they do have is generally less nutritious. In short, their right to food is violated.

The violation of the right to have food, then, is the central problem of food policy. Why is this right not secured? To deal with this question requires an exploration of the causes of hunger from both the supply and the demand sides; Lester Brown and Erik Eckholm's systemic analysis (1974) remains valid.

The supply side

Limited land. Roughly one acre of land is under cultivation for every person on Earth. In a gross sense, there is probably that much more land available to be cultivated. But to bring it under the plow is increasingly difficult, usually very costly, and more and more problematic because the agricultural infrastructure is not in place. Preparing the apparently large land reserves in, for example, the southern Sudan or the upper Amazon for more intensive food crop cultivation would entail incalculable financial, social, and environmental costs. In addition, some argue that the steady loss of prime cropland to erosion, pollution, and urbanization in the industrialized world—reflected over the years in reports of the European Community and the U.S. Department of Agriculture and more recently in China—is also a long-term threat to the productivity of the world food system.

Increasingly threatened water supply. Scarcity of water may prove to be an even more serious constraint than limited or disappearing cropland. Fresh water for agriculture is already in short supply and is being further depleted by siltation, pollution, and the drawing down of underground water tables. The long-range environmental impact of irrigation and other water-related technologies is a matter of increasing concern.

Energy. Even though petroleum, a major direct and indirect element in food production and distribution, appears to be in temporary surplus worldwide, its price remains at a level much higher than it was before the "oil shocks" of the early 1970s, and still high (though only about half the 1980 price) for low-income developing countries that do not produce oil and must import it for both industry and agriculture. The prices of nitrogen fertilizer and pesticides made from petroleum have also risen significantly. As a result, the cost of increasing yields has risen beyond the capacity of many small Third World producers, and food prices continue to climb beyond the reach of the neediest people.

Environmental degradation. Many of the poorest countries are under severe ecological stress, aggravated by the growing misuse of agricultural resources, energy (especially fuelwood), and cattle feed (forage and ground cover). Agricultural productivity in those regions is reduced, and the world is threatened with irreversible environmental losses. Poor countries, moreover, are generally not equipped with the infrastructure (roads, transport, communications, technology, research, etc.) or managerial capacity (often weakened by corruption) to cope with the problems of protecting the water, air, and forest systems that underpin the processes of food production.

Shortage or inappropriateness of technology. Technological progress has contributed much to human welfare and improved food systems; but despite the dramatic improvements in modern technology that have increased food production, the number of hungry people has not diminished. In most developing countries, agricultural technology has not been able to keep up with the increased purchasing power of the elites. As the income gap between rich and poor widens, food produced using capital-intensive technology alone may not solve the world's hunger problem, because those increasing numbers of poor people cannot afford either to use the technology or to buy its products. Rising income also shapes demand and tends to skew production away from foods consumed by the poor; international investment opportunities often do the same, as in the case of Brazil's shift to growing soybeans for the Japanese market at the expense of black beans, the dietary staple of poor people in Brazil. There is evidence, moreover, that inappropriate application of some costly technologies introduced to increase food production, especially heavy mechanization, irrigation, and increased chemical use, has worsened the nutritional status of the poor in developing countries by depriving them of both their staple diet and their livelihood. It cannot be assumed that the capital-intensive, resource-depleting agricultural technology that enables one U.S. farmer to feed seventy other people will work either economically or socially in other settings.

Inadequate research.   Agricultural research for and in developing countries, particularly that of the international institutes established and stimulated by private donors and coordinated through the World Bank (the Consultative Group on International Agricultural Research [CGIAR]), has unquestionably contributed in significant measure to boosting food production. Yet the bulk of this increasingly expensive research—90 percent of which takes place in and is concerned with production in the northern temperate zone—is devoted to commercial agriculture and the processing and marketing of cash crops. Relatively little agricultural research money is spent on tropical agriculture (except possibly for rice), subsistence food crops (rather than those for export), the study of nutritional implications of production patterns, or the development of production techniques helpful to small farmers and landless rural poor, who will have to produce more if food security is to be achieved.

Unpredictable weather.   Since 85 percent of the world's agricultural products are grown on rainfed land, the most decisive supply-side factor in the long run is the weather, which for the most part is neither predictable nor controllable. Although debate over the seriousness of the buildup of greenhouse gases in the atmosphere continues, there is some concern among scientists and others about such man-made weather modifications that could increase average temperatures over the next decades in the Northern Hemisphere—enough to weaken the climatic base that sustains the North's capacity to produce for export.

It is possible to adjust to some of these constraints: Substitutes can be found for fossil fuels and energy-saving techniques can conserve them; increased trade and stockpiling can guard against the effects of adverse weather conditions; and improved farming practices can increase yields and conserve moisture and soil resources. But it is very difficult to deal with all of the problems at once.

The demand side

Although there are some difficult ethical issues involved on the supply side of this problem—who should own what, who should plant what and when, what farming practices are acceptable, and who should decide in all

these cases—those on the demand side may be even more difficult.

Population growth.   The dramatic increase in the number of people in the world, of course, puts great stress on the world's food supply; as population grows, more food must be produced. As long as the world adds the equivalent in population of one Mexico per year and one China per decade, this problem will persist; 85 percent of population growth occurs in the developing world.

Where hunger and poverty prevail, experience suggests that population growth is, in general, likely to hold steady or increase. The main characteristics of high-population-growth societies are high infant mortality, low life expectancy, low literacy (especially among women), and the positive economic value of the surviving children to their families. People in very poor countries may have large numbers of children, because they need many births to ensure that some children survive to work the farm, carry on the family and its culture, and help the old. Population growth, however, is not the cause of hunger; on the contrary, both are symptoms of poverty and underdevelopment. Where economic development takes place, providing at least a minimum assurance of food and income, population growth rates tend to decline, though not always immediately.

Rising affluence.   In addition to the purely quantitative pressure of numbers exerted by population growth, even greater strain results from overconsumption by the affluent. As economic growth takes place in developing countries and more people increase their incomes and move beyond the subsistence level, stress mounts on available food supplies. While population growth puts a steadily growing and heavier quantitative (or absolute) burden on the food system in terms of sheer production requirements, rising affluence, because of the resulting differential consumption patterns, exerts a much more rapidly escalating pressure, which can be described as more qualitative (or relative). The middle-income countries' share of food imports has risen steadily, to the point where those countries comprise one of the largest segments of the world food import market. The consumption patterns of the affluent exert far greater pressure on the global resource base, in absolute and per capita terms, than those of the poor.

Household surveys by both public and private agencies indicate that the first increment of increased income often goes toward trying to improve the diet, which in most cases means shifting from tubers to grains, and then from grains to poultry and meat. This change places greater stress on the grain supply, because between two and seven pounds of grain are required to produce a pound of chicken, pork, or beef. Since the food supply in most food-deficit developing countries can generally be increased significantly (at least in the immediate future) only through imports, a larger proportion of their limited foreign exchange will be diverted from development programs to food purchases—as it has already been diverted to pay or service external debt. Not only is economic progress thus slowed but the poor remain unable to buy costly imported food and are thus bypassed by the economic growth that does take place, unless their country adopts policies to prevent such an outcome. Moreover, if a significant portion of the growth is attributable to agricultural exports like coffee, cocoa, fruits, and sugar, the irony is compounded, since so little of the earnings from the sale and processing of the cash crops accrues to those who produce and harvest them on land they do not own, but which could be used to raise crops for local consumption.

Inequitable social and political structures. It is clear from the work of Amartya Sen (1981) and others that the problems of food and hunger ultimately can be understood and relieved only in the broader, more fundamental context of development. The objective is to enable people to grow or buy the food they need, that is, to achieve food security. This is not famine relief but the reduction, and eventual elimination, of chronic hunger. It is in this sense that the food problem inexorably becomes a development problem, reflecting the political and economic arrangements within and among nations and in the global economy. Hunger is a symptom of the underlying social "diseases" of underdevelopment and injustice. People are hungry because they are poor, and they become and remain poor because they lack the power to choose otherwise; if they have the option, they generally will not choose leaders, structures, or policies that make or keep them poor.

Approaches to ethical analysis of food policy

As late as the 1970s, Anglo-American moral and political philosophy provided very little justification for aid to the undernourished people in foreign countries. Human-rights theorists favored traditional Western civil and political liberties but opposed substantive rights that demanded positive action on the part of government. Utilitarians, drawing on the vocabulary of the reform movements in eighteenth-century Britain, still held that the maxim "the greatest good for the greatest number" applied exclusively within the bounds of a single country where politicians worked for "the interest of the governed." Furthermore, international relations theory, based on principles of sovereignty and nonintervention, considered the relations between states to the general exclusion of the interests of populations (Beitz, 1979; Brown, 1977; O'Neill, 1985).

Confrontation with the issue of world hunger in the 1970s and 1980s, however, produced a number of significant shifts in philosophical premises concerning both human rights and the theory of international relations favorable to the interests of people in need. Philosophers began to turn their backs on traditional positions, objecting to so-called positive rights to government assistance for deprived persons (Shue, 1980). Political philosophers, moreover, repudiating customary arguments about the limits of political obligation, provided new arguments justifying standard assistance to afflicted populations on an international basis (Beitz, 1979).

These initiatives were anticipated in the religious community with articulation of a cosmopolitan political theory based on the promotion and defense of human rights, identification of "the universal common good" as a norm for political action (John XXIII, 1963), and specification of "the principle of solidarity" for aid from rich to poor nations (Paul VI, 1967).

By the mid-1990s moral philosophers formulated three views concerning world hunger and international food policy: subsistence rights and duties, global justice and development, and humanitarian aid. In addition, difficulties in reaching victims of starvation in situations of civil conflict have raised two specialized questions for the political ethics of humanitarian aid: (1) donors' right of access to affected populations, and (2) the obligation of "humanitarian intervention," with military means, if necessary, by the international community.

Subsistence rights and duties. The case for subsistence rights argues that some goods are necessary for the enjoyment of any other rights and so themselves are basic rights (Shue, 1980). Personal security would be one such right routinely recognized. Similarly, the right to subsistence qualifies as a basic right because without the satisfaction of the right to food people will fail to enjoy any of the other rights to which they are entitled.

A parallel argument for the right to "basic needs" claims that deprivation of subsistence needs erodes the minimal standards of decency and dignity to which human beings are entitled (Christiansen, 1982). "Decency" is understood as referring to a physical quality of life beneath which a person tends to be rejected or avoided by others; and "dignity" is defined as control over resources necessary for life so that a person can maintain personal and political freedom without manipulation by those who otherwise exercise control over the economy. On the same grounds, some argue for "relative equality" in economic life as a condition of political equality in democracies (Gutmann, 1980; Christiansen, 1980).

Along with the right to subsistence come corresponding duties incumbent on governments and citizens of all countries. These are: (1) the duty not to deprive; (2) the duty to prevent deprivation; and (3) the duty to aid the hungry (Shue, 1980). The duty not to deprive is a simple expression of the maxim of nonmaleficence, "do no harm." In practice, however, it may be far more difficult, calling for complex economic policy decisions, such as debt forgiveness, correction or elimination of structural adjustment programs (i.e., fiscal and budgetary reforms imposed on Third World countries by the International Monetary Fund as conditions of credit), and the shift from promoting cash crops to supporting agriculture for domestic consumption.

The duty of preventing deprivation entails developing cooperative institutions to prevent standard threats to food security. Such standard threats would include drought cycles, depletion of aquifers, and inappropriate farming techniques. In addition, they would also embrace natural disasters, such as catastrophic storms, and social disruptions, such as war or market failure. The duty of prevention requires sustained efforts to devise, implement, and support institutions and policies that would defend vulnerable populations against routine threats to subsistence. In response to the endemic, chronic hunger noted above, the duty of prevention would establish reliable means of access for the world's poor to the means of livelihood or, in times of crises, emergency relief.

Finally, the duty to aid the hungry entails providing emergency assistance when the standard provisions against hunger fail to satisfy the needs of victims in a particular crisis. As opposed to theories of humanitarian aid discussed below, however, the subsistence rights and duties theory places emphasis on establishing programs to prevent hunger in a routine way rather than treating emergency assistance as the primary means of ensuring food security.

Global justice and development. The duty to prevent hunger has required sustained reform of global economic and political institutions, which has led, in turn, to a rethinking of the applicability of principles of justice to international relations. In the past, international relations theory presented serious impediments to any conception of justice across national boundaries. The principle of sovereignty established the unqualified responsibility of governments for their own population. In effect, that meant citizens were subjects dependent on the goodwill and effectiveness of their political leaders without recourse to other political authorities when their basic social contract for basic welfare went unfulfilled. For their part, leaders of nations were committed to nonintervention in the affairs of other states. Aid might be offered on humanitarian grounds or out of political interest, but there were no reasons to sustain an obligation to protect people in general from severe deprivation, or to enjoin intervention where governments failed to guard their own people from starvation.

Cosmopolitan political theories, that is, those grounded in the universal rights of persons as opposed to state sovereignty, provide the foundation for principles of international justice (Beitz, 1979). According to such theories, the increasing economic interdependence of nations through communication, travel, and various technologies establishes conditions for modifying principles of sovereignty and nonintervention in the interest of justice among nations. (Parallel arguments have been made in theological sources [John XXIII, 1963]). Without ceasing to be citizens of their own countries, men and women are citizens of the world community, subject to a code of universal justice. These theories would contribute to the alleviation of world hunger by promoting equitable economic relations on a world scale.

Another defense of global justice in food policy argues that natural resources are randomly distributed and accordingly are inappropriately regarded, on the analogy with private property, as the exclusive possession of nations in which they are found (Brown, 1977). Because nations have done nothing morally deserving of these endowments, the argument runs, in the face of mass hunger or other grave deprivations, they are not justified in either maintaining exclusive control of resources or gaining exceptional profit from them. An analogous theological argument posits "the common purpose of created things" to be the livelihood and fulfillment of all of the members of the human family, urging that "no one is justified in keeping for his exclusive use what he does not need, when others lack necessities" (Paul VI, 1967, no. 23).

Critics of this view object because redistribution of wealth from nations of the North to those of the South does not ensure a just distribution of wealth within poor countries and destabilizes the necessary order in the international system (Tucker, 1977). Still others contend that the market remains the best solution to problems of deprivation and that attempts at building other global institutions in the name of justice will only lead to worsened economic conditions (Novak, 1984).

Humanitarian aid. Until the advent of subsistence rights and global justice theories, emergency food relief was justified on humanitarian grounds, and this continues to be the case among voluntary agencies engaged in emergency relief (Minear, 1991). Traditionally, humanitarianism has made two assumptions: (1) provision of emergency aid is an exceptional activity outside the normal structures of international politics, and (2) crisis relief is a matter of supererogation, proceeding from motives of charity or compassion rather than of accepted duty.

While humanitarianism customarily has been regarded as a secular version of the Christian virtue of charity, recent theology has tended to abandon the older firm distinction between justice and charity, which made justice obligatory and charity a matter of meritorious personal action. Instead, justice, which demands the construction of equitable international institutions to obviate most need for emergency aid between nations, is viewed as being informed by charity (Paul VI, 1967). In other words, charity, because of its zeal for the good and unity of the human family, is needed to effect justice (John Paul II, 1987).

1. *Right of access.* In the 1990s, private voluntary agencies and government offices concerned about political obstacles to relief efforts presented by host governments argued for increased immunity from extraneous considerations for humanitarian activities. A particularly important step in this direction has been a movement to assert the right of access for relief agencies to affected populations caught in areas of civil conflict (Minear, 1991). In this case, private humanitarian organizations, which frequently take the lead in providing aid to civilians in such situations, are effectively urging a limitation on the sovereignty of national governments. While maintaining a distinction between humanitarian aid and international justice, the assertion of such an immunity appears to share the assumption of subsistence rights and global justice theories, that is, the primacy of persons over states, which constitutes a revolutionary change in attitudes toward the political salience of human rights.

2. *Humanitarian intervention.* The notion of humanitarian intervention against massive violations of civilian rights by military forces has been a part of just-war theory since the mid-1970s (Walzer, 1977). The Gulf War (1991) and the crises in Somalia and Bosnia-Herzegovina (1992–1994), however, provided new meanings for the term. First used to describe the independent actions of voluntary organizations in providing relief without local government authorization, "humanitarian intervention" has been the term applied to missions of mercy by international organizations (e.g., U.N. agencies and the International Committee of the Red Cross) and governments not party to the conflicts, when assisting afflicted civilians in areas of armed strife.

Finally, in an effort that strained the traditional nonviolence and neutrality of relief operations and came close to just-war usage, humanitarian intervention, as in Somalia in 1992–1993, accepted the use of force by foreign powers to guard convoys and ensure distribution of relief supplies for civilians at risk. Once again the primacy of persons over states was affirmed.

Ethical questions

The prevalence of hunger and malnutrition (i.e., the food problem) reflects not only production shortfalls, lack of reserves, technological inadequacies, and climatic variations but also basic economic, social, and political structures and societal relationships. Programs concentrating on food alone will not solve the problem of food security. Sociopolitical obstacles to improving food availability often are even more intractable than

technical obstacles (except perhaps for the weather); they involve more variables and are more resistant to change. Policies concerning pricing, taxes, exchange rates, credit, debt repayment, movement of food within countries, research, extension services, and especially land tenure place the rural poor and small farmers at a disadvantage and act as disincentives to their production of food—which most analysts insist is necessary to solve the food problem. These are the people who must be involved in the development of new policies so that incomes can rise in a reasonably equitable manner to push demand upward and thereby increase food production to meet that demand; appropriate policies cannot be imposed directly from outside, although they can be supported.

Over the long term, demand-side considerations may give rise to more urgent ethical questions than those arising on the supply side. In other words, supply-side questions are mainly (not exclusively) technical and related to production, and therefore generally get economic answers. On the demand side, however, the problems (except perhaps for population growth) are more likely to be policy related, hence, more political: Who gets what? Under what conditions? And who decides? These are essential allocative considerations in ethics. Several food-policy questions arise in the context of a political theory of justice.

1. *Should food allocation be governed primarily by the market?* If the market, as organizing principle, is viewed as the most efficient means of securing more food for more people, the law of supply and demand will determine the allocation of food. Effective demand is measured in terms of money available to meet the price asked. Because a shortage of food will cause food prices to rise and thereby stimulate greater production and trade (the law of supply and demand), nothing (e.g., managing trade, limiting profits, regulating prices, and subsidizing purchases) should be done to interfere with the market mechanism. Market interventions (e.g., for aid or relief) would create an artificial scarcity and distort the system. In domestic situations, food would be provided to the needy by the state only as emergency relief. Internationally, it would be meaningless to encourage a curtailment of consumption in affluent countries, because that action would lessen demand, lower prices, and therefore reduce production. Prices do not reflect need, because need is measured not in terms of money available (i.e., "effective" demand) but of food required. Therefore, it is necessary to decide whether the market should be regulated—"distorted," economists might say—so that the allocation of food will respond to need. The answer is clearly affirmative if the central concerns are hunger and the true cost of hunger to society.

2. *Does the state have an obligation to feed the hungry?* This question raises the much larger issue of the ethical

character of overall public social policy. The extent of the obligation of the community to provide for the general welfare of all its people is the background for any discussion of the specific provision of food for those who, for one reason or another, are hungry. Feeding, of course, is not the only, or even the best, way to meet the longer-term needs of hungry people; helping them to grow or purchase food would represent authentic development.

3. *Should food aid be used as an instrument of foreign policy?* Although foreign aid programs, in terms of food or otherwise, have always had political as well as humanitarian motivations, the ethical answer here has to be no. The question really is whether food, which sustains life, should be treated like every other commodity. In practice, U.S. food aid, for example, has regularly been provided directly (via loans) to governments for strategic reasons; but donated food aid has generally been given to nongovernmental organizations (NGOs) or to the U.N. World Food Program on the basis of the latter's judgment of need. The question of how much either modality leads to dependency remains open.

4. *Should food relief today be limited because of more serious problems tomorrow?* Those who support triage or lifeboat ethics argue that food aid is counterproductive, because food aid encourages the poorer nations to postpone reforming their own food systems and allows the present generation to live and add more people to be fed in the future—an unendingly difficult task. The ethical implications are clearly problematic.

5. *Can some nations be classified as "expendable"?* Harsh as this question may seem, hard choices are made every day in many policy areas, including food policy—the Middle East versus sub-Saharan Africa, Southeast Asia versus Central America, eastern Europe versus developing countries. Guidelines for such decisions, some ethicists and others argue, should not weigh political factors more heavily than human needs. Racial, ethnic, cultural, and religious factors that might be considered in the decision should also be ethically evaluated.

6. *Is it appropriate to urge countries to grow food for export in order to service external debt?* The strong commitment of foreign-aid agencies to a conventional market-oriented development philosophy—"get the prices and exchange rates right, and development will follow"—frequently has led these agencies to insist that poor, often food-deficit countries export agricultural commodities in order to earn convertible currencies with which to service their external debts (which totaled nearly $1.8 trillion at the beginning of 1994) (World Bank, 1986). One outcome of implementing this policy in some countries has been to degrade further the diet of the poor, who are generally unable to grow or buy the basic foods they need.

7. *Is there an obligation to reduce consumption in more affluent societies?* The widening gap between rich and poor nations (and between rich and poor within nations) presents a strong ethical challenge. What is the morality of consumption patterns of the affluent in a world with so much hunger? Consumption of grain-fed beef and pork, wastage of food, profligacy in energy use, and so on, can strongly affect both the availability and the price of food all over the world. Some would argue that simpler lifestyles in the rich nations have become a moral imperative in order to facilitate more equitable distribution of the world's resources. Others counter that changes in individual consumption patterns would have little or no effect on distribution and that no one has a right to what another has legitimately earned.

8. *Do we, in this generation, have the right to deplete natural resources in our quest for food?* This question stems from the urgency of the increasingly recognized global threats to the environment. It raises questions of both intergenerational justice—"do we have the right to borrow from our children without their consent?"—and "creational" justice—"do we have the right to subordinate the rest of creation to our own use and comfort?" It is not likely that these two questions will be easily answered.

9. *What are the ethical implications of the continued (often subsidized) sale of arms and provision of military assistance to regimes and other groups engaged in violence against neighboring states or against their own people?* Military conflict increasingly has prevented hungry people from obtaining the food they need, and military expenditures divert resources from development. On the other hand, there is the related question (noted above) of the extent to which food donors have the right to violate state sovereignty in order to feed undernourished people.

Conclusion: Beyond food policy

Empirical observation confirms that the global food system has not succeeded in getting everybody fed and suggests that the market alone will not allocate food (or anything else) equitably. In order to discuss the basic food problem fully, it is necessary to look closely at the character of the global economic system and to deal with all forms of economic transfers—investment, trade, finance, and aid. This requires an examination of a global system operated mainly by its most powerful members—transnational corporations and financial institutions—in their own interests. Governments generally occupy no more than second place in the global market. There is no national or international accountability or control over the roughly $1 trillion that moves every day in that market, and there is little or no national affiliation or loyalty. Although these international corporations and banks may come to see helping the poor to be in their interest, especially in view of growing concern about the environment, so far they have not been impelled to significant action to empower the poor.

Nevertheless, because the world's chronic food crisis is likely to remain in the forefront of contemporary problems for the foreseeable future, the ethical issues raised by it are likely to face both decision makers and ordinary people. But the food crisis, together with the environmental crisis, can neither be discussed intelligently nor resolved reasonably without attention to such other public-policy matters as corporate business practices, the philosophy of bank lending, population prgrams, socioeconomic development plans, foreign assistance, trade and investment, and social values and priorities. The stance one takes toward the problem of getting the hungry fed will be part of one's overall social ethical stance and hence relates to a more general understanding of the obligation of the rich to the poor, the welfare role of the state, and the role of economic factors in human development.

DREW CHRISTIANSEN
MARTIN M. MCLAUGHLIN

Directly related to this entry is the entry INTERNATIONAL HEALTH. *For a further discussion of topics mentioned in this entry, see the entries* CLIMATIC CHANGE; ENVIRONMENTAL ETHICS; JUSTICE; LIFE, QUALITY OF; OBLIGATION AND SUPEREROGATION; POPULATION POLICIES; RIGHTS, *article on* SYSTEMATIC ANALYSIS; *and* UTILITY. *This entry will find application in the entries* AGRICULTURE; HEALTH POLICY, *article on* HEALTH POLICY IN INTERNATIONAL PERSPECTIVE; *and* SUSTAINABLE DEVELOPMENT. *For a discussion of related ideas, see the entries* AUTONOMY; BENEFICENCE; ETHICS, *articles on* SOCIAL AND POLITICAL THEORIES, *and* RELIGION AND MORALITY; *and* FREEDOM AND COERCION.

Bibliography

BEITZ, CHARLES R. 1979. *Political Theory and International Relations.* Princeton, N.J.: Princeton University Press.

BROWN, LESTER RUSSELL, and ECKHOLM, ERIK P. 1974. *By Bread Alone.* New York: Praeger.

BROWN, PETER G. 1977. "Food as National Property." In *Food Policy: The Responsibility of the United States in the Life and Death Choices,* pp. 65–78. Edited by Peter G. Brown and Henry Shue. New York: Free Press.

CHRISTIANSEN, DREW. 1982. "Basic Needs: Criterion for the Legitimacy of Development." In *Human Rights in the Americas: The Struggle for Consensus,* pp. 245–288. Edited by Alfred T. Hennelly and John Langan. Washington, D.C.: Georgetown University Press.

———. 1984. "On Relative Equality: Catholic Egalitarianism After Vatican II." *Theological Studies* 45, no. 4:651–675.

GUTMANN, AMY. 1980. *Liberal Equality.* Cambridge: At the University Press.

JOHN XXIII. 1992. [1963]. "Pacem in terris (Peace on Earth)." In *Catholic Social Thought: The Documentary Heritage.* Edited by David J. O'Brien and Thomas A. Shannon. Maryknoll, N.Y.: Orbis.

JOHN PAUL II. 1992. [1987]. "Sollicitudo rei socialis (On Social Concern)." In *Catholic Social Thought: The Documentary Heritage.* Edited by David J. O'Brien and Thomas A. Shannon. Maryknoll, N.Y.: Orbis.

MINEAR, LARRY. 1991. *Humanitarianism Under Siege: A Critical Review of Operation Lifeline Sudan.* Trenton, N.J.: Red Sea Press.

NOVAK, MICHAEL. 1984. *Freedom with Justice: Catholic Social Thought and Liberal Institutions.* San Francisco: Harper & Row.

O'NEILL, ONORA. 1985. *Faces of Hunger: An Essay on Poverty, Justice, and Development.* London: Allen and Unwin.

PAUL VI. 1992. [1967]. "Populorum progressio (On the Development of Peoples)." In *Catholic Social Thought: The Documentary Heritage.* Edited by David J. O'Brien and Thomas A. Shannon. Maryknoll, N.Y.: Orbis.

SEN, AMARTYA K. 1981. *Poverty and Famines: An Essay on Entitlement and Deprivation.* Oxford: At the Clarendon Press.

SHUE, HENRY. 1980. *Basic Rights: Subsistence, Affluence, and U.S. Foreign Policy.* Princeton, N.J.: Princeton University Press.

TUCKER, ROBERT W. 1982. *The Inequality of Nations.* New York: Basic Books.

U.N. CONFERENCE ON ENVIRONMENT AND DEVELOPMENT (UNCED). 1992. *Report of the United Nations Conference on Environment and Development (1992): Rio di Janeiro, Brazil. (Agenda 21).* New York: United Nations.

U.N. FOOD AND AGRICULTURE ORGANIZATION (FAO) CONFERENCE. 1993. *Agriculture: Towards 2010.* Rome: Author.

U.N. WORLD FOOD CONFERENCE. 1974. *The World Food Problem: Proposals for National and International Action.* Rome: United Nations.

U.S. COUNCIL ON ENVIRONMENTAL QUALITY. 1980. *The Global 2000 Report to the President: Entering the Twenty-First Century.* 3 vols. Washington, D.C.: U.S. Government Printing Office.

U.S. PRESIDENTIAL COMMISSION ON WORLD HUNGER. 1980. *Overcoming World Hunger: The Challenge Ahead.* Washington, D.C..: Author.

WALZER, MICHAEL. 1977. *Just and Unjust Wars: A Moral Argument with Historical Illustrations.* New York: Basic Books.

WORLD BANK. 1986. *Poverty and Hunger: Issues and Options for Food Security in Developing Countries.* Washington, D.C.: Author.

WORLD COMMISSION ON ENVIRONMENT AND DEVELOPMENT. 1987. *Report of the World Commission on Environment and Development: "Our Common Future."* New York: United Nations. Chaired by Gro Harlem Brundtland.

WORLD CONFERENCE ON AGRARIAN REFORM AND RURAL DEVELOPMENT (WCARRD). 1979. *Improving the Organization and Administration of Agricultural Development.* Rome: U.N. Food and Agriculture Organization.

FRANCE

See MEDICAL ETHICS, HISTORY OF, *section on* EUROPE, *subsection on* CONTEMPORARY PERIOD, *article on* SOUTHERN EUROPE.

FRAUD, THEFT, AND PLAGIARISM

Fraud in biomedical research usually refers to fabrication of data or plagiarism of others' works; less egregious offenses may be included under the rubric "misconduct." This entry discusses the context in which fraud occurs in biomedical research, the reason it is especially damaging to this enterprise, the pressures to commit fraud, and the response of the biomedical community, including its efforts to prevent fraud.

Biomedical research, like other scientific research, has as its goal discovering the truth about nature. Thus, truth is the stock-in-trade of research. This fact makes fraud especially damaging to the scientific enterprise, because it strikes at the heart of it. Furthermore, the way in which science advances requires that researchers be able to trust one another.

Scientific advances usually occur in small, incremental steps; often there are also missteps and false leads. Each step (or misstep) is communicated to the researcher's colleagues through professional meetings and papers published in scholarly journals. In this way, the entire research community can evaluate the work and build on it. The success of the overall enterprise depends on free and open communication and on bit-by-bit additions or corrections to the total body of knowledge. A journal publication does not contain all the data obtained by the researcher in a study or experiment; instead, the paper follows a rather rigid format in which the researcher describes his or her methods, reports the salient results, and analyzes and interprets them. To draw valid conclusions, it is essential to this process that the researcher be completely honest. Furthermore, the research community is entirely dependent on each researcher's account of his or her methods and results. Others can argue with the researcher's analysis or interpretation, but since they were not present when the experiment was done, they must trust the researcher to report honestly what was done and what results emerged. For this reason, peer review cannot be expected to detect fabrication; it deals with the quality of the work, not its honesty. Obviously, then, even rare instances of fraud are unacceptable. They damage the trust on which the system depends.

Many instances of fraud in science are recounted by William Broad and Nicholas Wade in *Betrayers of the Truth* (1982). For example, they suggest that Gregor Mendel, the father of genetics, committed fraud. The more recent cases, however, suggest an ordinariness to the phenomenon that is cause for new concern. Are large numbers of otherwise unexceptional researchers committing fraud on a more or less regular basis? Beginning in 1974, when it was discovered that William Summerlin, a researcher at Memorial Sloan-Kettering Cancer Center, had painted black spots on his experimental mice to simulate successful skin grafts, there has been a spate of well-publicized instances of fraud. Summerlin gave what has became a familiar excuse: He had been pressured by his supervisor to produce rapid results.

Many explanations have been offered for an increase in the number of highly publicized cases of biomedical fraud. Some researchers and commentators believe that it is simply a matter of numbers. Since World War II, there have been many more biomedical researchers than there were earlier, so there are inevitably more dishonest ones. This means, in absolute numbers, more cases of fraud, even though the prevalence may not have increased. Others believe that the context in which research is done has changed to create more pressure and, thus, more temptation to commit fraud and that the prevalence of fraud has therefore increased. Still others believe that the prevalence is probably the same as it always was but that the popular media are simply more interested in reporting it, so that the number of reported cases has increased in relation to the number that occur. There is no way to be certain which of these explanations is correct, but it is likely that they are all involved in the increasing attention to research fraud.

Changes in the context of biomedical research

In the United States, and to a lesser extent in Europe and Japan, biomedical research has changed dramatically in the last half of the twentieth century, in ways that almost certainly result in more cases of fraud. Before that time, research was carried out by a few devotees who were motivated primarily by curiosity or zeal and earned their living in other ways, often by teaching or in clinical practice. The rest of society was largely uninterested in their endeavors, and governments did not support them. During World War II, however, the practical potential of biomedical research became readily apparent to nearly everyone. For example, wartime advances in surgical techniques, new methods of transfusion of blood products, and the introduction of penicillin had immediate and dramatic impact not only on the individual soldier, but on the entire war effort. After the war, the United States—flushed with its successes and feeling its resources virtually limitless—committed itself to funding an extensive and rapidly growing biomedical research enterprise, mainly through the National Institutes of Health (NIH). Suddenly, what had once been an individualistic, somewhat eccentric pastime became a gigantic, publicly supported enterprise. Big Science was born.

With the advent of Big Science, there were not only many more people engaged in biomedical research, but they were careerists whose livelihood depended on their research. The motivation for their work was no longer just curiosity or zeal, but professional survival. Advancement within institutions and claims to continued funding by the NIH depended on demonstrating success. Since successful research is rather difficult to evaluate, particularly contemporaneously, it became commonplace to measure success in large part by the number of a researcher's publications in scholarly journals. Success in this context is often referred to as productivity, and it is assumed that each publication represents one scientific question answered and thus can be considered a unit of productivity. It should not be surprising, then, that some career researchers are greatly tempted to cut corners to produce publishable manuscripts as rapidly and frequently as possible. Furthermore, as research groups became larger and more far-flung, supervision of less experienced investigators became looser and more remote and it became easier for them to commit fraud. It is quite likely, therefore, that instances of fraud have become more frequent both because of the larger numbers of researchers and because of changes in the system that emphasize productivity. There is no way to know the true prevalence of fraud in biomedical research, however, partly because it is almost certain that many cases are never discovered.

By the mid-1970s, it became apparent that resources were not limitless, and this may have affected the public's attitude toward cases of fraud in biomedical research. The public, after all, was funding the lion's share of the huge biomedical-research establishment. With a new sense of limits, the public wanted its money to be well spent, and it became more alert to evidence of waste, including episodes of fraud. The media responded to the proprietary interest of the public in Big Science and the public's new propensity to be outraged when its trust was abused. Thus, another reason for the apparent increase in the prevalence of fraud in biomedical research was probably the increased media attention it received.

Types of misconduct.   As mentioned earlier, fraud usually refers to fabrication of the data in an experiment or to plagiarism of a paper. Summerlin was fabricating data. John Darsee, arguably the best known of the fabricators, invented not only data but entire experiments and the names of coauthors (Culliton, 1983). The most renowned of the recent plagiarists, Alias Al-

sabti, submitted under his name copies of other researchers' papers that had been published in obscure journals (Broad, 1980).

However, there are other deceptive practices in biomedical research that are probably a great deal more common than outright fabrication or plagiarism (Angell, 1983). These practices include "trimming" data, which means altering results to make them consistent, or "selecting" data, which means simply ignoring inconsistent or inexplicable results. Another deceptive practice is "duplicate publication," that is, reporting the same work in different journals. Usually neither publication refers to the other, contrary to scientific norms requiring authors to refer to other relevant work, and editors are not informed of the existence of the other paper, since most editors would not publish work if they knew it had already been published.

Finally, certain practices that involve an element of deception are so common as to be almost standard. These include deliberately dividing research studies into fragments that can be reported in separate papers; such fragments have been termed "least-publishable units" (Broad and Wade, 1982). Fragmentation is deceptive because the paper is usually presented as a single study. As the fragments have tended to grow smaller, the list of authors has tended to grow longer. Each author can then claim a publication. Often the list of authors includes individuals whose contributions fall far short of those usually associated with authorship. For example, someone may be listed as an author simply because he or she is the lab director, the chairman of the department, or even a junior colleague who needs encouragement. As the episodes of outright fraud became publicized in the 1980s, these other practices became more widely recognized.

Increasingly, the term "fraud" was abandoned for the broader, and legally less provocative, concept of "misconduct" (U.S. Department of Health and Human Services [DHHS], 1991). This has led to controversy between the Public Health Service and the National Academy of Sciences (NAS). The former favored the broad definition, which includes "other practices that seriously deviate from those that are commonly accepted within the scientific community for proposing, conducting, or reporting research," as well as fabrication, falsification, and plagiarism. The NAS preferred not to include "other practices," since the phrase is too vague to be meaningful and could be mischievously applied (Dresser, 1993). For example, it is possible that a researcher who used highly unusual methods would be accused of misconduct under this definition even if there were no question of dishonesty.

The question of the incidence of fraud—or, probably more to the point, the prevalence of researchers who commit fraud, since they seldom stop with one offense—is still being debated. Any estimate depends on an assessment of how often fraud occurs without being discovered. It also requires a guess as to whether fraud is more likely among the more "productive" researchers and whether a researcher who commits fraud is likely to do it only occasionally or habitually. Since the NIH began tracking allegations of fraud in research institutions receiving NIH funding—nearly all research institutions—it has confirmed fewer than 100 cases each year, in some years fewer than twenty. This amounts to less than 0.2 percent of the research projects funded. Broad and Wade, however, guess that for every case of major fraud that comes to light, a hundred or so go undetected, and that for each major instance, "perhaps a thousand minor fakeries are perpetrated" (Broad and Wade, 1982). If the data in a paper are internally consistent and plausible, there is no way to know whether they are fabricated. And if the results are relatively unimportant or consistent with the experiments of others, the work may never be replicated or even cited. Obviously, then, the exact prevalence of fraud in biomedical research is unknown and unknowable.

Why do researchers commit fraud?

The motives of those committing research fraud have been extensively debated. In general, there are two schools of thought about motives. According to one, fraudulent researchers are simply "bad apples," who turn up in small numbers in any endeavor. They commit fraud because of character flaws or psychological problems. There is not much to be done about them except to try to ferret them out of the system as quickly as possible.

The other school of thought sees fraudulent researchers as succumbing to an increasingly stressful system in which the demands for productivity are nearly impossible to meet. In particular, attention has been focused on the relentless pressure to publish to obtain positions, promotions, and funding. According to this view, those who commit fraud are merely those who crack first; the others could succumb at any time and, indeed, have often already succumbed in smaller ways, such as reporting their work in least-publishable units and engaging in honorary authorship. The answer to the problem, then, is to reform a faulty system, not to focus on the guilty researchers.

At first, in the late 1970s and early 1980s, the bad-apple school was predominant. In 1983, when the U.S. Congress held its first hearings on research fraud, representatives of the scientific community were quick to defend the system and characterize the fraudulent researchers, not the system, as defective. Efforts to deal with the problem focused on developing procedures for responding to allegations of fraud; few efforts attended to aspects of the *system* that may predispose researchers to commit fraud.

Responses to fraud

The need to develop uniform procedures for responding to allegations of fraud was clear. When John Darsee was discovered in the act of fabricating data in 1981, neither Harvard Medical School, the institution where the fraud took place, nor the NIH, the funding institution, had developed explicit procedures for responding to such a situation, and Darsee's superiors had little precedent to draw on in dealing with the situation. As with earlier episodes, they handled the situation in an ad hoc and hesitant way, largely accepting Darsee's claim that this was a single episode in an otherwise blameless career. He was for a time even permitted to continue to do research. Only later did it become clear that Darsee had committed fraud repeatedly, at Emory University as well as at Harvard, and that very little of his prolific work could be relied on (Culliton, 1983).

Largely in response to the Darsee case and the way in which it was handled, academic institutions and professional organizations, beginning with the Association of American Medical Colleges (AAMC) in 1982, began to develop explicit guidelines to apply in future cases (AAMC, 1982). Most guidelines were quite similar and had in common the following features: a preliminary inquiry within the institution to make certain the allegations were not frivolous; if the allegations were determined to be serious, a second formal investigation by persons outside the department of the accused, including persons outside the institution; protection of the rights of the whistle-blower as well as those of the accused; notification of the funding agency; if the accused was determined to be guilty of fraud, formal retraction of fraudulent publications. In 1985, the NIH published interim guidelines that would require all institutions receiving NIH funding to have in place similar procedures for dealing with allegations of fraud (NIH, 1986).

Preventing fraud.   By the mid-1980s, the biomedical research community had made great strides in responding to allegations of fraud. Attention then turned to the issue of preventing it. Gradually, the bad-apple theory of the cause of fraud gave way to a more complicated analysis that acknowledged the fault was partly within the system (Petersdorf, 1986; Institute of Medicine, 1989). Several aspects of modern biomedical research were examined. Since research studies were growing very large, with multiple collaborators, sometimes in multiple centers, it was no longer expected that all collaborators were familiar with all aspects of the work or even acquaintances of one another. This fact had made it possible for Darsee to fabricate work and attribute it to coauthors without their knowing about it (or, indeed, without their even existing). The fact that his name was buried among others, some quite senior and respected, made it less likely that the work would be doubted (Relman, 1983; Huth, 1983). In addition, some research centers (sometimes termed "research mills") were themselves also growing extremely large, and the lab directors were becoming increasingly remote from the relatively junior researchers who actually generated the data. Supervision, ethical as well as scientific, was therefore much looser, although at the same time it was understood that all researchers were to "produce."

The most important aspect of modern biomedical research to be linked with a predisposition to fraud, however, was the "pressure to publish" (Angell, 1986; Huth, 1992). Most of the well-known cases of fraud were committed by relatively junior researchers working in very large and productive departments in prestigious institutions. For example, Robert A. Good, Summerlin's supervisor, had published 342 papers (an average of sixty-eight per year) in the five years before Summerlin's fabrication (Woolf, 1986). To be successful in this environment meant achieving a very high rate of publication. Most observers believe that this pressure to publish leads to fraud in predisposed individuals. Thus, the bad-apple and faulty-system theories may both be partly correct.

In the late 1980s, attention turned toward reforming the system to make fraud less likely. A number of organizations issued guidelines calling for closer supervision of junior researchers, attention to ethics in training programs, and, perhaps most important, a limit to the number of publications considered when evaluating a researcher for promotion or funding (Institute of Medicine, 1989; Harvard University; 1992; Teich and Frankel, 1992; Council of Biology Editors, 1990). For the first time in biomedical research, then, it was proposed that fewer publications might be better than more (Angell, 1986). The regulations of the Department of Health and Human Services (DHHS) addressed many of these issues (U.S. DHHS, 1991). The NIH established an Office of Scientific Integrity to deal specifically with allegations of fraud in research funded by the NIH. In 1992, this was reconfigured as the Office of Research Integrity within the DHHS. In the meantime, two committees of the U.S. Congress—the House Committee on Government Operations (Subcommittee on Human Resources and Intergovernmental Relations) and the House Committee on Energy and Commerce (Subcommittee on Oversight and Investigations)—have undertaken investigations of allegations of fraud in biomedical research. These were begun in 1988 because of a widely held view that the research community had been un-

willing to police itself adequately. There certainly were grounds for such a view in the early 1980s. Obviously, fraud cannot be entirely eliminated in any human endeavor, but there are now procedures in place for investigating allegations of fraud and plans for reforming the system to make fraud less likely. That is perhaps the best we can hope for.

MARCIA ANGELL

Directly related to this entry is the entry RESEARCH, UNETHICAL. *For a further discussion of topics mentioned in this entry, see the entries* ANIMAL RESEARCH; BIOMEDICAL ENGINEERING; BIOTECHNOLOGY; COMMUNICATION, BIOMEDICAL, *article on* SCIENTIFIC PUBLISHING; CONFLICT OF INTEREST; GENETIC ENGINEERING; GENETICS AND HUMAN BEHAVIOR; PATENTING ORGANISMS; PHARMACEUTICS, *article on* PHARMACEUTICAL INDUSTRY; PROFESSION AND PROFESSIONAL ETHICS; RESEARCH ETHICS COMMITTEES; *and* RESEARCH METHODOLOGY. *For a discussion of related ideas, see the entries* ACADEMIC HEALTH CENTERS; COMMERCIALISM IN SCIENTIFIC RESEARCH; CONSCIENCE; LICENSING, DISCIPLINE, AND REGULATION IN THE HEALTH PROFESSIONS; RESEARCH, HUMAN: HISTORICAL ASPECTS; RESEARCH POLICY; TRUST; *and* WHISTLEBLOWING. *Other relevant material may be found under the entries* BIOETHICS EDUCATION, *article on* OTHER HEALTH PROFESSIONS; HEALTH OFFICIALS AND THEIR RESPONSIBILITIES; RESEARCH BIAS; SEX THERAPY AND SEX RESEARCH; *and* TECHNOLOGY.

Bibliography

ANGELL, MARCIA. 1983. "Editors and Fraud." *CBE [Council of Biology Editors] Views* 6:3–8.

———. 1986. "Publish or Perish: A Proposal." *Annals of Internal Medicine* 104, no. 2:261–262.

ASSOCIATION OF AMERICAN MEDICAL COLLEGES. AD HOC COMMITTEE. 1992. *The Maintenance of High Ethical Standards in the Conduct of Research.* Washington, D.C.: Author.

BROAD, WILLIAM J. 1980. "Would-Be Academician Pirates Papers." *Science* 208, no. 4451:1438–1440.

BROAD, WILLIAM J., and WADE, NICHOLAS. 1982. *Betrayers of the Truth.* New York: Simon & Schuster.

COUNCIL OF BIOLOGY EDITORS. EDITORIAL POLICY COMMITTEE 1990. *Ethics and Policy in Scientific Publication.* Bethesda, Md.: Author.

CULLITON, BARBARA J. 1983. "Coping with Fraud: The Darsee Case." *Science* 220, no. 4592:31–35.

DRESSER, REBECCA. 1993. "Defining Scientific Misconduct: The Relevance of Mental State." *Journal of the American Medical Association* 269, no. 7:895–897.

HARVARD UNIVERSITY SCHOOL OF MEDICINE. FACULTY IN MEDICINE. 1992. "Faculty Policies on Integrity in Science." Harvard University, Cambridge, Mass.

HUTH, EDWARD J. 1983. "Responsibilities of Coauthorship." *Annals of Internal Medicine* 99, no. 2:266–267.

———. 1992. "Pressures to Publish: Why and What to Do About It." *European Science Editing* 46:3–5.

INSTITUTE OF MEDICINE (U.S.). COMMITTEE ON THE RESPONSIBLE CONDUCT OF RESEARCH. 1989. *The Responsible Conduct of Research on the Health Sciences.* IOM-89-01. Washington, D.C.: National Academy Press.

NATIONAL INSTITUTES OF HEALTH (NIH). 1986. *Policies and Procedures for Dealing with Possible Misconduct in Science."* NIH Guide for Grants and Contracts, vol. 15, no. 11. Bethesda, Md.: Author.

PETERSDORF, ROBERT G. 1986. "The Pathogenesis of Fraud in Medicine." *Annals of Internal Medical Science* 104, no. 2: 252–254.

RELMAN, ARNOLD S. 1983. "Lessons from the Darsee Affair." *New England Journal of Medicine* 308, no. 23:1415–1417.

TEICH, ALBERT H., and FRANKEL, MARK S. 1992. *Good Science and Responsible Scientists: Meeting the Challenge of Fraud and Misconduct in Science.* Washington, D.C.: American Association for the Advancement of Science.

U.S. DEPARTMENT OF HEALTH AND HUMAN SERVICES (DHHS). PUBLIC HEALTH SERVICE. 1991. "Policies and Procedures for Dealing with Possible Scientific Misconduct in Extramural Research." *Federal Register* 56, no. 114(June 13):27383–27394.

WOOLF, PATRICIA K. 1986. "Pressure to Publish and Fraud in Science." *Annals of Internal Medicine* 104, no. 2:254–256.

FREEDOM AND COERCION

Freedom is a desirable component of human personalities, interpersonal relationships, and social and governmental arrangements, but the concept is difficult to define. To some, "What is freedom?" can seem a futile question (Arendt, 1968); but existentialists, pragmatists, linguistic analysts, deontologists, utilitarians, liberals, conservatives, and others have given many answers. Analyses of the idea of freedom and assessments of its value have sources in many disciplines. The great English poet John Milton's *Areopagitica* is a classic defense of freedom, and much other literature concerns itself with freedom (Bolt, 1962; Kazantzakis, 1953; Morrison, 1987).

Freedom is a complex notion, a family or cluster of ideas that applies to a wide range of phenomena. Isaiah Berlin said that there are more than 200 senses of the word "freedom" (Berlin, 1970). This entry concentrates on a few meanings that have, or that are easily mistaken to have, logical connections with "coercion."

Kinds of freedom

A number of ideas and terms that should be distinguished from freedom are often associated with it. "Liberty" seems at first to be synonymous with "freedom"; but we do not speak of an animal's liberty, although we may speak of its freedom. This suggests that freedom and liberty are not perfectly synonymous. Liberty refers primarily to political freedom, but there are many other kinds of freedom. Hanna Pitkin claims that liberty presumes a formal relationship with government (Pitkin, 1972); and Joel Feinberg defines liberty as "the absence of legal coercion" (Feinberg, 1984, p. 7), which means that options for individuals are left open by the state. "Liberation," as in "women's liberation" or "animal liberation," suggests a struggle to change the fixed values and practices of a culture. Being "at liberty" to do something means that we have no duty to refrain from it and have claims against others that they not interfere with our doing it (Feinberg, 1986). Point of view sometimes matters: Escaped prisoners say they are "free," while law enforcement officials say they are "at large." "A free country" can mean that no other country dominates it, but inside such a country individual persons may in fact be very unfree. One can feel unfree because of dependence on others. "Feeling free" denies feeling scrutinized, regulated, or out of control.

Freedom contrasts with restrictions. Limitations or constraints inhibit or negate different kinds of freedom, but only some kinds of restrictions are coercive. Some constraints are internal to persons, some external; some are negative, some positive. Joel Feinberg develops these distinctions into a four-way typology of constraints: internal negative, internal positive, external negative, and external positive (Feinberg, 1980). Respective examples of these constraints are weakness, fear, lack of money, and being handcuffed.

Positive external freedom. Positive external freedom consists in having the external means to achieve our ends and fulfill our desires or interests. It involves the availability of resources in the environment, such as schools open to all, or medical resources and personnel. Patients in great pain who desire medication may be fortunate to have compassionate doctors who give them the means to relieve pain; those with uncaring or inattentive doctors may be denied the means to pain relief and lack positive external freedom. A pregnant woman who wants an abortion but lacks the means to pay for it lacks the positive external freedom to have the abortion. Whether society should pay for abortions for the poor, thereby enhancing their positive external freedom, is highly controversial.

Isaiah Berlin (1970) and Frithjof Bergman (1977), among others, developed the distinction between internal and external freedom. They contend that the mere absence of external constraints and the presence of external means is not enough for freedom in the fullest sense. True freedom involves something internal to the person.

Negative internal freedom. Negative internal freedom is the absence of internal psychological or physiological obstructions that inhibit the fulfillment of goals, desires, and interests. Persons so overcome by temptation, rage, jealousy, or sexual passion that they temporarily lose control of themselves or those confused or overwhelmed by unconscious processes, psychoses, neuroses, compulsions, addictions, and other nonvoluntary character defects and disorders generally lack negative internal freedom. Genetic and neuromuscular conditions involving pain, weakness, or hyperactivity also constrain negative internal freedom. Should the idea of negative constraints include internally functioning physical processes that have external causes? The answer is not completely clear; but if it is affirmative, then negative internal freedom is also lacking if individuals are temporarily stupefied by alcohol or by recreational or psychotropic drugs; if they are more permanently brain damaged or retarded; if they lose independence as a result of a degenerative disease; or if they are controlled and their options reduced by lobotomies, psychosurgery, hypnosis, behavior modification, or indoctrination. Used skillfully with the informed, voluntary consent of patients, many psychotherapies can increase human freedom rather than reduce it. Sigmund Freud thought that increasing the freedom of patients was the major purpose of psychoanalysis.

Positive internal freedom.   Positive internal freedom consists in the effective presence of all internal factors that contribute to fulfilling one's goals, desires, and interests; to being self-reliant, one's own master; and to being in control of one's life. It requires the possession of certain elements of character, such as self-mastery—the ability to choose what to value, and having adequate mental resources and skills to choose rightly. Isaiah Berlin emphasized the presence of "my own, not other men's acts of will"; being "a subject, not an object"; being "moved by reasons, by conscious purposes, which are my own"; being "somebody, not nobody; a doer—deciding, not being decided for, self-directed, . . . conceiving goals and policies of my own and realizing them"; and being above all "conscious of myself as a thinking, willing, active being, bearing responsibility for my choices, and able to explain them by reference to my own ideas and purposes" (Berlin, 1970, p. 131). Being positively free is what most medical ethicists mean by being autonomous, or rationally autonomous.

Bergman's interpretation of positive internal freedom accentuates the ability to identify ourselves with our values and choices.

> An act is free if the agent identifies with the elements from which it flows; it is coerced if the agent dissociates himself from the element which generates or prompts the action. . . . Freedom is a function of identification and stands in a relationship of dependency to that with which a man

identifies. . . . The primary condition of freedom is the possession of an identity, or of a self—freedom is the acting out of that identity. (Bergman, 1977, p. 37)

Bergman shows how the idea of freedom may be incorporated by its bearer, how a self might predicate freedom of itself. Positive internal freedom is the self's identification with its actions, feelings, thoughts, with its own nature. Bergman identifies three main models of free self-identification. One is Platonic, one Aristotelian, and one fashioned after the protagonist in Fyodor Dostoyevsky's *Notes from the Underground* (Dostoyevsky, 1960). Each model has implications for how patients experience elements of the medical world—the doctor–patient relationship, informed consent, the nature of their maladies, and the role of treatment.

A Platonic self identifies only with the purely rational, narrowly defined as products of mind that can be shown to be coherent and consistent. An Aristotelian self identifies with rationality but also with having an animal nature, and does not dissociate from all of its impulses and idiosyncratic desires. Underground selves do not identify with much of anything—not with rationality nor with any of their own impulses. They are inconsistent and undirected and can never achieve positive freedom.

Many ethicists believe that freedom of will is an essential part of positive internal freedom. Free will involves more than a capacity for making choices, for there may be both free and unfree choices. Free choices are creative, originative, or "contracausal"; and choices are not free if completely determined by antecedently existing desires, beliefs, or other conditions. Being responsible for decisions and actions depends on whether they originate with us, as opposed to being programmed into us by heredity, physical or social environment, fate, or God, even if we are influenced by them (Edwards, 1969; Erde, 1978).

Isaiah Berlin calls attention to problematic features of positive freedom. The idea of positive freedom may be developed in a way that splits the notion of the self into a higher real or true self and a lower apparent or experiential self. Positive freedom belongs only to the real or true self and involves suppressing or eliminating the apparent self, thus turning people against themselves.

From the time of the Stoics, many philosophers identified the true self with reason, and thus freedom was control of or complete escape from desires and feelings. The ascetic strain in Christianity found these themes congenial. For Immanuel Kant, only the real, rational lawgiving self was free, not the apparent self given in experience. Georg W. F. Hegel identified being rational with being free. Jean-Jacques Rousseau (1950) distinguished what the majority actually wants, "the will of all," from what it would want if it were well enough informed and sufficiently intelligent, "the general will." Rousseau contended that the general will for the common good should be forced on unwilling members of society (Berlin, 1970). But who or what is the proper interpreter of the general will? Rousseau's ambiguous answer waffled between the vote of the majority and the vote of enlightened legislators; but it was only a short step from the latter to the opinions of the self-appointed paternalist experts.

When every person's true will is equated with the opinion of experts, positive freedom endangers negative freedom. Rousseau was willing to "force men to be free," which meant forcing them to obey laws expressing the general will for the common good. The enlightened expert would become the authentic spokesman for humanity's true, real, or general will (Berlin, 1970). Thus, by forcing men to be free, Rousseau meant forcing them to accept what experts (like himself, or enlightened legislators) believe to be best for them in ways that decrease their freedom of action. Such a theory of positive freedom enables elitists, paternalists, and totalitarians to turn freedom upon itself. Berlin says, "Once I take this view, I am in a position to ignore the actual wishes of men or societies, to bully, oppress, torture them in the name, and on behalf, of their 'real' selves . . . the free choice of [mankind's] 'true,' albeit often submerged and inarticulate, self" (1970, p. 133).

There are perplexities about the logical and moral structure of positive freedom, especially as it relates to other forms of freedom. In addressing some of these perplexities, Gerald MacCallum, Jr., proposes a schema for the concept of freedom. He follows Berlin's characterization of negative freedom as "freedom from" constraints, and of positive freedom as "freedom to" act because we have the necessary resources. MacCallum argues that both are aspects of a more complex, three-variable concept: "_____ is free from _____ to do (or omit, or be, or have) _____" (MacCallum, 1967). Statements about freedom that omit the terms indicated by any of the blanks are incomplete. "Joe is free to vote Democratic" fails to mention what Joe is free from (threats, prejudices, or previous promises).

MacCallum's analysis helps clarify the logic of the concept of freedom, but it seems incomplete. The fullest schema should incorporate the perspective of positive freedom, as in "_____ is free from _____ to do (have, etc.) _____ because (of) _____." The final blank makes a place for positive freedom. Consider: "Joe is free from prejudice to vote Democratic because he faced the influence of greed on the Republican way of thought." Here, having a reflective perspective fills in the final blank.

Some concepts of positive freedom may thus degenerate into a paternalistic or totalitarian elitism that ra-

tionalizes coercion of "inferiors" for their own good. To some theorists, negative external freedom for the masses is anathema (Popper, 1963). Dostoyevsky's Grand Inquisitor argues that most people lack both sufficient intelligence and fortitude (Dostoyevsky, 1960). The masses need a benevolent authoritarian because they are too weak to live with the horrible truth about suffering, death, and meaninglessness; they need miracles, mystery, and authority—a set of lies and enforced commands—in order to be happy. The Grand Inquisitor's paternalism is powerfully present in medicine's history, and the Inquisitor is an analogue for the physician in some models (Brody, 1991).

Negative external freedom. Negative external freedom is the absence of external pressures and constraints. It is the most obvious contrast with coercion. Freedom is external to the individual person in relationship to external constraints; it is negative in the absence of external constraints, some of which are coercive. Negative freedom and lack of positive external constraints are equivalent: both consist in the absence of external restraining forces. "Joe jumped freely" alleges that Joe was not pushed, threatened, or drunk. "Joy entered the mental hospital freely" denies that she was committed or coerced by governmental power or family pressures.

Negative external freedom is often called freedom of action, the ability to do what we want or choose to do, unencumbered by external restraints such as chains, shackles, walls, or jails or by external constraints such as laws, institutional prohibitions, or coercive pressures from other people. Absence of encumbrances usually correlates with increased options for choice.

Many species of positive external freedom are recognized and cherished. The First Amendment to the U.S. Constitution distinguishes and affirms many kinds of freedom of action—freedom of religion, freedom of speech, freedom of the press, freedom to assemble peaceably, and freedom to petition government for a redress of grievances. As kinds of freedom of action, these constitutionally guaranteed rights mean that government, as are other institutions and individual persons, is forbidden to interfere with our choice of religion, with expressing our thoughts, with our efforts to communicate beliefs, knowledge, and ideas through the press and other media, and so on. Yet, all these kinds of freedom of action have their limits even in law; none is absolute or without qualification.

Historically, many classes of individuals were externally unfree in a great variety of ways. The fullest enjoyment of external positive freedom in the United States was once limited to competent landowning white males, while severe restrictions were imposed on the freedom of action of females, slaves, nonwhites, minors, mentally disabled persons, the landless, and other disfavored groups. Gradually, as prejudices waned, usually after prolonged and bitter struggles, both the socially allowable scope and the kinds of freedom of action were extended. In the latter part of the twentieth century, freedom found new foci. The civil rights movement that began in the United States in the 1960s led to the women's liberation and gay rights movements; a similar revolution led to the end of apartheid in the Republic of South Africa in 1994. Worldwide, many groups advocate on behalf of animals. "Animal liberation" opposes killing animals for food or in medical experimentation and by hurtful uses in rodeos, zoos, and other forms of entertainment for humans. The scope of application for the concept of freedom of action is constantly evolving.

The value of freedom

What kind of value does freedom have? Philosophers distinguish between intrinsic values—things desirable for their own sake; instrumental values—things desirable as means to ends; and side constraints—things necessary for living together peacefully in a pluralistic society in which many people honestly disagree about values.

Positive internal freedom is perhaps the most plausible candidate for the status of an intrinsic good, for it consists of all the resources that constitute capable and responsible individual selfhood. Cherishing it for its own sake is prizing the fullness of our own unique individuality. Hedonistic utilitarians, who think that only pleasure is intrinsically good, are inconsistent if they value positive internal freedom as an end in itself. John Stuart Mill came very close to this inconsistency in his *On Liberty* (1947). As opponents see it, the fact that hedonistic utilitarians must treat even positive internal freedom as nothing more than a very great instrumental good for producing pleasure or happiness reveals a major inadequacy of their theory. Even if freedom is good in itself, Mill correctly noted the intrinsic satisfaction derived from acting freely.

Positive external freedom is by definition a means to other ends; and it would be peculiar, to say the least, if negativities or absences, whether those of internal or external freedom, are good in themselves. These forms of freedom seem more like instrumental conditions for the realization of the positive goods of life. All forms of freedom are immensely useful, indeed absolutely essential, in pursuing most human interests; but some freedom is also intrinsically good, most ethicists believe. Basic human welfare consists largely in being free in the fullest possible sense.

Ethicists like H. Tristram Engelhardt, Jr., emphasize the importance of negative external freedom as a side constraint, that is, as a "basic, minimum presupposition of ethics" to which all parties can commonly assent. It is the sole means for peaceable coexistence among persons in a pluralistic society who disagree about intrinsic values, including the value of freedom, but who are nevertheless committed to resolving disputes without resorting to force. A universal basic commitment to freedom generates a tolerant society in which many distinctive values and moral perspectives can flourish (Engelhardt, 1986). But do we have a common basic interest only in freedom?

Coercion and freedom of action

Can morally legitimate limits to freedom of action be identified and distinguished from illegitimate limits? Is coercion always illegitimate, or is it sometimes morally justified? To answer, we must have a clear concept of coercion. According to Tom Beauchamp and James Childress, "Coercion . . . occurs if and only if one person intentionally uses a credible and severe threat of harm or force to control another. The threat of force or punishment used by some police, courts, and hospitals in acts of involuntary commitment for psychiatric treatment is a typical form of coercion. Society's use of compulsory vaccination laws is another" (Beauchamp and Childress, 1994, p. 164). Beauchamp and Childress capture the core of the concept of coercion, as ordinarily understood. Coercion is a relationship between at least two persons. Coercers may be acting as private individuals, or they may be playing an institutional role like law enforcement officer or functionary of a court or hospital. Coercers intentionally threaten those coerced with harm if they do not bend to the coercer's will. Those coerced clearly perceive that they are being threatened. Coercion restricts freedom of action, not by reducing the alternatives available to those coerced but by increasing the cost of pursuing the alternatives that they favor (Feinberg, 1986). When thieves say, "Your money or your life," they present their victims with an unwelcome forced choice. Their clear preference for saving their lives is not eliminated, but the cost of doing so dramatically increases. As Joel Feinberg says, "In general, effective coercion closes the [combined] option of noncompliance *and* avoidance of the threatened cost, while keeping open either without the other" (Feinberg, 1986, p. 192). Coercion can be resisted, nearly always at a very high price.

Coercive pressures come in degrees, depending on how much the victim values and disvalues the options allotted by the coercer. Under certain circumstances, a patient might lose control and consent to treatment (invalidly), almost as a reflex. If a patient refuses to have a broken leg pinned and, in an attempt to change her mind, someone pulls on her leg without her consent, that is coercive if there is an implied threat to inflict more pain.

If this analysis of "coercion" is accepted, most constraints on freedom clearly do not count as coercion. Language is misused when anything that limits or constrains behavior is called coercive. If Beauchamp and Childress are right, only other agents can be coercers. Unless someone else deliberately deprives them of resources in order to control them, those who lack means to their ends are not coercively denied negative external freedom. Poor people who cannot afford to buy a new car are not coerced into carlessness by poverty itself. Poor women who cannot afford abortions are not coerced to have unwanted babies just because they are poor, and poor students who cannot afford advanced education are not coerced into a career choice. Internal constraints like rages, jealousies, passions, psychoses, neuroses, and so on definitely deprive persons of negative internal freedom; but these constraints are not coercive because they are not external, and there are not other persons making threats. Internal constraints that interfere with positive internal freedom are not coercive for the same reasons. External natural conditions like storms and earthquakes that constrain negative external freedom of action are not coercive because they are not agents, no matter how threatening they might be.

Some philosophers suggest additional qualifications of the analysis of coercion. The concept is fuzzy at the edges. Disagreements about where to draw lines and how to deal with borderline cases are inevitable and are usually settled by stipulation. Consider the following proposed modifications.

Can nonpersonal external things like natural processes count as coercers? Unlike Beauchamp and Childress, Feinberg thinks that they can; threatened rock slides and hurricanes may exert pressures that significantly increase the costs of pursuing their interests on those making decisions about whether to travel (Feinberg, 1986). Similarly, for those who think before acting, the risk of getting acquired immunodeficiency syndrome (AIDS) can significantly increase the cost of pursuing some sexual interests.

Must coercers use only the threat of force and not force itself? Like Beauchamp and Childress, Feinberg calls the actual use of force "compulsion" rather than "coercion" and insists that compulsion closes options, whereas coercion makes them more costly to pursue (Feinberg, 1986). However, others, like Michael D. Bayles (Pennock and Chapman, 1972) and the *Dictionary of the Social Sciences,* cited by J. Roland Pennock (Pennock and Chapman, 1972), have no difficulty in calling the actual use of force "coercion."

Must the mechanism of coercive pressure always be negative—like threats or the actual use of force? Or may the intentional use of intense positive pressures be coercive? Here there is much disagreement. Biomedical research on prisoners has been strictly supervised in the last few decades because prisons are considered to be highly coercive environments; protections for students, who are vulnerable to the graders' power, and for hospital patients, who are vulnerable to the physicians' power, issue from similar concerns.

If, to gain consent, vulnerable persons like prisoners, students, or patients are offered benefits or advantages to which they are not otherwise entitled, is that coercion, manipulation, or exploitation? When prisoners are enticed by drug companies to become subjects for testing new drugs by promises of better living conditions, early parole, more opportunities for entertainment, conjugal visits, and so on, are they thereby coerced into compliance in a manner that invalidates the voluntariness of informed voluntary consent? Besides coercion, deceit, exaggeration, manipulation, exploitation, enticement, or undue incentives may control persons and thereby invalidate informed voluntary consent. These incentives should be avoided by conscientious medical professionals. If anesthetized female patients are used without their knowledge or consent to teach medical students how to do pelvic examinations, these patients are not coerced, not conscious of a threat; but clearly they are wronged.

Are total institutions so inherently coercive that coercion invalidates voluntariness? The answer depends in part on the intensity or irresistibility of the positive inducements, but the crucial consideration is whether positive incentives, or only negative reinforcements, properly belong to the concept of coercion. Beauchamp and Childress (1994) exclude positive incentives, as do Robert Nozick (1969) and Bernard Gert (Pennock and Chapman, 1972). However, Feinberg clearly favors calling abnormally attractive offers coercive (Feinberg, 1986), as do Virginia Held (Pennock and Chapman, 1972) and Donald McIntosh (Pennock and Chapman, 1972). Those who include positive incentives in the concept of coercion usually argue that the crucial consideration is not whether the coercive mechanism is negative but whether it is the kind of thing that a normal or rational person might reasonably be expected to resist (Pennock and Chapman, 1972).

Morally acceptable and unacceptable uses of coercion

Is coercion always wrong or morally unacceptable? Beauchamp and Childress cite the use or threat of force by police, courts, and hospitals, and society's use of compulsory vaccination laws as typical examples of coercion; but they do not thereby mean to suggest that involuntary civil commitment and compulsory vaccination are morally wrong just because they are coercive. It is not always wrong to try to control others by coercive or other manipulative means.

Often there are valid moral justifications for using coercion. Parental coercion of children is inevitable at times, but not thereby wrong. Good laws, penalties for noncompliance, and proper enforcement mechanisms like the police, the courts, and the prisons exist for the sake of coercing lawless persons into behaving themselves. Coercive deterrents are perfectly in order when society confronts those who commit crimes such as murder, rape, or pillage. A defense force that is strong enough to be a credible and severe threat of harm to hostile nations serves a morally valid but coercive purpose. Rational persons do not want to live in a society without laws, police, prisons, and military protection; such a society would not last very long. Sometimes violent patients must be controlled coercively to protect other patients and members of the medical staff. Pedophiles and pyromaniacs do not live merely an "alternative lifestyle"; their predilections result in great harm to the persons and/or properties of others; and they must be deterred or stopped—coercively if necessary. With no qualms of conscience, college professors threaten students with bad grades to motivate them to improve their learning and performance; occasionally they promise better grades than earned in exchange for sexual and other favors.

Thus, using coercion is often, but not always, the morally right thing to do. Other human values besides freedom must be protected coercively. But when is coercion morally unacceptable? And how can we tell when it places morally unjustifiable limits on freedom?

We will consider a few of the most important and influential answers, beginning with the one accepted almost universally as most basic. In *On Liberty*, John Stuart Mill asked about the nature and limits of power that legitimately can be exercised over other individuals. He answered:

> The sole end for which mankind are warranted, individually or collectively, in interfering with the liberty of action of any of their number, is self-protection. . . . The only purpose for which power can rightfully be exercised over any member of a civilized community, against his will, is to prevent harm to others. His own good, either physical or moral, is not a sufficient warrant. (Mill, 1947, ch. 1)

Of course, the nature of "harm" and the relevant degree of its seriousness must be clarified, as Mill and others try to do (Feinberg, 1984, 1985, 1986).

Mill's "harm to others" principle justifies the use of coercion against those who would harm others, but not against those who would harm themselves, as long as they are competent adults "in the maturity of their faculties." Mill accepted a weak paternalism designed to protect children, minors, and people who are not "ca-pable of being improved by free and equal discussion" from self-harm. Unfortunately, the line between things that harm others and that harm the self is not always clearly drawn; many harms to the self often result in harms to others, as with drunk drivers; but this does not mean the distinction is useless.

Although Mill regarded the "harm to others" principle as the only consideration that legitimates coercive constraints on freedom of action, other ethicists propose additional liberty-limiting or coercion-legitimizing principles. Feinberg considers "the offense principle" that authorizes preventing serious offenses to others, the "legal paternalism" principle that would prevent self-harm by a competent self, the "legal moralism" principle that would prohibit inherently immoral conduct, and several others (Feinberg, 1984). He regards only the "harm to others" and "offense" principles to be valid (Feinberg, 1984).

Freedom, paternalism, and coercion in the practice of medicine

Many questions about negative freedom of action and its proper limits arise within the practice of medicine. Is it a legitimate restriction of the right to freedom of speech when government forbids medical professionals to inform patients about legal medical interventions that government officials oppose? What balances should be struck when physician freedom conflicts with patient freedom? Should medical professionals be free to abstain from providing services to which they have moral objections—like withholding nutrition and fluids from patients who will die without them, or participating in performing abortions? Should competent adult patients be free to choose among and refuse treatments? Should terminally ill patients be free to refuse all life-sustaining procedures, including nutrition and fluids? Should a pregnant woman be free to demand that any qualified physician give her an abortion at any time during pregnancy and for any reason? Does academic freedom give medical researchers the right to investigate all questions of interest, no matter what happens to patients, and without any restrictions at all? Should pro-life groups be free to protest on the grounds of, or just outside, abortion clinics? Should anyone, including prisoners and persons who are mentally ill or retarded, be free to decide whether to enroll as subjects in experiments? Should persons with AIDS be free to enter into drug trials earlier than standard enrollment practices permit? In which of these situations is freedom of action morally justified, and in which is it not? On what grounds, if any, should the freedom of action of patients or of medical professionals be restricted? Do any of these situations involve coercion, justified or unjustified? In which, if any, of these situations should freedom of action be restricted by the "harm to others" principle or the "offense to others" principle? Do other liberty-limiting principles apply to these situations?

Mill and many contemporary medical ethicists find that strong paternalistic medical uses of coercion against competent adults are morally unacceptable. Paternalists believe that they know what is best for others and act upon this belief. In medicine, valid consent must be informed, competent, and voluntary. The ideal of informed voluntary consent requires that patients' own judgments about what is beneficial or best for themselves should prevail. Being informed is incompatible with passively accepting that others, like doctors, always know best. Informing patients properly requires effective communication with them concerning the nature of the relevant medical proceedings, their risks, benefits, alternatives, and the right to refuse. Ignorance, deceit, and misinformation can interfere significantly with freedom. Being competent is incompatible with severe mental encumbrances. Being voluntary is incompatible with coercion and requires that patients have negative external freedom of action. Valid consent is uncoerced. Ties between freedom and medical ethics are ancient; but they have changed greatly since the Hippocratic Oath avowed that the sick, whether slave or free, would be treated for their own benefit—as determined by physicians.

Is there any place for paternalism in medicine? Is freedom such a great good or strong side constraint that competent patients must be free to make even costly mistakes? Since physicians usually determine who is and who is not competent, does not freedom-limiting paternalism inevitably creep back in when determining competency? One of the most difficult questions of medical ethics is whether competent adult patients should ever be coerced into being free on the basis of the paternalistic judgment that being free is in their best interests. If freedom is such a strong requirement, should it ever be temporarily diminished coercively for the sake of its long-run enhancement, especially when it can be predicted that patients are highly likely to express retrospective gratitude for such coercion?

Occasionally, extremely passive patients, or those weakened by disease and pain, do not want to know the medical options or to make treatment decisions for themselves, so they say to their doctors, "Just do what you think is best for me." When treatment decisions that will have an enormous impact on their future lives must be made, should doctors allow these patients to choose freely not to exercise their freedom? Some ethicists believe in positive internal freedom to the extent that they reject a free or autonomous renunciation of choice. Others hold that forcing people to be free is always an

unacceptable violation of their rights and selfhood (Feinberg, 1986).

Should doctors coercively threaten to withhold all treatment, including pain medication, from patients who abdicate freedom, until they are ready to act as responsible moral agents, to listen to a full explanation of the medical options, and to participate in making treatment decisions for themselves? Some ethicists insist that patients should not be allowed to abdicate being free moral agents, and that doctors are morally obligated to try to restore or enhance patients' freedom or autonomy—coercively if necessary (Komrad, 1983; Brock, 1983). Taking one side or another in this debate depends largely on one's judgment about whether the "real self" of the patients is present to refuse to exercise its autonomy, or whether in the future that self is likely to say, "Thank you, doctor, for coercing me into exercising my freedom!"

REM B. EDWARDS
EDMUND L. ERDE

For a further discussion of topics mentioned in this entry, see the entries ABORTION; AIDS; AUTHORITY; AUTONOMY; BEHAVIOR CONTROL; ETHICS, *especially the article on* SOCIAL AND POLITICAL THEORIES; HARM; HUMAN NATURE; OBLIGATION AND SUPEREROGATION; PAIN AND SUFFERING; PATERNALISM; PERSON; PSYCHOANALYSIS AND DYNAMIC THERAPIES; SUBSTANCE ABUSE, *especially the article on* ADDICTION AND DEPENDENCE; *and* UTILITY. *This entry will find application in the entry* SUICIDE. *For a discussion of related ideas, see the entries* POPULATION POLICIES, *especially the section on* STRATEGIES OF FERTILITY CONTROL; *and* RIGHTS.

Bibliography

ARENDT, HANNAH. 1968. *Between Past and Future: Eight Exercises in Political Thought.* Enl. ed. New York: Viking.

BEAUCHAMP, TOM L., and CHILDRESS, JAMES F. 1994. *Principles of Biomedical Ethics.* 4th ed. New York: Oxford University Press.

BERGMANN, FRITHJOF. 1977. *On Being Free.* Notre Dame, Ind.: University of Notre Dame Press.

BERLIN, ISAIAH. 1970. *Four Essays on Liberty.* London: Oxford University Press. The key essay is ch. 3, "Two Concepts of Liberty," originally published in 1958. Much of the early criticism of it is addressed in the book's introduction.

BOLT, ROBERT. 1962. *A Man for All Seasons: A Play in Two Acts.* New York: Vintage.

BREGGIN, PETER R. 1980. *The Psychology of Freedom: Liberty and Love as a Way of Life.* Buffalo, N.Y.: Prometheus.

BROCK, DAN. 1983. "Paternalism and Promoting the Good."

In *Paternalism*, pp. 237–260. Edited by Rolf Sartorious. Minneapolis: University of Minnesota Press.

BRODY, HOWARD. 1991. "The Chief of Medicine." *Hastings Center Report* 21, no. 4 (July/August):17–22.

BUCHANAN, ALLEN. 1978. "Medical Paternalism." *Philosophy and Public Affairs* 7, no. 4:370–390.

CULVER, CHARLES M., and GERT, BERNARD. 1982. *Philosophy in Medicine: Conceptual and Ethical Issues in Medicine and Psychiatry*. New York: Oxford University Press.

DEWEY, JOHN. 1989. *Freedom and Culture*. Buffalo, N.Y.: Prometheus.

DOSTOYEVSKY, FYODOR. 1960. *Notes from the Underground* and *The Grand Inquisitor*. New York: E. P. Dutton.

EDWARDS, REM B. 1969. *Freedom, Responsibility, and Obligation*. The Hague: Martinus Nijhoff.

ENGELHARDT, H. TRISTRAM, JR. 1986. *The Foundations of Bioethics*. New York: Oxford University Press.

ERDE, EDMUND L. 1978. "Free Will and Determinism." In vol. 2 of *Encyclopedia of Bioethics*, pp. 500–507. Edited by Warren T. Reich. New York: Macmillan.

FEINBERG, JOEL. 1980. *Rights, Justice and the Bounds of Liberty: Essays in Social Philosophy*. Princeton, N.J.: Princeton University Press.

———. 1984. *Harm to Others*. New York: Oxford University Press.

———. 1985. *Offense to Others*. New York: Oxford University Press.

———. 1986. *Harm to Self*. New York: Oxford University Press.

KANT, IMMANUEL. 1956. *Groundwork of the Metaphysics of Morals*. Translated by Herbert James Paton. New York: Harper & Row.

KAZANTZAKIS, NIKOS. 1953. *Zorba the Greek*. Translated by Carl Wildman. New York: Simon & Schuster.

KOMRAD, MARK S. 1983. "A Defense of Medical Paternalism: Maximizing Patients' Autonomy." *Journal of Medical Ethics* 9, no. 1:38–44.

MACCALLUM, GERALD C., JR. 1967. "Negative and Positive Freedom." *Philosophical Review* 76, no. 3:312–334.

MILL, JOHN STUART. 1947. *On Liberty*. Edited by Alburey Castell. New York: Appleton-Century-Crofts.

MORRISON, TONI. 1987. *Beloved: A Novel*. New York: Alfred A. Knopf.

NOZICK, ROBERT. 1969. "Coercion." In *Philosophy, Science and Method: Essays in Honor of Ernest Nagel*, pp. 441–472. Edited by Sidney Morgenbesser, Patrick Suppes, and Morton White. New York: St. Martin's Press.

———. 1974. *Anarchy, State, and Utopia*. New York: Basic Books.

PATTERSON, ORLANDO. 1991. *Freedom in the Making of Western Culture*. New York: Basic Books. This historical and sociological study presents some empirical research on how freedom is experienced or measured by individuals and some recent critiques of Isaiah Berlin.

PENNOCK, J. ROLAND, and CHAPMAN, JOHN W. 1972. *Coercion*. Chicago: Aldine Atherton.

PITKIN, HANNA F. 1972. *Wittgenstein and Justice: On the Significance of Wittgenstein for Social and Political Thought*. Berkeley: University of California Press.

POPPER, KARL R. 1963. *The Open Society and Its Enemies*. 4th ed., rev. New York: Harper & Row.

RAZ, JOSEPH. 1986. *The Morality of Freedom*. New York: Oxford University Press.

ROUSSEAU, JEAN-JACQUES. 1950. *The Social Contract* and *Discourses*. Translated by George Douglas Howard Cole. New York: E. P. Dutton.

WERTHEIMER, ALAN. 1987. *Coercion*. Princeton, N.J.: Princeton University Press.

FRIENDSHIP

The physician–patient relationship has traditionally been understood to be analogous to a friendship. Although modern medicine is characterized more by technical competence, increased specialization, and growing bureaucratization, and the relationship between patient and medical professional is less a friendship than an interaction between strangers, until recently friendship was judged the most fitting description of the doctor–patient relationship because the relationship was understood not primarily as an impersonal commercial transaction but as a special moral reality constituted by the distinctive needs of the patient. As an attempt to articulate the nature of the relationship between patients and medical professionals, particularly physicians but also nurses, hospital administrators, social workers, and clergy, the model of friendship was both descriptive and prescriptive; thus, it emphasized attitudes, dispositions, intentions, virtues, and qualities of character that ought to be present in physicians and patients alike (Illingworth, 1988).

Most important, friendship was judged an appropriate analogy of the physician–patient relationship because to some degree the relationship is characterized by the three marks of friendship: benevolence, mutuality, and a shared good (Wadell, 1989). Benevolence is primary because the good of the patient is the fundamental goal and central concern of medicine, taking precedence over all other considerations. Doctors and nurses are trained for the explicit purpose of benefiting others. Their principal commitment is to the health and well-being of patients, not research, professional advancement, or financial reward (Pellegrino and Thomasma, 1988). Just as a friend seeks another's good for that person's own sake, so the medical profession seeks the good of patients (Laín Entralgo, 1969). The patient–physician relationship is constituted by benevolence inasmuch as a person who has an illness he or she cannot relieve depends on the skills and generosity of another for healing (Pellegrino and Thomasma, 1988).

The second characteristic of friendship, mutuality, is also present in the doctor–patient relationship. Proper diagnosis, sound therapy, and healing require both the technical expertise and the care of physicians and nurses, and the ongoing cooperation and active participation of patients. Healing is not something physicians do alone; rather, it is a dynamic, interpersonal process in which patients must be intimately involved. No physician can heal without patients who are open, communicative, and trustworthy.

Mutuality stresses that friendships are partnerships in which people work together to achieve shared purposes (Wadell, 1989). Similarly, patients and medical professionals must collaborate if illness is to be overcome and health restored. The partnership between patients and their physicians and nurses will work only if each party is characterized by certain virtues. Patients must be truthful and communicative, cooperative (following a mutually agreed-upon treatment plan), trustworthy, and just (e.g., avoiding unwarranted lawsuits, making payments on time). In addition, medical professionals must be adequately skilled, loyal, compassionate, other-regarding, and self-effacing, lest self-interest weaken their primary commitment to serve the sick (Pellegrino and Thomasma, 1988).

The third mark of friendship is that it is constituted by shared goods and purposes. The shared good of medical friendship is restoring the patient's health; it is what physician, nurse, and patient are mutually seeking (James, 1989). However, the shared good can be extended to include secondary interests of physicians and nurses if the patient identifies with their desire to learn and become more skillful by caring for the patient, or if the patient embraces their interest in professional advancement.

Nonetheless, despite these similarities to other kinds of friendships, there are important differences. Medical friendships involve an unavoidable inequality in knowledge and technical skills between patients who are ill and medical personnel specially trained to care for them. There also is more distance and objectivity to medical friendships than is normally the case with other types of friendships. Although medical professionals are concerned for the well-being of patients, they must exercise sufficient detachment lest emotional involvement hinder the objectivity necessary for good diagnosis and treatment (Veatch, 1983). Unlike other friendships, the relationship between physicians and patients seldom extends beyond the specialized setting of the clinic or hospital, and may last no longer than the patient's need to be treated.

Because of these differences it is best to speak of the relationship between patients and their physicians as a "special-purpose" friendship (Fried, 1976). This ac-

knowledges not only the distinctive nature of the relationship but also its limited scope and purpose. The patient and the medical professional understand their respective roles and recognize that the parameters of the relationship are defined and limited by the specific crisis of illness. In this respect, medical friendships are akin to Aristotle's friendships of usefulness. In order to show that not all friendships are or need to be the same in duration or intensity, Aristotle distinguished friendships based on usefulness, friendships based on pleasure, and friendships based on character and virtue (Wadell, 1989). Like medical friendships, friendships of usefulness are relationships formed around common tasks or projects (in this case, healing) in which each person is useful to the other and needs the other to complete the task. There are clear limits to the relationship and well-defined expectations. Thus, patients normally would not expect to have virtue friendships (relationships formed around a mutual desire to become good) with their physicians, but would expect their physicians to be persons of integrity and good character, and would hope that they have virtue friendships with someone.

History of the friendship model

The description of the patient–physician relationship as friendship can be traced to the ancient Greeks and Romans, particularly the Stoic doctrine of the universal kinship of all humanity and the duty of people to show compassion to one another, especially the suffering; in this respect, medicine was an expression of philanthropy (Amundsen and Ferngren, 1983). Love for humanity (*philanthropia*) and for the art of healing (*philotechnia*) was at the heart of the physician's vocation (Laín Entralgo, 1969). Physicians befriended their patients by working to procure their good through healing and thus enable them to achieve the perfection of their human nature. This demanded a certain kind of character of the physician. He had to be compassionate, generous, attentive to the needs of the sick, available, and abidingly benevolent.

With the advent of Christianity, the model of friendship was integrated into a vision of faith. The physician's care for the sick was a function of discipleship, a most fitting imitation of Christ's concern for those in need and an expression of Christian love, or agape. The physician was motivated not only by love for others but also and most especially by love for God; doctoring was an act not only of benevolence but also of charity (*caritas*). Medicine was a ministry to those in need and an exemplary reflection of a divine love characterized by generosity, selflessness, and sacrifice (Amundsen and Ferngren, 1983). Here the meaning of benevolence broadened because the Christian physician was concerned not only about patients' physical well-being but their spiritual well-being as well. Since the physician's primary commitment was to Christ, and only secondarily to medicine, he was obliged to remind patients of their religious duties, particularly confessing their sins if their life was in danger (Laín Entralgo, 1969). This ministering to both physical and spiritual needs made the physician–patient relationship a Christian friendship (*amicitia christiana*). With the emergence of monasticism in the fourth and fifth centuries, medical care became centered in monasteries, which functioned as early hospitals or havens for the sick; and physicians were often monks selected by their abbots to exercise this special Christian ministry (Amundsen and Ferngren, 1983).

Friendship remained an apt description of the patient–doctor relationship through the first half of the twentieth century. There were many reasons for this. First, people tended to choose physicians whose religious, ethnic, and socioeconomic background was similar to their own. This was especially true in urban areas, where immigrants settled in the same neighborhoods. Second, popular culture presented a picture of the ideal physician as friendly, compatible, and approachable. People were encouraged to choose physicians who embodied these qualities, and physicians were taught that their personal style and character were indispensable in their relationship with patients (Rothman, 1991).

Third, prior to World War II the majority of doctor–patient encounters took place in the patient's home, not in an office or hospital (Rothman, 1991). The frequency of home visits not only brought greater intimacy to the patient–physician relationship but also gave patients and physicians much more opportunity to know and trust one another. Through these personal encounters, doctors could learn not only about their patients but also about their family background and general surroundings. Fourth, because diagnostic tools were more primitive, a physician had to listen attentively to patients' descriptions of their symptoms and experience of illness. Solid diagnosis depended on communication, careful attention to case history, and knowledge of the family's medical history (Rothman, 1991). Fifth, it was financially advantageous for a physician to be sensitive, caring, and compassionate because virtually the only way he could build his practice was by his patients' recommending him to their relatives and friends. What mattered to most people was not a physician's degrees or hospital affiliation, but that he was warm, friendly, and neighborly (Rothman, 1991).

After World War II the dynamics of the patient–physician relationship began to shift. Overall, these changes contributed to a distancing between patients and physicians, a lessening of trust, and a growing division between the lay world and the medical world (Rothman, 1991). There are several explanations for the change. First, after 1945 there was a sharp decline in the frequency of house calls. Patients met their doctor not in their home but at his office (Rothman, 1991). Second, the decline of general practitioners and the rise of medical specialists meant that the doctor was likely to be a stranger (Rothman, 1991). Third, the pace and rhythm of health care accelerated, becoming much more intense, hectic, and pressured. Physicians and nurses had much less time to spend with patients because they had more patients for whom to care, and the care itself had grown more complex and demanding (Rothman, 1991).

Fourth, although technological advances improved diagnosis, they depersonalized medical care. Earlier, solid diagnosis made detailed conversations with patients indispensable; now, improvements in technology made them largely superfluous (Rothman, 1991). Finally, the physician became less a friend and more a stranger because the lifestyle and culture of physicians grew increasingly specialized, remote, and enclosed. Patients felt alienated from doctors because they understood little of their language, their duties, or their world (Rothman, 1991). Collectively, these changes contributed to an overall deterioration in the patient–physician relationship. Trust declined while suspicion and wariness increased. The medical encounter became one more commercial transaction in which the doctor was a stranger and the patient a wary consumer (Rothman, 1991).

The physician as stranger

These changes in the patient–physician relationship have convinced many that the model of friendship no longer applies. This is not because physicians lack warmth and compassion, but because a "substantial portion of health care today is delivered in institutional settings where ongoing relationships or friendships are extremely difficult if not impossible" (Veatch, 1983, p. 196). A growing number of people receive health care not from familiar family doctors but from specialists, clinics, student health services, and hospital outpatient services. This, plus the increased mobility of Americans, challenges the assumption that the patient–doctor relationship ought to be modeled on friendship; the reality is that patients and physicians are much more likely to be strangers to one another (Veatch, 1983).

But the friendship model may also be unworkable because in a secular, pluralist society even the most basic conditions for friendship cannot be presumed. Friendship requires common values, shared beliefs, and mutually agreed-upon purposes (Wadell, 1989). Likewise, medical friendship requires at least minimal agreement on the purpose of health care, the goals of medicine, and the meaning of both suffering and healing in a person's life (Engelhardt, 1983). Such agreement is increasingly unlikely in a pluralist, fragmented society in which shared moral viewpoints are rare. The patient–physician relationship is ambiguous not only because each may know little about the other, but also because their values, beliefs, and convictions regarding fundamental issues of life and death may be radically dissimilar. The growing emphasis on free and informed consent as a way of negotiating an agreement between patients and physicians who are strangers underscores that the friendship model, however ideal, increasingly misdescribes the relationship (Engelhardt, 1983).

Others reject the friendship model because it mistakenly presumes most people want a friendship with their doctor. Some people want a more distanced relationship with their physician and would not want their doctor to presume they were seeking friendship (Illingworth, 1988). They are not looking for a friend but for competently delivered service (James, 1989). Others prefer the anonymity that comes when a doctor or nurse is a stranger, especially for medical procedures such as abortion, cosmetic surgery, and perhaps mental health therapy (Veatch, 1983). Finally, a more radical rejection of the friendship model sees it as a violation of patient autonomy, particularly when patients have no desire for friendship with their physicians (Illingworth, 1988).

Strengths of the friendship model

Although the relevance of the friendship model has been questioned, many are reluctant to abandon it completely. First, it is a reminder that medicine is not primarily a business but a calling. Along with law, ministry, and counseling, it is a moral profession that demands at least some sort of personal relationship with patients; its principal purpose is altruistic: to benefit and serve the needs of patients (Ladd, 1983). The friendship model appreciates what is distinctive about the medical profession because it recognizes it as a unique vocation and way of life dominated not by self-interest but by care and benevolence (Pellegrino and Thomasma, 1988).

Second, the friendship model affirms that healing must be holistic, addressing not only the physical dimensions of illness but the psychological, social, and spiritual elements as well (Pellegrino and Thomasma, 1988). If the goal of healing is not just to cure a disease but to treat the whole person, a physician or nurse must know a patient well enough to judge what this would entail; in this respect, the friendship model is an antidote to biological reductionism. Effective treatment must take into account the concrete individuality of the patient, because both illness and healing are eminently personal (Fried, 1976). Thus, biomedically correct ther-

apy is not sufficient for good treatment; rather, good treatment involves knowledge of what is unique to patients: their family and economic background, their social and cultural context, their values, desires, beliefs, and interests (Pellegrino, 1983). That healing must be done in the unique context of an individual's life recognizes that the benevolence at the heart of medicine must be personalized.

Third, describing the patient–medical professional relationship in terms of friendship acknowledges that good treatment includes not only sound diagnosis and therapy but also an affective element (Laín Entralgo, 1969). A skilled physician or nurse is not only technically competent but also sympathetic. He or she must have some imaginative grasp of what the patient is undergoing and of how both illness and treatment might affect the patient (Laín Entralgo, 1969). Too, because the alienating and disorienting experience of illness leaves a patient in special need of comfort and support, a truly skilled medical professional must be sensitive and compassionate (Drane, 1988).

Fourth, by stressing the moral equality of the medical professional and the patient, the friendship model avoids the extremes of paternalism and contractualism (James 1989). "Both doctor and patient must be free to make informed decisions and to act fully as moral agents. The values of both doctor and patient must be respected since each is a person deserving of respect as such" (Pellegrino and Thomasma, 1988, p. 34).

Fifth, the model of friendship both explains and legitimates the time, energy, and attention a doctor or nurse gives to a patient; in this respect, it responds to the charge of utilitarianism that the traditional patient–physician relationship is not always conducive to the greatest good of the greatest number (Fried, 1976). Theirs is a special relation in which the primary loyalty of physicians or nurses must be to their patients; thus, not only is their partiality justified but, because of the claim patients have on their care and concern, absolute impartiality would be a failure in benevolence.

Finally, to describe the patient–medical professional relationship as analogous to friendship underscores the central importance of a physician's or nurse's character. To be a good doctor or nurse, one not only must have scientific knowledge and technical skill, but also must be a person of integrity and virtue (Drane, 1988). The medical profession requires people who are honest, unselfish, caring, trustworthy, and just. Thus, although the emphasis in medical ethics is often on rights and duties, ultimately the best guarantee that the patient's interests will be served is the character and integrity of the health-care professional (Pellegrino and Thomasma, 1988).

PAUL J. WADELL

Directly related to this entry are the entries PROFESSIONAL–
PATIENT RELATIONSHIP; *and* FIDELITY AND LOYALTY.
*For a further discussion of topics mentioned in this entry,
see the entries* CARE, *article on* CONTEMPORARY ETHICS
OF CARE; LOVE; PATIENTS' RESPONSIBILITIES, *article on*
VIRTUES OF PATIENTS; *and* VIRTUE AND CHARACTER.
This entry will find application in the entry PROFESSION
AND PROFESSIONAL ETHICS. *For a discussion of related
ideas, see the entries* AUTONOMY; COMPASSION; EMO-
TIONS; HEALING; INFORMED CONSENT; METAPHOR AND
ANALOGY; RESPONSIBILITY; TRUST; UTILITY; *and* VALUE
AND VALUATION.

Bibliography

AMUNDSEN, DARREL W., and FERNGREN, GARY B. 1983.
"Evolution of the Patient-Physician Relationship: Antiquity Through the Renaissance." In *The Clinical Encounter:
The Moral Fabric of the Patient-Physician Relationship,*
pp. 3–46. Edited by Earl E. Shelp. Dordrecht, Netherlands: D. Reidel.

DRANE, JAMES F. 1988. *Becoming a Good Doctor: The Place of
Virtue and Character in Medical Ethics.* Kansas City, Mo.:
Sheed and Ward.

ENGELHARDT, H. TRISTRAM, JR. 1983. "The Physician-Patient
Relationship in a Secular, Pluralist Society." In *The Clinical Encounter: The Moral Fabric of the Patient-Physician
Relationship,* pp. 253–266. Edited by Earl E. Shelp. Dordrecht, Netherlands: D. Reidel.

FRIED, CHARLES. 1976. "The Lawyer as Friend: The Moral
Foundations of the Lawyer-Client Relation." *Yale Law
Journal* 85:1060–1089.

ILLINGWORTH, PATRICIA M. L. 1988. "The Friendship Model
of Physician/Patient Relationship and Patient Autonomy." *Bioethics* 2, no. 1:22–36.

JAMES, DAVID N. 1989. "The Friendship Model: A Reply to
Illingworth." *Bioethics* 3, no. 2:142–146.

LADD, JOHN. 1983. "The Internal Morality of Medicine: An
Essential Dimension of the Patient-Physician Relation-
ship." In *The Clinical Encounter: The Moral Fabric of the
Patient-Physician Relationship,* pp. 209–231. Edited by Earl
E. Shelp. Dordrecht, Netherlands: D. Reidel.

LAÍN ENTRALGO, PEDRO. 1969. *Doctor and Patient.* Translated
by Frances Partridge. New York: McGraw-Hill.

PELLEGRINO, EDMUND D. 1983. "The Healing Relationship:
The Architectonics of Clinical Medicine." In *The Clinical
Encounter: The Moral Fabric of the Patient-Physician Relationship,* pp. 153–172. Edited by Earl E. Shelp. Dordrecht, Netherlands: D. Reidel.

PELLEGRINO, EDMUND D., and THOMASMA, DAVID C. 1988.
*For the Patient's Good: The Restoration of Beneficence in
Health Care.* New York: Oxford University Press.

ROTHMAN, DAVID J. 1991. *Strangers at the Bedside: A History
of How Law and Bioethics Transformed Medical Decision
Making.* New York: Basic Books.

VEATCH, ROBERT M. 1983. "The Physician as Stranger: The
Ethics of the Anonymous Patient-Physician Relation-
ship." In *The Clinical Encounter: The Moral Fabric of the
Patient-Physician Relationship,* pp. 187–207. Edited by Earl
E. Shelp. Dordrecht, Netherlands: D. Reidel.

WADELL, PAUL J. 1989. *Friendship and the Moral Life.* Notre
Dame, Ind.: University of Notre Dame Press.

FUTURE GENERATIONS, OBLIGATIONS TO

Suppose it is true, as it seems to most of us, that history—or at least the pace of change—is accelerating.
People who live a normal life span today experience far
greater changes in history, in culture, and in surrounding landscapes than did their ancestors. In some sense
persons today are closer to their great grandparents than
they will be to their great grandchildren. If a moral dimension is added, and it is noted that human activities
drive the acceleration, it seems that choices made today—wittingly or unwittingly—alter the objects that
form the present context, and speed the arrival of a
"new" world in which the offspring of today's adults will
develop a culture meaningful to them, and hardly meaningful to their parents. Hence the "generation gap."

A new moral attitude

If actions today determine the shape of the future, how
can people escape moral responsibility when making
choices today that may cause great suffering in the future, or when choices made today might cut short the
duration of the human species? Surprisingly, this troubling idea has only recently led to serious soul-searching
among philosophers in the Western tradition, because
most Western thinkers have assumed, especially since
the Enlightenment and the industrial revolution, that
change is unavoidably progress. The idea that some
choices—to detonate nuclear weapons or to destroy rain
forests, for example—might irreversibly harm the future
has only recently and partly replaced the dominant idea
that change, on the whole, is development (Becker,
1934; Bury, 1928). Most discussions of this topic have
therefore proceeded from the assumption that the future
can be made better by making an appropriate bequest in
wealth, in techniques, in culture; but they have not
considered the question of whether future generations
might be irrevocably harmed (see, e.g., Golding, 1972;
Rawls, 1971). They have therefore addressed the question as one of benevolence rather than of strict obligations, and have searched mainly for a "just savings rate"
or a fair schedule of investment.

The idea that there is an obligation to act "sustainably" has ancient origins: The Hebrew prophet Ezekiel
warned against fouling the clean water and trampling
good pasture. But the idea of sustainable use had only

local applications until it became clear, toward the end of the twentieth century, that human activities have become a dominant factor in larger and larger "natural" dynamics (McKibben, 1989). Recent historical scholarship has rethought the impact of earlier cultures on natural systems, and scholars now agree that indigenous cultures, such as the Native Americans in North America, had far more impact (through fires, hunting, and so on) than was previously thought (see Cronon, 1983). Gary Nabhan (1982) reports that more bird and vegetative diversity was found in Mexican lands that were used continuously by indigenous tribes than was found in an otherwise comparable, professionally managed, preserve in the United States.

Traditional histories emphasized the primitivism of early cultures, as measured by their inability to control their environment. Before such accounts were revised, few questioned whether there was a need to worry about the bequest to the future. Why should currently existing humans modify their behavior to protect the well-being of their successors, even though those successors can never repay such a change? Or should it be assumed that future generations can be left to care for themselves? If there are moral obligations to care for the future, how far do they extend? Do generations in the future have a fair claim to a portion of limited resources, such as petroleum? If, as is hoped, the human species lasts far into the future, the morally acceptable share of the present generation seems tiny. If, on the other hand, Earth is, by the middle of the twenty-first century, destined to collide with a huge asteroid that will obliterate all complex life forms, these resources will have been foolishly "wasted" if they are meted out in tiny portions.

Past inattention to the future

Historically speaking, these questions have hardly been addressed directly because most theorists, under the influence of historical optimism and a strong form of moral individualism, have settled upon a simplifying assumption: that any generation can fulfill its obligations to the future by leaving the next generation, taken on the whole, better off than it (the older generation) was when it accepted responsibility from its predecessors. In this way, improvements and decrements to welfare are aggregated within generations and compared across generations, allowing the conclusion that while the present generation is undoubtedly using more than its share of resources, it will leave the next generation with both wealth and technological skill that more than compensate for lost mineral and other resources.

This assumption has two distinguishable elements. First, it assumes that moral obligations are by definition obligations to identifiable individuals who exist in the present (or who will exist in the next) generation. It rejects, for example, the idea that there are obligations to a deity or to the society/community, insisting that all obligations are owed to individuals who have identifiable interests. Second, it assumes that resource extraction and environmental degradation can be traded off against other sources of individual welfare; this latter idea is expressed in the economists' faith that for every resource there is an adequate substitute. The first of these assumptions shortens the horizon of moral concern and limits the group of individuals whose interest must be counted in moral reasoning; the second introduces a social, utilitarian-based calculus in which dollars and techniques are judged economic substitutes for resources and undegraded natural systems.

The assumption that limits concern for the future to maintaining the well-being of immediate posterity is supported by three arguments. The first is practical: the assumption makes obligations to the future more conceptually manageable. While this is an important argument, it is not convincing in itself. It should be accepted only if it allows for an adequate account of the complexities of real situations. An overly simple conceptual and moral map of intergenerational mores will not reveal the moral terrain on which decisions affecting the future are made.

A second, more theoretical argument is based on the economists' idea of a "discount rate." In their decision making, most people show a distinct preference for current satisfactions over future ones—they discount future benefits and costs by some factor across time (Lind, 1982). Any significant positive percentage rate of discount would reduce cost to future welfare toward zero in a generation or so. This understanding of future values expressed in present valuations (such as willingness to pay in the present for deferred welfare compensations in the future) has the advantage that decisions regarding the future can be treated as economic decisions based on present-dollar values. In this system of analysis, the present willingness to pay to protect the interests of the future must compete with other demands on resources. There should be a close connection between what is paid to uphold ideals for the future and the intensity with which the ideals are held. The economists' method is attractive because it allows comparison of the intensities of competing desires (Page, 1992). Even strong advocates of this mainstream economic approach to most environmental problems acknowledge that attempts to understand intergenerational equity severely strain the concepts and methods of present-dollar methodologies (see, e.g., Kneese and Schulze, 1985).

The first systematic writer on environmental ethics, John Passmore, has stated a third, highly theoretical and general argument in favor of the simplifying assumption (Passmore, 1974). He begins by noting that representatives of both utilitarianism and rights theories reach the same conclusion: "Our obligations are to *immediate* posterity." The argument achieves great generality because it rests on the common thread that unites all recent Western ethics—the assumption of "moral individualism," which states that all harms are harms to individuals. Accepting this individualistic principle as true by consensus, Passmore argues that there cannot be obligations to the distant future because it cannot be known what will harm the distant future. It cannot be known what the unborn will value, nor can it be known what new technological solutions will have made present worries obsolete. Passmore concludes that any Western ethic, being individualistic, must therefore neglect any harms to individuals who cannot be identified.

Problems of identification and distance

Passmore's position and that of Martin Golding (1972) gain credibility because no one has decisively solved the "identification problem": How can unknown and unknowable interests, rights, and values of the future be taken into account if the individuals who will experience and express those values cannot be identified? Worse, how can it be known if people will exist in the future and how many there will be? Philosopher Derek Parfit (1983) has posed the following paradox: Imagine two societies, one that uses natural resources profligately, with no thought for the future, and one that consciously acts as a good steward regarding natural resources, carefully husbanding them for future use. Since these different policies and attendant management regimes will rapidly change the context in which people act, their lives will take different paths, people will marry differently, and the persons who would have been born had the conservative policy been followed, will never exist. As for the person who actually comes into existence as a partial result of policy choices by those who are profligate, that person—provided life is still on the whole attractive—has no reason to complain against wasteful ancestors because they bestowed the gift of life on that person.

Parfit's Paradox contradicts the clear intuition of most people that severely lowering the future's standard of living is wrong. But it would be a mistake to dismiss it as a conceptual trick. Parfit's Paradox challenges the ability of present generations to identify any determinate persons who are owed obligations in the distant future, and apparently entails that no individualistic ethic can ever adequately conceptualize the idea of obligations to distant generations (Norton, 1982). Standard individual ethics, such as utilitarianism and rights theory, may not be able, in principle, to formulate a theory of long-term sustainability.

But presentism, the view that obligations can be only to immediate successors, seems inadequate to account for widespread and deeply felt intuitions. Suppose, for example, it is proposed that toxic wastes be sealed in metal drums that are guaranteed to last one century but are likely to deteriorate rapidly thereafter, causing severe and unpredictable health risks. Even though it would apparently be unobjectionable to the reductionistic, single-generation approach, environmentalists and other citizens take it as obvious that such storage is morally objectionable.

Several individualistic responses to these problems of the single-generation approach try to show that despite initial appearances, individualism can account for intuitions regarding obligations to the future. Perhaps the most straightforward of these approaches argues that while it cannot be known in detail what future people will want, there are basic human needs that there is every reason to believe any future human will experience, and that each generation has an obligation to maintain natural systems adequate to fulfill these future needs. For example, it might be thought that productive farmland is owed to future generations so that they can feed themselves, and a pollution-free environment that will not threaten their health, because food and health are likely always to be valued (Baier, 1984; Callahan, 1971). Whether this approach provides sufficient guidance to present policy depends on the extent to which common human values can be specified and whether particular resources can be identified as essential to all future humans.

Current research in the reductionistic tradition attempts to show that the single-generation approach can account indirectly for intuitions of long-term concern. If toxic disasters that will threaten later generations are created, for example, the children of the present generation face a more onerous task in protecting their offspring. This "ratcheting" approach explains that distant generations ought not to be harmed wantonly, for doing so harms the children of the present generation indirectly (Howarth and Norgaard, 1992). Whether this approach will prove useful in understanding obligations to distant generations is not yet clear. In the meantime, the ascendancy of global environmental problems (such as global warming, ozone layer depletion, and loss of biological diversity) ensures that discussions of environmental problems will involve judgments affecting many generations. It is doubtful whether the traditional, individualistic ethical frameworks can make sense of these long-term obligations. In particular, felt concerns for the future include not just whether individuals in the future will be able to satisfy their needs and desires; it is also hoped that they will share present values, and will project present culture and its values into the future.

The single-generation approach is only one of the many possible solutions to what can be called "the distance problem." How far into the future do moral obligations extend? Daniel Callahan (1971) explicitly rejects the reductionistic approach that limits all obligations to those owed to the next generation, avowing obligations to distant generations; but he provides no solution to the identification problem—that individuals or their needs cannot be identified past a generation or so.

Another approach rejects the individualistic formulation of the distance problem altogether, and treats obligations to the future as obligations to an organic society, which the conservative English philosopher and social critic Edmund Burke defined as "a partnership not only between those who are living, but between those who are living, those who are dead and those who are to be born" (Burke, 1955). According to this organicist view of society, there are obligations to the society that cannot be reduced to obligations to any individual members of it. It is therefore possible to define a sharp theoretical divide between individualistic approaches that limit obligations to identifiable individuals (and hence place a heavy burden of proof on obligations to protect the distant future) and those that recognize obligations to the society as a whole (and hence are more concerned about obligations to the distant future).

The two-tier approach

But the distance problem and the identification problem are not the only difficult problems in conceptualizing obligations to the future. Many of environmentalists' deepest concerns are based on a rejection of the economists' assumption that all resources are intersubstitutable. They reject reductionism and its concomitant attitude that all costs and benefits can be traded off across generations because certain irreversible changes that might be perpetrated, such as destroying species and natural systems like the rain forest or severely overheating the atmosphere, would represent unrecompensable harms to the future. This "two-tier," or "hybrid," approach to valuation recognizes, in addition to interchangeable units of welfare, certain moral constraints that limit behaviors that can severely harm the future (Page, 1977; Norton, 1992). This approach assumes that economic values should predominate in most decisions. However, in those cases where there is the threat of serious and irreversible harms, risky activities should be considered morally forbidden.

This two-tier approach to future values can be represented as in Figure 1, which plots the degree of irreversibility of a human-caused effect against its moral impact (Norton, 1992). Decisions that have risk of high impact—for example, loss of key processes in heavily used ecosystems, production of wastes that cannot be properly controlled in the future, perhaps heavy use of fossil fuels—must be guided by a moral value that trumps

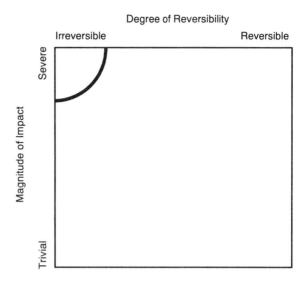

FIGURE 1   Risk decision square

After Norton, 1992, p. 102.

simple economic arguments. The key principle here may well be "the safe minimum standard of conservation," which presumes that resources should be saved, "provided the costs are bearable" (Ciriacy-Wantrup, 1952). According to Figure 1, decisions with a high degree of reversibility and decisions with trivial consequences for future generations—as well as those characterized by both—can be decided by ordinary economic reasoning. We can think of the "red area," in the upper left of the diagram, as containing decisions that risk unrecompensable harms to the future. Those decisions are therefore constrained by a moral principle of sustainability: each generation is obligated to use the earth, and especially the processes that sustain its productivity, so that future generations face options and possibilities as rich as the preceding generation had.

Economists and others who believe all resources are interchangeable can express their view by claiming the red area is empty. If all damages are compensable, then all are reversible if society is wealthy enough. So the diagram is a formalism, allowing a focus on the difficult problem of characterizing the decisions in the red area. Bryan Norton and Robert Ulanowicz (1992) have argued that the degree of irreversibility should be measured as the time that would be required to restore damage, once it has been done. Developing a scale to measure severity of effects may prove more difficult, although it seems plausible to map severity along a continuum ranging from catastrophe (destruction of ecosystems essential to human survival), for example, to minor inconveniences at the other extreme. Or it may be possible, as explained below, to calibrate the vertical axis as a measure of spatial scale—obligations become more stringent regarding activities that alter or degrade larger areas.

A covenant with the future

Edith Brown Weiss has developed a system of obligations expressed in the legal vernacular of planetary rights and obligations (Weiss, 1989). According to this view, there is a minimum level of equality owed to all generations and to people within generations. Arguing that intergenerational obligations are supported by all of the major religions of the world and are recognized in international law, Weiss interprets present obligations as owed to future generations as generations, not as individuals nor on a national basis. These obligations include protecting the natural and cultural heritage of future generations, which are considered elements in a "global commons." This important work could provide a legal framework for incorporating concern for the integrity and health of the ecosystems that provide the context of current human activities.

There is a growing legal tradition that emphasizes protecting natural systems; presumably, that means sustaining productive systems even if that necessitates severely curtailing some kinds of economic activities as too dangerous to the future. This approach, sometimes referred to as "contextualism" (Norton, 1991), recognizes that the value of human activities depends not only on their content but also on protecting their ecological context. This approach fits well with Weiss's idea of an intergenerational trust and provides a scientific elaboration of it.

Aldo Leopold, author of "The Land Ethic" (1949) and the intellectual father of "ecological medicine" (Callicott, 1992), recognized that the violence done to ecological systems is a function of human population size, the scale and the ubiquity of technologies applied, and the inherent resilience of the "land system" (Leopold, 1949; Norton, 1991). Leopold believed that human activities, especially "violent" ones that undermine the structure of the natural systems upon which those activities depend, are wrong because they induce illness in the land community. Since it often is not known how to fix problems once they are caused, he argued, it is better to practice preventive medicine.

Human population growth poses some of the most perplexing moral problems humans face today. At current rates of growth, human population doubles every thirty-nine years, since the annual rate of growth is about 1.8 percent (Ehrlich and Ehrlich, 1991). Great disparity, however, exists in the population growth rates across cultures and countries; highly industrialized countries of the North have passed through a demographic transition to lower birthrates, and the current rates of population growth in these countries will, if they con-

tinue, lead to population stabilization early in the twenty-first century. In less industrially developed nations of the South, however, the transition from high birthrates and high death rates to low birthrates and low death rates has stalled. Improved medicine and sanitation, and other factors, have resulted in lower mortality rates and rapid population growth. In some countries in which the death rate has been reduced as birthrates remain high, population growth is increasing exponentially.

While a few economists (such as Simon, 1981) argue that growing populations should be seen as an economic resource and see no reason to seek reduction of the birthrate, this is a minority position. The more widely accepted position is that human population growth is a serious problem, although there is considerable disagreement about the severity of the problem and the urgency of responses demanded. One group of theorists emphasizes the dangers of rapid population growth and the difficulties of attaining economic growth rates that will provide necessities in a timely fashion. These theorists would address the problem with rapid development of economic resources for the poorest members of the poorest societies, trying to move them through the demographic transition as rapidly as possible. This compassionate attitude is buttressed by felt responsibilities that result from exploitative and neocolonial practices visited by developed nations on less developed nations, and because debts owed to wealthy nations for past "development" projects in the less developed nations represent major impediments in the latter's path to development.

Another group of theorists argues on ecological and evolutionary grounds that population growth, if unchecked by disease and famine or by birth control, will grow until any feasible level of productivity will be inadequate (Ehrlich and Ehrlich, 1991). The only solution, they argue, is to reduce the birthrate immediately and rapidly through education, advocacy of family planning, and so forth. In an extreme form, this approach designates certain areas of the world as already hopelessly overpopulated, and advocates elimination of foreign aid to countries that do not reduce their birthrate immediately (Hardin, 1974). This "lifeboat ethic" argues that the obligation to reduce population growth is so urgent that coercive and invasive methods of birth reduction are justified.

Anyone who accepts that the population growth rate is a serious problem must face grave moral dilemmas, including those that arise because the individual right of families to control their reproduction is valued highly in almost all societies. This is one area where scientists and religious leaders are sharply divided; pronatalist values espoused by some religious leaders have come under attack by natural scientists who insist that, like all species, humans must live within the limits imposed by their natural environment.

Peter Vitouszek and colleagues (1986) calculated that humans now appropriate nearly 40 percent of the primary productivity of terrestrial ecological systems, meaning that only 60 percent of the productivity of biomass and usable energy produced by plants is available for the sustenance of the millions of species other than humans. Human procreative decisions may therefore determine whether any wild ecological systems will survive for more than a few decades. More and more of the larger and more spectacular vertebrates that give interest to wild places exist in precarious populations, and within decades may exist only in zoos and highly managed preserves.

Practical, if long-range, questions regarding limits to population have not been clarified by modern philosophers, who have been unable to reach any consensus on human reproductive ethics. For example, utilitarians have been unable to agree whether each generation has an obligation to maximize the sum of all future utility existing in all future generations, or to maximize the average total utility of individuals who in fact exist (Narveson, 1967). That is, the calculation of interests of future generations in utilitarian aggregations of happiness can be conceived in two different ways that lead to different results. According to the greatest total utility formula, the present generation should act to maximize *happiness* in the future (which might be achieved by having *many* people with modest levels of welfare), whereas the other approach assumes a population limit set by the availability of goods and services, and attempts to maximize the average welfare of this smaller group of welfare consumers. How these issues are resolved will determine which formulas should be used for calculating the interests of present and future generations. Very little consensus currently exists in favor of any particular foundation for obligations to the future.

Toward sustainability

In this survey of obligations to future generations, especially the obligation to live sustainably, there is much room for disagreement, and little substantive consensus on the nature, extent, and the strength of those obligations. Despite remaining disagreements regarding the exact foundations of obligations to the future, a broad moral and political consensus is emerging in favor of a sustainability ethic (Daly and Cobb, 1989; Norton, 1991; Costanza, 1991). Practically, this ethic will, for the foreseeable future, consist in the pursuit of goals that are supportable on a number of different theories. It seems likely that the protection of biodiversity for many future generations will remain a priority social value. As noted above, Edith Weiss has elaborated an intergenerational trust that rests on teachings common to all major religious traditions. Religious leaders and scientists, therefore, may unite behind an ethic of sustainability (Sagan, 1992) owed by each culture to its past and to its future—a sort of Burkean community—to protect the wonders of creative nature for all future generations. That moral obligation to sustainability can then be given more specificity by science. That common value, when buttressed by the apparent scientific impossibility of saving genes and species without saving their habitats, points toward an obligation to protect the *processes* of nature. These processes—of energy capture, transport, and transformation, for example—include the use of energy to maintain complex ecological structure; and it is the integrity of this complex structure that supports nature's creativity and self-healing powers. Nature is organized hierarchically, with smaller systems embedded in larger systems, and each level functions both as a whole and as a part of a larger system (Koestler, 1989).

In this hierarchical, systems view, adaptation—creative response to limitations and opportunities—is pervasive at all levels. Nature creates order by dissipating energy to maintain structure, providing relative stability within which smaller systems can adapt. The effectiveness of any behavioral adaptation, whether genetic or cultural, depends not just on the behavior but also on the context of the behavior. Adaptation is essentially relational in this sense—valued behaviors are good in their context—not good in an absolute sense. It follows that the destruction of the ecological and physical context of a society destroys cultural values, because culturally taught and learned behaviors get their meaning from the relatively stable environmental context that gave rise to them (Page, 1992). Protection of the landscape, the larger context that allows local adaptations and gives meaning to behaviors in their local conditions, therefore must be a priority goal of conservation.

The landscape-level dynamic depends upon the complex structure and organization that allow living systems to cheat the law of entropy, growing and developing, by collecting and using energy to maintain their complex processes on many levels and scales. In these complex, multiscalar processes, human activities, including economic ones, gain their meaning in a local context, or "bioregion." Protection of the cultural legacy can be achieved only if the natural legacy is protected. I therefore believe that the sustainability ethic will evolve to represent a multilevel conception of moral obligation. Individualist ethics, which governs the interactions among human persons, must be supplemented with a more communitarian and longer-range ethic that governs the relations between human populations and their larger context. Aldo Leopold referred to this expansion of the sense of scale, and the concomitant expansion in perception and values that will occur if human individual and cultural practices are truly placed within an ecological and physical context, as learning to "think like a mountain" (Leopold, 1949).

Conclusions

The process involved in developing a truly intergenerational ethic will involve, then, recognition of responsibilities to culture, to protect its context and its continuity, and, on a larger scale, to protect the future of the human species against rapid change in global conditions, such as climate and hydrological cycles. If that is so, the development of a consensus behind this change in thinking, perhaps based on a coalition of scientists and religious leaders, may result in a revolution in human activities that will affect the environments of the descendants of today's generations, even distant ones. What has emerged from the present argument, however, is that the development of this consensus, which seems well founded in ancient teachings of many religions, may require a reconsideration of some of the most cherished value assumptions of post-Enlightenment Western civilization, including the assumption that ethical systems can be built upon an exclusively individualistic foundation.

BRYAN G. NORTON

For a further discussion of topics mentioned in this entry, see the entries ECONOMIC CONCEPTS IN HEALTH CARE; ENVIRONMENTAL ETHICS; ENVIRONMENTAL POLICY AND LAW; ENVIRONMENT AND RELIGION; ETHICS; HARM; OBLIGATION AND SUPEREROGATION; POPULATION ETHICS; RIGHTS; SUSTAINABLE DEVELOPMENT; *and* UTILITY. *This entry will find application in the entries* AGRICULTURE; CLIMATIC CHANGE; *and* HAZARDOUS WASTES AND TOXIC SUBSTANCES. *For a discussion of related ideas, see the entries* BENEFICENCE; CONSCIENCE; HUMAN NATURE; JUSTICE; LIFE, QUALITY OF; *and* VALUE AND VALUATION.

Bibliography

BAIER, ANNETTE. 1984. "For the Sake of Future Generations." In *Earthbound: New Introductory Essays in Environmental Ethics*, pp. 214–246. Edited by Tom Regan. New York: Random House.

BECKER, CARL. 1934. "Progress." In vol. 12 of *Encyclopaedia of the Social Sciences*, pp. 495–499. Edited by Edwin R. A. Seligman and Alvin Johnson. New York: Macmillan.

BURKE, EDMUND. 1955 [1790]. *Reflections on the Revolution in France*. Library of Liberal Arts no. 46. Indianapolis: Bobbs-Merrill.

BURY, JOHN BAGNELL. 1928. *The Idea of Progress: An Inquiry into Its Origin and Growth*. London: Macmillan.

CALLAHAN, DANIEL. 1971. "What Obligations Do We Have to Future Generations?" *American Ecclesiastical Review* 144:265–280.

CALLICOTT, J. BAIRD. 1992. "Aldo Leopold's Metaphor." In *Ecosystem Health: New Goals for Environmental Management*. Edited by Robert Costanza, Bryan Norton, and Benjamin D. Haskell. Washington, D.C.: Island Press.

CIRIACY-WANTRUP, SIEGFRIED V. 1952. *Resource Conservation: Economics and Politics*. Berkeley: University of California Press.

COSTANZA, ROBERT, and WAIGNER, LISA, eds. 1991. *Ecological Economics: The Science and Management of Sustainability*. New York: Columbia University Press.

CRONON, WILLIAM. 1983. *Changes in the Land: Indians, Colonists, and the Ecology of New England*. New York: Hill and Wang.

DALY, HERMAN E.; COBB, JOHN B.; and COBB, CLIFFORD W. 1989. *For the Common Good: Redirecting the Economy Toward Community, the Environment, and a Sustainable Future*. Boston: Beacon Press.

EHRLICH, PAUL R., and EHRLICH, ANNE H. 1991. *The Population Explosion*. New York: Simon and Schuster.

GOLDING, MARTIN P. 1972. "Obligations to Future Generations." *Monist* 56, no. 1:85–99.

HARDIN, GARRETT. 1974. "Lifeboat Ethics—The Case Against Helping the Poor." *Psychology Today* 8, no. 4:38–43, 123–126.

HOWARTH, RICHARD B., and NORGAARD, RICHARD B. 1992. "Environmental Valuation Under Sustainable Development." *American Economic Review* 82, no. 2:473–477.

KNEESE, ALLEN V., and SCHULZE, WILLIAM D. 1985. "Ethics and Environmental Economics." In vol. 1 of *Handbook of Natural Resource and Energy Economics*, pp. 191–220. Edited by Allen V. Kneese and James L. Sweeney. Amsterdam: North Holland Press.

KOESTLER, ARTHUR. 1989. [1967]. *The Ghost in the Machine*. London: Arkana.

LEOPOLD, ALDO. 1949. *A Sand County Almanac, and Sketches Here and There*. Oxford: Oxford University Press.

LIND, ROBERT C. 1982. *Discounting for Time and Risk in Energy Policy*. Washington, D.C.: Resources for the Future.

McKIBBEN, BILL. 1989. "Reflections: The End of Nature." *The New Yorker*, September 11, pp. 47–105.

NABHAN, GARY P. 1982. *The Desert Smells like Rain: A Naturalist in Papago Country*. San Francisco: North Point Press.

NARVESON, JAN. 1967. "Utilitarianism and New Generations." *Mind* 76:62–72.

NORTON, BRYAN G. 1982. "Environmental Ethics and the Rights of Future Generations." *Environmental Ethics* 4, no. 4:319–337.

———. 1991. *Toward Unity Among Environmentalists*. New York: Oxford University Press.

———. 1992. "Sustainability, Human Welfare, and Ecosystem Health." *Environmental Values* 1:97–111.

NORTON, BRYAN G., and ULANOWICZ, ROBERT E. 1992. "Scale and Biodiversity Policy: A Hierarchical Approach." *Ambio* 21, no. 3:244–249.

PAGE, TALBOT. 1977. *Conservation and Economic Efficiency: An Approach to Materials Policy*. Baltimore: Johns Hopkins University Press.

———. 1992. "Environmental Existentialism." In *Ecosystem Health: New Goals for Environmental Management.* Edited by Robert Costanza, Bryan Norton, and Benjamin Haskell. Covelo, Calif.: Island Press.

PARFIT, DEREK. 1983. "Energy Policy and the Further Future: The Identity Problem." In *Energy and the Future,* pp. 166–179. Edited by Douglas MacLean and Peter G. Brown. Totowa, N.J.: Rowman and Littlefield.

PARTRIDGE, ERNEST, ed. 1981. *Responsibilities to Future Generations.* Buffalo, N.Y.: Prometheus.

PASSMORE, JOHN. 1974. *Man's Responsibility for Nature: Ecological Problems and Western Traditions.* New York: Scribner.

RAWLS, JOHN. 1971. *A Theory of Justice.* Cambridge, Mass.: Harvard University Press.

SAGAN, CARL. 1992. "To Avert a Common Danger." *Parade,* March 1, pp. 10–14.

SIKORA, R. I., and BARRY, BRIAN, eds. 1978. *Obligations to Future Generations.* Philadelphia: Temple University Press.

SIMON, JULIAN. 1981. *The Ultimate Resource.* Princeton, N.J.: Princeton University Press.

VITOUSZEK, PETER M.; EHRLICH, PAUL R.; EHRLICH, ANNE H.; and MATSON, PAMELA A. 1986. "Human Appropriation of the Products of Photosynthesis." *Bioscience* 36, no. 6:368–373.

WEISS, EDITH BROWN. 1989. *In Fairness to Future Generations: International Law, Common Patrimony, and Intergenerational Equity.* Tokyo: United Nations University.

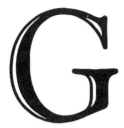

GENDER IDENTITY AND GENDER-IDENTITY DISORDERS

The term "gender" has a long etymological history in Latin roots signifying birth, race, and kind, and in Greek roots signifying birth, race, and family. In contemporary usage, the term generally signifies the male or female nature or identity of a person. That meaning, however, is more complex than might first appear. A satisfactory understanding of gender will contribute significantly not only to an understanding of gender-identity disorders but also to the ways in which the notion of gender is otherwise important to the theory and practice of medicine.

Despite the temptation to designate all human beings as either male or female, human sexual diversity is not easily confined by those simple categories. Human gender has at least chromosomal, hormonal, anatomical, psychic, and social components. Given the variability that is possible among such components, males are not all interchangeable replicas of one another, and neither are females. Neither are the male and the female always especially distinct from one another. The "male" and the "female" have fluid rather than fixed borders. For example, some human beings are born with an extra sex chromosome, resulting in XXY or XYY genetic complements; the former appear eunuchoid as adults and the latter appear male. In Turner's syndrome only a single X chromosome is present; individuals with this variation appear female though they will be infertile by reason of undifferentiated gonads. With regard to anatomy, some persons are born with both ovarian and testicular tissue or with ambiguous genitalia. Individuals within and between genders can vary, too, with respect to hormone traits that drive the development of bodily and behavioral traits. The range of human sexual traits extends even more widely in psychological qualities and social behavior inasmuch as cultural notions of masculinity and femininity—normative notions about how maleness and femaleness should be expressed—vary widely. Gender is thus a complex notion with both biological and cultural components.

Much contemporary feminist, anthropological, and gay and lesbian analysis has taken pains to differentiate biological components of sex and socially constructed components of gender. Attention to gender as an element of ethical analysis permits attention to matters that otherwise might be neglected: how notions of male and female are connected to matters of authority and power, how relations between genders are structured, how personal and social identities are constituted, and how justice may be analyzed in terms of gender. For instance, a number of scholars have shown that medicine has compromised women's interests. Women's lives have been medicalized much more than men's lives. Emotions, menstruation, and menopause, for example, have been subject to medical interpretations that have treated female traits as defects to be remedied (Apple, 1990). Women are often disproportionately hospitalized, medicated, and treated surgically, and they have been historically excluded from the professional practice of medicine (Walsh, 1977). Women also have been neglected in biomedical experimentation; consequently, biomedicine has assumed that males are an adequate research base for treating women and has ignored possible differences required in the health care of women. The treatment women have received often has been defined in relation to a gender "standard" based on male and female reproductive roles. Some feminist analysis has found that medical practices surrounding childbirth infantilize women (Laslie, 1982). Debates about "maternal–fetal" conflicts may mask a male valuation of children at the expense of the reproductive rights of women. Access to contraceptives, abortion, in vitro fertilization, and embryo implantation also have been criticized as exemplifying male mistrust of and hegemony over women (Smart, 1987). These examples make it clear that the theory and practice of medicine should not assume a neutral identity between the male and the female in the way health care is theorized or delivered.

What remains to be accomplished by greater attention to gender is the larger task of identifying ways in which biomedicine can accommodate the interests of persons regardless of gender-related differences and ways in which medicine can become less constrained by unjustifiable gender assumptions. This article takes up some of the representative ways in which the notion of gender is important to ethical analysis regarding gender identity, health, and sexual orientation.

Gender assignment

A newborn's gender is a matter of concern for both parents and physicians, but sometimes a child's traits do not permit an easy classification as male or female. Children may be born with irregular gonads or, as mentioned above, ambiguous genitalia and atypical chromosomal traits. Gender assignment refers to the decision made to designate a newborn as either male or female. The traits that are taken as establishing a child's "real" gender reflect not only the state of biomedical knowledge but also cultural and moral standards about what traits are most important in gender identities.

Tests to determine the presence of testes, ovaries, and levels of various hormones in children with ambiguous genitalia are now available to physicians, as are surgical techniques to construct female genitalia and methods of enlarging some exceptionally small penises. Such tests were not always available, and these same methods may not be available even now in some regions of the world. Historically, children were matched to one gender rather than another on the basis of physical resemblance or the presence or absence of testes and ovaries. Such methods could not, however, distinguish humans with true intersexed conditions (in which both testicular and ovarian tissue is present), and they failed to be sensitive to the complexity of human sexual iden-

tity. Chromosomal and hormonal tests offer another way of characterizing the gender of children, but such methods still may presuppose that a child's gender is given as either male or female. Testing of this kind assumes that human beings are bifurcated neatly into male and female, and that children with ambiguous gender need only be studied carefully in order to determine their place in that order.

Gender-assignment decisions and therapy, however, make it clear that gender can be as much a product of human choice as of biological traits. Use of the term "assignment" suggests that gender is conferred rather than discovered. Even if the opportunity for postnatal assignment of the gender of children is not routinely offered to parents, prevailing theories of medical management of ambiguously gendered children suggest that any child's gender is moldable through early application of medical and psychological methods (Money and Ehrhardt, 1972). That gender assignment consists of more than mere discovery of gender as it has been obscured by ambiguous anatomy or genetics makes clear gender's connections to cultural standards of masculinity and femininity.

Suzanne J. Kessler has identified a number of ways in which cultural ideals about the male, the female, and a dimorphically gendered society influence the practice of gender assignment (Kessler, 1991). She has described how gender-assignment decisions sometimes are made primarily on the basis of the expected size and function of a child's genitalia rather than on more complex assessments of genetic and endocrinological tests. Kessler thinks that children may be assigned as female if physicians and parents view them as having an inadequately sized penis, a view that not only reduces male gender to genital appearance but also perpetuates a notion of femaleness as a kind of failed maleness. There is no question that biogenetic features shape the sexuality and behavior of each and every individual, but it appears just as true that social and moral judgments also profoundly influence an individual's gender identity. This is to say that gender is not merely a function of chromosomal, hormonal, or anatomical traits. Acknowledging that social influences, often unconsciously, play a role in gender assignment requires resisting the view that gender is merely given in the raw material of human biology. Acknowledging these social influences also requires paying attention to the way in which sexist or other prejudicial views may guide decisions about a child's "real" gender.

Gender-identity disorders

Gender-identity disorders are discordances between one's felt gender and one's assigned gender. These discordances may be especially acute in regard to expectations about appropriate behavior for a particular gender.

Ordinarily, most persons experience themselves as male or female and express themselves in ways congruent with social expectations and roles accorded to that gender. At a very early age, however, small numbers of individuals discover themselves uncomfortable with the gender identity being imposed on them by virtue of their anatomy. This discomfort is not merely a sense of being inadequate in a particular gender role, it is discomfort with being identified as one gender rather than another. Such disorders range from comparatively mild discomfort to outright rejection of the designated gender.

Children may manifest gender disorders through rejection of stereotypic clothing or play activities, disavowal of actual anatomic characteristics, and, sometimes, assertions that they will grow up to be members of the opposite sex. The degree of severity varies, and some children eventually moderate or give up their determination to identify as members of the opposite sex. Rather more boys than girls with such childhood manifestations have homoerotic sexual orientations as adults, but neither males nor females usually retain in adulthood strong desires to be members of the opposite sex or beliefs that they are "trapped" in the wrong kind of body. Adolescents and adults, too, may have transient or lingering beliefs that they belong to the opposite sex, and in addition to declarations about the inappropriateness of their bodies and expected social roles, they may cross-dress, though not for purposes of sexual satisfaction and without the desire to achieve new anatomical sex characteristics. In the most extreme cases, however, some individuals retain a strong opposite-gender identification and do seek to conform their behavior and anatomy to the chosen gender. (This phenomenon of transsexualism is discussed in the next section.) Numerous and often competing theories have been offered to account for the occurrence of gender "dysphoria," as gender dissatisfaction has been called, and these theories variously suggest heritable traits, family dynamics, early physical illness, and early psychic events as among the causes (American Psychiatric Association (APA), 1987).

The nature of parental and health-professional response to gender dysphoria is of moral interest in a number of ways. It is interesting to note, for example, that the chief impairment attributed to gender-identity disorders is the generation of conflict between those affected and their peers and family. It is also recognized as impairing social and occupational functioning. While those affected may sometimes be depressed and may have other psychic disorders, many affected individuals claim that except for social difficulties, they are not especially disturbed by their felt gender preferences. The question may be posed, then, whose purposes treatment of gender-identity disorders serves.

Given a history in which moral preferences were sometimes encoded in psychiatric diagnoses, contemporary psychiatry has attempted to divest itself of responsibility for the enforcement of moral or political values. The APA has stated: "Neither deviant behavior, e.g., political, religious, or sexual, nor conflicts that are primarily between the individual and society are mental disorders unless the deviance or conflict is a symptom of a dysfunction in the person" that generates persistent stress, disability, or significant risk of suffering, death, pain, disability, or loss of freedom (1987, p. xxii). One may ask, in light of this definition, whether gender-identity treatments do in fact reinforce larger social expectations about appropriate gender identifications and behaviors. It may be replied that children and adolescents affected by gender dysphoria often face significant depression and restriction of opportunities as a result of their nonconforming beliefs and behaviors, and that for this reason treatment is morally appropriate because measures to protect a child from undue conflict and depression are a parent's prerogative. It does not follow, of course, that a parent might do anything at all in order to achieve a particular gender identity or behavior in a child. Insofar as social considerations are relevant to establishing the morality of a particular therapy, one would still need to consider the extent to which children and adolescents might be treated because they live in a society dominated by a view of mutually exclusive gender roles untrue to the diversity of human beings. The debate about the social influences on choices regarding gender dysphoria has thus far occurred primarily in relation to adults rather than children, and it will be profitable to consider the debate from perspectives on adult transsexualism.

Transsexualism

The term "transsexualism" was first used in the 1940s to describe adults who verbally and behaviorally identified themselves as male or female in contradiction to their anatomical sex and the behavior expected of that sex. (The term is to be distinguished from "transvestism," which describes persons who dress as members of the opposite sex but do not identify themselves as members of that gender. Some persons may dress thus for sexual satisfaction.) Historically, transsexuals were thought to suffer from psychological disorders, and some health-care practitioners still maintain this view. Transsexual therapy in the sense we know it today, however, more typically describes a range of surgical, hormonal, and psychological therapies whose goal is to conform anatomy, secondary sex characteristics, and behavior to those of the desired gender. Surgical efforts may involve mastectomy, the removal of penis and scrotum, the construction—to the extent this is possible—of a penis or vagina, and accompanying hormonal treatments to spur the appropriate characteristics in hair, voice tone, fat distribution, and so on. Such treatment cannot, however, achieve sexual fertility in the chosen gender. Various components of this therapy have been attempted since the 1930s. In the 1950s, Christine Jorgensen, formerly George, became famous as a male transsexed to a female. Since then the term "transgender therapy" has often been used to describe this overall type of therapy. It should be noted that transgender therapy does not impose a particular sexual orientation on an individual. A client who undergoes female transgender therapy, for example, may identify herself as lesbian or as heterosexual after the therapy. Certainly not all persons who consider themselves "trapped" in the wrong anatomy desire transgender therapy, given its costs and limitations. Neither do all persons who want such therapy qualify for it, since transsexualism may be accompanied by other psychic disorders that make the therapy unlikely to improve the lot of the person seeking it.

Transgender therapy has important implications for a person's legal and social standing in professional associations, entitlement to marry, legal rights to be recognized as a member of the chosen gender, and so on. Transsexed Renee Richards won the right to play in women's professional tennis, but other transsexuals have not been so successful in securing equivalent rights. Individuals undergoing such therapy often face legal difficulties insofar as they might violate laws regarding cross-dressing and the use of public washrooms. Prison housing also raises special problems, since persons in transgender therapy are especially vulnerable to contemptuous treatment and violence.

A number of ethical questions attend the practice of transgender therapy, especially since it challenges the expectation that congenital anatomy is gender destiny. First of all, there is the conceptualization of requests to be transgendered. Such requests presuppose that one's gender cannot be reduced to genitalia or chromosomal birthright. Indeed, to move away from seeing transsexualism as a psychological disorder is to acknowledge not only the separability of psychic identity and biological sex but also that some aspects of gender are subject to choice. Even if one acknowledges that gender is not reducible to any single trait, it does not automatically follow that transgender therapy and its surgery and lifelong hormonal treatments are ethically proper. One might object to transgender therapy from a natural-law perspective if one argued that such therapy violated that tradition's principle of bodily integrity because the significant bodily alterations do not confer an appropriate benefit important to other natural-law objectives. On the other hand, if one assumes that gender identity is not reducible to biological characteristics, it is possible to argue within the natural-law tradition, as Robert H. Springer has done, that transgender therapy serves an important moral good insofar as it protects psychic health (Springer, 1987).

Some feminist analysis has seen in transgender therapy the extension of patriarchal privilege insofar as male-to-female transgenderism is much more common than its opposite. Janice Raymond has argued that transgenderism trivializes women insofar as the therapy reduces femaleness to a trait that men may or may not adopt, as they wish. By contrast, but still in support of her argument about patriarchal privilege, she characterizes female-to-male transgenderism as an attempt to bypass constraints on female participation in male-dominated society (Raymond, 1979). Raymond does not call for a ban on transgender therapy, but she does believe that greater social accommodation of gender diversity in the context of a greater social emancipation of women would eliminate the incentives to transgender therapy, with its attendant evils.

Because the ratio of men to women who seek transgender therapy is not constant around the world, it is unclear that transgender therapy represents primarily male interests (Godlewski, 1988). It is also hard to see how persons suffering with gender dysphoria from an early age can be accurately described as choosing transgender therapy for trivial or trivializing reasons. Even if transgender therapy were fully implicated in the evils Raymond ascribes to it, she would be right to seek recourse for those evils in something other than a ban on the practice. It is certainly desirable to eradicate social evils, but there is no ethical principle maintaining that the only legitimate way to remove unwanted personal suffering is through the moral correction of the entire social order that may be causing or contributing to it. Utilitarian theory would lend support to the pursuit of the therapy. Utilitarian ethics not only advocates the greatest happiness for the greatest number of people; in John Stuart Mill's formulation it also relies on the libertarian principle, a principle of noninterference with individual pursuits insofar as they do not harm others. Attempting to find ways to conform bodily and behavioral traits to a felt psychic gender might promote the general good insofar as it leads to important biomedical advances in addition to whatever benefits it confers on particular individuals. Moreover, it is unclear that transgender therapy affects others in ways sufficiently harmful to justify foreclosing the option through legal or medical consensus. Nor would there be anything in an ethical approach like that of John Rawls, who relies on a kind of social contractarianism that would preclude the practice of transgender therapy (Rawls, 1971). Indeed, it would appear that in formulating the principles and policies by which a just society ought to be governed, his original social contractors would have to envisage a place for transsexuals and accommodate in principle their therapeutic interests.

That a therapy is morally acceptable, of course, does not by itself establish what priority it ought to have in a health-care system. Some persons seeking transgender therapy have found private insurers and government health programs unwilling to pay for it because, it is said, such therapy is akin to cosmetic treatment and is in any case experimental and unproven. In response to claims of this kind, Eric B. Gordon has argued that the therapy meets an important psychic need of some persons, that it can work, and that its limitations can be overcome with better standards of determining eligibility. Gordon therefore concludes that public funding of transgender therapy ought to be provided according to the merits of the case (Gordon, 1991). To the extent this argument is successful, it would appear to extend to private insurers who offer coverage for similar psychic disorders, though the terms of such coverage might exclude preexisting conditions or might limit the amount of money paid to any individual, regardless of condition.

Sexual-orientation therapy

At least since the coining of the term "homosexuality" in 1869, a broad array of techniques has been used with men and women to redirect sexual orientation from homosexuality to heterosexuality. Much of this therapy has been based on a strict identification of male and female with opposite-sex desire: Maleness means attraction to women, and femaleness means attraction to men. Departures from this gender norm have been treated in a variety of ways that include moral censure, legal sanction, and formal medical declarations of pathology (Bayer, 1987). Techniques used to achieve a therapeutic goal of heterosexuality have typically reflected prevailing treatment methods: various forms of behavioral therapy, drug and hormone treatment, surgery, and a wide variety of psychotherapies (Murphy, 1992). While some therapy has been well-meaning and carried out with professional integrity, there also has been involuntary treatment, gruesome castrations in the Nazi camps, and abusive chemical and electrical aversive therapies.

In 1973, the APA formally abandoned the view that homosexuality was necessarily pathological, a view it had held at least since its first formal diagnostic manual of 1952. The APA nevertheless maintains the diagnostic category "sexual-orientation distress" for those who suffer from unwanted sexual orientations. Though technically relevant to any sexual orientation, the diagnostic category is functionally limited to homosexuality, given the utter rarity of individuals professing distress from heterosexual orientation. Despite the formal declassification of homosexuality, some therapists still argue that homosexuality is pathological. Some other therapists wish to treat homosexuality, but they do not identify it as a disorder. These latter therapists approach homosexuality as an unwanted trait and justify their efforts as respecting the wishes of their clients. Some programs, for example, will enroll men and women only if they are "dissatisfied" with their sexual orientation (Schwartz

and Masters, 1984). Some therapists practice from a religious perspective. Recovery from sin rather than from disease is the goal of religious reorientation programs (Pattison and Pattison, 1980), and they use Bible study, prayer, and group socializing to inaugurate or restore heterosexuality. It remains a matter of debate whether the extinguishing of unwanted traits is a legitimate objective for medicine and whether sexual-orientation therapy reveals social flaws in the treatment of homosexuality generally. Sexual-orientation therapy is an important opportunity to consider what such therapy suggests about a society's understanding of gender, difference, suffering, and medical collusion with larger social injustices. In this latter regard, sexual-orientation therapy can prove ethically instructive as to how homosexuality comes to be problematized as a deficit to be remedied rather than as a difference to be cultivated and nurtured.

Some commentators have argued that sexual-orientation therapy is immoral because it contributes to social prejudice against gay men and lesbians. Many gay men and lesbians see efforts designed to bring about sexual reorientation as an example of continuing disregard for their lives and as a falsification and devaluation of the integrity and worth of homoeroticism. Gerald C. Davison has argued that the mere availability of such therapy encourages its use, thereby perpetuating oppressive views about homosexuality (Davison, 1976). By contrast, Frederick Suppe has pointed out that such an argument is conclusive only if the therapy presupposes that homosexuality is inherently inferior to heterosexuality and that such therapy is socially influential in perpetuating injustice. A program that treated homosexuality merely as an unwanted trait would not be susceptible to Davison's objections (Suppe, 1984). Even if such therapy does not contribute to social injustice directly, social injustice regarding homosexuality may be a spur to such therapy, whether homosexuality is conceived as inherently inferior or merely an undesired trait; pursuit of sexual-orientation therapy may be an artifact of social injustice rather than an injustice in itself (Murphy, 1991).

Reports of success in reorientation come most typically from psychoanalysts, behavior therapists, and religious programs. However, these reports of success have been criticized on the basis of methodological problems including small sample size, success standards that measure behavior change but not psychic readjustment, inadequacy of long-term assessment, and the uncontrolled nature of the studies. While there are reports of success in achieving heterosexual behavior and even heterosexual marriage, it is still unclear whether the therapies themselves have been responsible for those changes or whether and to what extent those changes will endure across a person's lifetime. Because of problems of these kinds, it is unclear that there is any generally effective therapy useful on randomly selected persons seeking sexual reorientation (Murphy, 1991). If this is so, it would follow that such therapy should be represented to patients or clients as experimental and unproven. In the past, some people were treated involuntarily for their homoerotic sexual orientation (Murphy, 1992). Certainly, any such coercive treatment could today only be seen as morally objectionable, given a principled respect for autonomous decision making in the absence of any consensus that homosexuality is a moral or medical evil.

Since homosexuality is not confined to adults, it is also germane to consider the ethics of therapy with children. Given a confluence of scientific reports about possible biogenetic origins of homosexual orientation in males (Hamer et al., 1993; Bailey and Pillard, 1991; LeVay, 1991), discussions about the control of the sexual orientation of children are likely to come into greater prominence. In the past, parents turned to punishment, moral exhortation, religious counsel, reform school, and even electroshock therapy in order to bring their children to heterosexuality. Certainly one may expect that discussion about the control of sexual orientation not only will raise questions about the ethics of experimentation with children but also will engage ethical questions about the extent to which parents may properly attempt to control the characteristics of children (Crocker, 1979; Murphy, 1990).

Conclusions

The meaning of gender has become a focal point for moral and political analysis both in medicine and in the culture at large. This analysis typically focuses on the ways in which the biology and the cultural construction of gender are intertwined. It asks whether and with what consequences male gender stands paradigmatically for all human beings and whether the male is not preferentially treated. It asks whether biologically and socially polarized notions of gender are adequate to express the range of human gender variability. It asks whether the presumption of heterosexuality is normative and valid for judging the nature and destiny of all persons. It makes clear that treating gender, social roles, and sexual orientation as undivided in nature often has led to injustices against women, intersexed beings, and gay men and lesbians. A simplistic conflation of the biological and social roles of both males and females renders much more difficult the task of identifying and interpreting those social presumptions and moral values that impose oppression and disadvantage on the basis of gender. Appreciating the importance of gender to ethical analysis will offer biomedicine the opportunity to serve human beings as the persons they are and want to be rather than as the persons invidious gender presumptions would have them be.

TIMOTHY F. MURPHY

Directly related to this entry are the entries SEXUAL IDENTITY; *and* SEXUAL DEVELOPMENT. *For a further discussion of topics mentioned in this entry, see the entries* BODY, *article on* SOCIAL THEORIES; CHILDREN, *especially the article on* MENTAL-HEALTH ISSUES; FEMINISM; HEALTH-CARE FINANCING; HEALTH AND DISEASE, *article on* SOCIOLOGICAL PERSPECTIVES; HOMOSEXUALITY; MENTAL ILLNESS, *article on* CONCEPTIONS OF MENTAL ILLNESS; NATURAL LAW; RESEARCH BIAS; SEXISM; SEX THERAPY AND SEX RESEARCH; SEXUALITY IN SOCIETY, *article on* SOCIAL CONTROL OF SEXUAL BEHAVIOR; UTILITY; *and* WOMEN, *especially the article on* HISTORICAL AND CROSS-CULTURAL PERSPECTIVES. *For a discussion of related ideas, see the entries* AUTONOMY; *and* VALUE AND VALUATION. *Other relevant material may be found under the entries* BEHAVIOR MODIFICATION THERAPIES; FAMILY; PSYCHOANALYSIS AND DYNAMIC THERAPIES; *and* SPORTS.

Bibliography

AMERICAN PSYCHIATRIC ASSOCIATION (APA). 1987. *Diagnostic and Statistical Manual of Mental Disorders (DSM-III-R)*. 3d ed., rev. Washington, D.C.: Author.

APPLE, RIMA D., ed. 1990. *Women, Health, and Medicine in America*. New York: Garland.

BAILEY, J. MICHAEL, and PILLARD, RICHARD C. 1991. "A Genetic Study of Male Sexual Orientation." *Archives of General Psychiatry* 48, no. 12:1089–1096.

BAYER, RONALD S. 1987. *Homosexuality and American Psychiatry: The Politics of Diagnosis*. 2d ed. Princeton, N.J.: Princeton University Press.

CROCKER, LAWRENCE. 1979. "Meddling with the Sexual Orientation of Children." In *Having Children: Philosophical and Legal Reflections on Parenthood*, pp. 145–154. Edited by Onora O'Neill and William Ruddick. New York: Oxford University Press.

DAVISON, GERALD C. 1976. "Homosexuality: The Ethical Challenge." *Journal of Consulting and Clinical Psychology* 44, no. 2:157–162.

GODLEWSKI, JULIAN. 1988. "Transsexualism and Anatomic Sex Ratio Reversal in Poland." *Archives of Sexual Behavior* 17, no. 6:547–548.

GORDON, ERIC B. 1991. "Transsexual Healing: Medicaid Funding of Sex Reassignment Surgery." *Archives of Sexual Behavior* 20, no. 1:61-74.

HAMER, DEAN H.; HU, STELLA; MAGNUSON, VICTORIA L.; HU, NAN; and PATTATUCCI, ANGELA M. L. 1993. "A Linkage Between DNA Markers on the X Chromosome and Male Sexual Orientation." *Science* 261, no. 5119: 321–327.

KESSLER, SUZANNE J. 1991. "The Medical Construction of Gender: Case Management of Intersexed Infants." *Signs* 16, no. 1:3–26.

LASLIE, ADELE E. 1982. "Ethical Issues in Childbirth." *Journal of Medicine and Philosophy* 7, no. 2:179–195.

LEVAY, SIMON. 1991. "A Difference in Hypothalamic Structure Between Heterosexual and Homosexual Men." *Science* 253, no. 5023:1034–1037.

MONEY, JOHN, and EHRHARDT, ANKE A. 1972. *Man and Woman, Boy and Girl: The Differentiation and Dimorphism of Gender Identity from Conception to Maturity.* Baltimore: Johns Hopkins University Press.

MURPHY, TIMOTHY F. 1990. "Reproductive Controls and Sexual Destiny." *Bioethics* 4, no. 2:121–142.

———. 1991. "The Ethics of Conversion Therapy." *Bioethics* 5, no. 2:123–138.

———. 1992. "Redirecting Sexual Orientation: Techniques and Justifications." *Journal of Sex Research* 29, no. 4: 501–523.

PATTISON, E. MANSELL, and PATTISON, MYRNA LOY. 1980. " 'Ex-Gays': Religiously Mediated Change in Homosexuals." *American Journal of Psychiatry* 137, no. 12:1553–1562.

RAWLS, JOHN. 1971. *A Theory of Justice.* Cambridge, Mass.: Harvard University Press.

RAYMOND, JANICE G. 1979. *The Transsexual Empire: The Making of the She-Male.* Boston: Beacon Press.

SCHWARTZ, MARK F., and MASTERS, WILLIAM H. 1984. "The Masters and Johnson Treatment Program for Dissatisfied Homosexual Men." *American Journal of Psychiatry* 141, no. 2:173–181.

SMART, CAROL. 1987. " 'There Is of Course the Distinction Dictated by Nature': Law and the Problem of Paternity." In *Reproductive Technologies: Gender, Motherhood, and Medicine,* pp. 98–117. Edited by Michelle Stanworth. Minneapolis: University of Minnesota Press.

SPRINGER, ROBERT H. 1987. "Transsexual Surgery: Some Reflections on the Moral Issues Involved." In vol. 2 of *Sexuality and Medicine,* pp. 233–247. Edited by Earl E. Shelp. Dordrecht, Netherlands: D. Reidel.

SUPPE, FREDERICK. 1984. "Curing Homosexuality." In *Philosophy and Sex,* pp. 391–420. New rev. ed. Edited by Ralph Baker and Frederick Elliston. Buffalo, N.Y.: Prometheus.

WALSH, MARY ROTH. 1977. *"Doctors Wanted: No Women Need Apply": Sexual Barriers in the Medical Profession, 1835–1975.* New Haven, Conn.: Yale University Press.

GENE MAPPING AND SEQUENCING

See GENOME MAPPING AND SEQUENCING.

GENE THERAPY

I. Strategies for Gene Therapy
   W. French Anderson
   Theodore Friedmann
II. Ethical and Social Issues
   Eric Juengst
   LeRoy Walters

I. STRATEGIES FOR GENE THERAPY

Most human disease results from an interaction of inborn genetic factors with environmental influences. Except in specific cases (e.g., surgery to remove an inflamed appendix, antibiotics to cure pneumonia), modern-day medical treatments do not cure diseases. Therapy only modifies the symptoms of a disease, thereby giving the body an opportunity to heal itself. If the body heals itself quickly, the ailment is called an "acute" disease; if the body cannot heal itself, the ailment is called a "chronic" disease. More definitive therapies are clearly needed.

With the advent of molecular biology in the 1960s and of the recombinant deoxyribonucleic acid (DNA) era in the early 1970s, concepts and tools began to appear for a rational kind of treatment: gene therapy. The revolutionary new concept underlying this approach is that effective treatment should correct the underlying genetic defect itself and not just its symptoms (Tatum, 1966; Sinsheimer, 1969; Aposhian, 1970; Davis, 1970; Freese, 1972; Anderson, 1972; Friedmann and Roblin, 1972; Morrow, 1976; Friedmann, 1976).

The first major impetus for this approach came from the clarification during the mid-1960s of the mechanisms by which some kinds of viruses are able to transform normal cells (that are growing in tissue culture) into tumor cells. Researchers found that after some of these "tumor viruses" infect cells, their own DNA becomes integrated into the DNA of the host cell, becoming a permanent and heritable part of the cell genome. At least some of the integrated viral genes continue to function (i.e., be expressed) stably and permanently in the cells and cause the cells to grow in an unregulated cancerlike fashion. In other words, these viruses carry out precisely the function that medical scientists wanted to emulate—to introduce foreign genes into cells in a way that allows the new genes to function. The difference is that the added genes would be meant to be therapeutic for the cell rather than to satisfy the needs of the invading virus.

In the early 1970s, the technical possibilities of the emerging field of molecular genetics and the developing awareness of molecular biology among those interested in human clinical disease led to the first tentative connections between molecular genetics and therapeutics. The clinical need for new and more effective treatments began to be discussed at scientific meetings, and the possible application of viruses to carry out clinically useful gene transfer was debated (Friedmann, 1983, 1990, 1992; Wolff and Lederberg, 1994). Since those early discussions, the technology of gene transfer has developed dramatically. Gene therapy is now being used in an attempt to treat a broad range of diseases including cancer, heart disease, genetic diseases, and AIDS. A new era of medicine has begun.

But along with this epochal change in the science and technology of medicine, a number of emerging moral, ethical, and public-policy issues have cast an aura of uncertainty on at least some of the genetic manipulations that are becoming feasible (Anderson and Fletcher, 1980; Fletcher, 1983, 1985; Walters, 1986, 1991). Although a reasonable consensus has emerged concerning the scientific, public-policy, and ethical aspects of somatic-cell gene therapy (i.e., treatment of just the "body" cells, not germ-line cells, of the patient), still unresolved are the ethical issues surrounding germ-line gene therapy and enhancement genetic engineering.

Strategies for gene therapy

The goal of gene therapy is to treat human diseases by correcting the genetic defects that underlie the genetic disorders or by adding new genes to some of the patient's cells in order to provide or bolster a therapeutic function (e.g., to help the immune cells fight cancer in the body).

There are three general approaches to genetic correction of human disease. The first, called ex vivo, involves the removal of cells from the patient, correction of the cells outside the body by the addition of the normal gene, and the subsequent return of the corrected cells to the patient in a way that allows the new function to be expressed and to ameliorate the disease. Most of the over one hundred currently approved gene-transfer clinical protocols use this approach.

The second approach, called in situ, introduces the new gene directly into the site of disease in the patient (e.g., into a cancer mass, or into the lining of the pulmonary tree in cystic fibrosis). The gene can be introduced either in the form of a virus vector or even as naked DNA.

The third approach, called in vivo, is less well studied than the other two methods because vectors have not been built that can be injected directly into the bloodstream and that will carry the therapeutic gene to the proper tissue in a safe and efficient manner. When an injectable vector is developed, however, then gene therapy will become as simple to administer as insulin or penicillin therapy is now.

Gene augmentation. All current gene-therapy clinical protocols are based on the concept of adding a normal gene to the genome rather than replacing or correcting the aberrant gene already present (Friedmann, 1989; Anderson, 1992; Miller, 1992; Mulligan, 1993). Implied in this approach are the notions that the newly added gene will be introduced into a location in the genome different from the site of the defective gene and that the expression of the new gene will override the effects of the aberrant gene (which will remain and continue to be expressed as it was before the genetic correction). This concept is likely to be valid for a large number of human disorders, especially for those caused by the absence of an enzymic function—the "loss of function" defects.

In cases in which the genetic defect underlying a disease is a "gain of function" defect (in which the very presence of the genetic error and its expression is damaging to normal cellular function), the simple addition of a normal copy of the involved gene might not have an ameliorative effect on the resulting disease. In such cases, means must be found to "turn off" or otherwise interfere with the expression of the defective gene. Approaches toward this goal are being developed and involve the use of "gene knockout" manipulations, "antisense" segments that interfere specifically with an individual gene, as well as other ingenious approaches.

Methods for gene transfer

Viral vectors. Agents exist in nature to carry out precisely the job that is needed for clinically useful gene transfer. These agents include the several classes of viruses that have evolved to introduce their genetic information into infected target cells and to allow those genes to become a permanent, heritable, and functional part of the host-cell genome. Not only have viruses evolved mechanisms to carry out this function, but they do so with very high efficiency. The newly introduced gene is, for all intents and purposes, a new cellular gene. Of course, viruses have their own evolutionary purposes for carrying out their genetic transfers, often producing deleterious effects on the infected cells. By finding ways to inactivate or remove the viral genes and replace them with the desired therapeutic genetic material, it has been possible to take advantage of the high efficiency of gene transfer by infectious viral agents to allow therapeutic applications.

These techniques were developed during the 1980s with several classes of viruses, including those that use DNA as well as those that use ribonucleic acid (RNA) as their genetic material. Because of the extensive work in the 1960s on the DNA-containing papova tumor viruses (such as SV40 and polyoma) and the discovery that they produce tumors by integrating their tumor-causing genes (oncogenes) into the genome of the infected cells, the earliest efforts for eventual clinical application of viral gene transfer centered around the development of disarmed and clinically useful delivery systems from these DNA viruses. Despite their initial promise, the small DNA-containing tumor viruses have not proven to be good models for clinically applied gene transfer.

In the case of the larger DNA viruses, such as the adenoviruses and herpes viruses, efficient vectors have recently been developed and, in the case of adenovirus, are presently being used to carry a normal copy of the cystic fibrosis gene into the lining of the pulmonary airways in patients with cystic fibrosis. Vectors derived from both adenoviruses and herpes viruses have the advantage of being able to introduce foreign genetic information into cells that are no longer replicating or are replicating very slowly, such as the neurons of the central and peripheral nervous systems, hepatocytes, and epithelial cells of the normal mammalian airway.

The majority of the over one hundred approved clinical protocols use retroviruses—agents that have an RNA genome and that make DNA copies of their genomes through the action of the enzyme "reverse transcriptase." The resulting DNA copy becomes integrated into the genome of the infected host cells and the genes carried by the viral DNA continue to be expressed in the cell, often stably and permanently, without any discernible damage to the cell.

In the early 1980s, techniques were developed for removing the potentially deleterious viral genes and replacing them with potentially therapeutic nonviral genes. During the subsequent few years, a number of workers demonstrated that such viruses were able to infect many of the important target cells involved in human genetic disease, including bone-marrow cells, hepatocytes, blood lymphocytes and other white cells, skin fibroblasts and keratinocytes, and vascular endothelial cells. Furthermore, it was shown that the expression of a newly introduced gene, transferred into genetically defective human cells via retroviral vectors, resulted in the correction of disease-specific defects in the cells. Through the work of many investigators, retroviral vectors have now reached a state of refinement and efficiency that satisfies most of the potential scientific, public-policy, and ethical concerns, and thus has allowed clinical application to proceed rapidly.

The first federally approved use of a retroviral vector in a human patient took place on May 22, 1989, at the Clinical Center of the National Institutes of Health (NIH) in Bethesda, Maryland. A 52-year-old man suffering from malignant melanoma received an infusion of his own immune blood cells (specifically, tumor-infiltrating lymphocytes [TIL]) into which had been inserted a marker (i.e., nontherapeutic gene). The purpose of the study was threefold: (1) to determine if gene transfer could be safely carried out in human patients; (2) to determine if gene-modified cells could be recovered from human patients; and (3) to determine if gene-marked TIL could be used to better understand how these cells combat cancer. All three of these objectives were realized (Rosenberg et al., 1990).

The first approved gene-therapy protocol began on September 14, 1990, also at the NIH. A four-year-old girl suffering from adenosine deaminase (ADA) deficiency (a genetic disease that produces a severe immunodeficiency disease) was given back her own immune cells (specifically her blood T lymphocytes) that had been corrected by inserting a normal copy of an ADA gene. At the time of gene therapy she had a very weak immune system, was constantly ill, and had to be quarantined to avoid contact with other children to protect her from common childhood infections that were potentially lethal for her. Within a few weeks after gene therapy began, her immune system showed improvement, and after several months she began living a relatively normal life (Culver et al., 1991; Anderson, 1992).

By the end of 1994, over one hundred gene-therapy/transfer clinical protocols had been approved worldwide. Most of them were in centers in the United States, but several protocols in Europe and Asia had been initiated. Most of these protocols used retroviral vectors to transfer the desired gene into a patient's cells ex vivo, followed by readministration of the modified cells to the patient. The target diseases for these protocols are discussed below.

Physical methods. There are a number of nonviral methods that can be used to transfer functional new "foreign" genes into defective human or other animal cells, but the efficiency of most of these procedures is low. The observation in the 1970s that the simple inorganic salt called calcium phosphate can form complexes with DNA and that the mixture is taken into cells provided a major impetus for molecular biologists to study mechanisms of gene expression in mammalian cells. However, even at its best, this procedure is very inefficient when compared with viral gene transfer.

In a clinical experiment attempted in 1980 by Martin Cline and his colleagues, the calcium phosphate gene-transfer approach was used in two patients suffering from thalassemia, a disease characterized by poor hemoglobin production resulting in severe anemia. Cline and his colleagues tried to introduce the normal beta globin gene into cells of the bone marrow in these two patients. In addition to the technical problems of poor efficiency of gene transfer and uncertainty over the appropriate target cells, the experiment had not been approved by Cline's university committees nor by the federal regulatory agencies with jurisdiction over human experimentation. The result was that Cline was punished by both his university (with loss of administrative responsibility) and by the federal government (by loss of grant support for his research). The experiment itself was unsuccessful. As a result of this unfortunate initial experience with gene therapy, clearer restrictions on the use of gene-transfer tools on human subjects were developed, including the establishment of the Human Gene Therapy Subcommittee under the Recombinant DNA Advisory Committee of the National Institutes of Health (Thompson, 1994).

Many modifications of physically mediated gene transfer have been made. Of particular interest are the methods that rely on the entrapment of the incoming DNA within lipid vesicles (liposomes) or other lipid complexes (lipofection). Another important technology is microinjection, in which the DNA is inserted directly into the nucleus of the target cell by means of a tiny glass needle. The primary use of microinjection has been in the production of transgenic mice and farm animals by inserting new genes into fertilized ova ex vivo and then placing the gene-modified ova into surrogate mothers for development.

Collectively, these methods have been used effectively in tissue-culture applications and in some animal studies. But even the improved efficiencies of these methods compared with previous ones have not allowed gene transfer to be carried out with sufficient ease and efficiency to permit human clinical application except for the use of liposomes and lipofection.

Tissue targeting.   In vivo delivery of genes for the correction of human disease will be carried out by introducing the corrective normal genes (carried in a viral or nonviral vector) directly into the bloodstream or into the appropriate organ or tissue in the body of the patient. Assuming that it would be unnecessary and possibly undesirable to introduce new genes into tissues that would not need to express the new function, the incoming therapeutic genetic information should be targeted specifically to those cells in which expression of a normal version of the gene is required.

There are at least two approaches to providing such tissue specificity. One approach would be to accept the notion that a delivery vector used in vivo, whether it be a virus or a physical reagent, might be somewhat nonspecific (i.e., "leaky" or promiscuous) in its recognition of target cells, while retaining the possibility of conferring tissue specificity onto genes by incorporating into the vector the appropriate promoters, enhancers, and other regulatory signals to allow expression only in selected target cells. Many such tissue-specific regulatory sequences have now been described, and in some cases they provide relatively tight tissue-specific gene expression.

The second potential approach to tissue specificity, which could be used in combination with the first, would be through the delivery of the therapeutic exogenous genes, in the form of viral vectors or a chemical reagent, only to the organ or tissue in which expression is desired. To deliver a gene specifically to the liver in an animal, one might be able to take advantage of the fact that cells of the liver, like the cells of probably all other organs, express "receptors" on their surface that are different from those found on other tissues. A variety of tissue-specific proteins and receptors are expressed on the surface of cells, and these molecules might eventually represent suitable targets for the design of tissue-specific vectors carrying therapeutic or toxic genes.

Sequence correction and gene replacement.
An ideal but presently impossible method of gene therapy would rely on the specific correction of a genetic error (i.e., mutation) responsible for a disease. For instance, one might imagine ways to correct specifically the genetic mutation responsible for sickle-cell anemia (a single base change in one position of the gene for the hemoglobin protein beta globin) without modifying any other positions in the genome. An extended version of this approach might be to remove larger portions of mutant genes or possibly even entire genes from disease-affected cells and to replace the mutant genetic information at this normal position in the genome with a normal copy of those genetic segments.

Until several years ago, there was no way to even begin carrying out this task. However, a number of geneticists have recently developed methods for making specific genetic changes at specific sites by "homologous recombination." This technique relies on a segment of normal gene, together with some attached genetic material, being introduced into defective animal cells that direct the incoming normal sequence to the correct location in the genome. Once the newly added normal sequence has found its proper site, normal cellular machinery carries out the steps that allow the normal sequence to replace the defective sequence. The efficiency of homologous recombination is still very low and not useful for clinical applications, but ultimately this will be a method of choice for genetic correction.

Disease targets.   There are a large number of diseases that are the subject of gene-therapy protocols. It should be pointed out that all the initial gene-therapy trials are designed to test safety and, as of late 1994, there were no side effects or adverse reactions recognized to have been caused by a transferred gene.

One might imagine that only the simple, single-gene disorders would be suitable candidates for gene therapy. Examples would be the six genetic diseases presently undergoing trials: ADA deficiency, cystic fibrosis, hemophilia, familial hypercholesterolemia, Gaucher's disease, and alpha-1 antitrypsin deficiency. However, geneticists are now beginning to discover the genetic components underlying some of the common human diseases that result from the faulty interactions of several genes. These disorders include diabetes, hypertension, coronary vascular disease and arteriosclerosis, most forms of cancer, and others. Surprisingly, the number of genes involved in these apparently complex trials may not be as great as previously thought, and there is now optimism that the genetic basis for these human disorders will become understood in the not-too-distant future.

Because of their genetic component, many of these complex diseases are now the subject of gene-therapy protocols. In fact, over 60 percent of all the presently approved clinical protocols are for the study and/or treatment of cancer. In addition, there are a number of gene-therapy protocols approved for the treatment of AIDS.

Since most human disorders are probably a reflection of the interaction of environmental conditions with genetic factors, it seems safe to say that genetic attacks on most human disease will eventually become possible.

Nontherapeutic genetic modification. In the early 1970s, the concept of gene therapy was entirely foreign to the realities of medicine. The necessary tools and techniques had not become available. For that reason, there was little urgency in defining the ethical, social, and public-policy issues that such genetic manipulations might produce. There are very few remaining technical, medical, public-policy, or ethical doubts concerning the justification for somatic-cell gene therapy for otherwise inadequately treated human disease. However, the same tools and techniques being developed for the therapy of human disease are also available for nontherapeutic genetic manipulation of human beings.

As with other innovative medical interventions, therapy is aimed at severe disorders that are universally viewed as errors that provide no benefit to the patient, family, or species, and thus are to be avoided or treated whenever possible. Our human inability to accept the harmful consequences of our human genetic legacy is the rationalization underlying medicine itself. Most medical, scientific, theological, and metaphysical traditions of both the Western and Eastern worlds accept the concept that, while human disease is a reflection of entirely normal and expected processes of nature, its appearance in the form of human disease and suffering is to be fought. There are certainly some traditions that hold that human happiness comes from an ability to accept natural processes. But despite that view, the alleviation of suffering caused by human disease is generally considered a moral good and even a moral imperative.

However, forms of medical treatment are occasionally directed toward less obvious pathological conditions, and, to a greater or lesser extent, our societies have come to accept medical approaches to these conditions as well as to more obvious pathological states. Medical intervention is already practiced for the enhancement of a variety of both disease-related and non–disease-related human traits. Plastic surgery is generally not condemned as unethical or unacceptable. Will the same attitude pertain to genetic approaches to the modification of non–disease-related human characteristics?

Compared with the acceptance of genetic correction of obvious "disease," arguments have been raised against enhancement genetic engineering, such as the use of gene manipulation to try to improve or enhance characteristics such as size, skin color, and intelligence. These characteristics certainly have major genetic components, and it therefore seems likely that they can and will become susceptible to genetic modification. To the extent that defects in these traits constitute truly damaging errors or disease, they ought to, and will, be treated with all the tools at our command. But to the extent that they are not errors but rather normal human variations, the pursuit of forms of enhancement genetic modification is fraught with risks for society.

What are the potential risks? They fall into three categories: medical, societal, and philosophical (Anderson, 1989, 1990).

Medical. Gene transfer could be medically hazardous in ways we cannot now predict. We understand very little about how the human body works. We know roughly how a simple gene operates, but we have only a limited conception of how body organs develop and function. Even though we do not understand how a human body is directed by its genes, we can now begin to change those genes. We know of the danger of disrupting a tumor suppressor gene or activating an oncogene. There might be other types of genes that could be inadvertently affected that would produce detrimental results. We can predict the risks of cosmetic surgery; we cannot predict, at present, the risks of genetic engineering.

The concern is that, at this point in the development of our scientific expertise, we do not have sufficient knowledge to risk gene transfer except where there is clear benefit, such as in the treatment or prevention of serious disease. It may be that there is very little risk from gene transfer. Experience from therapeutic protocols will provide that information.

Societal. Gene transfer for enhancement purposes would require moral decisions our society is not now prepared to make. Let us assume, while considering the following scenarios, that there are no medical risks at all from genetic engineering.

1. What if a human gene were cloned that could produce a brain chemical resulting in markedly increased memory capacity in monkeys after gene transfer? Insertion of the gene into patients with severe memory impairment resulted in marked improvement. Should a normal person be allowed to receive such a gene on request?

2. Should a prepubescent adolescent whose parents are both five feet tall be provided with a growth hormone gene on request?

3. Should a worker who is continually exposed to an industrial toxin receive a gene to provide resistance to this toxin at the worker's or the employer's request?

These scenarios suggest three problems that would be difficult for our society to resolve: What genes should be provided; who should receive a gene; and how to prevent discrimination against individuals who do or do not receive a gene.

What gene? There is general agreement that it would be ethically appropriate to use gene transfer for treatment of serious disease. But what distinguishes a serious disease from a "minor" disease or from a genetic variation? Does the absence of growth hormone that results in a growth limitation to two feet in height represent a serious disease? What about a limitation to a height of four feet? to five feet? Each observer might draw the lines between serious disease, minor disease, and genetic variation differently. But all can agree that there are extreme cases that clearly represent serious disease. Once one moves into the gray area beyond serious disease, it is difficult to ascertain any rational stopping point.

Who should receive? If the position is established that only patients suffering from serious diseases are candidates for gene insertion, then the issues of patient selection are no different from other medical situations: The determination is based on medical need within a supply-and-demand framework. But if the use of gene transfer extends to allowing a normal individual to acquire, for example, a memory-enhancing gene, profound problems could result. On what basis is the decision made to allow one individual, but not another, to receive the gene? Should it go to those best able to benefit society (the smartest)? To those most in need? To those with low intelligence? If so, how low? Will enhancing memory help a mentally retarded child? Should it go to those chosen by a lottery, or to those who can afford to pay? As long as our society lacks a significant consensus about these answers, the best way to make equitable decisions in such cases is to base them on the seriousness of the objective medical need rather than on the personal wishes or resources of an individual.

Discrimination? If individuals are carriers of a disease (e.g., sickle-cell anemia), would they be pressured to be treated? Would they have difficulty in obtaining health insurance unless they agreed to be treated? These are ethical issues also raised by genetic screening and by the Human Genome Project. But the concerns would become even more troublesome if there were the possibility for "correction" by the use of gene transfer. Finally, we must face the issue of eugenics, the attempt to make hereditary "improvements." The abuse of power that societies have historically demonstrated in the pursuit of eugenic goals is well documented. Might we slide into a new age of eugenic thinking by starting with small "improvements"? It would be difficult, if not impossible, to determine where to draw a line if enhancement engineering were to begin.

Philosophical. The power of genetic engineering forces us to reflect on the question: What does it mean to be human? Adding an occasional gene here and there is not going to alter who and what we are as a human race. But once again the "slippery slope" argument arises: If we draw no lines, if we accept that people have a right to make what they want of their lives, then we condone the right of humans to manipulate their ge-

nomes in the absence of any real knowledge of what they are doing. Might we add here and alter there until we become a society of chimeras, uncertain of who we are? Probably not. Humans adjust. Perhaps society a hundred years from now will consider genome manipulation as standard. But what that future society might do is not our concern. It is our responsibility to enter the genetic engineering era in as responsible a way as possible. Our society is relatively comfortable with the use of genetic engineering to treat individuals with serious disease. Until we have acquired far greater wisdom than we now have, it can be argued that gene transfer should never be used in attempts to make ourselves "better."

Germ-line genetic modification. The above discussion has centered around genetic modification of the somatic, nonreproductive cells in a patient's body. As long as the exogenous therapeutic gene is delivered only to the somatic cells of the patient, a therapeutic effect would be limited to the treated patient and would not affect progeny or future generations. Of course, it is known that foreign genes can, under some circumstances, be introduced into the reproductive (germ) cells of animals and expressed in future generations. Animals carrying foreign exogenous genes in their germ line (transgenic animals) have been produced using mice, rats, rabbits, and some domestic livestock, implying that the techniques for producing transgenic human beings are already available. In these studies, foreign genes are introduced into a fertilized egg either by direct microinjection or by injection with a viral vector. The resulting genetically modified embryo is returned to a surrogate female who then carries the pregnancy to term and delivers the genetically modified offspring.

This gene-transfer procedure is now standard in many molecular genetics laboratories. The technical problems that prevent attempts to carry out similar studies aimed at the production of genetically modified human beings are seen in the inefficiency and the major risks inherent to the procedure in animals (Anderson, 1984). In the case of the animal most readily available for study, the mouse, the appearance of transgenic animals even in the most experienced hands can be as low as 2 to 10 percent with the rest of the ova being damaged or killed. This high level of damage to ova constitutes, at present, an ethical barrier to human experiments.

The ethical discussion of germ-line gene therapy is well underway (Fowler et al., 1989; Lappé, 1991; Mauron and Thevoz, 1991; Zimmerman, 1991; Munson and Davis, 1992; Davis, 1992; Neel, 1993; Danks, 1994). It has been argued (Anderson, 1985; Fletcher and Anderson, 1992) that there are three criteria that need to be satisfied before it would be ethical to attempt germ-line gene therapy in humans:

1. Considerable experience (over a number of years) with somatic-cell gene therapy that clearly estab-

lishes the effectiveness and safety of treatment of so-matic cells

2. Adequate animal studies that establish the reproducibility, reliability, and safety of germ-line gene therapy, using the same vectors and procedures that would be used in humans

3. Public awareness and approval of the procedure since unborn generations will be affected. The gene pool is a joint possession of all members of society. Since germ-line therapy will affect the gene pool, the public should have a thorough understanding of the implications of this form of treatment. Only when an informed public has indicated its support, through the various avenues open for society to express its views, should clinical trials begin.

Conclusion

Gene therapy has the potential for providing mankind with enormous good. It is our responsibility to establish adequate safeguards to prevent abuses so that the full power of this technology can be realized by society.

W. FRENCH ANDERSON
THEODORE FRIEDMANN

Directly related to this article is the companion article in this entry: ETHICAL AND SOCIAL ISSUES. *For a further discussion of topics mentioned in this article, see the entries* EUGENICS; GENETICS AND ENVIRONMENT IN HUMAN HEALTH; HEALTH AND DISEASE; HUMAN NATURE; *and* JUSTICE. *For a discussion of related ideas, see the entries* GENOME MAPPING AND SEQUENCING; MEDICINE, PHILOSOPHY OF; *and* RISK. *See also the entries* BIOTECHNOLOGY; *and* TECHNOLOGY, *articles on* PHILOSOPHY OF TECHNOLOGY, *and* TECHNOLOGY ASSESSMENT.

Bibliography

ANDERSON, W. FRENCH. 1972. "Genetic Therapy." In *The New Genetics and the Future of Man*, pp. 109–124. Edited by Michael Pollack Hamilton. Grand Rapids, Mich.: William B. Eerdmans.

———. 1984. "Prospects for Human Gene Therapy." *Science* 226, no. 4673:401–409.

———. 1985. "Human Gene Therapy: Scientific and Ethical Considerations." *Journal of Medicine and Philosophy* 10, no. 3:275–291.

———. 1989. "Human Gene Therapy: Why Draw a Line?" *Journal of Medicine and Philosophy* 14, no. 6:681–693.

———. 1990. "Genetics and Human Malleability." *Hastings Center Report* 20, no. 1:21–24.

———. 1992. "Human Gene Therapy." *Science* 256, no. 5058:808–813.

ANDERSON, W. FRENCH, and FLETCHER, JOHN C. 1980. "Gene Therapy in Human Beings: When Is It Ethical to Begin?" *New England Journal of Medicine* 303, no. 22:1293–1297.

APOSHIAN, H. VASKEN. 1970. "The Use of DNA for Gene Therapy—the Need, Experimental Approach, and Implications." *Perspectives in Biology and Medicine* 14, no. 1: 987–1108.

CULVER, KENNETH W.; ANDERSON, W. FRENCH; and BLAESE, R. MICHAEL. 1991. "Lymphocyte Gene Therapy." *Human Gene Therapy* 2, no. 2:107–109.

DANKS, DAVID M. 1994. "Germ-Line Gene Therapy: No Place in Treatment of Genetic Disease." *Human Gene Therapy* 5, no. 2:151–152.

DAVIS, BERNARD D. 1970. "Prospects for Genetic Intervention in Man." *Science* 170, no. 2:1279–1283.

———. 1992. "Germ-Line Therapy: Evolutionary and Moral Considerations." *Human Gene Therapy* 3, no. 4:361–363.

FLETCHER, JOHN C. 1983. "Moral Problems and Ethical Issues in Prospective Human Gene Therapy." *Virginia Law Review* 69, no. 3:515–546.

———. 1985. "Ethical Issues In and Beyond Prospective Clinical Trials of Human Gene Therapy." *Journal of Medicine and Philosophy* 10, no. 3:293–309.

FLETCHER, JOHN C., and ANDERSON, W. FRENCH. 1992. "Germ-Line Gene Therapy: A New Stage of Debate." *Law, Medicine, and Health Care* 20, nos. 1–2:26–39.

FOWLER, GREGORY; JUENGST, ERIC T.; and ZIMMERMAN, BURKE K. 1989. "Germ-Line Gene Therapy and the Clinical Ethos of Medical Genetics." *Theoretical Medicine* 10, no. 2:151–165.

FREESE, ERNST, ed. 1972. *The Prospects of Gene Therapy.* Washington, D.C.: U.S. Government Printing Office.

FRIEDMANN, THEODORE. 1976. "The Future for Gene Therapy—a Re-evaluation." *Annals of the New York Academy of Science* 265:141–152.

———. 1983. *Gene Therapy: Fact and Fiction in Biology's New Approaches to Disease.* Cold Spring Harbor, N.Y.: Cold Spring Harbor Laboratory.

———. 1989. "Progress Toward Human Gene Therapy." *Science* 244, no. 4910:1275–1281.

———. 1990. "The Evolving Concept of Gene Therapy." *Human Gene Therapy* 1, no. 2:175–181.

———. 1992. "A Brief History of Gene Therapy." *Nature Genetics* 2, no. 2:93–98.

FRIEDMANN, THEODORE, and ROBLIN, RICHARD O. 1972. "Gene Therapy for Human Genetic Disease?" *Science* 175, no. 25:949–955.

LAPPÉ, MARC. 1991. "Ethical Issues in Manipulating the Human Germ Line." *Journal of Medicine and Philosophy* 16, no. 6:621–639.

MAURON, ALEX, and THÉVOZ, JEAN-MARIE. 1991. "Germ-Line Engineering: A Few European Voices." *Journal of Medicine and Philosophy* 16, no. 6378:649–666.

MILLER, A. DUSTY. 1992. "Human Gene Therapy Comes of Age." *Nature* 357:455–460.

MORROW, JOHN F. 1976. "The Prospects for Gene Therapy in Humans." *Annals of the New York Academy of Science* 265:13–21.

MULLIGAN, RICHARD C. 1993. "The Basic Science of Gene Therapy." *Science* 260, no. 5110:926–932.

MUNSON, RONALD, and DAVIS, LAWRENCE H. 1992. "Germ-Line Gene Therapy and the Medical Imperative." *Kennedy Institute of Ethics Journal* 2, no. 2:137–158.

NEEL, JAMES V. 1993. "Germ-Line Gene Therapy: Another View." *Human Gene Therapy* 4, no. 2:127–128.

Rosenberg, Steven A.; Aebersold, Paul; Cornetta, Kenneth; Kasid, Attan; Morgan, Richard A.; Moen, Robert; Karson, Evelyn M.; Lotze, Michael T.; Yang, James C.; Topalian, Suzanne L.; Merino, Maria J.; Culver, Kenneth; Miller, A. Dusty; Blaese, R. Michael; and Anderson, W. French. 1990. "Gene Transfer into Humans—Immunotherapy of Patients with Advanced Melanoma, Using Tumor-Infiltrating Lymphocytes Modified by Retroviral Gene Transduction." *New England Journal of Medicine* 323, no. 9:570–578.

Sinsheimer, Robert L. 1969. "The Prospect for Designed Genetic Change." *American Scientist* 57, no. 1:134–142.

Tatum, Edward L. 1966. "Molecular Biology, Nucleic Acids and the Future of Medicine." *Perspectives in Biology and Medicine* 10, no. 1:19–32.

Thompson, Larry. 1994. *Correcting the Code: Inventing the Genetic Cure for the Human Body.* New York: Simon and Schuster.

Walters, LeRoy. 1986. "The Ethics of Human Gene Therapy." *Nature* 320, no. 6059:225–227.

———. 1991. "Human Gene Therapy: Ethics and Public Policy." *Human Gene Therapy* 2, no. 2:115–122.

Wolff, Jon A., and Lederberg, Joshua. 1994. "An Early History of Gene Transfer and Therapy." *Human Gene Therapy* 5, no. 4:469–480.

Zimmerman, Burke K. 1991. "Human Germ-Line Therapy: The Case for Its Development and Use." *Journal of Medicine and Philosophy* 16, no. 6:593–612.

II. ETHICAL AND SOCIAL ISSUES

There are four possible types of human genetic intervention that can be performed on individuals. Such intervention can be targeted either toward an individual's somatic (nonreproductive) cells or toward germ-line (reproductive) cells. Similarly, the goal of genetic intervention may be the cure or prevention of disease or it may be the enhancement of human capabilities. These two pairs of alternatives can be represented schematically in a two-by-two matrix:

	Somatic	Germ-Line
Cure or Prevention of Disease	1	2
Enhancement of Capabilities	3	4

This article focuses on the first two of the four possible types of human genetic intervention.

Milestones in the public discussion of gene therapy

The years 1950 to 1969. In the first half of the twentieth century imaginative anticipations of the human genetic future appeared in the writings of J. B. S. Haldane (1924), Aldous Huxley (1932), and Hermann J. Muller (1935). A qualitatively new phase in the

public discussion began after World War II. Human genetics began to emerge as a distinct field; one concrete illustration of this emergence was the creation of a new journal, *The American Journal of Human Genetics,* in 1949. A decade later, the centennial of Charles Darwin's *The Origin of Species* gave biologists an opportunity to reflect on the past course of human evolution and on the likely future of the human race.

H. J. Muller's 1959 essay "The Guidance of Human Evolution" was almost certainly the most important stimulus to the genetic-intervention debate of the early 1960s. In the essay Muller, a classical geneticist, expressed doubt about the feasibility of "making direct alterations or substitutions of a desired kind in the genetic material itself" (Muller, 1959, p. 36). He expressed a strong preference for improving the human condition by the widespread, voluntary use of artificial insemination and other new reproductive methods. Muller's description of the human genetic load, or harmful mutations (Muller, 1950), and his self-consciously radical proposal for counteracting that load provided a major impetus for a series of conferences held in the 1960s (Hoagland and Burhoe, 1962; Wolstenholme, 1963; Sonnenborn, 1965; Roslansky, 1966). The important book by Theodosius Dobzhansky, *Mankind Evolving: The Evolution of the Human Species,* was also written at least in part as a response to Muller's views about the increasing burden of the human genetic load and to what Dobzhansky termed "Muller's bravest new world" (Dobzhansky, 1962).

The CIBA Foundation symposium held in London in November of 1962 on the theme "Man and His Future" provided an interesting snapshot of the then-prevailing views about human genetic intervention (Wolstenholme, 1963). At the symposium J. B. S. Haldane, Julian Huxley, Joshua Lederberg, and H. J. Muller (through a paper—he did not attend) shared ideas about both the goals and possible methods of deliberate genetic modification. Four strategies for achieving genetic change were considered by symposium participants: (1) voluntary artificial insemination using sperm from donors of "high genetic quality"; (2) direct intervention in the human germ-line to produce heritable changes; (3) genetic modification of somatic cells to achieve desired changes in the individual; and (4) clonal reproduction. Only the second and third of these techniques are pertinent to this article.

The CIBA Foundation symposium participants seemed to agree that germ-line intervention at the molecular level would be more difficult than the modification of somatic cells and that the enhancement of human capabilities would be more difficult than the cure of disease. The participants' anticipations of somatic-cell techniques are particularly interesting in the light of subsequent developments. J. B. S. Haldane envisioned "the deliberate provocation of mutations"; he also suggested that it might one day be possible to "synthesize new genes and introduce them into human chromosomes" or to "duplicate existing genes" for the same purpose (Haldane, 1963, p. 353). Joshua Lederberg asserted that "the ultimate application of molecular biology would be the direct control of nucleotide sequences in human chromosomes, coupled with recognition, selection, and integration of the desired genes . . ." (Lederberg, 1963, p. 265). Lederberg advocated that such techniques be employed either prenatally or in the early postnatal period to modify the phenotype (the external appearance) of the developing individual rather than its genotype (the genetic makeup) (Lederberg, 1963, p. 266).

The earliest extended commentary on the ethics of human genetic intervention was authored by theologian Paul Ramsey. In a lecture presented at a 1965 symposium (Roslansky, 1966), Ramsey saw parallels between Muller's pessimism about the human genetic load and a Christian understanding of history that acknowledges divine sovereignty. Ramsey argued that the Christian ethic should be oriented toward means rather than toward even the important end of preventing Muller's genetic apocalypse. The means of artificial insemination by donor (AID) advocated by Muller were viewed by Ramsey as ethically problematic because they would separate reproduction and the expression of love. On the other hand, Ramsey affirmed a belief in the potential value of "genetic surgery" to eliminate genetic defects, both in an individual and in the reproductive cells that would be passed on to future generations (Ramsey, 1966).

Between 1965 and 1969 the academic discussion of designed genetic change in humans abated somewhat. After H. J. Muller's death in 1967, Joshua Lederberg emerged as the most prominent scientist in the genetic engineering discussion. In Europe, Jesuit theologian Karl Rahner published a major essay entitled "On the Problem of Genetic Manipulation" in 1967. Despite the relative quiescence of academic debate, the first hints of political interest in human genetic intervention became evident in March of 1968, when Lederberg and Arthur Kornberg both testified before a U.S. Senate subcommittee considering Walter Mondale's proposal to establish a National Commission on Health Science and Society (U.S. Congress, 1968). Neither scientist saw a pressing need for a national commission to consider issues in genetic engineering. In fact, organ transplantation, the definition of death, and human experimentation received more attention at the hearings than did gene therapy. Meanwhile, molecular biologists made substantial progress, synthesizing a simple viral genome in 1967 (Goulian et al., 1967) and isolating important genes from the *E. coli* bacterium in 1969 (Shapiro et al., 1969). These successes and parallel developments in the

laboratory made the technically complex task of performing genetic surgery seem more feasible.

At an interdisciplinary symposium held in December 1969, biologist Bernard Davis summarized the prospects for genetic intervention in humans as of the end of the decade (Davis, 1970). Moral theologian James Gustafson responded to the Davis paper with a paper of his own, entitled "Genetic Engineering and the Normative View of the Human." In his paper, Gustafson noted Rahner's affirmation of the human capacity for self-creation (1967) and cautiously espoused "human initiative, human freedom (if you choose) to explore, develop, expand, alter, initiate, intervene in the course of life in the world, including his own life" (Gustafson, 1973, p. 57).

The years 1970 to 1978. In the 1970s the ethical discussion of human genetic intervention was overshadowed by debates about two related but distinct topics: the ethics of genetic testing and screening, and the potential biohazards of a new form of laboratory research—recombinant DNA research. Nonetheless there were important publications on gene therapy during this time. Paul Ramsey's 1965 essay was incorporated into a 1970 book entitled *Fabricated Man: The Ethics of Genetic Control* (Ramsey, 1970). Joseph Fletcher responded to Ramsey and other cautious commentators with an article and a book advocating the widespread and vigorous use of many new genetic and reproductive technologies (Fletcher, 1971, 1974).

The first symposium to foreshadow the 1980s discussion of human gene therapy was held in May 1971 under the aegis of the National Cathedral in Washington, D.C. At this symposium, physicians W. French Anderson and Arno Motulsky, lawyer Alexander Capron, and theologian Paul Ramsey discussed somatic-cell gene therapy in categories that continued to be relevant into the 1990s (Hamilton, 1972). Several other authors also contributed to the evolving ethical literature during the decade (Friedmann and Roblin, 1972; Motulsky, 1974; Lappé and Morison, 1976; Baltimore, 1977; Howard and Rifkin, 1977).

The years 1979 to 1985. The ethical discussion of human gene therapy took a decisively international turn at the end of the 1970s. The new phase of deliberation was initiated by a 1979 conference sponsored by the World Council of Churches. At the conference one working group focused its attention on "ethical issues in the biological manipulation of life." The group's final recommendation put forward what came to be the orthodox position on gene therapy during the 1980s—that somatic-cell gene therapy for the cure of disease (Type 1 in the matrix) is ethically acceptable, while germ-line intervention for prevention or cure of disease (Type 2) or enhancement of human capabilities (Types 3 and 4) is unacceptable (Abrecht, 1980, vol. 2).

In 1980 two U.S. developments stimulated the next stage of public debate. The first was a letter from leaders of Roman Catholic, Jewish, and Protestant religious groups to then-President Jimmy Carter. The letter argued that "we are rapidly moving into a new era of fundamental danger triggered by the rapid growth of genetic engineering" (U.S. President's Commission, 1982, p. 95). The second development was public disclosure in the *Los Angeles Times* of Martin Cline's unapproved gene-therapy experiments (Jacobs, 1980). One immediate response to the Cline study was a widely cited essay by W. French Anderson and John C. Fletcher entitled "Gene Therapy in Human Beings: When Is It Ethical to Begin?" (Anderson and Fletcher, 1980).

During the years 1981 and 1982, two major parallel studies of gene therapy were conducted, one in Europe by the Parliamentary Assembly of the Council of Europe, the other in the United States by a presidential bioethics commission. The culmination of these two study processes occurred in 1982. The Parliamentary Assembly acted first, adopting a position in favor of somatic-cell gene therapy in January 1982 (Council of Europe, 1982). On the question of germ-line intervention for the cure or prevention of disease, the Parliamentary Assembly opposed "tampering" with the human genetic heritage yet expressed an almost wistful hope that a list of legitimate target diseases for germ-line approaches might be drawn up. In November of the same year, at a congressional hearing, the U.S. President's Commission on Ethical Problems in Medicine and Biomedical and Behavioral Research released its report entitled *Splicing Life* (U.S. President's Commission, 1982; U.S. Congress, 1982). The major thrust of the report was to reassure the public that currently contemplated somatic-cell approaches were not qualitatively different from other widely accepted modalities of health care. In addition, the U.S. President's Commission put forward proposals for the public oversight of gene-therapy research.

From 1983 to 1985 major policy statements on gene therapy were compiled by various special committees in Denmark (Denmark, 1984), Sweden (Sweden, 1984), and what was then West Germany (Federal Republic of Germany, 1985). In addition, Pope John Paul II devoted a major lecture to the topic (John Paul II, 1983), and the Congressional Office of Technology Assessment in the United States produced an update of the 1982 *Splicing Life* report (U.S. Congress, 1984). All of these reports and the papal address were in agreement that somatic-cell gene therapy for the cure of disease was ethically acceptable.

A second development in the years 1983 through 1985 was the discussion and creation of a public review mechanism for human gene therapy protocols in the United States. In part as a response to the problems that had surrounded the Martin Cline study, and in part because of the recommendations in the *Splicing Life* report, the Recombinant DNA Advisory Committee (RAC) of the National Institutes of Health agreed to provide review before the studies were carried out with human subjects. In the summer of 1984 the RAC created a special working group to provide initial review of such proposals, and by 1985 the RAC's working group had developed and published guidelines for somatic-cell gene-therapy protocols called "Points to Consider" (National Institutes of Health [NIH], 1985). At the end of 1985 the RAC and its working group were poised, waiting for the first clinical protocol to be submitted for public review (Walters, 1991a).

The years 1986 to 1994.   After 1985, the public discussion of gene therapy was characterized by four important developments: (1) the proliferation of policy statements on gene therapy by nations and international organizations, resulting in the establishment of national guidelines and review processes in many countries; (2) the revival of the discussion of germ-line gene therapy in the wake of its universal proscription by those national guidelines; (3) the initiation of numerous gene-therapy protocols in the United States and several other nations; and (4) the expansion of the clinical applications of somatic-cell gene-therapy techniques beyond the treatment of paradigmatic genetic diseases like severe combined immunodeficiency to other areas of medicine. Each of these developments underscored ethical and social dimensions of gene therapy that continue to affect the evaluation of advances in genetic medicine.

Between 1986 and 1994 the number of national and international policy statements regarding the issues involved in human gene therapy increased dramatically. Particularly important were the 1987 German Committee of Inquiry report (cf. Sass, 1988), the statement by the European Medical Research Councils (1988), the 1989 Swiss Amstad Report (cf. Bourrit et al., 1989), the 1990 report from the Council for International Organizations of Medical Sciences (CIOMS) (Bankowski and Capron, 1991), the 1991 French National Ethics Committee's "Avis sur la thérapie génique" (France, 1991), the 1992 British Clothier Commission Report (Great Britain, 1992), and the final report of the Canadian Royal Commission on New Reproductive Technologies (Royal Commission, 1993). These reports reflected an international consensus that properly regulated research on somatic-cell gene therapy was appropriate to pursue. As a result, by 1994 a number of nations, including Australia, Canada, France, Italy, the Netherlands, Switzerland, and the United Kingdom had established national procedures for reviewing somatic-cell gene-therapy protocols.

The most important variation within the international response to gene therapy during this period occurred with the question of germ-line gene therapy. While no public group advocated the immediate pursuit of germ-line gene therapy, responses ranged from the legal prohibition of such research (Germany), to research moratoria on any human clinical trials (European Medical Research Councils), to calls for more policy discussion of the topic in anticipation of scientific progress (Bankowski and Capron, 1991).

These official expressions of caution in turn contributed to a resurgence in the academic and public discussion of germ-line gene-therapy research. Articles developing and defending the positive case for pursuing human germ-line gene therapy appeared in the mainstream bioethics literature (Zimmerman, 1991; Munson and Davis, 1992; Wivel and Walters, 1993). Public interest groups in the United States, following the lead of their European counterparts, released position statements condemning germ-line interventions in humans (Council for Responsible Genetics, 1992). This dialogue was facilitated by the founding, in 1990, of the journal *Human Gene Therapy*, which devoted space in each issue to articles addressing the ethical and regulatory aspects of gene therapy. The journal quickly became a principal locus of discussions of the merits of germ-line research and was quickly emulated by other journals, such as the British publication *Gene Therapy*.

These statements on and discussions of gene therapy emerged against a backdrop of vigorous scientific activity during this period. Early in 1990, Michael Blaese and W. French Anderson from the NIH introduced a proposal to treat severe combined immunodeficiency in children by means of somatic-cell therapy. This disease features the almost total inactivation of a child's immune system because of the malfunctioning of a single gene, which fails to produce an essential enzyme, adenosine diaminase (ADA). Between April and August of 1990, the NIH Recombinant DNA Advisory Committee examined the Blaese-Anderson protocol. Upon the approval of the protocol by the NIH director and the U.S. Food and Drug Administration, the experiment commenced in September 1990. The initial results from the study were quite encouraging. Meanwhile, the first European gene-therapy experiment (also for ADA deficiency) was initiated in Milan in 1992.

In part because of this early success, the numbers of human somatic-cell gene-therapy protocols reviewed and approved in the United States rose dramatically during the following years. By early 1994, a total of forty-nine human gene-therapy protocols had been approved by the RAC and reviewing such protocols had become the committee's primary mission, collapsing any distinction between the RAC and its "Human Gene Therapy Subcommittee."

Meanwhile, biomedical scientists were also taking the public discussion of gene therapy in another direction. Interestingly, only twelve of the first forty-nine RAC-approved gene-therapy protocols were intended to treat health problems that had been traditionally labeled as "genetic diseases." The range of clinical strategies utilizing recombinant DNA techniques expanded almost immediately to include a variety of gene-tagging and gene-transfer techniques that did not fit the traditional conception of gene therapy. By 1994 the public had learned about gene-transfer strategies to combat a variety of cancers, human immunodeficiency virus (HIV) infection, and arthritis (McGarrity, 1991), in addition to classic genetic diseases such as cystic fibrosis and Gaucher's disease (a disorder in which fats build up in the cells).

This expansion of the applications of gene transfer techniques had the effect of enmeshing gene-therapy protocols in much larger biomedical research contexts, which often involved their own ethical and social challenges. The fact that somatic-cell gene-transfer technologies were involved began to look like a side issue in the face of the other traditional questions of research ethics that gene transfer protocols faced. Thus, for example, this period saw the gene-therapy community begin to struggle with the translation of experimental interventions into clinical practice, through the provision of gene therapy as a form of innovative clinical care, outside the public research review process (Thompson, 1993). This development raised no issues peculiar to gene therapy, but it did return the discussion to the fundamental bioethical distinction between biomedical research and innovative clinical practice on which the RAC's gene-therapy review process was based.

Ethical issues in somatic-cell gene therapy

Because somatic-cell gene therapy is in many ways an extension of traditional medical approaches—especially the administration of drugs or biologics and cell or tissue transplantation—the ethical questions surrounding the practice closely parallel those that any innovative therapy must face. The major substantive ethical questions about gene therapy have to do with the anticipated benefits and risks of this new intervention, the selection of patient-subjects, the process of informing patient-subjects or their proxies, and the preservation of privacy and confidentiality.

The risk–benefit question examines the seriousness of the disease to be treated, the existence and effectiveness of alternative therapies, and the probable benefits and harms of the genetic approach. For gene-therapy protocols, this has also meant attempting to prepare for unforeseen as well as predictable risks in designing molecular genetic interventions. In particular, this concern has focused on anticipating possible risks involved in the delivery and integration of DNA into the subject's cells, including the risk of germ-line effects (Temin, 1990).

In the case of the Blaese-Anderson proposal to treat severe combined immunodeficiency in children, there was immediate agreement on the life-threatening character of the disease. For children with a matched sibling donor, a bone marrow transplant was often a permanently effective treatment. For other children there did exist an alternative but very expensive treatment: an enzyme treatment derived from cattle. However, the researchers argued that the genetic modification and reintroduction of a child's own T-lymphocytes might provide even greater benefit. The potential risks of genetically modified cells had been studied in mice and monkeys, as well as in the human subjects of a gene-marking study initiated in 1989. On the efficacy side, there were promising data from one study of mice performed in Milan, Italy.

The selection of patient-subjects was included as an ethical issue to be considered for reasons that stretch back to the early use of renal dialysis in Seattle, Washington. In the early 1960s, when renal dialysis was a scarce resource, a local review committee considered which patients with end-stage renal disease were the most fitting candidates for dialysis. In similar fashion, organ procurement agencies and transplant centers have, over time, developed guidelines for choosing among the large numbers of candidates for cadaver kidneys, hearts, and lungs. In the case of the Blaese-Anderson protocol, severe combined immunodeficiency caused by ADA deficiency was so rare that all children with the disorder who had no matched sibling donors were in principle eligible for the protocol. Yet, even within this group of eligible children, choices had to be made among children of different ages and differing disease severity.

The need for informed consent by patient-subjects is one of the central tenets of research ethics. Thus, it is no surprise that this issue would be considered in ethical discussions about gene therapy. A complicating factor with gene therapy is that the proposed intervention is technically at the cutting edge of research and requires that patient-subjects have at least a basic understanding of molecular biology. In the case of the Blaese-Anderson protocol, a basic knowledge of immunology was also important. Effective techniques for conveying complex technical information to laypeople do exist and should be employed in the consent process for these and all research protocols. One special issue in gene therapy is the fact that the subjects will often be in relatively desperate clinical circumstances, which can exert a powerful influence on the motivations of the subjects, their families, and their physicians. Since many potential gene-therapy subjects will be in quite vulnerable circumstances, extra

review precautions may be required to ensure that their participation is voluntary. Thus, the influence of clinical desperation needs to be taken into account.

The protection of privacy and confidentiality for the pioneer patient-subjects in gene-therapy research is also important. In other cases involving innovative therapy—for example, in the early heart transplants, the first birth after in vitro fertilization, and the use of a baboon heart in a child—a virtual media circus has surrounded both the subjects and the research team. A proper approach to patient-subjects will not isolate them from public view but will attempt to strike a balance between disclosure to an interested public and respect for their privacy.

Finally, as somatic-cell gene-therapy techniques begin to show promise within the confines of the research setting, the process of their translation into clinical use will raise issues. Concern to prevent the premature adoption of unvalidated genetic interventions will increasingly have to be weighed against the claims of patients seeking access to the clinical benefits that new techniques might offer.

These ethical considerations for human gene-therapy research are not unique to this practice. In fact, they can be viewed as derivations from, or approximations of, several venerable principles of biomedical ethics. The risk–benefit question is obviously related to the principle of beneficence. Both informed consent and the protection of privacy and confidentiality have their primary roots in the principle of autonomy. Fairness in the selection of patient-subjects is clearly an application of the principle of justice.

In addition to these substantive issues, there is an important procedural issue to be raised about gene therapy. Because special public concern seems to surround the genetic technologies, most countries have created national public review mechanisms to evaluate human gene-therapy protocols, at least during the early years of somatic-cell gene therapy. The result of this process has been both public education about and public confidence in this new approach to disease. It is possible that a similar approach would have been useful in the early years of past biomedical innovations, for example, cardiac transplantation and in vitro fertilization. In the future the evolving ethic of biomedical research may require a similar public review process for other major biomedical innovations, as a complement to the important work of local research ethics committees.

Ethical issues in germ-line gene therapy

The major difference between somatic-cell gene therapies and clinical techniques aimed at germ-line genetic intervention is that the latter would produce clinical changes that could be transmitted to the offspring of the person receiving the intervention. This simple difference is often the only consideration cited in the many official statements that endorse somatic-cell gene-therapy trials while proscribing or postponing research aimed at developing human germ-line gene-therapy techniques. Behind these official statements, however, lies a longer argument, revolving around four sets of concerns: scientific uncertainties; the need to use resources efficiently; social risks; and conflicting human rights concerns.

Scientific uncertainties.

Even the proponents of germ-line gene therapy agree that human trials under our current state of knowledge would be unacceptable. In order for gene-therapy techniques to be effective, the genes must be stably integrated, expressed correctly only in the appropriate tissues, and reliably targeted to the correct location on a chromosome. If the intervention cannot eliminate the parents' risk of transmitting the alleles (alternative forms of a gene that can be located at a particular site on the chromosome) they carry, or can only do so by substituting other genetic risks, its promise remains weak. Critics maintain that, given the complexity of gene regulation and expression during human development, germ-line gene-therapy experiments will always involve too many unpredictable long-term iatrogenic (physician-caused) risks to the transformed subjects and their offspring to be justifiable (Council for Responsible Genetics, 1993).

Proponents, however, respond that our current ignorance only justifies postponing human trials of germ-line therapy techniques until their promise can be improved. A more optimistic reading turns the argument around: To the extent that the barriers to effective therapy can be overcome, its promise should encourage research to continue. Proponents add that, by focusing on the obvious barriers to performing clinical trials today, critics of germ-line therapy ignore the fact that it will take further research to determine whether or not current barriers should ultimately dissuade society from contemplating clinical trials in the future (Munson and Davis, 1992).

Proponents bolster their technological optimism with an argument from medical utility: that germ-line gene therapy offers the only true cure for many diseases. If illnesses are understood to be, at root, "molecular diseases," then therapeutic interventions at any level above the causal gene can only be symptomatic. From this perspective, all gene therapies involving simply the addition of genes are palliative measures on the road to complete "gene surgery," which could involve the excision of the pathological alleles from the organism (Zimmerman, 1991).

Allocation of resources.

One common criticism of the argument from medical utility is that it betrays a reductionistic attitude that fails to appreciate approaches that could achieve the same ends more efficiently. Since it must become possible to identify target pre-embryos before their transformation, the argument goes, it would be more efficient to simply use the same techniques to identify healthy pre-embryos for implantation (Mauron and Thévoz, 1991). Many clinical geneticists argue that even our current methods of prenatal screening serve this function. Against these convenient, effective approaches, they conclude, germ-line gene-therapy techniques will never be cost-effective enough to merit high enough social priority to pursue.

One scientific rejoinder that is made to this argument is that screening will not help with all cases. Presumably, for example, as more beneficiaries of somatic-cell gene therapy survive to reproductive age, there will be more couples whose members are both afflicted with the same recessive disorder (Walters, 1991b). Gene-therapy strategies that affect the germ line may also be the only effective ways of addressing some genetic diseases, such as those with origins very early in development. And by preventing the transmission of disease genes, germ-line gene therapy would obviate the need for screening or costly and risky somatic-cell gene therapy in subsequent generations of particular families.

Social risks.

Proponents of germ-line gene-therapy research also can point out that screening prevents genetic disease only by preventing the birth of the patients who would suffer from it. This, they point out, is a confusion of therapeutic goals that runs the long-term risk of encouraging coercive eugenic practices and tacitly fostering discrimination against those with genetic disease. By attempting to prevent disease in individuals rather than selecting against individuals according to their genotype, proponents argue, germ-line gene therapy would allow us to maintain our commitment to the value of moral equality in the face of biological diversity (Catholic Health Association, 1990).

Critics reply to this that, on the contrary, it is germ-line gene therapy that has the more ominous social implications, by opening the door to genetic enhancement. One line of argument recalls the historical abuses of the eugenics movement to suggest that, to the extent that the line between gene therapy and enhancement would increasingly blur, germ-line interventions would be open to the same questions about the proper vision of human flourishing that eugenics faced. Even those who dispute the dangers of the "slippery slope" in this context take pains to defend the moral significance of the distinction "between uses that may relieve real suffering and those that alter characteristics that have little or nothing to do with disease" (Fletcher, 1985, p. 303).

Proponents must then argue that appropriate distinctions between these different uses can be confidently drawn (Anderson, 1989), and point out that the same eugenic challenges already face those engaged in preimplantation screening or prenatal diagnosis (Fowler et al., 1989).

Human rights concerns.   Finally, however, some critics argue that the focus of germ-line gene therapy on the embryonic patient has other implications that foreclose its pursuit: If the primary goal of the intervention is to address the health problems of the pre-embryo itself, germ-line gene therapy becomes an extreme case of fetal therapy, and the pre-embryo gains the status of a patient requiring protection. Germ-line therapy experiments would involve research with early human embryos that would have effects on their offspring, effectively placing multiple human generations in the role of unconsenting research subjects (Lappé, 1991). If the pre-embryo is given the moral status of a patient, it would be very hard to justify the risks of clinical research that would be necessary to develop the technique. For example, would pre- or postimplantation screening be allowed in order to determine which attempts were successful?

This objection to human germ-line gene therapy research is couched in several ways. For the Europeans, it is often interpreted as the right to one's genetic patrimony (Mauron and Thévoz, 1991); germ-line gene-therapy interventions would violate the rights of subsequent generations to inherit a genetic endowment that has not been intentionally modified (Knoppers, 1991). For advocates of people with disabilities, this concern is interpreted in terms of the dangers to society's willingness to accept their differences (Asch, 1989). Interestingly, some feminists join this position as well, out of a concern for the impact on women of taking the pre-embryo too seriously as an object of medical care (Minden, 1987).

Proponents can offer several responses to these concerns. One is to argue that germ-line gene therapy is a reproductive health intervention aimed at the parents, not the fetus (Zimmerman, 1991). Its goal is to allow the parents to address their reproductive risks and have a healthy baby, in cases where the parents' own views of preimplantation screening prohibit preimplantation screening and selective discard of an embryo (Cook-Deegan, 1990). In taking this position, proponents acknowledge moral uncertainty over the status of the pre-embryo and defend parental requests for germ-line intervention as falling within the scope of their reproductive rights. Their argument is that, as a professional policy, medicine should continue to accept, and respond to, a wide range of interpretations of reproductive health needs by prospective parents, including requests for germ-line gene therapy (Fowler et al., 1989).

Conclusion

No other biomedical intervention in history has received as much international and interdisciplinary attention as human gene therapy (Fletcher, 1990). Three points of striking consensus have emerged from that global discussion:

The first point is that somatic-cell gene-therapy research does not constitute a major break with medical therapeutics, but that this technique should be regulated through public review processes. As somatic-cell gene-therapy techniques branch off into different medical domains, this policy raises hard questions about how seriously to take the public's involvement.

The second point of consensus is that current concerns about clinical risks and biohazards, research involving pre-embryonic subjects of uncertain moral status, and long-range social risks make human experimentation with germ-line interventions unacceptable for the time being. Beyond that, the discussion is flourishing about whether germ-line interventions could ever be ethically acceptable and, if so, under what circumstances.

The third point of consensus is less often directly stated but is nonetheless implied in much of the literature; it also animates the international discussion of these techniques. That is the view that gene therapy, both somatic and germ-line, should be evaluated solely as a clinical tool employed on behalf of presenting patients, and not as a eugenic public-health device designed to benefit the population. In contemporary political argot, genetic medicine should continue to be an empowering, not an exclusionary science. It should continue to be about helping living people address their individual health problems, and not about protecting the "gene pool" or society from the ebb and flow of human alleles in populations.

ERIC JUENGST
LEROY WALTERS

Directly related to this article is the companion article in this entry: STRATEGIES FOR GENE THERAPY. *Also directly related is the entry* GENETIC ENGINEERING, *article on* HUMAN GENETIC ENGINEERING. *For a further discussion of topics mentioned in this article, see the entries* EUGENICS; EUGENICS AND RELIGIOUS LAW, *articles on* JUDAISM, *and* CHRISTIANITY; EVOLUTION; *and* GENETICS AND ENVIRONMENT IN HUMAN HEALTH. *For a discussion of research ethics, see the entries* FETUS, *article on* FETAL RESEARCH; INFORMED CONSENT, *article on* CONSENT ISSUES IN HUMAN RESEARCH; PRIVACY AND CONFIDENTIALITY IN RESEARCH; *and* RESEARCH POLICY. *For a discussion of related ideas, see the entries* GENETICS AND THE LAW; GENETIC TESTING AND SCREENING; GENOME MAPPING

Mapping and Sequencing; Health and Disease; *and* Reproductive Technologies, *articles on* artificial insemination, *and* ethical issues.

Bibliography

Abrecht, Paul, ed. 1980. *Faith and Science in an Unjust World: Report of the World Council of Churches' Conference on Faith, Science, and the Future.* 2 vols. Philadelphia, Pa.: Fortress Press.

Anderson, W. French. 1989. "Human Gene Therapy: Why Draw a Line?" *Journal of Medicine and Philosophy* 14, no. 6:681–693.

Anderson, W. French, and Fletcher, John C. 1980. "Gene Therapy in Human Beings: When Is It Ethical to Begin?" *New England Journal of Medicine* 303, no. 22:1293–1297.

Asch, Adrienne. 1989. "Reproductive Technology and Disability." In *Reproductive Laws for the 1990s*, pp. 69–124. Edited by Sherrill Cohen and Nadine Taub. Clifton, N.J.: Humana Press.

Baltimore, David. 1977. "Genetic Engineering: The Future—Potential Uses." In *Research with Recombinant DNA: An Academy Forum*, pp. 237–240. Washington, D.C.: National Academy of Sciences.

Bankowski, Zbigniew, and Capron, Alexander, eds. 1991. *Genetics, Ethics and Human Values: Human Genome Mapping, Genetic Screening and Gene Therapy.* Geneva: Council for International Organizations of Medical Sciences (CIOMS).

Bourrit, Bertram; Mandofia, Maria; Mauron, Alex; and Thévoz, Jean-Marie. 1989. "Analyse de l'Argumentation Ethique du Rapport Amstad." *Bulletin des Médicines Suisses* 70:1823–1828.

Catholic Health Association of the United States. 1990. *Human Genetics: Ethical Issues in Genetic Testing, Counseling, and Therapy.* St. Louis, Mo.: Author.

Cook-Deegan, Robert Mullan. 1990. "Human Gene Therapy and Congress." *Human Gene Therapy* 1:163–170.

Council of Europe. Parliamentary Assembly, Thirty-Third Ordinary Session. 1982. "Recommendation 934 (1982) on Genetic Engineering." In *Texts Adopted by the Assembly*, January 26, 1982 (22nd Sitting). Strasbourg: Author.

Council for Responsible Genetics. Human Genetics Committee. 1993. "Position Paper on Human Germ Line Manipulation (Fall, 1992)." *Human Gene Therapy* 4, no. 1:35–37.

Davis, Bernard D. 1970. "Prospects for Genetic Intervention in Man." *Science* 170, no. 964:1279–1283.

Denmark. Indenrigsministeriet. 1984. *Fremskridtets Pris.* Copenhagen: Indenrigsministeriet.

Dobzhansky, Theodosius. 1962. *Mankind Evolving: The Evolution of the Human Species.* New Haven, Conn.: Yale University Press.

European Medical Research Councils. 1988. "Gene Therapy in Man: Recommendations of European Medical Research Councils." *Lancet* 1, no. 8597:1271–1272.

Federal Republic of Germany. Arbeitsgruppe. 1985. *In-Vitro–Fertilisation, Genomanalyse und Gentherapie.* Bonn: Bundesminister der Justiz und Bundesminister für Forschung und Technologie.

Fletcher, John C. 1985. "Ethical Issues in and Beyond Prospective Clinical Trials of Human Gene Therapy." *Journal of Medicine and Philosophy* 10, no. 3:293–309.

———. 1990. "Evolution of Ethical Debate About Human Gene Therapy." *Human Gene Therapy* 1, no. 1:55–68.

Fletcher, Joseph. 1971. "Ethical Aspects of Genetic Controls: Designed Genetic Changes in Man." *New England Journal of Medicine* 285, no. 14:776–783.

———. 1974. *The Ethics of Genetic Control: Ending Reproductive Roulette.* Garden City, N.Y.: Anchor.

Fowler, Gregory; Juengst, Eric T.; and Zimmerman, Burke K. 1989. "Germ-line Gene Therapy and the Clinical Ethos of Medical Genetics." *Theoretical Medicine* 10: 151–165.

France. Comité Consultatif National d'Ethique pour les Sciences de la Vie et de la Santé. 1991. "Avis sur la thérapie génique." *Human Gene Therapy* 2, no. 4:329.

Friedmann, Theodore, and Roblin, Richard O. 1972. "Gene Therapy for Human Genetic Disease?" *Science* 175, no. 25:949–955.

Goulian, Mehran; Kornberg, Arthur; and Sinsheimer, Robert L. 1967. "Enzymatic Synthesis of DNA, 24. Synthesis of Infectious Phage Phi-X-174 DNA." *Proceedings of the National Academy of Sciences* 58, no. 6:2321–2328.

Great Britain. Committee on the Ethics of Gene Therapy. 1992. "Report of the Committee on the Ethics of Gene Therapy." *Human Gene Therapy* 3, no. 5:519–523.

Gustafson, James M. 1973. "Genetic Engineering and the Normative View of the Human." In *Ethical Issues in Biology and Medicine*, pp. 46–58. Edited by Preston N. Williams. Cambridge, Mass.: Schenkman.

Haldane, J. B. S. 1924. *Daedalus; or, Science and the Future.* New York: E. P. Dutton.

———. 1963. "Biological Possibilities for the Human Species in the Next Hundred Years." In *Man and His Future: A CIBA Foundation Volume*, pp. 337–361. Edited by Gordon Wolstenholme. London: J. & A. Churchill.

Hamilton, Michael Pollack, ed. 1972. *The New Genetics and the Future of Man.* Grand Rapids, Mich.: William B. Eerdmans.

Hoagland, Hudson, and Burhoe, Ralph W., eds. 1962. *Evolution and Man's Progress.* New York: Columbia University Press.

Howard, Ted, and Rifkin, Jeremy. 1977. *Who Should Play God? The Artificial Creation of Life and What It Means for the Future of the Human Race.* New York: Dell.

Huxley, Aldous. 1932. *Brave New World.* London: Chatto and Windus.

Huxley, Julian. 1963. "The Future of Man—Evolutionary Aspects." In *Man and His Future: A CIBA Foundation Volume*, pp. 1–22. Edited by Gordon Wolstenholme. London: J. & A. Churchill.

Jacobs, Paul. 1980. "Pioneer Genetic Implants Revealed." *Los Angeles Times*, October 8, 1980, pp. 1, 26.

John Paul II. 1983. "The Ethics of Genetic Manipulation." *Origins* 13, no. 23:385, 387–389.

JUENGST, ERIC T. 1990. "The NIH 'Points to Consider' and the Limits of Human Gene Therapy." *Human Gene Therapy* 1, no. 4:425–433.

KNOPPERS, BARTHA MARIA. 1991. *Human Dignity and Genetic Heritage: A Study Paper Prepared for the Law Reform Commission of Canada.* Ottawa: Law Reform Commission of Canada.

LAPPÉ, MARC. 1991. "Ethical Issues in Manipulating the Human Germ Line." *Journal of Medicine and Philosophy* 16, no. 6:621–639.

LAPPÉ, MARC, and MORISON, ROBERT S., eds. 1976. "Ethical and Scientific Issues Posed by Human Uses of Molecular Genetics." *Annals of the New York Academy of Sciences* 265:1–208.

LEDERBERG, JOSHUA. 1963. "Biological Future of Man." In *Man and His Future: A CIBA Foundation Volume*, pp. 263–273. Edited by Gordon Wolstenholme. London: J. & A. Churchill.

MAURON, ALEX, and THÉVOZ, JEAN-MARIE. 1991. "Germ-Line Engineering: A Few European Voices." *Journal of Medicine and Philosophy* 16, no. 6:649–666.

McGARRITY, GERARD J. 1991. "The Metamorphosis of Gene Insertion and Gene Therapy." *Human Gene Therapy* 2, no. 1:3–4.

MINDEN, SHELLEY. 1987. "Patriarchal Designs: The Genetic Engineering of Human Embryos." In *Made to Order: The Myth of Reproductive and Genetic Progress*, pp. 102–109. Edited by Patricia Spallone and Deborah Lynn Steinberg. Oxford, U.K.: Pergamon Press.

MOTULSKY, ARNO G. 1974. "Brave New World?" *Science* 185, no. 4152:653–663.

MULLER, H. J. 1935. *Out of the Night: A Biologist's View of the Future.* New York: Vanguard Press.

———. 1950. "Our Load of Mutations." *American Journal of Human Genetics* 2, no. 2:111–176.

———. 1959. "The Guidance of Human Evolution." *Perspectives in Biology and Medicine* 3:1–43.

———. 1963. "Genetic Progress by Voluntarily Conducted Germinal Choice." In *Man and His Future: A CIBA Foundation Volume*, pp. 247–262. Edited by Gordon Wolstenholme. London: J. & A. Churchill.

MUNSON, RONALD, and DAVIS, LAWRENCE. 1992. "Germ-Line Gene Therapy and the Medical Imperative." *Kennedy Institute of Ethics Journal* 2, no. 2:137–158.

NATIONAL INSTITUTES OF HEALTH (U.S.). 1985. "Recombinant DNA Research; Request for Public Comment on 'Points to Consider' in the Design and Submission of Human Somatic-Cell Gene Therapy Protocols." *Federal Register* 50, no. 14:2940–2945.

RAHNER, KARL. 1967. "Zum Problem der genetischen Manipulation." In *Schriften zur Theologie*, vol. 8, pp. 286–321. Einsiedeln, Switzerland: Benziger Verlag.

RAMSEY, PAUL. 1966. "Moral and Religious Implications of Genetic Control." In *Genetics and the Future of Man*, pp. 107–169. Edited by John D. Roslansky. New York: Appleton-Century-Crofts.

———. 1970. *Fabricated Man: The Ethics of Genetic Control.* New Haven, Conn.: Yale University Press.

ROSLANSKY, JOHN D., ed. 1966. *Genetics and the Future of Man: A Discussion of the Nobel Conference Organized by Gustavus Adolphus College, St. Peter, Minnesota, 1965.* New York: Appleton-Century-Crofts.

ROYAL COMMISSION ON NEW REPRODUCTIVE TECHNOLOGIES (CANADA). 1993. *Proceed with Care—Final Report.* Ottawa, Canada: Ministry of Supply and Services.

SASS, HANS-MARTIN. 1988. "A Critique of the Enquete Commission's Report on Gene Technology." *Bioethics* 2, no. 3:264–275.

SHAPIRO, JIM; MACHATTIE, LORNE; ERON, LARRY; IHLER, GARRET; IPPEN, KARIN; and BECKWITH, JON. 1969. "Isolation of Pure *lac* Operon DNA." *Nature* 224:768–774.

SONNENBORN, T. M., ed. 1965. *The Control of Human Heredity and Evolution.* New York: Macmillan.

SWEDEN. SOCIALDEPARTEMENTET. GEN-ETIKKOMMITTÉN. 1984. *Genetisk Integritet.* Statens Offentliga Utredningar, vol. 88. Stockholm: Author.

TEMIN, HOWARD M. 1990. "Safety Considerations in Somatic Gene Therapy of Human Disease with Retrovirus Vectors." *Human Gene Therapy* 1, no. 2:111–123.

THOMPSON, LARRY. 1993. "Should Dying Patients Receive Untested Genetic Methods?" *Science* 259, no. 5094:452.

U.S. CONGRESS. HOUSE COMMITTEE ON SCIENCE AND TECHNOLOGY. SUBCOMMITTEE ON INVESTIGATIONS AND OVERSIGHT. 1982. *Human Genetic Engineering.* Washington, D.C.: U.S. Government Printing Office.

———. OFFICE OF TECHNOLOGY ASSESSMENT. 1984. *Human Gene Therapy.* Washington, D.C.: Author.

———. SENATE SUBCOMMITTEE ON GOVERNMENT RESEARCH. 1968. *National Commission on Health Science and Society.* Washington, D.C.: U.S. Government Printing Office.

U.S. PRESIDENT'S COMMISSION FOR THE STUDY OF ETHICAL PROBLEMS IN MEDICINE AND BIOMEDICAL AND BEHAVIORAL RESEARCH. 1982. *Splicing Life: A Report on the Social and Ethical Issues of Genetic Engineering with Human Beings.* Washington, D.C.: U.S. Government Printing Office.

WALTERS, LEROY. 1991a. "Human Gene Therapy: Ethics and Public Policy." *Human Gene Therapy* 2, no. 2:115–122.

———. 1991b. "Ethical Issues in Human Gene Therapy." *Journal of Clinical Ethics* 2, no. 4:267–274.

WIVEL, NELSON A., and WALTERS, LEROY. 1993. "Germ-Line Gene Modification and Disease Prevention: Some Medical and Ethical Perspectives." *Science* 262, no. 5133: 533–538.

WOLSTENHOLME, GORDON, ed. 1963. *Man and His Future: A CIBA Foundation Volume.* London: J. & A. Churchill.

ZIMMERMAN, BURKE K. 1991. "Human Germ-Line Therapy: The Case for Its Development and Use." *Journal of Medicine and Philosophy* 16, no. 2:593–612.

GENETIC ASPECTS OF HUMAN BEHAVIOR

See GENETICS AND HUMAN BEHAVIOR.

GENETIC COUNSELING

I. Practice of Genetic Counseling
   Barbara Bowles Biesecker
II. Ethical Issues
   Robert F. Murray, Jr.

I. PRACTICE OF GENETIC COUNSELING

Genetic counseling may be described as the interaction between a health-care provider and patient or family member on concerns about the birth of a child with medical problems, reproductive testing options, a family history of ill health, or the diagnosis of an inherited condition. There are over four thousand genetic conditions, chromosome disorders, and birth abnormalities that can result in miscarriage, stillbirth, death early in life or problems in childhood or adulthood. Those who seek this medical and psychological counseling service ask questions and have concerns about why a condition occurred, the chances that it may occur again in the future, and how they may be helped to cope with uncertainty, risk, or other ramifications of a diagnosis. These services are often provided by a team of clinical genetics specialists (physician geneticists and master's-level genetic counselors) in a medical genetics clinic within a hospital or in an outreach setting. Attention is paid to the medical, educational, and emotional needs of patients and their family members related to genetic conditions.

This article reviews the history of genetic counseling, the training of genetic counselors, and the practice standards and values inherent in the goal of nondirective counseling.

Genetics evaluation and counseling services

An accurate diagnosis must be established to address patients' needs. This is true even if the person seeking counseling is not affected with a genetic condition. The diagnosis of the patient or relative(s) in question determines the inheritance pattern in the family and thus the risk information that is provided. The diagnosis may be determined from family history information, pregnancy history, medical records, clinical examination, or test results. The physician geneticist on the team typically performs this diagnostic aspect of genetic counseling. Medical and pediatric geneticists are physicians who have completed special postresidency fellowships in clinical genetics. Their expertise is to recognize rare patterns of physical features unique to particular genetic disorders; interpret molecular, biochemical, or chromosomal test results; and recommend management of related medical concerns.

The educational component of genetic counseling includes a wide range of information that stems from the diagnosis, including the inheritance pattern, the risk of recurrence, medical management or surveillance, prognosis, schooling needs, support groups, financial issues, reproductive options, and potential inherited and emotional ramifications to members of the patient's family. Genetic counselors and clinical geneticists are trained to address this spectrum of concerns, and most often, both participate in this portion of counseling sessions.

The psychosocial counseling component explores patients' emotional responses to the information discussed. It is provided in a supportive and nonjudgmental manner. Discussion of genetic conditions or risks often elicits feelings of lowered self-esteem, guilt, shame, loss, and blame, either on the part of patients or their family members. Genetic counseling in its most specific sense describes the psychodynamic process that occurs within a counselor–client relationship based on trust and rapport. The relationship borrows from clinical psychology its basic assumption that the client is capable of caring for his or her own emotional well-being. Exploration of the implications of genetic disorders assists clients in adjusting their expectations, coping with difficulty, and facing dilemmas. Empathic elucidation of the client's feelings conveys respect and benevolence and is not intended to be persuasive. Thus, the relationship is best described as client-oriented. Master's degree–level genetic counselors, in particular, have expertise in this aspect of genetic counseling.

History

To appreciate the current standard of practice in genetic counseling, it is important to outline its history. In the United States, academic geneticists (nonphysicians), most of whom did not study humans, were the pioneers in addressing queries from affected family members about their risk of specific genetic conditions. From the early 1900s in Europe, Great Britain, and the United States, and particularly in the late 1930s and early 1940s in Nazi Germany, the practice of eugenics was widespread. This included the mass elimination of certain populations as well as forced sterilization of the mentally impaired. Because of their concerns about these eugenic practices, academics in subsequent years resisted providing childbearing advice to those who sought their expertise. This laid the groundwork for patient autonomy in reproductive decision making that has evolved over subsequent decades. This evolution of genetic counseling has been described as consisting of three paradigm shifts, from eugenics, to preventive medicine, and finally to psychologically oriented counseling (Kessler, 1979).

As human genetics developed into an academic field and medical information became available about inherited conditions, physician geneticists and smaller numbers of clinical Ph.D. geneticists became the primary communicators of information related to genetic conditions. Departments of Human Genetics became established in the 1940s and 1950s and led to the development of medical subspecialties. Practicing clinicians came to recognize the time-consuming and psychologically demanding aspects of communicating emotionally volatile information to families and began to involve nurses and social workers in the provision of services. Thus, a team approach to counseling ensued, yet nurses and social workers, at that time, had no formal education in genetics.

Training and certification of genetic counselors

The first master's degree–level genetic counseling graduates entered the field in the early 1970s and became integrated into a clinical practice team alongside medical geneticists. There are now more than 1,300 of these health-care professionals throughout the United States and smaller numbers of nurses and social workers who have specialized in the area of clinical genetics. The vast majority of counselors are Caucasian females, and programs are actively recruiting applicants from diverse ethnocultural backgrounds (Rapp, 1988). As of 1994, eighteen master's degree graduate programs exist, including four clinical-nurse specialist programs. Two of these programs are in Canada, one is in South Africa, and one is in Great Britain.

Persons who pursue genetic counseling often have undergraduate degrees in both biology or chemistry and the social sciences. Most successful applicants have participated in a community counseling endeavor prior to entering graduate school. Graduate programs are typically two years long and entail clinical, biochemical, and molecular genetics coursework coupled with psychology, public health, biomedical ethics, and social work. Genetic counseling students are trained in a variety of clinical settings throughout their studies; thus, there is a large experiential component to their education. Most programs limit the number of students enrolled to less than ten per year because this aspect of genetic counseling training is closely supervised and labor intensive. A master's degree in human genetics or genetic counseling is awarded.

In the past, the American Board of Medical Genetics has certified master's-level genetic counselors, as well as medical geneticists and several types of Ph.D.-trained geneticists. As of 1993, in the United States, genetic counselors are certified by the newly established American Board of Genetic Counseling (ABGC). Eligibility for certification requires stringent academic preparation as well as experience in counseling individ-

uals for a variety of indications and in divergent settings. The ABGC also plans to certify graduate programs in genetic counseling in order to uphold professional standards for training and practice.

Standard of practice

Sheldon Reed (1974) stressed the importance of utilizing the term "counseling" in referring to this clinical genetics practice in an effort to distinguish it from genetic advice giving (eugenics). Reed also emphasized that patient autonomy in decision making (particularly with regard to reproduction) should be respected and upheld. A definition of genetic counseling, subsequently published by the American Society of Human Genetics Ad Hoc Committee on Genetic Counseling in 1975, emphasized the educational component to the service and thus, the importance of an effective communication process (Epstein et al., 1975). It implies (but does not state) the central dogma of genetic counseling, nondirectiveness, by describing patient autonomy in terms of individuals choosing their own course of action.

The term "nondirectiveness" was widely adopted in the genetic counseling literature in the mid-1970s. Although use and interpretation of the term varies dramatically, "nondirective" was borrowed from the writings of the psychologist Carl Rogers to describe a noneugenic counseling process. Rogers first coined the term in 1942 to describe his psychotherapeutic approach of not advising, interpreting, or guiding his clients. The concept led to confusion in the field of clinical psychology as Rogers realized that his very presence in a relationship had many "directive" aspects. By 1978, he had adopted the term "person-centered" to describe his therapeutic approach (Rogers, 1978). Clinical geneticists and genetic counselors often use the term to describe various aspects of their practice, but there has been debate about whether genetic counseling can be nondirective (Bartels et al., 1993).

Nondirectiveness should not be interpreted to mean that genetic counseling is value-neutral. Geneticists have long recognized that their values and ideas often are not identical to those of their patients. Rather, geneticists and counselors are explicit about certain values, such as the patient's role in making his or her own decisions, particularly about childbearing. It is impossible for geneticists and counselors to know with any certainty what they would do if they were faced with others' circumstances. In one international survey, clinical geneticists identified patient autonomy as one of the most important values in the provision of services (Wertz and Fletcher, 1988).

Nondirectiveness was never intended to suggest a lack of provider bias. Biases are inherent to being human, and providers bring their own biases to the therapeutic relationship. The expression and discussion of such biases often may occur in a counseling session. Their acknowledgment actually defines genetic counselors as client-oriented. A common bias among counselors, for instance, is the assumption that clients are capable of self-growth following a tragic event or personal struggle. They value self-development, privacy, knowledge, and emotional revelation, and their relationship with their clients depends on their use or expression.

Genetic counseling clearly has directive components. The education of patients is directive insofar as the counselor imparts certain information to the client. Since clients often come seeking such information, this activity is necessarily directed. Medical management and referrals to support groups or agencies are explicitly directive. A refusal to offer a carrier test to a minor or to offer prenatal testing for fetal sex selection are further examples of directive activities. Genetic counseling may even involve making recommendations.

There are also implicitly directive components to the counseling relationship conveyed through body language, emphasis, and time spent. These directive factors, however, do not diminish the need for client-oriented psychological counseling and autonomous decision making regarding reproduction. These aspects of genetic counseling are critical to the standard of practice often termed "nondirective." As Rogers discovered, the professional relationship does serve as a potent influence on the client; thus, what is reinforced by the counselor are the feelings and reactions expressed by the client without interpretation or judgment. The client is therefore empowered in his or her own central ability to develop further within the relationship. This approach defines a standard for practice. Because genetic counseling is a client-oriented service and inherently flexible, critics have stated that no standard of practice exists. This stems from confusing an outcome-based practice (eugenics) with a process-based standard (client-centered counseling).

The National Society of Genetic Counselors adopted, in 1991, a code of ethics that outlines guidelines for the practice of master's-trained counselors. The code is based on an ethical framework called the ethics of care and addresses many of the important components of the relationship between the counselor and client. The following section discusses in more detail the ethical issues governing genetic counseling service provision.

Goals of counseling

The overall goal of genetic counseling is to reduce human emotional suffering or struggle related to genetic conditions and to address clients' concerns. Clinical ge-

netics professionals who claim to know better than their patients what are "correct" or "good" decisions are practicing in direct conflict with the objective of patient-centered care. There is a critical need for research to evaluate the effectiveness of genetic counseling in addressing clients' needs and concerns. Previous investigation into the effectiveness of genetic counseling has often been limited to patients' retention of information, specifically risk factors (Sorenson et al., 1981). Although risk education is an important component of genetic counseling, families frequently do not make rational decisions based on critical interpretation of numbers. Outcomes for families are highly complex and it is often their psychological and social circumstances that determine their decision making and coping. Patients' expectations and desires, their interpretations of services, and their degree of satisfaction are all important sources of information to shape the approach and success of genetic counseling.

Conflicts arise in the provision of clinical genetics services when issues of serving the public good are introduced as a desired outcome. Genetic services are patently eugenic if the goal is to reduce the incidence of genetic disease. Several international genetic-screening programs exist that boast "successful" outcomes defined as the reduction of children affected with certain genetic disorders (by abortion or restricted matings). Such screening programs do not promote client-centered decision making and autonomy as important outcomes and may or may not include genetic counseling as a component of the service (Andrews et al., 1994). In addition, in times of increasing competition for health-care resources, it becomes increasingly difficult to justify expensive counseling services designed to help clients make autonomous, informed decisions. Pretest education and counseling are critical components of any genetic-testing or population-screening program. Without upholding this as a rigid practice guideline, clinical genetics professionals risk reverting to the tragedies of eugenic programs.

Settings

Genetic counseling occurs most often in obstetrical and pediatric genetics clinics. At least half of all genetic counselors practice some degree of prenatal genetic counseling. Typically this entails discussion with a woman or couple of their family histories and potential risks to a developing baby. Prenatal counseling usually involves decisions regarding the use of available testing options. When a test result indicates there is a problem or potential problem, then more extensive counseling ensues. Prenatal services are offered through university hospitals, private hospitals, and, increasingly, in private clinics or offices. Testing options may include amniocentesis, chorionic villus sampling, ultrasound, or preimplantation diagnosis. These techniques allow an opportunity to perform biochemical, cytogenetic, visual, or molecular evaluation on a developing fetus that may provide information about the likelihood that a genetic disorder or birth defect has occurred. None of these methods guarantees the arrival of unimpaired children, and the occurrence of many disorders is impossible to predict prior to delivery or onset of symptoms.

Because many birth abnormalities are unpredictable, pediatric clinics are also frequent settings for genetic counseling services. Most of these clinics are located in academic hospitals and focus on families' questions about the cause of a child's physical or mental maldevelopment. The sessions may address diagnostic, prognostic, or psychosocial issues. Certain chromosome or DNA testing (by obtaining a blood sample) may assist in making the diagnosis, but the essence of the evaluations is thorough physical examination and history taking. Emotional issues related to the child's prognosis often take precedence over more immediate issues, such as current school needs.

The financial aspects of genetic counseling services have significant impact on service delivery. Genetic counseling is primarily a cognitive endeavor that is labor intensive. Counseling services historically have been reimbursed by third-party payers at a lower rate than medical services, particularly those involving a laboratory test. Prenatal testing procedures and accompanying laboratory services are one aspect of genetic services that has proved reimbursable. This differential creates conflicts of interest for geneticists and counselors, who often face administrative pressures to balance the expenditures of clinic services. It is incumbent upon both providers to ensure that financial needs are not met by directing patients toward more significantly reimbursable services.

In the United States, genetic services disproportionately serve persons with third-party coverage or who have other means to pay for services. Attempts have been made, initially by the federal government and subsequently by state governments, to support statewide genetic services for the geographically and economically underserved. Such programs have met with variable success. Many states provide funds for geneticists to travel periodically to outreach settings, such as public-health-department clinics, in more rural areas. Most often these services are pediatric genetic services since prenatal genetic services are time-dependent and require special equipment for patients who choose testing.

Genetic services have been described as a luxury, particularly in comparison to the significant need for more basic health services, such as, in the United States, prenatal care. In addition, racial minorities are underserved, as they are in most medical settings in the United States. More equitable genetic service delivery occurs in countries in which there is socialized medicine. Yet national health services place more emphasis on public-health outcomes and less on autonomous decision making and costly counseling services (Wertz and Fletcher, 1988). This suggests there will be challenges to the current mode of delivering genetic services if the United States adopts a similar health-care system in the future.

Future considerations

It is not currently possible, nor will it be possible in the future, for geneticists or genetic counselors to provide genetic counseling services to every person whose life is, or may be, touched by a genetic condition. The Human Genome Project in the United States, beginning in 1989, and genome research internationally have led to rapid identification of genes involved in the causation not only of single gene disorders, but also of more common diseases such as diabetes, cardiovascular disease, and cancer. With an abundance of new genetic tests expected, some aspects of genetic services must be integrated into primary-care settings. Because there are insufficient numbers of counselors and clinical geneticists to provide appropriate pretest education and counseling, new models of service delivery are needed.

Many of the education components to genetic counseling are and will continue to be provided not only by genetics specialists, but also by nurses and primary-care physicians. Education will need to be increasingly supplemented by interactive computer programs, videotapes, and written materials. The more complex the ramifications of genetic testing, or the more directly related to reproductive options, the more desirable it is that genetic counselors and medical geneticists play a role in the education and counseling in order to maintain the high standards of practice and noneugenic goals that currently govern genetics practice. Also, when the majority of patients' psychological needs stem from a genetic condition, genetic counseling by a certified counselor will continue to be desired. With significant professional education efforts and elegantly designed referral or triage mechanisms, services may be enhanced in the future. A significant goal for genetics providers is to more thoroughly meet the needs of a wider spectrum of the population with a broader array of services.

A variety of providers can and should respond to the increasing needs. Here, appropriate referral mechanisms will play an important role. For instance, if genetic testing becomes available to assist in predictions of cardiovascular disease, these tests may be offered in a primary-care physician's office. A nurse may provide the background information on what genetic information may be gleaned from the test and then what type of prevention program may be designed in conjunction with the results. There would seem to be little need for referral for genetic counseling in this scenario, or for other medical management uses of testing where the emotional issues are less likely to be profound.

On the other hand, cystic fibrosis gene testing illustrates the potential complexities of genetic testing. Test results can be ambiguous, there may be reproductive ramifications, and improvements in treatment of the disorder have increased longevity and quality of life. Even if cystic fibrosis carrier testing is offered in primary-care physicians' offices, the education component needs to be thorough and balanced; and referral for genetic counseling when the results indicate someone is a gene carrier will remain important.

When genetic testing becomes increasingly utilized as a tool for medical management, and not merely as a means to obtain risk information, there is likely to be less psychological turmoil for patients. Carrier testing or presymptomatic testing for a serious, late-onset disorder, however, illustrates the need for client-oriented counseling. As the number and background of professionals providing genetic tests expand, there is a greater potential threat to autonomous, well-informed decision making. The maintenance of the current high standard of practice for genetic counseling is a key issue in considering the consequences of the diffusion and proliferation of these services.

BARBARA BOWLES BIESECKER

Directly related to this article is the companion article in this entry: ETHICAL AND SOCIAL ISSUES. *For a further discussion of topics mentioned in this article, see the entries* AUTONOMY; CARE; COMPASSION; EMOTIONS; *and* VALUE AND VALUATION. *For a discussion of related ideas, see the entries* EUGENICS; GENETIC TESTING AND SCREENING, *especially the articles on* PREIMPLANTATION EMBRYO DIAGNOSIS, *and* PRENATAL DIAGNOSIS; HOSPITAL, *article on* MODERN HISTORY; INFORMATION DISCLOSURE; PROFESSIONAL–PATIENT RELATIONSHIP, *articles on* SOCIOLOGICAL PERSPECTIVES, *and* ETHICAL ISSUES; *and* PROFESSION AND PROFESSIONAL ETHICS.

Bibliography

ANDREWS, LORI; FULLARTON, JANE; HOLTZMAN, NEIL; and MOTULSKY, ARNO, eds. 1994. *Assessing Genetic Risks: Implications for Health and Social Policy.* Washington, D.C.: National Academy Press.

BARTELS, DIANNE M.; LEROY, BONNIE S.; and CAPLAN, ARTHUR L., eds. 1993. *Prescribing Our Future: Ethical Challenges in Genetic Counseling.* New York: Aldine de Gruyer.

EPSTEIN, CHARLES J.; CHILDS, BARTON; FRASER, F. CLARKE; McKUSICK, VICTOR A.; MILLER, JAMES R.; MOTULSKY, ARNO G.; RIVAS, MARIAN; THOMPSON, MARGARET W.; SHAW, MARJORY W.; and SLY, WILLIAM S. 1975. "Genetic Counseling." *American Journal of Human Genetics* 27, no. 2:240–242.

EVANS, MARK I., ed. 1993. "Reproductive Genetic Testing: Impact upon Women—NIH Workshop, Bethesda, MD, November 21–23, 1991." *Fetal Diagnosis and Therapy* 8, suppl. 1. Special Issue.

KESSLER, SEYMOUR, ed. 1979. *Genetic Counseling: Psychological Dimensions.* New York: Academic Press.

MARKS, JOAN H.; HEIMLER, AUDREY; REICH, ELSA; WEXLER, NANCY; and INCE, SUSAN, eds. 1989. *Genetic Counseling Principles in Action: A Casebook.* Birth Defects Original Article Series, vol. 25, no. 5. White Plains, N.Y.: March of Dimes Birth Defects Foundation.

PALMER, SHANE. 1992. "Guiding Principles, Resolutions, Clarify Stance." *Perspectives in Genetic Counseling: Newsletter of the National Society of Genetic Counselors* 14, no. 1:1, 4–5.

RAPP, RAYNA. 1988. "Chromosomes and Communication: The Discourse of Genetic Counseling." *Medical Anthropology Quarterly,* n. s., 2, no. 2:143–157.

REED, SHELDON C. 1974. "A Short History of Genetic Counseling." *Social Biology* 21, no. 4:332–339.

ROGERS, CARL. 1978. "The Formative Tendency." *Journal of Humanistic Psychology* 18, no. 1:23–26.

SORENSON, JAMES R.; SWAZEY, JUDITH P.; and SCOTCH, NORMAN A. eds. 1981. *Reproductive Pasts, Reproductive Futures: Genetic Counseling and Its Effectiveness.* Birth Defects Original Article Series, vol. 17, no. 4. New York: Alan R. Liss.

WERTZ, DOROTHY C., and FLETCHER, JOHN C. 1988. "Attitudes of Genetic Counselors: A Multinational Study." *American Journal of Human Genetics* 42, no. 4:592–600.

II. ETHICAL ISSUES

Genetic counseling is a complex communication process that takes place between a genetic counselor and one or more counselees, also called clients. It may involve a single encounter lasting 30 to 60 minutes or multiple encounters over months or years. The type and duration of the encounter is determined by the nature of the condition that led to the encounter. This includes whether the condition under discussion is genetic or nongenetic, the mode of inheritance, and the severity of the disorder, including its prognosis. Therapeutic and reproductive implications play a significant role as well as the counselor's evaluation of the effectiveness of the counseling encounter.

Effective and helpful genetic counseling should be guided by several ethical principles and human values judged by most workers in the field to be of vital importance (Wertz et al., 1990). These include autonomy; beneficence and nonmaleficence; confidentiality; veracity and truth-telling; and informed consent. It is also crucial that varied cultural and ethnic factors be taken into account. The professional code of ethics for genetic counselors should also be considered (Palmer, 1992).

Since genetic counseling usually occurs in medical settings such as clinics, medical centers, or private offices, the ethical values that currently prevail in medical and nursing practice should also play a role in genetic counseling. These principles or values influence different aspects of the counseling process to different degrees. Their influence may also vary according to the cultural background, ethnicity, or religious beliefs of the counselees and their families. The latter factors should receive serious attention, since cultural, religious, or ethnic differences can profoundly influence the relative weight given to one value or principle over another. This is especially true when counseling involves individuals from other countries (Wertz et al., 1990). Counselees from the so-called Third World may cherish religious tenets and ethical values drastically different from those of the Jewish and Christian faiths that inform so much of Western medical ethics (Fisher, 1992).

Autonomy and nondirectiveness

A major facet of the counseling process, and one important goal of a successful counseling process, is a course of action (or inaction) that is determined according to the best available evidence. Genetic counselors generally agree that this decision should be made by the counselee, and that it should be made freely and without coercion (Fraser, 1974; Ad Hoc Committee on Genetic Counseling, 1975). Counselors want to avoid, to the extent possible, being accused of "playing god" and to resist any temptation to practice eugenics, the process of manipulating genes in order to "improve" genetic makeup. The manipulation is accomplished by directing the counselees about what reproductive decisions they should or should not make. This is inappropriate because respect for autonomy should be a predominant ethical value guiding the counseling process and its outcome. This is the clear consensus of genetic counselors from all over the world (U.S. President's Commission, 1983; Wertz and Fletcher, 1988).

If counselees are to make autonomous decisions, they must be fully informed about the disorder in question, free of coercion, aware of all the possible choices, and have access to any facilities and/or services to implement their decision. In its purest sense and with only rare exceptions, the nature of the decision is not an issue as long as the counselee has decided that such a decision is in her or his best interest. In this model of counseling the counselor makes every effort to be "nondirective," that is, to refrain as much as possible from providing any suggestion directly or indirectly to the counselee as to what decision she or he should make (Fraser, 1974,

1979; Hsia, 1979). No counselor can be totally unbiased and without any interest in the decision that is made. However, the aim in counseling is to create "an accepting psychologic climate" and thereby the possibility of a nondirective relationship (Antley, 1979).

An ethical dilemma may arise for the counselor if the counselee wants to make a decision that will have what the counselor strongly feels are mostly negative consequences. For example, a man and a woman are both affected by a serious homozygous recessive disorder (e.g., sickle-cell anemia) and are advised that all their children will be similarly affected. After being counseled, and with full knowledge of the genetic consequences, they decide to have their own biological children. This kind of decision is called dysgenic by some, because it has the potential of resulting in an increase in the number of deleterious genes in the next generation. This will be true if the couple has more than two children and they in turn live to reproduce in an environment where these genes have no selective advantage. Some counselors feel that the counselor may be justified in not honoring the principle of nondirectiveness because the net reproductive effect is likely to produce more harm than benefit (Yarborough et al., 1989). It further results in a situation in which children who are destined to live a life of pain and suffering are knowingly brought into the world. Furthermore, there is the possibility of genetic harm to this population if this practice becomes more common. These harms must be balanced against the benefit to these parents of having their own biological children, even if these children are much more likely to suffer or to die an early death.

The counselor who feels that the principle of nondirectiveness ought not be violated under any circumstances should at least explore with the counselees the psychosocial and emotional reasons that led them to this decision. The counselor should assist them in a careful and deliberate examination of the benefits and harms that may effect them and their offspring (Kessler, 1979). Strong arguments have been advanced suggesting that by applying the principle of beneficence, the counselor is justified in attempting to persuade counselees to reconsider their decisions in certain cases without violating the rule of nondirectiveness (Yarborough et al., 1989).

Beneficence/nonmaleficence: Whose needs come first?

When the counselee is trying to balance the benefits and harms of a particular decision against one another, there may be a tendency to emphasize the benefits over the harms. In some cases, the benefit or beneficence for the counselee(s) may mean maleficence or harm for the child. If parents who know they will have a child with a serious genetically determined disease decide to go ahead because they believe they have a "right to bear children," they may benefit in having their own biological children. At the same time they might not be judged "responsible parents" because they may not have given serious enough consideration to the suffering and discomfort their offspring will suffer. Even if this factor has been considered, the parents may justify their decision on the religious grounds that they are merely following the dictates of a higher power, leaving it to God to determine whether or not they have children.

In some cases it may be difficult for counselor and counselee to agree on what constitutes a benefit and what a harm, since such determinations are often rather subjective, governed primarily by the counselee's values. For example, abortion of an affected fetus might be considered a benefit to some and harmful to others, depending on whose needs are considered primary. Providing information that there is a high probability that a counselee at risk to inherit a serious genetically determined disease of late onset has in fact inherited it might seem a beneficent act by some who value knowledge of any sort, and a maleficent or harmful act by others who value information only when it leads to the prevention or correction of harm. In the tension between these contrasting ethical principles, medical ethical tradition suggests that nonmaleficence should be weighted more heavily than beneficence in cases where they are in conflict. This position is consistent with the maxim of *primum non nocere*, first do no harm (Beauchamp and Childress, 1989), since providing information without clear benefit has the potential for causing social and emotional harm.

Veracity and truth-telling in genetic counseling

A major part of the genetic counseling process is the exchange of information about the medical and family history provided by the counselee and comprehensive genetic and medical information about the disease in question provided by the counselor (Fraser, 1974; Hsia, 1979). The counselee needs accurate information, including the correct diagnosis, in order to choose a beneficial course of action. Truth-telling is an essential ingredient of the relationship between genetic counselors and counselees. Part of the trust that exists between them is based on this virtue. As a consequence, the genetic counselor should provide truthful, accurate, and complete information to the counselee concerning the genetic disorder being considered.

On some occasions the genetic counselor might have very good reasons for violating this important trust. Failure to tell the truth will most often involve withholding information rather than lying. But the counselor bears the burden of justifying failure to tell the whole truth. This is the case even if the counselor is keeping back some information until a time when it may be more readily received, that is, when the counselee is judged to be better prepared to accept negative information and its attendant consequences. Some reasons that might be given for holding back information include:

1. The information, if transmitted, is likely to cause permanent damage to the self-image of the counselee or result in a serious or severe emotional reaction. This is the case when a female is found to have an XY sex chromosomal constitution rather than the normal XX sex chromosomes.
2. Refraining from transmitting the information will not have a significant effect on the options open to the counselee or her or his family nor will it compromise any therapy the counselee or the family should receive.
3. The counselee has a history of serious depression and the information, if fully given, has a good chance of exacerbating the depression with a significant risk of suicide.
4. The information reveals evidence that the putative father in a family is not the biological father of a particular child; if this information is provided, it is likely to lead to the breakup of the family and the child will no longer have a father.
5. A young man or woman has been found to be a presymptomatic carrier of a late-onset, autosomal (related to chromosomes that are common to both sexes), dominant condition and does not want a fiance to be told because it is feared she or he might break off the relationship.

The latter two cases, in which information is withheld from third parties, raise the question of the counselor's obligation or "duty to warn" others who might be affected by the presence of the genetic condition in a spouse or significant other. For some counselors, the "right to know" or the "duty to warn" provides strong justification for telling the whole truth at all times during the counseling process, regardless of the potential consequences. At the same time, a minority of counselees feel they have a right "not to know." These people would rather not be told about a serious genetic condition of late onset, especially if there is no effective therapy or other maneuver that will forestall its onset or significantly reduce its symptoms. If counselees do not wish to know about their incurable condition, the information may nevertheless have to be placed in the medical record so that future health-care givers will be alert to the counselee's status. The information can also be provided if counselees should change their minds. In general, genetic counselors will withhold information only where there is a strong likelihood for serious harm to the family or to the self-image or status of the individual (Wertz et al., 1990).

Confidentiality and the control of genetic information

Medical genetics is more concerned with the family than almost any other medical subspecialty. As part of the evaluation of a clinically significant genetic disorder, the genetic counselor is required to collect detailed family data and record it in the form of a "pedigree." This enables the counselor and the medical geneticist to determine whether there is a pattern of occurrence in the family consistent with control by a single gene of major effect (often referred to as a "Mendelian" gene). The pedigree may also provide information that may indicate the presence of inherited chromosomal structural rearrangements called translocations. More often than not, the pedigree information is insufficient to make this determination. But when it does demonstrate the presence of an inherited defect, this knowledge can have serious, even grave, implications for the other genetically related members of the family. This is especially true when one is dealing with conditions that demonstrate autosomal or X-linked dominant or X-linked recessive modes of inheritance, because inheritance of a single mutant gene on an X or non-X chromosome can cause the full-blown clinical disorder.

Under the medical model that governs medical geneticists and genetic counseling, the counselee has the status of a patient. All information relative to his or her case is covered by the guarantee of privacy and confidentiality that is required of health professionals (Beauchamp and Childress, 1989). The medical geneticist or genetic counselor should get permission from the counselee to contact other family members to inform them that they are at risk for a serious genetically determined disorder. In general, this is not a problem; most counselees readily consent to having their relatives contacted or are willing to do this themselves. But in at least two instances the genetic counselor may face an ethical dilemma concerning the release of information to third parties.

1. The disorder is *not* treatable and can be diagnosed by prenatal diagnosis, so a couple at risk could theoretically avoid the birth of an affected child; or individuals at risk for this might wish to take special predictive tests and use the knowledge to get their affairs in order or in other ways to alter their life situation.

2. The disorder *is* treatable and can be cured or can have the symptoms and any complications significantly reduced by safe and readily available therapy; or the expression of the disorder can be prevented if it is detected before the symptoms have appeared.

The obligation to maintain confidentiality of patient records and genetic information obtained in a medical setting is not absolute and may be breached when there is adequate justification. The exceptions may be invoked only if there are extenuating or overriding personal or social circumstances. The State of Texas statute on confidentiality, for example, allows confidential information to be disclosed if there is the probability of imminent physical injury to the patient or others (Andrews, 1987). In the case of genetic disorders, the most compelling argument for breaching confidentiality besides those instances where it is required by law is the protection of third parties from harm (Andrews, 1987). In ethical terms this is sometimes cited as "the duty or obligation to warn" when there is a clear or imminent danger.

In the cases shown above, there would appear to be clear justification for breaching confidentiality in the second case but not in the first. In the first example, useful information might be provided to third parties, but there is no evidence of harm because the condition identified is not treatable. In the second example, the fact that there is a treatment or a method of preventing the condition means that failure to warn would result in harm to a third party. Since the burden of justification would be on the genetic counselor to show that the harm, however, conceived, is correctable or preventable, it makes sense not to breach confidentiality in instances where the potential harm is not clearly defined. The U.S. President's Commission for the Study of Ethical Problems in Medicine and Biomedical and Behavioral Research regarding confidentiality provided four conditions under which the requirements of confidentiality can be overridden and genetic information released to relatives or their physicians (1983).

Revealing genetic information, especially in cases of presymptomatic diagnosis, has other important implications for the counselee's eligibility for health insurance and possibly for life insurance. Depending on the condition involved, such information if revealed can also affect employability and opportunities for promotion. There is always a significant risk that sensitive information, if released, may find its way to individuals or agencies that might harm the counselee in the future.

Informed consent in genetic counseling

Since a major component of genetic counseling is communication of information, and since the counselee is encouraged to make her or his own decision, problems or conflicts with informed consent are unusual. Informed consent is especially relevant in the counseling process when a procedure may result in potentially harmful or ambiguous outcomes, for example:

1. in connection with prenatal diagnosis, when the counselee or woman who is to undergo the test needs to understand its risks, benefits, errors, and limitations;
2. as a prelude to presymptomatic testing for a serious disorder without available treatment or methods of prevention, where a positive result can have profound implications for the individual's future life;
3. in connection with participation in a research protocol in which there may be questions about the future use of data or tissue or blood (especially DNA) in future studies or in the search for other genetic markers.

Ethnic and cultural influences

The population of the United States and many other industrialized nations is becoming more diverse. It is estimated that by the year 2010 nearly one-third of the population of the United States will be made up of minorities. Genetic counseling that promotes individual autonomy and is consistent with the ethical values discussed here will require that counselors be aware of and responsive to a wide and growing range of ethnic and cultural variations among those who are now and will be seeking genetic counseling (Fisher, 1992). Conflicts are almost certain to arise when the values and decisions of the ethnically and/or culturally different counselees conflict with those of the counselors and the Western values derived from Jewish and Christian sources that in general govern the decision-making process. The value systems that have been used traditionally in counseling will probably have to be applied in significantly different ways if the process and outcome of counseling is to be helpful and effective.

ROBERT F. MURRAY, JR.

Directly related to this article is the companion article in this entry: PRACTICE OF GENETIC COUNSELING. *For a further discussion of topics mentioned in this article, see the entries* AUTONOMY; BENEFICENCE; CONFIDENTIALITY; INFORMATION DISCLOSURE; *and* INFORMED CONSENT. *For a discussion of related ideas, see the entries* DNA TYPING; EUGENICS; FAMILY; FREEDOM AND COERCION; GENETIC TESTING AND SCREENING, *especially the article on* PRENATAL DIAGNOSIS; MEDICAL INFORMATION SYSTEMS; PROFESSIONAL–PATIENT RELATIONSHIP; RISK; *and* VALUE AND VALUATION.

Bibliography

AD HOC COMMITTEE ON GENETIC COUNSELING. AMERICAN SOCIETY OF HUMAN GENETICS [Charles J. Epstein, Chairman]. 1975. "Genetic Counseling." *American Journal of Human Genetics* 27, no. 2:240–242.

ANDREWS, LORI B. 1987. *Medical Genetics: A Legal Frontier.* Chicago: American Bar Foundation.

ANTLEY, RAY M. 1979. "The Genetic Counselor as Facilitator of the Counselee's Decision Process." In *Genetic Counseling: Facts, Values and Norms,* pp. 137–168. Edited by Alexander M. Capron, Marc Lappé, Robert F. Murray, Jr., Tabitha M. Powledge, Sumner B. Twiss, and Daniel Bergsma. National Foundation–March of Dimes Birth Defects Original Article Series, vol. 15, no. 2. New York: Alan R. Liss.

BEAUCHAMP, TOM L., and CHILDRESS, JAMES F. 1989. *Principles of Biomedical Ethics.* 3d ed. New York: Oxford University Press.

FISHER, NANCY L. 1992. "Ethnocultural Approaches to Genetics." *Pediatric Clinics of North America* 39, no. 1: 55–64.

FRASER, F. CLARKE. 1974. "Genetic Counseling." *American Journal of Human Genetics* 26, no. 5:636–659.

——. 1979. "Introduction: The Development of Genetic Counseling." In *Genetic Counseling: Facts, Values and Norms,* pp. 5–15. Edited by Alexander M. Capron, Marc Lappé, Robert F. Murray, Jr., Tabitha M. Powledge, Sumner B. Twiss, and Daniel Bergsma. National Foundation–March of Dimes Birth Defects Original Article Series, vol. 15, no. 2. New York: Alan R. Liss.

HSIA, Y. EDWARD. 1979. "The Genetic Counselor as Information Giver." In *Genetic Counseling: Facts, Values and Norms,* pp. 169–186. Edited by Alexander M. Capron, Marc Lappé, Robert F. Murray, Jr., Tabitha M. Powledge, Sumner B. Twiss, and Daniel Bergsma. National Foundation–March of Dimes Birth Defects Original Article Series, vol. 15, no. 2. New York: Alan R. Liss.

KESSLER, SEYMOUR. 1979. "The Genetic Counselor as Psychotherapist." In *Genetic Counseling: Facts, Values and Norms,* pp. 187–200. Edited by Alexander M. Capron, Marc Lappé, Robert F. Murray, Jr., Tabitha M. Powledge, Sumner B. Twiss, and Daniel Bergsma. National Foundation–March of Dimes Birth Defects Original Article Series, vol. 15, no. 2. New York: Alan R. Liss.

PALMER, SHANE. 1992. "Guiding Principles, Resolutions, Clarify Stance." *Perspectives in Genetic Counseling: Newsletter of the National Society of Genetic Counselors* 14, no. 1:1, 4–5.

U.S. PRESIDENT'S COMMISSION FOR THE STUDY OF ETHICAL PROBLEMS IN MEDICINE AND BIOMEDICAL AND BEHAVIORAL RESEARCH. 1983. *Screening and Counseling for Genetic Conditions.* Washington, D.C.: Author.

WERTZ, DOROTHY C., and FLETCHER, JOHN C. 1988. "Attitudes of Genetic Counselors: A Multinational Study." *American Journal of Human Genetics* 42, no. 4:592–600.

WERTZ, DOROTHY C.; FLETCHER, JOHN C.; and MULVIHILL, JOHN J. 1990. "Medical Geneticists Confront Ethical Dilemmas: Cross-Cultural Comparisons Among Eighteen

Nations." *American Journal of Human Genetics* 46, no. 6:1200–1213.

YARBOROUGH, MARK; SCOTT, JOAN A.; and DIXON, LINDA K. 1989. "The Role of Beneficence in Clinical Genetics: Nondirective Counseling Reconsidered." *Theoretical Medicine* 10, no. 2:139–149.

GENETIC DIAGNOSIS

See GENETIC TESTING AND SCREENING.

GENETIC ENGINEERING

I. Animals and Plants
   Bernard E. Rollin
II. Human Genetic Engineering
   Robert Wachbroit

I. ANIMALS AND PLANTS

In April 1988, the U.S. Patent Office announced that it "now considers non-naturally occurring non-human multicellular living organisms, including animals, to be patentable" (U.S. Congress, Office of Technology Assessment, 1989, p. 12). One year later, the first animal patent was issued to Harvard University for a mouse that was genetically engineered to be highly susceptible to developing tumors, a trait rendering it useful for various aspects of cancer research. The DuPont Corporation then produced the patented mouse in large numbers for commercial distribution.

Although legislation and court decisions had provided for patenting of plants and, in 1980, of microorganisms, concerns about these "lower" life forms had not seized the public imagination as did the patenting of "higher" animals. One of the few consensus conclusions that emerged among people concerned about genetic engineering after the animal patenting decision was that the issues surrounding the genetic engineering of animals were too complex to be decided by bureaucratic fiat from the Patent Office; rather, they had to be adjudicated as a matter of public policy by the U.S. Congress. Precisely what the moral and prudential issues were, however, was by no means clear, and people found it very difficult to separate moral issues from purely emotional ones.

Religious criticism

Some of the strongest negative responses to genetic engineering of animals seem to be expressed in the dictum encapsulated in numerous variations on the culturally pervasive Frankenstein myth: "There are certain things humans were not meant to know, do, or meddle with." Such a view is predicated on the notion that genetic engineering of animals is *intrinsically* wrong, regardless of what effects it might have—that is, that genetic engineering of animals is wrong even if it produces significant benefit and little or no actual or potential harm. This sort of position is most frequently advanced from a theological perspective, and is generally enunciated with little argument to buttress or even explicate the claim. For example, a statement signed by twenty-four religious leaders from a variety of faiths affirms that "the gift of life from God, in all its forms and species, should not be regarded solely as if it were a chemical product subject to genetic alteration and patentable for economic benefit" (Crawford, 1987, p. 480). Unfortunately, the statement fails to provide any argument as to *why* this perspective should not be adopted; presumably it is believed to be self-evident.

In the same vein, one can find condemnations of the placing of human genetic material in animals, as was done in the case of the human growth hormone gene being inserted into pigs to produce animals of greater size. The statement cited above, for example, asserts that "the combining of human genetic traits with animals . . . raises unique moral, ethical, and theological questions, such as the sanctity of human worth" (Statement of 24 Religious Leaders). Again, no elucidation or clarification is presented, nor was any subsequently forthcoming. It should be noted that not all religious voices oppose genetic engineering of animals on such grounds. For example, in 1982 the U.S. President's Commission for the Study of Ethical Problems in Medicine and Biomedical and Behavioral Research, responding to a formal request from representatives of the Catholic, Protestant, and Jewish faiths to look at the social and ethical issues pertaining to genetic engineering, issued a monograph entitled *Splicing Life: A Report on the Social and Ethical Issues of Genetic Engineering with Human Beings.* In the section on religious concerns, the report stressed that there seem to be no legitimate intrinsic religious objections to genetic engineering, pointing to the long theological tradition in the biblical religions that teaches that human beings are "cocreators" of the world, along with God.

A third example of an alleged ethical problem unsupported by explication or argument concerns the violation of "species integrity" effected by genetic engineering. Such claims simply assume that transmutation of species at the hands of humans is inherently wrong, and that fixed, immutable species are the building blocks of nature, as they were for those who accepted the classical idea of the Great Chain of Being. These points require much support, as modern biology rejects the fixed notion of species, and humans have been altering plant and animal species significantly for much of history. If genetic engineering is an activity continuous with what humans have perennially done, the burden is on the critic to show why effecting the same result through a different technology represents a morally relevant difference.

Potential risks

In sum, then, though such claims are politically significant, they do not, in the form we have described, represent clear moral questions. It is, however, possible to develop them into more obvious moral questions by rephrasing them in terms of the possible direct risks to humans and to the environment that could result from genetic engineering of animals.

Proponents of genetic engineering often argue that risks can be anticipated and controlled. But proper assessment of risk requires levels of knowledge far in excess of that currently available in the field, where we can *do* more than we can *know*, as is often the case with powerful new technologies; nuclear power provides an example that cannot easily be ignored.

Potential dangers emerging from genetic engineering of animals obviously stem from the rapidity with which such activity can introduce wholesale change in organisms. Traditional "genetic engineering" was done by selective breeding over long periods of time, allowing ample opportunity to observe the untoward effects of narrow selection of isolated characteristics. With the techniques currently available, however, scientists are doing their selection "in the fast lane."

First, unanticipated consequences may affect the organism that is being rapidly changed. The apparent characteristic being genetically engineered may have unsuspected implications. For example, when wheat was genetically engineered for resistance to blast, a form of blight, that characteristic was looked at in isolation and the genetic basis for this resistance was encoded into the organism. The wheat's backup gene for general resistance, however, was ignored. As a result, the new organism was very susceptible to all sorts of viruses that, in one generation, mutated sufficiently to devastate the crop.

Second, the isolated characteristic being engineered into the organism may have unsuspected harmful consequences to humans who interact with the organism— for example, people who consume the resultant life form, if it is a food animal. One can imagine genetically engineering, for example, faster growth in beef cattle in such a way as to increase certain levels of hormones that, when increased in concentration, turn out to be carcinogens for human beings over a period of years.

The key issue here is that one can genetically engineer traits in animals without a full understanding of the mechanisms involved in expression of traits in the organism or, for that matter, without knowing all that is affected by the gene in question, with resulting disaster. These possibilities suggest caution in such engineering until one has at least a reasonable sense of the physiological mechanisms affected.

A second set of risks replicates and amplifies problems inherent in selection by breeding. These include narrowing of a gene pool, the tendency toward genetic uniformity, the emergence of harmful recessive gene traits, the loss of hybrid vigor, and, of course, the greater susceptibility of organisms to devastation by pathogens (microorganisms that cause disease), as has been shown in some genetically engineered crops.

A third set of risks arises from the fact that in certain cases, when one changes animals, one thereby alters the pathogens to which they are host. This can occur in two ways. First, in genetically engineering for resistance to a given pathogen in an animal, one unwittingly could create an environment in the animal favorable to a natural mutation of that pathogenic microbe to which the modified animal would not be resistant. These new organisms then could be infectious to these or other animals, or to humans.

One possible example of this sort of reaction has been discussed regarding the so-called SCID mouse developed as a model for AIDS (Marx, 1990). These animals are genetically engineered to possess a human immune system and are then infected with the AIDS virus. Some researchers suggest that in such a mouse, the AIDS virus could become more virulent and infectious by interacting with native mouse viruses, thereby taking on new characteristics such as becoming transmissible by contact with the airborne virus. For similar reasons the National Institutes of Health, which had developed a different mouse model for AIDS, took extraordinary precautions to assure that the experimental mice could not accidentally escape.

Even if one were to genetically alter an animal without specifically changing its immune system, one might inadvertently alter the pathogens to which it is host indirectly by changing the microenvironment where they live. This, in turn, could result in these pathogens becoming dangerous to humans or other animals. Thus, for example, in altering agricultural animals such as cattle by genetic engineering, one runs the risk of affecting the pathogenicity of the microorganisms that inhabit the organism in unknown and unpredictable ways. The more precipitous the change, the more difficult it is to estimate the effects on the pathogens.

A fourth set of risks is ecological, associated with the possibility of radically altering an animal and then having it escape into an uncontrolled environment. While this might seem to be a minimal danger when dealing with intensively maintained and strictly confined cattle, chickens, or laboratory animals, it could pose a real problem with extensively managed and loosely confined sheep or cattle, as well as with rodents or rabbits that may escape despite ordinary precautions. Experience teaches us that the dangers of releasing animals into a new environment cannot be estimated, even with species whose characteristics are well known. Witness the uncontrollable proliferation of rabbits and cats released in Australia and of the mongoose in Hawaii, as well as our inability to deal with accidental release of killer bees. Ignorance of what could happen with newly engineered creatures is even more certain. A scientifically sound but fictional account of such a scenario can be found in Michael Crichton's 1990 novel, *Jurassic Park*.

A fifth set of risks is also environmental. By now, we are all familiar with the threat to global and regional ecosystems posed by agricultural expansion in Third World countries. Slash-and-burn techniques deployed in order to provide grazing land for cattle has led to desertification in Africa and dramatic loss of species in South America. What effect would genetic engineering have on these pernicious pursuits? The answer is not clear. It could be argued in favor of genetic engineering that our ability to genetically adapt animals and plants to indigenous conditions would halt such practices while allowing for economic growth. However, it is equally plausible to suggest that such technology could augment plunder of the environment by foisting animals on all sorts of hitherto undisturbed areas with unimaginable consequences. Once again, it is difficult to foresee such risks.

A sixth set of risks derives from potential military application of such technology. It is not difficult to imagine the sorts of weapons that could be created by using animals as carriers to infect populations with human pathogens.

Finally, the patenting of genetically engineered animals poses socioeconomic risks. For example, many farmer groups anticipate that small family farmers might be forced to acquire expensive patented animals in order to compete with large corporations and could well be forced out of business. This, in turn, might strengthen the ever-increasing tendency of large agribusiness to monopolize the food supply. One cannot predict the resultant effects on consumers or on the social fabric.

Proponents of genetic engineering of animals respond to the enumeration of risks by suggesting mechanisms for minimizing such risks. Such mechanisms include strict confinement of genetically engineered farm and laboratory animals, strictly limited experimental release of such nondomestic animals as fish, and genetically engineering such traits into the animals as metabolic deficiencies that can be met only by human-supplied diets, so that the animals could not survive in the wild. Proponents also list numerous potential bene-

fits of genetic engineering. Genetically engineered animals could, for example, increase productivity of food and fiber. Such was the point in developing the "super pig" and "super chicken," which are a good deal larger than normal animals. Development of such animals could boost economic growth and help the nation producing the animals to compete in world trade. Genetic engineering could minimize environmental damage by fitting animals to hitherto nonproductive environments. And through what has been called "molecular pharming," mammals can be genetically engineered to produce in their milk biologically active drugs and chemicals that are rare or expensive. Goats have already been developed that secrete TPA, a drug used to dissolve blood clots, in their milk. Proponents also stress the value of genetically engineered animals to biomedicine. Such animals can, in theory, model a variety of diseases and conditions. Most notably, they can be used as high-fidelity models of human genetic disease, some of the most devastating and untreatable diseases afflicting people. In addition, they can be used to study the safety and efficacy of gene therapy employed to treat these diseases.

Proponents of genetic engineering of animals also argue that it is simply not feasible to ban genetic engineering of animals. Unlike other potentially dangerous technologies, such as nuclear technology, genetic engineering can be done relatively cheaply and easily. A ban in a given country would simply drive the technology to places without a ban, and would jeopardize effecting any meaningful regulatory framework. It could also harm a country's ability to compete economically.

Protecting animal welfare

The entire set of risk-related issues discussed above represents a mixture of moral and prudential issues that ultimately involve weighing risks and benefits. Another significant moral issue associated with genetic engineering of animals, however, has received relatively little attention. This is the issue of the possible pernicious effects of genetic engineering on animals themselves. Since human benefits can, and will likely, exact a cost in animal suffering, and there is no benefit to humans militating in favor of controlling that suffering, the task of protecting such animals will be formidable.

The current tendencies in genetic engineering of animals, if unchecked and unregulated, will engender a significant degree of animal suffering, especially in the two areas that will dominate the genetic engineering of animals: agriculture and biomedicine.

In agriculture, attempts to engineer animals have largely focused on increasing productivity. Emphasis has been placed on increasing the size of pigs and chickens by insertion of modified genes controlling growth. While greater growth has indeed been achieved, significant suffering has been engendered, for example, in the form of arthritis and joint problems in the feet and legs, for the structural strength of the extremities does not increase in proportion to the extra weight. Based on the development of confinement systems in industrialized agriculture, it is clear that if the pain, suffering, and disease of the animals does not interfere with economic productivity, they are ignored. Hence the existence of "production diseases" endemic to confinement agriculture. Most important, there are no legal or regulatory constraints on what can be done to animals in pursuit of increasing agricultural productivity, either in agricultural research or in industry. Given the absence of such constraints and the historical willingness of industrialized agriculture to sacrifice animal welfare for productivity, the moral problem inherent in genetically engineering animals for production agriculture is obvious.

The probability of generating suffering in animals developed for biomedical research is even more dramatic. Until now biomedical science has lacked animal "models" of many devastating human genetic diseases. Genetic engineering of animals containing the genetic defects responsible for the human diseases certainly will be eagerly undertaken by the research community as soon as it is technically possible to do so. While such high-fidelity models may well reduce the number of animals used in research, the defective animals themselves will suffer greatly, since the genetic diseases they replicate often involve symptoms of tragic severity.

One of the first such models attempted was a mouse containing the genetic basis for Lesch-Nyhan disease, whose most horrible symptom involves an irresistible impulse for the patient to self-mutilate—typically to bite off lips and fingers—unless restrained. There is no cure or treatment for this disease, and patients rarely live beyond the third decade. In the case of the Lesch-Nyhan mouse, though the genetic basis for the disease was successfully created in the mouse, the animal did not exhibit symptoms. It is widely believed, however, that the technical problems preventing success in creating symptomatic "models" of such diseases will be solved within a decade.

The creation of animal "models" by genetic engineering could represent a breakthrough in the study of and cure for genetic disease in humans. To accomplish this goal, however, entails a dramatic moral problem. Great numbers of animals would live lives of excruciating pain and suffering. Although society is indeed in the process of debating new ethical standards to elevate the treatment of animals, it does not yet appear prepared to sacrifice significant potential human benefits for the sake of animal welfare. In 1985, U.S. federal legislation specified that pain and suffering in research animals should be controlled unless it is impossible to do so, as when the object of the research is pain or suffering or, more frequently, when one cannot control the pain and suffering without compromising the goal of the research. The problem, however, is that for the genetic diseases in question, whose adverse manifestations are chronic, no methods exist for controlling the pain and suffering in humans or in the animals. Presumably, the animals will be used for a significant portion of their lives; anesthesia for long periods is not technically feasible. The problem of controlling suffering in such genetically engineered models of disease has never been addressed by the research community.

It is clear, therefore, that unrestricted genetic engineering of animals is certain to produce significant and perhaps unprecedented degrees of animal suffering in agriculture and biomedicine. While genetic engineering can certainly secure benefits for animal welfare—for example, by genetically engineering disease resistance into animals, as has already been accomplished with chickens—the costs in pain and suffering to the animals, delineated above, represent a moral issue that is probably the most significant of all the questions raised by genetic engineering.

The regulatory imperative

A total ban on genetic engineering of animals does not appear to be practicable. Those in society concerned about the ethical and prudential issues seek a prolonged moratorium on animal patenting to discourage the development of genetically engineered animals while society deliberates the issues involved. Whether or not such legislation is enacted, such deliberation is essential in order to provide a rational basis for implementing a viable regulatory framework for controlling and minimizing both the risks to human beings and the environment and the animal suffering that accompany the development of this powerful new technology.

The genetic engineering of plants has provoked far less controversy in society. In the first place, humans are accustomed to the dramatic manipulation of plants to the point of creating new species—the tangelo, for example. Indeed, it is estimated that 70 percent of grasses and 40 percent of flowering plants represent new species created by humans through hybridization and other means of artificial selection. On the other hand, the insertion of animal genes into plants, as has been done with the insertion of flounder genes into tomatoes to prevent freezing, elicits a negative reaction from a substantial portion of the public. This reaction seems to be less a concern about intrinsic wrongness of such manipulation than a fear of dangers resulting from consuming the product.

Thus, when genetic engineering of plants is assessed by the same categories used to discuss genetic engineering of animals, one encounters different results. There is relatively little emphasis on the intrinsic wrongness of such engineering, and virtually no concern about plant welfare, since few people believe that plants are sentient. The bulk of social concern arises from possible untoward consequences of such engineering on humans and on the environment. The latter, especially, represents a legitimate concern, since there are many extant examples of plants moving into unintended environments with detrimental effects—for example, the disruption of native growth along waterways by Russian olive trees.

BERNARD E. ROLLIN

Directly related to this article is the companion article in this entry: HUMAN GENETIC ENGINEERING. *For a further discussion of topics mentioned in this article, see the entries* AGRICULTURE; ANIMAL RESEARCH; ANIMAL WELFARE AND RIGHTS, *especially the article on* ETHICAL PERSPECTIVES ON THE TREATMENT AND STATUS OF ANIMALS; *and* PAIN AND SUFFERING. *For a discussion of related ideas, see the entries* ECONOMIC CONCEPTS IN HEALTH CARE; ENVIRONMENT AND RELIGION; GENE THERAPY; GENETICS AND THE LAW; RISK; *and* VALUE AND VALUATION. *See also the* APPENDIX (CODES, OATHS, AND DIRECTIVES RELATED TO BIOETHICS), SECTION V: ETHICAL DIRECTIVES PERTAINING TO THE WELFARE AND USE OF ANIMALS.

Bibliography

CRAWFORD, MARK. 1987. "Religious Groups Join Animal Patent Battles." *Science* 237, no. 4814:480–481.

CRICHTON, MICHAEL. 1990. *Jurassic Park: A Novel.* New York: Knopf.

FOX, MICHAEL W. 1992. *Superpigs and Wondercorn: The Brave New World of Biotechnology and Where It All May Lead.* New York: Lyons & Burford.

KUEHN, MICHAEL R.; BRADLEY, ALLEN; ROBERTSON, ELIZABETH J.; and EVANS, MARTIN J. 1987. "A Potential Model for Lesch-Nyhan Syndrome Through Introduction of HPRT Mutations into Mice." *Nature* 326, no. 6110: 295–298.

MARX, JEAN. 1990. "Concerns Raised About Mouse Models for AIDS." *Science* 247, no. 4944:809.

REGAN, TOM. 1983. *The Case for Animal Rights.* Berkeley: University of California Press.

ROLLIN, BERNARD E. 1981. *Animal Rights and Human Morality.* Buffalo, N.Y.: Prometheus.

———. 1986. "'The Frankenstein Thing': The Moral Impact of Genetic Engineering of Agricultural Animals on Society and Future Science." In *Genetic Engineering of Animals: An Agricultural Perspective,* pp. 285–297. Edited by J. Warren Evans and Alexander Hollaender. New York: Plenum.

———. 1989. *The Unheeded Cry: Animal Consciousness, Animal Pain, and Science.* Oxford: Oxford University Press.

———. 1991a. "Federal Laws and Policies Governing Animal Research: Their History, Nature, and Adequacy." In *Biomedical Ethics Reviews, 1990,* pp. 195–227. Edited by James M. Humber and Robert F. Almeder. Clifton, N.J.: Humana.

———. 1991b. "Transgenic Animals—Science and Ethics." In *The Experimental Animal in Biomedical Research,* vol. 2. Edited by Bernard E. Rollin and M. Lynne Kesel. Boca Raton, Fla.: CRC Press.

SCRIVER, CHARLES R.; BEAUDET, ARTHUR L.; SLY, WILLIAM S.; and VALLE, DAVID, eds. 1989. *The Metabolic Basis of Inherited Disease.* 6th ed. New York: McGraw-Hill.

SINGER, PETER. 1990. *Animal Liberation.* 2d ed. New York: New York Review of Books.

Statement of 24 Religious Leaders Against Animal Patenting. N.d. Foundation on Economic Trends, Washington, D.C.

U.S. CONGRESS. OFFICE OF TECHNOLOGY ASSESSMENT. 1989. *Patenting Life—Special Report.* Vol. 5 of *New Developments in Biotechnology.* Washington, D.C.: Author.

U.S. PRESIDENT'S COMMISSION FOR THE STUDY OF ETHICAL PROBLEMS IN MEDICINE AND BIOMEDICAL AND BEHAVIORAL RESEARCH. 1982. *Splicing Life: A Report on the Social and Ethical Issues of Genetic Engineering with Human Beings.* Washington, D.C.: Author.

II. HUMAN GENETIC ENGINEERING

"Human genetic engineering" refers to the genetic modification of human beings using the techniques of modern biotechnology. Nearly all commentators have argued for caution in proceeding with the development of human genetic engineering, but there are significant differences in the nature of the concerns that these commentators have raised. This article begins by discussing some of the conceptual distinctions and empirical assumptions that have formed the background of most discussions in this area. It then proceeds to examine the ethical arguments and problems that are central to such discussions.

Empirical assumptions and conceptual distinctions

Genetic causation and determinism. Geneticists commonly draw a distinction between the genetic endowment of an organism (the organism's *genotype*) and the characteristics that the organism manifests (its *phenotype*). This distinction arises from an awareness that there is no simple relation between individual genes and characteristics, and, more specifically, that genes do not *determine* characteristics. The phenotype is the product not only of the genotype but also of a complex interaction between genotype and environment. Whether the interaction between genotype and environment de-

termines the phenotype is a matter of some controversy. Some geneticists have argued that important random events occur during the development of an organism, so that no claim of determinism can be made (Lewontin, 1991).

These points should be borne in mind when assessing the discussion concerning human genetic engineering. The general aim of human genetic engineering is to modify particular human characteristics. However, we are still a long way from knowing which human characteristics can be modified through genetic intervention. It may turn out that the causal relationship between some human characteristics and genes is extremely complex or is dependent upon significant random events occurring during development. If this is the case, then modifying the genes is not a feasible or possible way of modifying such characteristics. One of the central aims of genetic research is to understand the relationship between genotype and phenotype. It remains to be seen whether as a matter of biology *any* of the characteristics that have been frequently mentioned in the discussions about human genetic engineering—such as memory, intelligence, character, moral sentiments—can be modified by genetic manipulation. As a result, except for analyses concerning treatment of certain diseases, most of the discussions so far have tended to be abstract and hypothetical in their speculations regarding what genetic engineering will be able to accomplish.

Therapy versus enhancement.   Several writers have framed their discussion of human genetic engineering by distinguishing genetic interventions that aim at *therapy*—the cure or prevention of disease—from those that aim at the *enhancement* of human traits or abilities. ("Enhancement" is understood here quite broadly, so that the distinction between therapy and enhancement will appear mutually exclusive and exhaustive: thus, "correcting" a feature that is undesirable or falls below some norm would count as an enhancement as long as that feature was not associated with a disease.) The motive for invoking this distinction is a belief that the two kinds of intervention differ in their moral acceptability, or in the moral considerations that enter into a judgment of their acceptability. Specifically, writers who uphold the distinction argue that engineering aimed at enhancements is morally more problematic or requires more justification than engineering aimed at therapy (Anderson, 1985, 1989).

The contrast between engineering aimed at therapy and engineering aimed at enhancement is reminiscent of the contrast between "negative eugenics" and "positive eugenics" that informed discussions about human genetics earlier in the twentieth century. Negative eugenics, it was argued, aims at improving the species by eliminating bad genetic material, whereas positive eugenics serves this aim by promoting good genetic material (Kevles, 1985). If there is a substantive point to be made by using the terminology of "therapy" versus "enhancement" rather than the older terminology of "negative" versus "positive" eugenics—a point that goes beyond an attempt to dissociate, by linguistic means, human genetic engineering from the disastrous history of the eugenics movement—then that point might be that the goal of human genetic engineering is to improve the individual, not the population or the species. This dissociation, however, cannot be complete. Even if the motivation focuses on the individual, the appeal can be broad and thus the effect can easily be populational (Proctor, 1992).

In any case, the modern contrast between therapy and enhancement plainly points to the contrast between health and disease. Whether genetic intervention to increase the height of an individual who would otherwise grow to be four feet, ten inches counts as therapy or as enhancement depends upon whether being four feet, ten inches is considered to be a disease (or the result of a disease). The contrast between health and disease, however, is controversial in itself, both with regard to where the *boundary* between them ought to be drawn and on what *basis* it is properly constituted. The difficulty of locating the boundary between health and disease raises the issue of how useful the contrast between therapy and enhancement can be. But difficulties remain even if we put controversial borderline cases to one side and consider only conditions that are universally recognized as serious diseases. For example, no one disputes that AIDS is a serious disease. Should genetically engineering a resistance to AIDS be considered therapy—because it aims at preventing disease—or enhancement—because it aims at producing a trait (an enhanced immune system) that human beings do not normally possess (Engelhardt, 1990)? Indeed, for any case where genetic engineering is employed to deal with a *nongenetic* disease, it is unclear whether that response should be considered therapy or enhancement.

The question of what constitutes the basis for distinguishing between health and disease raises the issue of to what extent the distinction between health and disease, and so the distinction between therapy and enhancement, is the result of social and political pressures. If these distinctions are understood to be socially constructed, then the claim that engineering aimed at therapy is morally less problematic is open to doubt.

Ethical arguments

The ethical concerns that have been raised regarding human genetic engineering can be divided into two groups—those that have attended primarily to the possible *results* (products) of genetically engineering people, and those that have attended primarily to the *means* (process) that genetic engineering represents. The first group focuses on such questions as: What kind of people could there be? How are we to assess the harms, benefits, and risks in having genetically engineered human beings? The second group focuses on the ethical propriety of using *genetic* techniques to alter people.

The following discussion will be confined to these general ethical questions. Sometimes the concerns raised about human genetic engineering have more to do with the specific context in which it might be pursued rather than with the engineering itself. For example, as has been noted, human genetic engineering is easily associated with eugenics. Eugenics, in turn, has often been associated with governmental policies that involve morally troubling procedures: forced sterilization, compulsory abortions, forced matings. The moral questions surrounding such procedures can obscure the general question of whether genetic modification of people is morally justifiable in itself. Important as they are, questions about specific policies will be put to one side in this discussion, since human genetic engineering does not need to be tied to any such coercive state actions (Glover, 1984).

Assessing the results. It is not at all difficult to point to possible genetic modifications that would have disturbing biological and social consequences. First, there is a good deal that we do not know when we insert new genes into a complex organism. Perhaps the result is something far more dangerous than we can manage. For example, some might think that genetic engineering to increase memory capacity would be good. But perhaps by altering that trait we would thereby make an individual emotionally unstable or interfere with some other beneficial trait.

Second, injustices and unfair discriminations based on biological differences (as in racism and sexism) are all too familiar. These harms could well be perpetuated on the basis of biological differences that result from genetic engineering. For example, if the availability of human genetic engineering becomes a matter for market forces to decide, then differences in economic class may become biologically entrenched. The rich not only may be healthier, they also may be brighter, stronger, prettier, and so on.

Finally, we should note the nefarious uses that could be made of human genetic engineering. Commentators have often expressed fears about the creation of a group of people we can easily enslave, or of a "super race" who can easily enslave us. This last possibility has captured the imagination of several modern writers, not only in such famous antiutopian literature as Aldous Huxley's *Brave New World* (1932) but also in C. S. Lewis's image of one generation enslaving all future generations by having the power to make its descendants what it pleases (Lewis, 1947).

Nevertheless, despite all these possible harms, it is not difficult to imagine possible modifications that would be extremely beneficial. There is room for improvement in human beings. We try to increase people's mental abilities, control their aggressive tendencies, and enhance their moral sentiments. Until now we have pursued these goals through education and social and political institutions. If we could achieve some of these results more effectively through genetic engineering, why shouldn't we?

Without denying the possibility of beneficial results, several commentators have argued that we should proceed with caution, carefully weighing the harms against the benefits in each case. Each proposed modification must be critically scrutinized so that we can achieve the benefits of human genetic engineering without inviting disaster (Glover, 1984; Engelhardt, 1984).

This response, of course, raises many of the standard questions attached to any harms-versus-benefits approach: What items are we weighing when we look at the harms and benefits? Should we look only at physical harms and benefits (such as physical pain and pleasure), or should we include possible economic and social gains or losses, or even more complex values? How do we weigh harms against benefits when these attach to different individuals or generations? Who should decide which trade-offs are acceptable?

As difficult as these questions are, they are not peculiar to human genetic engineering: the same questions arise in many areas of health policy. We should, however, note a striking problem regarding the distribution of the benefits of human genetic engineering. The problem arises because the idea of genetic manipulation challenges our understanding of what constitutes a just distribution of goods.

The general problem of distributive justice may be stated as follows: How ought the various social goods (such as power and wealth) be distributed in the face of obvious inequalities in the distribution of natural goods (intelligence, vigor, beauty, and the like)? The goal is to achieve some form of "social equality" (for example, equality of opportunity) despite "natural inequalities."

However, if we can control natural inequalities such as those in intelligence or strength through genetic engineering, what is the goal of a just distribution? Should natural inequalities in intellectual endowment be any more tolerated than social inequalities in educational opportunities? Is there a morally significant distinction between natural and social goods, so that natural inequalities should be viewed differently from social inequalities?

Some writers have objected to the case-by-case, weighing-the-harms-against-the-benefits approach, claiming that in a broad class of cases—those involving positive human genetic engineering, if not human genetic engineering in general—we run the risk of losing our humanity. This loss is not simply a harm that needs to be weighed against the benefits; the loss of our humanity would undermine any alleged benefit of genetic engineering (Kass, 1985).

Concern over a loss of our humanity is often presented in vague terms, perhaps intentionally so (Anderson, 1985). No one has suggested that there are specific genes for humanity, nor is there a consensus about what human traits constitute humanity. If the loss of our humanity could be identified as a specific harm resulting from specific genetic alterations, then it would seem that this harm is one of many possible harms—of great weight and significance, to be sure—that should be included when we weigh the benefits against the harms. Often, however, the loss of our humanity is presented as a loss that would occur without our realizing it, as if being aware of such a loss would require the exercise of precisely those qualities of humanity that we were losing. According to this objection, therefore, there should be a ban: We are not wise enough, or invulnerable enough, to engage in activities such as genetic engineering.

An important challenge this objection faces is to explain what kind of norm the preserving of our humanity reflects. If it is a norm that reflects a particular culture, taste, or tradition, then the appeal to "our" humanity has little persuasive force. Basing a ban on that kind of norm would seem too much like imposing on all future generations the parochial concerns of a few. If the norm reflects a norm in nature, a different set of problems arises. The modern scientific understanding of nature does not recognize anything like a norm of humanity that has intrinsic moral significance or that has any absolute moral claim on us (Engelhardt, 1990). Consequently, this approach has the daunting task of having to challenge and revise our scientific understanding of nature (Kass, 1985).

Assessing the means.   Some objections to human genetic engineering have not focused on any particular consequence or harm. The objection is not so much against altering human characteristics as against *using genetic technology* to alter human characteristics. These objections tend, therefore, to be broad objections to the very idea of genetically engineering human beings.

One common objection to this effect is expressed in claims that we are "playing God" or that we are arrogantly interfering with "God's plan." This point of view is often exemplified in the titles of popular books on

genetic engineering: *Who Should Play God?* (Howard and Rifkin, 1977) and *Playing God* (Goodfield, 1977). This type of argument has generally received the following reply: First, as an argument for a general prohibition, it would apply with equal force to such activities as public-health management or medicine in general. Curing people who would otherwise die before they reach reproductive age can have a profound effect on later generations. Why should genetic engineering be any more a matter of arrogant interference than prenatal care? Second, the objection rests on controversial assumptions. There is certainly no agreement among religious leaders that we understand God's plan and therefore know what constitutes interference with that plan (U.S. President's Commission, 1982).

A secular but in some ways similar objection proceeds by first noting the distinction between *somatic* and *germ-line* genetic engineering—the distinction between genetic modifications that are not inheritable and those that are. The objection then proceeds to state that germ-line genetic engineering should be prohibited because it is interfering with the wisdom of evolution (Chargaff, 1976). Our genetic makeup is the result of natural selection taking place over a vast amount of time. By altering the human genome without understanding why it evolved in the way it did, we run the risk of, for example, deleting a gene we suppose to be harmful but the benefit of which we come to realize only too late.

Consider, in this light, the case of sickle-cell anemia. Sickle-cell disease results from a point mutation in the gene that produces hemoglobin. This mutation alters the hemoglobin so that the blood cells become distorted ("sickled"); to what degree depends upon the presence of unaffected hemoglobin. Although in heterozygotes there is little tendency toward sickling, in homozygotes there is a significant amount of sickling, which results in the production of blood cells that cannot transport oxygen into tissues. Despite the severity of the disease, we can give an evolutionary explanation for the presence of sickle-cell anemia among black Africans: In its heterozygote state, the mutation offers some protection against *falciparum* malaria. Thus, although the gene is linked to a disease, it does in certain circumstances confer a benefit. Perhaps, so the objection goes, there are hidden benefits in other "harmful" genes. Until we have a better understanding of human evolution, we should not alter human genes.

A common reply to this objection is to point out, once again, that medicine and public-health efforts in general can have profound evolutionary consequences. Moreover, when it comes to evolutionary change, it may well be (to paraphrase Henry David Thoreau) that we sit as many risks as we run. Having evolved in a particular way does not ensure our future survival. Some species have become extinct because they were unable to adapt promptly or adequately to their changing environment. For all we know, our future survival may depend upon our genetically engineering humans in response to sudden environmental changes (Jackson and Stich, 1979).

Conclusion

Human genetic engineering raises profound challenges to ethics in general and bioethics in particular. Many claims and arguments in ethics rest upon distinctions such as social goods versus natural goods, enhancements versus corrections, harms versus benefits. It is precisely these distinctions that may be altered by genetic engineering; thus, the task of moral assessment must be pursued with particular care. Under the impetus of human genetic engineering, we may need to rethink many of our moral concepts and theories.

ROBERT WACHBROIT

Directly related to this article is the companion article in this entry: ANIMALS AND PLANTS. *Also directly related are the entries* MEDICAL GENETICS; GENE THERAPY; GENETIC COUNSELING; GENETIC TESTING AND SCREENING; GENETICS AND ENVIRONMENT IN HUMAN HEALTH; GENOME MAPPING AND SEQUENCING; *and* REPRODUCTIVE TECHNOLOGIES, *article on* CRYOPRESERVATION OF SPERM, OVA, AND EMBRYOS. *For a discussion of the ethics of genetic engineering, see the entries* EUGENICS; EUGENICS AND RELIGIOUS LAW; EVOLUTION; FUTURE GENERATIONS, OBLIGATIONS TO; GENETICS AND HUMAN SELF-UNDERSTANDING; HEALING; HEALTH AND DISEASE; LIFE; SOCIAL MEDICINE; *and* VALUE AND VALUATION. *Other relevant material may be found under the entries* BIOMEDICAL ENGINEERING; *and* BIOTECHNOLOGY.

Bibliography

ANDERSON, W. FRENCH. 1985. "Human Gene Therapy: Scientific and Ethical Considerations." *Journal of Medicine and Philosophy* 10, no. 13:275–291.
———. 1989. "Human Gene Therapy: Why Draw a Line?" *Journal of Medicine and Philosophy* 14, no. 6:681–693.
CHARGAFF, ERWIN. 1976. "On the Dangers of Genetic Meddling." *Science* 192:938, 940.
ENGELHARDT, H. TRISTRAM. 1984. "Persons and Humans: Refashioning Ourselves in a Better Image and Likeness." *Zygon* 19, no. 3:281–295.
———. 1990. "Human Nature Technologically Revisited." *Social Philosophy and Policy* 8, no. 1:180–191.
GLOVER, JONATHAN. 1984. *What Sort of People Should There Be?* New York: Penguin.
GOODFIELD, JUNE. 1977. *Playing God: Genetic Engineering and the Manipulation of Life.* New York: Harper & Row.
HOWARD, TED, and RIFKIN, JEREMY. 1977. *Who Should Play God? The Artificial Creation of Life and What It Means to the Future of the Human Race.* New York: Dell.
HUXLEY, ALDOUS. 1932. *Brave New World: A Novel.* Garden City, N.Y.: Doubleday, Doran.
JACKSON, DONALD A., and STICH, STEPHEN P., eds. 1979. *The Recombinant DNA Debate.* Englewood Cliffs, N.J.: Prentice-Hall.
KASS, LEON. 1985. *Toward a More Natural Science: Biology and Human Affairs.* New York: Free Press.
KEVLES, DANIEL J. 1985. *In the Name of Eugenics: Genetics and the Uses of Human Heredity.* New York: Knopf.
LEWIS, C. S. 1947. *The Abolition of Man: Or, Reflections on Education with Special Reference to the Teaching of English in the Upper Forms of Schools.* New York: Macmillan.
LEWONTIN, RICHARD. 1991. *Biology as Ideology: The Doctrine of DNA.* New York: Harper.
PROCTOR, ROBERT N. 1992. "Genomics and Eugenics: How Fair Is the Comparison?" In *Gene Mapping: Using Law and Ethics as Guides,* pp. 57–93. Edited by George J. Annas and Sherman Elias. New York: Oxford University Press.
U.S. PRESIDENT'S COMMISSION FOR THE STUDY OF ETHICAL PROBLEMS IN MEDICINE AND BIOMEDICAL AND BEHAVIORAL RESEARCH. 1982. *Splicing Life: A Report on the Ethical Issues of Genetic Engineering with Human Beings.* Washington, D.C.: U.S. Government Printing Office.

GENETICS, MEDICAL

See MEDICAL GENETICS.

GENETICS AND ENVIRONMENT IN HUMAN HEALTH

Human beings have always noted the physical and mental resemblance of children to their parents. Heredity was easily accepted as the principal explanation of physical characteristics. In contrast, nature/nurture and genetics/environment debates raged about what caused human diseases and particularly about how intelligence, temperament, criminality, alcoholism, and psychiatric disorders developed. One side argued that human nature could not be changed appreciably, while others argued that it could—and therefore advocated what they considered optimal physical and psychological conditions for good health. During the nineteenth century, supernurturists espoused the anti-Darwinian view of Lamarck that the environment influenced heredity directly; such a view reappeared in the Soviet Union in the 1930s—a position that was thoroughly discredited by the 1960s when the Soviets decided to restore research in genetics.

In recent years a much more productive concept has emerged, namely, the interaction of genetic and environmental factors. Genes are sequences of DNA in our twenty-three pairs of chromosomes in each nucleated cell. Genes specify the sequence of proteins, which are the main effector molecules of our cells, serving as enzymes (catalysts), structural molecules (like collagen), antibodies to fight off infections, and binders of oxygen or vitamins or chemicals (prescribed medicines or chemicals from the environment). Environmental factors include social and familial environment, intrauterine environment, cigarette smoking, alcohol, other substance abuse, stress, and exposures to chemical, physical, and biological agents. Some environmental exposures (ultraviolet light, X rays, certain industrial chemicals) cause damage to the DNA, or mutations, which alter gene function as well as the structure and function of the protein specified by that gene. Many such mutations are of little consequence. Others may lead to disease or become a basis for natural selection and evolution.

There are many examples of gene-environmental interactions. Skin color is largely genetic, but it is also influenced by sun exposure. Body weight and obesity reflect food intake and energy expenditure as well as genetic determinants. For infectious diseases, such as malaria and tuberculosis, genetic determinants affect the severity of illness and likelihood of dying. A drug having no side effects at usual doses in most individuals may cause severe symptoms in a person with an unusual form of one of the enzymes that metabolize the drug. Without the exposure to the drug, the variant would be innocuous.

In the 1920s, Herman J. Muller noted the adverse effects of ionizing radiation on genes and chromosomes and became concerned about the resulting deleterious effects on human health. He predicted similar effects from chemicals though there was little interest in chemically mediated genetic effects until about thirty years later. Both ionizing radiation and chemicals can produce mutations and chromosomal aberrations in human cells, including the germ cells (eggs and sperm). Mutations—changes in the genes—also may occur randomly during the complex replication of DNA and division of cells.

All humans carry several recessive genes for potentially serious diseases. Recessive genes are those which must occur in double dose (from both parents) in order to cause any effect; a single dose of the recessive gene in a carrier of that gene is innocuous except for the X chromosome in males (who have only one X chromosome). So-called dominant genes cause effects when present in single dose and are transmitted from just one parent. In addition, we have numerous gene variants; most appear to have no apparent functional effect, others may make us more or less susceptible to various specific diseases or specific environmental exposures. The Human Genome Project will accelerate the finding of such genes.

Role of genetic tests in assessing risks for environmental exposures in human disease

All living things interact with multiple environments. The physical environment—temperature, humidity, sunlight, altitude—often sets boundaries crucial to development of new species and individual behaviors. The biological environment includes myriad "pests" or parasites, which kill, injure, or cause illnesses in organisms they make their targets or hosts. From time immemorial, the resulting infectious diseases have accounted for most human illnesses and deaths. Various epidemics remind us we must not be complacent about infectious agents, including HIV/AIDS, new hepatitis viruses, "slow viruses" associated with degenerative neurological and joint diseases, and a newly discovered *Chlamydia* organism that causes pneumonia and might even be involved in coronary heart disease.

Rachel Carson's *Silent Spring* (1962) and the emergence of the environmental movement worldwide focused attention on hazards to ecosystems and to human health from chemicals. Many of these agents have been introduced to control biological hazards in agriculture or to assure safe drinking water. Others are utilized in industry and commerce and promoted in such company slogans as "Better Living Through Chemistry." Of more than four million chemicals listed by the American Chemical Society, about 70,000 are widely used in modern society as pharmaceuticals, pesticides, cosmetics, food additives, and industrial and commercial agents.

Essentially all new chemicals and some older chemicals must be tested for potential toxicity to humans and other living things before they can be approved for sale. Thus, the U.S. Food and Drug Administration requires extensive animal and clinical testing of new drugs, vaccines, and medical devices, and of old drugs proposed for new uses, as well as animal testing for food additives and cosmetics. Under the pesticide laws and the Toxic Substances Control Act of 1976, the U.S. Environmental Protection Agency requires toxicity testing data for all new chemicals proposed for sale. The Occupational Safety and Health Administration, Consumer Product Safety Commission, Department of Agriculture, and Department of Transportation, and their state and local counterparts, also have responsibilities for control of chemical hazards.

Risks from environmental agents are related to the dose or level of exposure as well as to intrinsic potency of the agent and susceptibility of the person exposed. In general, the highest exposures are in patients receiving potent drugs or radiation as medical treatments and in workers manufacturing or cleaning up chemicals in various operations. Therefore, it is logical and efficient to investigate potential risks to human health in patients and in workers with known exposures to specific agents.

Studies of risks to the general population from contamination of groundwater or from air pollution, consumer products, or hazardous waste sites are far more difficult because the levels of exposure are typically much lower and the likelihood of adverse effects is similarly reduced.

Chemical exposures may cause immediate toxicity to the skin, eyes, lungs, heart, liver, nervous system, reproductive organs, or other target sites in the body. Some effects may be unrecognized at first, including mutations in specific genes that might lead to cancer or birth defects, or be passed on to future generations. Repeated exposures at relatively low doses may have cumulative toxic effects; examples are impairment of brain function and reduction of IQ by lead from the air, drinking water, or paint chips, and fibrosis and lung failure from breathing asbestos fibers or silica dust. For ethical reasons and to meet regulatory requirements, companies that develop new chemicals perform or contract for extensive testing to identify and characterize their potential hazards to health. Tests can detect mutagenic effects on bacterial and mammalian cells and birth defects, cancers, and organ-specific effects in animals.

Mutations are at the heart of the multistage process of carcinogenesis (cancer formation) and may cause various genetic diseases and birth defects. Thus, using genetic techniques to detect mutagenic chemicals is an efficient way to screen for potential cancer or genetic disease risks. The most commonly used test, the Ames test, measures mutation rates in *Salmonella* bacteria. Of course, bacteria may not metabolize chemicals the same way our bodies do, and they do not have plasma proteins to carry bound chemicals to specific organs. A new generation of tests combines in vivo exposures in whole animals with in vitro assays of effects on chromosomes, genes, and organ functions in laboratory tests. Such assays offer short testing times and relatively low cost, compared with lifetime exposures of rats or mice.

Lifetime rodent bioassays now cost more than $1.5 million per chemical and take up to five years to organize, perform, and analyze. Since standard studies utilize fifty animals in each group (sex, species, dose), statistical certainty is quite limited, and often there are wide confidence limits regarding the effects being tested. A maximally tolerated dose, rather than that to which human populations are exposed, is used to try to detect any effects. Two particular controversies center on interpretation of the rodent lifetime bioassay.

First, cell damage at the "maximally tolerated dose" may trigger compensatory responses leading to cancers that would not occur at the much lower doses more representative of human exposures. However, if lower doses were tested, the probability of detecting true carcinogenic effects in reasonable numbers of animals would be reduced at least proportionately. Second, present regulatory policy aims to prevent worst-case estimates of one additional case of cancer per million persons exposed to a specific chemical. Many living organisms produce potent toxins—part of their survival equipment against natural predators; these plant toxins and food constituents have been inadequately tested. If our aim is to protect human health, we should know more about all our chemical risks, not just those arising from industrial activities. We should recognize that the long-feared epidemic of cancer related to post-World War II production of industrial and agricultural chemicals has not materialized, if one corrects for the major effects of cigarette smoking as well as for aging of the population since cancers increase with aging.

Per one million Americans, 23 percent (230,000) currently die of various cancers. Evidence of environ-

TABLE 1. Percent of Total Cancer Risk Attributed to Various Factors

Class of Factors	Best Estimate	Range of Estimates
Tobacco	30	25–40
Alcohol	3	2–4
Diet	35*	10–70*
Food Additives	<1	0–2
Reproductive/Sexual Behavior	?	1–15
Occupation	4	2–8
General Pollution	2	<1–3
Consumer products	<1	<1–2
Medicines/medical products	1	0.5–3
Geophysical factors (sunlight, e.g.)	3	2–4
Infection	10	1–?
Psychological and other causes	?	?

*Least certain; note the wide range of estimates
Source: Doll, 1981.

mental, and therefore preventable, causes of cancer in humans is tabulated in Table 1.

Ecogenetics: Host variation in susceptibility to chemicals

Humans vary remarkably in their responses to chemical exposures and, therefore, in their risks of adverse effects. Such variation may reflect differences in sex, age, nutrition, lifestyle decisions to smoke cigarettes or drink alcoholic beverages, recreational exposures to similar or other chemicals, occupational exposures, and use of protective gear or medicines. In addition, the variation may reflect inherited differences in metabolism of specific chemicals and in vulnerability of target sites for the chemical's actions in the body. These inherited differences and their influence on the effects of exposures to environmental agents are the subject of the field of ecogenetics. Biochemical and molecular techniques are being used to develop markers of host susceptibility as well as markers of exposure and of preclinical effects.

To cause cancer, mutations, or birth defects, many chemicals must be activated by enzymes to intermediates that attack DNA. Other enzyme systems detoxify potentially toxic compounds. Genetic variation in biotransformation steps can put different people at different risks from similar exposures. When such genetic variants occur with frequencies greater than 1 percent in a given population, they are termed polymorphisms.

For example, cytochrome P450 enzymes form a family of dozens of related enzymes with distinct and overlapping characteristics. Amidst the complexity, however, one specific P450 enzyme (debrisoquine 4-hydroxylase) is responsible for marked variation in the metabolism of more than thirty drugs. From an environmental point of view, we may ask whether people who are "poor metabolizers" and "extensive metabolizers" of these pharmaceuticals have similar differences in handling chemicals from the general environment. Several studies indicate they do.

There is an excess of extensive metabolizers of debrisoquine among lung-cancer patients who have smoked. This result fits the hypothesis that extensive metabolizers would be more effective than poor metabolizers at activating cancer-causing chemicals found in cigarette smoke; extensive metabolizers may, therefore, have a greater risk of lung cancer. Lung cancers are by far the leading cancer killer in both men and women, accounting for 27 percent of cancer deaths and 6 percent of all deaths in the United States, and possible variation in risk of lung cancer for different people is therefore important.

Until recently, distinguishing poor and extensive metabolizers of debrisoquine required administering debrisoquine or another drug, then collecting and analyz-

ing urine samples. Besides the inconvenience, results can be influenced by diet and medications. A technique that relies on multiplication of DNA from white blood cells now can detect most individuals characterized as poor metabolizers. (The 1993 Nobel Prize in chemistry was awarded for development of the DNA multiplication technique, the polymerase chain reaction [PCR] which is used in these tests and has wide applications in biology, forensic testing, medicine, and ecogenetics.)

Deficiency in the enzyme glutathione-S-transferase (GST) may be another important predisposing factor in development of cancers. About 45 percent of Caucasians lack detectable activity of a particular form of GST. Several studies testing GST in blood samples or in lung tissue suggest GST-deficient smokers are at higher risk, presumably because this enzyme detoxifies carcinogenic chemicals. Thus, GST-normal smokers are partially protected against lung cancer, but more study is needed. Interesting related findings have come from animal studies. High GST activity is a very important protective factor against liver cancer from aflatoxin (a toxin from fungi that grow on peanuts and corn). Big differences in GST activity explain a long-puzzling observation that rats develop tumors from doses of aflatoxin that have no effect at all on mice; mice have much higher GST activity than rats. GST activity in human liver specimens more closely resembles that of rats, especially at low aflatoxin exposures like those in diet or environment. So humans are at risk from aflatoxin-contaminated foods.

Polymorphic variation of the liver enzyme N-acetyl transferase (NAT) accounts for marked differences in blood levels of several drugs, including the antituberculosis drug isoniazid, after standard doses. Half the Caucasian and black populations have the slow acetylator phenotype (the form of the gene and enzyme with lower activity) associated with higher levels of still-active drug and a propensity to adverse effects. The same detoxification mechanism metabolizes several other chemicals, including the potent human bladder carcinogens beta-naphthylamine, benzidine, and 4-aminobiphenyl, former mainstays of the dyestuff industry worldwide. People who are slow acetylators are at higher risk for bladder cancer, as expected from the hypothesis that they would be less able to detoxify these potent carcinogens by acetylation to inactive products. DNA probes are now available to assay this kind of genetic variation in peripheral blood cells rather than having to administer a test drug and measure metabolites in urine.

These ecogenetic phenomena may apply to all kinds of diseases, not just cancers. For example, the common organophosphorus pesticide, parathion, is converted to its toxic intermediate, paraoxon, by the P450 system and then inactivated by a circulating plasma enzyme, paraoxonase. About half of the Caucasian population has low paraoxonase activity. For similar exposures, people with lower activity of this enzyme are likely to be at higher risk for neurologic toxicity and take longer to recover. Recent success in cloning the paraoxonase gene will facilitate ecogenetic studies of pesticides.

Ecogenetics: Nutrition and infectious diseases

Genetic variation is important in nutritional studies of such major dietary components as saturated fats, cholesterol, milk, and iron.

High blood cholesterol levels are related both to diet and to inherited variation in several genes affecting the proteins that carry fat (lipoproteins) and their cell receptors. Cholesterol- and fat-reducing diets and drugs can reduce coronary heart disease deaths and heart attacks, at least in middle-aged men. However, responses to diet and drugs may differ among people with several different genetic causes of high levels of fat components in the blood.

Milk is a fascinating subject in anthropology. The milk sugar, lactose, must be metabolized by the enzyme lactase to release its energy. If it is not metabolized, lactose in the intestinal tract causes bloating, irritation, diarrhea, and sometimes internal bleeding. With very rare exceptions, infants have intestinal lactase activity. After weaning (i.e., after two years of age), most children in the world stop making the lactase enzyme. For a long time, this did not present a problem because children would no longer be sucking or drinking milk after the age of two. But since milk from goats and cows has become a prominent food in the past 8,000 years, differences have arisen among human populations. Among people of African, Asian, and Native American ancestry, more than 90 percent still deactivate the lactase gene and cannot metabolize the lactose sugar in milk, while about 90 percent of Caucasians have retained the lactase gene and, therefore, tolerate milk in their diets without problems. Due to the high prevalence of protein deficiency and milk's very good protein value, powdered milk has been shipped to many Third World countries and to Native American reservations, only to have many recipients refuse to drink the milk; some of them have used the powdered milk to paint their adobes. Before the milk-associated diarrhea was understood, these behaviors were ridiculed. Now we realize that many people were unable to digest the milk. We must ask, on a populationwide basis, how to balance a mild state of ill health produced by drinking milk against a more severe state of ill health caused by protein deficiency, particularly in children.

Chronic anemias due to iron deficiency are a major health problem throughout the world. Iron can be supplied inexpensively by fortification of flour. However, it is known that a small percentage of individuals—varying in different populations—carry genes (for types of anemia called thalassemias or for an iron metabolism disorder known as hemochromatosis) that make these individuals absorb iron excessively. Thus, these people might be injured by additional dietary intake of iron in bread. The utilitarian notion of doing the most good for the largest number has been challenged, with a call for (expensive) diagnostic testing to identify those at risk from excess iron ingestion. Nevertheless, supplementation has proceeded in many countries.

In human history, infectious diseases were major selective factors in survival of various populations. Our knowledge is greatest for the role of malaria. Vivax malaria infection found in West Africa occurs only in individuals who have certain blood group antigens (known as Duffy antigens) on their red blood cells; the malaria-causing parasite uses these molecules as portals of entry into red blood cells, where the parasite multiples. Surviving black populations have Duffy-negative cells, which the parasite cannot enter. For falciparum malaria, which is often lethal in childhood, several genetic "defects" of the red blood cell, such as sickle-cell trait, thalassemia trait, and glucose-6-phosphate dehydrogenase deficiency, all slow multiplication of the parasite and, if present, confer an advantage in survival. For many other common genetic diseases, such as cystic fibrosis, the selective factors in human history that led to the relatively high frequency of this gene (5 percent of the Caucasian population are gene carriers) are altogether unknown.

Bioethical issues about ecogenetics

Ecogenetics is still in its infancy as a scientific field, yet numerous important ethical issues have been anticipated and must be addressed before any potential tests should be used to screen workers or populations. Before the extensive development of biochemical genetics, J. B. S. Haldane published in *Heredity and Politics* (1938) the concept that those who are susceptible to potter's bronchitis—a common problem in British potters—might be protected or excluded from work in that occupation. Identification, exclusion, stigmatization, and discrimination that can result from knowledge of genetic risk factors for disease raise moral and ethical issues of great potential importance. Labeling is an ethical issue. Susceptibility to one kind of chemical does not predict susceptibility to chemicals with unrelated metabolism or structure. Thus, no one should be branded as "hypersusceptible" to chemical exposures on this basis. Justice may be impaired if carriers of currently unknown predisposing traits go undetected due to scientific ignorance, while those whose predisposing traits can be detected might be subjected to discriminatory action. Many genes occur with markedly different frequency in different ethnic or racial groups. Therefore, targeted testing or screening programs could lead to controversy because particular ethnic and racial groups are involved disproportionately. Quantitative assays of enzyme activity always have overlap between noncarriers and carriers of a gene affecting enzyme activity, thereby causing false identification of carriers. The new DNA probe techniques should reduce these problems, but negative publicity about the interpretation of DNA fingerprinting for use in courts of law heightens fears about genetic databanks and their potential misuse by scientists, government, insurance companies, or employers.

Useful tests for genetic predispositions to particular environmental chemicals could lead to better diagnosis, more informed regulations, and targeted preventive approaches, but knowledge of variations in susceptibility must not diminish our commitment to reduce exposures in the environment for all workers. Ironically, as we do reduce exposures enough to protect most of the population, genetic variations in general will account for a larger proportion of the remaining risk among those exposed.

Even when risk factors are very well established, the cause of a disease in a specific individual may be uncertain. The well-recognized interaction of cigarette smoking with workplace asbestos exposure in causing lung cancer reveals scientific uncertainties and legal and ethical problems in determining causation and responsibility in individual cases. In other situations, scientific evidence may be misused. For example, the U.S. Air Force denied African-Americans with sickle-cell trait access to the Air Force Academy on the uninvestigated presumption that they would be at increased risk for inflight complication and fatal accidents, and that such risk would be significant compared with all the other reasons for such accidents.

A few observers feel genetics currently is overemphasized in biomedical research and may constitute a "back door to eugenics." Others point to many well-known environmental factors that are neglected and argue that environmental factors can be manipulated more easily. Concern with genetics is said to detract from the emphasis on simple public-health and medical measures that should be the mainstay of management of disease. Still others counter that disease management will be most efficient and rational when mechanisms of disease are better understood and medical efforts can be directed at the fraction of the population most at risk. Thus, medicine and public health ultimately will both benefit.

Much work needs to be done to elucidate genetic risk profiles for various diseases as we move into the era of genetic medicine. In the meantime, both the population-wide approach, with emphasis on environmental measures, and the genetic approach that aims to identify individuals at highest risk, can be advocated. For example, it is recommended that the entire population follow a prudent diet that avoids excess fat, cholesterol, and salt. At the same time, appropriate tests may identify those at highest risk of developing coronary heart disease and high blood pressure and therefore most readily motivated to change their diets.

The very small fraction of the health budget spent on genetic counseling, prenatal diagnosis, and genetic screening can certainly be justified in developed countries. Developing nations face different public-health priorities. Most resources need to be directed to alleviate and prevent infectious diseases and high infant mortality. Of course, common genetic diseases like sickle-cell anemia and thalassemias might well warrant genetic public-health services in some developing countries.

Although much early impetus for genetic testing arose in the context of occupational exposures to specific workplace chemicals, the recognition of genetic factors predisposing to common diseases—especially coronary heart disease—has raised the specter of employers and insurers testing for these common traits, leading to discriminatory hiring or promotion practices based on a statistical probability that individuals will develop predicted health problems. So as not to deny employees information that might be useful to explain their illnesses or devise individual preventive actions, scientifically sound screening tests should be offered, we believe, on a strictly voluntary, confidential basis through third parties unassociated with employers or insurers. Such programs will have to overcome healthy skepticism that such information can be kept confidential in a computerized world.

GILBERT S. OMENN
ARNO G. MOTULSKY

Directly related to this entry are the entries GENETICS AND HUMAN SELF-UNDERSTANDING; LIFESTYLES AND PUBLIC HEALTH; *and* OCCUPATIONAL SAFETY AND HEALTH. *For a further discussion of topics mentioned in this entry, see the entries* ENVIRONMENTAL POLICY AND LAW; GENETIC TESTING AND SCREENING; HAZARDOUS WASTES AND TOXIC SUBSTANCES; *and* HEALTH PROMOTION AND HEALTH EDUCATION. *For a discussion of related ideas, see the entries* ANIMAL RESEARCH; ENVIRONMENTAL ETHICS; EVOLUTION; GENETIC COUNSELING; GENETICS AND RACIAL MINORITIES; GENOME MAPPING AND SEQUENCING; INTERNATIONAL HEALTH; JUSTICE; *and* UTILITY.

Bibliography

AMES, BRUCE N. 1979. "Identifying Environmental Chemicals Causing Mutations and Cancer." *Science* 204, no. 4393:587–593.

AMES, BRUCE N.; PROFET, MARGIE; and GOLD, LOIS S. 1990. "Dietary Pesticides (99.99% of All Natural)" and "Nature's Chemicals and Synthetic Chemicals: Comparative Toxicology." *Proceedings of the National Academy of Sciences* 87, no. 19:7777–7786.

CARSON, RACHEL. 1962. *Silent Spring.* Boston: Houghton Mifflin.

DOLL, RICHARD, and PETO, RICHARD. 1981. "The Causes of Cancer: Quantitative Estimates of Avoidable Risks of Cancer in the United States Today." *Journal of the National Cancer Institute* 66, no. 6:1191–1308.

DUSTER, TROY. 1990. *Backdoor to Eugenics.* New York: Routledge.

EICHELBAUM, MICHAEL, and GROSS, A. S. 1990. "The Genetic Polymorphism of Debrisoquine/Sparteine Metabolism Clinical Aspects." *Pharmacology and Therapeutics* 46, no. 3:377–394.

GRANDJEAN, PHILIPPE. 1991. *Ecogenetics: Genetic Predisposition to the Toxic Effects of Chemicals.* New York: Routledge, Chapman and Hall/World Health Organization.

HALDANE, JOHN BURDON SANDERSON. 1938. *Heredity and Politics.* New York: W. W. Norton.

INTERNATIONAL AGENCY FOR RESEARCH ON CANCER. IARC WORKING GROUP ON THE EVALUATION OF CARCINOGENIC RISKS TO HUMANS. 1987. *IARC Monographs on the Evaluation of Carcinogenic Risks to Humans. Overall Evaluation of Carcinogenicity: An Updating of IARC Monographs vols. 1–42, Suppl. 7.* Lyons, France: Author.

MOTULSKY, ARNO G. 1978. "Bioethical Problems in Pharmacogenetics and Ecogenetics." *Human Genetics,* suppl. 1:185–192.

———. 1989. "Societal Problems in Human and Medical Genetics." *Genome* 31, no. 2:870–875.

———. 1992. "Nutrition and Genetic Susceptibility to Common Diseases." *American Journal of Clinical Nutrition* 55, no. 6, suppl.:1244S–1245S.

MOTULSKY, ARNO G., and BRUNZELL, JOHN D. 1992. "The Genetics of Coronary Atherosclerosis." In *The Genetic Basis of Common Diseases,* pp. 150–169. Edited by Richard A. King, Jerome I. Rotter, and Arno G. Motulsky. New York: Oxford University Press.

NATIONAL RESEARCH COUNCIL (U.S.). COMMISSION ON LIFE SCIENCES. BOARD ON ENVIRONMENTAL STUDIES AND TOXICOLOGY. COMMITTEE ON BIOLOGIC MARKERS. SUBCOMMITTEE ON REPRODUCTIVE AND NEURODEVELOPMENTAL TOXICOLOGY. 1989a. *Biologic Markers in Reproductive Toxicology.* Washington, D.C.: National Academy Press.

———. COMMITTEE ON DIET AND HEALTH. 1989b. "Implications for Reducing Chronic Disease Risk." In *Diet and Health: Implications for Reducing Chronic Disease Risk,* pp. 85–98. Washington, D.C.: National Academy Press.

OMENN, GILBERT S., and LAVE, LESTER B. 1988. "Scientific and Cost-Effectiveness Criteria in Selecting Batteries of Short-term Tests." *Mutation Research* 205, nos. 1–4: 41–49.

OMENN, GILBERT S., and MOTULSKY, ARNO G. 1978. "'Ecogenetics': Genetic Variation in Susceptibility to Environmental Agents." In *Genetic Issues in Public Health and Medicine,* pp. 83–111. Edited by Bernice H. Cohen, Abraham M. Lilienfeld, and Pien-Chien Huang. Springfield, Ill.: Charles C. Thomas.

OMENN, GILBERT S.; OMIECINSKI, CURTIS J.; and EATON, DAVID L. 1990. "Eco-genetics of Chemical Carcinogens." In *Biotechnology and Human Genetic Predisposition to Disease: Proceedings of a UCLA Symposium Held at Steamboat Springs, Colorado, March 27–April 3, 1989,* pp. 81–93. Edited by Charles R. Cantor, C. Thomas Caskey, Leroy E. Hood, Daphne Kamely, and Gilbert S. Omenn. New York: Wiley-Liss.

U.S. CONGRESS. OFFICE OF TECHNOLOGY ASSESSMENT. 1983. *The Role of Genetic Testing in the Prevention of Occupational Disease.* Washington, D.C.: U.S. Government Printing Office.

———. 1991. *Medical Monitoring and Screening in the Workplace.* Washington, D.C.: U.S. Government Printing Office.

VOGEL, FRIEDRICH, and MOTULSKY, ARNO G. 1986. *Human Genetics, Problems and Approaches.* 2d ed. Berlin: Springer-Verlag. (3d ed. in press, 1995.)

GENETICS AND HUMAN BEHAVIOR

I. Scientific and Research Issues
   Glayde Whitney
II. Philosophical and Ethical Issues
   Richard A. Shweder

I. SCIENTIFIC AND RESEARCH ISSUES

One of the most difficult topics in philosophy and ethics is how to deal with individual differences. Why are some people good while others are evil by any standard? Why are some people smart, enthusiastic, and energetic while other people are severely mentally impaired? What makes someone crazy by any definition; alcoholic versus not alcoholic; or a murderer, arsonist, or upright citizen?

Not only are there individual differences, there are also average differences among various groups of individuals. People can be sorted into groups on the basis of many traits, and behavioral differences may be seen among the groups. People concerned with ethics and philosophy may sometimes have difficulty handling individual differences, and even more difficulty with group differences. In recent years discussions of group differences have become increasingly politically contentious. Nevertheless, group differences in behavior exist and are well documented; indeed, some are obvious to any impartial observer.

Consider sex differences. Among sexually mature humans, sexual aggression is almost exclusively a male-instigated behavior; cases of a woman raping a man are virtually unheard of. Indeed, physically assaultive crime is predominantly a male endeavor (Wilson and Herrnstein, 1985; Ellis and Hoffman, 1990). Consider an even more sensitive example, the link between race, sex, age, and crime. It is rare, for instance, to hear of an elderly woman mugging a stranger on the street or being the perpetrator of a murder. Group and individual differences in behavior are real, whether or not people wish to acknowledge them.

In order to understand the present status of our knowledge of genetics and human behavior, we must be careful not to confuse some issues of politics (or philosophical and ethical preferences) with some issues of scientific knowledge. Individual behavioral differences theoretically may result from different genetic inheritance. Just as one person inherits red hair and another person inherits blond hair, one person might inherit a genetic constitution that causes a certain brain chemistry predisposing that person to violent, impulsive criminal behavior (an example will be discussed further on). Charges of genetic determinism, sexism, racism, or political incorrectness in regard to investigation of genetic causes of behavior are political concepts, not scientific ones.

Early in the twentieth century, theories of genetic influence on behavior were popular. Then a number of political events occurred that resulted in many people becoming philosophically, ethically, and politically opposed to theories of genetic influences on human behavior. These historical developments include (1) the rise of Nazism in Germany, with scientifically incorrect theories of genetic determinism of racial differences; (2) the rise of Marxist-Leninism in the Soviet Union, with scientifically incorrect theories of environmental determinism of individual differences; (3) the elaboration of the civil rights movement in the United States, with scientifically incorrect theories denying the reality of individual differences (Whitney, 1990a). The political controversies (some continuing today) are so fundamentally important to society that many people are very sensitive about scientific knowledge concerning genetics and behavior (Davis, 1986; Pearson, 1991), making them unable to accept a differentiation between scientific and political inquiry.

In scientific investigations of individual differences, scientists attempt to discover the causes of individual differences, whatever they may be. Investigations of human behavior are perhaps always close to ethical concerns. However, many scientists believe that true knowledge of causes is important and in itself is ethically neutral. It is important to separate scientific knowledge from what a society decides to do with that knowledge.

There is a somewhat complicated history of philosophical misunderstanding of genetic science that has been covered by many people. Basically, what happened earlier in the twentieth century is that some influential people concerned about social reform and the betterment of mankind made the mistake of thinking that "genetically caused" meant a condition would be impossible to change. In their political writings they argued that if a condition was caused by the environment, then the condition would be easy to change if society wanted to change it (Degler, 1991). Thus, for many, "genetic" came to be associated with notions of social stagnation and cruel "social Darwinism," and "social" or "environmental" came to be associated with desirable social change and improvement of living conditions.

The fallacy is a simple one: "environmental cause" does not mean "easily changed," and "genetic cause" does not mean "unchangeable." Yet the misunderstandings resulting from this fallacy continue today. For example, it is "politically correct" today to claim that most social ills are caused by social conditions, and it is quite "politically incorrect" to maintain that some social realities might be caused by genetic conditions. It is often viewed as acceptable to suggest that conditions of poverty and social disorganization cause crime and stupidity. It is much less acceptable to suggest that genetic dispositions to impulsive criminality and stupidity might cause much poverty and social disorganization.

Most scientists interested in genetics and human behavior argue that knowledge of causes is important regardless of political or ethical pronouncements. At one time one could be burned at the stake for suggesting that the Earth was round rather than flat. Today scientists are sometimes attacked for suggesting that some socially important differences among people might be caused by genetic differences.

Methods of study

A scientific approach to individual differences in behavior begins with a consideration of their fundamental causes. In scientific theory all causes of individual differences in human behavior can be placed in one of two categories: environmental effects or inherited (genetic) effects. Environmental effects include all experiences that could be different between two people and thereby influence their different growth and behavior, including nutrition, schooling, parental behavior, disease and accidents, and so forth. Genetic effects stem from inherited differences in the DNA, the basic material of the genetic code, which can cause two people to develop differently. It is a postulate of the scientific approach that all causes of individual differences can be understood as arising from either environment or genetic inheritance.

The main technical problem in understanding the role of genetics in human behavior is that genetic origin and rearing environment usually covary (go together) with human subjects. Children get their genes from their biological parents. Those same parents usually raise their children. If children then grow up to resemble their parents, and children of different parents grow up to be different, is it because of the shared genes or the shared environments? Somehow the scientist must overcome the usual family covariation of genes and environment in order to discover if inheritance (genetic differences) or environmental effects cause the individual differences in behavior that we see around us. Most of the general methods used to discover and separate genetic and environmental influences on behavior can be placed in one of three categories: (1) adoption method; (2) twin method; (3) genetic pattern method. These can be best understood by describing their application with real examples.

The major psychosis of schizophrenia presents many philosophical, ethical, and political dilemmas. It has many symptoms but can generally be characterized by sensory and cognitive hallucinations (for example, hearing voices of people who are not present, and experiencing delusional thoughts and beliefs). At the present time there is neither a medical cure for nor means of preventing schizophrenia, although the symptoms can often be treated. The existence of schizophrenia presents serious ethical issues to society because it is relatively common and often severely incapacitating.

Schizophrenia affects about 1 percent of the general population and about 10 to 15 percent of the biological children of a person with schizophrenia. If both parents have schizophrenia, about 40 percent of the children develop schizophrenia. This "familiality" (tendency to run in families) has been known for a long time.

Two major theories developed about the cause of schizophrenia. One was that it resulted from bizarre child-rearing behavior. According to this theory, if parents were inconsistent in their treatment of a child, then the child would grow up with a poor grasp on reality and, in extreme cases, develop the social withdrawal, hallucinations, and delusional thought that characterize schizophrenia. Because mothers traditionally spend more time with children than do fathers, this family-environment-cause theory became known as the theory of the schizophrenogenic mother ("genic" means "causing"). The second main theory about the cause of schizophrenia was that it was largely a genetic condition. The genetic theory was that if a person inherited a certain gene or set of genes, then that person would be susceptible to developing schizophrenia. If the person did not inherit the necessary genes, then the person would not develop schizophrenia.

A major problem with deciding between these two scientific theories about the cause of schizophrenia is that in most families, the parents who raise the children are also the genetic parents of the children. The source

of the parenting and the source of the genes are the same, so simply observing that schizophrenia runs in families does not reveal anything about its cause. It was widely documented that strange parental behavior often occurred in families that produced schizophrenic children. But there was no clear interpretation for that observation. Did the strange behavior of the parent cause the schizophrenia of the child? Or was the preschizophrenic child abnormal enough to cause the disruption in the family? Or did the strange behavior of the parent and the schizophrenia of the child result from the genes that they shared?

Adoption method.   The adoption method provides a way for the scientist to separate environmental parenting from genetic parenting. If scientists can find sets of biological (genetic) parents and their children who were separated at birth, then they will be able to look at the effect of genes without the added confusion of a shared family environment. Also, if they can study sets of adoptive parents and the children they have adopted, then they can look at the effects of the parenting behavior—the home environment—without the confusion of shared genes. Thus the adoption method provides an effective way to separate genetic from environmental causes.

Leonard Heston reported the first modern adoption study of schizophrenia in 1966. He found that the adopted-away offspring of schizophrenic mothers, when raised in nonschizophrenic families, had a lifetime incidence of schizophrenia of about 16 percent; this outcome was essentially identical to that of natural offspring raised by a schizophrenic biological parent. Further, about half of the adopted-away children of schizophrenic mothers displayed some sort of psychiatric or criminal problems as adults.

Later studies excellently summarized by Irving Gottesman and Dorothea Wolfgram (1991) have confirmed and extended Heston's findings. Genes, not prenatal environment, are implicated because the results are about the same when the biological schizophrenic parent is the father. Being raised in a family environment that includes the bizarre behavior of schizophrenics does not induce schizophrenia in individuals without the predisposing genes. Schizophrenic genes appear to be necessary but are not alone always sufficient for the onset of the psychosis. This is most clearly illustrated by the incidence of schizophrenia among twins.

Twin method.   The twin method is another important approach that helps a scientist decide between an interpretation of genetic causation or an interpretation of environmental causation. The basic logic of the twin method is straightforward. Twin pairs are one or the other of two types: identical or fraternal.

Identical twins (also called monozygotic, that is, one zygote) are genetically identical. They are created when one egg is fertilized by one sperm, giving rise to one individual. When, very early in development, that one individual divides into two separate embryos, the result is identical twins. Identical twins are genetically identical because early in development they actually were one individual. If the individual differences for any trait (such as eye color or schizophrenia) were 100 percent caused by genes, then identical twins should be identical for that trait. Fraternal twins (also called dizygotic, that is, two zygotes) are created when two separate eggs are each fertilized by a different sperm. Fraternal twins are thus genetically just like any other full siblings. They have both parents in common; they just happen to have been conceived and born at the same time. On average, full siblings, including fraternal twins, share half their genes. Since identical twin pairs share all their genes whereas fraternal twin pairs share half their genes, the essence of the twin method is to compare identical and fraternal twins. If a pair of identical twins are more similar to one another than are fraternal twins, that is strong evidence that the trait under consideration is influenced by the genes.

With regard to schizophrenia, members of identical twin pairs are concordant (that is, both show the condition) much more frequently than are members of fraternal twin pairs. That finding is consistent with the theory of genetic causation of schizophrenia. However, when one member of an identical twin pair is schizophrenic, the other twin is also schizophrenic in only about 50 percent of the pairs. An incidence of 100 percent would be expected if genes were the whole story.

Twin pairs are called "discordant" when one twin shows the trait and the other twin does not. When identical twins who are discordant for schizophrenia have children, the risk for the offspring is about 10–15 percent whether the parent is the twin with schizophrenia or the twin without it. The identical twin who does not display schizophrenia transmits the susceptibility to the child every bit as much as does the twin with blatant schizophrenia. Such transmission in the absence of schizophrenic behavior is further strong evidence for genetic transmission of susceptibility. What the causal factors are, in addition to the proper genes, is unknown. And although genes are clearly necessary for schizophrenia, exactly what the condition consists of genetically is unknown. Theories range from suggesting a single gene that disrupts brain chemistry, to suggesting that the simultaneous inheritance of many genes (at least more than two) is necessary in order to induce susceptibility to schizophrenia (Gottesman and Wolfgram, 1991).

Genetic pattern method. The third commonly used method is to look for genetic patterns of transmission for traits of interest. The genetic pattern method comes from almost a century of research into basic genetics. It has been discovered and repeatedly demonstrated that some basic patterns of inheritance are widely shared by plants and animals, including humans. If a trait of interest shows a pattern of occurrence that is identical to a known genetic pattern, that increases the likelihood that the new trait is influenced by genes. However, it is important to understand that consistency with a genetic pattern does not *prove* genetic causation. Further evidence confirmed by other methods is necessary for proof.

In order to illustrate the genetic pattern method with real human behavior examples, it is necessary to review some basic genetics. There are perhaps as many as 100,000 different genes. For creatures, like humans, that reproduce sexually, each individual has two copies of most genes, one from the mother and one from the father. Different copies of the same gene are called alleles. A particular allele may be dominant or recessive. The allele is said to be dominant if its effect is seen when only one copy is present. An allele is said to be recessive if two copies must be present in order to show the effect. In order to show a recessive characteristic, the individual must inherit copies of the same allele from the mother and from the father. To be a "carrier" of a genetic trait means that an individual has one copy of a recessive allele that causes the trait. With that we can illustrate some genetic patterns.

Dominant traits

Single-gene dominant inheritance means that only one copy of the allele is necessary to display the condition; thus everyone with the allele will display the condition. If the allele is rare in the population, then most individuals with the condition will have one copy of the dominant allele; their other allele for that gene will be the recessive allele. Huntington's disease is a well-known example of a dominant genetic disease. The disease's symptoms include degeneration of the nervous system, usually beginning in middle age, that results in death. In this devastating disease, as the nervous system degenerates, there is usually a gradual loss of intellectual ability and emotional control. The genetic pattern shown by Huntington's is that of a condition caused by a rare single dominant gene. Since affected people have one copy of the dominant disease gene and one copy of a recessive gene (for "normal nervous system"), half of their offspring develop the disease if they live long enough. Huntington's never skips a generation. Since the gene is dominant, the person who inherits it will manifest the disease (if he or she lives long enough). If one full sibling has the condition, there is a 50–50 chance that any other sibling will also get the disease.

Recessive traits

In contrast to dominant conditions, recessive conditions show a very different pattern of occurrence. To reiterate, essentially, "recessive" means that both copies of the gene must be of the same form (the same allele) in order to show the condition. Two parents, neither of whom shows a trait, can have a child affected by a recessive trait (this happens if both parents are carriers of one copy of the recessive allele; the child thus has two copies, one from each parent, and manifests the condition). Recessive traits can "skip generations" because parents and their offspring can carry one copy of the recessive gene and not display the associated trait. In the population there are many recessive genes that cause various abnormal conditions. Each particular recessive allele may be rare, but since there are many of them, their combined impact on a population can be substantial.

Among humans, a classic example of recessive inheritance is the condition of phenylketonuria (PKU). Individuals with PKU usually are severely mentally impaired. Most never learn to talk; many have seizures and display temper tantrums. PKU is a form of severe mental retardation that is both genetic and treatable. It is genetic in that it is caused by a recessive genetic allele. Without two copies of that particular allele, a person will not develop the set of symptoms, with mental impairment, that is characteristic of PKU. However, following scientific knowledge of the details of PKU, a treatment became available. It was discovered that the recessive gene prevents the normal metabolism of a substance that is common in food. Therefore many normal foods are toxic to the individual with two PKU alleles. Providing a special diet that is low in the offending substance can prevent or minimize the nervous system damage that leads to the profound intellectual disabilities of untreated PKU individuals.

The example of PKU demonstrates that inherited (genetic) conditions can be treated. Knowledge of specific causation can result in effective treatment. This is an extremely important point ethically and philosophically because it is often misunderstood and misinterpreted. This is why it was stated earlier that "genetic determinism" is a political, not a scientific, concept.

Today, well over 100 different genes are known for which relatively rare recessive alleles cause conditions that include among their symptoms severe mental impairment. The rapidly developing knowledge of basic genetic chemistry, from molecular genetics to biotechnology and the Human Genome Project, which is mapping human genes, holds out the hope that we may soon be able to treat many more of these devastating genetic conditions effectively.

Sex-linked traits

Not everyone has two copies of each gene. For genes that are technically "sex-linked" (genes in the X chromosome), women have two copies while men have only one copy. The basic biology of human chromosomal sex determination is that the vast majority of normal women have two copies of the X chromosome. The vast majority of normal men have only one copy of the X chromosome. Instead of a second X chromosome, men have one copy of the Y chromosome. The X chromosome is a relatively large chromosome that contains many genes. The Y chromosome is one of the smallest chromosomes and contains relatively few genes. From this it follows that there are many genes (those on the X chromosome) for which women normally have two copies but men normally have only one copy. Also, there are some genes on the Y chromosome for which men normally have one copy and normal women have no copies.

One gene on the Y chromosome is sometimes called the tdf gene (testes determining factor) because early in embryological development, it causes the beginning of sexual differentiation of the male. Many of the anatomical and behavioral differences between the sexes can ultimately be traced to the effect of this one gene.

On the X chromosome there are many alleles that act as recessives in women (females need two copies to show the effect) but as dominant genes in men (males have only one copy of the X-linked allele, so they show its effect). Many more men than women will display the trait caused by a sex-linked recessive allele because every man with one copy of the allele will show the trait, but women need two copies of the same X-linked allele in order to show the trait.

Red/green color blindness and hemophilia are two well-known examples of sex-linked recessive conditions. Both can influence behavior in important ways. Although many affected men are not aware that they are color-blind until they are scientifically tested, that does not mean the condition is without effect on their behavior. Red/green color-blind men tend to confuse shades of red and green; to many, both appear brownish. Color blindness can have effects ranging from the humorously trivial to quite important. Color confusion can result in mismatched socks and weird shirt-slack combinations, or confusion of traffic signals (which is why the relative position of red/green traffic lights is standardized) and port/starboard lights on ships. A survey in Minnesota suggested that even with mandatory hunter orange clothing, it was a bit more dangerous to go hunting with a color-blind companion (Foltz, 1962).

It has been suggested that the sex-linked recessive hemophilia allele has had an influence on world history. Among European royalty, a number of the male descendants of Queen Victoria have been hemophiliacs. Did the worrisome effects of this "bleeding disease," which affected the tsarevich Alexei of Russia, contribute to the political downfall of the Romanov dynasty? One source of Rasputin's influence was his ability to calm the tsarevich during bleeding episodes (Vogel and Motulsky, 1979).

There is also a sex-linked recessive allele that apparently affects the likelihood of impulsive aggression. Biochemically, the X-linked allele affects an important chemical in the brain called monoamine oxidase (which is also involved in the effects of amphetamines and cocaine on the brain). All males known to have the particular X-linked allele display rather low intelligence and impulsive acting out. The impulsive criminal behaviors are reported to be most often triggered by anger, and the acts committed are out of proportion to the provocation. Behaviors noted include attacks with deadly weapons, such as stabbing a prison guard with a pitchfork, attempting to run over a complaining boss with a car, forcing women to undress at knifepoint. Some affected males are arsonists. Others have engaged in incestuous rape, exhibitionism, and voyeurism. Unaffected males and women from the same families are reported to be normal (Bruner et al., 1993).

The bioethical dilemmas facing modern society are starkly illustrated by the study of genetic influences on aggressive and criminal behavior. At essentially the same time that Han Bruner and his colleagues were publishing their scientific study, political pressure was being exerted in the United States to stifle such research. A scientific conference had been planned for October 1992 on the topic "Genetic Factors in Crime." One of the sponsors providing money for the conference was the National Institutes of Health (NIH). Under political pressure, the NIH first froze its support and then effectively prevented the conference by withdrawing support. As reported in *Science,* "the Congressional Black Caucus, among other mostly African-American critics, argued it was racist to suggest the existence of links between genes and crime" (1993, p. 619). Nancy Touchette (1993) points out that favorable scientific review had led NIH to support the conference on genetics and crime. It was strictly political pressure that led to its cancellation. Are there topics that are too controversial to be subjected to rational discourse and scientific investigation? Today it is common to hold up to ridicule the antiscientific nonsense of the Middle Ages while at the same time pretending to know the causes of some of today's most intractable social problems. A review of the substantial evidence concerning race differences in criminal behavior and possible genetic influences is available elsewhere (Whitney, 1990b).

Intelligence

There are more data about the inheritance of intelligence than about any other complex behavioral characteristic of humans. The notion of substantial genetic influences on individual variation in intelligence remains controversial even after almost a century of investigation.

Intelligence testing grew out of a societal problem: the failure of "universal education." When universal public education was first implemented in France during the latter half of the nineteenth century, it failed. Not everyone who went to school acquired an education. Alfred Binet and others invented intelligence tests in order to aid in the prediction of school performance (Boring, 1957; Fancher, 1985). Despite the controversies that continue to swirl around the applications of "standardized testing," intelligence tests remain among the best predictors of school performance (Jensen, 1980), and the original problem persists.

The level of intellectual functioning (abstract reasoning, ability to perform complex cognitive tasks, score on tests of general intelligence, IQ) is a strongly heritable trait. In 1963 Nikki Erlenmeyer-Kimling and Lissy Jarvik summarized the literature dealing with correlations between the measured intelligence of various relatives. After eliminating studies based on specialized samples or employing unusual tests or statistics, they reviewed eighty-one investigations. Included were data from eight countries on four continents spanning more than two generations and containing over 30,000 correlational pairings. The overview that emerged from that mass of data was unequivocal. Intelligence appeared to be a quantitative polygenic trait, that is, a trait influenced by many genes, as are such physical characteristics as height and weight.

The results did not suggest that environmental factors were unimportant. Rather, genetic variation was quite important. The less sensitive trait of height (or weight) can be used to illustrate this distinction. It is well known that an individual's height (or weight) can be influenced by nutrition. Inadequate diets during development can result in reduced height (or weight). The average height of whole populations has changed with changes in public health and nutrition. Yet at the same time, individual differences in height (or weight) among the members of a population are strongly influenced by heredity. In general, taller people tend to have taller children across the population as a whole, and the relative height of different people is strongly influenced by their genes. And that also appears to be the case with intelligence. The Erlenmeyer-Kimling and Jarvik survey data suggested that about 70 percent of the variation among individuals in measured intelligence was due to genetic differences. The remaining 30 percent of the variation was due to unspecified (and still unknown) environmental effects.

Thomas Bouchard and Matt McGue (1981) provided an updated summary of the world literature on intelligence correlations between relatives. They summarized 111 studies, fifty-nine of which had been reported during the seventeen years since the Erlenmeyer-Kimling and Jarvik review of 1963. Bouchard and

McGue summarized 526 familial correlations from 113,942 pairings. The general picture remained the same. Roughly 70 percent of normal-range variation was attributable to genetic differences and about 30 percent appeared to be due to environmental effects.

Much is known about the genetics of mental retardation and learning disabilities. The most common single causes of severe general learning disabilities are chromosomal anomalies (having too many or too few copies of the many genes that occur together on the abnormal piece of chromosome). Among the many chromosomal anomalies that include mental retardation as a symptom, trisomy 21 is the cause of Down's syndrome, and the fragile X condition may by itself account for most, if not all, of the excess of males among people with severe learning disabilities (Plomin et al., 1990). A large number of rare single-gene mutations, many of them recessive like the PKU example already discussed, induce metabolic abnormalities that severely affect nervous system function and thus lead to mental retardation. Because the specific alleles involved are individually rare and recessive, such abnormalities of metabolism can cause learning-disabled individuals to appear sporadically in otherwise unaffected families (Vogel and Motulsky, 1979). The new molecular genetic technology holds future therapeutic promise for many learning disabilities.

Personality

Dimensions of personality tend to be familial (Eaves et al., 1989). Modern studies of twins and adoptees suggest that for adults, some major dimensions are influenced by differences in family environments, and some are not. For the dimension of extroversion, which encompasses such tendencies as sociability and impulsivity, genetic factors account for about 40 percent to 60 percent of the variation among adults in different studies. About 50 percent of the variation is environmental in origin. But, surprisingly to many people, none of the variation among adults appears to be related to environmental differences among families.

For neuroticism, which taps such traits as anxiousness (a characteristic state of anxiety), emotional instability, and anxious arousability (a tendency to react with anxiety to events), 30 percent to 40 percent of the adult variation appears to be caused by genetic differences, and again none of the variation is from environmental differences that are shared by members of the same family. In contrast, social desirability, which measures a tendency to answer questions in socially approved ways, a tendency to want to appear accepted by and acceptable to society, does not show evidence of genetic causation. Essentially all of the measurable variation in social de-

sirability appeared to be environmental, with about 20 percent due to family environment.

Some authors, including Robert Plomin, John DeFries, and Gerald McClearn in their 1990 textbook, suggest that because extroversion and neuroticism are general factors involved in many other personality scales or dimensions, most of the others also show moderate genetic variation. As an example, a twin study (Tellegen et al., 1988) involving eleven personality scales found genetic influence of various degrees for them all. On average across the eleven personality scales, 54 percent of the variation was attributable to genetic differences among the people, and 46 percent to environmental differences.

Tendencies toward affective (mood) disorders, including psychotic depression and bipolar disorder (manic-depression), also are clearly influenced genetically. A lack of familial co-occurrence has established the separateness of schizophrenia from the affective psychoses. Unipolar depression and bipolar affective disorder do co-occur; in addition, there may be a genetically influenced major depressive syndrome distinct from manic-depression. The affective disorders probably include a diversity of genetic conditions.

Other traits

Although data are sparse for many traits, modern studies are revealing genetic involvement in many conditions of importance to society. Robert Plomin and colleagues (1990) point out that the best single predictor of alcoholism is alcoholism in a first-degree biological relative. Alcoholism clearly runs in biological families. Severe alcoholism affects about 5 percent of males in the general population; among male relatives of alcoholics, the incidence is about 25 percent. The incidence remains about the same for adopted-away sons of male alcoholics. However, biological children of nonalcoholics are not at increased risk for alcoholism when raised by alcoholic adoptive parents.

Both adoption and twin studies of adult criminality suggest genetic involvement for serious crimes against persons and for property crimes. Large-scale adoption studies have suggested a genetic distinction between crimes associated with alcoholism and criminality not associated with alcoholism. Interestingly, socioeconomic status was found to be an interaction variable. Low socioeconomic status of the adoptive home was associated with an increased incidence of adult criminality only when the biological parent was also criminal or alcoholic (Whitney, 1990b).

In addition to twin studies that indicate obesity is highly heritable, a large adoption study of obesity among adults found that family environment by itself had no apparent effect. In adulthood, the body-mass index of the adoptees showed a strong relationship to that of their biological parents. However, there was no relationship between weight classification of adoptive parents and the adoptees. The relation between biological parent and adoptee weight extended across the spectrum, from very thin to very obese. Once again, cumulative effects of the rearing home environment were not important determinants of individual differences among adults (Stunkard et al., 1986).

Conclusion

To an extent that is truly surprising, even to many of the scientists conducting the studies, research indicates pervasive influences of genetics on human behavior. To a large extent many of the psychological differences among people are proving to be strongly affected by genetic differences. Intellectual ability, anxiousness, tendency to react with depression, impulsive violence, weight, height, hair color, and a host of other traits are strongly influenced by our genes. Genetic determinism? Of course not. But neither is it the simplistic environmental determinism that was so popular among academics only a few years ago. For instance, hair color, which is inherited, is not "genetically determined"; sophisticated coloring agents are readily available.

Understanding and accounting for individual and group differences requires an assessment of many of the mainstream philosophical and scientific theories that attempt to understand human behavior. In an excellent review of much behavior genetic research, David Rowe (1994) starts out by stating that "most people" believe that how children are raised has much to do with the differences in the way they turn out. Parents' behavior is thought to be a crucial determinant of the adult behavior of their children. He suggests that in important respects this widespread belief may be wrong. He points out that it would not be the first time in history that whole cultures, both laypeople and experts, had been wrong in their beliefs. The theory of a flat Earth at the center of the universe would not have gotten us to the moon, and environmental determinist theories of human behavior have not yet solved most of our social problems.

GLAYDE WHITNEY

Directly related to this article is the companion article in this entry: PHILOSOPHICAL AND ETHICAL ISSUES. *Also directly related are the entries* GENE THERAPY; GENETIC COUNSELING; GENETIC ENGINEERING; GENETICS AND ENVIRONMENT IN HUMAN HEALTH; GENETICS AND HUMAN SELF-UNDERSTANDING; GENETICS AND THE LAW; GENETICS AND RACIAL MINORITIES; GENOME MAPPING AND SEQUENCING; EUGENICS; *and* MEDICAL GENETICS. *For a further discussion of topics mentioned in this article, see the entries:* ACTION; ADOPTION; EMOTIONS; FAMILY; MENTAL ILLNESS; NATIONAL SOCIALISM; RACE AND RACISM; SEXISM; *and* SUBSTANCE ABUSE, *especially the article on* ALCOHOLISM. *For a discussion of related ideas, see the entries* BEHAVIORISM; BIOLOGY, PHILOSOPHY OF; FEMINISM; GENDER IDENTITY AND GENDER-IDENTITY DISORDERS; HOMICIDE; HOMOSEXUALITY; PUBLIC HEALTH; *and* SEXUAL IDENTITY.

Bibliography

BORING, EDWIN G. 1957. *A History of Experimental Psychology.* 2d ed. New York: Appleton-Century-Crofts.

BOUCHARD, THOMAS J., JR., and McGUE, MATT. 1981. "Familial Studies of Intelligence: A Review." *Science* 212, no. 4498:1055–1059.

BRUNER, HAN G.; NELEN, MARCEL R.; VAN ZANDVOORT, PEITER; ABELING, NICO G. G. M.; VAN GENNIP, ALBERT H.; WOLTERS, ERIK C.; KUIPER, MICHAEL A.; ROPERS, HANS HILGER; and VAN OOST, BERNARD A. 1993. "X-Linked Borderline Mental Retardation with Prominent Behavioral Disturbance: Phenotype, Genetic Localization, and Evidence for Disturbed Monoamine Metabolism." *American Journal of Human Genetics* 52, no. 6:1032–1039.

DAVIS, BERNARD D. 1986. *Storm over Biology: Essays on Science, Sentiment, and Public Policy.* Buffalo, N.Y.: Prometheus.

DEGLER, CARL N. 1991. *In Search of Human Nature.* New York: Oxford University Press.

EAVES, LINDEN J.; EYSENCK, HANS J.; and MARTIN, NICK G. 1989. *Genes, Culture, and Personality: An Empirical Approach.* San Diego, Calif.: Academic Press.

ELLIS, LEE, and HOFFMAN, HARRY, eds. 1990. *Crime in Biological, Social and Moral Contexts.* New York: Praeger.

ERLENMEYER-KIMLING, NIKKI, and JARVIK, LISSY F. 1963. "Genetics and Intelligence: A Review." *Science* 142, no. 3598:1477–1479.

FANCHER, RAYMOND E. 1985. *The Intelligence Men.* New York: W. W. Norton.

FOLTZ, DONALD E. 1962. "Speaking Out." *Saturday Evening Post,* October 13, p. 8.

GOTTESMAN, IRVING I., and WOLFGRAM, DOROTHEA L. 1991. *Schizophrenia Genesis: The Origins of Madness.* New York: W. H. Freeman.

GROSS, BARRY R. 1990. "The Case of Philippe Rushton." *Academic Questions* 3, no. 4:35–46.

HESTON, LEONARD L. 1966. "Psychiatric Disorders in Foster Home Reared Children of Schizophrenic Mothers." *British Journal of Psychiatry* 112, no. 489:819–825.

HOLDEN, CONSTANCE, ed. 1993. "NIH Kills Genes and Crime Grant." *Science* 260, no. 5108:619.

JENSEN, ARTHUR. 1980. *Bias in Mental Testing.* New York: Free Press.

PEARSON, ROGER. 1991. *Race, Intelligence and Bias in Academe.* Washington, D.C.: Scott-Townsend.

PLOMIN, ROBERT; DEFRIES, JOHN C.; and MCCLEARN, GERALD E. 1990. *Behavioral Genetics: A Primer.* 2d ed. New York: W. H. Freeman.

ROWE, DAVID C. 1994. *The Limits of Family Influence: Genes, Experience, and Behavior.* New York: Guilford Press.

STUNKARD, ALBERT J.; SØRENSEN, THORKILD I. A.; HANIS, CRAIG; TEASDALE, THOMAS W.; CHAKRABORTY, RANAJIT; SCHULL, WILLIAM J.; and SCHULSINGER, FINI. 1986. "An Adoption Study of Human Obesity." *New England Journal of Medicine* 314, no. 4:193–198.

TELLEGEN, AUKE; LYKKEN, DAVID T.; BOUCHARD, THOMAS J., JR.; WILCOX, KIMBERLY J.; SEGAL, NANCY L.; and RICH, STEPHEN. 1988. "Personality Similarity in Twins Reared Apart and Together." *Journal of Personality and Social Psychology* 54, no. 6:1031–1039.

TOUCHETTE, NANCY. 1993. "Genetics and Crime: It's Not Over Till It's Over." *Journal of NIH Research* 5, no. 6: 32–34.

VOGEL, FRIEDRICH, and MOTULSKY, ARNO G. 1979. *Human Genetics: Problems and Approaches.* New York: Springer-Verlag.

WHITNEY, GLAYDE. 1990a. "A Contextual History of Behavior Genetics." In *Developmental Behavior Genetics: Neural, Biometrical and Evolutionary Approaches,* pp. 7–24. Edited by Martin E. Hahn, John K. Hewitt, Norman D. Henderson, and Robert Benno. New York: Oxford University Press.

———. 1990b. "On Possible Genetic Bases of Race Differences in Criminality." In *Crime in Biological, Social, and Moral Contexts,* pp. 134–149. Edited by Lee Ellis and Harry Hoffman. New York: Praeger.

WILSON, JAMES Q., and HERRNSTEIN, RICHARD J. 1985. *Crime and Human Nature.* New York: Simon and Schuster.

II. PHILOSOPHICAL AND ETHICAL ISSUES

It is not the aim of this article to enter into any of several controversies that have been provoked by eugenic thinking, or to draw strong conclusions about the facts of nature and nurture, or to seek some kind of "biosocial" synthesis of opposite views (see Duster, 1990; Gould, 1981; Kevles and Hood, 1992; Nelkin and Tancredi, 1992; Suzuki and Knudtson, 1992; Lewontin, 1992). It is not the aim of this article to critique various models and conceptualizations of "heritability" or "kin selection" (Hamilton, 1964; Lewontin, 1976; Plomin, 1986).

It is not the aim of this article to assess the evidence in behavioral genetics and behavioral science for or against various kinds of genetic and environmental explanations of "altruistic" behavior, of gender differences, or of individual and group differences in health, intelligence, character, or criminality (Bem, 1993; Bowman and Murray, 1990; Elia, 1988; Herrnstein, 1990; Loehlin et al., 1975; Maccoby, 1974; Plomin, 1986; Rossi, 1977; Scarr, 1987; Wilson and Herrnstein, 1986). It is not the aim of this article to explain why adopted chil-

dren are treated differently from blood kin, or why identical twins do not have the same fingerprints (Lewontin, 1992), or why identical twins reared together in the same home are less similar in their personalities and behavioral dispositions than one might suppose (Plomin and Daniels, 1987), or why heritability estimates derived from studies using an adoption design do not converge with heritability estimates derived from studies using a twin design (Plomin et al., 1990).

It is not the aim of this article to debate the cogency of various naturalistic and nonnaturalistic "resolutions" of the mind–body problem (Adams, 1987; Dennett, 1991; McGinn, 1991; Popper and Eccles, 1977), or to explain or explain away the appearance and function of "consciousness," "intentionality," and "free will" in the material world (see Churchland, 1986; Flanagan, 1992). It is not the aim of this article to reconsider the problem of universals, or the concept of innateness, or to address the Neoplatonic implications ("all learning is reminiscence") of the increasingly popular idea that "online" mental structures are not so much constructed as selected from a complex array of preexisting forms (Gazzaniga, 1993; Piatelli-Palmarini, 1989; Werker, 1989).

The aim is quite otherwise—to raise questions, as did Arthur Caplan in his earlier *Encyclopedia of Bioethics* contribution, "Genetic Aspects of Human Behavior: Philosophical and Ethical Issues," about the type of social order, understood as a moral order, that is most compatible with certain presumed facts about human nature, including our ability to alter our essential nature.

Historical background

The phoenix of eugenic thinking has risen up out of the pyres of the 1930s and 1940s, and its resurrection in our culture is nearly complete. Whether one toasts this regeneration of interest in the quality of each person's "natural" endowment or dreads it, it is hard to deny that eugenic thinking is very much with us today.

Not since the time of Sir Francis Galton in the late nineteenth and early twentieth centuries have so many prominent scientists held (and occasionally expressed) the view that successful people and their offspring do better in life because they have better genes, and that ethnic, racial, social class, and gender differences in, for example, health, intelligence, criminality, and interpersonal sensitivity are best understood in genetic terms (Freedman, 1979; Herrnstein, 1990; Jensen, 1969; Scarr, 1987; Wilson and Herrnstein, 1985). Not since Galton's time has there been such a strong undercurrent of informed opinion in our culture willing to "essentialize," "substantialize," or "naturalize" human abilities, mental capacities, behavioral dispositions, and life prospects (Buss, 1989; Degler, 1991; Gazzaniga, 1993; Symons, 1979; Wilson, 1975). Many people are willing to view everything from shyness to the ability to learn languages to the proneness to suffer from a particular physical or mental disease as the product of a genetic inheritance that can be analyzed alternatively at the level of the individual, the family, the social group, or the species.

Not since Galton's time have so many intellectuals been open to the findings of behavioral genetics and willing to accept the conclusion drawn by researchers like Thomas Bouchard and his colleagues in their study of identical twins reared in different home environments that "for almost every behavioral trait so far investigated, from reaction time to religiosity, an important fraction of the variations among people turns out to be associated with genetic variation" (Bouchard et al., 1990, p. 224). Not since Galton's time have the halls of science, medicine, industry, and government been so alive with the voices of ethically minded eugenicists eager to make the world a better place through selective alterations in the genetic endowment of particular members of our species (see Duster, 1990; Kevles and Hood, 1992; Lewontin, 1992).

Many people find these developments morally appealing. Eugenic thinking appeals to them because it brings to mind the image of a caring physician saving "defective" babies from Tay-Sachs disease or assisting a particular ethnic group in alleviating the suffering caused by some heritable disease to which that community is especially prone. Eugenic thinking excites their rational intuitions about the values of self-improvement, beneficence, protection of the vulnerable, justice, and control, while linking progress to something else that is good, the growth of knowledge. It appeals to them because they hope that one day, in the not-too-distant future, advances in science and genetic engineering will provide everyone with the means to be well-born. They picture a future in which human beings have created the secular equivalent of a heaven on earth. They surmise the progressive evolution of our species and suppose a state of organic grace in which everyone is free and equal, happy, healthy, responsible, and in the top 1 percent of the class.

Other people find the recurrence of eugenic thinking morally obnoxious. They think that the idea that "people do well in life because they have better genes" is a self-serving ideology designed to divert the community from promoting equality in the distribution of relevant human "goods," wealth, property, and education rather than genetic resources. They believe that successful individuals and groups are successful because they work long and hard at the things they do and because they have opportunities (financial resources, good coaching) to be successful. They are suspicious of scientific findings of genetically determined racial, ethnic, or class differences in school performance, criminality, or any

other behavioral disposition or human ability. They view such "findings" as a loathsome expression of a dark desire to indict socially oppressed groups with the sin of inherent inferiority. In the context of a real world ripe with communal conflicts based on "ancient hatreds," they are made anxious by eugenic thinking. They remember the pyres of the 1930s and 1940s, and a time and a place when the utopian ideals of the government and its scientists, doctors, jurists, and intellectuals were not so humanitarian and egalitarian. They view eugenic thinking as a scourge.

The aim of this article is to understand these divergent moral intuitions about the implications of eugenic thinking by examining the qualities an action, policy, or practice must exhibit to make it right or good. One major view in moral philosophy argues that it is our beliefs about nature, including human nature, that set the standard for moral evaluation. Plato and Aristotle held this view when they asked whether monarchy or slavery or the institution of the family was in accord with human nature. Thomas Hobbes, Niccolò Machiavelli, Immanuel Kant, and Jean-Jacques Rousseau held this view. The challenge of eugenic thinking, like the challenge of moral philosophy itself, is that it raises provocative questions about the type of social order, understood as a moral order, that is most compatible with certain presumed or imagined facts about human nature, including our ability to choose to alter certain aspects of our essential nature. Should we exercise this ability, and if so, how?

Eugenic thinking: Galton's moral crusade

In 1865 Sir Francis Galton coined the expression "nature–nurture" in an essay entitled "Hereditary Talent and Character" published in *MacMillan's Magazine*. In 1883 he started using the word "eugenics," a Greek word meaning "well-born." By the turn of the twentieth century, the Greek word and the coined expression had become associated with an influential moral crusade whose aim was to increase the stock of basic human goods—intelligence, civility, and health—through the application to human beings of scientific principles of plant and animal breeding.

In 1911, the year Galton died, a veritable Who's Who of enlightened, ethically sensitive intellectuals, scientists, and politicians—among them Charles Eliot, president of Harvard University, Winston Churchill, and the British social reformers Sidney and Beatrice Webb—could be counted among those who were convinced that the aims of the eugenicists were noble and true, and that, through the intelligent application of scientific knowledge, we could increase the value of our collective genetic inheritance and rid the population of diseased bodies, wicked souls, and dull minds.

Eugenic thinking conjoins three types of theories: a theory of organic nature, a theory of human nature, and a theory of moral duty. The theory of organic nature asserts that the essence of an organism's nature (including its abilities, behavioral dispositions, and life prospects) is material (based in its genes). The theory of human nature asserts that since human beings are organisms, therefore individual and group similarities and differences in abilities, behavioral dispositions, and life prospects can be understood in material (genetic) terms. The theory of moral duty asserts that human beings can and ought to manage their own care and progress by altering their material nature. At the heart of eugenic thinking, then, there is a perceived ethical obligation to nurture our nature (our genetic resources) and to construct a social and political environment that makes it possible to bend nature in the direction of human values and ideals.

In Galton's time the only eugenic means to the moral end of promoting health, civility, and intelligence was regulation of the reproductive process via selective breeding and the crude all-or-nothing procedure of sterilization. In the United States, the forced sterilization of people with dull and criminal minds became legal in 1907 in the state of Indiana, and many other states followed suit. Judicial wisdom later upheld the constitutionality of sterilization laws ("Three generations of imbeciles is enough!" ruled Oliver Wendell Holmes, Jr., in 1927 in the U.S. Supreme Court decision *Buck vs. Bell*). But the ethical underpinnings of the case in favor of forced sterilizations had already been articulated by a voice of even greater authority, that of Galton's famous cousin, Sir Charles Darwin.

In *The Descent of Man*, Darwin expressed his concerns about the future of the genetic capital of our species in the following terms:

> We build asylums for the imbecile, the maimed and the sick, we institutionalize poor laws; and our medical men exert their utmost skill to save the life of everyone to the last moment. Thus the weak members of civilized societies propagate their kind. No one who has attended to the breeding of domesticated animals will doubt that this must be highly injurious to the race of man. Both sexes ought to refrain from marriage, if they are in any marked degree inferior in body or mind, but such hopes are Utopian and will never be partially realized until the laws of inheritance are thoroughly known. (quoted in Degler, 1991, pp. 41–42)

The implicit ethical logic of Darwin's argument seemed especially appealing to Galton and other eugenicists of his time. Indeed, the underlying logic of the argument—third-party effects, the social cost of unregulated individual choice, the social benefits of expert regulation—has from time immemorial seemed appealing to many ethicists and scientists. Twenty-five hundred years ago, in *The Republic*, Plato developed a rationale for state regulation of marriage choices. Social benefits, he argued, accrue from ensuring that individuals maximize the fit between their biologically inherited behavioral inclinations and their socially inherited occupational responsibilities.

Eugenics: The idea of the "primordial" in everyday thought

Any attempt to comprehend the "official" return of eugenic thinking in the late twentieth century must acknowledge the historical and cross-cultural pervasiveness of the idea of the "primordial" in everyday thought. The idea of the primordial is that people who are similar, proximal, emotionally and morally bonded to each other, or related as (or "as if") members of the same family are linked to each other by a common substance (e.g., "blood" and "bone"). It is the idea that what living things do is an extension of what they are, which is material or substantive, at least to some extent. Some social scientists have argued that the idea of "shared substance" and the tendency to equate "code with substance" and "fellow feeling" with "shared substance" is a fundamental feature of the human mind (Fiske, 1991).

Few of us are entirely free of this type of primordial or eugenic thinking in some aspect of our daily lives. Much of this thinking seems innocent or even beneficent, like breeding greyhounds to run fast or Tibetan terriers to be loyal, screening fetuses for defects, searching for the gene responsible for a dreaded disease, maintaining official records on the ethnic or racial distribution of lactose malabsorption or sickle-cell anemia, or wondering which characteristics of our mates (beauty, intelligence, self-confidence, a dislike of pudding) are likely to be reproduced in our children. In each case we reveal an intellectual inclination to substantialize the nature of life and of living things.

Yet, although few of us are entirely free of eugenic thinking in everyday life, our eugenic reasoning rarely displays the marks of generality and consistency that we associate with a philosophy of life or an intellectual doctrine. In the United States, where human beings typically reproduce unregulated by any conscious system of eugenic control, it is commonplace to deliberately and systematically breed dogs, cows, horses, plants, and almost anything that is alive, except human beings. In India, on the other hand, where marriages are typically arranged by older (and as they believe, wiser) relatives, eugenic calculations are explicit and pervasive in the mating of human beings, while dogs, plants, and cattle reproduce unregulated by any conscious system of eugenic control. In everyday life, both cultures are eugenic, but not consistently so, and the two cultures do not display a eugenic regard for the same types of living things.

By conjoining a materialist theory of organic nature with a materialist theory of human nature with an interventionist theory of moral duty, Galton's eugenic thinking was more consistent and doctrinaire than everyday thought. Although there are significant elements of primordial thinking in everyday life, relatively few people are consistently eugenic in their thinking about these matters. To canvas everyday thought is to discover shards of eugenic thinking that do not coalesce into an integrated pattern.

For example, some people think that animal nature is essentially material (genetic) but that there is in the essence of human nature something more, something non-natural or spiritual. Some people extend this dualistic thinking to nonhuman animals, to their pets or, in the case of some vegetarians, to any living creature that nurses its young. (In India, among strict vegetarians, any species that has gender is prohibited as food because anything that has gender is thought to be a potential vehicle for an immortal reincarnating soul.)

Others think that human nature is essentially material (genetic), but they do not think that individual and group differences are part of human nature. Still others think that even if all similarities and differences between animals, human and nonhuman, are essentially material (genetic), human beings should not be so eager to bend nature to their will, and they dread the Faustian consequences of "playing God."

Some people think "playing God" is all right, as long as the God is a relatively minor deity with limited powers of control. They do not mind ceding to individuals, or even relatives, the right to influence marriage choices or the right to decide to abort a "defective" fetus, but they would not want to extend that right to a bureaucracy or to the state. And they worry about the limits of parental rights to mold the essential nature of an offspring and to act as guardian for its "interests." It is one thing—and "obviously good"—to alter the genetic code of a child so it will not be born with Down syndrome. It is quite a different thing—and not so obviously good—to genetically engineer a child to be patriotic and pious, or to redesign its genetic code so that the child lacks the capacity to experience "negative" emotions such as sorrow, anger, and fear. In everyday life, even those people who are totally at ease with the idea that everything about human and nonhuman animals and their behavior is material ("in the genes") may find themselves raising questions about the proper limits of rational planning and systems of control for managing human fate.

Indeed few people in everyday life are uniform or consistent in their thinking about the particular aspects of human nature to which eugenic doctrines might be applied. Height, skin color, sickle-cell anemia, and lactose intolerance? Sure. Intelligence? Well, maybe. Alcoholism, shyness, and fear of heights? I don't know. Morality, religious preference, musical interests, and a distaste for puddings? Really? Is that what the scientists say?

The recurrence of Galton's dream

Despite the prevalence of "primordialist" thinking in everyday life, Darwin's logic and Galton's movement experienced a setback during the 1920s, 1930s, and 1940s in the United States. The waning of the official influence of eugenic reasoning in the social, political, and scientific context of the Franklin D. Roosevelt presidency is a complex story (Degler, 1991). Suffice it to say that eugenic thinking temporarily lost its grip on the official and popular imagination even before it became associated with the evils of the Third Reich, the Nazi sterilization and extermination programs and experiments in the breeding of an Aryan "super-race."

Soon after World War II, however, the wind shifted again—back toward the eugenic ideas advocated by Galton and Darwin. Indeed, as we approach the turn of yet another century, the National Institutes of Health and the Department of Energy of the United States have committed nearly a billion dollars of public funds to the Human Genome Project in a state-sponsored effort to seek scientific knowledge of the material essence of human nature (Kevles and Hood, 1992).

This recent recurrence of a fascination with eugenic ideas has been stimulated, at least in part, by technological and scientific developments on various fronts. Major advances have occurred in the isolation and identification of genetic markers and in the screening of genetic defects and autosomal recessive disorders (recessive genes that are harmless to a single carrier yet are dangerous for an offspring if paired across both parents) like cystic fibrosis, sickle-cell anemia, and Tay-Sachs disease. There has been progress in the cloning of human genes and the application of recombinant DNA. Indeed, it has now become commonplace in the popular press to headline research findings in biochemistry and to feature stories about the latest discovery of a "long-sought" gene that is the cause of some dreaded disease. The stories invariably conclude with a visionary litany: "Scientists say that this discovery could lead to new therapies and even a cure."

Technological capacity to control and manipulate the human reproductive process has also expanded. Through sperm banking, in vitro fertilization, and artificial insemination, the means are at hand for the selective breeding of human excellences. Galton's dream of ridding the world of pathology and defective specimens through biochemistry has come to seem like a pending reality.

Each of these scientific and technological advances carries with it an atmosphere thick with moral implications. Information garnered through genetic screening makes it possible to abort fetuses doomed to a life of pathology and devastating disease. Yet it also has implications for decisions about marriage, childbearing and abortion, and for the control and regulation of these things by individuals or organizations with third-party interests and worries about social costs (e.g., insurance companies, the state). That a "public health policy" can be a moral minefield becomes apparent when one reads recommendations like this one from Linus Pauling:

> There should be tattooed on the forehead of every young person a symbol showing possession of the sickle-cell gene or whatever other similar gene, such as the gene for phenylketonuria in a single dose. If this were done, two young people carrying the same seriously defective gene in a single dose would recognize this situation at first sight, and would refrain from falling in love with one another. It is my opinion that legislation along this line, compulsory testing for defective genes before marriage, and some form of semi-public display of this possession, should be adopted. (Pauling, 1968)

Advances in extracorporeal fertilization make it possible for the egg of one woman to be fertilized in vitro and then gestated in the womb of another woman, a boon for some couples. Yet our very capacity to separate the identity of the "mother" as genitor (the person who contributes the egg) from the "mother" as gestator (the person who contributes the womb and goes through the labor of birth) raises new and difficult moral questions hitherto never imagined, except perhaps in mythology, in nightmares, or by Dr. Seuss.

Who is the "natural" mother of the child, the mother who lays the egg or the one who hatches it, the mother who contributes the genetic substance or the one who brings it to term? Imagine the effect on family life and on our sense of responsibility for the young when the notion of "shared substance" linking parent to child goes the way of "miasmas" and "ethers" and other notions that we now view as archaic. Imagine a world in which it is commonplace, through technological innovations, to redesign from scratch the genetic codes contributed by the genitors of a fetus, or to dispense with the need for genitors entirely. At that point the distinction between "natural offspring" and "adopted child" is likely to disappear. Perhaps that will be for the good, and everyone will come to view the old distinction as invidious and feel highly motivated to care for everyone else's children the way they once selectively cared for their own. Or perhaps the waning of the primordial idea of kith and kin, of kindred and kind, will lead to a disastrous weakening of the bond between generations and a diminishment in the inclination of adults to sacrifice for the young. Unintended consequences can be a worry when one has the power of "God" without divine foresight.

Many moral uncertainties and anxieties accompany technological change, and not every change in technological capacity is unequivocally an "advance." For example, the technologies associated with in vitro fertilization and cloning have even led one biological anthropologist to imagine a future world in which human cloning is commonplace and women are no longer needed for reproduction. "Why," she asks, "would the Nobel Prize–winning sex let the sex with the boring, meaningless lives eat up half the food if they are no longer needed for reproductive purposes?" (Elia, 1988, p. 272). To anticipate a battle of the sexes over scarce resources, and to fear gender genocide as the unintended consequence of the growth of knowledge, may seem extreme. Nevertheless, "slippery-slope" and "unintended-consequence" arguments abound in considerations of the ethics of bending the material essence of human beings to our own wills. (See Glover, 1984, for a series of philosophical arguments against slippery-slope reasoning and in favor of intelligent and moral human answers to the question, "What sort of people should there be?")

The current fascination with eugenic thinking—and, for some, the sheer horror of it all—cannot and should not be understood without an analysis of the moral, political, and social implications of advances in science and technology at particular times and in particular places and for particular individuals or groups of individuals within a society. Research on recombinant DNA, for example, holds out the promise that a "defective" fetus might one day, through human intervention, be transformed into an "excellent" fetus. Yet qualities of excellence such as "health," "civility," and "intelligence" are relatively abstract qualities; those in power versus those out of power, or those from different cultural or subcultural traditions, may disagree substantially on how such qualities should be defined. Whoever has the power to define a human excellence in such cases will have the capacity to alter human fate. Within any complex, nonegalitarian society composed of diverse ethnic and racial groups (such as the United States), that power and the presumed authority on which it rests are likely to be contested.

The question of what constitutes "defective" genetic material is going to impose itself on public policy debates with a force comparable to debates about affirmative action, the right to life, and the morality of capital punishment. The issue will not go away. Simple or inexpensive biomedical technologies will be used if they make it possible to eliminate "defective" genetic material without also eliminating "positive" genetic material or the potential for future reproductive success. They will be used even if they are illegal.

Advances in amniocentesis, for example, have made it possible to include gender among the potential criteria of a "defective" baby and to make abortion decisions accordingly. In South Asia and among many Americans and American residents of South Asian origin, what counts as a "defective" baby is, at times, gender-based. Given the financial burdens associated with the practice of dowry transfers at marriage, mothers who have already given birth to several girls are highly motivated to have a son. Consequently, in some clinics in India 95 percent of elected abortions involve a female fetus. If this practice of selective female abortion were to become widespread it would result in a relative scarcity of females, which, from a narrow economic point of view, ought to increase the perceived value of women which, ironically, might weaken the dowry system or at least increase the status of women in society. This is a difficult case for "pro-choice" advocates, many of whom are inclined to argue, somewhat inconsistently, that it is ethically acceptable to abort a healthy fetus that is unwanted but ethically unsound to abort a female fetus that is healthy, whether it is wanted or not. The difficulties are likely to grow. If detailed "personal" information about the characteristics of the fetus is made available in the first trimester of pregnancy, the argument that the fetus is not a person is going to seem increasingly questionable. Should such information be suppressed? Eugenic thinking is going to raise many challenging questions about the fabric of our constitutional liberties.

Twenty-five hundred years after Plato's *The Republic* and 100 after Galton named the movement, eugenic thinking is very much with us. Eugenic thinking, whether it is concerned with individual and group differences in the distribution of inherited human excellences, or with an agenda for the alteration of the material essence of a single human being or a whole species, carries with it a set of provocative and controversial normative implications, which moral philosophers have a responsibility to address.

How our moral intuitions will be given historical and cultural definition in the light of eugenic thinking remains to be seen. Human nature is at least complicated enough to have two sides; we live, as Kant suggested, in "two worlds," a noumenal world and a phenomenal world. In the noumenal aspect of our nature, we are all free and equal, we recognize and respect each other as autonomous persons (or "spirits"), and we have high regard for all that is implied by the idea of autonomy. In the phenomenal aspect of our nature, however, we are unequal, and our autonomy is compromised to varying degrees. We are unequal in our material resources (both genetic and financial), in our motivations, in our bargaining power, in our foresight, in our vulnerability to duress, in the opportunities we are likely to have, given our location within the social order, and in our very capacity to act as autonomous agents.

There is thus an inherent tension in our nature and no easy reconciliation of noumenal and phenomenal claims. If we try to enforce noumenal liberty and equality in the phenomenal world, we introduce too many degrees of regulation and authoritarian control (communism, the "iron cage" of the bureaucratic liberal state), which is inconsistent with the very autonomy we seek to protect. If we fail to enforce nuomenal liberty and equality in the phenomenal world, we banish the "right" and the "good" from the natural world. If we throw up our hands and try to transcend or escape the phenomenal world in gnostic revulsion over the bleak absence of the divine in nature, we abandon society for the cave. Morality is a compromise we strike between these two inherently conflictual sides of our nature for the sake of a life in a social order that has some semblance of decency. And precisely because morality is a compromise it is composed of plural goods and obligations that cannot be reconciled or reduced to a single thing.

In the West, the current compromise between the noumenal and phenomenal sides of human nature is the "liberal expectancy," the moral idea of "equal life prospects." But the idea of "equal life prospects" is an abstract idea that needs to be filled in, implemented, and made relevant in the light of our beliefs about the sources of difference in the world, and in the light of what it is possible for us to accomplish technologically, and what is possible for us to afford.

Many classical societies of old subscribed to the idea of "god-gifts" (inherited qualities of excellence, a natural telos) and of a divine plan for their unequal distribution in the phenomenal world. They never considered the possibility that the state might level the genetic playing field. Their expectancy was that each person should have the opportunity to realize the full potential of his or her natural endowment, whatever that endowment might be. It was also their expectation that the fruits or products realized by each person, fulfilling his or her own peculiar nature, would be valued and esteemed by everyone else in society. In this way a balance was achieved between the moral qualities of self-improvement, fairness, respect, and community. That is what it meant for inherited differences to be part of a divine plan. That is what our liberal democracy will have to achieve if we are to convince ourselves and our offspring that our science, technology, and social and political institutions are really an extension of the mind of God.

RICHARD A. SHWEDER

Directly related to this article is the companion article in this entry: SCIENTIFIC AND RESEARCH ISSUES. *For a further discussion of topics mentioned in this article, see the entries* EUGENICS; GENETIC ENGINEERING, *article on* HUMAN

GENETIC ENGINEERING; GENETICS AND ENVIRONMENT IN HUMAN HEALTH; *and* HEALTH PROMOTION AND HEALTH EDUCATION. *For a discussion of related ideas, see the entries* AUTONOMY; GENE THERAPY; GENETIC COUNSELING; GENOME MAPPING AND SEQUENCING; JUSTICE; MEDICAL ETHICS, HISTORY OF, *section on* THE AMERICAS, *article on* UNITED STATES IN THE TWENTIETH CENTURY; PUBLIC HEALTH, *article on* PHILOSOPHY OF PUBLIC HEALTH; *and* VALUE AND VALUATION. *Other relevant material may be found under the entries* ABORTION, *section on* CONTEMPORARY ETHICAL AND LEGAL ASPECTS, *article on* CONTEMPORARY ETHICAL PERSPECTIVES; GENETICS AND HUMAN SELF-UNDERSTANDING; LIFE; *and* NATURE.

Bibliography

ADAMS, ROBERT MERRIHEW. 1987. "Flavors, Colors and God." In *The Virtue of Faith and Other Essays in Philosophical Theology*, pp. 243–262. New York: Oxford University Press.

BEM, SANDRA LIPSITZ. 1993. *The Lenses of Gender: Transforming the Debate on Sexual Inequality*. New Haven, Conn.: Yale University Press.

BOUCHARD, THOMAS, JR.; LYKKEN, DAVID T.; McGUE, MATTHEW; SEGAL, NANCY L.; and TELLEGEN, ANKE. 1990. "Sources of Human Psychological Differences: The Minnesota Study of Twins Reared Apart." *Science* 250, no. 4973:223–228.

BOWMAN, JAMES E., and MURRAY, ROBERT F., JR. 1990. *Genetic Variation and Disorders in Peoples of African Origin*. Baltimore: Johns Hopkins University Press.

Buck v. Bell. 1927. 274. U.S. 200.

BUSS, DAVID M. 1989. "Conflict Between the Sexes: Strategic Interference and the Evocation of Anger and Upset." *Journal of Personality and Social Psychology* 56:735–747.

CHURCHLAND, PATRICIA SMITH. 1986. *Neurophilosophy: Toward a Unified Science of the Mind-Brain*. Cambridge, Mass.: MIT Press.

DEGLER, CARL N. 1991. *In Search of Human Nature: The Decline and Revival of Darwinism in American Social Thought*. New York: Oxford University Press.

DENNETT, DANIEL C. 1991. *Consciousness Explained*. New York: Little, Brown.

DUSTER, TROY. 1990. *Backdoor to Eugenics*. New York: Routledge.

ELIA, IRENE. 1988. *The Female Animal*. New York: Henry Holt.

FISKE, ALAN PAGE. 1991. *Structures of Social Life: The Four Elementary Forms of Human Relations: Communal Sharing, Authority Ranking, Equality Matching, Market Pricing*. New York: Free Press.

FLANAGAN, OWEN J. 1992. *Consciousness Reconsidered*. Cambridge, Mass.: MIT Press.

FREEDMAN, DANIEL G. 1979. *Human Sociobiology: A Holistic Approach*. New York: Free Press.

GAZZANIGA, MICHAEL S. 1993. *Nature's Mind: The Biological Roots of Thinking, Emotions, Sexuality, Language, and Intelligence*. New York: Basic Books.

GOULD, STEPHEN JAY. 1981. *The Mismeasure of Man*. New York: W. W. Norton.

HAMILTON, WILLIAM D. 1964. "The Genetic Evolution of Social Behavior." *Journal of Theoretical Biology* 7, no. 1: 1–52.

HERRNSTEIN, RICHARD J. 1990. "Still an American Dilemma." *Public Interest* 98:3–17.

JENSEN, ARTHUR R. 1969. "How Much Can We Boost IQ and Scholastic Achievement?" *Harvard Educational Review* 39, no. 1:1–123.

KEVLES, DANIEL J., and HOOD, LEROY, eds. 1992. *The Code of Codes: Scientific and Social Issues in the Human Genome Project*. Cambridge, Mass.: Harvard University Press.

LEWONTIN, RICHARD C. 1976. "The Analysis of Variance and the Analysis of Causes." In *The IQ Controversy: Critical Readings*, pp. 179–193. Edited by Ned J. Block and Gerald Dworkin. New York: Pantheon Books.

———. 1992. "The Dream of the Human Genome: Doubts About the Human Genome Project." *New York Review of Books* 39, no. 10 (May 28):31–40.

LEWONTIN, RICHARD C.; ROSE, STEVEN; and KAMIN, LEON J. 1984. *Not in Our Genes: Biology, Ideology and Human Nature*. New York: Pantheon.

LOEHLIN, JOHN C.; LINDZEY, GARDNER; and SPUHLER, JAMES N. 1975. *Race Differences in Intelligence*. San Francisco: W. H. Freeman.

MACCOBY, ELEANOR, and JACKLIN, CAROL NAGY. 1974. *The Psychology of Sex Differences*. Stanford, Calif.: Stanford University Press.

McGINN, COLIN. 1991. *The Problem of Consciousness*. Oxford: Basil Blackwell.

NELKIN, DOROTHY, and TANCREDI, LAURENCE. 1992. *Dangerous Diagnostics: The Social Power of Biological Information*. New York: Basic Books.

PAULING, LINUS. 1968. "Reflections on the New Biology." *UCLA Law Review* 15, no. 2:267–272.

PIATTELLI-PALMARINI, MASSIMO. 1989. "Evolution, Selection and Cognition: From 'Learning' to Parameter Setting in Biology and in the Study of Language." *Cognition* 31, no. 1:1–44.

PLOMIN, ROBERT. 1986. *Development, Genetics and Psychology*. Hillsdale, N.J.: L. Erlbaum.

PLOMIN, ROBERT; CHIPUER, HEATHER M.; and LOEHLIN, JOHN C. 1990. "Behavioral Genetics and Personality." In *Handbook of Personality: Theory and Research*, pp. 225–243. Edited by Lawrence Pervin. New York: Guilford Press.

PLOMIN, ROBERT, and DANIELS, DENISE. 1987. "Why Are Children in the Same Family So Different from Each Other?" *Behavioral and Brain Sciences* 10, no. 1:1–16.

POPPER, KARL R., and ECCLES, JOHN C. 1977. *The Self and Its Brain*. New York: Springer-Verlag.

ROSSI, ALICE S. 1977. "A Biosocial Perspective on Parenting." *Daedalus* 106, no. 2:1–31.

SCARR, SANDRA. 1987. "Three Cheers for Behavioral Genetics: Winning the War and Losing Our Identity." *Behavior Genetics* 17, no. 3:219–228.

SUZUKI, DAVID, and KNUDTSON, PETER. 1992. *Genetics: The Ethics of Engineering Life*. Rev. ed. Cambridge, Mass.: Harvard University Press.

Symons, Donald. 1979. *The Evolution of Human Sexuality.* New York: Oxford University Press.

Werker, Janet F. 1989. "Becoming a Native Listener." *American Scientist* 77, no. 1:54–59.

Wilson, Edward O. 1975. *Sociobiology: The New Synthesis.* Cambridge, Mass.: Harvard University Press.

Wilson, James Q., and Herrnstein, Richard. 1985. *Crime and Human Nature.* New York: Simon and Schuster.

GENETICS AND HUMAN SELF-UNDERSTANDING

Sherlock Holmes once asked his friend and colleague Dr. Watson, "Did you notice the remarkable thing about the dog which barked in the middle of the night?" Watson replied, "I heard no dog barking in the middle of the night." Holmes's response to this was characteristic: "That was the remarkable thing."

And about the influence of genetics on human self-understanding the most remarkable thing is not that there has been absolutely no influence at all, but that that influence has been, and remains, so small and limited. The present entry, therefore, in the main will deal with the implications for human self-understanding of the discoveries of the geneticists, and with some of the sometimes extraordinarily widespread and stubborn refusals to take proper account of those discoveries. Little can be said about their extremely limited actual influence.

There is, however, one area in which genetic discoveries are already of enormous perceived importance for all those immediately concerned. Genetic defects in the fetus are with increasing frequency construed as indications for abortion. Consider, for instance, the case of the island of Sardinia, a strongly traditional Roman Catholic society in which until very recently many children were born with inherited anemia. Nevertheless, "Nine-tenths of couples at risk of having an affected child now know this, and when the woman becomes pregnant nine-tenths of them choose to end pregnancies which would have produced a genetically damaged infant" (Jones, 1993, p. 60). Although this is immediately a matter of a practical application rather than of any sort of theoretical self-understanding, in the longer term—if it becomes possible to produce "designer babies" by predetermining their genetic makeup—the impact upon human self-understanding is bound to be enormous.

Genetic facts ignored or outright repudiated

The system of hereditarian ideas that in the twentieth century have won by far the most numerous and powerful converts, and led to the most catastrophic consequences, was developed long before there was any concept of the gene. Nor did many of those converts, if any, later display much concern over the fact that the developing science of genetics provided no basis whatsoever for their cherished racial doctrines. The seminal figure here was a Frenchman, Arthur de Gobineau (1816–1882), who is now called "the Father of Racism." His master idea was that of a supposedly superior "Aryan" stock, which alone possessed true civilizing potential. That stock, he believed, had been irrevocably debilitated by miscegenation and was now under threat from lesser white elements within Europe and still more destructive nonwhite hordes beyond.

These ideas, mediated through Gobineau's friendship with Richard Wagner and his Bayreuth circle, had an immediate appeal in imperial Germany. British-born Houston Stewart Chamberlain (1855–1927), who had married Wagner's youngest daughter, acquired German nationality on the eve of World War I. He became a personal friend of Kaiser Wilhelm II and was recruited as an official propagandist for the German cause, a cause he presented as an attempt—made by the nation that was "manifestly superior" to all others in art, music, literature, philosophy, and science—to dominate the European heartland.

Chamberlain's magnum opus was *Die Grundlagen des 19ten Jahrhunderts* (*Foundations of the Nineteenth Century*, 1899). A monstrous book, it is a mixture of contorted pseudohistory and fanatical Germanic mysticism, presenting the world as a stage for a Manichaean conflict between an "Aryan" principle of good and the "Jewish" principle of evil. In October 1923, Adolf Hitler and Alfred Rosenberg visited Wagner's Haus Wahnfried, where they immediately recognized and accepted Chamberlain as the prophet and seer of the future Third Reich (Bullock, 1962). There is no reason to doubt that Alfred Rosenberg, official philosopher of the National Socialist German Workers' Party, considered his own *Der Mythus des 20ten Jahrhunderts* (*The Myth of the Twentieth Century*), published in 1934, to have been erected upon *Foundations of the Nineteenth Century*.

Another tradition also originated long before genetics emerged as a science. Again the founding father was a Frenchman, albeit one writing a century earlier than Gobineau. Claud-Adrien Helvétius (1715–1771) was a philosopher and one of the Encyclopedists. In his *De l'Esprit* (*Concerning Mind*, 1758) he maintained that "All men are born equal in mental capacity; the manifold differences that seem so conspicuous result from nothing but the inequalities in men's social condition and opportunities." The book was, for reasons that are irrelevant here, condemned by the Sorbonne, and publicly burned. Fifteen years later, in his *De l'Homme* (*Concerning Man*), the watchword of Helvétius became "l'éducation peut tout" (education can do everything).

Whereas the tradition stemming from Gobineau simply ignored the claims of genetic science, in its boldest form the tradition descending from Helvétius denies outright that there are or could be any relevant findings about hereditary factors in the production of different mental capacities. As his later statement makes clear, the prime purpose of this denial was to clear the way for a doctrine and program of environmental absolutism, according to which we are all, in all things, completely creatures of our several and usually different environments. The presumably unfulfillable promise of that program was epitomized in a famous behaviorist boast: "Give me a dozen healthy infants, and my own world to bring them up in, and I'll guarantee to take any one at random and train him to become any type of specialist you like to select—doctor, lawyer, merchant, soldier, sailor, beggar-man or thief" (Watson, 1925, p. 104).

Helvétius limited his environmentalism to the development of mental capacities. The author of the article "Behaviorism" for the *Encyclopaedia of the Social Sciences*, writing in the late 1920s, put no such limitations upon his contention that "At birth human infants, regardless of their heredity, are as equal as Fords" (Kallen, 1931, p. 498).

This assertion, as it stands, is so flagrantly false that we have to construe it as tacitly taking some crucial qualification for granted. For whereas it used to be notorious that customers could have their Model T in any color they wished, so long as they wanted it black, babies come in a variety of skin pigmentations. They also come in two sexes. Furthermore, whereas skin pigmentations are paradigmatically skin-deep, there are other physiological differences extending to the deeper structure. So perhaps we should charitably construe Kallen as contending not that there are in fact no discernible differences, since very obviously there are; but that these observed differences, along with all other genetically determined differences, however obvious or however far from obvious, are actually unimportant and/or irrelevant.

There are two common mistakes. The first is to assume that anything innate must be manifest at birth. That is quite wrong. For instance, although human males do not display facial hair on the delivery table, they do begin to do so, in an extremely wide range of environments, in their early teens. The second mistake is to assume that it is possible to determine a priori that some difference is too small to be relevant and important. This is a point that can be most effectively enforced by drawing an example from the natural rather than the social sciences. Even though the difference between the two natural isotopes of uranium is only three neutrons—about 1 percent of the atomic weight of uranium—those three neutrons make the difference between being able and being unable to sustain an explosive chain reaction.

Even supposing that all human beings were at birth as similar to one another as Model T Fords, it still would not necessarily follow that our innate human nature could, given the appropriate environment, be molded into any shape desired. To establish this possibility decisively in any particular case—and it is, surely, only case by particular case that this could be done—it is necessary to show that molding of the kind desired has on some occasion actually been achieved. For, as Aristotle rightly remarks, the argument from actuality to possibility always goes through. That is, if anything is actual, then it must be possible.

It was in hopes of establishing just how completely the behavior of adolescents is shaped by the cultures in which they have been socialized that in 1925 Franz Boas—a protagonist of nurture in the great nature/nurture controversy of the 1920s—sent his doctoral student Margaret Mead to the South Seas. Her mission resulted in the publication three years later of the all-time anthropological best-seller *Coming of Age in Samoa*, significantly subtitled *A Psychological Study of Primitive Youth for Western Civilization* (Mead, 1928).

Although Mead's findings have been discredited (Freeman, 1983, 1991)—many of the most exciting were the diametric opposite of the truth—there can be no question that in its day (a day lasting several decades) her book had a very substantial influence upon a great many people's self-understanding. That substantial influence, however, was not exercised against the acceptance of the discoveries of geneticists but, rather, through a reaction against the perceived threat arising from their previous and possible future discoveries. The threat was to the protagonists of nurture in the nature/nurture controversy. They maintained that the prime determinant of all human behavior is the environment, whereas their opponents contended that, on the contrary, it is our innate nature.

Implications of basic general facts of human genetics

An exploration of the true implications of genetic discoveries for a late-twentieth-century understanding of human nature must begin from a statement of two fundamental and complementary facts.

The first of these is the fact of genetic diversity. Except for identical twins—monozygotic (one-egg) as opposed to dizygotic (two-egg) twins—no two people who have ever lived or ever will live have been, are, or will be built on the same genetic plan; the chance that any particular existing array of particular genes either has occurred in the past or will occur in the future is for all practical purposes nil. Furthermore, this genetic uniqueness is compounded by environmental uniqueness, because the phenotypic expression is conditioned at every step in development by environmental forces that are forever changing: Even identical twins become different persons because, during intrauterine life and increasingly after birth, they are exposed to different environmental conditions.

Leo Loeb, whose life's work was a study of biological individuality, put this first fundamental fact into an evolutionary perspective: "We find, phylogenetically, a progressively increasing complexity in the activities of organisms and increasing differences between members of the same species, an increasing individualization which reaches its highest development in man" (quoted in Williams, 1979, p. 45).

The second fundamental and complementary fact is that, along with this enormous genetic diversity *as individuals*, we nevertheless have *as a species*—presumably because our species evolved so recently—an equally remarkable genetic homogeneity: "This means that if, after a global disaster, only one group—the Albanians, the Papuans or the Senegalese—survived, most of the world's genetic diversity for functional genes would be preserved. . . . Other creatures vary much more from place to place. . . . The difference between the highland and the lowland populations of the mountain gorilla a few miles apart in central Africa is more than that between any two human groups" (Jones, 1993, p. 51).

To deduce normative and prescriptive conclusions directly from such purely factual and neutrally descriptive premises would be to commit the naturalistic fallacy. (This fallacy is perhaps most commonly committed in attempts to derive such normative conclusions directly from allegations about human nature or from statements of laws of nature.)

We cannot, therefore, validly deduce from the facts of genetic homogeneity any doctrine of the moral unity of humankind. Nevertheless, it does become very awkward to insist, in the face of these facts, that there are fundamental and innate differences between Greeks and barbarians or between blacks and whites that justify treating members of such contrasting groups in importantly different ways. Again, while we cannot validly deduce any prescriptive conclusions from the facts of genetic diversity, these facts are very congenial to people who want to maximize the number and variety of alternatives between which individuals can choose. For they make it likely that a variety of different alternatives will be chosen by the variety of different individuals. Similarly, were it not for this diversity of talents and inclinations, the possibilities of a wealth-creating division of labor combined with a free and effective market for labor would not be nearly so great as they in fact are (Williams, 1979).

To those for whom a main, if not the supreme, political objective is raising (or reducing) everyone to the same equal condition, the facts of our genetic diversity must constitute a formidable embarrassment: "For . . . a thoroughgoing egalitarian . . . inequality that derives from biology ought to be as repulsive as inequality that derives from early socialization" (Jencks et al., 1972, p. 73). Presumably under pressure of that embarrassment, the distinguished social scientist who wrote the sentence just quoted refrained from speculating about the eventual, no doubt extremely long-term, possibilities of reproducing human populations by big-batch clonings, and instead proceeded to discuss approaches to the ideal of "cognitive equality" (Jencks et al., 1972, pp. 54, 109). Thanks to the general genetic diversity and the limited intellectual capacities of many, the cost of realizing this ideal might be universal, nearly total nescience.

These same facts of genetic diversity and genetic homogeneity are comfortably conformable with the rights claims of the American Declaration of Independence; and this notwithstanding that those claims have sometimes been misunderstood to have been grounded upon a denial of that diversity. Certainly the signers of that document held it "to be self-evident, that all men are created equal. . . ." But there is no full stop at the word "equal." For, as Abraham Lincoln once explained, the signers "did not intend to declare all men equal in all respects. They did not mean to say that all men were equal in color, size, intellect, moral development, or social capacity. They defined with tolerable distinctness in what respects they did consider all men created equal—certain inalienable rights, among which are life, liberty and the pursuit of happiness." These equal rights, therefore, are grounded not in any mistakenly assumed equality of ability or inclination but in our common humanity; not, as we might say, in our genetic uniformity but in our genetic homogeneity.

Implications of genetic facts about individuals and collectives

Thomas Jefferson—the man who, thanks to his "peculiar felicity of expression," was asked to draft the Declaration of Independence—was under no illusions about equal talents. On the contrary: In his sole published book, *Notes on the State of Virginia*, he developed a scheme for a fiercely selective system of primary education, in the course of which "twenty of the best geniuses will be raked from the rubbish annually." After six further years of schooling, ten of those twenty "are to be chosen, for the superiority of their parts and dispositions," and sent to study "at William and Mary College (Jefferson, 1955 [1787], p. 143; cf. pp. 137–142).

In this, as no doubt in many other ways, Jefferson was by today's standards in the highest degree "politically incorrect." Certainly Sir Andrew Huxley—a great-grandson of Thomas Henry Huxley—was in his 1977 Presidential Address to the British Association for the Advancement of Science constrained to speak of "the assumption of equal inherited ability as something which . . . does not require experimental evidence . . . and which it is politically wicked to question." He went on to complain: "There is in fact a taboo on openminded investigation . . . at least as strong as the resistance in Darwin's day to questioning the authority of the Bible." This taboo appears to be stronger in the United States, where the media systematically misrepresent what seems to be the contrary if largely tacit consensus of the researchers (Snyderman and Rothman, 1988; cf. Fletcher, 1991). If and insofar as the truth is that inherited abilities are extremely unequal, then any such failure or refusal to take account of the genetic facts must contribute substantially to human self-misunderstanding.

Nor is there any reason to believe that Jefferson, having rejected the notion that talent is distributed equally among individuals, would nevertheless have been content to concede that among different collections of unequally talented individuals, such unequal talents are always distributed in the same way. He would not, for instance, have accepted uncritically the categorical pronouncement issued in 1965 by the U.S. Department of Labor: "Intelligence potential is distributed among Negro infants in the same proportion and pattern as among Icelanders or Chinese, or any other group. . . . There is absolutely no question of any genetic differential."

Whether or not that pronouncement is true, there is no question that it does not follow from the previously quoted assertion "that if, after a global disaster, only one group . . . survived, most of the world's genetic diversity for functional genes would be preserved." For even if all the genetic diversity was preserved—even if, that is, at least one single specimen of every functional gene was preserved—this would not begin to show that the distribution within the surviving group was the same as that within all those others that, by the hypothesis, did not survive.

On the other hand, the truth of that assertion about the survival of most, if not all, "the world's genetic diversity for functional genes" does carry some practically important implications. In the first place, it means that to be true, statements about the genetically determined abilities or inclinations of particular subsets of the total human population must be statements about averages rather than categorical statements to the effect that either all or no members of that subset are either able to do this or are strongly inclined to do that. From statements about the average characteristics of any set, it is impossible immediately to infer any conclusion about the characteristics of a particular member of that set. Thus, from the statement that the members of some set are on average five feet, nine inches tall, we are certainly not licensed to infer that any single member of that set is either five feet nine inches tall or is of any other particular height.

The practical importance of this elementary logical truth is that people cannot properly be ruled out of consideration for appointments on the ground that some set to which they belong is on average deficient in characteristics essential in those appointments. So we can be reassured that even if that pronouncement by the U.S. Department of Labor were shown to be false, and so long as the assertion about the survival of most, if not all, of "the world's genetic diversity" for fundamental genes was known to be true, this falsification would not provide any justification whatsoever for hostile discrimination against the members of any of the subsets concerned.

But, granted that that assertion is indeed known to be true, we still need to appreciate something that holds for differences on average between sets of all sorts. We have here another of those cases in which what seems comparatively small can turn out to make a very large difference. For where a characteristic is normally distributed—as is the case with most characteristics measured by psychologists—a difference between two averages of only a single standard deviation will produce quite dramatic changes in the numbers at the extremes. Take, for instance, the much-measured characteristic of IQ, which certainly is both normally distributed and at least in part genetically determined. And suppose that we have two sets of people differing by one standard deviation in respect of that characteristic. Then, all other things being equal, we should expect—absent either substantial hostile discrimination or gross social disadvantage—that the set with the higher average IQ will by comparison be heavily overrepresented in whatever sorts of occupations and achievements demand very high IQs. On the same assumptions we should also expect that set to be correspondingly underrepresented among those rated, by whatever are the prevailing standards, as educationally subnormal (ESN). In this area, as in others, the operation of policies founded upon false assumptions can have extremely disturbing, unintended consequences (Jensen, 1972).

The challenge of sociobiology

Any consideration of the influence of genetics upon human self-understanding has to attend to E. O. Wilson's *Sociobiology: The New Synthesis*, "sociobiology" being defined as "the systematic study of the biological basis of all social behaviour" (Wilson, 1975, p. 4). In the final chapter of an earlier treatise, *The Insect Societies*, Wilson had envisaged that "the same principles of population biology and comparative zoology," which had "worked so well in explaining the rigid systems of the social insects, could be applied point by point to vertebrate animals" (Wilson, 1971).

In the case of human societies this application will apparently involve a takeover by evolutionary genetics. For

> Sociology *sensu stricto* . . . still stands apart from sociobiology because of its largely . . . nongenetic approach. . . . Taxonomy and ecology . . . have been reshaped entirely . . . by integration into neo-Darwinist evolutionary theory—the "Modern Synthesis" as it is often called—*in which each phenomenon is weighed for its adaptive significance and then related to the basic principles of population genetics.* (Wilson, 1975, p. 4; emphasis added)

This particular statement, however, concludes cautiously: "Whether the social sciences can be truly biologicized in this fashion remains to be seen."

In subsequent writings Wilson has been less cautious and more explicit in his reductionist ambitions. The issue at stake is the extent to which human cultures, and the behaviors that are a part of them, can be accounted for by "genetic determinism." Thus, in his treatise *On Human Nature*, Wilson stresses that it is on the interpretation of this "key phrase" that "the entire relation between biology and the social sciences depends" (Wilson, 1978, p. 55).

The final chapter of *Sociobiology: The New Synthesis* gets off to a splendid start with this sentence: "Let us now consider man in the free spirit of natural history, as though we were zoologists from another planet completing a catalog of social species on Earth." Suppose that we actually do begin in this way, as Wilson in fact did not. Then the first peculiarity we have to pick out is, surely, the extended period between birth and maturity, the incomparable capacity for learning, and the importance of learned (as opposed to instinctual) behavior.

This unrivaled capacity for learning—together with its instrument and expression, developed language—provides our species with a serviceable substitute for the (genetic) inheritance of acquired characteristics. It is this serviceable substitute for the (genetic) inheritance of acquired characteristics that constitutes the first threat to the project for a reductionist human sociobiology. For it makes it impossible fully to understand the workings of human societies, as it is certainly not impossible to understand those of insect societies, without constantly taking account of their pasts as well as of the previously acquired information stocks to which their members have access. (What is peculiar to our species, it must be emphasized, is not the exogenetic [nongenetic] transmission of specific possible behaviors from one generation to the next, as such, but the enormous number and variety of possible behaviors that, thanks to the hypertrophy of the human brain and to the presumably concurrent and connected development of language, can now be transmitted exogenetically.)

No doubt this "unrivaled capacity for learning," like all our other innate capacities and dispositions, is itself genetically determined. But—and here we come to the second of the peculiarities that threaten the project for a reductionist sociobiology—the directions to which *we* turn such capacities, and how far *we* inhibit or pursue such inclinations, is not already determined by our genes. It is instead for us to decide. For we are creatures of a kind whose members are all, to a greater or lesser extent, agents; and insofar as we are, we can and cannot but make choices between alternative courses of action. Agents as such always could have done, and could do, other than they did or will do—in a strong sense that can, and perhaps can only, be explained ostensively.

Presumably there are in some nonhuman mammals embryonic developments on these lines, just as there certainly are, in several species other than ours, cases of the exogenetic inheritance of the acquired characteristic of a learned behavior. In both instances, however, the prehuman anticipations of what has in our species become a vastly extended and elaborately sophisticated development appear to be comparatively minor. It is this second peculiarity of our species, even more than the first, that makes the human sciences irreducibly different from the natural sciences. Wilson does in his own way recognize the reality of choice. But, once again, he fails to appreciate its revolutionary and relevant significance.

The issue at stake is the extent to which cultures, and the behaviors that are a part of them, can be explained in terms of a "genetic determinism." It is on the interpretation of this "key phrase," as Wilson stresses, that "the entire relation between biology and the social sciences depends" (Wilson, 1975, p. 532). So, as an example of an organism whose behavior is genetically "predestined," he instances the mosquito: "The mosquito is an automaton," with "a sequence of rigid behaviors programmed by the genes to unfold swiftly and unerringly from birth to the final act of oviposition" (Wilson, 1978, p. 55).

Wilson then offers one of an abundance of possible examples of a "restricted," as opposed to a "rigid," behavior, in which "the genes have their way unless specifically contravened by conscious choice." Yet it will not do, as Wilson does, to leave it at that. For whenever genes have causally necessitated their—shall we say owners, or subjects, or whatever else?—to have not uncontrollable reflexes but inhibitable and controllable desires or dispositions or orientations or inclinations, then this must open the possibility that choice will intervene to contravene.

A scientific Calvinism?

In 1932, in an essay published under what would now be deemed a provocative title, *The Inequality of Man*,

J. B. S. Haldane, at that time Britain's leading geneticist, told how his distinguished predecessor William Bateson had, during World War I, lectured about innate differences. A Scottish soldier commented: "Sir, what you're telling us is nothing but scientific Calvinism."

Haldane then proceeded to develop this theme by reference to *Crime as Destiny: A Study of Criminal Twins* (Lange, 1931). This book, which Haldane thought might one day be seen as "the most important . . . of this century," reported the results of a study of pairs of brothers at least one of whom was incarcerated in a south German jail. Of the 428 nontwin brothers of prisoners, only about one in twelve had a record of criminal imprisonment.

Of the sixteen undoubtedly dizygotic twins, only two of the incarcerated men had criminal brothers, and in one of these cases one brother was a habitual criminal while the other, after engaging in criminal behavior for one year, had been law-abiding for the following fifteen. So the record of the dizygotic twins seems very similar to that of the nontwin brothers.

But the case of the thirteen monozygotic pairs was very different. Ten of these pairs were both criminals. The stories of these ten pairs are told in great detail, and the behavioral resemblances of each set of twins are often extraordinarily close. Haldane, echoing Lange, construed these findings as counting against a doctrine of the freedom of the will. They tend to show that most, if not all, "of those moral decisions that land us in jail or otherwise are predetermined."

So what do these and similar, more recent findings, including the claims about supposedly "criminal" chromosomes, actually tend to show? Since there is no reference here, either explicit or implicit, to a creator God, these findings can at most be compatible with (without in any way providing positive support for) the specifically theological doctrine of predestination—a doctrine that, though commonly identified with Calvin and Calvinism, was in fact substantially shared by Thomas Aquinas, Martin Luther, and other classical theologians. It is important to be clear about this. For the doctrine is that specifically theological one that carries the infinitely appalling implication that we are all creatures of an omnipotent creator God who secretly makes us behave in ways that, absent gratuitous exercises of divine grace and forgiveness, must earn the punishment of eternal torment.

Do such genetic findings, considered in an entirely secular and this-worldly context, constitute anything more than an approach to a genetic explanation of something that everyone knew to be the case long before there was such a thing as a science of genetics or any science at all—namely, that most of us have some, though by no means in everyone the same, natural inclinations? Surely they do not even begin to show that

none of our behaviors are—to reemploy Wilson's terminology—"restricted" as opposed to "rigid." The former behaviors are those in which agents are strongly inclined to behave in particular ways yet could do differently if they so chose.

It is necessary to distinguish more from less fundamental senses of "having a choice" and "could have done otherwise." When Martin Luther protested before the Diet of Worms, "Here I stand. I can no other. So help me God," he was not asserting that he had been afflicted with a general paralysis that left him physically incapable of withdrawing to his Saxon refuge. In the more fundamental sense he certainly could have done that, but for him any such alternative was intolerable. When some unfortunate businessman receives from a "godfather" an "offer he cannot refuse," we may say that he has no choice but to sign a document transferring his property to the Organization. But the fact that in the more fundamental sense he did have a choice can be brought out by comparing his situation with that of the treacherous Mafioso who without warning is gunned down from behind. And to anyone who nevertheless tries to deny that those who, in this fundamental sense, did have choices and could have done otherwise, what can be said but that those expressions are definable only by reference to the sorts of situations to which they are conventionally applied? For how can we understand what is meant by "having a choice" or "being able to do other than we do" if not by reference to the sorts of situations to which we have learned to apply such expressions as "He had a choice" or "She could have done something else"?

ANTONY FLEW

Directly related to this entry are the entries BIOLOGY, PHILOSOPHY OF; HUMAN NATURE; EVOLUTION; *and* GENETICS AND HUMAN BEHAVIOR. *For a discussion of related ideas, see the entries* BIOTECHNOLOGY; EUGENICS; GENE THERAPY, *article on* ETHICAL AND SOCIAL ISSUES; GENOME MAPPING AND SEQUENCING; *and* RACE AND RACISM.

Bibliography

BULLOCK, ALAN. 1962. *Hitler: A Study in Tyranny*. Rev. ed. Harmondsworth, U.K.: Penguin.

CHAMBERLAIN, HOUSTON STEWART. 1910. *Foundations of the Nineteenth Century*. Translated by John Lees. London: John Lane.

FLETCHER, RONALD. 1991. *Science, Ideology and the Media: The Cyril Burt Scandal*. New Brunswick, N.J.: Transaction.

FREEMAN, DEREK. 1983. *Margaret Mead and Samoa: The Making and Unmaking of an Anthropological Myth*. Cambridge, Mass.: Harvard University Press.

————. 1991. "There's Tricks i' th' World: An Historical Analysis of the Samoan Researches of Margaret Mead." *Visual Anthropology Review* 7, no. 1:103–128.

GOLDBERG, STEVEN. 1977. *The Inevitability of Patriarchy.* 2d ed. London: Temple-Smith.

HALDANE, J. B. S. 1932. *The Inequality of Man.* Harmondsworth, U.K.: Penguin.

JEFFERSON, THOMAS. 1955. [1787]. *Notes on the State of Virginia.* Edited by William Peden. Chapel Hill: University of North Carolina Press.

JENCKS, CHRISTOPHER; SMITH, MARSHALL; ACLAND, HENRY; BANE, MARY JO; COHEN, DAVID; GINTIS, HERBERT; HEYNES, BARBARA; and MICHELSON, STEPHEN. 1972. *Inequality: A Reassessment of the Effect of Family and Schooling in America.* New York: Basic Books.

JENSEN, ARTHUR R. 1972. *Genetics and Education.* London: Methuen.

JONES, STEVE. 1993. *The Language of the Genes: Biology, History, and the Evolutionary Future.* London: HarperCollins.

KALLEN, HORACE M. 1931. "Behaviorism." In vol. 2 of *Encyclopaedia of the Social Sciences*, pp. 495–498. New York: Macmillan.

KITCHER, PHILIP. 1985. *Vaulting Ambition: Sociobiology and the Quest for Human Nature.* Cambridge, Mass.: M.I.T. Press.

LANGE, JOHANNES. 1931. *Crime as Destiny: A Study of Criminal Twins.* Translated by Charlotte Haldane. London: Allen & Unwin.

MEAD, MARGARET. 1928. *Coming of Age in Samoa: A Psychological Study of Primitive Youth for Western Civilization.* New York: William Morrow.

SNYDERMAN, MARK, and ROTHMAN, STANLEY. 1988. *The IQ Controversy: The Media and Public Policy.* New Brunswick, N.J.: Transaction.

WATSON, J. B. 1925. *Behaviorism.* New York: W. W. Norton.

WILLIAMS, ROGER J. 1979. *Free and Unequal: The Biological Basis of Individual Liberty.* Indianapolis: Liberty Press.

WILSON, EDWARD O. 1971. *The Insect Societies.* Cambridge, Mass.: Harvard University Press.

————. 1975. *Sociobiology: The New Synthesis.* Cambridge, Mass.: Harvard University Press.

————. 1977. "Biology and the Social Sciences." *Daedalus* 106, no. 4: 127–140.

————. 1978. *On Human Nature.* Cambridge, Mass.: Harvard University Press.

GENETICS AND THE LAW

The interaction of genetics with law is driven by the powerful information that can be discerned about individuals by genetic testing. In general, genetic data can be divided into two broad categories: information that determines identity or biological relationship, and information that has diagnostic or predictive value about one's health or the health of one's potential children. As we have entered an era where genetic testing can make definitive statements about identity and discern critical facts about health, it is crucial that societies develop rules to regulate the use of these data. The possibility that genetically engineered organisms could create biohazards also has stimulated much public discourse and some legal activity.

Advances in genetics have stimulated legislative interest and judicial attention for several decades. Analysis of how legal systems use genetic (and other scientific) information to help order society suggests that too often lawmakers and judges are not provided with an adequate technological primer to enable them to properly use new knowledge. Lawmakers and judges need routine access to institutions that can neutrally and competently evaluate genetic data. Work performed by the Office of Technology Assessment for Congress is an apt model.

Courts have long recognized the value of biological markers to determine identity. Blood-group analysis was first used more than fifty years ago to exclude wrongfully accused males in paternity disputes; subsequently, human leukocyte antigen (HLA) testing and, since 1986, deoxyribonucleic acid (DNA) based approaches, have been used widely in Europe and the United States in both civil and criminal proceedings to determine alleged familial relationships or to decide whether biological samples from crime scenes match those from a particular individual. DNA forensics has revolutionized the investigation of violent crimes (Committee on DNA Technology in Forensic Science, 1992).

The legislative and executive branches of governments have often been eager (sometimes too eager) to translate advances in genetic knowledge into progressive public-health policy. During the first half of the twentieth century, now-repudiated eugenic theories that claimed a factual foundation in genetics were used to rationalize the involuntary sterilization of institutionalized retarded and mentally ill persons in the United States and several European countries, particularly Germany (Reilly, 1991). Since the early 1960s the United States and European nations have conducted mass genetic screening of newborns to detect rare but ameliorable forms of genetically caused mental retardation. During the 1970s the first carrier-screening programs were launched, often with government support, to identify otherwise healthy individuals who carried particular disease genes placing them at high risk of bearing a child with a recessive disorder if the child were conceived with a person who carried the same disease gene.

The unprecedented ability to learn genetic facts about individuals creates a fundamental tension between the right to privacy and the competing interests of the state and other social institutions. In the United States and in many other nations there is a constitutional right to privacy. Many of the U.S. Supreme Court opinions that initially articulated this right arose from challenges to the state's power to restrict access to contraception and abortion (*Roe* v. *Wade*, 1973), areas of crucial importance to genetic counseling.

Fueled by the Human Genome Project—a federally funded effort begun in 1991 to map and, ultimately, to sequence every human gene—the array of clinically useful genetic tests will increase substantially in coming years. This has raised fears of genetic discrimination. As is demonstrated by the introduction of involuntary eugenic sterilization in the People's Republic of China, genetic information can be used to limit fundamental rights. In the United States and Europe, some are concerned that genetic data will be used to rationalize discriminatory treatment by insurers, employers, and other social institutions. No technologically advanced nation has yet fully explored the social consequences of having a large amount of genetic information available about its citizenry.

Who should have access to genetic information?

The most important legal issue that arises from our growing power to read the genetic code is summarized in a single question: Who should have access to genetic information about ourselves? The response each society develops will reflect the dimensions of the individual's right of privacy, which vary widely. In the United States, Canada, the European Union, Australia, and Japan, discussion of the need to develop rules on the acquisition, storage, and control of genetic information is underway and guidelines are beginning to emerge.

Genetic testing raises challenging privacy conflicts between individuals. Depending on the context, spouses, parents, children, siblings, and even members of one's extended family may have powerful claims to know genetic facts about an individual. For example, when a physician determines that a child is suffering from a genetic disorder, that information may be extremely important to the reproductive planning of the child's aunts and uncles. If the child's parents refuse to communicate with relatives, are there circumstances that would justify the decision by the physician to warn relatives? The common-law expectation that the physician–patient encounter will be conducted in confidence offers some guidance about how to regulate the flow of genetic information within families (Andrews, 1987), but novel questions remain. For example, how should a physician respond to a request for genetic testing from an identical twin? There is virtually no case law concerning the duty of an individual to share genetic information with relatives, but this topic has been explored by several national committees (e.g., U.S. President's Commission for the Study of Ethical Problems in Medicine and Biomedical and Behavioral Research, 1983; Committee

on Assessing Genetic Risks, 1994) that have strongly valued the protection of personal privacy, while acknowledging that situations might arise that would justify a disclosure to a third party.

Beyond the family, genetic information may be of interest to public-health authorities, insurers, employers, school systems, child welfare agencies, law enforcement officials, the courts, and the military. In the United States there is growing discussion about whether existing legislation and common law are sufficient to guide the nonclinical uses of genetic data, such as in the underwriting practices of insurers, the hiring practices of employers, and by adoption agencies (McEwen and Reilly, 1992) so as to minimize improper discrimination based on genotype. Constitutional law, especially in determining the limits on state action to further the public health, is relevant to the implementation of mass genetic screening programs and the development of DNA data banks.

The decision to undergo genetic testing

In democratic societies an individual has the right to determine whether or not he or she will undergo genetic testing. The exception, now widespread in the Western world, is newborn screening; these programs test infants for several rare, severe, treatable genetic diseases, usually without giving parents an opportunity to decline. In the United States compulsory newborn screening has never been challenged in court, but would likely be upheld as a valid exercise of the public-health power. However, state-based compulsory screening to identify children with genetic conditions that are not associated with obvious disease are less likely to pass constitutional muster.

Informed consent

In noncompulsory situations, decisions about whether to undergo genetic testing are governed by the doctrine of informed consent, derived from case law and medical literature that developed largely in the United States from the 1960s on (U.S. President's Commission, 1982a). The term "informed consent" first appeared in the case law in 1957 (*Salgo* v. *Leland Stanford Jr. Univ. Bd. of Trustees*), and the concept was developed at length three years later by the Supreme Court of Kansas (*Natanson* v. *Kline*, 1960).

An informed choice presumes that the individual has had an opportunity to become educated about the relevant issues. At a minimum, the physician or genetic counselor should inform the individual about the nature and purpose of the test, any significant risks associated with it, and foreseeable problems that may arise from undergoing the procedure or learning the result (*Canter-*

bury v. *Spence,* 1972). The individual should be informed that test results could discern that assumed biological relationships are incorrect (e.g., nonpaternity or undisclosed adoption). Some commentators advocate informing persons that the presymptomatic diagnosis of disease or recognition of increased risk for a serious disorder could compromise access to health and life insurance and restrict employment opportunities (Billings et al., 1992).

Liability for failure to inform about relevant genetic tests

Most of the litigation concerning genetic information has focused on whether or not a physician owed a duty to warn a patient that she was at increased risk for having a child with a serious genetic disorder. This litigation has given rise to the concepts of "wrongful birth" and "wrongful life." The notion of wrongful life arose in a discussion of whether children should have legal recourse for the stigmatization of illegitimacy; the concept of wrongful birth was developed from about 1975 to 1985 as a number of court decisions (e.g., *Becker* v. *Schwartz,* 1978) and law review articles considered the dimensions of a physician's duty to inform women about reproductive risks (Capron, 1979).

In the United States most jurisdictions will not permit children with birth defects to bring wrongful-life lawsuits against physicians. Such suits typically allege a failure to warn parents about a reproductive risk that subsequently occurred. Judges have been unwilling to permit the child plaintiff in a wrongful-life suit to argue that but for the warning that a physician failed to give, he or she would not have been born. To do so would require the jury to measure the value of an impaired life (due to a serious birth defect) against nonexistence.

In contrast, many jurisdictions do permit wrongful-birth lawsuits brought by the parents of children with birth defects, arguing that the physician's failure to warn breached a duty of care and deprived them of an opportunity to avert the birth of an affected child. If a jury decides that such a duty exists, that the physician breached it, and that an injury occurred, then the jury must decide the damages. Virtually all jurisdictions permit the jury to calculate the special costs of raising a child with the particular disorder; some permit additional damages to be awarded to the parents for loss of economic productivity, and a few permit damages to be awarded for emotional harm (Andrews, 1987).

The availability of ever more genetic tests, some intended to diagnose only mild to moderately severe disorders, will eventually define the limits of the duty to warn. It is likely that actions for wrongful birth will be limited to situations where the physician knew or should have known of the availability of a test for parents who have a significantly increased risk of bearing a child with a serious disease that manifests at birth or in childhood.

Regulation of genetic services

In many nations, education and counseling about genetic disorders is provided through a network of state-supported family-planning clinics. For example, pursuant to Article 20 of its Eugenic Protection Law (1949), in Japan every local government must set up a Eugenic Protection Counseling Center. In 1989 there were 836 such centers, most staffed by the Japan Family Planning Association and subsidized by the Ministry of Health and Welfare. The law lists more than twenty hereditary disorders for which abortion may be permitted, but does not have a general provision to cover elective termination of any fetus with a serious hereditary disorder (Takagi, 1991).

In the United States during the 1980s, a federal rule prohibited federally funded family-planning clinics from counseling about abortion. This had a chilling effect on discussions about genetic screening and testing as well. The rule survived constitutional attack (*Rust* v. *Sullivan,* 1991), but was rescinded by an executive order in 1993.

A growing number of nations have limited the use of certain technologies that are relevant to clinical genetics. Alarmed by the use of amniocentesis and karyotyping to identify fetal sex and abort females, India has prohibited prenatal sex selection. Germany, Austria, and Switzerland have forbidden surrogate pregnancies, and France has ruled that the surrogacy contract is unenforceable. These nations also prohibit embryo donation. Preimplantation diagnosis for X-linked disorders is permissible (Knoppers and Le Bris, 1993).

In the United States perhaps the first federal law pertaining to genetic services was the Sickle Cell Anemia Control Act, which in 1972 made funds available to state-based voluntary screening programs that provided access to appropriate genetic counseling. The federal statute, which reduced concerns about poorly drafted state legislation, stimulated a wave of interest in disease-specific legislation. In 1973 the National Cooley's Anemia Control Act appropriated $11 million to support state and local screening programs for beta-thalassemia, an incurable, fatal blood disease of childhood. The Department of Health, Education and Welfare then developed a comprehensive approach to genetic services.

The most significant federal legislation pertaining to the provision of genetic services in the United States was the National Sickle Cell Anemia, Cooley's Anemia, Tay-Sachs, and Genetic Diseases Act, which amended Title XI of the Public Health Service Act. During fiscal 1978, the first year in which funds were appropriated, the Bureau of Maternal and Child Health (MCH) divided $6.8 million about evenly between genetic services grants to individual states and the funding of sickle-cell screening and education clinics. In 1983 MCH began using Title XI dollars to support regional genetic networks that operate under the aegis of a Council of Regional Networks for Genetic Services. Since 1985 MCH has supported the development of newborn screening programs for sickle-cell anemia.

Advances in molecular genetics have spawned a new interest in DNA-based diagnostics. This in turn has raised concerns, particularly among academically based physicians and state regulatory officials, about the quality of the testing services that laboratories will provide. A few states, notably New York and California, have well-developed approaches to evaluating and monitoring genetic testing laboratories, but most do not. A committee of the Institute of Medicine has concluded that the Clinical Laboratories Improvement Act of 1988 and the Medical Devices Act of 1976 grant the Food and Drug Administration sufficient authority to oversee DNA diagnostic facilities, but that the relevant regulations have not yet been applied to these new labs (Committee on Assessing Genetic Risks, 1994).

Until the early 1990s, most genetic testing was performed in medical centers, and most individuals had assistance from genetic counselors. In the United States these counselors had master's-degree training and obtained certification from the American Board of Medical Genetics. No state required that genetic counselors be licensed. In the future most counseling will be done by persons without such specialized training. This raises the need to develop alternative training programs and mechanisms to ensure competence.

Newborn screening.   Beginning in 1962 with the first law to mandate newborn screening for phenylketonuria (PKU), a disease leading to brain damage and mental retardation, there has been a steady growth of state-operated, population-based newborn screening in the Western world. In the United States every state participates in newborn screening, most as mandated by state law. The programs were originally aimed at identifying children with treatable inborn errors of metabolism; they now include screening for sickle-cell anemia and (in a few states) congenital adrenal hyperplasia, two other disorders where early diagnosis can be lifesaving.

Screening statutes and regulations typically mandate testing, but exempt children whose parents object on religious grounds. In a few states, notably Maryland, the parent is routinely given an opportunity to refuse the test. A report by the Institute of Medicine has concluded that newborn screening can be safely and efficiently conducted on a voluntary basis, and has recommended that new tests be added only when pilot studies have confirmed their potential benefit (Committee on Assessing Genetic Risks, 1994).

Carrier screening.   Carrier screening is intended to identify otherwise healthy persons who, depending upon whom they marry, may be at high risk for having children with a severe genetic disorder. In the United States population-based screening programs have been undertaken to identify carriers for sickle-cell anemia and Tay-Sachs disease. Since its start in the mid-1970s, Tay-Sachs screening has been community based, conducted without state intervention, and highly utilized by the Ashkenazi Jewish population in which the disease is relatively common. In contrast, sickle-cell screening programs were often implemented by law. Between 1970 and 1972 twelve states and the District of Columbia enacted statutes that mandated carrier screening of African-Americans, usually by tying it to entry into the public schools or to obtaining a marriage license. Most state laws failed to offer pretest education or to provide access to genetic counseling. Concerns about genetic discrimination provoked a strong outcry from the African-American community and led to corrective federal legislation (Reilly, 1975).

Voluntary mass screening for beta-thalassemia has been conducted in Sardinia, Cyprus, and Greece. In 1975 geneticists in Sardinia initiated a screening program, heavily endorsed by prominent social institutions, that has had a remarkable impact. By 1991 more than 167,000 people had been tested and about 90 percent of carrier couples had been identified. The vast majority of at-risk couples chose prenatal diagnosis; most of the women with affected fetuses had them aborted. In fifteen years the number of children born with beta-thalassemia in Sardinia declined by 90 percent (Cao, 1991).

The cloning of the cystic fibrosis gene in 1989 sparked debate over the criteria that should be met before mass carrier screening could be offered. One in twenty-five white persons of northern European extraction is a carrier. In England several population-based cystic fibrosis screening programs have been introduced regionally, and a large voluntary effort was undertaken in Denmark. In the United States there is general agreement that population-based cystic fibrosis screening efforts must be voluntary, preceded by adequate education, and anchored to the availability of competent genetic counseling.

Prenatal screening.   Prenatal genetic screening is widely practiced in the United States and Europe. In the United States it is now standard practice for physicians to inform women who will be thirty-five at the time of delivery that they are at a relatively high risk (1 in 270) for having a fetus with Down syndrome. The age of thirty-five was chosen based on studies showing that among women thirty-four and under who had amniocentesis, the risk of miscarriage after the procedure was greater than the risk of bearing a child with Down syndrome. The requirement that women be informed is not statutorially imposed; it reflects clinical consensus and court decisions.

Screening programs that measure the concentration of alpha-fetoprotein (AFP) in maternal serum (MS) to identify women at increased risk of having a child with a neural tube defect (anencephaly or spina bifida) were first used in England and Wales in the 1970s (U.K. Collaborative Study, 1977). In the United States from 1978 to 1983, the Food and Drug Administration hesitated to license the test reagents for sale in interstate commerce. Opponents of licensing argued that the test generated too many false positives, that some laboratories would perform it inaccurately, and that adequate counseling would not be available to assist women in understanding the results. For a time the American Medical Association opposed routine prenatal screening of maternal serum alpha-fetoprotein (MSAFP) (Council on Scientific Affairs, 1982). In 1983 the FDA withdrew a conservative proposal that would have sharply limited use of the reagents, setting the stage for widespread use. In 1986 California enacted a law that required physicians to inform women about the availability and purpose of MSAFP screening, but through 1993 only the District of Columbia had enacted a similar rule. About 70 percent of women in California chose to be tested (Cunningham and Kizer, 1990).

During the late 1980s in the United States, MSAFP screening grew rapidly. This was partly the result of reports on successful screening experiences, but a bulletin published by the legal department of the American College of Obstetricians and Gynecologists warning physicians of a liability risk if they did not inform their patients about the test also had a substantial impact. The rapid growth of MSAFP testing stimulated the American Society of Human Genetics to develop a policy statement on laboratory practices (American Society of Human Genetics, 1987). California controls this technology by limiting testing to six regional laboratories within the state. Elsewhere most MSAFP tests are performed by commercial laboratories operating under standard state public health and federal Clinical Laboratory Improvement Act licenses.

Clinical standards of practice evolve as physicians gain experience with new diagnostic or therapeutic methods. In contrast, medicolegal standards of care develop jurisdiction by jurisdiction as appellate courts consider arguments about whether an act or omission breached a duty owed to a patient. The duty of the physician to inform women who will be thirty-five or older at delivery of the age-associated risk of Down syndrome, and of the existence of a test to diagnose that condition in the fetus, is well established. With the exception of California, where they are statutorily required to do so, it is not yet clear whether physicians have a legal duty to inform pregnant women about MSAFP screening, but

it is likely to become established. Similarly, neither the medical literature nor court decisions suggest that there is a duty to inform women about the "triple marker" screen to detect fetuses with Down syndrome; but, given the growing use of this test, courts could decide that physicians have a duty to inform women about it.

During the late 1980s and 1990s a number of feminist scholars scrutinized prenatal screening and testing. They challenged others to reconsider whether prenatal screening confers a net social benefit, to assess its impact on persons with developmental disabilities, and to reflect on how it affects the very notion of pregnancy (Lippman, 1991). MSAFP screening, for example, has been criticized because of a high false positive test rate that generates anxiety in women who initially test positive but turn out on further testing not to be carrying an affected fetus (Press and Browner, 1993).

Laws to curb genetic discrimination

There is growing concern that genetic data acquired to assist in the resolution of a clinical problem or in the course of screening might be used in nonclinical contexts that may harm the economic or social interests of the individual or his or her relatives. The origins of this concern can be traced to the eugenics movement that flourished in the 1920s and 1930s, during which many states in the United States and some European nations enacted involuntary sterilization laws targeting institutionalized persons. U.S. immigration law from 1921 until 1968 favored entry by immigrants from northern and western Europe over eastern and southern Europe, a pattern rationalized in part by eugenic beliefs (Reilly, 1991).

During the early 1970s in the United States, some persons who participated in sickle-cell screening programs and were found to be carriers experienced employment discrimination. For a short time a few life insurance companies placed persons with sickle-cell trait outside the normal risk pool (Reilly, 1975). This led several states to enact legislation that specifically forbade the use of sickle-cell testing to determine insurability and employability.

Concerns about genetic discrimination as a consequence of screening and testing have grown among geneticists since the mid-1980s (Billings et al., 1992). The possibility that genetic data could be used to deny individuals access to health insurance has become a major topic (Task Force on Genetic Information, 1993).

In 1989 Representative John Conyers introduced the Human Genome Privacy Act. It was reintroduced in 1990 (H.R. 2045, 1991), and hearings were held in 1991, but the bill, which pertained only to the protection of genetic data derived through the use of federal funds, did not become law. Since 1991 several states have considered, and some have adopted, laws that specifically prohibit the use of genetic data in certain contexts, usually underwriting life insurance or hiring. Wisconsin prohibits employers from requiring or administering a genetic test without first obtaining the subject's prior written informed consent. California forbids insurers from charging discriminatory rates to persons solely because they carry a disease allele that may be associated with disability in their offspring. Montana forbids life insurers from refusing applicants on the basis of a "specific chromosomal or single-gene genetic condition" (McEwen and Reilly, 1992).

The enactment of the Americans with Disabilities Act (ADA) of 1990, which covers persons who can demonstrate that they have been discriminated against because they are perceived to be disabled, has raised the possibility that otherwise healthy persons who carry a gene that will eventually cause a disease or increase their risk of becoming ill may invoke the law to seek redress of employment discrimination (Gostin, 1991). The courts will ultimately decide the scope of coverage. One court has held that severe obesity, a genetically influenced condition, may qualify for protection under Section 504 of the Rehabilitation Act, which uses the same definition of disability as does the ADA.

Genetic discrimination in determining access to health insurance is a problem of significant size only in the United States and South Africa, nations that have not provided guarantees to their citizens of universal access to a basic package of health care. In the United States the problem is further exacerbated by the federal Employee Retirement Income Security Act (ERISA), which permits employers to self-insure and thereby circumvent state regulations intended to provide coverage for individuals at higher than average risk (McGann v. H & H Music Co., 1991).

Regulation of human genetic research

Accelerating efforts to find the genes that contribute to particular illnesses has led the Office for Protection from Research Risks (OPRR) of the National Institutes of Health to issue guidelines for use by local institutional review boards (IRBs) in their assessment of grant applications that would involve genetic testing of human subjects. Although they are advisory in nature, the OPRR guidelines shape the conduct of research and have substantial regulatory weight. They stress that the decision to participate in human genetic research requires an informed consent, that subjects must have access to adequate genetic counseling, and that participants must be told that should they enter and then withdraw from a study, the researcher is not required to purge existing data or destroy cell lines or DNA derived from them. The OPRR has instructed local IRBs that in gathering family histories, investigators may seek information that

is routinely available from other public sources (such as names and addresses), but may not seek nonpublic information, for example, about illnesses or adoptions, a position that could impede data gathering (Office for Protection from Research Risks, 1993).

Regulation of the introduction of new life forms into the environment

The ability to recombine DNA from widely divergent species raised the possibility that genetic engineering could create serious biohazards. In 1973 the National Academy of Sciences formed a committee to evaluate the safety of this research. The committee called for a voluntary moratorium until safety issues could be evaluated, and recommended that the National Institutes of Health (NIH) establish a committee to oversee the evaluation and develop guidelines for conducting the research. After extensive discussions at the International Conference on Recombinant DNA Molecules held in Asilomar, California, leading scientists issued a statement of principles that advocated stringent research practices until safety issues had been fully explored (Berg et al., 1975).

In 1976 the newly formed Recombinant DNA Advisory Committee (RAC) of the NIH published its first guidelines, focusing on laboratory safety and containment issues. As the evidence mounted that safety concerns were not as dangerous as had been feared, the guidelines were relaxed. The RAC guidelines have been widely replicated by other federal agencies, state and local governments, universities, the industrial community, and other nations (Committee on Scientific Evaluation of the Introduction of Genetically Modified Micro-Organisms and Plants into the Environment, 1989).

Requests to field-test microorganisms were first proposed to the RAC in the early 1980s. In 1983 the RAC approved the first such test (to determine if a genetically engineered bacteria could protect plants against frost damage). This prompted a legal challenge, arguing failure to comply with the National Environmental Protection Act (NEPA). A federal district court ruled that the RAC approval process required assessment of an environmental impact statement; an appelate court reversed the requirement of an impact statement, but upheld the injunction pending NEPA review.

During the 1980s Congress held several hearings on the environmental release of genetically engineered organisms, but it did not enact new legislation. In 1986 the Office of Science and Technology Policy (OSTP) issued the Coordinated Framework for Regulation of Biotechnology, which identified the agencies responsible for approving biotechnology products and their respective jurisdictions for regulating planned introductions (OSTP, 1986). It concluded that existing laws were sufficient to regulate release issues. In the 1980s, as experience with controlled environmental releases of genetically modified microorganisms and plants mounted, reports by the National Academy of Sciences, the Office of Technology Assessment, and the General Accounting Office concluded that there was no significant evidence that the environmental release of organisms modified by recombinant DNA constituted unique hazards (Committee on Scientific Evaluation of the Introduction of Genetically Modified Micro-Organisms and Plants into the Environment, 1989).

During the early 1990s economic and safety issues arose over requests to the FDA to license the use of recombinant bovine somatotropin (growth hormone) as a means to improve milk production by dairy cows. After a full review, the FDA licensed the hormone, which is chemically identical to the naturally occurring substance. This was the first of many genetically engineered agricultural products that will enter the marketplace. Despite the evidence that bioengineered milk poses no discernible risk, it is likely that it and other food products will be labeled, partly out of an effort to respect religious traditions concerning food purity.

DNA forensics

During the 1980s molecular biologists developed techniques to compile a unique DNA profile of every human being (except for identical twins), a technology that has fostered a revolution in forensic science (Jeffreys et al., 1985). Law enforcement officials in England first used DNA evidence to resolve violent crimes in 1986, and the techniques are now used in many nations. In the United States since 1987, DNA evidence has been widely used, usually in the prosecution of rape. In these cases DNA is extracted from semen, blood, or other tissue found at a crime scene and compared to DNA taken from a suspect. The evidence has usually been admitted after a *Frye* hearing, a proceeding by which a judge decides whether the evidence in question is based on theories and practices that have reached general acceptance in the relevant scientific community. Courts in jurisdictions that follow the more liberal Federal Rules of Evidence, which permit the judge to admit any information that is relevant and not unduly prejudicial, also admit this evidence.

The introduction of DNA forensic evidence occurred as courts in the United States followed the lead of European courts in permitting the use of human leukocyte antigen (HLA) testing to inculpate accused males in civil paternity suits. DNA-based paternity testing evidence has since been admitted in many states (Committee on DNA Technology in Forensic Science, 1992).

In 1989 controversy erupted over a number of aspects of how DNA evidence was generated. The core

problem has been to determine the likelihood that a crime scene sample could match that taken from a randomly selected individual—in essence, the chance of erroneously convicting the wrong suspect. The debate over this question turns on statistical arguments over whether DNA markers are inherited independently through the generations and uncertainty as to their distribution in different ethnic groups. After reviewing objections from expert witnesses, several courts have refused to permit the use of DNA evidence (e.g., *Commonwealth v. Curnin,* 1991), but most are convinced of its utility.

In 1992 a committee of the National Academy of Sciences recommended that the independence of the DNA markers should not be assumed. The committee suggested that until the statistical argument was resolved, experts testifying in court should limit themselves to stating whether or not a DNA profile of tissue found at the crime scene that matched the profile of the suspect was or was not present in a randomly selected data base of DNA samples. If it was not, then the expert could state, for example, that among a population of 300 randomly selected white males not one had a DNA profile like that of the suspect (Committee on DNA Technology in Forensic Science, 1992). The committee's recommendation has been criticized for being overly cautious.

In 1993 the U.S. Supreme Court, considering the question of standards of admissibility of scientific evidence for the first time, held that the *Frye* standard was too restrictive, and that the judge, applying the Federal Rules of Evidence, must decide whether the evidence offered was based on a sufficiently solid scientific basis (*Daubert v. Merrill Dow Pharmaceuticals, Inc.,* 1993). This decision may ease the debate over the admissibility of DNA-based forensic evidence. Scientific consensus over the proper statistical approach in using DNA evidence to make statements about identity will eventually be achieved. DNA evidence will continue to be widely used, for it constitutes a powerful means to exonerate wrongfully suspected individuals and to support the prosecution of perpetrators.

DNA banks

By 1993 eighteen states had enacted laws that require convicted felons (typically, those convicted of sexual offenses) to provide a tissue sample prior to parole. DNA extracted from these samples is being used to create a reference base with which to compare biological samples taken from rape victims or from crime scenes. Because of the high rate of recidivism among sexual offenders, the possibility that a crime scene sample will be found to match a sample in a state data base is reasonably high, especially since investigators will be able to query all state data bases through a system organized by the Federal Bureau of Investigation. In 1993 murders in Minnesota and Virginia were solved by comparing crime scene samples to DNA profiles located in data bases compiled on felons before parole. DNA data bases composed of samples from unidentified bodies and of samples from unknown persons found at crime scenes are also being established. In the former case comparison of the banked DNA and DNA from relatives of a missing person may conclusively identify the remains; in the latter case sample comparisons may indicate whether a series of rapes are the work of one or several criminals (McEwen and Reilly, 1994).

A federal appellate court has held that taking DNA samples from convicted felons prior to parole does not violate the Fourth Amendment prohibition against unreasonable searches (*Jones* v. *Murray*, 1992). Further constitutional challenges are likely to argue that DNA data-banking laws should not require tissue samples from convicted felons who have no history of crimes against the person.

The collection and storage of DNA samples from large populations, possibly even entire populations, is likely to occur routinely in coming years. The two rationales for such an undertaking are to create a DNA data base for identification purposes and to promote the scientific study and clinical use of genetic information, particularly in regard to preventing the onset of genetically influenced diseases. The U.S. military collects tissue samples on new recruits. Researchers in many nations have established small DNA banks in the course of searching for disease genes. As of the mid-1990s, this conduct was unregulated, but concern for the interests of the individuals whose samples are stored suggests that it is likely that the state will eventually regulate academically based and commercial DNA storage facilities (Annas, 1993).

Gene therapy

In the United States, experiments in which recombinant DNA is introduced into cells of a human subject with the intent of modifying a gene are regulated by the NIH Guidelines for Research Involving Recombinant DNA molecules (National Institutes of Health, 1984), and its subsequent amendments. In Canada the Medical Research Council Standing Committee on Ethics in Experimentation has taken a similar approach, one that requires both local and national review.

Research to treat disease by the reintroduction of genetically modified cells or the use of DNA sequences as drugs, "somatic-cell therapy," has been fully reviewed by several national commissions (U.S. President's Commission, 1982b), and Congress has held hearings about it. The civic, religious, scientific, and medical groups that have studied the topic have concluded that this therapy does not present unique ethical problems (Office of Technology Assessment, 1984). Commentators in Canada and the European Medical Research Councils have also concluded that the therapy is not fundamentally different from other medical therapies ("Gene Therapy," 1988).

Unlike somatic-cell therapy, in which the impact of the intervention is limited to an individual patient, germ-line therapy—the manipulation of the genome in cells that are the progenitors of egg or sperm cells—affects the patient's descendants. This fact, coupled with the concern that genetic engineering may someday permit germ-line enhancement—the introduction of DNA sequences intended to increase the likelihood of having a child with desired traits rather than to avert disease—has provoked much concern. Religious and civic groups have urged a ban on such germ-line manipulations, and the RAC has stated that it would not approve proposals to do research intended to further this goal in humans. The Parliamentary Assembly of the Council of Europe has recommended that the Committee of Ministers provide in the European Convention on Human Rights an explicit recognition of the right to a genetic inheritance that has not been artificially interfered with, unless it is in accord with principles that are compatible with respect for other human rights, language that would permit interventions to prevent disease (Knoppers, 1991).

The individual human genome and the collective human gene pool deserve special protection. We have entered an era in which relatives, insurers, employers, school systems, and the state may be able to acquire ever more genetic information about individuals. We must ensure that genetic testing confers benefits rather than causing injuries. The means to accomplish this will almost certainly be legislation that reasonably subordinates the interests of third parties in the data to the individual's right to privacy. We also possess the power, through massive environmental pollution, to threaten our gene pool and those of other species. We must act as responsible caretakers, a duty that demands a global vision.

PHILIP R. REILLY

Directly related to this entry are the entries CONFIDENTIALITY; DNA TYPING; INFORMATION DISCLOSURE; *and* PRIVACY IN HEALTH CARE. *For a further discussion of topics mentioned in this entry, see the entries* EUGENICS; GENETIC COUNSELING; GENETIC ENGINEERING; GENETICS AND ENVIRONMENT IN HUMAN HEALTH; GENETIC TESTING AND SCREENING; INFORMED CONSENT; *and* MEDICAL GENETICS. *For a discussion of related ideas, see the entries* ABORTION, *section on* CONTEMPORARY ETHICAL AND LEGAL ASPECTS, *article on* LEGAL AND REGU-

LATORY ISSUES; GENETICS AND RACIAL MINORITIES; GENOME MAPPING AND SEQUENCING; HEALTH SCREENING AND TESTING IN THE PUBLIC-HEALTH CONTEXT; PROFESSIONAL–PATIENT RELATIONSHIP; *and* RACE AND RACISM. *See also the entries* FUTURE GENERATIONS, OBLIGATIONS TO; *and* RISK.

Bibliography

AMERICAN SOCIETY OF HUMAN GENETICS. 1987. "Policy Statement for Maternal Serum Alpha-Fetoprotein Screening Programs and Quality Control for Laboratories Performing Maternal Serum and Amniotic Fluid Alpha-Fetoprotein Assays." *American Journal of Human Genetics* 40, no. 2:75–82.

ANDREWS, LORI B. 1987. *Medical Genetics: A Legal Frontier.* Chicago: American Bar Foundation.

ANNAS, GEORGE J. 1993. "Privacy Rules for DNA Databanks: Protecting Coded 'Future Diaries.'" *Journal of the American Medical Association* 270, no. 19:2346–2350.

Becker v. Schwartz. 1978. 46 N.Y.2d 401, 386 N.E.2d 807, 413 N.Y.S.2d 895.

BERG, PAUL; BALTIMORE, DAVID S.; BRENNER, SIDNEY; ROBLIN, RICHARD O.; and SINGER, MAXINE F. 1975. "Summary Statement of the Asilomar Conference on Recombinant DNA Molecules." *Proceedings of the National Academy of Sciences U.S.A.* 72, no. 6:1981–1984.

BILLINGS, PAUL R.; KOHN, MEL A.; DE CUEVAS, MARGARET; BECKWITH, JONATHAN; ALPER, JOSEPH S.; and NATOWICZ, MARVIN R. 1992. "Discrimination as a Consequence of Genetic Testing." *American Journal of Human Genetics* 50, no. 3:476–482.

Canterbury v. Spence. 1972. 464 F.2d 772, 150 U.S. App.D.C. 263 (D.C. Circuit).

CAO, ANTONIO. 1991. "Antenatal Diagnosis of B-Thalassemia in Sardinia." In *Genetics, Ethics and Human Values: Human Genome Mapping, Genetic Screening and Gene Therapy* (Proceedings of the 24th CIOMS Round Table Conference), pp. 72–79. Edited by Z. Bankowski and Alexander M. Capron. Geneva: CIOMS.

CAPRON, ALEXANDER M. 1979. "Tort Liability and Genetic Counseling." *Columbia Law Review* 79, no. 4:618–684.

COMMITTEE ON ASSESSING GENETIC RISKS, INSTITUTE OF MEDICINE. 1994. *Assessing Genetic Risks: Implications for Health and Social Policy.* Washington, D.C.: National Academy Press.

COMMITTEE ON DNA TECHNOLOGY IN FORENSIC SCIENCE, NATIONAL RESEARCH COUNCIL. 1992. *DNA Technology in Forensic Science,* p. 27. Washington, D.C.: National Academy Press.

COMMITTEE ON SCIENTIFIC EVALUATION OF THE INTRODUCTION OF GENETICALLY MODIFIED MICRO-ORGANISMS AND PLANTS INTO THE ENVIRONMENT, NATIONAL RESEARCH COUNCIL. 1989. *Field Testing Genetically Modified Organisms: Framework for Decisions.* Washington, D.C.: National Academy Press.

COMMITTEE FOR THE STUDY OF INBORN ERRORS OF METABOLISM, NATIONAL RESEARCH COUNCIL. 1975. *Genetic Screening: Programs, Principles, and Research.* Washington, D.C.: National Academy of Sciences.

Commonwealth v. Curnin. 1991. 409 Mass. 218, 565 N.E. 2d 440.

COUNCIL ON SCIENTIFIC AFFAIRS, AMERICAN MEDICAL ASSOCIATION. 1982. "Maternal Serum Alpha-Fetoprotein Monitoring." *Journal of the American Medical Association* 247, no. 10:1478–1481.

CUNNINGHAM, GEORGE C., and KIZER, KENNETH W. 1990. "Maternal Serum Alpha-Fetoprotein Screening Activities of State Health Agencies: A Survey." *American Journal of Human Genetics* 47, no. 6:899–903.

Daubert v. Merrill Dow Pharmaceuticals, Inc. 1993. 125 L.Ed. 2d 469, 113 S. Ct. 2786.

"Gene Therapy in Man: Recommendations of the European Research Councils." 1988. *Lancet* 2, no. 8597:1271–1272.

GOSTIN, LARRY. 1991. "Genetic Discrimination: The Use of Genetically Based Diagnostic and Prognostic Tests by Employers and Insurers." *American Journal of Law and Medicine* 17:109–144.

Human Genome Privacy Act. 1991. H.R. 2045, 102d Cong., 1st sess., April 24.

JEFFREYS, ALEC J.; WILSON, VICTORIA; and THIEN, SAMUEL L. 1985. "Individual-Specific 'Fingerprints' of Human DNA." *Nature* 316, no. 6023:75–79.

Jones v. Murray. 1992. 962 F2d 302 (4th Cir.).

KNOPPERS, BARTHA M. 1991. *Human Dignity and Genetic Heritage: Study Paper Prepared for the Law Reform Commission of Canada.* Ottawa: Law Reform Commission of Canada.

KNOPPERS, BARTHA M., and LE BRIS, SONYA. 1993. "Ethical and Legal Concerns: Reproductive Technologies 1990–1993." *Current Opinion in Obstetrics and Gynecology* 5, no. 5:630–635.

LIPPMAN, ABBY. 1991. "Prenatal Genetic Testing and Screening: Constructing Needs and Reinforcing Inequities." *American Journal of Law and Medicine* 17, nos. 1–2: 15–50.

McEWEN, JEAN E., and REILLY, PHILIP R. 1992. "State Legislative Efforts to Regulate Use and Potential Misuse of Genetic Information." *American Journal of Human Genetics* 51, no. 3:637–647.

———. 1994. "A Review of State Legislation on DNA Forensic Data-Banking." *American Journal of Human Genetics* 54, no. 6:941–958.

McGann v. H & H Music Co. 1991. 946 F2d. 401 (5th Circ.).

Natanson v. Kline. 1960. 186 Kan. 393, 350 P.2d 1093; 187 Kan. 186, 354 P.2d 670.

NATIONAL INSTITUTES OF HEALTH. 1984. "Guidelines for Research Involving Recombinant DNA Molecules." *Federal Register* 49, no. 227:46266–46291.

———. OFFICE FOR PROTECTION FROM RESEARCH RISKS. 1993. *Protecting Human Research Subjects: Institutional Review Board Guidebook.* Washington, D.C.: U.S. Government Printing Office.

PRESS, NANCY A., and BROWNER, C. H. 1993. "Collective Fictions: Similarities in Reasons for Accepting Maternal Serum Alpha-Fetoprotein Screening Among Women of Diverse Ethnic and Social Class Backgrounds." *Fetal Diagnosis and Therapy* 8, suppl. 1:97–106.

REILLY, PHILIP R. 1975. "Genetic Screening Legislation." In *Advances in Human Genetics V*, pp. 319–376. Edited by Harry H. Harris and Kurt Hirschhorn. New York: Plenum Press.

———. 1991. *The Surgical Solution: A History of Involuntary Sterilization in the United States.* Baltimore: Johns Hopkins University.

Roe v. Wade. 1973. 410 U.S. 113.

Rust v. Sullivan. 1991. 111 S. Ct. 759.

Salgo v. Leland Stanford, Jr. Univ. Bd. of Trustees. 1957. 154 Cal. App. 2d 560, 317 P. 2d 170.

TAKAGI, K. 1991. "Genetic Screening-Policymaking Aspects." In *Genetics, Ethics, and Human Values* (Proceedings of the 24th CIOMS Conference), pp. 117–131. Edited by Z. Bankowski and Alexander M. Capron. Geneva: CIOMS.

TASK FORCE ON GENETIC INFORMATION AND INSURANCE, NATIONAL INSTITUTES OF HEALTH–DEPARTMENT OF ENERGY WORKING GROUP ON ETHICAL, LEGAL, AND SOCIAL IMPLICATIONS OF HUMAN GENOME RESEARCH. 1993. "Genetic Information and Health Insurance." Bethesda, Md.: U.S. National Center for Human Genome Research.

U.K. COLLABORATIVE STUDY ON ALPHA-FETOPROTEIN IN RELATION TO NEURAL-TUBE DEFECTS. 1977. "Maternal Serum-Alpha-Fetoprotein Measurement in Antenatal Screening for Anencephaly and Spina Bifida in Early Pregnancy." *Lancet* 1, no. 8026:1323–1332.

U.S. OFFICE OF SCIENCE AND TECHNOLOGY POLICY. 1986. "Coordinated Framework for Regulation of Biotechnology: Announcement of Policy; Notice for Public Comment." *Federal Register* 51, no. 23:23302–23350.

U.S. OFFICE OF TECHNOLOGY ASSESSMENT. 1984. *Human Gene Therapy: Background Paper.* Washington, D.C.: Author.

U.S. PRESIDENT'S COMMISSION FOR THE STUDY OF ETHICAL PROBLEMS IN MEDICINE AND BIOMEDICAL AND BEHAVIORAL RESEARCH. 1982a. *Making Health Care Decisions: The Ethical and Legal Implications of Informed Consent in the Patient-Practitioner Relationship.* Washington, D.C.: Author.

——— 1982b. *Splicing Life: A Report on the Social and Ethical Issues of Genetic Engineering with Human Beings.* Washington, D.C.: Author.

———. 1983. *Screening and Counseling for Genetic Conditions: A Report on the Ethical, Social and Legal Implications of Genetic Screening, Counseling and Education Programs.* Washington, D.C.: U.S. Government Printing Office.

GENETICS AND RACIAL MINORITIES

People are not born equal, nor do they live or die equal. Religion, race, class, and nationality have been a perennial source of stigmatization and discrimination. Racial minorities (herein abbreviated "minorities") are particularly at risk. In this entry, minorities are categorized as subset populations of a state that have relatively little power and are discriminated against. Hence, the white minority population of South Africa is not a minority, even though numerically they are a minority. Examples of minorities include the Ainu and Koreans of Japan, Australian Aborigines, the Palestinians in Israel, the Catholics in Northern Ireland, Africans and Algerians in France, Africans and their descendants and Asian Indians in Great Britain; and, in the United States, African-Americans, Hispanics, peoples of Asian-Pacific Islander and American Indian-Alaskan Native origin, and the poor.

Jews in the United States are not included here as a racial minority because Jews are not a race. Judaism is a religion and includes such disparate peoples as the Falasha of Ethiopia and Yemenites and Jews of Iraq, Iran, and China. Reference, however, will be made to Tay-Sachs disease screening in Jews in the United States for the purpose of comparison.

Distribution of genetic diseases among minority and nonminority groups

Diabetes is divided into insulin-dependent diabetes mellitus (IDDM) or Type I, and non–insulin-dependent diabetes mellitus (NIDDM) or Type II (Bowman and Murray, 1990). Type I diabetes is uncommon in tropical regions, and accordingly is less common in Africans than in African-Americans, but the prevalence of Type I diabetes is higher in European Americans than in African Americans. The reverse is true with Type II diabetes, which has a higher frequency in African Americans than European Americans.

Certain Asian, Pacific, and Amerindian populations are at increased risk of Type II diabetes. The Pima Indians of the United States have one of the highest world frequencies (35 percent of the adult population) (Polednak, 1989). As one would expect, Type II diabetes is higher in Mexican Americans (because of their Amerindian component) than in Anglo-Americans. Unfortunately, in Mexican Americans the incidence of diabetes-related end-stage renal disease is greater than that predicted from their excess of Type II diabetes. The disease also has an earlier age of onset, greater severity, and poorer control of diabetes than that of other groups (Polednak, 1989). Unfortunately, the higher morbidity and mortality of diabetes in the Mexican American group could also be a reflection of inadequate medical care. The ethical consequences of the market health care system and poverty in the United States are once more quite evident.

Let us now look at screening and prenatal programs for hemoglobins in Canada, Italy, and Cuba. A population survey in Vietnam is also mentioned because many

Vietnamese populations form minority communities in the United States.

H. Granda and colleagues (1991) conducted an extensive nationwide sickle hemoglobin screening program in Cuba, which involved education, couples at risk counseling, and prenatal diagnosis. Blood was obtained from mothers when they attended for prenatal care. If the mother was positive for sickle hemoglobin, couples were given an appointment at a genetics center, where fathers were tested and counseled. The counseling was nondirective and decisions were made by the couples. The author indicated that about one hundred children with sickle-cell disease (HbSS or HbSC) are expected to be born yearly in Cuba. In 1989 this number was reduced by about 30 percent. "Ninety-eight affected fetuses were found. In seventy-two cases the pregnancy was terminated" (p. 153).

James Bowman and colleagues (1971) studied red cell enzyme variation and hemoglobins in populations of Vietnam. The prevalence of glucose phosphate dehydrogenase deficiency was lowest in the Sedang, the Vietnamese, and the Rhade. The highest prevalence of glucose-6-phosphate dehydrogenase deficiency was in the Stieng (0.153). The lowest frequencies of hemoglobin E were in the Vietnamese and the Sedang, and the highest in the Stieng (0.365). Unfortunately, it was not possible to test for alpha thalassemia or beta thalassemia, hereditary markers that are known to be in high frequency in these populations. These studies point to the difficulty of screening for hemoglobins and thalassemias in the United States in these populations. Ethnic groups and language must be identified and appropriate educational and counseling material and counselors with a variety of languages must be required for first generation peoples from Vietnam.

Charles Scriver and colleagues (1984) described a beta-thalassemia disease prevention program in communities in Quebec at highest risk. The populations were of Greek, Italian, Asian, and Oriental, and French Canadian descent. A total of 6,748 persons were screened from December 1979 to December 1982 using MCV/Hb A$_2$ indices. This group included 5,117 senior high school students with a participation rate of 80 percent. (In Canada, parental permission is not needed for screening of students.) The prevalence of beta-thalassemia carriers was 4.7 percent, with a tenfold variation among the various ethnic groups. A total of 60 carriers and 120 unaffected individuals were surveyed. Eleven fetal diagnoses were performed during the study period, either by fetoscopy and globin chain analysis or by amniocentesis and DNA analysis. There was one spontaneous abortion following fetoscopy and seven live births. The economic cost of the program (cost per case prevented) was $6,700, which was slightly less than the average cost of treatment of one patient in one year. A preprogram survey showed that even though 88 percent of those ascertained favored a program, only 31 percent considered fetal diagnosis an acceptable option. Nevertheless, when faced with the actual decision, *all of the couples at risk* took the option of fetal diagnosis.

These figures resemble those found by Rowley and colleagues (1991) for Southeast Asians in the United States, but are unlike those for blacks in a prenatal diagnosis program, all of whom stated that they could not terminate a pregnancy for any reason. Other important facts emerged. The couples who were at risk claimed that they would not have considered pregnancy without the availability of fetal diagnosis. Only one couple with an affected fetus refused abortion. The authors concluded that their findings indicated acceptance of the program, relative absence of stigmatization of carriers, acceptance of the efficacy of fetal diagnosis, and cost-effectiveness.

Extensive surveys for abnormal hemoglobins and thalassemias have been reported in Italy (Tentori and Marinucci, 1983). This analysis will concentrate, however, on the outcome of a screening program for the prospective prevention of thalassemia in the province of Latium, Italy. The average frequency of heterozygous alpha- or beta-thalassemia was 2.4 percent. This figure was ascertained from a study of 289,763 students. In a region of 17,000 km^2, a single center was able to examine about 50,000 students per year, which is about 80 percent of all intermediate school children. In this region, couples at risk of childbearing age since 1980 were analyzed. Some of these couples (51 out of 161) had already had an affected child and came to the center during or before a new pregnancy, but the majority (110 out of 161) had no affected children and came for counseling before conception as a consequence of the school screening program. Of the 94 prospective couples, 35 were former students identified in the school screening program or through one of their close relatives. From January 1980 to April 1983, 37 of the 110 prospective couples became pregnant and 6 of 31 monitored pregnancies had a homozygous fetus that was aborted. Further evidence was given to show that the population approved of the screening program and at-risk couples accepted prenatal diagnosis and abortion.

At this point some comparisons may be made from the international experience. Evidently, in the most Catholic of countries, Italy, prenatal diagnosis for thalassemia was accepted to such an extent that if generalizations can be made from this study, the disease may be expected to almost disappear in the next generation. The acceptance of prenatal diagnosis is also high in Canada among populations at risk for thalassemia. It would appear that at present, the black minority population in the United States is most reluctant to accept prenatal diagnosis and abortion. The reasons have not been documented. Education, religion, suspicion of the health-care system are all conjecture, and not supported by other statistics. The U.S. National Center for Health Statistics in 1990 recorded that in the white population there were 17.5 abortions in 1973 and 30.0 abortions in 1987 per 1,000 live births. Blacks were classified in the "all other" group and undoubtedly consisted of the majority. In this population there were, per 1,000 live births, 28.9 abortions in 1973 and 55.7 in 1987. The figures that show black women aborting fetuses at a higher rate than white women are inconsistent with those that show black women declining to abort fetuses with sickle-cell disease. This suggests a need for further study.

Eugenics

A major scientific and pseudoscientific weapon for discrimination against minorities has been eugenics, a political, economic, and social policy that espouses the reproduction of the "fit" over the "unfit" (positive eugenics) and discourages the birth of the "unfit" (negative eugenics) (Haller, 1963; Ludmerer, 1972). Sir Francis Galton (1871) introduced the word *eugenics* in nineteenth-century Great Britain. He documented the concentration of genius and high achievement in his family and in families of his peers, and disparaged the intellectual abilities of the "masses," and even the peoples of nations such as Spain and France.

The "fit" and "unfit" have been variously defined. The earlier eugenics movement in the United States targeted as "unfit" individuals with epilepsy, criminals, crippled and deformed peoples; persons who were mentally defective, or who had low intelligence; patients with communicable diseases such as syphilis, tuberculosis, or leprosy; alcoholics and drug abusers; poor people; and Eastern European immigrants to the United States. The Nazis marked Jews, Gypsies, and other so-called non-Aryan peoples as individuals who were incurably mentally defective. In the heyday of eugenics, sterilization, infanticide, euthanasia, or a variety of "final solutions" were tools for the prevention or elimination of the "unfit" (Haller, 1963; Ludmerer, 1972).

But who are the "unfit" today, and how are they dealt with? Today, scientific advances in prenatal diagnosis—with the option for abortion—have broadened the "unfit" base to identify early in pregnancy fetuses with hereditary disorders such as Tay-Sachs disease, neural tube defects, Down syndrome, sickle-cell anemia, and cystic fibrosis. These fetuses are placed in the unfit category because abortion is offered as an option in genetic counseling. If they were not "unfit," abortion would not be offered. There also have been repeated attempts to link genetics with abusers of alcohol or drugs and with perpetrators of violent crime since the beginning of the eugenics movement in the United States.

However, "white collar" criminal activities such as embezzlement, insider trading in the stock market, and the savings and loan associations' siphoning of hundreds of millions of dollars from their members have not been objects of study, which suggests that classism, or racism, or both are contributory factors to the linking of genes with crime. Neil Holtzman and Mark Rothstein (1992) perceptively alluded to an example of the selectivity of eugenicists. They quoted Lancelot Hogben's (1938) reference to hemophilia in the royal families of Europe: "No eugenicist has publicly proposed sterilization as a remedy for defective kingship" (p. 457).

Consequently, eugenics is invariably directed to those minorities who have relatively little power, without regard to race, ethnic group, or religion. This entry does not classify most middle- and upper-class African-Americans as minorities because pressures on health-care resources place the poor in all populations at risk for genetic discrimination.

There also operates what could be called "passive eugenics." Passive eugenics is the societal acceptance of infant and maternal mortality rates in the United States that exceed those of any industrialized country. Passive eugenics is an inequitable system of health care. A recurring shibboleth, "health-care resources are scarce," is incomplete. Health-care resources are scarce only for the poor. A society that passively accepts deaths by preventable social and economic inequities will also tolerate the discouragement of the birth of children with "preventable" genetic disorders.

Mandatory sterilization

To compound the problem, at least thirteen states (Reilly, 1991) still have mandatory sterilization laws on their books, all under the aegis of the police power of the State, and affirmed by the landmark Supreme Court decision of *Buck* v. *Bell* (1927), which legalized mandatory sterilization for eugenic reasons. Carrie Buck was alleged to be the feebleminded mother of a feebleminded child. She was a ward of the State Colony of Virginia for Epileptics and the Feeble-Minded. Carrie Buck's mother was also confined to the same institution and was said to be feebleminded. James E. Coogan (1953) disputed the diagnoses of both Carrie Buck and her daughter. J. H. Bell was the superintendent of the State Colony and had been looking for a test case in order to prevent the birth of mentally deficient children by mandatory sterilization. Even though Carrie Buck's attorney was appointed by those who wanted Carrie Buck sterilized, he eloquently warned, in part, "A reign of doctors will be inaugurated and in the name of science new classes will be added, even races may be brought within the scope of such regulation, and the worst form of tyranny practiced" (Reilly, 1991, p. 87). While Carrie Buck's attorney was predicting the dangers of compulsory sterilization, Hitler and his colleagues were laying the groundwork for National Socialism with the earlier eugenics movement in the United States as a model (Ludmerer, 1972). In their rush to judgment, it is likely that those who were intent on sterilizing Carrie Buck were also guided by prejudice against the poor. Dr. Harry Laughlin's "expert" testimony in Virginia against Carrie Buck substantiates this premise. Laughlin asserted, "These people belong to the shiftless, ignorant, and worthless class of anti-social whites of the South" (Coogan, 1953, p. 45). The most powerful condemnation of eugenics is revealed in Laughlin's statement. The poor are also selectively affected by passive eugenics. Consequently, the "slippery slope" from passive to active eugenics may be an inexorable continuum.

The police power of the state

The police power of the state is based on utilitarian ethics in that the Supreme Court in *Munn* v. *Illinois* (1877) supported a fundamental precept of both democratic and totalitarian societies: The private interests of the individual must be subservient to the public interest. The threat of eugenics today lies not in blatant criminal behavior like that associated with Nazi Germany but in subtle social and political precepts. In fact, some of the court decisions that may lead to eugenics are even based on liberal ethical views of autonomy, and the right to privacy as found in *Roe* v. *Wade* (1973). Discrimination is cryptic, however, even in the field of ethics, which like economics, provides principles for the allocation of "scarce resources." The canon of "scarce resources," like so-called just wars, is repeated by countless philosophers, but both doctrines have killed millions of innocent people through the centuries. In this discussion of the relationship of ethics to eugenics, it is important to remember a major thesis of this presentation: All propositions that have been used to foster eugenics were not necessarily developed with eugenic intent.

Immanuel Kant

Eugenics is incompatible with Immanuel Kant's dictum that one should treat humanity always as an end and never as a means (Kant, 1964). He maintained that the supreme principle of morality cannot be obtained by studying generalizations from examples derived from experience. Examples cannot replace moral principles and they cannot be a foundation on which moral principles are derived.

Utilitarianism

If minorities accept utilitarianism as a philosophy, it subjects them to "the greatest good for the greatest number." But here is the dilemma: To reject this concept would be to negate marriage laws, compulsory vaccination for communicable diseases, seat belt laws, and most public health measures.

John Rawls and "a theory of justice"

"People are poor because they have defective genes" is a recurring catch phrase. John Rawls (1978) is particularly concerned about the disadvantaged members of society and has developed an important theory of justice in an attempt to resolve some of the major objections to utilitarianism. In so doing he examined a social contract mechanism, which in a way was an outgrowth of previous social contracts outlined by John Locke (1632–1704), Jean-Jacques Rousseau, and Kant. Rawls argued that justice denies that the loss of freedom for some is compensated by a greater good shared by others. A just society not only is designed to foster the good of its members but also is regulated by a public impression of justice.

The heart of Rawls's theory is that the participants must begin under a veil of ignorance. If one were to know in advance one's position in society, it would be the unusual person who would choose a position that jeopardizes his or her self-interest. Rawls provides examples: "[I]f a man knew he was wealthy, he might find it rational to advance the principle that various taxes for welfare measures be counted unjust; if he knew that he was poor, he would most likely propose the contrary principle. "To represent the desired restrictions one imagines a situation in which everyone is deprived of this sort of information" (pp. 18–19). Since utilitarianism espouses the sacrifice of some persons in order to promote the happiness of others, or the majority, Rawls's precepts are patently in opposition to utilitarianism and to eugenic proscriptions against minorities.

Situation ethics

Joseph Fletcher (1979) fostered situation ethics as more useful in resolving moral dilemmas. He postulated that moral judgments are made by following one of two choices: rule ethics or situation ethics. Rule ethics involves what one ought to do. A priori examples are various divine command philosophies or deontological ethics as espoused by Kant. In situation ethics, the agent is central. It is up to the individual to judge what is best under the circumstances and make a decision. This is the a posteriori approach—collect the facts; examine the circumstances; look at the individual, the family, the economic circumstances, society and any other factors that may bear on the situation. One seeks, as in utilitarianism, the greatest good for the greatest number. A correct decision in one situation may be nonsensical in another. As Fletcher pointed out, physicians are probably more comfortable with situation ethics, for its precepts are what the clinician subscribes to in daily practice. Most physicians do not judge what is best for their patients according to Kant's "categorical imperative."

With the advent of new technology, considerable attention is directed to the question: "What is a person?" Fletcher believed that in order for one to qualify as human, or a person, the following criterion should be taken into account: minimum intelligence (an IQ of less than 40 places the individual in the questionable category; an IQ of less than 20 indicates that the individual is not a person). To quote an aphorism from Fletcher, "*Homo* is indeed *sapiens,* in order to be *Homo* (Fletcher, 1979, p. 12). A person is judged by the following attributes: self-awareness; self-control; a sense of time; a sense of futurity; a sense of the past; the capability to relate to others; concern for others; communication; control of existence; curiosity; change and changeability; balance of rationality and feeling; idiosyncrasy; being idiomorphous, a distinctive individual; neocortical function (pp. 12–16). It follows that if an individual is not a person he or she is "unfit" and a eugenic target.

Albert Blumenthal

Albert Blumenthal (1977) exceeded the fondest hopes of the eugenics movement in the United States in the 1920s:

> There are no intrinsic moral rights, hence people do not have an inherent moral right to reproduce. The unborn child has a moral right not to be born to parents who have serious genetic deficiencies or who are likely to be unable or unwilling to care for him so that he can develop into a good citizen. Other people have moral rights not to be burdened by obligations to care for the children which improvident, neglectful and incompetent parents produce and by the deficient adults which these children so often become. (pp. 203–204)

Blumenthal felt that all prospective parents should be licensed according to their parental fitness: some "to reproduce but not to rear children, others to rear but not to reproduce and still others both to beget and rear children." Parents licensed for all functions should be free of serious genetic defects and dysfunctional habits, should love children, should be knowledgeable about nutrition, child psychology, and education, and should be able to provide sufficient economic support. The state would determine a couple's permissible number of children.

Critical theory

Critical theory, critical legal theory, and critical social science (Unger, 1986; Kairys, 1982) have meaningful implications for minorities but for some reason are not alluded to in publications on ethical issues in genetics. Humans are dominated and oppressed because they un-

critically accept social roles allotted to them. Established power and organizations shape people's lives because they are accepted as given, beginning in the elementary schools and continuing throughout formal education. Critical theory forces an analysis of the sources of power. But even this may be impossible. People are confronted with repeated dilemmas brought about by a latticework of interrelated events and objects over which they have no control. Critical science questions that an increase in human power over nature will produce human betterment or progress. A major tenet is that power is differentially distributed and frequently used by those who possess it to oppress those who are powerless. Consequently, an increase in scientific knowledge may not rebound to the welfare of the less powerful in a society. Indeed, it may be used to dominate them. In addition to branches of the state and federal governments, the Church, universities, medical centers, scientific, social, economic, political, and philosophical organizations, the Institute of Medicine, the American Medical Association, the American Hospital Association, and many other self-appointed authorities are often major sources of power—and more often, the oppressors.

David Kairys (1982) disagreed with the ideal model that a particular legal mode of reasoning or analysis characterizes the legal process. Kairys further related that the economic decisions that shape our society and affect our lives on the most basic of social issues are not made democratically, or even by our elected government officials. The law is not neutral, value free, or independent of and unaffected by social and economic relations, political forces, and cultural phenomena. The law enforces and legitimizes dominant social and power relations without a need for or the appearance of control from outside and by individuals who *believe in their own neutrality* (a most dangerous situation for the powerless) and the myth of legal reasoning. It is most difficult to counter individuals who do not know that they are harmful. Furthermore, in the United States at least, the law is a highly respected force for the perpetuation of existing power. Accordingly, the law confers a legitimacy on a social system and ideology that is dominated by a corporate elite that cloaks itself under the mantle of science, with an occasional reference to God.

Public policy

What is public policy? From early childhood we are taught that the "people" decide in a democracy. A contradictory view is that public policy is merely what those who have power decide. Even morality has been placed in this category. Variations of this theme are ancient and recur throughout history. In Book I of Plato's *Republic,* the Sophist, Thrasymachus, maintained that laws serve only to protect the interest of those in power. A Marxist view (Lavine, 1984) is that morality is contrived and dictated by the ruling elite to control the masses: All morality is class morality. Scholars of the Critical Legal Issues Movement (Unger, 1986) profess that the law is not neutral, but is guided and dictated by political considerations. Accordingly, some expressions like common values and public policy—though sacrosanct to some—have disparate interpretations. Needless to say, this view of the law and public policy has ominous implications for those who believe that eugenics is dead. It should also be a reminder to geneticists that they may be only minor players in the determination of public policy.

The police power of the state

Eugenic precepts in the United States are embedded in constitutional rights. The landmark Supreme Court decision of *Munn* v. *Illinois* (1877) established that the private interests of the individual must be subservient to the public interest, and formed the basis for the constitutionality of such diverse edicts as mandatory vaccination, and seat belt and sterilization laws. In short, whatever the state deems critical for the public good is supported by the umbrella of the police power of the state, provided, of course, that the law does not negate the Constitution. Paradoxically, the doctrine that the private interests of the individual must be subservient to the public interest is similar in both totalitarianism and democracy. Consequently, eugenics may prosper under disparate systems of government.

The police power of the state also invades marriage and the family. Family definitions and marriage restrictions open the door to eugenics because many of the prohibitions against marriage—particularly those against consanguineous mating—are far less defensible, genetically, than the mating of carriers with identical traits for genetic disorders. The banning of consanguineous mating facilitates the interdiction of mating of carriers for sickle-cell disease, Tay-Sachs disease, cystic fibrosis, and eventually the mating of carriers of several thousand genetic disorders, once the techniques for early diagnosis in utero are developed.

The expanding field of prenatal diagnosis could not have been developed without the landmark Supreme Court decision of *Roe* v. *Wade* (1973), which established the right of a woman to have an abortion—under certain conditions. This decision was preceded by *Griswold* v. *Connecticut* (1965), which established the right *not* to procreate. Although abortion is legal, the Supreme Court decisions of *Maher* v. *Roe* (1977) and *Harris* v. *McRae* (1980) and the Congressional legislation known as the Hyde Amendment affirmed that even if abortion is legal—under certain conditions—the state has no obligation to pay for it.

Health-care inequity

As noted earlier, laws and practices with eugenic implications are often designed for other purposes. For instance, universal health care may operate to discourage the birth of children with genetic defects, because of their perceived burden on public funds. Limits to state support of children born of mothers who are on welfare is a policy that has eugenic implications for poor mothers who repeatedly bear children with "preventable" genetic disorders. Scientific advances in genetics create a fertile ground for eugenics, because inequities in the delivery and costs of health care have led to plans for additional rationing of health care under the rubric of broadening the base of the U.S. market health-care system to include those 37 million Americans who are merely bystanders to decent preventive health care and health. If health-care resources are indeed scarce for the poor, economic pressures to reduce health-care costs may one day restrict the birth of children with "preventable" severe genetic disorders by indirect coercion or by mandatory legislative and court prohibitions. Accordingly, eugenics may reenter public policy under the guise of "limited resources." The recurring theme of "limited resources" coincides with an explosion of scientific advances in genetic testing from ova to spermatozoa, from blastulae to fetal and trophoblastic cells in pregnant women, to fetuses, to newborns, to children, and to adults. Blastulae are embryos in the early stages of development in which a vesicle is surrounded by a single layer of cells. One of these cells may be extracted and studied for genetic defects without harm to the developing embryo.

Wrongful birth, wrongful life

Once scientific advances become part of the public domain, the courts have invariably supported their use, and expect patients to be made aware of them. Accordingly, failure to inform patients of medical advances has been a source of litigation in the form of wrongful birth and wrongful life suits. One of the first wrongful life cases, *Gleitman* v. *Cosgrove* (1967), rejected a woman's plea that she would not have borne a child blinded by rubella if she had known that rubella early in pregnancy could affect the fetus. The reason for the rejection of her argument was that abortion was illegal, and therefore the physician was under no obligation to suggest an illegal act. Even though abortion is now legal under certain conditions, the Supreme Court has decreed that the state is under no obligation to fund abortions for poor women (*Harris* v. *McRae*, 1980). Nevertheless, the states generally pay for voluntary (indirect coercive) sterilization for poor women. Accordingly, sterilization as an option to prevent future children with genetic disorders now has a more scientific rationale, but, as always, will disproportionately be limited mainly to poor women.

Wrongful birth and wrongful life decisions have formed the basis for litigation to ensure that women will be informed of the availability of genetic and other tests in early pregnancy, and to alert women of the risk of bearing a child with a genetic or other disorder. Wrongful life and wrongful birth litigation led also to assaults on the autonomy of women. Women are now at risk of incarceration for fetal abuse and of discrimination in the workplace, under the aegis of protection of the fetus. The rights of the fetus are often pitted against maternal duties and rights. It even has been suggested that charges of genetic neglect may follow women who elect to bear children affected with preventable congenital and genetic disorders (Shaw, 1984), a policy which patently would be eugenic. Pregnant women who drink alcohol or who are cited for drug abuse have been censured, and even incarcerated (Tanne, 1991). Fetal abuse is equated with child abuse. It is inescapable, however, that there is no greater fetal abuse than abortion. Accordingly, family, community and societal pressures could open a path to eugenics by questioning the discretion of women who elect to have children with preventable genetic disorders. Not surprisingly, since risk analysis is a major factor in insurance and employment, recent advances in genetic prediction may be taken into account in considerations for health, life insurance, and employment. Interestingly, even though the Americans with Disabilities Act of 1990 was passed to protect disabled persons from the private insurance system, the act specifically does not interfere with state laws that allow insurance companies to place restrictions on claims from disabled persons (Natowicz et al., 1992).

Interestingly, the right-to-life (anti-choice) and the opposing pro-choice movements may serve as a needed balance. Paradoxically, these opponents serve as buffers to eugenics. The right-to-life movement opposes abortion, a modern tool to eliminate the "unfit," but the pro-choice movement fosters autonomy and freedom for the women to choose or not choose abortion, and if autonomy prevails, society will not be able to mandate abortion.

Genetic testing

In the early 1970s many mistakes were made in genetic testing programs for sickle hemoglobin. These mistakes led to state-mandated screening, insurance company and employee discrimination, and widespread stigmatization (Bowman, 1977). It may be widely believed that genocide and other motives were responsible for the mandatory laws and discrimination of carriers for sickle hemoglobin (Bowman, 1977). However, it has been asserted that the principal reasons for discriminatory laws

and insurance restrictions of carriers of sickle hemoglobin were misinformation in brochures from the National Institutes of Health; pressure for the use of a solubility test by the Ortho Pharmaceutical Company; the proliferation of black community organizations in sickle hemoglobin screening programs with improper educational materials; inadequate testing procedures; and little or misinformed counseling. Further, most, if not all, of the state and District of Columbia mandatory sickle hemoglobin laws were instigated by black physicians, state legislators, or community groups. Jews, on the other hand, knew their history and its tragic consequences in Nazi Germany. *All* programs for Tay-Sachs disease were voluntary, and directed by experienced geneticists, with the cooperation of rabbis and the community (Kaback and O'Brien, 1973).

The lessons to be learned from sickle-cell screening in the black community and Tay-Sachs disease screening in the Jewish community include (1) involving the community first in any widespread genetic screening program; (2) contacting religious and community leaders, physicians, insurance companies, and other concerned parties in a program of community education so as to minimize misinformation, with its discriminatory and stigmatizing consequences; and (3) emphasizing voluntary genetic screening instead of mandated state laws. There have never been recommendations for either federal or state mandatory programs for Tay-Sachs disease. As of mid-1994, however, mandatory newborn screening for sickle hemoglobin was the law in over thirty-nine states in order to decrease morbidity (incidence of disease) and mortality early in life from pneumococcal disease (bacterial pneumonia) by the early introduction of prophylactic penicillin.

Counseling

All publications on genetic counseling emphasize the importance of education of the community before genetic screening is instituted, as well as accurate testing and counseling that is sensitive to the racial, class, and religious characteristics of the community (Bowman and Murray, 1990). Whenever possible, counselors should be of the same ethnic group as the counselees. Language is important. Today, efforts are made to produce educational and counseling material in the language of the counselees. This may be impossible, particularly when dealing with communities such as those from Vietnam and Laos, where many languages are used. Other writers such as Peter Rowley, Starlene Loader, Carol Sutera, Margaret Walden, and Alyssa Kozyra (1991) found that in a prenatal diagnosis program obstetricians were reluctant to provide education before pregnant woman were tested for hemoglobins. Such practice is contrary to accepted practice in genetic programs. It is paternalistic and denies autonomy to the pregnant woman, placing her at risk for stigmatization for employment, life, and health insurance, without her consent. On the other hand, in the real world of practice in a busy obstetrician's office, other means of counseling may have to be found, such as ethnically relevant educational materials, recordings, and office or home videos.

A recapitulation and challenge

The prospects of eugenics are anathema to most geneticists and ethicists. Nevertheless, consider the plight of poor women in the United States. Several states have decreased benefits for parents receiving Aid to Families with Dependent Children (AFDC) (Jencks, 1992). For example, in 1951, Georgia became the first state to deny welfare grants to more than one illegitimate child of a welfare mother. Louisiana followed in 1960 by denying public assistance to 23,000 children born out of wedlock on the same basis. Twelve states supported punitive action against those who might in the future conceive a child out of wedlock, and some even attempted to mandate the imprisonment or sterilization of women who bore more than one child out of wedlock (Solinger, 1992). The Supreme Court decision of *Dandridge v. Williams* (1970) restricted total state Aid for Dependent Children (AFDC) to a maximum of $250 per month per family, no matter how large the family. The state of Wisconsin in 1992 embarked on an "experiment" in which a limit would be placed on public funding of women on welfare who bear children out of wedlock; New Jersey has decided not to increase AFDC recipient benefits if a woman has a child while on welfare (Jencks, 1992). President Bill Clinton suggested during his campaign that no one be allowed to collect AFDC for more than two years (Jencks, 1992). As a follow up, Clinton gave Wisconsin permission to impose a two-year limit on indigent families with children. One may conclude that if legislators are so draconian as to attempt to mandate incarceration or sterilization for women who have more than one child out of wedlock, poor women who have children with "preventable severe genetic disorders" are at risk for mandatory sterilization or other coercive means to prevent the birth of such children.

In summary, scientific, economic, social, and legal forces may eventually restrict the birth of children with severe genetic disorders, particularly those who are members of poor racial groups. The scientific advances include developments in prenatal diagnosis and the eventual deciphering of the human genome. The legal precedents are based on the police power of the state (the doctrine that the private interests of the individual must be subservient to the public interest), mandatory sterilization laws, and the legalization of abortion. The social pressures include the dictum that health-care re-

sources are scarce and the fact of widening gap between the haves and the have-nots.

Today, however, we are concerned not only with those with genetic disease who may be stigmatized as unfit but also with individuals who carry a single dose (carriers) of a genetic defect, which causes little if any effect. Since all people have at least five recessive genes, all of us are at risk for having "unfit" children. Five recessive genes may, however, be just the tip of the iceberg. When the human genome is mapped, many more potentially harmful genes—recessive and otherwise—may be unveiled in each of us. Consequently, in this day of rapid advances in genetics, we all are potentially able to pass "unfit" disorders to the next generation. Since we are all in the same position, scientific advances in the understanding of the human genome *may* be one of the best defenses against subjecting minorities to eugenic discrimination. We rarely discriminate against those who are "like ourselves."

JAMES E. BOWMAN

Directly related to this entry are the entries EUGENICS; GENETIC TESTING AND SCREENING; *and* RACE AND RACISM. *For a further discussion of topics mentioned in this entry, see the entries* GENETIC COUNSELING; HEALTH-CARE FINANCING, *especially the articles on* MEDICARE, *and* MEDICAID; HEALTH POLICY, *article on* POLITICS AND HEALTH CARE; MATERNAL–FETAL RELATIONSHIP, *articles on* ETHICAL ISSUES, *and* LEGAL AND REGULATORY ISSUES; *and* PUBLIC POLICY AND BIOETHICS. *For a discussion of ethical theories and concepts mentioned in this entry, see the entries* AUTONOMY; CASUISTRY; ETHICS, *article on* NORMATIVE ETHICAL THEORIES; JUSTICE; *and* UTILITY. *For a discussion of related ideas, see the entries* ABORTION, *section on* CONTEMPORARY ETHICAL AND LEGAL PERSPECTIVES; GENETICS AND ENVIRONMENT IN HUMAN HEALTH; GENOME MAPPING AND SEQUENCING; LAW AND BIOETHICS; NATIONAL SOCIALISM; *and* PUBLIC HEALTH, *articles on* HISTORY OF PUBLIC HEALTH, *and* PHILOSOPHY OF PUBLIC HEALTH.

Bibliography

BLUMENTHAL, ALBERT. 1977. *Moral Responsibility: Mankind's Greatest Need—Principles and Practical Applications of Scientific Utilitarian Ethics.* 2d ed. Santa Ana, Calif.: Rayline Press.

BOWMAN, JAMES E. 1972. "Mass Screening Programs for Sickle Cell Crisis." *Journal of the American Medical Association* 222, no. 13:64.

———. 1977. "Genetic Screening Programs and Public Policy." *Phylon* 38:117–142.

———. 1991. "Prenatal Screening for Hemoglobinopathies." *American Journal of Human Genetics* 48, no. 3:433–438.

BOWMAN, JAMES E.; CARSON, P. E.; FRISCHER, H.; POWELL,

R. D.; COLWELL, E. J.; LEGTERS, L. J.; COTTINGHAM, A. J.; BOONE, S. C.; and HISER, W. W. 1971. "Hemoglobin and Red Cell Enzyme Variation in Some Populations of the Republic of Vietnam with Comments on the Malaria Hypothesis." *American Journal of Physical Anthropology* 34, no. 3:313–324.

BOWMAN, JAMES E., and MURRAY, ROBERT F., JR. 1990. *Genetic Variation and Disorders in Peoples of African Origin.* Baltimore: Johns Hopkins University Press.

Buck v. Bell. 1927. 274 U.S. 200, 47 S. Ct. 584.

COOGAN, JOHN E. 1953. "Eugenic Sterilization Holds Jubilee." *Catholic World* 177, no. 1057:44–49.

Dandridge v. Williams. 1970. 397 U.S. 471, 25 L. Ed. 491, 90 S. Ct. 1153.

FLETCHER, JOSEPH. 1979. *Humanhood: Essays in Biomedical Ethics.* Buffalo, N.Y.: Prometheus.

GALTON, FRANCIS. 1871. *Hereditary Genius: An Inquiry Into Its Laws and Consequences.* New York: B. Appleton.

Gleitman v. Cosgrove. 1967. N.J. 22, 227 A.2d 689, 22 ALR 3d 1411.

GRANDA, H.; GISPERT, S.; DORTICOS, A.; MARTIN, M.; CUADRAS, Y.; CALVO, M.; MARTINEZ, G.; ZAYAS, M. A.; OLIVIA, J. A.; and HEREDERO, L. 1991. "Cuban Programme for Prevention of Sickle Cell Disease." *Lancet* 337, no. 8734:152–153.

Griswold v. Connecticut. 1965. 381 U.S. 479, 14 L. Ed. 2d 510, 85 S. Ct. 1678.

HALLER, MARK H. 1963. *Eugenics: Hereditarian Attitudes in American Thought.* New Brunswick, N.J.: Rutgers University Press.

Harris v. McRae. 1980. 448 U.S. 297, 65 L. Ed. 2d 784, 100 S. Ct. 2671.

HOLMES, STEVEN A. 1994. "Federal Government Is Urged to Rethink Its System of Racial Classifications." *New York Times,* July 8, p. A9.

HOLTZMAN, NEIL A., and ROTHSTEIN, MARK A. 1992. "Eugenics and Genetic Discrimination." *American Journal of Human Genetics* 50, no. 3:457–459.

JENCKS, CHRISTOPHER. 1992. *Rethinking Social Policy: Race, Poverty, and the Underclass.* Cambridge, Mass.: Harvard University Press.

KABACK, MICHAEL M., and O'BRIEN, J. S. 1973. "Tay-Sachs: Prototype for Prevention of Genetic Disease." *Hospital Practice* 8, no. 3:107–116.

KAIRYS, DAVID, ed. 1982. *The Politics of Law: A Progressive Critique.* New York: Pantheon.

KANT, IMMANUEL. 1964. *Groundwork of the Metaphysic of Morals.* Translated by H. J. Paton. New York: Harper & Row.

LAPPÉ, MARK; GUSTAFSON, JAMES M.; and ROBLIN, RICHARD O. 1972. "Ethical and Social Issues in Screening for Genetic Disease. A Report from the Research Group on Ethical, Social and Legal Issues in Genetic Counseling and Genetic Engineering of the Institute of Society, Ethics and the Life Sciences." *New England Journal of Medicine* 286, no. 21:1129–1132.

LAUGHLIN, HARRY H. 1930. *The Legal Status of Eugenical Sterilization: History and Analysis of Litigation Under the Virginia Sterilization Statute. Supplement to the Annual Report of the Municipal Court of Chicago for the Year 1929.* Chicago: Fred J. Ringley.

LAVINE, THELMA Z. 1984. *From Socrates to Sartre: The Philosophic Quest.* New York: Bantam Books.

LUDMERER, KENNETH M. 1972. *Genetics and American Society: A Historical Appraisal.* Baltimore: Johns Hopkins University Press.

Maher v. Roe. 1977. 432 U.S. 464, 53 L. Ed. 2d 484, 97 S. Ct. 2376.

Munn v. Illinois. 1877. 94 U.S. 113, 24 L. Ed. 77.

NATOWICZ, MARVIN R.; ALPER, JANE K.; and ALPER, JOSEPH S. 1992. "Genetic Discrimination and the Law." *American Journal of Human Genetics* 50, no. 3:465–475.

POLEDNAK, ANTHONY P. 1989. *Racial and Ethnic Differences in Disease.* Oxford: Oxford University Press.

RAWLS, JOHN. 1958. "Justice as Fairness." *Philosophical Review* 67, no. 2:164–194.

REILLY, PHILIP R. 1991. *The Surgical Solution: A History of Involuntary Sterilization in the United States.* Baltimore: Johns Hopkins University Press.

Roe v. Wade. 1973. 410 U.S. 113 L. Ed. 2d 147, 93 S. Ct. 705.

ROWLEY, PETER T.; LOADER, STARLENE; SUTERA, CAROL J.; WALDEN, MARGARET; and KOZYRA, ALYSSA. 1991. "Prenatal Screening for Hemoglobinopathies. I. A Prospective Regional Trial." *American Journal of Human Genetics* 48, no. 3:439–446.

SCRIVER, CHARLES R.; BARDANIS, MARIETTA; CARTIER, LOLA; CLOW, CAROL I.; LANCASTER, GERALD A.; and OSTROWSKY, JULIA T. 1984. "β-Thalassemia Disease Prevention: Genetic Medicine Applied." *American Journal of Human Genetics* 36, no. 5:1024–1038.

SHAW, MARGERY W. 1984. "Conditional Prospective Rights of the Fetus." *Journal of Legal Medicine* 5, no. 1:63–116.

SOLINGER, RICKIE. 1992. *Wake Up Little Susie: Single Pregnancy and Race Before Roe v. Wade.* New York: Routledge.

TANNE, JANICE HOPKINS. 1991. "Jail for Pregnant Cocaine Users in U.S." *British Medical Journal* 303, no. 6807:873.

TENTORI, L., and MARINUCCI, M. 1983. "Hemoglobinopathies and Thalassemias in Italy and Northern Africa." In *Distribution and Evolution of Hemoglobin and Globin Loci: Proceedings of the Fourth Annual Comprehensive Sickle Cell Center Symposium on the Distribution and Evolution of Hemoglobin and Globin Loci at the University of Chicago, October 10–12, 1982.* Edited by James E. Bowman. New York: Elsevier Publishing.

UNGER, ROBERTO MANGABEIRA. 1986. *The Critical Legal Studies Movement.* Cambridge, Mass.: Harvard University Press.

GENETIC TESTING AND SCREENING

I. Preimplantation Diagnosis
    Alan H. Handyside
II. Prenatal Diagnosis
    Mark I. Evans
    Mordecai Hallak
    Mark P. Johnson

I. PREIMPLANTATION DIAGNOSIS

The detection of genetic defects that cause inherited disease in human embryos before implantation (preimplantation diagnosis) has a number of advantages for couples known to be at risk of having affected children (Handyside, 1992). The main advantage is that selection of unaffected embryos for transfer to the uterus means that any resulting pregnancy should be normal. It eliminates the possibility of terminating by conventional methods at later stages a pregnancy diagnosed as affected. Another advantage relates to the use of superovulation and in vitro fertilization (IVF) for access to embryos at the early stages. Superovulation increases the number of eggs that reach maturity in a single reproductive cycle. After IVF, an average of five or six embryos can be screened simultaneously, increasing the chance of identifying unaffected embryos. Although several IVF cycles may be necessary, since pregnancy rates average only one in three to four embryo transfers (Hardy, 1993), establishing a normal pregnancy may in many cases take less time than following a series of terminations of affected pregnancies diagnosed at later stages.

For deoxyribonucleic acid (DNA) analysis, cells are removed or biopsied from each embryo at about the eight-cell stage, early on the third day after insemination. The DNA analysis is then carried out, if possible within eight to twelve hours, and unaffected embryos are transferred to the uterus later the same day. The embryos are apparently unharmed by this process since the cells have not become specialized at this early stage (Hardy et al., 1990). As an alternative, the first polar body (a small nondividing cell produced during egg formation and containing one set of discarded chromosomes) is removed from eggs before fertilization to test (indirectly) whether the egg itself has inherited the genetic defect from women carriers (Verlinsky et al., 1990). Preconception diagnosis may be ethically more acceptable to those opposed to the manipulation of human embryos. However, it is limited to the analysis of maternal genetic defects, is less efficient, and has so far failed to establish a pregnancy after diagnosis.

To date, pregnancies (and in some cases births) have been achieved mainly after preimplantation diagnosis to identify the sex of embryos and to transfer females in couples at risk of diseases affecting only boys (Handyside et al., 1990). However, specific diagnosis of embryos affected by cystic fibrosis (Handyside et al., 1992) and several other diseases has recently been achieved. This is accomplished by amplifying DNA specific for the male Y chromosome or for the cystic fibrosis gene, for example, from the single cells biopsied from each embryo. In principle, similar strategies can be used for the detection of almost any genetic defect that has been characterized at the DNA level (Hardy and Handyside, 1992). Examples include Duchenne muscular dystrophy, Tay-Sachs disease, hemophilia A and B, beta-thalassemia, sickle-cell disease, alpha$_1$-antitrypsin deficiency, and Lesch-Nyhan syndrome. Another technique for identifying the sex of embryos is the use of fluorescent DNA probes that recognize the sex chromosomes. This approach also enables embryos with abnormal numbers of chromosomes to be identified in carriers of chromosome abnormalities or in older women at increased risk of Down syndrome (Griffin et al., 1991, 1992).

The ethical issues raised by preimplantation diagnosis are concerned first, with the manipulation of human preimplantation embryos and second, with the use of this approach to screen for genetic defects that would not justify terminating established pregnancies. Ethical objections to the manipulation of human preimplantation embryos are generally based on the view that there is in principle no difference between an eight-cell embryo, for example, and a midgestation fetus or a child. They are all human individuals, and since informed consent is not possible, should not be interfered with. On this basis, terminating an affected pregnancy in midgestation is no more or less acceptable than discarding affected preimplantation embryos. The opposing view draws a sharp distinction between these stages of a human's development and consequently argues that the ethical constraints are different at each stage. In this case, manipulation of early embryos to remove cells for genetic analysis is acceptable; some would argue that discarding affected embryos is preferable to termination at later stages. Even after normal conception with fertile couples, it is known that many fertilized embryos are often lost before implantation because they have gross genetic, usually chromosomal, defects (Burgoyne et al., 1991).

The other ethical issue arises out of the possibility that preimplantation diagnosis might be used to screen for genetic characteristics associated with only mild non–life-threatening conditions, for example, for the health of the individual, or indeed, simply for physical characteristics. Examples of milder inherited conditions include detection of the premutation predisposing to the fragile X syndrome, hereditary blindness or deafness, and Huntington disease, which causes dementia in later life. In these cases, the principle that a couple has the right to choose prenatal screening may still be a sufficient safeguard. After all, a couple is unlikely to elect IVF and preimplantation diagnosis unless they feel strongly about the effects of any condition and often know firsthand exactly what is involved because they already have affected children or relatives. Of more concern is the identification of single genes, segregating in families, that predispose to cancer or heart disease. Also, with so much worldwide effort directed toward mapping the human genome, fears have been expressed about the use of preimplantation diagnosis to yield "designer babies." This is not a realistic prospect, however, since it overlooks the fact that even with complete knowledge of the human genome, geneticists would be able to identify embryos with the desired characteristics only if the parents had passed on the right combination of genes.

Preimplantation diagnosis is rapidly becoming an established procedure and many clinics will be starting their own programs over the next few years. In the United Kingdom, legislation regulates the use of any procedure involving human fertilization and embryo manipulation, including preimplantation diagnosis. The alteration of an embryo's genes, for example, even for gene therapy or for cloning of embryos, is illegal. In addition, all IVF clinics must be licensed by a government-appointed authority with both specialist and nonspecialist members. This authority has the power to withhold a license if a clinic has not demonstrated minimum standards of competence or if the proposed purpose is not considered ethically or otherwise justified. For example, the authority does not allow the identification of an embryo's sex simply to allow couples to choose the sex of their child. It is important that similar initiatives be taken in other countries to ensure that clinics have the necessary expertise to attempt preimplantation diagnosis and prevent its misuse.

ALAN H. HANDYSIDE

Directly related to this article are the other articles in this entry: PRENATAL DIAGNOSIS, NEWBORN SCREENING, CARRIER SCREENING, PREDICTIVE AND WORKPLACE TESTING, LEGAL ISSUES, *and* ETHICAL ISSUES. *Also directly related is the entry* GENETIC COUNSELING. *For a further discussion of topics mentioned in this article, see the entries* ABORTION; EUGENICS, *especially the article on* ETHICAL ISSUES; FETUS; GENOME MAPPING AND SEQUENCING; LIFE; MEDICAL GENETICS; PERSON; *and* REPRODUCTIVE TECHNOLOGIES, *especially the articles on* SEX SELECTION, *and* IN VITRO FERTILIZATION AND EMBRYO TRANSFER. *For a discussion of related ideas, see the entry* MARRIAGE AND OTHER DOMESTIC PARTNERSHIPS.

Bibliography

BURGOYNE, PAUL S.; HOLLAND, K.; and STEPHENS, R. 1991. "Incidence of Numerical Chromosome Anomalies in Human Pregnancy Estimation from Induced and Spontaneous Abortion Data." *Human Reproduction* 6, no. 4: 555–565.

GRIFFIN, DARREN K.; HANDYSIDE, ALAN H.; PENKETH, RICHARD J.; WINSTON, ROBERT M.; and DELHANTY, JON D. 1991. "Fluorescent In-Situ Hybridization to Interphase Nuclei of Human Preimplantation Embryos with X and Y Chromosome Specific Probes." *Human Reproduction* 6, no. 1:101–105.

GRIFFIN, DARREN K.; WILTON, LEANDER J.; HANDYSIDE, ALAN H.; WINSTON, ROBERT M.; and DELHANTY, JON D. 1992. "Dual Fluorescent in Situ Hybridization for Simultaneous Detection of X and Y Chromosome-Specific Probes for the Sexing of Human Preimplantation Embryonic Nuclei." *Human Genetics* 89, no. 1:18–22.

HANDYSIDE, ALAN H. 1992. "Preimplantation Diagnosis of Genetic Defects." In *Infertility: Proceedings of the Twenty-Fifth Study Group of the Royal College of Obstetricians and Gynaecologists*, pp. 331–344. Edited by James O. Drife and Alexander A. Templeton. London: Springer-Verlag.

HANDYSIDE, ALAN H.; KONTOGIANNI, ELENA H.; HARDY, KATE; and WINSTON, ROBERT M. 1990. "Pregnancies from Biopsied Human Preimplantation Embryos Sexed by Y-Specific DNA Amplification." *Nature* 344, no. 6268:768–770.

HANDYSIDE, ALAN H.; LESKO, JOHN G.; TARIN, JUAN J.; WINSTON, ROBERT M. L.; and HUGHES, MARK. 1992. "Birth of a Normal Girl After in Vitro Fertilization and Preimplantation Diagnostic Testing for Cystic Fibrosis." *New England Journal of Medicine* 327, no. 13:905–909.

HARDY, KATE. 1993. "Development of Human Blastocysts in Vitro." In *Preimplantation Embryo Development*, pp. 184–199. Edited by Barry D. Bavister. New York: Springer-Verlag.

HARDY, KATE, and HANDYSIDE, ALAN H. 1992. "Biopsy of Cleavage Stage Human Embryos and Diagnosis of Single Gene Defects by DNA Amplification." *Archives of Pathology and Laboratory Medicine* 116, no. 4:388–392.

HARDY, KATE; MARTIN, KAREN L.; LEESE, HENRY J.; WINSTON, ROBERT M.; and HANDYSIDE, ALAN H. 1990. "Human Preimplantation Development in Vitro Is Not Adversely Affected by Biopsy at the 8-Cell Stage." *Human Reproduction* 5, no. 6:708–714.

VERLINSKY, YURY; GINSBERG, NORMA; LIFCHEZ, A.; VALLE, J.; MOISE, J.; and STROM, CHARLES M. 1990. "Analysis of the First Polar Body: Preconception Genetic Diagnosis." *Human Reproduction* 5, no. 7:826–829.

II. PRENATAL DIAGNOSIS

Modern prenatal diagnosis began in the late 1960s and early 1970s with the development of laboratory techniques for the culturing of amniotic fluid cells (Fuchs and Riis, 1956; Steele and Breg, 1966). As with many new technologies, priority was given to patients believed to be at highest risk—and, in this case, those willing to consent to abortion if an abnormality were detected. Before the risks of prenatal diagnosis were known and the resource was very scarce, this priority was understandable, but it is now an unacceptable standard of care in the United States (Eden and Boehm, 1990). Since the literature on prenatal diagnosis is vast, the interested reader is referred to other materials (Evans, 1992; Evans et al., 1989; Fleischer et al., 1991).

Reproductive risks and indications

From 2 to 4 percent of all infants are born with a serious defect. If minor defects are included, the rate can reach 8 to 10 percent. Of serious abnormalities, approximately half are genetic. The remainder can be attributed to drugs, alcohol, infections, or other nongenetic causes.

The following are indications for offering prenatal diagnosis: (1) advanced maternal age—at age twenty-five, a woman has a 1 in 476 risk of having a baby with a chromosome abnormality; at age thirty, the risk is 1 in 385; at age thirty-five it is 1 in 192, and at age forty it is 1 in 66 (Evans, 1992); (2) a genetic history of abnormalities; (3) belonging to an ethnic group known to be at risk (e.g., sickle-cell disease in African-American patients, Tay-Sachs disease in Jewish patients); (4) previous poor reproductive outcomes, including infants born with birth defects; (5) a family history of infants with birth defects; (6) multiple miscarriages; (7) documentation in a current pregnancy of a problem, such as an abnormal maternal serum alpha-fetoprotein screen or an abnormal ultrasound.

Advanced maternal age is still the most common indication for prenatal diagnosis; worldwide, it accounts for more than 90 percent of all prenatal diagnostic procedures. Although it is a standard of care in the United States to inform pregnant women over the age of thirty-five as to the availability of prenatal diagnosis, the choice of that age as the cutoff is entirely arbitrary (ACOG, 1987). In fact, the risk of a child with a chromosome abnormality begins to increase prior to age thirty, then continues to rise at an accelerated rate (Hook et al., 1983).

Couples who already have had a child with Down syndrome or another chromosomal abnormality face a recurrence risk of 1 percent or more in each subsequent pregnancy (Stene et al., 1984). They are candidates for prenatal diagnosis regardless of age.

A known cytogenetic abnormality (i.e., a balanced translocation) in one of the parents is a less frequent but important indication for prenatal diagnosis (Boue and Gallano, 1984). Such balanced translocations typically come to light after the birth of a child with an "unbalanced" chromosomal rearrangement. Parental balanced translocations may also be uncovered as part of the diagnostic evaluation of multiple spontaneous first-trimester abortions.

Some abnormalities are significantly linked to certain ethnic groups. For example, Tay-Sachs disease is seen mostly in Ashkenazi Jews, sickle-cell anemia in African-Americans, and beta-thalassemia in Mediterranean peoples.

A previous child or first-degree relative with a neural tube defect is an indication for amniocentesis. Such a defect is inherited in a multifactorial pattern. A couple who has had a child with anencephaly or meningomyelocele faces approximately a 3 percent risk of having a second affected child. At least 90 percent of open defects (those in which there is communication between the subarachnoid space and the amniotic cavity) can be detected by measurement of alpha-fetoprotein in the amniotic fluid. Amniotic fluid acetylcholinesterase is also elevated in the presence of these defects and has proven to be a very useful diagnostic adjunct.

Women who have had elevated serum alpha-fetoprotein levels on two occasions during pregnancy, and whose gestational timing has been confirmed by ultrasound examination, are at markedly increased risk of having a child with a neural tube defect and are candidates for amniocentesis for definitive diagnosis.

Procedures for prenatal diagnosis

There are three basic approaches to identifying fetal defects: visualization, analysis of fetal tissues, and laboratory studies (see Table 1).

Visualization. The application of ultrasonographic methods to the study of human anatomy has had a tremendous impact on all areas of medicine. The development of high-resolution, real-time scanners has

TABLE 1.   Methods Used for Prenatal Diagnosis

I. *Visualization*
   Noninvasive
      Ultrasonography
   Invasive
      Embryoscopy
      Fetoscopy
      Endoscopy

II. *Analysis of Fetal Tissues*
   Amniocentesis
   Chorionic villus sampling
   Cordocentesis (fetal blood sampling)
   Skin biopsy
   Liver biopsy
   Muscle biopsy

III. *Laboratory Studies*
   Cytogenetics
   Biochemical
   DNA

made it possible to visualize essentially any part of the fetal anatomy in exquisite detail (Romero et al., 1988; Fleischer et al., 1991).

Second-trimester ultrasound examinations are performed in 30 to 50 percent of all pregnancies in the United States, frequently in the obstetrician's office. More detailed examinations are best performed by ultrasonographers with special interest and expertise in fetal anatomy, pathology, and physiology. Prenatal diagnosis may be most successful when a particular defect is sought. A thorough examination includes a variety of measurements to assess intrauterine growth and gestational age, and to identify skeletal disproportions. In addition, each part of the fetal anatomy (face, intracranial structures, chest, heart, abdomen, genitourinary system, and extremities) is examined in detail.

Analysis of fetal tissues.   Because visualization techniques do not provide genetic information about the fetus, amniocentesis or chorionic villus sampling may be indicated where a fetus is at risk for genetic abnormality.

Amniocentesis.   Transabdominal amniocentesis (needle puncture of the uterus) is the most widely used invasive technique for prenatal diagnosis because of the wealth of information that can be derived by studying cells in the amniotic fluid and the fluid itself.

Amniocentesis should be performed by an obstetrician skilled in the technique. It is commonly performed with ultrasonographic guidance (Benaceraff and Frigoletto, 1983; Romero et al., 1985), although many thousands of procedures have been performed without it. In skilled hands an adequate sample is obtained on the first attempt in over 99 percent of cases, and successful fluid cell cultures are established in 98 to 99 percent of these. The major risk of amniocentesis is fetal loss. In the 1976 National Institute of Child Health and Human Development study the rate of loss (spontaneous abortion, fetal deaths in utero, and stillbirths) was 3.5 percent in the subjects and 3.2 percent in the controls; after adjustment for maternal age, the rates were 3.3 percent and 3.4 percent, respectively. This loss rate of approximately 1 in 200 is widely believed to have decreased in major centers to about 1 in 300.

With increasing experience and confidence of needle placement under ultrasound guidance, it has become possible to perform amniocentesis earlier and earlier. Motivated by the desirability of completing prenatal diagnostic studies as early as possible, and by the limited availability of chorionic villus sampling (CVS) in many areas, several prenatal diagnosis programs have begun offering amniocentesis as early as 10 to 14 weeks' gestation. Limited experience in the last few years suggests that the safety of the procedure will likely become comparable with that of traditional amniocentesis, but long-term outcome studies are not yet available.

Early amniocentesis still does not enable chromosome analysis or biochemical analyses to be performed as quickly as they can be after a chorionic villus sample. However, it may be useful in some twin pregnancies (if there is a single fused placenta or if sampling both fetuses may not be possible by CVS) or other circumstances in which CVS is contraindicated.

Chorionic villus sampling.   Although amniocentesis has proven to be very safe and highly reliable, the desirability of a procedure that can provide information prior to eighteen or twenty weeks' gestation is obvious. Although the decision to terminate a pregnancy is rarely (if ever) easy, it is perhaps more easily made earlier in pregnancy.

Chorionic villus sampling (CVS) is a first-trimester alternative to amniocentesis. The chorionic villi are the forerunners of the placenta and can be obtained by aspiration, usually between nine and twelve weeks' gestation. The most common technique relies entirely on ultrasound guidance. A metal sound is introduced through the internal cervical os to chart the path for the catheter on the ultrasound, and to determine the degree of curvature between the cervical canal and the placenta. A malleable catheter (usually plastic with an aluminum guide) one to two millimeters in diameter is then bent to permit easy passage through the cervix and maneuvering to the implantation site. The tip of the instrument is advanced through as much of the placenta as possible. The metal guide is removed, a 20 cc syringe is attached to the catheter, and suction is applied. The catheter is then slowly pulled back, with some rotation, to increase tissue aspiration. The villi that are torn from the chorion are taken up in tissue culture medium and examined under the dissecting microscope to determine the adequacy of the sample. An adequate sample is successfully obtained on the first attempt by an experienced operator in 85 percent of cases, and after two attempts in 98 percent of cases. Alternatively a needle can be passed transabdominally into the placenta, and villi then aspirated. The choice of approach (transcervical or transabdominal) depends on placental location and the experience of the operator. The ability to utilize both approaches is necessary for optimum efficiency and safety. Use of transabdominal CVS does increase with advancing gestational age, which is a function of placental accessibility. After fourteen weeks' gestation most procedures are performed transabdominally, since the placenta gains bulk and moves away from the cervix.

As with amniocentesis, there has been great concern about the risk of spontaneous abortion or fetal injury as a result of CVS. The first major problem in determining the loss rate, however, was differentiating the true procedure-related losses (added) from the spontaneous losses. Overall, the fetal loss rate after a normal ultrasound at eight to ten weeks has been estimated to be 1.4 to 2.7 percent. However, the spontaneous abortion rate increases with maternal age (and other factors, such as tobacco and alcohol consumption). Since 80 to

90 percent of CVSs are performed in women over the age of thirty-five, the spontaneous abortion rate at this age (4.0–4.3%) is also more relevant than lower spontaneous risks in younger women.

Published data on the safety and efficacy of CVS have begun to emerge, but reflect data two to three years old (Cole, 1987; Wilson et al., 1989; Rhoads et al., 1989; Jackson et al., 1992). Most studies showed no statistical difference between procedure-related fetal loss and spontaneous losses. Patients are usually informed, however, that CVS is believed to carry between a 1 percent and a 0.5 percent risk of fetal loss due to the procedure.

Laboratory studies. Neural tube defects (spina bifida and anencephaly) occur in about one in 700 white and one in 1,000 black pregnancies. Amniocentesis to measure alpha-fetoprotein (AFP) and sometimes acetylcholinesterase (fetal enzymes found in higher elevations when the fetus is affected) is used for the definitive diagnosis for patients at high risk. However, the vast majority (about 95%) of all infants with neural tube defects are born to couples unaware of any increased risk. Thus, inherent in a program to detect the vast majority of neural tube defects is the necessity to test *all* pregnancies. Clearly it is impossible to offer amniocentesis to all patients. Thus, the concept of testing for AFP in maternal serum (MSAFP testing) was developed in the mid-1970s (Brock et al., 1973). For neural tube defects, approximately 3 percent of patients will have either one blood test with very significantly elevated MSAFP or two tests, both of which are slightly elevated. Of these patients, ultrasound will find an obvious explanation for the elevations in approximately half the cases: twins, anencephaly, severe neural tube defect, or, most commonly, incorrect assessment of gestational age. The remaining 1.5 percent of patients are offered a genetic amniocentesis. In most large programs the detection rate for abnormalities is approximately 5 percent of patients who have the amniocentesis.

The chance of finding that babies born with chromosome anomalies such as Down syndrome tended to have lower-than-normal MSAFP values has led to a reevaluation of assessment of genetic risk (Cuckle et al., 1984; Merkatz et al., 1984). The definition of a low MSAFP is a value at which the adjusted risk for the given patient is equal at least to the risk of a thirty-five-year-old, regardless of her actual age. Through this test, thousands of women thought to be low risk have been identified as high risk and offered amniocentesis.

The potential benefits of mass screening for chromosomal abnormalities are obvious. If only women thirty-five years of age and older were offered amniocentesis or CVS, only about 12 to 20 percent of chromosome abnormalities would be detected. MSAFP, when properly performed, raises the detection rate to between 40 and 50 percent. In an effort to increase the detection rate beyond 40 to 50 percent, there has been research looking for additional serum markers.

There are vociferous arguments as to the best combination of markers, but the trend is toward multiple markers and attempts to move screening into the first trimester. It is very likely that the specifics, timing, and efficacy of screening will change rapidly in the next several years.

Ethical implications

It has become a fundamental tenet of genetics that there is no linkage between the offering of prenatal diagnosis, the documentation of fetal abnormalities, and the decision of whether to have an abortion. *Prenatal diagnosis is for the purpose of providing information to couples about what they can expect.* Even for couples who would not under any circumstances consider termination of pregnancy, the knowledge gained can be extremely valuable. In the vast majority of cases, general levels of anxiety can be considerably decreased, since a normal result will be found. In the event that an abnormality is detected, the patients then have the ability at least to be prepared for what is coming, and perhaps significantly to alter the way in which the obstetrical care of the patient is handled. For example, patients with ventral wall defects such as omphaloceles or gastroschises are best delivered in a tertiary-care center where an immediate repair of the defect can be undertaken. Patients with neural tube defects are best delivered by cesarean section, to avoid trauma to the open neural tube, which appears to decrease motor function. Fetuses with lethal disorders, such as trisomy 18, can be managed conservatively. Over 50 percent of fetuses with undiagnosed trisomy 18 have been delivered by emergency cesarean section, only to have the baby die and thus to have subjected the mother to a futile major operation.

The use of screening technologies, such as routine ultrasound and maternal serum alpha-fetoprotein screening, has brought many couples to prenatal diagnosis who otherwise would never have been seen. This is important from a public-health viewpoint, since if prenatal diagnosis were offered only to women age thirty-five or older, less than 20 percent of all chromosome abnormalities would be detected. The use of such tests as MSAFP screening was originally met with considerable skepticism and anxiety by women who previously were considered low risk and suddenly shifted to being high risk. However, after several years of experience, patients have learned to cope with the alteration in anxiety and, by and large, to undergo the further testing necessary to clarify their situations. In most cases these patients return to a lower state of anxiety with diagnoses of normal pregnancy.

Obstetricians have long held the concept of having two patients—mother and fetus. Only in recent years, with the advent of ultrasound and fetal treatments, has the distinction between mother and fetus become generally understood—elevating the standing of the fetus ethically and sometimes legally. Predictably, there are sometimes conflicts of interest between the two that have profound legal and ethical implications.

MARK I. EVANS
MORDECAI HALLAK
MARK P. JOHNSON

Directly related to this article are the other articles in this entry: PREIMPLANTATION DIAGNOSIS, NEWBORN SCREENING, CARRIER SCREENING, PREDICTIVE AND WORKPLACE TESTING, LEGAL ISSUES, *and* ETHICAL ISSUES. *For a further discussion of topics mentioned in this article, see the entries* FETUS; MATERNAL–FETAL RELATIONSHIP, *especially the article on* MEDICAL ASPECTS; *and* RISK. *For a discussion of related ideas, see the entries* ABORTION; CONFLICT OF INTEREST; GENETICS AND RACIAL MINORITIES; *and* RACE AND RACISM.

Bibliography

AMERICAN COLLEGE OF OBSTETRICIANS AND GYNECOLOGISTS (ACOG). 1987. "Antenatal Diagnosis of Genetic Disorders." *Technical Bulletin* no. 108.

———. 1991. "Triple Screening." *Technical Bulletin* no. 97.

BENACERAFF, BERYL R., and FRIGOLETTO, FREDERICK D. 1983. "Amniocentesis Under Continuous Ultrasound Guidance: A Series of 232 Cases." *Obstetrics and Gynecology* 62, no. 6:760–764.

BOUE, ANDRÉ, and GALLANO, PAUL. 1984. "A Collaborative Study of the Segregation of Inherited Chromosome Structural Rearrangements in 1356 Prenatal Diagnoses." *Prenatal Diagnosis* 4 (spec. 155):45–67.

BROCK, DAVID J. H.; BOLTON, ALAN E.; and MONAGHAM, JAMES M. 1973. "Prenatal Diagnosis of Anencephaly Through Maternal Serum Alpha-Fetoprotein Measurements." *Lancet* 2, no. 7835: 923–926.

CANADIAN COLLABORATIVE CVS-AMNIOCENTESIS CLINICAL TRIAL GROUP. 1989. "Multicentre Randomized Clinical Trial of Chorionic Villus Sampling and Amniocentesis: First Report." *Lancet* 1, no. 8628:1–6.

COLE, HELENE M., ed. 1987. "Diagnostic and Therapeutic Technology Assessment (DATTA). Chorionic Villus Sampling." *Journal of the American Medical Association* 258, no. 24:3560–3563.

CUCKLE, HOWARD S.; WALD, NICHOLOS J.; and LINDENBAUM, ROBERT H. 1984. "Maternal Serum Alpha-Fetoprotein Measurements: A Screening Test for Down Syndrome." *Lancet* 1, no. 8383:936–929.

EDEN, ROBERT D., and BOEHM, FRANK H., eds. 1990. *Assessment and Care of the Fetus: Physiological, Clinical, and Medicolegal Principles.* Norwalk, Conn.: Appleton & Lange.

EVANS, MARK I., ed. 1992. *Reproductive Risks and Prenatal Diagnosis.* Norwalk, Conn.: Appleton and Lange.

EVANS, MARK I.; FLETCHER, JOHN C.; DIXLER, ALAN O.; and SCHULMAN, JOSEPH D., eds. 1989. *Fetal Diagnosis and Therapy: Science, Ethics and the Law.* Philadelphia: Lippincott.

FLEISCHER, ARTHUR C.; ROMERO, ROBERTO; MANNING, FRANK A.; JEANTY, PHILLIPÊ; and JAMES, ALAN E., JR., eds. 1991. *The Principles and Practice of Ultrasonography in Obstetrics and Gynecology.* 4th ed. Norwalk, Conn.: Appleton and Lange.

FUCHS, FRITZ, and RIIS, PAUL. 1956. "Antenatal Sex Determination." *Nature* 177, no. 4503:330.

HOOK, ERNEST B.; CROSS, PHILLIP K.; and SCHREINEMACHERS, DINA M. 1983. "Chromosomal Abnormality Rates at Amniocentesis and in Live Born Infants." *Journal of the American Medical Association* 249, no. 15:2034–2038.

JACKSON, LAIRD G.; ZACHARY, JULIA M.; FOWLER, SARAH E.; DESICK, ROBERT J.; GOLBUS, MITCHELL S.; LEDBETTER, DAVID H.; MAHONEY, MAURICE J.; PERGAMENT, EUGENE; SIMPSON, JOE LEIGH; BLACK, SUSAN; and WAPNER, RONALD J. 1992. "A Randomized Comparison of Transcervical and Transabdominal Chorionic Villus Sampling." *New England Journal of Medicine* 327, no. 9:594–598.

MERKATZ, IRWIN R.; NITOWSKY, HAROLD M.; MACRI, JAMES N.; and JOHNSON, WALTER E. 1984. "An Association Between Low Maternal Serum Alpha-Fetoprotein and Fetal Chromosomal Abnormalities." *American Journal of Obstetrics and Gynecology* 148, no. 7:886–894.

NATIONAL INSTITUTE OF CHILD HEALTH AND HUMAN DEVELOPMENT NATIONAL REGISTRY FOR AMNIOCENTESIS STUDY GROUP. 1976. "Midtrimester Amniocentesis for Prenatal Diagnosis: Safety and Accuracy." *Journal of the American Medical Association* 236, no. 13:1471–1476.

RHOADS, GEORGE G.; JACKSON, LAIRD G.; SCHLESSELMAN, SARAH E.; DE LA CRUZ, FELIX F.; DESNICK, ROBERT J.; MITCHELL, GOLBUS S.; LEDBETTER, DAVID H.; LUBS, HERBERT A.; MAHONEY, MAURICE J.; PERGAMENT, EUGENE; SIMPSON, JOE LEIGH; CARPENTER, ROBERT J.; ELIAS, SHERMAN; GINSBERG, NORMAN A.; GOLDBERG, JAMES D.; HOBBINS, JOHN C.; LYNCH, LAUREN; SHIONO, PATRICIA H.; WAPNER, RONALD J.; and ZACHARY, JULIA M. 1989. "The Safety and Efficacy of Chorionic Villus Sampling for Early Prenatal Diagnosis of Cytogenetic Abnormalities." *New England Journal of Medicine* 320, no. 10:609–617.

ROMERO, ROBERTO; JEANTY, PHILLIPÊ; REECE, E. ALBERT; GRANNUM, PETER; BRACKEN, MICHAEL; BERKOWITZ, RICHARD; and HOBBINS, JOHN C. 1985. "Sonographically Monitored Amniocentesis to Decrease Intraoperative Complications." *Obstetrics and Gynecology* 65, no. 3: 426–430.

ROMERO, ROBERTO; PILU, GIANLUIGI; JEANTY, PHILLIPÊ; GHIDINI, ALESSANDRO; and HOBBINS, JOHN C., eds. 1988. *Prenatal Diagnosis of Congenital Anomalies.* Norwalk, Conn.: Appleton & Lange.

STEELE, MARK W., and BERG, W. ROY, JR. 1966. "Chromosome Analysis of Human Amniotic Fluid Cells." *Lancet* 1, no. 7434:383–385.

STENE, JON; STENE, EEVA; and MIKKELSEN, MARGARETA. 1984. "Risk for Chromosome Abnormality at Amniocentesis Following a Child with a Non-Inherited Chromosome Aberration." *Prenatal Diagnosis* 4 (spec. 155): 81–95.

WALD, NICHOLAS J.; CUCKLE, HOWARD S.; DNESEM, JAMES W.; NANCHAHAL, KIRAN; ROYSTON, PATRICK; HADDON, JAMES E.; KNIGHT, GEORGE J.; PALOMAKI, GLENN E.; and CANICK, JACOB A. 1988. "Maternal Serum Screening for Down Syndrome in Early Pregnancy." *British Medical Journal* 297, no. 6653:883–887.

III. NEWBORN SCREENING

Phenylketonuria (PKU) is a genetic disease that, if undetected and untreated, can lead to often severe mental retardation. Each parent of the affected child carries a single PKU gene in his or her sex cells, giving the parents a one-in-four chance in every pregnancy of conceiving a child with this recessively inherited disorder. Carrier status is not harmful to the parents. The affected condition of the child, however, produces a biochemical defect in the body's ability to metabolize phenylalanine, an amino acid essential to nutrition. The result is a markedly increased level of phenylalanine and brain damage due to this accumulation or to an organic by-product of the body's abnormal biochemical processing of phenylalanine (Scriver, 1990).

The course of PKU can be altered by treating with a special diet low in biochemical and clinical phenylalanine, which controls the biochemical abnormalities (Hudson, 1970; Smith, 1970). Nevertheless, when this diet begins after mental retardation is present, the mental retardation cannot be reversed.

The need to initiate diet before mental retardation appears led to newborn screening for PKU. This was developed in the early 1960s by Robert Guthrie (Guthrie and Ada, 1963) as a test to measure phenylalanine in a dried blood specimen. The specimen was collected by pricking the newborn's heel with a lance and blotting the drops of blood on filter paper. These dried blood spots were sent to a laboratory for testing. This process resulted in the rapid and early diagnosis of PKU in the infant and could be followed quickly by initiation of the diet. Soon after development of the test, all fifty states in the United States and many countries throughout the world began routine screening for PKU in newborn infants (Therrel, 1987). In this early period, mistakes were made in a general rush toward newborn screening. A 1975 report of the National Research Council's Committee for the Study of Errors of Inborn Metabolism concluded that "hindsight reveals that screening programs for phenylketonuria were instituted before the validity and effectiveness of all aspects of treatment, including appropriate dietary treatment, were thoroughly tested" (p. 2).

Biomedical research led to tests and treatment for other genetic and partially genetic disorders besides PKU and these were gradually added to mandatory screening programs (Seashore, 1990). Among these disorders were (1) galactosemia, a disorder affecting the body's ability to process galactose, which comes from the lactose of milk; (2) congenital hypothyroidism, an endocrine disorder that results from aberrant development or function of the thyroid gland; and (3) sickle-cell disease, a genetic abnormality in hemoglobin, a component of human blood, that can cause serious crises and death even before one year of age. Most states have laws that require newborn screening for one or more of these three disorders. Some states also screen for other rare genetic disorders of metabolism. The American Academy of Pediatrics (1992) recommends that blood samples be taken from all infants prior to their discharge from the hospital; most states assign this duty to the hospital.

Technical and ethical issues

More than four million babies are born in the United States each year. Public policy, embodied in state laws and Federal programs (National Institutes of Health, 1987), increasingly recognizes that newborn screening tests play an important role in safeguarding child health and development. The ethical principle at work behind such laws obligates society and its members to prevent harm wherever possible. Newborn screening is the use of knowledge to prevent serious harm in cases where parents may be completely unaware of their genetic risks. In this framework, newborn genetic screening is a medical act in the context of preventive medicine, intended to be followed by medical intervention for the benefit of the newborn. A medical act creates a relationship with obligations between the participants, that is, the states, laboratories, physicians, and the parents (Knoppers and Laberge, 1990).

Technical issues. Challenging technical and ethical issues arise in newborn screening. Technical issues begin with accuracy and precision of testing. Large numbers of samples need to be tested quickly and inexpensively. Whether the laboratories where samples are tested should be centralized or dispersed depends on population size and density; it also depends on the availability of experts to perform and interpret several tests requiring state-of-the-art knowledge in measuring metabolites (PKU) and enzymes (galactosemia), and identifying proteins (sickle hemoglobin). Other important technical issues involve reporting, tracking, and monitoring the outcomes of treatment. States and nations differ as to whether all results or only abnormal results must be reported to attending physicians. Variation also exists in whether reports must be sent to the child's pediatrician, the physician in the hospital who authorized the test, or the hospital itself.

States also vary in strategies to track affected children, whose families may move several times. Following those treated for PKU through their reproductive years is important, because a female treated for PKU needs to resume the diet therapy before becoming pregnant, or the fetus can suffer serious brain damage (Koch et al., 1993). Some states have PKU and other registries, but some do not. The outcomes of treatment need to be monitored to assure a high degree of certainty that newborn screening is effective and to develop new treatment strategies. These outcome studies also broaden knowledge of these genetic disorders.

Ethical issues.   Ethical problems in newborn screening have to do with access, informed consent of parents, confidentiality and privacy, and the interests of third parties. Unfairness of access results from policy and resource allocation decisions. Where a child happens to be born may determine whether an infant is screened for a given disorder. Attaining an adequate and ethically valid informed consent is a complex process under any circumstances, but especially in the context of labor and childbirth, with their attendant anxieties and pressures. The state of Maryland tried to adopt a voluntary ("opt-in") approach to newborn screening, with a required informed-consent process for parents (Holtzman et al., 1983). Other states take either a strictly mandatory approach or legally permit an informed refusal ("opt-out") to newborn screening; if parents are advised of this option during the perinatal period, they may choose not to participate.

The privacy and confidentiality of the parents and the child need to be respected, a difficult task in the context of computerized record keeping and electronic access to information. Third parties with legitimate interests include both family members and insurers expected to cover treatment costs resulting from a disorder discovered through a screening program. Other family members who may be unaware of their genetic risks have a need to know that cannot be given priority unless the parents choose to cooperate and release the information. Agencies responsible for tracking affected children must zealously guard the privacy of these children.

The future of newborn screening

As the Human Genome Project unfolds, difficult ethical and public policy challenges will face newborn screening programs (Seashore, 1991). The blood spots on Guthrie cards are an excellent source of DNA that can be easily stored. New approaches to DNA testing will make it possible to identify the molecular basis for many more genetic conditions and also whether the child is a carrier of recessive genes. Issues of privacy will become increasingly significant because so much more can be known about each individual. Some of the information available will not predict disease but will bear upon such sensitive areas as susceptibility to diseases and personality traits.

Ought societies encourage research in these directions, especially in the case of conditions that cannot now be treated or are only of indirect or no immediate benefit to the child? Such questions are appropriate for professionals involved with newborn screening (Knoppers and Laberge, 1990) and at the highest level of national bioethics consideration. The answers potentially affect the well-being of every child screened at birth.

Margaretta R. Seashore

Directly related to this article are the other articles in this entry: Preimplantation diagnosis, prenatal diagnosis, carrier screening, predictive and workplace testing, legal issues, *and* ethical issues. *Also directly related to this article are the entries* Gene Therapy; Genetic Counseling; Genetic Engineering; Genetics and Environment in Human Health; Genetics and Human Behavior; Genetics and Human Self-Understanding; Genetics and the Law; Genetics and Racial Minorities; Genome Mapping and Sequencing; Eugenics; Medical Genetics; *and* Infants, *especially the article on* medical aspects and issues in the care of infants. *For a further discussion of topics mentioned in this article, see the entries* Confidentiality; Family; Harm; Laboratory Testing; Privacy in Health Care; Public Health; *and* Public Policy and Bioethics. *For a discussion of related ideas, see the entries* Abuse, Interpersonal, *article on* child abuse; Autonomy; Beneficence; Conflict of Interest; Fetus; Future Generations, Obligations to; Health Promotion and Health Education; Health Screening and Testing in the Public-Health Context; Information Disclosure; *and* Life.

Bibliography

American Academy of Pediatrics. Committee on Genetics. 1992. "Issues in Newborn Screening." *Pediatrics* 89, no. 2:345–349.

Guthrie, Robert, and Ada, Susi. 1963. "A Simple Phenylalanine Method for Detecting Phenylketonuria in Large Populations of Newborn Infants." *Pediatrics* 32, no. 3:338–343.

Holtzman, Neil A.; Faden, Ruth R.; Chwalow, A. Judith; and Horn, Susan D. 1983. "Effect of Informed Parental Consent on Mothers' Knowledge of Newborn Screening." *Pediatrics* 72, no. 6:807–812.

Hudson, Frederick P.; Mordaunt, Virginia L.; and Leahy, Irene. 1970. "Evaluation of Treatment Begun in First Three Months of Life in 184 Cases of Phenylketonuria." *Archives of Diseases in Childhood* 45, no. 239:5–12.

KNOPPERS, BARTHA MARIA, and LABERGE, CLAUDE M., eds. 1990. *Genetic Screening: From Newborns to DNA Typing.* Amsterdam: Excerpta Medica.

KOCH, RICHARD; LEVY, HARVEY L.; MATALON, REUBEN; ROUSE, BOBBYE; HANLEY, WILLIAM; and AZEN, COLLEEN. 1993. "The North American Collaborative Study of Maternal Phenylketonuria." *American Journal of Diseases of Childhood* 147:1224–1230.

NATIONAL INSTITUTES OF HEALTH. OFFICE OF MEDICAL APPLICATIONS OF RESEARCH. 1987. *Newborn Screening for Sickle Cell Disease and Other Hemoglobinopathies,* vol. 6, no. 9. Bethesda, Md.: Author.

NATIONAL RESEARCH COUNCIL. COMMITTEE FOR THE STUDY OF INBORN ERRORS OF METABOLISM. 1975. *Genetic Screening: Programs, Principles, and Research.* Washington, D.C.: National Academy of Sciences.

SCRIVER, CHARLES R.; KAUFMAN, SEYMOUR; and WOO, SAVIO L. C. 1990. "The Hyperphenylalaninemias." In *The Metabolic Basis of Inherited Diseases,* 6th ed., pp. 495–546. Edited by Charles R. Scriver, Arthur L. Beaudet, William S. Sly, and David Valle. New York: McGraw-Hill.

SEASHORE, MARGARETTA R. 1990. "Neonatal Screening for Inborn Errors of Metabolism: Update." *Seminars in Perinatology* 14, no. 5:431–438.

SEASHORE, MARGARETTA R., and WALSH-VOCKLEY, CATHERINE. 1991. "Introduction: New Technologies for Genetic and Newborn Screening." *Yale Journal of Biology and Medicine* 64, no. 1:3–7.

SMITH, ISABEL, and WOLFF, O. H. 1974. "Natural History of Phenylketonuria and Influence of Early Treatment." *Lancet* 2, no. 7880:540–544.

THERREL, B. L., ed. 1987. *Advances in Neonatal Screening.* Amsterdam: Excerpta Medica.

IV. CARRIER SCREENING

Carriers are people in whom one copy of a gene varies from the normal. Since carriers also have one normal copy of the same gene, they do not ordinarily exhibit symptoms of a genetic disorder. Sometimes the variant (mutant) gene is beneficial for the carrier. Having one gene that causes some, but not all, red blood cells to take a sickle shape protects the carrier from malaria. Having two such genes, however, leads to a severe, painful blood disorder called sickle-cell anemia.

There are two types of carriers. First, carriers of genes for autosomal recessive (AR) disorders have one normal and one variant gene at the same place on one of the forty-four autosomes (chromosomes common to both sexes). The normal gene takes precedence over the variant gene, so the carrier has no symptoms. The carrier can transmit only one copy of the variant gene to children. The children cannot have the disorder unless they receive a second copy of the variant gene from the other parent. If two carriers mate, each of their children has a one-in-four chance of having the disorder. Examples of AR conditions are cystic fibrosis (CF), which

affects lungs and digestion, greatly shortens life expectancy, and is found primarily among whites of European descent; sickle-cell anemia, a blood disorder with severe, painful crises, found primarily among people of African descent, though it also occurs in Mediterraneans and Asians; beta-thalassemia, a blood disorder causing anemia and early death, found among people of Mediterranean, African, and Asian descent; and Tay-Sachs disease, a disorder leading to profound mental retardation and death before age five, found primarily among people of eastern European (Ashkenazic) Jewish descent. In the United States, an estimated one in twenty-five whites carries a gene for CF, one in ten or eleven African-Americans carries sickle-cell trait, and one in thirty-one Ashkenazic Jews carries a gene for Tay-Sachs disease. Beta-thalassemia is a major world health problem. In Cyprus, one person in eight is a carrier, and in Sardinia, one couple in eighty is a carrier-carrier couple with a one-in-four risk, with each pregnancy, of having an affected child.

Second, carriers of X-linked recessive disorders are women with a variant gene on one of their two X (sex-determining) chromosomes. The woman, although not ordinarily affected herself, has a 50 percent chance of transmitting the variant gene to each child. Daughters receive a normal gene on the X chromosome from their father and are not usually affected. Since males have only one X chromosome, sons who inherit one copy of the variant gene will have the disorder. Examples of X-linked disorders are Duchenne muscular dystrophy, which usually confines a boy to a wheelchair by the age of ten and leads to death by the mid-teens, and fragile X syndrome, a leading cause of mental retardation.

The stated purpose of carrier testing and carrier screening is to inform potential parents of their genetic status so that they can make informed reproductive decisions. A couple who are both carriers of an AR disorder may decide not to marry, or to adopt, to use artificial insemination by a noncarrier donor, to have prenatal diagnosis and selectively abort affected fetuses, or simply to take their one-in-four chance of having a child with the disorder. A woman carrying an X-linked disorder might consider adopting, using an egg from a noncarrier donor, using a surrogate mother, having prenatal diagnosis and selective abortion, or taking her chances of having an affected son.

From a public-health point of view, especially in nations with national health insurance, the purpose of screening is to avoid the births of children with serious, costly, or untreatable disorders. Cost–benefit calculations are used to justify national screening programs.

Testing differs from screening. The word "testing" usually describes procedures performed at the request of individuals or families known to be at high risk, such as the siblings of persons with CF. Testing should always be voluntary (Wertz and Fletcher, 1989). Screening is a public-health concept. It applies to entire populations or to subsets of populations (e.g., pregnant women, newborns, or job applicants) without a known family history of a disorder. Screening may be voluntary or mandatory. The U.S. President's Commission (1983) recommended that all screening be voluntary, with the exception of newborns if, and only if, early treatment will benefit the newborn. Some believe that newborns should be screened, in the absence of available treatment, primarily to identify and inform parents of their carrier status before they conceive another child. Any such screening should be voluntary and should be carried out only after full information and informed consent. Mandatory or routine screening solely to identify carriers could lead to coercive eugenics.

Ordinarily no benefit is gained from testing or screening children for carrier status before they reach reproductive age. Testing at younger ages can lead to stigmatization and a poor self-image, or test results may be forgotten. Testing is best carried out in the context of reproduction, but preferably before marriage or pregnancy, so that people will have the maximum range of choices.

Testing and screening should be preceded by full information about the disorder and the various decisions, including the possibility of abortion, that an individual or couple may face if found to carry the gene. Screening in the absence of full information and support from the community can lead to misunderstanding and to accusations of genocide. The sickle-cell screening introduced in the United States in the early 1970s as the first public-health genetics program is an example of a poorly designed endeavor with little effect on reproductive decisions. In contrast, a Tay-Sachs screening program introduced with the support of Jewish community leaders led to 90 percent reduction in the births of children with Tay-Sachs, mostly through use of prenatal diagnosis (U.S. President's Commission, 1983; U.S. Congress, Office of Technology Assessment, 1992a). Orthodox Jewish communities, which opposed abortion but favored arranged marriages, developed a system for premarital carrier testing that would enable a rabbi to declare a match unsuitable if both persons were carriers while preserving individuals' anonymity. Carrier screening programs for beta-thalassemia in Cyprus and Sardinia and among Cypriots in London have reduced the births of affected children by 90 to 97 percent, largely through prenatal diagnosis (Cao et al., 1989; Angastiniotis, 1990; Modell and Petrou, 1988). Most people in these communities had seen children with thalassemia and wished to avoid it. The Greek Orthodox and Roman Catholic churches, while not approving abortion, did not condemn women who did not carry affected fetuses to term. In Cyprus, the church requires carrier testing before marriage but does not prohibit marriages between carriers.

In the next few years, CF testing of pregnant women will probably become routine. CF carrier screening in the general population, however, could be introduced only after extensive education of the target population, and only after ongoing pilot screening programs demonstrated public interest and lack of adverse effects. It is also possible that new treatments for CF will diminish public interest.

Fragile X may be the next major carrier test offered. Eventually carrier testing may become possible for predispositions to cancer and heart disease (Holtzman, 1989). These are multifactorial diseases (partly genetic, partly environmental), so risks will be less exact than with AR or X-linked disorders.

Protection of privacy is the primary ethical issue. Health insurers have misused information to deny coverage to families at risk of having children with costly disorders (U.S. Congress, Office of Technology Assessment, 1992b, 1992c). Employers have required carrier testing (notably for sickle-cell trait) as a precondition of hiring, even though there is usually no proven link between carrier status and susceptibility to occupational hazards (U.S. Congress, Office of Technology Assessment, 1990). Carrier testing has been applied disproportionately to ethnic groups new to an industry (Draper, 1991). Sometimes carriers become objects of discrimination. In the 1970s the U.S. Air Force Academy rejected candidates with sickle-cell trait. The Italian army rejects carriers of beta-thalassemia. To avoid discrimination, access to information by insurers, government agencies, and employers should be forbidden by law.

Carriers have ethical obligations of disclosure to family members. They should tell close blood relatives that the relatives may also be carriers. If a couple intends to have children, the carrier should tell the spouse or partner. If a carrier refuses to tell a partner and they intend to have children, the professional should be legally permitted to inform the partner.

ANTONIO CAO

Directly related to this article are the other articles in this entry: PREIMPLANTATION DIAGNOSIS, PRENATAL DIAGNOSIS, NEWBORN SCREENING, PREDICTIVE AND WORKPLACE TESTING, LEGAL ISSUES, *and* ETHICAL ISSUES. *Also directly related are the entries* FUTURE GENERATIONS, OBLIGATIONS TO; HEALTH SCREENING AND TESTING IN THE PUBLIC-HEALTH CONTEXT; *and* MEDICAL GENETICS. *For a further discussion of topics mentioned in this article, see the entries* CONFIDENTIALITY; EUGENICS; GENETIC COUNSELING; *and* GENETICS AND RACIAL MINORITIES. *For a discussion of related ideas, see the entries*

ABORTION; HEALTH-CARE FINANCING; RACE AND RACISM; *and* REPRODUCTIVE TECHNOLOGIES, *articles on* ARTIFICIAL INSEMINATION, *and* SURROGACY.

Bibliography

ANGASTINIOTIS, M. 1990. "Cyprus: Thalassemia Programme." *Lancet* 336, no. 8723:1119–1120.

CAO, ANTONIO. 1987. "Results of Programmes for Antenatal Detection of Thalassemia in Reducing the Incidence of the Disorder." *Blood Reviews* 1, no. 3:169–176.

CAO, ANTONIO; ROSATELLI, C.; GALANELLO R.; MONNI, G.; OLLA, G.; COSSU, P.; and RISTALDI, M. S. 1989. "The Prevention of Thalassemia in Sardinia." *Clinical Genetics* 36, no. 5:277–285.

DRAPER, ELAINE. 1991. *Risky Business: Genetic Testing and Exclusionary Practices in the Hazardous Workplace.* Cambridge: At the University Press. Describes how carrier testing has been used to exclude racial and ethnic minorities from industries. Employers favor preemployment testing; unions oppose it.

HOLTZMAN, NEIL A. 1989. *Proceed with Caution: Predicting Genetic Risks in the Recombinant DNA Era.* Baltimore: Johns Hopkins University Press. Describes scientific and societal aspects of increased use of genetic testing in the future, especially for common diseases such as cancer. Comprehensive and insightful.

MODELL, BERNADETTE, and PETROU, M. 1988. "Review of Control Programs and Future Trends in the United Kingdom." *Birth Defects* 23(5B):433–442. March of Dimes Birth Defects Foundation. Describes thalassemia carrier testing among London Cypriots.

U.S. CONGRESS. OFFICE OF TECHNOLOGY ASSESSMENT. 1990. *Genetic Monitoring and Screening in the Workplace.* OTA-BA-455. Washington, D.C.: U.S. Government Printing Office.

———. 1992a. *Cystic Fibrosis and DNA Tests: Implications of Carrier Screening.* OTA-BA-532. Washington, D.C.: U.S. Government Printing Office.

———. 1992b. *Genetic Counseling and Cystic Fibrosis Carrier Screening: Results of a Survey.* OTA-BP-BA-97. Washington, D.C.: U.S. Government Printing Office.

———. 1992c. *Genetic Tests and Health Insurance: Results of a Survey.* OTA-BP-BA-98. Washington, D.C.: U.S. Government Printing Office.

U.S. PRESIDENT'S COMMISSION FOR THE STUDY OF ETHICAL PROBLEMS IN MEDICINE AND BIOMEDICAL AND BEHAVIORAL RESEARCH. 1983. *Screening and Counseling for Genetic Conditions: A Report on Screening, Counseling, and Education Programs.* Washington, D.C.: U.S. Government Printing Office.

WERTZ, DOROTHY C., and FLETCHER, JOHN C. "An International Survey of Attitudes of Medical Geneticists Toward Mass Screening and Access to Results." *Public Health Reports* 194:35–44.

WERTZ, DOROTHY C.; JANES, SALLY R.; ROSENFIELD, JANET M.; and ERBE, RICHARD W. 1992. "Attitudes Toward the Prenatal Diagnosis of Cystic Fibrosis: Factors in Decision-making Among Affected Families." *American Journal of Human Genetics* 50:1077–1085. A study of 227 New England families reports that attitudes toward abortion were the strongest predictors of use of carrier testing.

V. PREDICTIVE AND WORKPLACE TESTING

The origin of the concept of genetic testing of workers and job applicants is generally attributed to J. B. S. Haldane, who wrote in 1938 in *Heredity and Politics* that the prevention of potter's bronchitis might be achieved by excluding from such work those at special risk to develop the condition. In the 1960s, Herbert Stockinger, then at the National Institute for Occupational Safety and Health, published several articles speculating about genetic traits that might predispose exposed workers to greater risk. When several large companies responded to employee requests for on-site company-sponsored sickle-cell trait-screening programs in the late 1970s, newspaper stories highlighted worker worries that those found to have sickle-cell trait would be transferred out of certain types of jobs to lower paying jobs, or forced out of work altogether.

There is justifiable concern that genetic testing and labeling of individuals may lead to discrimination in hiring, loss of job security, and even "a biologic underclass" (Nelkin and Tancredi, 1989). Furthermore, there is fear that emphasis on the susceptibility of some workers and removal of such workers might substitute for the improvement of workplace conditions for all, whereas both U.S. regulations and English and American common law require employers to provide "a safe and healthful workplace." The Occupational Safety and Health Act of 1970 instructs the Occupational Safety and Health Administration (OSHA) to set health standards so that, within technological feasibility, no worker, even if exposed at the level of the standard for a full working lifetime, would suffer any adverse effect.

Types of genetic testing in the workplace

Genetic testing may be undertaken in the work setting for several reasons. The first is for diagnosis of the underlying cause of a specific medical condition. The ethical imperative for such testing is similar to testing in the differential diagnosis of any other condition and may be highlighted by the poignant question, "Why me, doctor? You say I'm ill due to exposures on the job, but I'm no less careful than anyone else, and no one else has this problem. Why am I affected?"

The second kind of testing is called monitoring of exposures and early effects, or genetic toxicology, the study of effects of exposures on the genes. The genetic traits are biomarkers for specific job-related exposures and effects. Such genetic markers are a subset of markers that include measures of the concentrations of workplace chemicals, nutritional status, smoking status, lung function, and liver function. Such testing is required by law for those known to be exposed to lead, for example. The usefulness of some genetic tests has been investigated in exposed workers; both chromosomal changes and mutation rates in blood lymphocytes have been studied in relation to irradiation and chemical exposures on the job. This type of testing is only as good as the reliability and validity of the test and its appropriateness to the setting, as is true for many nongenetic tests.

The third type of genetic testing is called screening, to detect inherited predispositions to disease or to other adverse responses from otherwise well-tolerated exposures related to the job. This field is called ecogenetics, addressing the common interaction of inherited and environmental factors in disease. There are numerous relevant examples. Some genetic traits directly affect the activation or the detoxification of chemicals entering the body. Other inherited variation affects the sites of action of chemicals in the cells of particular organs, like the kidneys, liver, or lungs. The examples include chemicals prescribed as pharmaceutical agents, pesticides, air pollutants, food additives or contaminants, and certain infectious agents, such as malaria organisms. The test may measure the gene itself, an approach that is certain to grow with the new technologies and extensive mapping of genes in the Human Genome Project. Or the test may measure protein products of the gene, namely specific enzymes, receptors, binding proteins, or hemoglobin. The DNA test in a person should need to be done only once, since the genes do not change. The protein tests determine the gene expression, or phenotype, which may change over time, depending upon the pattern of gene expression in various tissues and the role of chemical inducers or other modifiers.

Finally, genetic screening might be directed at determining predisposition to such common diseases as heart disease, high blood pressure, diabetes, cancers, kidney disease, and nervous system or behavioral disorders. Because employers in this country's medical-care system bear most of the high and rapidly rising cost of employment-based health insurance, they have a strong incentive to reduce their financial risks from catastrophic or chronic illnesses. Employers may do so either by helping workers practice disease prevention and health promotion or by not hiring or not retaining workers with high-risk profiles for such illnesses, or both. It is certain that the identification of numerous gene markers for predisposition to common diseases from the spinoffs of the Human Genome Project will have the greatest application in this fourth type of testing.

So long as employers or individuals are risk-rated for health insurance costs, employers and insurance companies will seek people with lower projected health costs to employ and insure. Physicians and genetic counselors are all too familiar with cases in which insurance companies have canceled, restricted, or denied life, health, disability, mortgage, or auto insurance for patients or family members. Many of these decisions were ill informed. Some were based on carrier status rather than on homozygous inheritance of a recessive gene (a double dose of the abnormal gene carried by both carrier parents). Others were based on textbook descriptions of the most severe manifestations of quite variable dominant conditions. Sometimes there was confusion of genetic and nongenetic causes of similar-sounding diagnoses. The insurer has little incentive to take the risk of any uncertainty and generally will not be concerned about losing occasional clients or families.

Types of genetic monitoring in the workplace. These tests identify and quantify chromosomal aberrations, sister chromatid exchange frequencies (a measure of chromosome repair), or mutations in blood cells or sperm. As summarized by the Office of Technology Assessment of the U.S. Congress (1983, 1990), chromosome tests have been performed with workers exposed to ionizing radiation, arsenic, benzene, epichlorohydrin, ethylene oxide, phosphine, lead, cadmium, zinc, pesticides, and vinyl chloride monomer. Arsenic and benzene, as well as ionizing radiation, induce increased frequencies of long-lived chromosome aberrations, but chromosome methods are not sufficiently sensitive to be useful at low-dose exposures consistent with regulatory standards. There is an extensive literature with background values for abnormalities of chromosomes examined under the microscope per 100 cells in unexposed workers, for example from 0.1 to 3.0 for chromosome breaks, from 0.1 to 6.7 for breaks of a chromosome strand, and from 0.2 to 8.5 for any aberration. The ranges across studies are clearly quite wide, making studies of small numbers of exposed workers difficult to interpret.

Other kinds of tests can be used to monitor human exposure to mutation-causing agents (mutagens), either by measurement of the chemical or measurement of DNA damage presumably due to the chemical exposure. Mutagens have been measured in urine, feces, and blood. Some mutagens and carcinogens that combine chemically with DNA or with hemoglobin can be measured in blood cells. Germ cell damage can be tested in sperm. At the present time, little such monitoring is being done on a routine basis, due to the difficulties of validating and interpreting the results.

Genetic screening in the workplace. There is very little genetic testing and especially very little genetic screening being done to identify risks from specific chemical exposures in the workplace. In the 1960s and 1970s there was some screening for sickle-cell trait in African-Americans and for two other red-blood-cell traits (glucose-6-phosphate, dehydrogenase (G6PD) deficiency, and thalassemia trait) that were and are thought to predispose individuals to anemia ("low blood") upon chemical exposure in those with the inherited trait, especially in these examples, people of Mediterranean ancestry. For these well-characterized traits and several other clearly inherited traits listed below, it is essential to ask a series of logical questions: What is the evidence that specific workplace exposures put people with the particular trait at higher risk of some illness? What is the prevalence of the trait in various populations? How reliable and inexpensive are the tests for detection of the trait? What is the relationship between the trait and a particular disease? What proportion of the risk of the disease is accounted for by the trait? Are there differences between women and men? How significant is the "disease"? How treatable or reversible? Is the testing complicated by multiple forms of the gene? In general, we don't know nearly enough yet to answer most of these questions (Holtzman, 1989).

We then need to ask which chemicals might be of special hazard in relation to genetic differences among people. Some clues emerge from chemicals used as prescribed medications. We know that people receiving certain drugs have different plasma concentrations, different metabolic pathways, and different responses in the body due to inherited differences in metabolism or at target sites in the body's cells. Chemicals to which we are exposed by air or water pollution or food contamination or workplace activities may be chemically related to these drugs and may have analogous variation in effects in people.

Red-blood-cell disorders. Many medicines can cause breakdown of red blood cells (hemolytic anemia) in men of Mediterranean ancestry (such as Greeks, Italians, and Jews). This phenomenon can be traced to a deficiency of an enzyme coded for by a gene on the X chromosome. (Women have two X chromosomes and are protected by one normal gene; men have only one X chromosome, so they show the effects of an X chromosome recessive gene.) Many substances in industry are known to cause hemolytic changes when tested on blood cells in the laboratory and were thought to present undue risk to G6PD-deficient men. However, only a few compounds seem to have any effect in people (TNT in explosives, naphthalene in mothballs, naladixic acid in an antibiotic), and these have not been investigated extensively.

Sickle-cell trait was long considered to predispose to destruction of red blood cells and painful sickle crises under conditions of oxygen deprivation, as at high altitude without an oxygen supply. This presumption was based on studies of sickle-trait cells outside the body in the laboratory and a report of a death in an African-American soldier in mountain climbing maneuvers. The U.S. Air Force used such information in the early 1970s to exclude African-Americans with sickle-cell trait from flight training. Since such training is integral to the program at the U.S. Air Force Academy, African-Americans were excluded from enrollment at the Air Force Academy. No risk assessment was performed to justify such decisions. In 1980, the Air Force civilian leadership in the Carter administration overruled such practices after a full scientific review. In 1981, the Reagan administration reinstated severe restrictions, tied arbitrarily to the percent of the hemoglobin that is sickle-type hemoglobin in men with sickle-cell trait. Somewhat similar presumptions have been made about risks to army personnel in high-altitude maneuvers. Similarly, industrial chemical exposures have been shown to cause adverse effects at a higher rate in men or women with sickle trait.

Rare individuals with extreme deficiency of a certain red-blood-cell enzyme (NADH dehydrogenase) are known to be vulnerable to cyanosis ("turning purple"), due to oxidation of the iron atom in hemoglobin. Carriers of a single dose of this gene are at increased risk for cyanosis, headaches, and shortness of breath from certain drugs. Though the same susceptibility probably applies to industrial exposures to related chemicals, no industrial exposures that cause cyanosis have been linked specifically to this inherited trait.

Traits influencing cancer risk. Enzymes known to activate certain chemicals to become cancer causing, and other enzymes known to detoxify such chemicals, have common variants in human populations. These variants are associated with differences in function and therefore in levels of the carcinogens from any given dose or exposure. Four such enzyme systems will be described briefly here.

A common variation of an enzyme in the liver (N-acetyl transferase) accounts for marked differences in blood levels of the antituberculosis drug, isoniazid, after standard doses. Half the Caucasian and African-American populations have the type of that enzyme associated with higher levels of still-active drug and a propensity to adverse effects. This same detoxification system also metabolizes several chemicals known to cause cancer of the urinary bladder (beta-naphthylamine, benzidine, and 4-amino biphenyl). These chemicals were mainstays of the chemical dyes industry, and many bladder cancers have occurred in former workers in that industry. People who have the low-activity form of the enzyme have been proved to be at higher risk for bladder cancer, as predicted. Until recently, testing required administration of a sulfa drug, isoniazid, or caffeine and measurement of metabolites in blood and urine; now a DNA probe assay is available. For the thousands of workers who were exposed in past decades, testing might be helpful.

Among the dozens of related enzymes called cytochrome P450 monooxygenases, one specific P450 is responsible for marked variation in metabolism of more than thirty pharmaceuticals. So called "extensive metabolizers" are at higher risk of lung cancer, presumably due to greater activation of chemicals in cigarette smoke. No ties to industrial exposures have yet been identified. A DNA probe test is now available.

All cells in the body have enzymes called glutathione-S-transferases (GSTs); they detoxify some of the same compounds that are activated by the P450 enzymes. A common variant of GST-lacking activity appears to make those people more susceptible to smoking-induced lung cancers. Both enzyme and DNA tests are available. Again, there is no industrial exposure yet related to this common inherited trait of partial enzyme deficiency.

Susceptibility to a common pesticide, parathion, offers another example. Parathion is activated in the liver by the P450 enzymes and then detoxified in the blood by a circulating plasma enzyme. About half of the Caucasian population has a form of the detoxifying enzyme with low activity. For similar exposures, pesticide applicators or nearby residents with low activity would be expected to be at higher risk for symptoms of pesticide poisoning and would take longer to recover. Testing is feasible.

Proposed criteria for prudent development of job-related genetic tests

Development and validation of genetic tests for job-related exposures must be carried out in the context of fully responsible compliance with required and desirable engineering and process controls on exposures so as to protect all workers. Such control of exposures will always be necessary for the many various predispositions for which no tests have been developed anyway. Research and careful, open decision making must precede routine screening. Research can be undertaken only with the full understanding by all parties of what will be done, what might be learned, who will have access to the results and who will not, and what criteria might be applied if screening were to be considered later. In general, involvement of third-party research and testing organizations, including university research groups, is far preferable to research undertaken by the employer or insurer. The employee must have confidence that individual results will be protected from the employer and insurer. A widely cited set of criteria for potential screening follows (Omenn, 1982):

1. validation of a cost-effective test, with full delineation of false-positives, false-negatives, and predictive value of the test for the trait and for the associated disease state;
2. prevalence of the trait in at least 5 percent of the target population in order to warrant undertaking testing in what are generally rather small worksite populations;
3. a 3 to 10 times increased risk of the disease in those with the trait;
4. full agreement on third-party conduct of the testing, with anticipation of the various uses of the results;
5. confidence that management, with cooperation of labor, is controlling exposures at least to the regulatory requirements and, further, to the extent technologically and economically feasible.

Ethical implications of predictive genetic testing in the workplace

Most at jeopardy in workplace genetic predictive testing is the autonomy of the worker. Workers often distrust the motives and competence of the employer or the insurer to make disinterested, fair decisions about the relevance and significance of a "predisposing trait." On what scale is the predisposition to be judged? How is the employer to defend exclusionary decisions, even taken in the name of protecting the worker, when the motive may include also protecting the employer from higher medical or workers' compensation costs? How can the employer claim to be acting fairly when there are surely many other predisposing inherited traits not yet discovered, or not presently testable? And yet, what is the employer's defense when plaintiffs' attorneys or the Occupational Health and Safety Administration may confront an employer with injured workers and ask, "Did you do all that you could, with available knowledge, to protect your workers and to identify and notify them of any undue risks?"

In order to meet a reasonable standard of beneficence or even nonmaleficence the employer should engage workers or their representatives at every step of considering, planning, organizing, conducting, and evaluating research aimed at developing any screening or predictive testing program. Industrywide studies will often be required; such a model was developed twenty years ago by the United Rubber Workers, several companies, and the schools of public health at Harvard and North Carolina. For more than twenty years the State of Washington's Department of Labor and Industries has worked with the State Labor Council, the Association of Washington Businesses, the State Medical Association, and the University of Washington School of Public Health to develop worksite investigations and share information broadly. These models provide a basis for genetic studies, but few have been done to date.

Because genetic traits often occur with different frequencies in different ethnic or racial populations, there is a political problem that certain types of tests might be associated with particular populations and be perceived to lead to possible stigmatization or economic disadvantage. In this article, examples have been cited involving predominantly African-Americans or those of Mediterranean ancestry. Discrimination against women has occurred in certain industries, such as lead battery plants, in efforts to protect against risk to fetuses of pregnant women. However, those companies were instructed by the courts that providing a safe and healthful workplace must include lowering exposures enough to be safe for pregnant women. Obviously, it is improper to consider all women potentially pregnant, or to require women to be infertile or sterilized in order to be "safe" from such exposures, since it is likely that risks to the women and to men, as well, are being neglected in the focus on the fetus. While we have cited some genetic conditions which might make men more likely to be susceptible than women, we have no well-established examples in which women would be at higher risk because of inherited traits that are more common in women than in men.

If companies offer to finance testing on a voluntary, confidential basis, they must persuade their employees that the third-party organization conducting the tests has the competence to do the work properly and the capacity to ensure confidentiality for the worker and for the worker's relatives, since genetic tests do give information that may be revealing about relatives. Otherwise, many of the requirements of relevance, significance, confidentiality, and proper interpretation for the individual apply to all kinds of medical tests, not just genetic tests. But too often the reduction in charges leads to more out-of-pocket cost to the patient, so the worker and the worker's family are in a difficult position. Workers are also at risk of losing their health insurance if the employer lays them off and of having difficulty getting new coverage if they do find another job. These issues, of course, are part of the overall national debate on reforming our medical-care system.

One of the elements of health reform involves challenging every individual to take better care of her or his health and to practice prevention. Predictive genetic testing is a modern tool for health promotion and disease prevention, identifying those who might be most helped by early diagnosis or primary prevention of specific diseases. Workers should not be denied convenient access to high-quality testing if they want such testing; however, such testing should be organized on a voluntary and confidential basis. Voluntary, confidential testing for HIV (the virus causing AIDS) would be a far more appropriate model than the employer-dominated testing for use/presence of illegal drugs.

If employment-based health-promotion programs expand, as projected, workers may even use collective bargaining to demand access to such services, financed by employers. Such voluntary services can be compatible with ethical principles of autonomy, beneficence, nonmaleficence, and justice, as well as legal precepts under the Occupational Safety and Health Act, the National Labor Relations Act, the Rehabilitation Act of 1973, and the Americans with Disabilities Act of 1990, as discussed by the U.S. Congress Office of Technology Assessment (1983, 1990) and the AAAS/ABA report (1992).

Conclusion

It is remarkable how little predictive genetic testing has been carried out in worksites or by employers. In fact, there may be relatively few situations in which the five criteria listed above can be met at present. The long-standing tension between labor and management, particularly in the United States, over responsibility for ensuring a safe and healthful workplace has made worker populations unattractive to researchers seeking to identify genetic traits of importance for specific chemical exposures on the job. Scientists do not want their research to be caught up in labor/management disputes, and occupational health and safety agencies have invested little or no funding in such research, even though the laws governing these agencies require them to set standards to protect even the least susceptible.

It is a fact that workplace exposures to known hazardous chemicals are being reduced quite dramatically. The variation in risk from such remaining exposures will come mostly from accidents causing unexpected higher exposures and from differences among people in responses to low-level exposures.

Meanwhile, there is a widening phenomenon of reliance by companies on third-party medical and counseling services. This practice will enhance the prospect that unions and individual workers can find a mechanism for testing of interest to the workers without fear that employers will gain access to the information and use the information arbitrarily in making hiring and promotion or retention decisions.

It is certain that genetic screening for common diseases will develop more rapidly than genetic screening for susceptibility to effects from workplace chemicals. DNA diagnostic tests are under development in many academic and biotechnology company laboratories. These tests aim to detect propensity to coronary heart disease, breast cancer, prostate cancer, lung cancer, manic depressive illness, high blood pressure, diabetes, and many other common conditions. Most of these conditions are associated with high medical-care costs. Cost containment may put a premium on proper use of such tests, with decisions being made jointly by employers and employees or their representatives.

GILBERT S. OMENN

Directly related to this article are the other articles in this entry, especially the articles on CARRIER SCREENING, LEGAL ISSUES, *and* ETHICAL ISSUES. *Also directly related is the entry* OCCUPATIONAL SAFETY AND HEALTH. *For a further discussion of topics mentioned in this article, see the entries* CONFIDENTIALITY; ECONOMIC CONCEPTS IN HEALTH CARE; GENETICS AND THE LAW; HAZARDOUS WASTES AND TOXIC SUBSTANCES; HEALTH-CARE FINANCING; HEALTH POLICY, *article on* POLITICS AND HEALTH CARE; *and* RISK. *For a discussion of related ideas, see the entries* AUTONOMY; BENEFICENCE; GENETICS AND RACIAL MINORITIES; GENOME MAPPING AND SEQUENCING; HEALTH PROMOTION AND HEALTH EDUCATION; HEALTH SCREENING AND TESTING IN THE PUBLIC-HEALTH CONTEXT; RACE AND RACISM; RESEARCH POLICY, *article on* SUBJECT SELECTION; *and* SEXISM.

Bibliography

AMERICAN ASSOCIATION FOR THE ADVANCEMENT OF SCIENCE/ AMERICAN BAR ASSOCIATION, NATIONAL CONFERENCE OF LAWYERS AND SCIENTISTS. 1992. *The Genome, Ethics and the Law: Issues in Genetic Testing.* A report of a conference on the ethical and legal implications of genetic testing. Washington, D.C.: American Association for the Advancement of Science.

HALDANE, J. B. S. 1938. *Heredity and Politics.* New York: Norton.

HOLTZMAN, NEIL A. 1989. *Proceed with Caution: Predicting Genetic Risks in the Recombinant DNA Era.* Baltimore: Johns Hopkins University Press.

MOTULSKY, ARNO G. 1978. "Bioethical Problems in Pharmacogenetics and Ecogenetics." *Human Genetics* suppl. 1:185–192.

NELKIN, DOROTHY, and TANCREDI, LAURENCE. 1989. *Dangerous Diagnostics: The Social Power of Biological Information.* New York: Basic Books.

OMENN, GILBERT S. 1982. "Predictive Identification of Hypersusceptible Individuals." *Journal of Occupational Medicine* 24, no. 5:369–374.

OMENN, GILBERT S.; OMIECINSKI, CURTIS J.; and EATON, DAVID E. 1990. "Eco-genetics of Chemical Carcinogens." In *Biotechnology and Human Genetic Predisposition to Disease,* pp. 81–93. Edited by Charles R. Cantor; C. Thomas Caskey; Leroy E. Hood; Daphne Kamely; and Gilbert S. Omenn. New York: Wiley-Liss.

STOKINGER, HERBERT E., and MOUNTAIN, JOHN T. 1963. "Tests for Hypersusceptibility to Hemolytic Chemicals." *Archives of Environmental Health* 6:57–64.

U.S. CONGRESS. OFFICE OF TECHNOLOGY ASSESSMENT. 1983. *The Role of Genetic Testing in the Prevention of Occupational Disease.* Washington, D.C.: U.S. Government Printing Office.

———. 1990. *Genetic Monitoring and Screening in the Workplace.* Washington, D.C.: U.S. Government Printing Office.

VI. LEGAL ISSUES

"Genetic screening" refers to programs designed to canvass populations of healthy individuals to identify those with genotypes that place them or their offspring at high risk for disease or defect. "Genetic testing" refers to diagnostic procedures offered to individuals or families who are at increased risk for developing specific disorders or for bearing affected children. This article provides an overview of U.S. law governing newborn screening, prenatal screening, carrier screening, and occupational screening programs; it then discusses access to genetic testing, malpractice, informed consent, confidentiality and disclosure issues, and special testing situations. It also discusses laws governing DNA forensic testing and the regulation of DNA forensic data banks.

Legal issues in genetic screening

Newborn screening. The vast majority of states require the screening of infants for treatable inborn errors of metabolism, particularly phenylketonuria (PKU) (Andrews, 1985). Although most states make such screening compulsory, many permit parental refusal on religious or other grounds. Some statutes explicitly make newborn screening voluntary, but it often is done without obtaining informed consent.

Mandatory newborn screening programs have not been constitutionally challenged, but they would probably be upheld based on the state's police power—the same power that justifies vaccination and disease reporting requirements. The courts might recognize a limited right to refuse newborn screening under the First Amendment, which protects freedom of religious belief, and in accord with the right of parents to make decisions about rearing children without unnecessary state interference. The likelihood that a child who is not screened will actually be affected with an inborn error of metabolism (assuming there is no family history for the disorder) is extremely low (1:10,000), and the risk associated with a refusal of screening is significantly less than the risks inherent in many other decisions about children that parents normally make.

Prenatal screening. Prenatal screening is intended to detect genetic (or genetically influenced) disorders in fetuses. Obstetricians routinely inform certain groups of women about specific genetic tests, such as fetal karyotyping for women who will be 35 or older when they deliver and who therefore have an increased likelihood to be carrying a fetus with Down syndrome. Except for laws that require Rh testing, however, no state at present mandates any type of prenatal screening (Powledge and Fletcher, 1979). Were a state to enact such a law—for example, mandatory screening for maternal serum alpha-fetoprotein (now routinely used to identify women at increased risk of having a child with a neural tube defect)—a court would probably strike it down as an impermissible invasion of a pregnant woman's physical integrity and a violation of her constitutional right of privacy.

California and the District of Columbia have mandated that health-care workers inform pregnant women of the availability of prenatal screening for neural tube defects; the women are free either to undergo or to refuse the procedure (Cal. Health and Safety Code, 1991; District of Columbia Laws, 1985).

Carrier screening. Carrier screening generally involves testing healthy people to determine whether they are carriers of genes for recessive disorders, in order to provide them with information about potential childbearing risks. Since the early 1970s the Ashkenazi Jewish population has operated a number of highly successful, community-based, voluntary screening programs to identify carriers of the gene for Tay-Sachs disease. Also during the 1970s, a number of states enacted sickle-cell testing statutes to identify carriers of the sickle-cell trait. Many of these were based on erroneous clinical assumptions, targeted inappropriate groups (for example, children entering public schools), and made no provision for counseling or confidentiality (Reilly, 1977). These laws led to public outcry, resulting in the enactment of corrective federal legislation (National Sickle-Cell Anemia Control Act of 1972). Today, several states explicitly forbid using sickle-cell test information to make decisions about employment and related matters.

Much attention has centered on whether to develop population-based screening for the cystic fibrosis gene. Given the high frequency of the gene and increasingly accurate test methods, genetic counselors and physicians may soon begin to inform persons of reproductive age about this test. This could alter the prevailing standard of care—what "reasonable practitioners" should do—in effect requiring physicians and genetic counselors to inform patients about the test.

Occupational screening. Genetic screening can also occur in employment settings. If low-cost predictive tests become available to identify persons genetically predisposed to common chronic diseases such as cancer, diabetes, and coronary artery disease, some employers concerned about spiraling health costs may try to screen out high-risk workers. Industrial employers may also seek to detect those with heightened susceptibilities to the adverse effects of exposure to certain chemicals (*International Union, UAW v. Johnson Controls, Inc.*, 1991). Although very few companies currently operate screening programs, recent surveys suggest that a number of large companies would be interested in the eventual im-

plementation of genetic screening programs (U.S. Congress, Office of Technology Assessment, 1991).

There are legal restrictions on the extent to which employers may ask prospective and current employees to submit to genetic tests. Both the Rehabilitation Act of 1973, applicable to federal agencies, and the Americans with Disabilities Act of 1990 (ADA), applicable to private employers, specifically prohibit preemployment inquiries about health or disability status. While an employer may make an offer of employment contingent on genetic testing, the testing must be required of all applicants, and cannot be performed until after the offer has been made. In addition, employers who use genetic testing to exclude current workers from their jobs must offer them alternative employment.

Legal issues in genetic testing

Access to genetic testing services. In the United States, while the federal government plays a role in determining access to genetic services by funding some genetics programs, the states bear primary responsibility for providing genetic services. Some states directly provide or subsidize genetic services and have comprehensive statutes or regulations with commissions or advisory boards to oversee service delivery and the use of genetic data. Other states take a piecemeal approach, with laws that refer to only a limited set of genetic conditions or that merely require giving applicants for marriage licenses educational materials about particular disorders. Most states have no statutes relating to genetic services (apart from their newborn screening laws), apparently providing such services, if at all, only in reliance on a general constitutional mandate to provide for the health of their population. No state's failure to provide access to adequate genetic services has yet been legally challenged.

Canada and the European nations have significantly greater control over access to services through national health policies and programs. For example, the Norwegian Parliament has placed legal restrictions on access to prenatal diagnosis, strictly limiting the procedure to women over age thirty-eight or those with other specific medical indications (Fletcher and Wertz, 1989). Similarly, in Japan the Eugenic Protection Act has the effect of limiting rather than encouraging the use of genetic testing.

Malpractice and the duty to warn. Advances in genetic testing and counseling alter the standard of care expected of health-care professionals. Malpractice lawsuits have been brought, particularly against obstetricians, alleging breaches of the duty to warn (that is, failure to alert individuals or couples of their increased risk of a fetus with a genetic disease) (Elias and Annas,

1987). These negligence suits fall into two major categories: wrongful birth claims brought by parents of children born with genetic diseases who were not alerted to the risk, and wrongful life claims brought on behalf of children with genetic diseases (Wright, 1978).

Most jurisdictions recognize at least a limited cause of action for wrongful birth, with the major conceptual struggle involving the calculation of damages once negligence is established. However, most courts have rejected wrongful life claims, refusing to weigh the value of nonlife (the consequence of abortion) against the value of a "defective existence." A few states have enacted statutes that prohibit parents from filing wrongful life suits on behalf of their children or that forbid children from suing their parents for wrongful life. Advances in genetic testing will probably lead to novel negligence suits—for instance, claims for "wrongful abortion" based on an erroneous diagnosis of genetic disease in a fetus that, after termination, proves not to have been affected.

The requirement of informed consent. The consent of the patient is a prerequisite to genetic testing. This requires explaining to the patient, prior to the test, the nature and scope of the information to be gathered, the significance of positive test results, the nature of the disease in question, and, if relevant, the risks involved in procreation and the availability of reproductive alternatives (Andrews, 1987). To this list may soon be added the duty to warn about the possible interests of insurers and employers in test results. This process allows patients to weigh the benefits of testing against the possible risks, reduces misunderstandings, and minimizes potential legal liability.

In some situations (where a routine blood sample is taken from a pregnant woman for a battery of tests), consent to a particular genetic test may arguably be implied. For both ethical and legal reasons, however, eliciting a subject's full informed consent is ordinarily the proper course.

The advent of presymptomatic testing of persons at risk for Huntington disease and other disorders that depend on the participation of several family members for diagnosis (linkage testing) raises the question of whether one individual may compel another to submit to genetic testing. Although there exists no case law directly on this point, it is unlikely that a court would compel a relative to undergo such testing. To do so would be inconsistent with the concept of protecting bodily integrity and would violate the principle of informed consent.

Obtaining informed consent to genetic testing of children or adults who lack legal competency generally requires that a parent or guardian decide by proxy. However, legitimate conflicts between parent and child may arise. In general, as the child matures, his or her views should be given more weight. Many states have statutes

that authorize the provision of some types of medical care to adolescents without parental consent. Some may protect health-care professionals from liability for testing or counseling an adolescent where the parents oppose such action.

Stringent informed consent procedures are required for genetic testing in research settings. The U.S. Department of Health and Human Services has promulgated regulations applicable to all federally funded research with human subjects. These regulations provide explicit guidelines for ensuring that participation in the research is voluntary and that the research risks are minimized.

Confidentiality of genetic information. There is a strong presumption in clinical practice that medical information should remain confidential. Nonetheless, state laws addressing this subject are riddled with exceptions authorizing disclosure in a variety of circumstances. Moreover, except for a handful of statutes relating to birth defects registries, sickle-cell anemia, and a few other diseases, these laws were not drafted to consider the familial nature of genetic information. Although some statues make wrongful disclosure of DNA-based data held by state agencies a criminal offense, individuals must rely primarily on traditional common law tort and contract principles to obtain redress for confidentiality breaches.

Disclosure to relatives. Physicians and genetic counselors frequently acquire genetic information from one patient that may be extremely important to other family members. This raises the question of whether there is a right—or even an obligation—to disseminate such information to a patient's relatives despite the general presumption of medical confidentiality. Disclosing the results of a genetic test stored in a person's medical record is different from compelling him or her to be tested, because it involves no invasion of bodily integrity. Disclosure of genetic data within families also does not typically expose patients to the type or degree of harm from which the common law of privacy traditionally has sought to protect people. In addition, the potential benefit of the information to a relative can sometimes be substantial.

Case law provides no specific guidance on the circumstances under which genetic data may be disclosed to a relative over a patient's objection. The 1983 U.S. President's Commission for the Study of Ethical Problems in Medicine and Biomedical and Behavioral Research took the position that confidentiality may be overridden where (1) reasonable efforts to elicit consent to disclosure by the test subject have failed; (2) there is a high probability both that harm will occur if the information is not disclosed and that the disclosure can be used to avert that harm; and (3) the disclosure is made in as limited a manner as is reasonably possible (U.S.

President's Commission, 1983). This approach is consistent with judicial reluctance to impose liability against physicians who warn individuals that their spouses or potential spouses have serious infectious diseases.

The question of whether a health-care professional in some circumstances must disclose genetic data to a patient's relatives has never been decided in court. The recognition of a possible obligation to breach confidentiality to protect third parties derives in part from a 1976 California case holding that a psychotherapist had a duty to warn a woman that the therapist's patient had threatened her life when the therapist should have had reason to believe that the threat would be carried out (*Tarasoff* v. *Regents of the University of California*, 1976). Some argue that this case suggests there is a duty to warn a patient's blood relatives about important facts that may affect their health or reproductive plans. Others contend that the risk of someday parenting a child with a genetic disease is not analogous to an immediate threat of violence.

Disclosure to spouses.   Physicians and genetic counselors may discover nonpaternity in the course of genetic testing. The majority view has long been that disclosing the fact of nonpaternity to a husband is likely to cause more harm to the family than good (Andrews, 1987). Of course, selective nondisclosure stands in conflict with the expectation of both wife and husband that they will be told the truth. The current approach requires redefining the "client" (in whose best interests the health-care professional must act) as the couple rather than as two separate individuals. This may be sound ethical reasoning, but it lacks solid legal foundation.

Disclosure outside families.   Unlike disclosure within families, where the damage caused by the disclosure, compared with the benefit, is likely to be relatively small, disclosure of genetic data to other third parties can seriously harm individuals. Life, health, and disability insurers, employers, educational institutions, law enforcement agencies, the military, and other institutional entities routinely acquire genetic data through their review of medical records and communications with physicians. The risk thus arises that individuals will be mislabeled, stigmatized, or discriminated against on the basis of real or perceived differences in their genetic constitution (Gostin, 1991). When genetic information begins to be stored in large data banks, the risk of additional abuses will be magnified.

A proposed federal bill, the "Human Genome Privacy Act" (1991), sought to address this problem by limiting third-party disclosure of genetic information without the consent of the individual to whom the data relates. That bill was not enacted. Bills considered in several states would specifically prohibit the disclosure of genetic information to insurers and employers. Currently, however, few explicit legal safeguards exist to ensure that genetic data, once gathered, will not fall into the hands of third parties who will use it for nonmedical reasons.

Although no European nation has yet enacted a law that directly addresses the problem of genetic discrimination, in its 1991 report a committee convened by the Council of Europe recommended studying this issue (Council of Europe, 1991). In 1990 the Danish Parliament adopted a resolution that advocated a ban on the use of genetic data in employment decisions.

In the United States the Rehabilitation Act of 1973 and the Americans with Disabilities Act of 1990 (ADA) prohibit employment discrimination against otherwise "qualified" handicapped persons, and it is arguable that these statutes (along with similar state laws) can be interpreted to prohibit most types of genetic discrimination in employment. However, the extent to which the ADA will prove a means of redressing genetic discrimination must await judicial interpretation.

In this regard the U.S. Supreme Court decision that restricting the working of women of childbearing age in dangerous environments because of the risk of injury to their fetuses constitutes unlawful sex discrimination under Title VII of the Civil Rights Act of 1964 is important (*International Union, UAW* v. *Johnson Controls, Inc.*, 1991). Title VII, which also prohibits employment discrimination based on race, religion, and pregnancy, may be invoked in genetic discrimination lawsuits by women and members of minority racial groups where certain genetic conditions are unusually prevalent.

Fewer safeguards exist to prevent life, health, or disability insurers from refusing to write policies or rating applicants on the basis of genetic test results. A health maintenance organization, under general contract law principles, may presumably require submission to genetic testing as a condition of entry into a plan or exempt particular genetic diseases from coverage. A number of states have considered legislation to curtail genetically discriminatory underwriting practices, but few such laws have been passed.

Because much health insurance at present is tied to employment, complex relationships exist among the many laws regulating employers and insurers. For example, the ADA exempts insurance companies from its reach, leaving them free to discriminate against applicants based on perceptions of genetic risk. An employer may not, however, use the existence of genetically discriminatory insurance practices as a pretext for refusing to hire, for firing, or for taking other adverse action against an applicant or employee.

Special testing situations.   A few laws concerning adoption recognize the importance of acquiring a full family history from the child's biological parents and of sharing that information with the adoptive parents at the time of placement. A situation may arise where genetic information derived from a biological parent could be important to the health of an adopted child, or vice versa, years after the adoption (American Society of Human Genetics, 1991). A legal justification may exist for breaching secrecy so that the appropriate agency may contact the adoptive family, or biological parent, and communicate the data. Alternative reproductive methods, such as artificial insemination or surrogate motherhood, can give rise to similar testing and disclosure problems.

DNA forensics.   In recent years the discovery that certain short repetitive sequences of DNA vary greatly in length among individuals (except for identical twins) has become the basis for DNA-based identification technologies. This has had an extraordinary impact on criminal law. It is now possible to create a DNA profile of biological specimens from a crime scene and compare it with a similar profile prepared from the blood of a suspect or from biological specimens found in the suspect's possession. If these two samples do not match, the finding tends to exonerate the individual; if they match, the finding may be powerful evidence of the suspect's presence at the crime scene (U.S. Congress, Office of Technology Assessment, 1990; National Research Council, 1992). DNA identification evidence is widely used in both European and U.S. courts. The decision by the Pentagon to collect blood from military recruits to create a repository upon which DNA analysis could be used to resolve most personnel identification issues arising out of combat indicates the value of this technology.

DNA identification technology—also known as "DNA fingerprinting"—has stimulated a wave of genetic testing laws. In the United States a number of states have enacted laws that require blood samples to be taken from convicted felons at parole. The DNA profiles prepared from this blood will be stored and used as a data bank against which DNA samples from future crime scenes can be compared. Felon DNA data banks are premised on the high rate of recidivism, especially for rape. Federal legislation is pending that would provide federal funds to support DNA-based forensic laboratories that meet certain quality control standards and establish privacy standards for forensic DNA data banks (DNA Identification Act of 1991).

The impact of abortion law.   Resolution of the many legal issues generated by the increasing use of genetic screening and testing will be determined by an evolving societal discourse. The enactment by some states of laws that sharply limit access to abortion and the possibility that the U.S. Supreme Court will continue to interpret conservatively the constitutional right of privacy regarding abortion are important aspects of this dialogue. Laws have been enacted in a few states that deprive women of the abortion option even where tests indicate that the fetus is likely to have a serious genetic disorder. The U.S. Supreme Court has upheld federal regulations that prevent physicians in federally funded facilities from discussing abortion with their patients, thus affecting their ability to provide genetic counseling that includes consideration of prenatal diagnosis (*Rust v. Sullivan*, 1991). Although the Supreme Court has reaffirmed the decision in *Roe v. Wade* (1973) recognizing a woman's right to choose an abortion before fetal viability, it has upheld a variety of other restrictions on the procedure's availability (*Planned Parenthood of Southeastern Pennsylvania v. Casey*, 1992).

Conclusion

Genetic testing and screening raise numerous legal issues, and are likely to be the focus of much legal activity—in both the courts and the legislatures—well into the future. Apart from the abortion debate, the primary areas of activity involving genetics are likely to be legislative efforts to regulate the conditions under which genetic data—and DNA itself—may be acquired, stored, studied, and used. A related area will probably focus on the passage of laws designed to prevent genetic discrimination. Here, the current debate over national health insurance is likely to assume increasing importance. National health insurance will mitigate, although not completely resolve, some of the difficult legal issues that genetic screening and testing raise.

JEAN E. MCEWEN
PHILIP R. REILLY

Directly related to this article are the other articles in this entry: PREIMPLANTATION DIAGNOSIS, PRENATAL DIAGNOSIS, NEWBORN SCREENING, CARRIER SCREENING, PREDICTIVE AND WORKPLACE TESTING, *and* ETHICAL ISSUES. *Also directly related are the entries* DNA TYPING; GENETICS AND THE LAW; *and* HEALTH SCREENING AND TESTING IN THE PUBLIC-HEALTH CONTEXT. *For a further discussion of topics mentioned in this article, see the entries* ABORTION; AUTONOMY; CONFIDENTIALITY; DISABILITY, *article on* LEGAL ISSUES; HARM; INFORMATION DISCLOSURE; INFORMED CONSENT; *and* RISK. *This article will find application in the entry* PRIVACY IN HEALTH CARE. *For a discussion of related ideas, see the entries* ADOPTION; FAMILY; FETUS, *article on* PHILOSOPHICAL AND ETHICAL ISSUES; FUTURE GENERATIONS, OBLIGATIONS TO; GENETICS AND RACIAL MINORITIES; HEALTH POLICY, *article on* POLITICS AND HEALTH CARE; INFANTS; RACE AND RACISM; *and* SEXISM. *Other relevant material may be found under the entries* GENOME MAPPING AND SEQUENCING; HEALTH-CARE RESOURCES, ALLOCATION OF; JUSTICE; MEDICAL GENETICS; MEDICAL INFORMATION SYSTEMS; *and* REPRODUCTIVE TECHNOLOGIES, *articles on* ARTIFICIAL INSEMINATION, *and* SURROGACY.

Bibliography

Americans with Disabilities Act. 1990. Pub. L. no. 101-336, 104 Stat. 376.

AMERICAN SOCIETY OF HUMAN GENETICS. SOCIAL ISSUES COMMITTEE. 1991."American Society of Human Genetics Social Issues Committee Report on Genetics and Adoption: Points to Consider." *American Journal of Human Genetics* 48, no. 5:1009–1010.

ANDREWS, LORI B. 1985. *State Laws and Regulations Governing Newborn Screening.* Chicago: American Bar Foundation.

———. 1987. *Medical Genetics: A Legal Frontier.* Chicago: American Bar Foundation.

California Health and Safety Code. 1991. §289.7.

Civil Rights Act. 1964. Title VII. 42 U.S.C. §2000e, et seq.

COUNCIL OF EUROPE. AD HOC COMMITTEE OF EXPERTS ON BIOETHICS. 1991. "Final Activity Report (Project IX.4) of the Intergovernmental Programme of Activities for 1991." Brussels: Author.

District of Columbia Laws. 1985. §6–312.

DNA Identification Act. 1991. S.1355. 102d Cong. 1st sess. (June 11).

ELIAS, SHERMAN, and ANNAS, GEORGE J. 1987. *Reproductive Genetics and the Law.* Chicago: Year Book Medical Publishers.

FLETCHER, JOHN C., and WERTZ, DOROTHY C., eds. 1989. *Ethics and Human Genetics: A Cross-Cultural Perspective.* Berlin: Springer-Verlag.

GOSTIN, LARRY. 1991. "Genetic Discrimination: The Use of Genetically Based Diagnostic and Prognostic Tests by Employers and Insurers." *American Journal of Law and Medicine* 17, nos. 1–2:109–144.

Human Genome Privacy Act. 1991. H.R. 2045. 102d Cong. 1st sess. (April 24).

International Union, UAW v. Johnson Controls, Inc. 1991. 111 S.Ct. 1196.

NATIONAL RESEARCH COUNCIL. 1992. *DNA Technology in Forensic Science.* Washington, D.C.: National Academy Press.

National Sickle-Cell Anemia Control Act. 1972. Pub. L. no. 92-294, 86 Stat. 136 (1975).

Planned Parenthood of Southeastern Pennsylvania v. Casey. 1992. 112 S. Ct. 2791.

POWLEDGE, TABITHA, and FLETCHER, JOHN. 1979. "Guidelines for the Ethical, Social and Legal Issues in Prenatal Diagnosis." *New England Journal of Medicine* 300:168–172.

Rehabilitation Act. 1973. Pub. L. no. 93-112, 87 Stat. 355 (1988).

REILLY, PHILIP R. 1977. *Genetics, Law and Social Policy.* Cambridge, Mass.: Harvard University Press.

Roe v. Wade. 1973. 410 U.S. 113.

Rust v. Sullivan. 1991. 111 S. Ct. 1759.

Tarasoff v. Regents of the University of California. 1976. 17 Cal. 3d 425, 131 Cal. Rptr. 14, 551 P.2d 334.

U.S. CONGRESS. OFFICE OF TECHNOLOGY ASSESSMENT. 1990. *Genetic Witness: Forensic Uses of DNA Tests.* Washington, D.C.: U.S. Government Printing Office.

———. 1991. *Medical Monitoring and Screening in the Workplace: Results of a Survey.* Washington, D.C.: U.S. Government Printing Office.

U.S. PRESIDENT'S COMMISSION FOR THE STUDY OF ETHICAL PROBLEMS IN MEDICINE AND BIOMEDICAL AND BEHAVIORAL RESEARCH. 1983. *Screening and Counseling for Genetic Conditions: A Report on the Ethical, Social, and Legal Implications of Genetic Screening, Counseling, and Education Programs.* Washington, D.C.: U.S. Government Printing Office.

WRIGHT, ELLEN. 1978. "Father and Mother Know Best: Defining the Liability of Physicians for Inadequate Genetic Counseling." *Yale Law Journal* 87:1488–1515.

VII. ETHICAL ISSUES

The ethical issues raised by genetic testing and screening fall into three major categories: issues concerning education and counseling; problems involving confidentiality; and issues of justice. This entry discusses four main applications of genetic testing and screening: prenatal screening, including preimplantation embryo diagnosis; diagnosis of genetic disorders in newborns; identifying individuals who are at risk of having children with symptomatic genetic disorders; and the use of genetic information by employers and insurers.

Special moral features

There is a tendency to regard the ethical issues raised by genetic testing and screening as new and fundamentally different from those raised by other kinds of health care. Although the ethical concerns raised by genetic testing and screening are not entirely novel, there are a number of factors inherent in genetics that should heighten our sensitivity to the human values involved. Seven factors deserve mention.

Prophecy precedes cure. In the foreseeable future, genetics is likely to give us the ability to predict diseases long before it will help us to prevent, treat, or cure them. Huntington disease and sickle-cell disease are two of many examples.

Ambiguities in the concept of genetic disease. Presymptomatic testing, which can uncover incipient genetic disease before any symptoms appear, and carrier testing, which can aid in the search for genes in potential parents who might have offspring with a specific disease, challenge our everyday notions of disease. The prospect of prenatal testing for late-onset diseases such as Alzheimer's disease or Huntington disease poses an interesting conceptual question: Should we regard as ill a fetus or person who is likely to develop symptomatic disease in forty to seventy years? Individuals who carry a gene for a recessive disease generally are not themselves affected but may have affected children: Do such carriers have a genetic disorder? Also, people may wish that their offspring not have certain genetically determined traits, including eyes or hair of a certain color, or an undesired sex. What limits, if any, should be placed on parents' power to determine their offspring's characteristics?

Concepts of genetics and of risk are poorly understood. The public and, to a distressing extent, health professionals have a poor grasp of the basics of genetics, of probability, and of risk. Because so many of the putative benefits from genetic information hinge on understanding basic genetics and risk probabilities, it is imperative to ensure that the public and the experts to whom they will turn have the knowledge they need.

Emphasizing racial and ethnic differences. An emphasis on genetic differences is at the same time an emphasis on the differences among racial and ethnic groups. History is replete with examples of presumed racial or ethnic differences that were used as excuses to treat people badly. Especially when attention turns to the genetics of socially significant behaviors and traits, such as propensity toward violence or intellectual capacity, there will be temptations to claim that there are differences among groups, and that those differences are genetic in nature. When such differences are used as reasons for treating people differently or as explanations for enduring inequalities, the potential for injustice is great.

Genetics and personal identity. Our genetics affect our identity by influencing our physical attributes and traits, and our propensities toward disease. Genetics also ties us to our ancestors and our descendants, who shape the persons we are. Genetic inheritance is intimately connected with our personal identity.

Genetic information is also information about others. The information that one is a carrier of or afflicted with a genetic disease is also information relevant to one's biological relations, who may also be carriers or at risk of the same disease. A sister could receive the unwanted knowledge that she and her children are at risk of a serious genetic disease because a genetic test revealed her brother to be at risk of the same disease. Confidentiality can be difficult to maintain within a family, especially with certain forms of genetic testing that require obtaining tissue samples from biological relatives of the person being tested.

A disproportionate burden on women. In carrier screening programs especially, though potentially also in presymptomatic screening, women typically bear a disproportionate burden. They often are tested first, with men tested later if at all; when decisions are made whether to continue a pregnancy, women must bear the direct consequences, whatever choice is made.

One of the most important distinctions between genetic testing technology and other areas of medical diagnosis is the gap between the ability to identify the molecular basis for a genetic condition and the ability to do something about it. This gap is due to our current lack of understanding of how genes function in their complex interactions with other genes and the intracellular and extracellular environments. This discrepancy between diagnostic abilities and treatment abilities raises a number of ethical issues in different applications of screening and testing.

Our technology allows us to detect sequences of DNA that are associated with medical conditions. But locating an abnormal gene is only the first step in understanding the condition. The function of the gene must then be determined. Next, the connection between the alteration of the normal gene and the dysfunction at the cellular and tissue level must be worked out. Finally, the connection between cell and tissue dysfunction and the problems experienced by the affected person must be appreciated. The full understanding of a disease may be greatly enhanced by DNA technology, but genes are only part of the full story. While it is not necessary to fully understand a disease before effective treatments can be developed, much more must be learned than what genetic technology alone can tell us.

Perhaps the best illustration of this gap is sickle-cell anemia. This genetic condition is well understood (although not fully understood) at the genetic, cellular, and tissue levels, but there is little that medicine has been able to offer affected individuals beyond supportive care. Therefore, genetic technology will give medicine some powerful tools to diagnose conditions at a molecular level, and some critical information that will unravel the mysteries of many diseases, but we should recognize that years of hard work will be necessary before patients can be offered effective treatments based on this knowledge.

From an ethical perspective, this means that the benefits of genetic testing and screening for many conditions will be indirect—focusing on preventive measures in many cases. This contrasts with medical testing for such conditions as strep throat, coronary artery disease, and breast cancer, where the results of the test may result in immediate interventions to ameliorate or cure the condition. For genetic testing and screening of untreatable conditions, a more subtle ethical balancing of the benefits and risks must be undertaken. This is particularly true because many preventive measures require lifestyle changes. Human behavior is remarkably difficult to alter. This problem is illustrated in the efforts to find a gene associated with alcoholism. It has been suggested that if such a gene were to be found, we could test adolescents for the gene and counsel those who were positive to avoid alcohol. While reasonable on the surface, we must recognize that changing the behavior of teenagers (or anyone else) through warnings about health risks has not been very successful. If preventive measures rely heavily on long-term behavior changes, we must look carefully at whether predictive testing and screening offer real benefits.

There is enormous pressure to bring discoveries in molecular genetics into the clinical realm. This pressure, combined with our limited knowledge of human biology, will encourage an initial focus on disease prevention rather than on treatment. The pursuit of prevention in the absence of treatment for many genetic conditions raises a number of important ethical issues in genetic testing and screening.

Education and counseling

Enabling informed choice is a principal goal of many clinical applications of genetic technology. Particularly in prenatal screening, carrier screening, and presymptomatic testing and screening, individuals may be interested in their genetic status in order to make decisions about reproduction, lifestyle changes, or other personal plans. The results of genetic tests often have profound implications for people's lives; therefore, a reasonable understanding of the results is essential. In addition, technical limitations of the tests require that patients and physicians be appropriately educated about the possibilities of false positive or false negative results. Appropriate education and counseling of both health professionals and the public are an important part of any screening and testing service.

The sickle-cell and the Tay-Sachs screening programs illustrate the influence of education and counseling on the efficacy and acceptance of a program (U.S. President's Commission, 1983). The confusion between sickle-cell disease and sickle-cell trait led to unnecessary screening, inappropriate fears, and discrimination. The Tay-Sachs program was more carefully instituted with efforts to foster broad community understanding and support in its early stages.

Unfortunately, the general level of education in human genetics is relatively poor for both the medical profession and the lay public. This raises significant concerns, since there are too few trained genetic counselors to fully support the use of new genetic technology (Holtzman, 1988). Expanding the use of testing or screening beyond experimental protocols may significantly increase the risk of misuse and harm. For example, the early protocols for presymptomatic testing for Huntington disease entailed five to six sessions for counseling prior to providing diagnostic information, and subsequent follow-up for one to two years. Now that testing for Huntington is commercially available, there is no assurance that patients are being appropriately counseled and supported. The potential influence of genetic information on crucial decisions in patients' lives requires that screening and testing be performed in an environment that ensures informed decisions, emotional support, and available guidance.

Confidentiality

The personal nature of genetic information makes confidentiality a particularly important consideration in genetic testing and screening. Results of tests that reveal probabilities about future health may hold significant interest for an individual's family, employer, and health and life insurance companies, all of whom may claim a "right to know." The injustice of discrimination from the disclosure of genetic status may result from misunderstanding information. Again, the sickle-cell screening program is a prime example: Asymptomatic carriers of the gene were often labeled as ill or potentially ill, and deprived of insurance and job opportunities. In the future, disclosure of genetic information to certain institutions, such as employers or insurance companies, may be more carefully regulated by legislation to prevent discrimination.

Disclosure of health information in private relationships is less amenable to regulation. Reproduction raises some of the thorniest issues of confidentiality. Does a spouse have a right to know a mate's genetic status in order to make an independent, informed decision about reproduction? This issue has been discussed in the context of Huntington disease (Shaw, 1980), although the problem may become more common as screening and testing capabilities expand. A problem of confidentiality also arises in prenatal diagnosis and newborn testing when nonpaternity is discovered. Disclosure of this information to the husband may be devastating to the family, yet this information may be important for the husband's future reproductive choices. Some genetic counselors maintain confidentiality in this circumstance by deception, through the suggestion that the child's condition is due to a new mutation and that the husband will not be at risk of fathering a similarly affected child in the future. These dilemmas are an inherent part of pursuing genetic information.

Issues of justice

Justice becomes an issue for genetic testing and screening in two ways: access to genetic services and the allocation of health-care resources. Most, though not all, accounts of justice in health care make the *need* for such care a crucial factor in deciding what constitutes a just distribution of health care.

To the extent that genetic testing and screening become valued for their contribution to human well-being and the satisfaction of human need, access to them and to other health services to which they provide entry will become a matter of justice. To the extent that such tests and services are linked to human well-being but are made available on some basis other than need—for example, to those who can afford them—injustice will arise. Genetic services are likely to be treated like other health-care services. A health-care system that does not provide equitable access to most services is unlikely to do so for genetic services. The problem, then, is with injustice in the health-care system itself, not with genetics alone.

No society has unlimited resources to spend on genetic testing, screening, and other services. Just as genetics must compete for resources with other forms of health care, so health care must compete with other sectors of each nation's economy, including such social goods as education, housing, and food. Large-scale genetic screening programs, such as screening for carriers of cystic fibrosis (CF), could be very expensive. One study estimates a cost of U.S. $2.2 million for every CF birth avoided (Wilfond and Fost, 1990). Genetic screening and testing have no claim to primacy for health-care resources. One concern is that the combination of enthusiasm over genetics resulting from the Human Genome Project and the rapid development of tests by commercial laboratories will result in much broader testing than is medically advisable, ethically sound, or fiscally prudent.

Preimplantation embryo diagnosis and prenatal screening

There are a number of ethical issues in prenatal diagnosis that can be distinguished from the ethics of abortion more generally considered. Merely asking "To whom should prenatal diagnosis be offered?" raises a complex set of considerations. Traditionally, prenatal diagnosis has been offered to those in specific "high risk" groups, such as older mothers and those with a family history of congenital or genetic impairments. But "high risk" is itself a value-laden concept. For example, a pregnant woman thirty-five years of age has one chance in 300 of bearing a child with Down syndrome, while a thirty-year-old woman has a risk of one in 900. It is not clear why the thirty-five-year-old woman should be considered "high risk" based on these numbers alone. Conversely, it is not clear why a thirty-year-old woman's interest in amniocentesis should be discouraged with the argument that "maternal anxiety" is an inappropriate indication.

Defining when prenatal diagnosis is considered "indicated" has two components. The first is deciding what risk levels for serious conditions justify discussing prenatal screening. An emerging example is the question of whether to offer carrier screening for CF to African-Americans, whose risk is significantly less than for Caucasians but not zero. Do considerations of justice require us to provide full information about disease states and risk levels to all, or is it justified to restrict disclosure to those in whom screening would be cost-effective? How should cost-effectiveness be determined?

The second issue is to define conditions that are sufficiently severe to warrant prenatal diagnosis. Prenatal diagnosis for sex selection is an extreme example, but there are a host of genetic conditions that have less-than-severe health implications and/or a later age of onset. In an international survey of genetic counselors,

Dorothy Wertz and John Fletcher (1989) found substantial variation between nations on the discussion with prospective parents of "low-burden" disorders, such as Turner syndrome and XYY. Professionals will need to develop more explicit standards for when to inform patients about genetic risks, and when to provide prenatal diagnostic services. Our answer as a society may depend on how much control we believe parents should have over the genetic composition of their children.

The guiding principle in genetic counseling, at least in the United States, has been autonomous choice—a value promoted by nondirective counseling. However, a number of important questions have been raised about the degree of autonomy that exists in prenatal screening and diagnostic services. The very availability of these services, in conjunction with society's ambivalent attitude toward those with disabilities, may carry an implicit message to couples about appropriate or responsible behavior during pregnancy (Lippman, 1991). Within the context of the patient–counselor relationship, nondirective counseling may be undermined by unintended verbal cues that promote the counselor's values on the use of prenatal diagnostic services (Rothman, 1986; Duster, 1990).

Finally, some call for explicit "guidance" on decisions about selective abortion. Margery Shaw draws the analogy of child abuse in claiming that knowingly giving birth to a seriously impaired child could be considered negligent fetal abuse by the parents (Shaw, 1980). She suggests that courts and legislatures should develop standards by which parents will be held accountable for the genetic health of their children.

There is also an important emerging set of issues in prenatal diagnosis that does not relate to selective abortion. As our therapeutic measures improve, we will be able to treat a wider variety of genetic and congenital conditions in utero with fetal surgical techniques and, perhaps, gene therapy. If these approaches pose a risk or burden to the mother, a conflict will arise between responsibility to treat the fetus and respect for the autonomous refusal of the mother. Fortunately, the typical desire of parents to promote the welfare of their children despite personal sacrifice should make such conflicts rare.

Neonatal screening

Newborn screening is largely uncontroversial when used to detect conditions that pose a serious threat to the welfare of the child but can be ameliorated through early intervention. This is the case with such conditions as PKU, hypothyroidism, and sickle-cell disease. For other conditions, the benefit of early detection remains unclear. Examples here include maple syrup urine disease and galactosemia, both of which may produce serious harm or death shortly after birth, before the results of screening tests are available. In such cases, the burdens of mass newborn screening need to be more carefully considered. One of the burdens of screening is false positive and false negative results that occur with all tests that are not 100 percent sensitive and specific. For many of the present techniques, false positives outnumber true positives by ten to one. Repeat testing is then required to identify those who are truly affected.

False positives may harm parents by creating anxiety that may not be dispelled entirely by subsequent testing and counseling (Holtzman, 1991). In addition, there is a small but potential risk that the physician will misinterpret the results and begin unnecessary and potentially harmful treatments. In general, documentation of the extent of these problems in newborn screening has been poor.

A second set of issues arises when newborn screening techniques allow the identification of newborn carriers of genetic conditions, as well as those affected with the disease. This is presently the case with sickle-cell disease. Should parents be informed of the infant's carrier state in order to warn them that they may be at risk of having a future child with the disease? In essence, this is using newborn screening as a surrogate method of parental carrier screening.

On the one hand, this information about the infant may be useful for the child when he or she is considering reproduction in the future, and some parents will be alerted that future children are at risk. On the other hand, the difficulty in explaining the distinction between the carrier state and the disease may confuse many parents, leaving them with the impression that their infant is not healthy. In addition, questions should be raised about screening parents (without consent) through an unconsenting infant when the parents themselves could be directly offered carrier screening.

Finally, newborn screening programs raise the issues of freedom of choice and informed consent by parents. In the United States, newborns are generally screened within state-run programs that are designed to obtain blood from all newborns within a few days of delivery (Clayton, 1992). In only one state (Wyoming) is there any legislative requirement for informed consent. A few states will permit refusal of testing on religious grounds, and a few others permit refusal for any objections raised by the parents. In most circumstances, screening is done routinely, with little discussion of the pros and cons with the parents. Some commentators believe mandatory screening for PKU is justified on the basis of the substantial benefit for infants who are detected and promptly treated, particularly given the minimal risks involved in the blood test (Faden et al., 1982). Other commentators argue that the risk to an individual child is remote (PKU occurs in approximately one in fourteen thousand infants), and that voluntary screening is likely to be as effective as mandatory programs, as long as ad-

equate informed consent is provided (Annas, 1982). The appropriate role of government in providing genetic testing and screening is clearly at issue here. All of these issues are likely to be the subject of debate as the number of genetic conditions detectable in the newborn expands.

Carrier screening

Ethical issues raised by carrier screening include the possibility of coerciveness, the risks of focusing on at-risk populations, the need to create acceptable choices, and the consequences of introducing new tests.

Though most carrier screening is voluntary, some programs have relied on formal or subtle coercion. By June 1974, seven states in the United States mandated screening for sickle-cell trait (National Research Council, 1975). The U.S. screening program for Tay-Sachs disease has been criticized for more subtle forms of coercion, such as community pressure on individuals and couples (Goodman and Goodman, 1982). In Cyprus, the Church of Cyprus requires couples who wish to marry to be tested for the beta-thalassemia gene. The policy appears to have drastically reduced the number of children born with the disease (Angastiniotis et al., 1986). If, as seems likely, screening programs that might save money, like the one in Cyprus, are developed, the possibility of some degree of coerciveness grows.

Screening programs directed at populations at risk can be more efficient than screening the general population. Such targeting, however, can create its own ethical problems. Sickle-cell carrier screening in the United States was directed at people of African heritage. Some in the African-American community saw the program as a thinly disguised effort at eugenics. Recent programs in CF carrier screening focus on women likely to bear children. Though a woman can contribute only one of the two copies of the gene necessary to cause CF, programs have chosen to target women's reproductive capacity, compelling them to bear the heavier share of the burdens of testing.

Carrier screening can result in unacceptable choices available to people found to carry a disease gene. Individuals may have the option of choosing a mate who is not also a carrier, choosing not to have children, or, if the techniques are available, using prenatal testing and possibly abortion for affected fetuses. How acceptable each of these options is will depend on the individual's own life plans and ethical convictions, and on the practices and laws of his or her particular culture. Carrier screening programs should be designed to ensure that they provide ethically acceptable choices for people in that culture.

Whether new tests to identify carriers result in more benefit or harm depends upon many factors. A common means to manage such new technologies has been to have experts set a standard of good practice, taking into account the relevant factors. Shortly after the test for CF carriers was introduced, such a standard was articulated, calling for use of the test only in specific, limited circumstances (Beaudet et al., 1990). In contrast, commercial biotechnology companies might find it in their interest to promote the widest possible use of new tests. Finding ways to minimize the harms of premature use and overuse of carrier screening tests will be a priority for the future.

Predictive testing in the workplace and insurance

The idea of using genetic tests to identify individuals with heightened susceptibility to workplace exposures was introduced in 1938 by the eminent geneticist J. B. S. Haldane. Haldane's goal was to reduce the incidence of workplace-induced illness and death—a familiar public-health aspiration. The greatest ethical difficulties such screening poses are its potential coerciveness, its use as an alternative to reducing hazardous exposures, and the possibility that people of disfavored ethnic or racial groups might be disproportionately denied employment (Murray, 1983).

Workplace genetic screening, if imposed on workers and prospective workers by employers, would give employers intimate and potentially very important information about individuals that the individuals themselves might not have. It could, alternatively, force unwanted information on people. If most people would choose to work elsewhere if their health was at special risk in a particular work environment, and if they had a choice, virtually all of the benefits of a coercive program could be obtained with a voluntary program.

Employers might view screening out susceptible workers as a less expensive option than purchasing safer equipment or changing manufacturing processes or work practices. The specter of racism hangs over the discussion of workplace genetic screening, principally because the only publicized case involved African-American workers tested for sickle-cell trait.

In the mid-1980s a new rationale for workplace genetic testing emerged. Although its putative public-health purpose had not materialized, in part because hazardous exposures were diminishing and epidemiologic evidence linking genes to exposures to disease was lacking, a new potential use emerged. The ever-increasing cost of health care in the United States, much of it borne by employers, prompted people to think of ways to trim costs. Hiring workers unlikely to become ill or disabled, if screening could identify them, might be an attractive means of saving money. Genetic tests that predict the likelihood of common—and expensive—diseases such as coronary artery disease, cancer, and stroke

were suggested as one way of accomplishing this. If such testing were widely used, it could result in substantial numbers of people becoming essentially unemployable. In contrast to genetic testing for susceptibility to workplace disease, there is no intent to reduce the incidence of disease and early death in screening for nonworkplace diseases. There is no evidence at this time of widespread genetic screening by employers, but that may be because the tests have been too expensive to make such screening cost-effective. As the price of testing drops, the incentive to use genetic tests may grow.

Genetic tests that predict risks for common diseases have other potential applications with substantial ethical problems. Insurance may well be affected. As individuals learn more about their own genetically predicted health risks, their insurance-purchasing behavior is likely to change in a pattern known in the industry as "adverse selection"—those most likely to file a claim are most likely to buy insurance. Insurers argue that "actuarial fairness" requires that every person pay according to his or her particular risks (Clifford and Iuculano, 1987). This notion of fairness appears to work well enough in dealing with commercial insurance, such as policies for oil tankers. It is less obviously appropriate for health, disability, or life insurance (Daniels, 1990). Reassessments of the social purpose of each form of insurance and of underwriting will help clarify what role, if any, predictive genetic testing ought to play.

Conclusions

The widespread ignorance and misunderstanding about genetic disorders make it important to include adequate education and counseling as a constitutive part of genetic testing and screening programs. The sensitivity of genetic information and the fact that genetic information about an individual is also information about biological relatives mean that great care and thought need to be given to confidentiality when genetic information is generated. Finally, there must be continual vigilance to guard against unjust misuse of genetic information against individuals or groups of people.

THOMAS H. MURRAY
JEFFREY R. BOTKIN

Directly related to this article are the other articles in this entry: PREIMPLANTATION DIAGNOSIS, PRENATAL DIAGNOSIS, NEWBORN SCREENING, CARRIER SCREENING, PREDICTIVE AND WORKPLACE TESTING, *and* LEGAL ISSUES. *Also directly related are the entries* GENE THERAPY; GENETIC COUNSELING; GENETIC ENGINEERING; GENETICS AND ENVIRONMENT IN HUMAN HEALTH; GENETICS AND HUMAN BEHAVIOR; GENETICS AND HUMAN SELF-UNDERSTANDING; GENETICS AND THE LAW; GENETICS AND RACIAL MINORITIES; GENOME MAPPING

AND SEQUENCING; EUGENICS; and MEDICAL GENETICS. *For a further discussion of topics mentioned in this article, see the entries* ABORTION; AUTONOMY; BEHAVIOR CONTROL; CONFIDENTIALITY; FAMILY; FETUS; FREEDOM AND COERCION; HARM; HEALTH-CARE FINANCING; HEALTH-CARE RESOURCES, ALLOCATION OF; HUMAN NATURE; INFORMED CONSENT; JUSTICE; OCCUPATIONAL SAFETY AND HEALTH, *article on* TESTING OF EMPLOYEES; PERSON; PRIVACY IN HEALTH CARE; PRIVILEGED COMMUNICATIONS; PROFESSIONAL–PATIENT RELATIONSHIP; RACE AND RACISM; RIGHTS; RISK; *and* WOMEN, *article on* HEALTH-CARE ISSUES. *For a discussion of related ideas, see the entries* EUGENICS AND RELIGIOUS LAW; FERTILITY CONTROL; HEALTH SCREENING AND TESTING IN THE PUBLIC-HEALTH CONTEXT; MARRIAGE AND OTHER DOMESTIC PARTNERSHIPS; MATERNAL–FETAL RELATIONSHIP; PUBLIC HEALTH; *and* REPRODUCTIVE TECHNOLOGIES.

Bibliography

ANGASTINIOTIS, MICHAEL; KYRIAKIDOU, SOPHIA; and HADJIMINAS, MINAS. 1986. "How Thalassemia Was Controlled in Cyprus." *World Health Forum* 7, no. 3:291–297.

ANNAS, GEORGE J. 1982. "Mandatory PKU Screening: The Other Side of the Looking Glass." *American Journal of Public Health* 72, no. 12:1401–1403.

CLAYTON, ELLEN WRIGHT. 1992. "Screening and Treatment of Newborns." *Houston Law Review* 29, no. 1:85–148.

CLIFFORD, KAREN A., and IUCULANO, RUSSEL P. 1987. "AIDS and Insurance: The Rationale for AIDS-Related Testing." *Harvard Law Review* 100, no. 7:1806–1825.

DANIELS, NORMAN. 1990. "Insurability and the HIV Epidemic: Ethical Issues in Underwriting." *Milbank Quarterly* 68, no. 4:497–525.

DRAPER, ELAINE. 1991. *Risky Business: Genetic Testing and Exclusionary Practices in the Hazardous Workplace.* Cambridge: At the University Press.

DUSTER, TROY. 1990. *Backdoor to Eugenics.* New York: Routledge.

FADEN, RUTH R.; HOLTZMAN, NEIL A.; and CHWALOW, A. JUDITH. 1982. "Parental Rights, Child Welfare, and Public Health: The Case of PKU Screening." *American Journal of Public Health* 72, no. 12:1396–1400.

GOODMAN, MADELEINE J., and GOODMAN, LENN E. 1982. "The Overselling of Genetic Anxiety." *Hastings Center Report* 12, no. 5:20–27.

HOLTZMAN, NEIL A. 1988. "Recombinant DNA Technology, Genetic Tests, and Public Policy." *American Journal of Human Genetics* 42:642.

———. 1991. "What Drives Neonatal Screening Programs?" *New England Journal of Medicine* 325, no. 11:802–804.

LIPPMAN, ABBY. 1991. "Prenatal Genetic Testing and Screening: Constructing Needs and Reinforcing Inequities." *American Journal of Law and Medicine* 17, nos. 1–2: 15–50.

MURRAY, THOMAS H. 1983. "Warning: Screening Workers for Genetic Risk." *Hastings Center Report* 13, no. 1:5–8.

NATIONAL RESEARCH COUNCIL. COMMITTEE FOR THE STUDY OF INBORN ERRORS OF METABOLISM. 1975. *Genetic Screening: Programs, Principles, and Research.* Washington, D.C.: National Academy of Sciences.

NELKIN, DOROTHY, and TANCREDI, LAURENCE R. 1989. *Dangerous Diagnostics: The Social Power of Biological Information.* New York: Basic.

ROTHMAN, BARBARA KATZ. 1986. *The Tentative Pregnancy: Prenatal Diagnosis and the Future of Motherhood.* New York: Penguin.

SHAW, MARGERY W. 1980. "The Potential Plaintiff: Preconception and Prenatal Torts." In *Genetics and the Law II,* pp. 225–232. Edited by Aubrey Milunsky and George J. Annas. New York: Plenum.

TASK FORCE ON GENETIC INFORMATION AND INSURANCE. 1993. *Genetic Information and Health Insurance.* Bethesda, Md. National Institutes of Health.

U.S. PRESIDENT'S COMMISSION FOR THE STUDY OF ETHICAL PROBLEMS IN MEDICINE AND BIOMEDICAL AND BEHAVIORAL RESEARCH. 1983. *Screening and Counseling for Genetic Conditions: A Report on the Ethical Implications of Genetic Screening, Counseling, and Education Programs.* Washington, D.C.: Author.

WERTZ, DOROTHY C., and FLETCHER, JOHN C., eds. 1989. *Ethics and Human Genetics: A Cross-Cultural Perspective.* Heidelberg: Springer-Verlag.

WILFOND, BEN S., and FOST, NORMAN. 1990. "The Cystic Fibrosis Gene: Medical and Social Implications for Heterozygote Detection." *Journal of the American Medical Association* 263, no. 20:2777–2783.

WORKSHOP ON POPULATION SCREENING FOR THE CYSTIC FIBROSIS GENE. 1990. "Statement from the National Institutes of Health Workshop on Population Screening for the Cystic Fibrosis Gene." *New England Journal of Medicine* 323, no. 1:70–71.

GENITAL MUTILATION

See CIRCUMCISION, *article on* FEMALE CIRCUMCISION.

GENOME MAPPING AND SEQUENCING

Biomedical research was transformed in the 1980s by human genetics, which was itself transformed by molecular biology during the same period. New techniques to construct maps of the human chromosomes lay at the center of these transformations. While for decades those studying genetic disease engaged in searches for disease-associated genes, technological advances in the 1980s shifted the scale to the full complement of genes—the genome. Advancing techniques to study deoxyribonucleic acid (DNA) directly opened new frontiers for genetic exploration.

Genetics is largely a twentieth-century science. The term itself was not used until the first decade of the twentieth century. Genetics grew out of theoretical and experimental work that observed how characters, or traits, were inherited from generation to generation. The Austrian monk Gregor Mendel performed masterful experiments on inheritance in plants during the 1860s, but this work remained obscure, in part because its relevance to the central biological questions of the day—evolution and natural selection—did not become clear for many decades. The rediscovery of Mendel's principles at the turn of the twentieth century was the first of many giant strides taken by geneticists.

Mendel posited elements that conferred inheritance of characters. During the first two decades of the twentieth century, many investigators found that these elements, dubbed "genes," are embodied as physical units in chromosomes. Chromosomes are structures in the cell nucleus that become visible when cells are stained with specific dyes. The exact chemical nature of chromosomes was unknown then, as was the physical constitution of genes. The aggregate term "genome" refers to all the genetic material in the chromosomes, containing a species' full complement of genes. Genes are sorted differently among offspring but stably inherited once sorted, subject only to rare changes known as mutations. Inheritance of genes physically embodied as parts of chromosomes explains how the genetic makeup of a species can remain stable while mutations and occasional gene shuffling provide the variation necessary for natural selection.

The physical structure of genes began to emerge in the 1940s and 1950s. In 1944 Oswald Avery, Colin MacLeod, and Maclyn McCarty found that deoxyribonucleic acid (DNA) is the chemical that confers inheritance in the pneumococcal bacterium. James Watson and Francis Crick discovered the structure of DNA in 1953. DNA consists of a long chain of four constituent bases—adenine (A), cytosine (C), guanine (G), and thymine (T). These bases are linked into long molecular chains, millions of bases in length, by a sugar and phosphate backbone. It was immediately apparent that genetic instructions are encoded in the order of As, Cs, Gs, and Ts. The DNA chains are packaged as chromosomes in cell nuclei. Genes are physical stretches of DNA among the chromosomes.

Much of the progress in genetics was based on the study of viruses, bacteria, fruit flies, yeast, and other organisms. In the 1980s, many of the techniques that enabled genetics to advance in other organisms became applicable to humans. The ability to control crossbreeding and to observe multiple generations greatly expedited work on model organisms. Indeed, all the organisms whose genetics was relatively advanced had short reproductive cycles and were amenable to controlled mating, features not available in humans. Analyzing human genetics in the same detail as other organisms required technologies to trace precisely the inheritance of small chromosome regions through human pedigrees.

Human genetics long centered on the collection and documentation of pedigrees that suggested inheritance of diseases. Archibald Garrod applied Mendel's theoretical constructs to human disease, suggesting that some diseases were caused by aberrant genes inherited from one's parents (Garrod, 1909). He postulated that changes in the genetic substance (not yet known to be DNA)—mutations—could cause aberrant gene products, which could in turn disturb normal metabolism and cause disease. Certain diseases were passed as Mendelian traits.

Victor McKusick published the first catalog of human Mendelian disorders in 1966. The catalog grew to several thousand entries in subsequent editions over the next twenty-five years (McKusick, 1990). Initial entries were based principally on pedigree data suggesting a genetic causation. The number of conditions in the catalog grew consistently, but the elaboration of details about existing entries was even more impressive. The refinements included the chromosomal location of genes associated with familial conditions, the cloning of those genes, and in many cases a detailed understanding of disease mechanisms. During the 1980s, the direct molecular analysis of DNA, tracing chromosome regions through human pedigrees, became a dominant strategy in human genetics.

Gene maps

The central thrust of human genetics was finding disease-associated genes. The process typically involved several steps, each requiring a different kind of map. All genetic maps ultimately refer to the DNA constituting the chromosomes, but different maps are used for different purposes.

Genetic linkage maps establish the relative position of genetic markers, detectable DNA sequences, along the chromosomes. "Genetic linkage" refers to the inheritance of one trait along with another. A map of detectable variations using standard markers can be used to trace the inheritance of chromosome regions. By correlating the inheritance of chromosome regions to the inheritance of characters, such as specific genetic diseases, the approximate location of a gene can be determined. This narrows the chromosomal region whose DNA must be thoroughly scrutinized to look for the gene, and brings to bear the precise tools of direct DNA analysis. Genetic linkage is thus a bridge from the study of inherited characters that run in human families to the realm of molecular genetics.

A landmark 1980 paper described how DNA sequence differences among individuals could be used to construct a genetic map of the entire human genome (Botstein et al., 1980). A genetic linkage map could be assembled by systematically searching for minor sequence differences. DNA sequence differences occur once in every 200 to 1,000 bases when comparing any two persons, on average. The variation is minuscule in comparison with the size of the genome, but millions of these generally "silent" differences can, in theory, be detected. The vast majority have no observable effects, but they can nonetheless be used as chromosome markers. The key is to find regions of the genome likely to differ among individuals in a family.

A parent passes only one of each pair of chromosomes to each child. A sequence difference that distinguishes the two copies of chromosome 7 inherited from the mother, for example, can identify which copy of that chromosome went to which children. If the father has yet another two variations at the same marker site, then the copy of chromosome 7 coming from each parent can be unequivocally traced through the family.

If a disease is consistently inherited along with a marker for a specific chromosome region among individuals in many different families, it is quite likely that a gene in that region causes the disease in those individuals. Chromosome marker studies were used to locate the cystic fibrosis gene in an early success story of modern human genetics. Children who developed cystic fibrosis consistently inherited a different chromosome 7 from their parents than did their unaffected siblings. The specific region of chromosome 7 containing the gene was narrowed by studying many different families (Knowlton et al., 1985; Tsui et al., 1985; Wainwright et al., 1985; White et al., 1985). Genetic linkage to a region on chromosome 7 began an intense investigation of the DNA from that region in search of the gene. The next step was to clone DNA taken from children with the disease, and to compare it against DNA lacking the mutation. This process involved construction of a different kind of map, a physical map of ordered DNA clones, and extensive use of direct DNA sequence comparisons (Kerem et al., 1989; Riordan et al., 1989; Rommens et al., 1989).

Physical mapping is a critical element in the direct analysis of DNA from a chromosome region. The most generally useful form of a physical map is a set of ordered clones that contain DNA spanning an entire region of the chromosome. The chromosomal DNA is, in essence, fragmented into a size that can be copied in yeast or bacteria. The fragments are replicated manifold and then reassembled. A contiguous map of a chromosome region is complete when the DNA from any part of the entire region is contained in at least one such clone whose order is known relative to others on the map.

Ultimately, when a gene has been located to a region between genetic markers A and B on a genetic linkage map, investigators will know that the DNA between markers A and B is contained in clones 12,312 through 12,543, for example.

During the 1970s, biologists began to map DNA directly from the entire genomes of viruses and bacteria, and learned the enormous power of working from this molecular foundation. The genetics of viruses, bacteria, fruit flies, yeasts, nematodes, and mice were particularly sophisticated. Among these, yeasts and nematodes emerged as the prototypes for the Human Genome Project—starting from the structure of chromosomal DNA and progressing toward the underlying biology.

Yeasts live as single cells whose genes are enclosed in a cell nucleus, in contrast to bacteria and viruses, which lack a cell nucleus. The yeast genome contains over twelve million base pairs, roughly one-fourth of one small human chromosome. Since many genes are shared among all organisms, the study of yeast is a rapid and efficient way to test their functions (Botstein and Fink, 1988).

Caenorhabditis elegans is a soil-dwelling nematode. If molecular genetics is the reductionist core of biology, *C. elegans* is the reductionists' paradise. Sydney Brenner explicitly selected it in the early 1970s, to study the biological complexity of development and behavior. Its small size, rapid reproductive cycle, relatively small number of cells, and nearly transparent cell body make *C. elegans* an ideal model to study the development of multiple organs, including the nervous system. Enormous energy was invested over more than two decades to build up the informational base for nematode biology. The lineage of every cell was traced, and the interconnections among the cells of the nervous system were mapped (Sulston, 1983; Sulston and Brenner, 1974; Sulston and Horvitz, 1977; Sulston et al., 1983; White et al., 1986). The genome of its six chromosomes, containing approximately one hundred million base pairs, is in aggregate roughly comparable to a single human chromosome.

In the mid-1980s, groups in the United States and Europe began the task of fragmenting the entire genomes of yeast and *C. elegans,* cloning the fragments, and reconstructing the order of DNA fragments into maps of their entire genomes (Coulson et al., 1986; Olson et al., 1986). Decades of work had produced mutant strains in both organisms, whose biology was under intense study. Strains of yeast had well-characterized metabolic defects, for example, whose genes were precisely known. In *C. elegans*, there were mutations in which specific cell types failed to develop. The effects from loss of the cell could be directly observed, and correlated with specific genetic defects. Genes corresponding to these mutations could be directly mapped. Mapping the entire genome was intended to make this process far more efficient. The Human Genome Project grew, in part, from a desire to have similarly powerful physical maps to study human disease and normal physiology.

DNA sequencing is a physical mapping at its ultimate resolution. DNA sequence is, in a genetic sense, the territory to be mapped. Most information in chromosomes is contained in the order of bases that make up the DNA chains. In the mid-1970s, two groups independently discovered how to determine the sequence of DNA bases (Maxam and Gilbert, 1977; Sanger, 1988). As techniques became faster and less costly, the power of DNA sequence information as an analytical tool became apparent. Three individuals independently proposed to determine the DNA sequence of the entire human genome (that is, a reference sequence to be used for study, not the entire genome of a particular individual) (DeLisi, 1988; Dulbecco, 1986; Sinsheimer, 1989). Proposals to sequence the human genome provoked a controversy.

The Human Genome Project grew from the ensuing debate. The original proposals for DNA sequencing were broadened to encompass physical and genetic linkage maps, to analyze nonhuman organisms as models of human genetics, and to emphasize the development of new technologies for DNA analysis and its interpretation (Cook-Deegan, 1991). In the first five-year plan for the project, the goals of finding and mapping chromosomal markers for linkage studies and of assembling large-scale physical maps became primary. The ultimate goal almost imperceptibly shifted from a complete sequence to a complete structural catalog of genes in humans and selected nonhuman organisms.

The products of the Human Genome Project thus included not only maps of humans and other organisms but also new technologies for direct analysis of DNA. This included technologies to derive DNA sequence information, emphasizing automation and robotics. Just as important, it also included new computer methods to analyze map and sequence information, and complex pedigrees. Data bases to store the structural data had to be enlarged and refined, and made accessible to a broader range of users.

Genetic analysis extends well beyond the diseases inherited according to simple Mendelian patterns. Molecular genetic techniques can in some cases grab a molecular handle on diseases that otherwise elude study. Most common diseases have genetic forms. Atherosclerosis, arthritis, Alzheimer's disease, hypertension, diabetes mellitus, immune disorders, and many kinds of cancer at least occasionally run in families. When such inheritance is Mendelian (explained by a single gene), then finding that gene establishes one link in the causal chain leading to disease. Families with a single-gene form of disease may be rare, but they provide a valuable glimpse of molecular mechanisms. The mechanism found in one family may disclose clues about the cause of more common forms of the same disease. With complete genetic maps, finding the genes responsible for Mendelian traits is, theoretically, a matter of persistence. Molecular genetics should eventually find a gene whose function can be studied directly.

Complete genetic maps also enable investigators to search for multiple genes that must work in concert to produce disease. Hypertension and insulin-dependent diabetes are two diseases in which constellations of genes are at play. Many common diseases will similarly be explained as genes interacting with other genes and environmental factors. The study of animal models reveals specific genes that influence the course of a disease, that increase or diminish the risk of developing symptoms, or that point to specific environmental insults involved in disease expression. Genetic maps of various kinds are thus becoming essential tools in biomedical research.

Science policy issues

Resource allocation emerged as the first science policy issue facing those who wished to pursue genome mapping and sequencing. Consensus that genetic maps and technology development were important did not extend to agreement on how important the Human Genome Project was relative to other biomedical research opportunities. Whether the Human Genome Project deserved specific additional funding became the central question. The initial response of the biomedical research community was concern that the Human Genome Project would detract from other research by siphoning off monies better devoted to undirected basic research.

Three advisory groups convened to consider this question all reached the same conclusion: that a systematic mapping and sequencing program was likely to be far less costly and more powerful in the long run than a less organized effort (Health and Environmental Research Advisory Committee, 1987; National Research Council, 1988; U.S. Congress, 1988). Each of these committees reached a consensus that genetic strategies were becoming central to all biomedical research, and the work entailed in the Human Genome Project would have to be done eventually. The argument boiled down to a shared belief that mapping and sequencing at the scale of entire genomes was progressing with sufficient speed to justify a concerted research program. Constructing maps and developing technologies in an organized fashion would prove far more efficient than hoping that complete maps would emerge from thousands of uncoordinated searches for individual genes.

The three committees used somewhat different methods to project budget needs, but all agreed on the need for a project of roughly fifteen years' duration and approximately $200 million annual budget. Efficiency of resource allocation was invoked as the principal justification for the Human Genome Project. Those promoting the project argued that it would not displace other science of equal merit, but instead would free up resources by making available maps and technologies that would otherwise be assembled haphazardly and inefficiently. The question was not whether to construct maps and develop technologies but, rather, how to organize the effort and how quickly to proceed. These arguments convinced those in Congress and the executive branch, who allocated dedicated funds for genome mapping and sequencing programs.

The debate first surfaced in the United States, and the first formal reports were American in origin. The U.S. Department of Energy commenced its Human Genome Initiative in fiscal year 1987, and was joined by the National Institutes of Health in 1988. Italy also began a genome project in 1988; the United Kingdom and the Soviet Union followed suit in 1989. (The Soviet program was transferred to the Russian Republic in 1991 and 1992.) These efforts were soon joined by genome research programs of the European Community and the United Nations Educational, Scientific, and Cultural Organization (UNESCO). France, the Netherlands, and Denmark also mounted human genome programs by the end of the 1980s. In Japan, the Ministry of Education, Science and Culture began a human genome program in 1989. The Japanese Science and Technology Agency supported a pilot project to automate DNA sequencing beginning in 1981. In 1988 and 1989, this was augmented and expanded into a genome mapping and sequencing effort. The Ministry of Health and Welfare began a program aimed at human genetic diseases during this period, and the Ministry of International Trade and Industry seriously considered joining the fray. Scientists in several Latin American countries formed a collaborative network. Scientists in Canada, Australia, New Zealand, the People's Republic of China, and other nations petitioned their governments to implement human genome research programs.

This profusion of programs pursued similar but somewhat different goals. The Danish program, for example, was an incremental augmentation of ongoing disease-oriented research, while the U.S. efforts were largely focused on map construction and technology development. The Soviet genome budget funded much of all molecular biology in the U.S.S.R., while the U.S. program constituted less than 2 percent of the National Institutes of Health research budget. The budgets also varied widely, from a few million dollars to over one hundred million dollars in the United States. The programs were, moreover, administered by many different agencies and organizations with largely independent planning and advisory processes. While the ends were

largely similar, the means were disparate. The purpose of the Human Genome Project was to produce information tools that contained information from many different sources. Genetic linkage maps, physical maps, and DNA sequencing information would be contributed by thousands of laboratories throughout the world, but transforming this information into useful maps and data bases required collective efforts.

The main argument for organized work at the scale of entire genomes was its efficiency. Such efficiency necessitated more systematic organization of effort than existed in most biomedical research. Coordination thus emerged as a central policy concern—interagency coordination within countries and international collaboration around the globe. Most European countries centralized their research in ministries. The more decentralized organization in the United States and Japan raised greater barriers to coordination. In the United States, the Department of Energy and the National Institutes of Health jointly forged a five-year plan, intended to be revised every three to four years, and a coordinated planning apparatus (U.S. Department of Health and Human Services and U.S. Department of Energy, 1990). Coordination of the Japanese ministries was more informal.

Orchestrating collaboration across international borders proved more difficult. The Human Genome Organization (HUGO) was formed in April 1988 specifically to mediate international cooperation, and to harness various national programs into a coherent team. The task proved more difficult than its founding scientists anticipated. HUGO, intended to be a "United Nations of the human genome," in the words of founding president Victor McKusick, instead resembled the League of Nations—more a congeries of independently planned national efforts than the hoped-for coherent plan. The principal coordination mechanisms remained ad hoc arrangements among national programs and private philanthropic organizations, publication in the open scientific literature, and periodic international meetings, as in fields in biomedical research.

Social policy issues

Policymakers and the general public welcomed the possibility of understanding many diseases through genetics but greeted the genetic revolution with some trepidation. Public support was strong for biomedical research, and genome mapping promised to expedite biomedical research. Print, radio, and television news media reported a long succession of successful hunts for disease genes and the genesis of the Human Genome Project. Most of the coverage was quite favorable, but there were nagging doubts about potential misuse of the new technologies.

In the United States, many issues stemming from progress in human genetics were left to fester in the absence of a national forum in which to discuss issues related to bioethics. The National Commission for the Protection of Human Subjects of Biomedical and Behavioral Research operated from 1973 to 1978, laying a foundation for human subjects' protection. The National Commission demonstrated a welcome ability to mediate debate over difficult policy questions that involved scientific, legal, and social issues. The Ethics Advisory Board within the Department of Health, Education and Welfare was transiently active from 1978 to 1980. Its role included reviewing specific protocols that raised ethical or legal issues or that required waivers of usual human subjects' regulations. The U.S. President's Commission for the Study of Ethical Problems in Medicine and Biomedical and Behavioral Research operated from 1980 until 1983. A successor to the National Commission, its principal function was to serve as a national forum to discuss policy issues. The U.S. President's Commission issued two prescient reports on genetics, a 1982 report on recombinant DNA research and gene therapy and a 1983 report on genetic screening and counseling.

In 1985, Congress established the Biomedical Ethics Board and Biomedical Ethics Advisory Committee as congressional successors to the U.S. President's Commission. A report on implications of human genetics was the first of three mandated activities for the new body. Its structure was modeled on the Office of Technology Assessment, and it operated briefly from 1988 to 1989; then it ran aground on the shoals of abortion politics. While none of its mandated studies dealt directly with abortion, several topics nonetheless touched on interests of groups on both sides of the extremely divisive abortion debate. In March 1989, senators on the Biomedical Ethics Board found themselves completely deadlocked, and the Biomedical Ethics Advisory Committee could not operate in the face of this paralysis. Its ability to expend funds was terminated six months later, and its statutory authorization expired September 30, 1990.

Leaders of the effort to create the Human Genome Project recognized the need for national attention to social, legal, and ethical issues as scientific planning proceeded. The National Research Council report and the Office of Technology Assessment report stressed the need for a mechanism to address the social implications of applying knowledge gained through genome mapping and sequencing (National Research Council, 1988; U.S. Congress, Office of Technology Assessment, 1988). The Department of Energy took preliminary steps to support ethical analysis of its research program as early as 1986, but these failed to translate into specific grants or research activities for several years. At a September 1988 press conference to announce that he

would direct an office for human genome research at the National Institutes of Health, James D. Watson indicated that part of that program's budget should be dedicated to analysis of ethical, legal, and social issues. Following a Senate hearing in October 1989, the Department of Energy followed suit, and the joint NIH-DOE Working Group on Ethical, Legal, and Social Issues (ELSI) was established, chaired by Nancy Sabin Wexler.

ELSI was responsible for providing advice to both the NIH and DOE on research strategies, and for sponsoring a program of activities to promote outreach and public education and to produce policy options for Congress and the executive branch to consider. Within a year, the ELSI programs more than doubled the direct federal support of bioethics, then doubled it again by the end of fiscal year 1990.

The ELSI program was an unprecedented effort by a scientific research initiative to analyze its impact on social issues. The program, established by executive fiat, was quickly ratified by Congress. Once formulated, the strategy quickly spread abroad. The genome mapping and sequencing programs sponsored by Italy, France, the European Community, the Russian Republic (originally the Soviet Union), UNESCO, and Japan all explicitly included a component devoted to analysis of social and ethical issues. The British program was alone in being focused solely on the science, although even in the United Kingdom, the private Neufield Council evinced an interest in bioethical issues related to genome research. With the creation of the ELSI program, government science agencies acknowledged responsibility not only to support science but also to assess its social impact. This reflected a shifting social contract in which the biomedical research enterprise was increasingly expected to account for itself.

Most of the social policy issues posed by genome mapping and sequencing arose from application of knowledge or new technologies rather than in the conduct of research. Many of these application areas are briefly summarized here. The main effect of mapping and sequencing technologies was to accelerate the pace of the advance of human genetics. They also expedited the development of analytical methods useful in medicine and forensic science. The same techniques used to construct maps in most cases could be readily translated into new methods for DNA-based diagnosis, or to identify individuals by analyzing their DNA.

The first wave of concern stemmed from policy problems that had arisen in the 1960s and 1970s, when genetic screening for phenylketonuria and sickle-cell disease began. By producing vastly greater detail about the human genome and by augmenting diagnostic technologies, genome mapping and sequencing raised the prospect of more widespread genetic testing and screening. The ethical and legal concerns related to genetic testing centered on the confidentiality of information about individuals' disease susceptibility or other genetic data. The core issue was genetic discrimination; identifying the genes that caused disease, and discovering technologies to detect them, threatened discrimination against those carrying particular genes. Opportunities for discrimination abound when individuals at risk seek jobs, health insurance, life insurance, and other social benefits.

The ability to identify individuals by sampling their DNA enabled forensic uses of DNA tests. Genetic markers were useful not only in tracing the inheritance of chromosomal regions through families but also could serve as unique genetic identifiers, except in the case of identical twins. (Identical twins should, in theory, be genetically identical except in cells undergoing DNA rearrangement during development.) DNA testing could thus be used to establish paternity or to investigate violent crime (Committee on Forensic Uses of DNA Tests, 1992; U.S. Congress, Office of Technology Assessment, 1991). One common application, for example, was to compare sperm taken from a rape victim against DNA from a suspect in the crime. Another was to analyze hair and blood samples at the scene of a murder, and to look for matches with a suspect's DNA. DNA typing even became part of a human-rights investigation, when DNA sequencing of variable regions was used to trace possible genetic relationships between grandmothers and the children of parents who had been tortured and murdered in Argentina. These children had been separated from their families, and geneticists aspired to reunite the families (King, 1991). On the other hand, the forensic uses of DNA testing that grew from these powerful techniques of DNA analysis raised questions of civil liberties, due process of law, and international exchange of information between governments with widely differing criminal-justice codes and human-rights standards.

Public concern grew not only from applications of genetic technology but also from the troubled history of human genetics. Geneticists labored under the long shadow of eugenics. A wave of enthusiasm about prospects for human genetics crested in the 1920s and 1930s, as genetics entered the mainstream of science. The nascent field of human genetics became inextricably entangled in the parallel political movement that led to eugenic policies such as mandatory sterilization, immigration restriction, and antimiscegenation statutes. The eugenics movement started in the United Kingdom and the United States, and eventually merged with the racial hygiene movements in Nazi Germany and elsewhere (Adams, 1990; Gallagher, 1990; Kevles, 1985; Lifton, 1986; Muller-Hill, 1988; Proctor, 1988; Smith and Nelson, 1989).

Human molecular genetics historically grew from the molecular biological study of nonhuman organisms, on the one hand, and the study of human genetic disease, on the other. Medical genetics reacted strongly against eugenic ideology in the postwar era. The ethical norms of medical genetics were widely shared throughout the world (Wertz and Fletcher, 1989). Respect for the views of clients produced the ideal of "nondirective counseling" and explicit rejection of coercive social policies such as those espoused by eugenicists. Molecular biology concerned itself primarily with the detailed mechanisms of biology, and came to confront broad social issues only when molecular genetics began to find application in humans.

Molecular genetics might have more scientific depth than the facile interpretations of pedigree data that undergirded most eugenic thinking, but the public harbored a healthy skepticism about the facile prognostications of scientific elites, particularly regarding human genetics. While molecular genetics might prove more scientifically robust than eugenics, its potential for social mischief remained potent. The degree to which gene-mapping efforts provoked genetic discrimination and imposition of social stigma hinged on how accurately genetic tests could predict important characteristics of individuals.

Eugenic policies presumed genetic determinism. Eugenic ideology viewed genes as powerful determinants of behavior, intelligence, perception, athletic ability, moral stature, and even social class. Socially desirable or undesirable characteristics were foreordained at the time of conception. In the late 1970s and into the 1980s, debate about sociobiology rekindled this decades-old debate about nature versus nurture. Genetic determinism provoked a vigorous reaction. Geneticists concerned about the past abuses of human genetics rejected the central claims of strong genetic determinism, viewed correlations between genes and behavioral traits with great skepticism, and found policy implications of deterministic genetics particularly suspect (INSAN, 1984; Lewontin et al., 1984).

Molecular genetics focused on elucidating causal chains and physiological mechanisms, and was thus inclined to reductionist explanations of detailed molecular phenomena. It was, on its face, inclined to determinism. Molecular genetics aspired to explain behavior, and made some progress toward this end by illuminating behavior mutant organisms of the sea hare *Aplysia*, fruit flies, nematodes, and mice. It was clear that molecular defects could inhibit development of the nervous system, impede the transmission of neural impulses, and cause behavioral changes. This was a far cry, however, from establishing the primacy of genetics in determining behavior. Indeed, the complexity of behavior made it likely that the genetic dissection of most functions in the nervous system would be more readily understood as highly complex networks of genetic and nongenetic factors rather than linear causal chains.

Medical genetics in the postwar era explicitly rejected the coercive social policies of eugenics and concentrated on nondirective counseling to individual clients. Controversies about genetic determinism and sociobiology concerned principally those studying population genetics and evolution rather than medical genetics. Many human geneticists and molecular geneticists were largely oblivious to the social history of eugenics and the ongoing nature–nurture debate. Medical geneticists had traditionally concerned themselves primarily with Mendelian diseases, and were only beginning to deal with conditions in which the genetic basis was less clear. They were bewildered by claims that their science had inherent eugenic intentions. When a debate began about how the fruits of the Human Genome Project would be distributed and controlled, however, the project was ineluctably drawn into the cross fire.

The technologies of DNA sequencing and mapping made the discovery of new genes faster and more straightforward. Starting from genetics, however, turned the normal course of research on its head, since investigators were starting from genes of unknown function and looking for functional correlations, rather than starting from a known protein and looking for the genes encoding it.

This reversal of traditional research strategies induced confusion about how to interpret patent law. Exactly how did map and sequence information influence what could be patented? If one had, for example, sequenced all or part of a gene but had no idea what it did, could the gene's sequence nonetheless be patented? If so, a rapid survey of gene-bearing regions linked to a patenting strategy was central to developing new pharmaceutical and agricultural products using biotechnology. If genes of unknown function were not patentable, how would private biotechnology, pharmaceutical, agricultural, and other private firms protect their investments in research and development? Yet commercial attachments to such work might hinder the free exchange of scientific data. Genetic data were the essence of international genome mapping efforts; maps were constructed from collective data pooled from around the world. The new technologies thus raised a thorny and controversial issue that could be resolved only through a welter of legal activity, including patent applications, approvals or rejections of patent claims, litigation over patent infringements, possible new patent legislation, and accumulated judicial interpretations of patent law and DNA technologies.

ROBERT MULLAN COOK-DEEGAN

Directly related to this entry are the entries MEDICAL GENETICS; GENE THERAPY; GENETIC ENGINEERING; GENETIC COUNSELING; GENETIC TESTING AND SCREENING; PATENTING ORGANISMS; *and* GENETICS AND ENVIRONMENT IN HUMAN HEALTH. *For a further discussion of topics mentioned in this entry, see the entries* FUTURE GENERATIONS, OBLIGATIONS TO; HEALTH-CARE RESOURCES, ALLOCATION OF, *article on* MACROALLOCATION; HEALTH SCREENING AND TESTING IN THE PUBLIC-HEALTH CONTEXT; PUBLIC HEALTH; RESEARCH, HUMAN: HISTORICAL ASPECTS; *and* RESEARCH POLICY. *For a discussion of related ideas, see the entries* BIOLOGY, PHILOSOPHY OF; EUGENICS; EUGENICS AND RELIGIOUS LAW; EVOLUTION; GENETICS AND HUMAN SELF-UNDERSTANDING; HEALTH AND DISEASE; LIFE; TECHNOLOGY; *and* VALUE AND VALUATION. *Other relevant material may be found under the entries* BIOMEDICAL ENGINEERING; BIOTECHNOLOGY; COMMERCIALISM AND SCIENTIFIC RESEARCH; *and* MULTINATIONAL RESEARCH.

Bibliography

ADAMS, MARK B., ed. 1990. *The Wellborn Science: Eugenics in Germany, France, Brazil, and Russia.* New York: Oxford University Press.

AVERY, OSWALD T.; MACLEOD, COLIN M.; and McCARTY, MACLYN. 1944. "Induction of Transformation by a Desoxyribonucleic Acid Fraction Isolated from Pneumococcus Type III." *Journal of Experimental Medicine* 79: 137–158.

BOTSTEIN, DAVID, and FINK, GERALD R. 1988. "Yeast: An Experimental Organism for Modern Biology." *Science* 240:1439–1443.

BOTSTEIN, DAVID; WHITE, RAYMOND L.; SKOLNICK, MARK; and DAVIS, RONALD W. 1980. "Construction of a Genetic Linkage Map in Man Using Restriction Fragment Length Polymorphisms." *American Journal of Human Genetics* 32:314–331.

COMMITTEE ON FORENSIC USES OF DNA TESTS. 1992. *Forensic Uses of DNA Testing.* Washington, D.C.: Commission on Life Sciences, National Research Council, National Academy of Sciences.

COOK-DEEGAN, ROBERT MULLAN. 1991. "The Genesis of the Human Genome Project." In *Molecular Genetic Medicine,* vol. 1, pp. 1–75. Edited by Theodore Friedmann. San Diego: Academic Press.

COULSON, ALAN; SULSTON, JOHN; BRENNER, SYDNEY; and KARN, JONATHAN. 1986. "Toward a Physical Map of the Genome of the Nematode *Caenorhabditis elegans.*" *Proceedings of the National Academy of Sciences* 83:7821–7825.

DELISI, CHARLES. 1988. "The Human Genome Project." *American Scientist* 76:488–493.

DULBECCO, RENATO. 1986. "A Turning Point in Cancer Research: Sequencing the Human Genome." *Science* 231:1055–1056.

GALLAGHER, HUGH GREGORY. 1990. *By Trust Betrayed: Patients, Physicians, and the License to Kill in the Third Reich.* New York: Henry Holt.

GARROD, ARCHIBALD E. 1909. *Inborn Errors of Metabolism.* Oxford: Oxford University Press.

HEALTH AND ENVIRONMENTAL RESEARCH ADVISORY COMMITTEE. 1987. *Report on the Human Genome Initiative.* Washington, D.C.: Office of Energy Research, U.S. Department of Energy.

INSAN. 1984. *Designer Genes: IQ, Ideology, and Biology.* Petaling Jaya, Selangor, Malaysia: Instituto Analisa Sosial.

KEREM, BAT-SHEVA; ROMMENS, JOHANNA M.; BUCHANAN, JANET A.: MARKIEWICZ, DANUTA; COX, TARA K.; CHAKRAVATI, ARAVINDA; BUCHWALD, MANUEL; and TSUI, LAP-CHEE. 1989. "Identification of the Cystic Fibrosis Gene: Genetic Analysis." *Science* 245:1073–1080.

KEVLES, DANIEL J. 1985. *In the Name of Eugenics.* Berkeley: University of California Press.

KING, MARY-CLAIRE. 1991. "An Application of DNA Sequencing to a Human Rights Problem." In *Molecular Genetic Medicine,* vol. 1, pp. 117–131. Edited by Theodore Friedmann. San Diego: Academic Press.

KNOWLTON, ROBERT G.; COHEN-HAGUENAUER, ODILE; VAN CONG, NGUYEN; FREZAL, JEAN; BROWN, VALERIE A.; BARKER, DAVID; BRAMAN, JEFFREY C.; SCHUMM, JAMES W.; TSUI, LAP-CHEE; BUCHWALD, MANUEL; and DONIS-KELLER, HELEN. 1985. "A Polymorphic DNA Marker Linked to Cystic Fibrosis Located on Chromosome 7." *Nature* 318:381–382.

LEWONTIN, RICHARD C.; ROSE, STEVEN; and KAMIN, LEON J. 1984. *Not in Our Genes.* New York: Pantheon.

LIFTON, ROBERT JAY. 1986. *The Nazi Doctors.* New York: Basic Books.

MAXAM, ALLAN M., and GILBERT, WALTER. 1977. "A New Method for Sequencing DNA." *Proceedings of the National Academy of Sciences* 74:560–564.

MCKUSICK, VICTOR A. 1990. "Foreword to the Ninth Edition." In his *Mendelian Inheritance in Man,* pp. xi–xxix. Baltimore: Johns Hopkins University Press.

———. ed. 1966. *Mendelian Inheritance in Man.* Baltimore: Johns Hopkins University Press.

MULLER-HILL, BENNO. 1988. *Murderous Science.* New York: Oxford University Press.

NATIONAL RESEARCH COUNCIL. 1988. *Mapping and Sequencing the Human Genome.* Washington, D.C.: National Academy Press.

OLSON, MAYNARD V.; DUTCHIK, JAMES E.; GRAHAM, MADGE Y.; BRODEUR, GARRETT M.; HELMS, CYNTHIA; FRANK, MARK; MACCOLLIN, MIA; SCHEINMAN, ROBERT; and FRANK, THOMAS. 1986. "Random-Clone Strategy for Genomic Restriction Mapping in Yeast." *Proceedings of the National Academy of Sciences* 83:7826–7830.

PROCTOR, ROBERT N. 1988. *Racial Hygiene: Medicine Under the Nazis.* Cambridge, Mass.: Harvard University Press.

RIORDAN, JOHN R.; ROMMENS, JOHANNA M.; KEREM, BAT-SHEVA; ALON, NOA; ROZMA-HEL, RICHARD; GRZELCZAK, ZBYSZKO; ZIELENSKI, JULIAN; LOK, SI; PLAVSIC, NATASA; CHOU, JIA-LING; DRUMM, MITCHELL L.; IANNUZZI, MICHAEL C.; COLLINS, FRANCIS S.; and TSUI, LAP-

CHEE. 1989. "Identification of the Cystic Fibrosis Gene: Cloning and Characterization of Complementary DNA." *Science* 245:1066–1072.

ROMMENS, JOHANNA M.; IANNUZZI, MICHAEL C.; KEREM, BAT-SHEVA; DRUMM, MITCHELL L.; MELMER, GEORG; DEAN, MICHAEL; ROZMAHEL, RICHARD; COLE, JEFFREY L.; KENNEDY, DARA; HIDAKA, NORIKO; ZSIGA, MARTHA; BUCHWALD, MANUEL; RIORDAN, JOHN R.; TSUI, LAP-CHEE; and COLLINS, FRANCIS S. 1989. "Identification of the Cystic Fibrosis Gene: Chromosome Walking and Jumping." *Science* 245:1059–1065.

SANGER, FREDERICK. 1988. "Sequences, Sequences, and Sequences." *Annual Review of Biochemistry* 57:1–28.

SINSHEIMER, ROBERT. 1989. "The Santa Cruz Workshop, May 1985." *Genomics* 5:954–956.

SMITH, J. DAVID, and NELSON, K. RAY. 1989. *The Sterilization of Carrie Buck.* Far Hills, N.J.: New Horizon Press.

SULSTON, JOHN E. 1983. "Neuronal Cell Lineages in the Nematode *Caenorhabditis elegans.*" *Cold Spring Harbor Symposia on Quantitative Biology* 48:443–452.

SULSTON, JOHN E., and BRENNER, SYDNEY. 1974. "The DNA of *Caenorhabditis elegans.*" *Genetics* 77:95–104.

SULSTON, JOHN E., and HORVITZ, H. ROBERT. 1977. "Post-Embryonic Cell Lineages of the Nematode *Caenorhabditis elegans.*" *Developmental Biology* 56:110–156.

SULSTON, JOHN E.; SCHIERENBERG, E.; WHITE, J.G.; and THOMPSON, J. N. 1983. "The Embryonic Cell Lineage of the Nematode *Caenorhabditis elegans.*" *Developmental Biology* 100:64–119.

TSUI, LAP-CHEE; BUCHWALD, MANUEL; BARKER, DAVID; BRAMAN, JEFFREY C.; KNOWLTON, ROBERT; SCHUMM, JAMES W.; EIBERG, HANS; MOHR, JAN; KENNEDY, DARA; PLAVSIC, NATASA; ZSIGA, MARTHA; MARKIEWICZ, DANUTA; AKOTS, GITA; BROWN, VALERIE; HELMS, CYNTHIA; GRAVIUS, THOMAS; PARKER, CAROL; REDIKER, KENNETH; and DONIS-KELLER, HELEN. 1985. "Cystic Fibrosis Locus Defined by a Genetically Linked Polymorphic DNA Marker." *Science* 230:1054–1057.

U.S. CONGRESS. OFFICE OF TECHNOLOGY ASSESSMENT. 1988. *Mapping Our Genes—Genome Projects: How Big? How Fast?* OTA-BA-373. Washington, D.C.: U.S. Government Printing Office. Reprint. Baltimore: Johns Hopkins University Press.

———. 1991. *Genetic Witness: Forensic Uses of DNA Tests.* OTA-BA-438. Washington, D.C.: U.S. Government Printing Office.

U.S. DEPARTMENT OF HEALTH AND HUMAN SERVICES and U.S. DEPARTMENT OF ENERGY. 1990. *Understanding Our Genetic Inheritance: The First Five Years, FY 1991–1995.* DOE/ER-0452P. Springfield, Va.: National Technical Information Service.

U.S. PRESIDENT'S COMMISSION FOR THE STUDY OF ETHICAL PROBLEMS IN MEDICINE AND BIOMEDICAL AND BEHAVIORAL RESEARCH. 1982. *Splicing Life.* Washington, D.C.: Author.

———. 1983. *Screening and Counseling for Genetic Conditions.* Washington, D.C.: U.S. Government Printing Office.

WAINWRIGHT, BRANDON J.; SCAMBLER, PETER J.; SCHMIDTKE, JORG; WATSON, EILA A.; LAW, HAI-YANG; FARRALL,

MARTIN; COOKE, HOWARD J.; EIBERG, HANS; and WILLIAMSON, ROBERT. 1985. "Localization of Cystic Fibrosis Locus to Human Chromosome 7cen-q22." *Nature* 318:384–385.

WATSON, JAMES D., and CRICK, FRANCIS, H. C. 1953. "Genetical Implications of the Structure of Deoxyribonucleic Acid." *Nature* 171:737–738.

WERTZ, DOROTHY C., and FLETCHER, JOHN C. eds. 1989. *Ethics and Human Genetics: A Cross-Cultural Perspective.* New York: Springer-Verlag.

WHITE, JOHN G.; SOUTHGATE, EILEEN; THOMPSON, J. NICHOL; and BRENNER, SYDNEY. 1986. "The Structure of the Nervous System of the Nematode *Caenorhabditis elegans.*" *Philosophical Transactions of the Royal Society of London* B314:1–340.

WHITE, RAYMOND L.; WOODWARD, SCOTT; LEPPERT, MARK; O'CONNELL, PETER; HOFF, MARK; HERBST, JOHN; LALOUEL, JEAN-MARC; DEAN, MICHAEL; and VANDE WOUDE, GEORGE. 1985. "A Closely Linked Genetic Marker for Cystic Fibrosis." *Nature* 318:382–384.

GERMANY

See MEDICAL ETHICS, HISTORY OF, *section on* EUROPE, *subsection on* CONTEMPORARY PERIOD, *article on* GERMAN-SPEAKING COUNTRIES AND SWITZERLAND. *See also* NATIONAL SOCIALISM.

GLOBAL WARMING

See CLIMATIC CHANGE.

GREAT BRITAIN

See MEDICAL ETHICS, HISTORY OF, *section on* EUROPE, *subsection on* NINETEENTH CENTURY, *article on* GREAT BRITAIN; *see also the subsection on* CONTEMPORARY PERIOD, *articles on* UNITED KINGDOM, *and* REPUBLIC OF IRELAND.

GREECE

See MEDICAL ETHICS, HISTORY OF, *section on* EUROPE, *subsection on* ANCIENT AND MEDIEVAL, *article on* GREECE AND ROME, *and subsection on* CONTEMPORARY PERIOD, *article on* SOUTHERN EUROPE. *See also* EASTERN ORTHODOX CHRISTIANITY.

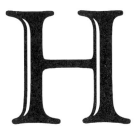

HANDICAPPED PERSONS

See DISABILITY; *and* MENTALLY DISABLED AND MENTALLY ILL PERSONS.

HARM

Health professionals are confronted with many different forms of harm suffered by their patients. Obviously, preventing, alleviating, or eliminating harm that results from disease is the proper goal of practicing medicine. Also, harm is a key concept in general ethics—as indicated by the fact that prohibitions against inflicting harm on others supposedly belong to the principles of any moral code. Moreover, taking care—by both action and omission—that others do not suffer harm is often regarded as the substantive and motivational core of morality. Hence it does not come as a surprise that in medical ethics, too, harm is an important concept. The Hippocratic tradition established *primum non nocere* (above all, do no harm) as the physician's most important rule of conduct. Almost any ethical disagreement in medicine could be formulated in a way that involves an appeal to choose or avoid one harm that must be balanced against other instances of harm, other values, or other duties.

However, harm is also a vague concept; in and of itself it does not provide much moral guidance. What counts as harm varies greatly, as do the scope and relative importance of the prescription to do no harm.

Conceptual questions

An instance of harm may be assessed with reference to kind, degree, and duration. Risk assessment, not considered here, also includes the probability of harm's occurrence. According to the *Oxford English Dictionary,* harm is "evil (physical or otherwise) as done to or suffered by some person or thing; hurt, injury, damage, mischief." As far as harm is relevant to moral deliberation, however, this broad concept must be restricted. First, harm should be understood as person- (or animal-) regarding, that is, as consisting of events or states of affairs that are negative for someone—as expressed in Joel Feinberg's definition of harms as "setbacks to interest" (Feinberg, 1984, p. 31). As long as the sticky question of what counts as interests remains open, the concept of harm is still neutral to various ethical theories. Problems start with determining who counts as a bearer of interests; for instance, embryos (as potential persons?), the deceased or permanently unconscious (as former persons?), or animals. These issues, although obviously important for evaluating abortion, transplantation, abating-treatment decisions, or animal protection, will not be pursued here.

A further restriction, one that reflects ordinary language usage, will be to understand harm as a normative concept, such that harmful actions are prima facie—though not necessarily on balance—morally wrong. This has several implications. First, it limits the realm of harm to what can in principle be influenced by humans. It would not make sense to deliberate morally about ineluctable evils, deplorable though they may be.

However, linking harm to human agency obviously makes it subject to limits of variable human knowledge and technology.

Second, understanding harm as a normative concept requires it to be of significant disvalue to its "victim." Although harm is conceptually complementary to benefit (interest satisfaction), not just any loss or lack of benefit is to count as harm. Along the scales of both numbers and degrees of interest satisfaction, there are numerous positions of submaximal satisfaction (disbenefits) that it seems inappropriate to call "harms." There is thus an asymmetry between harm and benefit, as acknowledged by ordinary moral discourse, in the sense that harm pertains exclusively to the basics of well-being. It may be wrong to prevent someone from obtaining a luxury good, but that does not make such prevention a harm. Other arguments elucidating this asymmetry emphasize that harm has or leads to distinct phenomenal qualities of bodily or psychological painfulness and suffering, which is not true for all instances of lacking benefit (e.g., Noddings, 1989), or that pity for someone's experience of harm is a motivation distinct from other forms of benevolence (e.g., Sidgwick, 1907).

Thus conceived, nonharming takes moral precedence over providing those benefits the lack of which does not count as harm. Such asymmetry between harm and benefit has been traditionally acknowledged (e.g., Mill, 1861), but a more systematic focus on harm is a rather recent development (a notable exception being Jeremy Bentham's 1789 taxonomy of "pains" by sources, kinds, and circumstances) of "applied" ethics with an eye to some concrete moral rules. Where the whole of morality (for instance, for John Stuart Mill) or at least some of its rules aim at the improvement of people's well-being, concrete efforts must first focus on the most important impediments to well-being, that is, on existing harm.

Morally relevant harms, then, are those avoidable instances of evil that (1) consist in significant setbacks to someone's interests and therefore ought to be avoided if possible, (2) unless outweighed by conflicting moral obligations, or by requiring extremely demanding sacrifices from particular agents. The second aspect, to be dealt with in the final section of this entry, indicates possible agent-centered limits to a duty of nonharming. The first aspect treats harm as a purely consequentialist concept, that is, one that is neutral in regard to both identity of agent and type of action—that is, to possible restrictions of aspect (2). This understanding requires a more exact consideration of harm's nature and of how to determine "significance" as the criterion distinguishing between harm and other instances of lacking benefit. Obviously, certain basic differences between moral theories will influence what their proponents understand as (normatively) "significant" lacks of benefit. Thus, those who argue for far-reaching moral obligations to promote other people's well-being are likely to have higher standards of "significance" than do proponents of only minimal moral responsibility for others' well-being. Other disagreements may regard only the classification of particular lacks of benefits, without resulting in disagreement on what is morally right. A moral theory, for instance, that reduces all moral obligations to the one obligation of lessening harm (that is, negative utilitarianism, the least harm for the greatest number of people) might tend to employ a broader concept of harm than does a theory that acknowledges an additional obligation of beneficence. Both theories might, however, agree on the scope of moral obligation.

Inflicting harm needs to be distinguished from "wronging," that is, the violation of legitimate moral claims (Feinberg, 1984). Consider, for instance, the debate over medical paternalism. Is a physician ever justified in alleviating or preventing harm to a competent patient against his or her will (say, transfusing a Jehovah's Witness who would otherwise die)? Antipaternalists, all agreeing that the patient would be unduly wronged, can argue from an inherently subjective understanding of harm, thereby precluding the possibility of involuntary benefit to the patient. Or they can argue that on balance the patient would be harmed by a reduced sense of self-determination. Or they can hold that the wrong of infringing autonomy outweighs a physician's duty to prevent harm. Conflation of wronging and harming would blur these distinctions.

Medical ethics obviously is concerned with those instances of harm that are likely to occur in the context of medical practice. According to causes, one must distinguish here between those harms that occur without medical practice and are what the latter aims against (e.g., bodily and mental incapacities) and those harms that occur due to medical interventions (e.g., side effects, perhaps the preservation of life of miserable quality). According to kind, one has to distinguish between those harms that can be described as specifically disease-linked (e.g., pain, physical or mental incapacities, or premature death) and those harms that may occur due to psychosocial aspects of medical practice (e.g., patients' anxiety, mistrust, annoyance). For convenience, we will refer to all of these instances of harm as "medical harms"—evaluating which, however, raises both fundamental questions of harm in general and problems specific to medicine.

Problems with harm in medicine

Harm assessment within medicine occurs in two different contexts: in evaluating interventions for individual patients and in evaluating the justice of resource distribution in health care. A crucial question in both contexts is whether there are objective criteria for evaluating harm. If such criteria could be found, they might justify a physician's overriding a patient's "harmful" preference. Moreover, they could be adduced in surrogate decision making for noncommunicating patients, as well as in matters of allocative justice (where it becomes crucial to evaluate medical interventions in terms of their comparative tendencies to avoid or alleviate net harm).

As to the more precise nature of harm, most authors now agree that there is an irreducible plurality of harms. By slightly modifying common classifications (see Griffin, 1986), one can distinguish between viewing harm as (1) a significant setback only to existing wants or desires, possibly after procedural safeguards have been met (e.g., death due to nonresuscitation would be harmful only to a patient who would—if informed and asked— not consent to such nontreatment), or as (2) a significant setback also to wants that are assumed to obtain under various idealized conditions (e.g., death due to nonresuscitation would be harmful also to a consenting patient who lacks the desire to be resuscitated only because he or she does not realize that resuscitation would *not* be a very painful intervention), or as (3) a significant setback also to interests that are want-independent (e.g., death due to nonresuscitation would be harmful to a patient, regardless of whether he or she wants it). Position (3) can plausibly be called inconsistent, because it both defines harm as directed to someone and makes the content of harm completely independent of this someone's desires. Hence, without necessarily influencing substantive judgment on what is morally wrong, this conceptual position seems inadmissible.

Although another position, (4) that harm is some negative mental state (like experiencing pain or despair) rather than some negative state of the world (frustration of wants), opens complex philosophical questions, it can be neglected here. For practical purposes, proponents of (4), too, must rely on some indicator of negative mental states, and thus again face the choice between existing and idealized wants, that is, between (1) and (2) as a practical position. The fundamental distinction between "want regard" and "ideal regard" (as a precision of subjective versus objective concepts of interest) was introduced by Brian Barry (1990) in political philosophy. In that area, lack of autonomy in forming one's wants is less obviously a danger than it is in medicine, where patients can so easily be ill informed, manipulated, or otherwise incompetent when forming their preferences. Therefore, at least certain procedural safeguards—such as standards of informed consent—are not inconsistent with "want regard" in medicine. Other safeguards, like elevating standards for patient competence to a level commensurate with the expected harm that would result from acting in accordance with patient choice (e.g., Buchanan and Brock, 1989), cross over into "ideal re-

gard." Forcing a Jehovah's Witness to be transfused, using the argument that she would want it if she were not bound to her irrational belief system, clearly puts harm assessment under some ideal-regarding constraint.

A common argument in favor of taking harm as an objective concept stresses the broad consensus in what "rational persons desire to avoid for themselves" (Culver and Gert, 1982, p. 70). Reference to the obvious consensus about the desirability of avoiding disease, disability, pain, premature death, and suffering, presupposed in daily medical work, is familiar from the debate over concepts of disease (Culver and Gert, 1982). To concur on this point does not imply acknowledging universal standards for all sorts of harm. Rather, pain, disability, and premature death are seen as universal harms simply in being setbacks to very basic interests, the satisfaction of which is instrumental to practically all conceptions of the good life. It would, of course, not come as a surprise to find this true for many kinds of harm, in contrast to mere lack of benefits.

However, most problems with medical harm start with the need to compare two instances of harm: alternative treatment courses or alternative resource distributions. Such comparative judgments are needed on kinds of harm (e.g., pain versus addiction; premature death versus disfigurement; disease versus a restricted lifestyle) and on how much, when, and for how long harm is to be accepted, and for what purpose. At least implicit comparative evaluations of (risks of) harm and benefit are involved in virtually any treatment decision or medical indication (Veatch, 1991). Here, more fundamental disagreement may start: Some authors emphasize the great variability in comparative harm assessment, pointing to its relatedness to the context of each patient's irreducibly personal or parochial conception of the good life (e.g., Engelhardt, 1986; Veatch, 1991). This position has nurtured so-called autonomy-centered medical ethics, which considers the assessment of harms and benefits to be the patients' business only. In contrast to this position, other scholars want to keep at least some objective ground for evaluations: medical interventions should, according to them, be determined futile not by patients but by professional standards whenever they appear to be disproportionately harmful and thus "not reasonable" (Brody, 1992); or they see interpersonal variability in ranking harm—though it exists—as not predominant and therefore not ruling out a beneficence-centered medical ethics.

Certain other kinds of harm that medicine is liable to produce, however, raise no problems of either qualitative or quantitative subjective assessment. In particular, the work of feminist ethicists (e.g., Nodding, 1989; Warren, 1992) and physician-ethicists (e.g., Cassell, 1991; Pellegrino and Thomasma, 1988) has created a new awareness of widely neglected kinds of harm to patients that occur in daily medical practice: anxiety, alienation, helplessness, loss of self-control, and mistrust of the technophile orientation of modern medicine and its proponents. Such harms can be reduced or avoided when caregivers are humane and sympathetic.

Finally, harm may occur as a setback to patients' higher-level "critical interests" (Dworkin, 1993) in living a life they consider good. Notably, decisions about one's time and manner of dying are likely to relate to such highly personal, critical interests. Focusing on these would involve yet another conceptual enlargement of (modern) medical harm.

How to handle pluralist harm assessment

Undeniably, different people have very different notions of what "medical harm" would be for themselves or for others. Autonomy-centered medical ethics has seen its task as spelling out procedures to foster a "morality of mutual respect" (Engelhardt, 1986) and patients' self-determination. This approach leads to particular concern for informed consent, policies for advance directives, substituted judgment, and so on. A contrasting approach urges that instead of inviting radical individualism in assessing medical harm, we redetermine medicine's substantive goals. Daniel Callahan (1991), for example, argues that such individualism results in net harm to all by consuming too many resources for marginal benefits and setting wrong priorities in our lives. Stressing the importance of expectations and cultural presumptions in determining what individuals view as harm, Callahan hopes to find arguments acceptable to the whole of society—in favor, for instance, of decreasing individual expectations for life-prolonging treatment in old age.

Other authors concur that individualistic harm assessment is the wrong paradigm for medicine: "Moral atomism" is viewed as impoverishing medical practice socially and morally, that is, as giving up grounds on which a sense of community and good decision making should develop (Pellegrino and Thomasma, 1988). Others see "moral atomism" as leading to a waste of physicians' power to assist patients in pursuing their goals (Brody, 1992, p. 50) or as leading to paralysis in crucial policy questions, such as how to determine the best treatment interests of incompetent patients (Emanuel, 1991). Ezekiel Emanuel opts for communitarian healthcare settings, where groups of patients and physicians shape medicine according to their shared assessment of harms and benefits; others are confident that the consensus on harm in the context of medicine is substantial (Pellegrino and Thomasma, 1988; Cassell, 1991; Brody, 1992). They see the main problem in "the view that the physician respects autonomy by taking a negative, hands-off stance" (Brody, 1992), which they argue ought to be given up in favor of assisting patients, in a critical and trustworthy manner, to assess harms and benefits.

Harm-referring duties: Nonmaleficence and beneficence

Some scholars in ethics formulate a distinct duty of nonmaleficence, expressing a prohibition on actions with foreseeably harmful effects. Others, however, include this prohibition as part of a duty of beneficence. This, and whether such obligation is construed as a prohibition on causing net harm to someone (such that, say, shooting a murderer to save the life of his three victims would not be maleficent), or on harming itself (the shooting would be maleficent, though perhaps justified), is a question of terminological and classificatory preference. The duty of nonmaleficence is still indeterminate under any of these descriptions, not only because they reintroduce the problems of harm assessment but also because they are silent about permissible limits and trade-offs.

Harm and benefit can result from actions that vary with (a) the generic mode (commission vs. omission, such as active killing vs. letting die); (b) causal mode (infliction vs. nonremoval vs. nonprevention, such as killing vs. not saving a drowning person vs. not preventing a murder); or (c) intentional mode (intending vs. merely foreseeing vs. not even foreseeing the consequence, such as killing by murder vs. killing by pain relief vs. killing by accident).

A simple-act consequentialist ethical theory would prescribe avoidance of harm regardless of these distinctions, but it might want to spell out some agent-centered constraints: Certain actions, although morally laudable, are not required of the agent; for example, a therapist need not risk his own death in treating a violent patient. Proponents of deontologic ethics might want to add further constraints related to distinctions (a), (b), and (c) above (e.g., set up a prohibition on active killing).

Again, in any ethical theory, harm sometimes ought not be prevented or removed from one patient because of other overriding duties (e.g., to remove still greater harm from another or to respect patient self-determination). However, there are many different views as to what counts as overriding duty. Between the two extremes—understanding nonmaleficence as the trivially indeterminate principle "avoid harm (whatever that is) unless it is outweighed" or having as many specified duties as there are different normative theories—attempts have been made to give a more specific meaning to nonmaleficence without leaving the middle ground of broader consensus. Recognizing a distinct principle of nonmaleficence is fairly common in medical (in contrast to general) ethics. It is meant to guide actions by caregivers in those situations that are most likely to produce harm. This tailoring, which is influenced by normative perspectives, explains formal and substantial differences among medical ethical perspectives in what is understood as nonmaleficence in health care.

Tom Beauchamp and James Childress, for instance, turn to the four duties of beneficence originally distinguished by William Frankena (1973) according to both a distinction between harm and benefit, and to the action's causal mode, (b) above: (1) not to inflict harm, (2) to prevent harm, (3) to remove harm, (4) to promote good. However, they subsume (1) under nonmaleficence and (2)–(4) under beneficence (Beauchamp and Childress, 1989). The difference between negative and positive duties (i.e., duties of omission versus duties of commission)—again depending on aspects of causality—is thus introduced as a distinguishing criterion between both duties. Beauchamp and Childress do not, however, take this classification as such to be normatively decisive; rather, they intend to capture ordinary language usage, mirroring the empirical fact that noninfliction of harm often is achievable at lower cost to the agent than is obeying positive duties. It is in this sense that nonmaleficence takes precedence.

Along these lines, Allen Buchanan and Dan Brock have suggested that appeals to nonmaleficence in medicine be understood as specific reminders: in Hippocratic times, not to forget that some treatments were only burdensome and not beneficial; in our time, to correct "for professional biases toward over-treatment of non-communicating patients in conditions of great risk or profound uncertainty" (Buchanan and Brock, 1989, p. 256). These reminders pay attention to medicine's (increasing) potential not only to benefit patients but also to inflict harm upon them.

The duty of nonmaleficence may conflict with the autonomy of patients who request treatment that physicians consider harmful (e.g., unjustified surgery, futile chemotherapy, or drugs). With an eye to precisely this conflict, H. Tristram Engelhardt, Jr., understands the duty of nonmaleficence as a justification to limit patients' self-determination (Engelhardt, 1986).

A prohibition on killing patients is often taken to be the most prominent (negative) duty of medical nonmaleficence, death being a major harm for most people. For reasons of consistency, however, actions such as actively killing a patient can be called maleficent only if "passively" withholding or withdrawing life support is likewise seen to produce harm. Important though distinctions (a) or (b) above might be as deontological constraints, they could never turn a benefit (being allowed to die) into a harm (being killed). This is well observed by the controversial Roman Catholic doctrine of double effect, according to which, for example, indirect euthanasia can be justified in spite of the resulting harm (death), since death is not intended but merely foreseen as a by-product of beneficent painkilling (distinction (c) above).

In summary, there is a remarkable tension between harm's undisputed importance in medical ethics and the numerous different ways in which it comes to be con-

ceptualized, thus mirroring the plurality of existing ethical approaches.

BETTINA SCHÖNE-SEIFERT

For a further discussion of topics mentioned in this entry, see the entries AUTONOMY; BENEFICENCE; BIOETHICS; CARE; COMPASSION; DEATH AND DYING: EUTHANASIA AND SUSTAINING LIFE; DISABILITY; DOUBLE EFFECT; ETHICS, *especially the article on* NORMATIVE ETHICAL THEORIES; HEALTH AND DISEASE, *especially the article on* THE EXPERIENCE OF HEALTH AND ILLNESS; MEDICAL CODES AND OATHS; OBLIGATION AND SUPEREROGATION; PAIN AND SUFFERING; PATERNALISM; RISK; UTILITY; *and* VALUE AND VALUATION. *This article will find application in the entries* ABORTION; ANIMAL RESEARCH; ANIMAL WELFARE AND RIGHTS; DEATH; ORGAN AND TISSUE PROCUREMENT; *and* SUICIDE. *For a discussion of related ideas, see the entries* DEATH, ATTITUDES TOWARD; FIDELITY AND LOYALTY; HEALTH CARE, QUALITY OF; IATROGENIC ILLNESS AND INJURY; INFORMATION DISCLOSURE; INFORMED CONSENT; INJURY AND INJURY CONTROL; *and* LIFE, QUALITY OF. *See also the* APPENDIX (CODES, OATHS, AND DIRECTIVES RELATED TO BIOETHICS), SECTION II: ETHICAL DIRECTIVES FOR THE PRACTICE OF MEDICINE; SECTION III: ETHICAL DIRECTIVES FOR OTHER HEALTH PROFESSIONS; SECTION IV: ETHICAL DIRECTIVES FOR HUMAN RESEARCH; *and* SECTION V: ETHICAL DIRECTIVES PERTAINING TO THE WELFARE AND USE OF ANIMALS.

Bibliography

BARRY, BRIAN. 1990. [1965]. *Political Argument: A Reissue with a New Introduction.* Berkeley: University of California Press.

BEAUCHAMP, TOM L., and CHILDRESS, JAMES F. 1989. *Principles of Biomedical Ethics.* 3d ed. New York: Oxford University Press.

BENTHAM, JEREMY. 1963. [1789]. *An Introduction to the Principles of Morals and Legislation.* New York: Hafner.

BRODY, HOWARD. 1992. *The Healer's Power.* New Haven, Conn.: Yale University Press.

BUCHANAN, ALLEN E., and BROCK, DAN W. 1989. *Deciding for Others: The Ethics of Surrogate Decisionmaking.* New York: Cambridge University Press.

CALLAHAN, DANIEL. 1991. *What Kind of Life: The Limits of Medical Progress.* New York: Simon & Schuster.

CASSELL, ERIC J. 1991. *The Nature of Suffering: And the Goals of Medicine.* New York: Oxford University Press.

CULVER, CHARLES M., and GERT, BERNARD. 1982. *Philosophy in Medicine: Conceptual and Ethical Issues in Medicine and Psychiatry.* New York: Oxford University Press.

DWORKIN, RONALD. 1993. *Life's Dominion: An Argument About Abortion, Euthanasia, and Individual Freedom.* New York: Knopf.

EMANUEL, EZEKIEL J. 1991. *The Ends of Human Life: Medical*

Ethics in a Liberal Polity. Cambridge, Mass.: Harvard University Press.

ENGELHARDT, H. TRISTRAM, JR. 1986. *The Foundations of Bioethics.* New York: Oxford University Press.

FEINBERG, JOEL. 1984. *Harm to Others.* New York: Oxford University Press.

FRANKENA, WILLIAM K. 1973. *Ethics.* 2d ed. Englewood Cliffs, N.J.: Prentice-Hall.

GRIFFIN, JAMES. 1986. *Well-Being: Its Meaning, Measurement and Moral Importance.* Oxford: At the Clarendon Press.

MILL, JOHN STUART. 1979. [1863]. *Utilitarianism.* Indianapolis, Ind.: Hackett.

NODDINGS, NEL. 1989. *Women and Evil.* Berkeley: University of California Press.

PELLEGRINO, EDMUND D., and THOMASMA, DAVID C. 1988. *For the Patient's Good: The Restoration of Beneficence in Health Care.* New York: Oxford University Press.

SIDGWICK, HENRY. 1966. [1907]. *The Methods of Ethics.* 7th ed. New York: Dover.

VEATCH, ROBERT M. 1991. *The Patient-Physician Relation: The Patient as Partner, Part 2.* Bloomington: Indiana University Press.

WARREN, VIRGINIA L. 1992. "Feminist Directions in Medical Ethics." In *Feminist Perspectives in Medical Ethics,* pp. 32–45. Edited by Helen Bequaert Holmes and Laura M. Purdy. Bloomington: Indiana University Press.

HAZARDOUS WASTES AND TOXIC SUBSTANCES

Developed nations such as the United States annually use more than 60,000 hazardous chemicals in their agricultural and manufacturing processes. Because at least 10,000 of them are introduced each year, often we know very little about their effects on humans and the environment. When we began massive use of such chemicals, we did not realize that by the 1970s, human breast milk would become more contaminated with toxins than any allowable manufactured foods. We did not realize that measurable amounts of DDT would appear in the polar ice caps. We did not realize that, because of their long lifetimes, many hazardous chemicals would be able to migrate from their present waste sites and would threaten persons living thousands of years in the future. On the whole, we have assumed that dangerous chemicals are "innocent until proved guilty." Because we do very little sophisticated epidemiological testing and rarely take account of food-chain and synergistic effects, thousands of chemicals have become both important to our agricultural and manufacturing processes and ubiquitous in our environment. Hence, it is often difficult to prove that any one chemical is responsible for specific harms, even when we know that it is theoretically able to cause many "statistical casualties."

Hazardous wastes, byproducts of manufacturing, scientific, medical, and agricultural processes, have at least one of four characteristics: ignitability, corrosivity, reactivity, or toxicity (Wagner, 1990). Hazardous substances become wastes only when they have outlived their economic life. They include solvents, electroplating substances, pesticides such as dioxin, and radioactive wastes. Toxic substances, a subset of hazardous substances, have the characteristic of toxicity: the ability to cause serious injury, illness, or death.

Many persons became aware of the threat of hazardous wastes and toxic substances when Rachel Carson (1962) wrote *Silent Spring,* one of the earliest warnings of the dangers of pesticides, or when Michael Brown (1980) wrote his spellbinding account of hundreds of cancers, genetic damage, and birth defects near Love Canal, New York, and other waste sites. Indeed, hazardous-waste management has become one of the most serious environmental problems facing the world. In the United States alone, more than five billion pounds of toxic chemicals are released each year into air, water, and land. Approximately 80 percent of hazardous waste has been dumped into thousands of landfills, ponds, and pits. It has polluted air, wells, surface water, and groundwater. It has destroyed species, habitats, and ecosystems. It also has caused fires, explosions, direct-contact poisoning, and numerous cases of cancer, genetic harms, and birth defects.

In part to protect workers and the public from the dangers associated with hazardous substances, the U.S. Congress passed laws such as the 1954 Atomic Energy Act; the 1975 Hazardous Materials Transportation Act; the 1976 Resource Conservation and Recovery Act (RCRA); the 1976 Toxic Substances Control Act (TSCA); the 1977 Clean Water Act; the 1977 Clean Air Act; and the 1980 Comprehensive Environmental Response, Compensation, and Liability Act known as CERCLA or Superfund (Dominguez and Bartlett, 1986). These laws include provisions that require monitoring pollutants, reporting spills, preparing manifests describing particular wastes, and special packaging for transporting specific types of hazardous materials. The Clean Air Act regulates smelter emissions, for instance, and the Clean Water Act regulates mining-caused water pollution (Young, 1992). RCRA was passed to fill a statutory void left by the Clean Air Act and the Clean Water Act, which require removal of hazardous materials from air and water but leave the question of the ultimate deposition of hazardous waste unanswered. Although RCRA addresses the handling of such waste at current and future facilities, it does not deal with closed or abandoned sites. CERCLA focuses on hazardous-waste contamination when sites or spills have been abandoned; through penalties and taxes on hazardous substances, CERCLA provides for cleaning up abandoned sites.

Despite laws that govern dangerous substances, the use of toxic substances and the management of hazardous wastes raise ethical issues that have not been adequately addressed by existing regulations. Most of these ethical questions are related either to the equity of risk distribution or to the assessment and management of societal risks. The equity issues include siting, rights of future generations, workers' rights, free and informed consent, compensation, and due process. Questions about risk assessment and management include appropriate ethical behavior under conditions of uncertainty, where to place the burden of proof regarding alleged harms involving hazardous substances, and workers' and the public's right to know.

Equity issues

Those who can afford to avoid hazardous wastes and toxic substances typically do so. Those who cannot are usually poor or otherwise disadvantaged. For this reason, public and workplace exposure to such hazards raises questions of intergenerational, geographical, and occupational equity. Intergenerational-equity problems deal with imposing risks and costs of hazardous wastes and toxic substances on future persons. Geographical-equity issues have to do with where and how to site waste dumps or facilities using toxic substances. Occupational-equity problems focus on whether to maximize the safety of the public or of the people who work with hazardous materials because we often cannot protect both groups at once. For example, effective decontamination and safety assurance at waste sites typically require more worker exposure to toxins but reduce public risk. Using mechanical or nonhuman decontamination and safety procedures, however, is safer for workers but usually increases public risk because such procedures are less effective than those controlled closely by people (see Kasperson, 1983; Shrader-Frechette, 1993).

Intergenerational equity requires us to ask whether we ought to mortgage the future by imposing our debts of buried (or stored) hazardous wastes on subsequent generations. Current plans for future U.S. government storage of high-level radioactive waste, for example, require the steel canisters to resist corrosion for as little as 300 years. Nevertheless, the U.S. Department of Energy admits that the waste will remain dangerous for longer than 10,000 years. Government experts agree that, at best, they can merely limit the radioactivity that reaches the environment, and that "there is no doubt that the repository will leak over the course of the next 10,000 years" (Shrader-Frechette, 1993). To saddle our descendants with the medical and financial debts of such waste, much of which is extremely long-lived, is questionable at best: We have received most of the benefits from the use of industrial and agricultural processes that create hazardous wastes, whereas future persons will bear most of the risks and costs. This risk/cost–benefit asymmetry suggests that, without good reasons or compensating benefits, future generations ought not be saddled with their ancestors' debts (Shrader-Frechette, 1993). Moreover, any alleged economies associated with storage of hazardous waste are, in large part, questionable because of economists' practice of discounting future costs (such as deaths) at some rate of x percent per year. For example, at a discount rate of 10 percent, effects on people's welfare twenty years from now count only for one-tenth of what effects on people's welfare count for now. Or, more graphically, with a discount rate of 5 percent, a billion deaths in 400 years counts the same as one death next year. A number of moral philosophers, such as Derek Parfit, have argued that use of a discount rate is unethical, because the moral importance of future events, like the death of a person, does not decline at some x percent per year.

Another issue related to intergenerational equity is what sort of criteria might justify environmentally irreversible damage to the environment, such as that caused by deep-well storage of high-level nuclear waste. On the one hand, irreversible management schemes for nuclear waste, because they are premised on the nonretrievability of the waste, theoretically impose fewer management burdens on later generations, but they also preempt future choices about how to deal with the hazards. On the other hand, schemes that are reversible, because they are premised on the retrievability of the waste, allow for wider choices for future generations, but they also impose greater management burdens. If we cannot do both, is it ethically desirable to maximize future freedom or to minimize future burdens? The technical problems associated with storing long-lived hazardous waste for centuries are forcing us to take a great gamble with the freedom and the security of future persons. We are gambling that our descendants will not breach the waste repositories through war, terrorism, or drilling for minerals; that groundwater will not leach out and transport toxins; and that subsequent ice sheets, faulting, seismic activity, and geological folding will not uncover the wastes.

Using and storing toxins also raises questions of spatial or geographical equity. One such issue is whether it is fair to impose a higher risk (of being harmed by seepage from a hazardous-waste dump, for example) on persons just because they live in a certain part of the community. Or, is it ethical for people in one area to receive the benefits of products created by using toxic substances, while people in another area bear the health risks associated with living near a hazardous-waste dump or an industry employing toxic material? How does one site hazardous facilities equitably, and how does one transport toxic substances safely (see English, 1992)?

Questions about the equity of risk distribution are central to the issue of managing toxic substances because thousands of persons—such as the 1984 victims of the Union Carbide toxic leak in Bhopal, India—have already died as a consequence of exposure to hazardous substances. Economic comparisons of alternative chemical technologies and different waste sites typically ignore the externalities (or social costs) such as the inequitable distribution of health hazards and the risk–benefit asymmetries associated with using toxic substances or managing hazardous wastes. Geographical and intergenerational inequities are typically "external" to the benefit–cost schemes used as the basis for public policy. Consequently, decision makers almost always ignore such externalities (Shrader-Frechette, 1985).

The most serious problems of geographical equity in the distribution of risks associated with dangerous substances arise because developed nations often ship their toxic chemicals and hazardous wastes to developing countries. One-third of U.S. pesticide exports, for example, are products that are banned for use in the United States. These exports are annually responsible for 40,000 pesticide-related deaths, mainly in developing nations (Shrader-Frechette, 1991). Likewise, the United Nations estimates that as much as 20 percent of the hazardous waste produced in developed nations is sent to other countries where health and safety standards are virtually nonexistent. The Organization of African Unity has pleaded with member states to stop such traffic, but corruption and crime have kept the waste transport going (Moyers, 1990). Indeed, exporting toxic substances and hazardous wastes may be the current version of the infant-formula problem. During the last three decades of the twentieth century, U.S. and multinational corporations have profited by exporting infant formula to developing nations and by encouraging young mothers not to nurse their children. They have been able to do so only by extremely coercive sales tactics and by misleading persons in developing countries about the relative merits and dangers of the exports.

Some of the greatest risks associated with toxic substances and hazardous wastes, whether in developed or developing nations, are borne by workers. One of the main questions of occupational equity is whether it is just to impose higher health burdens on workers in exchange for wages. Is it fair to allow persons to trade their health and safety for money? This question is particularly troublesome in the United States, because many other countries—such as the Scandinavian nations, Germany, and the former Soviet Union—have standards for occupational exposure to risks from toxins that are just as stringent as standards for public exposure. The United States, however, follows the alleged "compensating wage differential (CWD)" of Adam Smith, presupposing that wages compensate workers for increased occupational exposures to toxic substances. As a consequence, U.S. regulators argue that, in exchange for facing higher risks than the public faces from toxic substances, workers receive higher wages that compensate them for their burden. Other countries do not accept the economic theory underlying the CWD and argue for equal health standards, for making public and worker exposure norms the same (Shrader-Frechette, 1991).

Consent and right to know

One reason critics question the theory underlying the CWD is its presupposition that, by virtue of accepting certain jobs, workers exposed to serious hazards give free, informed consent to the risks. Yet, from an ethical point of view, those most able to give free, informed consent—those who are well educated and who have many job opportunities—are usually unwilling to do so. Those least able to give genuine consent to a risky workplace or neighborhood—because of their lack of education or information and their financial constraints—are often willing to give alleged consent.

The 1986 U.S. Right-to-Know Act requires owners or operators of sites using hazardous materials to notify the Emergency Response Commission in their state that toxins are present at a facility. However, at least three factors suggest that this law may fail to ensure full conditions for the free, informed consent of persons likely to be harmed by some hazardous substance. First, owners or operators (rather than a neutral third party) provide the information about the hazard. Often those responsible for toxic substances and hazardous wastes do not inform workers and the public of the risks they face, even after company physicians have documented serious health problems. Employers in the chemical industry, for example, frequently spend money on genetic screening to exclude susceptible persons from the workplace rather than to monitor their health on the job (Draper, 1991). Second, the existence, location, and operational procedures of dangerous facilities are likely things to which citizens and workers have not given free, informed consent in the first place. Third, mining is not included among the industries required to report their toxic emissions to state and federal regulators. For example, Utah's Bingham Canyon Copper Mine, owned by Kennecott Copper, ranks fourth in the nation in total toxic releases, yet it and other mining companies do not report their releases (Young, 1992).

Sociological data reveal that, as education and income rise, people are less willing to accept either hazardous facilities or risky jobs; those who do so tend to be poorly educated or financially strapped. The data also show that the alleged CWD does not operate for poor, unskilled, minority, or nonunionized workers. Yet these are precisely the people most likely to have risky jobs, such as handling nuclear wastes. In other words, the very persons *least* able to give free, informed consent to occupational risks are precisely those who *most* often work in risky jobs (Shrader-Frechette, 1993).

At the international level, a similar situation occurs. The persons and nations least able to give free informed consent to the location of facilities for using or storing toxic substances are typically those who most often bear such risks. Hazardous wastes shipped abroad, for example, are usually sent to countries that will take them at the cheapest rate, and these tend to be developing nations that are often ill informed about the risks involved. In 1989, the United Nations passed a resolution requiring any country receiving hazardous waste to give consent before it is sent. Because socioeconomic conditions and corruption often militate against the exercise of free informed consent, however, it is questionable whether the U.N. resolution will have much effect (Shrader-Frechette, 1991).

Industries' offers of financial benefits—for storing hazardous waste in a developing nation or in an economically depressed community—create a coercive context in which requirements for free informed consent are unlikely to be met. Likewise, high wages for desperate workers who agree to take risky jobs may jeopardize their legitimate consent. In such contexts, we must admit either that our classical ethical theory of free informed consent is wrong or that our laws and regulations fail to provide an ethical framework in which those most affected by hazardous substances can give free informed consent to the risk.

Given the many consent-related problems relevant to risk from hazardous substances, a crucial issue is: Who should give consent? Liberty and grass-roots self-determination require local control of whether a hazardous facility is sited in a particular area. Yet, equality of consideration for people in all regions and minimizing overall risk often require federal control. Should a particular community be able to veto the location of a hazardous facility, even though that site may be the best in the country and may provide the most equal protection of all people? Or should the national government have the right to impose such risks on a local community, even against the wishes of that group?

On the one hand, federal jurisdiction is more likely to protect the environment, to avoid the tragedy of the commons, to gain national economies of scale, and to avoid regional favoritism. Federal jurisdiction is also more likely to provide compensation for victims of spillovers from another locale and to facilitate the politics of sacrifice by imposing equal burdens on all. On the other hand, local jurisdiction is more likely to promote diversity, to offer a more flexible vehicle for experimenting with waste regulations, and to enhance citizens' auton-

omy and liberty. Local jurisdiction also is likely to encourage cooperation through participation in decision making, to discourage some kinds of inequitable federal policies, and to help avoid many violations of rights.

Compensation

Current U.S. laws do not typically provide for full exercise of due-process rights by those who may have been harmed by toxins or hazardous wastes. Many of the companies that handle dangerous substances do not have either full insurance for their pollution risk or adequate funds to cover their liability themselves. RCRA and CERCLA, however, require such companies both to show that they are capable of paying at least some of the damages resulting from their activities and to clean up their sites. Because enforcement of liability and coverage provisions of these laws is difficult, many hazardous-waste industries often operate outside the law. Furthermore, most insurers have withdrawn from the pollution market, claiming that providing such coverage carries the risk of payments for claims that would bankrupt them.

Just as insurers fear potentially large liability claims in cases involving hazardous-waste substances, so do members of the public. For example, in 1987 when the U.S. Congress chose Yucca Mountain, Nevada, as the likely site for the world's first permanent facility for high-level nuclear waste, local residents and the state asked for unlimited, strict-liability coverage for any nuclear-waste accident or incident. The U.S. Department of Energy response to the citizens, solidified by the 1957 Price-Anderson Act, was that the government would allow the waste facility to bear only limited liability. Consequently, the U.S. nuclear program, including radioactive-waste management, has operated under a government-imposed limit for liability coverage. This limit, designed to protect the nuclear-waste industry from bankruptcy caused by accidents, is less than 3 percent of the government-calculated costs of the April 1986 Chernobyl nuclear catastrophe, and Chernobyl was not a worst-case accident (see Shrader-Frechette, 1993).

Limits on government or industry liability for hazardous-waste and toxic-substance incidents are problematic for several reasons. First, liability is a well-known incentive for appropriate, safe behavior. Second, refusal to accept full and strict liability suggests that hazardous- and radioactive-waste sites are not as safe as the government maintains they are. Third, if government officials may legally limit due-process rights, then, in the case of an accident at a hazardous-waste facility, the main financial burdens will be borne inequitably by accident victims rather than by the perpetrators of the hazard. Fourth, because much less is known about the dangers from hazardous wastes and toxic substances than about more ordinary risks, full liability seems a reasonable requirement. And finally, the safety record of hazardous facilities, in the past, has not been good. Every state and every nation in the world have extensive, long-term pollution from toxins. Even in the United States, the government has been one of the worst offenders. A congressional report has argued that cleaning up the hazardous and radioactive wastes at government weapons facilities would cost more than $300 billion (U.S. Congress, 1983; Shrader-Frechette, 1993). Such problems argue for citizens' rights to full liability.

Uncertainty, human error, and the burden of proof

Inadequate compensation for victims of toxins, inequitable distribution of the risks associated with hazardous wastes, and the uncertainties and potential harm associated with such substances provide powerful arguments for reducing or eliminating exposure to them. To decrease exposures and to move "beyond dumping," however, we must have market incentives for reducing the volume of toxic substances and hazardous wastes (Piasecki, 1984; Higgins, 1989). To reduce the volume of these threats, we must know exactly what effects they cause, and we must make risk imposers accountable for their behavior. Ensuring accountability is not easy. Adequate tests for medical responses to low-level chemical exposures require samples of thousands of persons, because so many toxic substances produce health effects synergistically, because there are many uncertainties about actual exposure to hazardous substances, because the effects of such exposure often are unknown (Ashford and Miller, 1991), and because phenotypical characteristics among individuals often vary by a factor of 200. All four variables cause extreme differences in humans' responses to toxins.

Uncertainties about exposure and about the consequences of exposure to hazardous substances are compounded by the fact that the industries that produce toxic substances and hazardous wastes—and that profit from them—usually perform the required tests to determine toxicity and health effects. Pesticide-registration decisions (about allowing use of the chemicals) in the West, for example, are tied to a risk–benefit standard that combines scientific and economic evidence. Because industry does most or all of the testing, and because environmental and health groups are forced to show that the dangers outweigh the economic benefits of a particular pesticide, there is much uncertainty about the real hazards actually faced by workers and consumers. As a consequence, virtually no groups want toxic substances or hazardous wastes used or stored near

them. Hence the protest: "Not in my backyard"—NIMBY.

NIMBY responses also arise as a consequence of public mistrust of human institutions for controlling hazardous wastes and toxic chemicals. All dangerous technologies are unavoidably dependent upon fragile, sometimes short-lived, human institutions and human capabilities. Faulty technology, after all, did not cause the injuries and deaths at Three Mile Island, Bhopal, Love Canal, or Chernobyl. Human error did. Human error and misconduct also may be the insoluble problem with using toxic substances and managing hazardous wastes. According to risk assessors, 60 to 80 percent of industrial accidents are due to human mismanagement or corruption (Shrader-Frechette, 1993). For example, at the nation's largest incinerator for hazardous wastes, run by Chemical Waste Management, Inc., in Chicago, a 1992 grand jury found evidence of criminal conduct, including deliberate mislabeling of many barrels of hazardous waste. They also discovered deliberate disconnection of pollution-monitoring devices. More generally, corruption in the waste-disposal industry has been rampant in the United States ever since the 1940s, when the Mafia won control of the carting business through Local 813 of the International Brotherhood of Teamsters. In the mid-1990s, three Mafia families still dominated hazardous-waste disposal and illegal dumping: the Gambino, Lucchese, and Genovese/Tiere crime groups (see Szasz, 1986). Given the potential for human error and corruption, citizens are frequently skeptical regarding whether hazardous and toxic substances will be handled safely, with little threat to workers or to the public.

Because of scientific unknowns and uncertainties about human behavior and corruption, several moral philosophers have argued that potentially catastrophic situations—involving hazardous wastes and toxic substances—require ethically conservative behavior (Cranor, 1993; Shrader-Frechette, 1991; Ashford and Miller, 1991). Such situations often require one to choose a "maximin" decision rule, to avoid situations with the greatest potential for harm, as John Rawls (1971) has argued. Ethical conservatism, in a situation of uncertainty, also may require society to place the burden of proof—regarding risk or harm—on the manufacturers, users, and disposers of hazardous substances, rather than on their potential victims. This, in turn, may mean that we will need to reform our laws governing so-called "toxic torts" (Cranor, 1993).

Given the longevity and the catastrophic potential of many toxic substances and hazardous wastes, we may need to reevaluate the human and environmental price we have paid for our economic progress. Although our society may not be able to avoid use of certain toxic substances and disposal of some hazardous waste, it is clear that we need to maximize the equity with which we distribute the risks associated with such threats. We also need to guarantee, so far as possible, that potential victims of toxins are informed about the risks they face and that they freely consent to avoidable risk impositions. Finally, we ought to ensure that those put at risk from toxic substances and hazardous wastes are compensated, so far as possible, for harm done to them. Because of numerous uncertainties about their effects, and because of the catastrophic potential and the longevity of many hazardous materials, our behavior regarding them ought to be ethically conservative.

KRISTIN SHRADER-FRECHETTE

Directly related to this entry are the entries ENVIRONMENTAL ETHICS; ENVIRONMENTAL HEALTH; ENVIRONMENTAL POLICY AND LAW; FUTURE GENERATIONS, OBLIGATIONS TO; JUSTICE; UTILITY; *and* RISK. *For a further discussion of topics mentioned in this article, see the entries* AGRICULTURE; OCCUPATIONAL SAFETY AND HEALTH, *article on* ETHICAL ISSUES; SUSTAINABLE DEVELOPMENT; TECHNOLOGY, *articles on* PHILOSOPHY OF TECHNOLOGY, *and* TECHNOLOGY ASSESSMENT. *Other relevant material may be found under the entries* FOOD POLICY; HARM; INFORMATION DISCLOSURE; INFORMED CONSENT, *articles on* HISTORY OF INFORMED CONSENT, *and* MEANING AND ELEMENTS OF INFORMED CONSENT; *and* PUBLIC HEALTH, *article on* DETERMINANTS OF PUBLIC HEALTH. *See also the* APPENDIX (CODES, OATHS, AND DIRECTIVES RELATED TO BIOETHICS), SECTION VI: ETHICAL DIRECTIVES PERTAINING TO THE ENVIRONMENT.

Bibliography

ASHFORD, NICHOLAS A., and MILLER, CLAUDIA. 1991. *Chemical Exposures: Low Levels and High Stakes.* New York: Van Nostrand Reinhold.

BROWN, MICHAEL H. 1979. *Laying Waste: The Poisoning of America by Toxic Chemicals.* New York: Pantheon.

CARSON, RACHEL. 1962. *Silent Spring.* Boston: Houghton Mifflin.

CRANOR, CARL F. 1993. *Regulating Toxic Substances: Philosophy of Science and the Law.* New York: Oxford University Press.

DOMINGUEZ, GEORGE S., and BARTLETT, KENNETH G., eds. 1986. *Hazardous Waste Management.* Boca Raton, Fla.: CRC Press.

DRAPER, ELAINE. 1991. *Risky Business: Genetic Testing and Exclusionary Practices in the Hazardous Workplace.* Cambridge: At the University Press.

EBENRECK, SARAH. 1983. "A Partnership Farmland Ethic." *Environmental Ethics* 5, no. 1:33–45.

ENGLISH, MARY R. 1992. *Siting Low-Level Radioactive Waste Disposal Facilities: The Public Policy Dilemma.* New York: Greenwood.

GREENBERG, MICHAEL R., and ANDERSON, RICHARD F. 1984. *Hazardous Waste Sites: The Credibility Gap.* New Brunswick, N.J.: Center for Urban Research.

HIGGINS, THOMAS E. 1989. *Hazardous Waste Minimization Handbook.* Chelsea, Mich.: Lewis.

KASPERSON, ROGER, ed. 1983. *Equity Issues in Radioactive Waste Management.* Cambridge, Mass.: Oelgelschlager, Gunn, and Hain.

LA DOU, JOSEPH. 1992. "First World Exports to the Third World: Capital, Technology, Hazardous Waste, and Working Conditions: Who Wins?" *The Western Journal of Medicine* 156, no. 5:553–554.

MOYERS, BILL D. 1990. *Global Dumping Ground: The International Traffic in Hazardous Waste.* Washington, D.C.: Seven Locks Press.

NORDQUIST, JOAN. 1988. *Toxic Waste: Regulatory, Health, International Concerns.* Santa Cruz, Calif.: Reference and Research Services.

PARFIT, DEREK. 1985. *Reasons and Persons.* New York: Oxford University Press.

PIASECKI, BRUCE, ed. 1984. *Beyond Dumping: New Strategies for Controlling Toxic Contamination.* Westport, Conn.: Quorum.

PIASECKI, BRUCE, and DAVIS, GARY A. 1987. *America's Future in Toxic-Waste Management: Lessons from Europe.* Westport, Conn.: Quorum.

POSTEL, SANDRA. 1987. *Defusing the Toxics Threat: Controlling Pesticides and Industrial Waste.* Washington, D.C.: Worldwatch Institute.

RAWLS, JOHN. 1971. *A Theory of Justice.* Cambridge, Mass.: Harvard University Press.

SAMUELS, SHELDON W. 1986. *The Environment of the Workplace and Human Values.* New York: Liss.

SHRADER-FRECHETTE, KRISTIN. 1985. *Science Policy, Ethics, and Economic Methodology: Some Problems of Technology Assessment and Environmental-Impact Analysis.* Dordrecht, Netherlands: D. Reidel.

———. 1991. *Risk and Rationality: Philosophical Foundations for Populist Reforms.* Berkeley: University of California Press.

———. 1993. *Burying Uncertainty: Risk and the Case Against Geological Disposal of Nuclear Waste.* Berkeley: University of California Press.

SZASZ, ANDREW. 1986. "Corporations, Organized Crime, and the Disposal of Hazardous Waste: An Examination of the Making of a Criminogenic Regulatory Structure." *Criminology* 24, no. 1:1–27.

U.S. CONGRESS. 1983. *Hazardous Waste Disposal: Hearings Before the Subcommittee on Investigations and Oversight of the Committee on Science and Technology, U.S. House of Representatives, Ninety-Eighth Congress, First Session, March 30–May 4, 1983.* Washington, D.C.: Government Printing Office.

WAGNER, TRAVIS P. 1990. *Hazardous Waste Identification and Classification Manual: The Identification of Hazardous Waste Under RCRA and the Classification of Hazardous Waste Under HMTA.* New York: Van Nostrand Reinhold.

WYNNE, BRIAN, ed. 1987. *Risk Management and Hazardous*

Waste: Implementation and the Dialectics of Credibility. New York: Springer-Verlag.

YOUNG, JOHN. 1992. *Mining the Earth.* Washington, D.C.: Worldwatch Institute.

HEALING

Health and wholeness

Healing is an action whose goal is the restoration of health. The English word "health" literally means "wholeness" and "to heal" means "to make whole." Ancient Greek had two words generally translated as "health": *hygieia*, meaning "a well way of living," and *euexia*, meaning "good habit of body." Leon Kass (1985) notes that the English and both Greek words for health are totally unrelated to all the words for disease, illness, and sickness. This is also true for German, Latin, and Hebrew. In addition, the Greek terms for health, unlike the English, are unrelated to all the verbs for healing. Health for the ancient Greeks was a state or condition unrelated to, and prior to, both illness and healers. The English emphasis on wholeness, Kass also notes, is comparatively static and structural, implying a whole distinct from all else and complete in itself and connoting self-sufficiency and independence. The Greek terms, in contrast, stress the functioning of the whole, and not only its working but its working well. Kass sums up this Greek understanding of health by defining it as a natural as opposed to a moral norm that reveals itself in activity as a standard of bodily excellence or fitness. It is the well-working of the organism as a whole, an activity of the living body in accordance with its specific excellences.

The work of healing in Western culture is the proper activity of the profession of medicine. Howard Brody (1987) calls medicine a craft in which scientific knowledge is applied to particular patients for the purpose of "a right and good healing action," employing the now-classic phrase of Edmund Pellegrino (1982). Unlike the Greek, the English language sets up a relationship between medicine, whose business is healing, and health that is problematic. Kass states the problem this way: Health and only health is the doctor's proper business; but health, understood as well-working wholeness, is not the business only of doctors.

Health as equilibrium. A less formal starting point than Kass's from which to examine the relationship between health and medicine is Pellegrino's definition of health as a state of accommodation, defined in different terms by each person (Pellegrino, 1982). We feel healthy, he says, when we have found an equilibrium between our already-experienced shortcomings and our aspirations and have adjusted our goals to the gap between them. This means that health cannot be understood apart from a person's life history, or to use José Ortega y Gasset's phrase, one's "personal project" (1963, p. 45). Healing, according to this definition of health, occurs when a new equilibrium is found between one's hopes and one's failures that can be incorporated into one's personal project. As such, healing must be based on an authentic perception of the experience of illness in the particular person.

The context of healing. It follows that for an action of someone who professes to heal to be a right and good healing action, it must be situated in the context of a personal history so as to restore the direction of a personal project. This requires that a dialogue be established between healer and patient whose goal is the creation of a common ground of meaning shared by the healer and the patient. How extensive that common ground must be to constitute a right and good healing action is open to question. In taking a medical history, physicians have traditionally tended to restrict the province of illness to the "facts of diseases," leaving unexplored the "fact of illness"—that is, the physical, psychological, and moral vulnerability the patient suffers in the attack on his or her very being that Pellegrino calls "the ontological assault of illness" (1982). However, this concentration on facts and diseases does not result from simple, unreflective traditionalism. Rather, it has enabled the profession of medicine to set very definite limits to the boundaries of healing and thereby to maintain control over the responsibilities that physicians take upon themselves as healers.

The boundaries of healing. The attempt by physicians such as Pellegrino to enlarge the boundaries of what counts as healing has often produced frustration and anger. For example, Franz J. Ingelfinger, in a classic editorial in the *New England Journal of Medicine*, rebukes those who would expand medical treatment to include families, not just individuals: "The curious idea is abroad that the doctor should be a factotum of health. By some singularity of reasoning, his role as healer is disparaged, and the words 'care, not cure' are becoming as tiresome as 'death with dignity'" (Ingelfinger, 1976, p. 565). He continues by lamenting that if the doctor is insensitive to the "multiple environmental conditions that threaten our mental and physical selves, he is regarded as failing the holistic image that many—both lay and medical—wish to impose on the physician" (Ingelfinger, 1976, p. 565). Ingelfinger concludes by asserting that the physician's primary concern, in spite of utopian claims to the contrary, should be sickness, not overall health; medicine should concentrate on "scientifically accurate diagnosis and treatment."

The nature of healing. The resistance of physicians such as Ingelfinger to what they regard as an unwarranted expansion of their role in society signals a fundamental disagreement within Western society about the nature of healing. Holistic approaches to medicine challenge traditional assumptions about who can be called a healer, what the goal of healing should be, and, most important, who can say what constitutes a right and good healing action: the healer or the one to be healed. Those who take positions like Ingelfinger's insist that only those who engage in "scientifically accurate diagnosis and treatment" deserve to be called healers, that healing aims at the cure of disease, and that the healer's profession alone can determine what constitutes a right and good healing action.

Those who disagree with these assumptions often attack their opponents as simply "uncaring." Victor Kestenbaum, however, argues that the point of departure and method, not the lack of feeling, is the real issue (1982). By distinguishing between caring and curing and limiting medicine to the latter, Ingelfinger and his colleagues take as normative the physician's perception of illness, shaped by the method of science, and then seek to derive global professional obligations from it. Thus they cut the phenomenon of illness to fit a prior conception of role and discourse. Pellegrino, Kestenbaum notes by way of contrast, starts with illness as experienced by the patient and derives professional obligations from the distinctly human dimensions of being ill and in distress. The responsibilities of the healer follow from the complexity and scope of the phenomenon of illness, not from the self-declared duties of the profession.

The healing profession

In the 1950s Pedro Laín Entralgo observed that "the curative activity of the physician is always determined by the reality of the human being towards which it is directed, that is, by the 'personal' conditions of the disease and of the patient" (1956, p. xv). Pellegrino believes that this accommodation to the reality of the patient follows from the promise that the medical profession, in the person of the physician, makes to the patient: "The promise of help that shapes the nature of every healing act and defines the requirements for successful healing—even when cure is not possible" (1982, p. 160). But, Pellegrino notes, considerable confusion exists between doctor and patient about what healing means. Physicians, he says, often fail to comprehend what the patient understands by the promise of healing; patients often fail to understand what the physician thinks he or she is promising. Physicians, in response, are moving toward a restricted sense of promise, emphasizing technical competence, whereas patients expect not only competence but compassionate help as well. The wider the gap between professional promises and lay expecta-

tions, the more difficult becomes the collaboration between physician and patient to discover the equilibrium that constitutes genuine healing. As the gap increases, Pellegrino also notes, patients will be more tempted to seek alternatives to the "medical model" and lose the benefits of scientific competence.

Competence and compassion. Healing requires, Pellegrino insists, both competence (in scientifically accurate diagnosis and treatment) and compassion (the capacity to enter into the experience of illness with the patient). Competence is a necessary but not sufficient condition of healing. Healing "must be shaped at every step by the purposes of the healing acts—by the good of the person who is ill—his bodily good, of course, but also his concept of health, his value system, and his sense of the kind and quality of life he thinks is worthwhile" (Pellegrino, 1982, p. 161). Pellegrino sums this up by declaring that the physician therefore has the obligation to protect the moral agency of the patient, to enhance it even in the face of the special vulnerabilities of being ill.

This protection of the moral agency of the patient lies at the heart of compassion; it is essential to the performance of a right and good healing action. Healing thus requires that the conversation between physician and patient encompass more than what can be accommodated by scientifically accurate medical language. As Jay Katz has observed, despite the quantity of words overflowing patients' medical charts, the world shared by doctor and patient is often one of profound silence, offering not the humaneness of shared understanding but the humaneness of services silently rendered (Katz, 1984).

The silent world of medicine

Yet modern scientific medicine owes its success to silence of a sort, a disbelief in words that Laín Entralgo traces to two tenets of the Hippocratic school of medicine. First, the latter rejected the use of words as a therapeutic tool; medicinal remedies were preferred to exorcism, which relied on the curative power of "fine words used in the manner of charms" (Laín Entralgo, 1956, p. 47). In addition, Hippocratic physicians trusted the patient's symptoms to reveal the causes of disease and dismissed the patient's own words about the source of his or her condition as unreliable opinion.

The clinical gaze. Michel Foucault (1973), in his discussion of the antecedents of modern medicine, discovers a similar kind of silence in the "clinical gaze," a reorganization of medical perception that took place in the eighteenth century. Disease ceased to be perceived as an alien force inserted into the body and subject to the words of exorcism; instead, disease was the body itself, become diseased. Healing became the task of deciphering corporal space, a work of seeing instead of speaking. The model physician is Hippocrates, who applied himself only to observation, despising all preconceived systems that might bias the observer. This clinical gaze flourishes only in the relative silence of theories, imaginings, and whatever serves as an obstacle to the sensible immediate. In addition, when physicians question the patient, they question only what they can see—the body become diseased—and only in the language proposed by the body. All other languages, including that spoken by the patient, must fall silent before the absolute silence of observation. Within this double silence, Foucault says, things seen can be heard at last, and heard solely by the virtue of the fact that they are seen. It is in this sense that "the clinical gaze has the paradoxical ability to hear a language as soon as it perceives a spectacle" (Foucault, 1973, p. 108).

The conversation that emerges from this double silence is an interior dialogue that the observer has with him- or herself, not a dialogue with the object of gaze. In the context of the physician–patient encounter, the language describing what the physician has seen gives structure to the encounter, not any language the patient might speak. The profundity of this silence derives from its absoluteness: Not only must the patient keep quiet about theories and imaginings that might relate to his or her illness, absolutely nothing the patient says can have any significance for the physician because no language can exist that has priority over the language of observation. This muting of the patient's own voice gives rise to what Foucault calls "the great myth of a pure Gaze that would be pure Language: a speaking eye" (Foucault, 1973, p. 114). What it sees, it gathers and organizes; and as it sees, and sees more clearly, it speaks and teaches. The speaking eye becomes "the servant of things and the master of truth" (Foucault, 1973, p. 115).

The language of curing.   Secretiveness, or what Foucault terms "esotericism," arises from this model for the physician–patient relationship because, as Foucault observes, one sees the visible (the true) only because one knows the language. Unlike Molière's physicians, who spoke Latin merely in order not to be understood, Foucault's clinicians speak openly about that which anyone can see but only they can understand, because through the language of clinical description they have the means to see and hear at the same time, having access to a language that masters the visible. At this point, the earlier epistemological silence (Foucault's "double silence") that results from a constriction of perception changes into the silence of which Jay Katz speaks, a silence made even more baffling and profound by having as its vehicle a multitude of words that make every pretense of being understandable.

In effect, this model of medical perception insists that healing cannot be spoken or even thought of apart from the language of curing, that is, scientifically accurate diagnosis and treatment. This clinical perception and its promise of truth tend to overshadow all other claims to truth, reducing the promise to help those who suffer illness to the promise to be scientifically competent. Attempting to expand that visual horizon—particularly in the direction of the perspective of the patient—risks introducing an unacceptable noise into the silence of the medical clinic, an unwelcome and meaningless distraction from the work of curing.

Healing and cultural reality

Healing, of course, is a much broader cultural phenomenon than that encompassed by Western scientific medicine. Admittedly, the success of Western medicine at curing has helped justify its claim to be the model for healing in the world today. Yet, as Eric Cassell notes, "the success of medicine has created a strain: the doctor sees his role as the curer of disease and 'forgets' his role as healer of the sick, and patients wander disabled but without a culturally acceptable mantle of disease with which to clothe the nakedness of their pain" (Cassell, 1976, p. 51). This strain also appears in the way patients perceive their physicians. Western culture has conferred upon doctors the role of the care of the sick; but although doctors' role as the curers of disease is clear, their role as healers remains obscure. The latter role, Cassell adds, depends less on their ability to provide a scientifically accurate explanation of their patient's illness than to provide an explanation consistent with the culture of the patient. The reality that counts is cultural reality, and the system used by the healer or doctor need be accurate only in terms of the culture in which it is being used, for it serves to explain illness. The importance of the healer's explanation, Cassell insists, cannot be overemphasized.

The healing relationship.   As Cassell sees it, the healer's knowledge, imparted to the patient, helps move the world of illness from the unknown to the rational world. This knowledge allows the patient to "work on" the illness and to make an essential link between conscious process and body process that, Cassell says, marks the "educated" patient. Such healing is not cognitive alone. In addition to educating the patient, healers also play an active physical part in providing a link between symbolic reason and the body: They use their hands. Cassell calls this the "tenderness phenomenon," as important as education in the process of healing. He associates this phenomenon with parenting, and, in this sense, healers serve as parents. In addition to other aspects of the parental role, we transfer to them the right to lay hands on us, to be tender to us, and to pass through our territorial defenses.

The connectedness that underlies the tenderness phenomenon works in both directions. Healer and sufferer become exquisitely sensitive to one another; each can sense the feelings of the other. If healers can accept that the feelings they have can come from the patient, they can use their own feelings in the presence of the patient to provide a vital link with the patient's interior emotional state that is otherwise closed to the clinical observer. Cassell emphasizes that the ability of healers to establish this connectedness with the patient is not an exception to the role of healer but is rather an integral part of the healing function. It shatters the silence of which Katz writes, and substitutes for clinical detachment the "constant will of one trying to recognize" (Brody, 1992, p. 263).

Establishing this connectedness does not make of the healer a great person but does place both healer and patient in the presence of a deep human mystery that is greater than both of them. It is to be present at a creation that Elaine Scarry likens to the rediscovery of language: "Physical pain is not only itself resistant to language but also actively destroys language, deconstructing it into the pre-language of cries and groans. To hear those cries is to witness the shattering of language. Conversely, to be present when the person in pain rediscovers speech and so regains his powers of self-objectification is almost to be present at the birth, or rebirth, of language" (Scarry, 1985, p. 172).

Explanation, education, and connectedness form the core of Cassell's understanding of the healing relationship. The problem with the scientific explanation of illness is not that it is incorrect, since, as Cassell notes, "we know that it need not be correct, since for most of the history of medicine it has not been correct" (Cassell, 1976, p. 128). Put differently, the virtue of scientifically accurate diagnosis and treatment does not lie in its correctness. The fact that it seems correct does not entitle it to stand as the only and sufficient explanation of illness. Although science has been empowered by Western culture to dictate diagnosis and disease categories, Cassell notes that it has little or nothing to say about sick persons, their behavior, patient–healer communication, and so on. "If the whole point of the clinical encounter is to decide what is the right and the good thing to do for a specific patient, then traditional medical theory is sorely lacking" (Cassell, 1991, p. 6).

The power of the healer

Although he recognizes the limitations of traditional medical theory, Cassell does not intend to belittle or dismiss the role that the scientific explanation of disease has in Western culture or the promise it holds for the world. He wishes, in fact, to acknowledge its power: "The therapeutic power of the doctor–patient relationship grows in importance as the technology of cure becomes more powerful" (Cassell, 1991, p. 69). Yet, unfortunately, even as the importance of the relationship between doctor and patient grows under the stimulus of technology, so does the isolation of the patient, who becomes lost in a maze of tests, procedures, and treatment teams. To disregard this relationship only adds insult to the injury inflicted by isolation. "It has been one of the most basic errors of the modern era in medicine to believe that patients cured of their diseases—cancer removed, coronary arteries opened, infection resolved, walking again, talking again, or back home again—are also healed; are whole again" (Cassell, 1991, p. 69). What has been forgotten, he says, is that technology itself has no power—humans acquire power by employing the technology.

The importance of power in the therapeutic relationship has been explored at length by Howard Brody (1992). He analyzes the healer's power in three components: Aesculapian, charismatic, and social. The healer acquires Aesculapian power by virtue of training in the craft of healing. The power is impersonal, transferable to any other healer of comparable skill and experience. Charismatic power is founded on the healer's personal qualities and character and cannot be readily transferred. It is independent of the disciplinary knowledge and skill belonging to Aesculapian power. Social power arises from the social status of the healer within a particular society. It derives its authority in part from the implied contract between the healing profession and society that empowers the profession to determine truth in regard to illness.

The power to heal involves a complex interplay among all three kinds of power; it is a mistake, Brody notes, to limit the power of healing to Aesculapian power alone. Any discussion of what constitutes a right and good healing action must entail an exploration of the proper use of the other forms of power that the healer possesses. These forms of power risk what Brody calls "the dark side of the force." This is "a lust, half childish, half sadistic, to use whatever power we might have to victimize others less powerful, and to enjoy it— to glory in the fact that they and not we are the victims, and to escape for a moment into the fantasy that since we can avoid their victimhood through our power, we are invulnerable and need never again feel fear" (Brody, 1992, p. 21).

The virtue of compassion. Healers can find the antidote to the dark side of the force by acknowledging the feelings of vulnerability and weakness that arise in them as they face the patient. They can do this only if they are open to the experience of being ill and in distress. To do this effectively, Brody says, healers need more than to be told they have an obligation to be open; they need to develop the virtue of compassion, an internalized habit of character that becomes an instinctive attitude of openness and vulnerability.

A major irony in the healer–patient relationship emerges here. To be compassionate in response to the suffering of the patient is itself a powerful act of healing. In showing compassion, the healer empowers the patient in a way that merely curing disease cannot. Curing disease eliminates a threat to bodily function and integrity; alleviating suffering, without which healing is a mere charade, restores the sufferer's connections with humanity and the ability to make sense of his or her own life. Yet, Brody says, this act of empowerment is possible only to the extent that the healer is willing to adopt a position of relative powerlessness, to acknowledge that the patient's suffering has incredible power over her or him and that it is impossible to remain unchanged in the face of it.

Shared power.   Western medical training urges compassion as a duty of the profession but at the same time warns, "Don't get too involved." Brody interprets this warning as a form of false reassurance that the power to heal does not entail the felt powerlessness of compassion. This denial of the power that the patient's suffering has over the physician is a rejection of the concept of shared power, which Brody states is the essential element in the ethical use of power. This denial also betrays a fundamental misperception of power as a zero sum game, that is, the belief that anything that increases the power of the patient within the healing relationship must necessarily decrease the healing power of the physician.

This "competitive" notion of power conforms to the type of moral reasoning that Carol Gilligan discovered among non-minority males in North American culture. The dominant male culture emphasizes the importance of finding the rules that govern a relationship and then selecting courses of action in keeping with the rules, even if such devotion to rules means sacrificing someone's interests to the considerations of abstract justice (Gilligan, 1982). She counters with a type of moral reasoning common to the women she studied: They tend to focus on the nuances of personal relationships and seek solutions that protect the interests of all affected parties and that avoid bringing harm to anyone.

Restructuring the power of healing.   Following the lead of Gilligan, other voices have appealed to an understanding of moral relationships from the perspective of women, such as Nel Noddings (1984), whose work on caring has influenced nursing ethics (Bishop and Scudder, 1991); and Virginia Warren (1989), who applies a feminist point of view to the conduct of med-

ical ethics itself. Although these critics represent a wide range of opinion on the means to be used and even on the foundational reasons for doing so, most of them would agree with Susan Sherwin that there is a need to develop conceptual models for restructuring the power associated with healing and to clarify how "excessive dependence can be reduced, how caring can be offered without paternalism, and how health services can be obtained within a context worthy of trust" (Sherwin, 1992, p. 93). Sherwin notes with approval that, for many mainstream medical ethicists, compassion is frequently claimed to be more compelling than justice, a tendency she finds especially common in the contribution of physicians to medical ethics.

If this need for compassion is admitted, the significant question then becomes, What can allow a physician to experience the powerful suffering of a patient in a way that encourages the physician to share power and therefore to become not only a curer but also a healer? What is needed is a way for healers, and physicians in particular, to experience the felt reality of shared power without seeing it as a betrayal of their Aesculapian power, no matter how evident in this process its limitations may appear to become.

The limits of Aesculapian power.   The strategy employed by many patient advocacy groups of leaving physicians' Aesculapian power undisturbed while severely restricting their social and charismatic power avoids the issue by ceding to physicians their chosen territory. Such an approach abandons the project of power sharing and attempts to render the healer–patient relationship "doctor-proof" by segregating Aesculapian power from the other forms of power. This strategy errs because it assumes that "we can wring morally acceptable actions out of any physician no matter how good or bad his motives if only we have the right rules for him to follow" (Brody, 1992, p. 55). As feminist critics have noted, this strategy endorses the "masculine" assumption that solving moral problems means discovering the right rules while leaving intact the existing power relationships. It cannot succeed because, as Brody points out, it mistakenly presumes that the healer's power comes in two neatly differentiated categories: power that helps fight illness, and power that can be used to violate patient's rights. But no such easy distinction is possible because the same powers can be easily redirected for good or ill.

The realization of shared power can take place only if those who profess to heal acknowledge responsibility for all the forms of power they possess. They must be reassured that owning up to their charismatic and social power does not imply that their Aesculapian power is fraudulent, although it may require them to admit that something like the placebo effect is present in almost every healing encounter (Brody, 1992). For physicians to profess to heal requires the realization that their Aesculapian power, despite the warrant of its scientific accomplishments, is limited in both its scope and effectiveness. Curing does not ensure healing, and healing is possible even if there cannot be cure; nor is every human ill subject to cure. Such an admission, however, does not exempt those who profess to heal from attending to the needs of the poor, the oppressed, or those victimized by war, prejudice, and despotism. It only reminds them that their social and charismatic powers alone have authority in these difficult areas.

Aesthetic distance.   Compassion, lest it degenerate into codependency, does need to maintain a certain strength and thus a certain distance from the plight of the sufferer. Brody characterizes this distance as aesthetic rather than emotional; it resembles the reader's approach to a work of fiction (Brody, 1992). To regard the suffering patient as a text, attended to at an aesthetic distance, still permits and even encourages intense emotional involvement. In reading the text presented by the sufferer, the healer must maintain in his or her imagination that separate vantage point from which the experience of the sufferer can be reinterpreted and reconnected to the broader context of culture and society.

Healing and community

Healing reconnects the sufferer both to the self and to the world. The final and perhaps least appreciated aspect of healing is the need for this reconnection to take place in the context of a community, a need as real for the healer as it is for the sufferer. Healing requires from the healer a commitment over time to become a person capable of compassion and therefore of healing, who has the deep knowledge of how to fuse power and powerlessness, strength and vulnerability. This openness to vulnerability required of healers is more than a simple disposition to the notion of vulnerability. As Brody notes, there is a difference between being "disposed" to something and striving over time to become something. It is the latter that is the mark of virtue.

In cultivating compassion as a professional virtue, healers must be willing to be formed by a compassionate community, "confident that they will receive empathic compassion and support from each other as they attend to the sufferings of their patients" (Brody, 1992, p. 267). In this arena, Brody ruefully notes, implicit issues of power have most stood in the way of the profession's reform. The self-imposed image of the physician as a powerful, scientific, objective individual, he says, works against the development of any effective peer support system. But it also cripples the physician's ability to be present to those in pain, which, as Stanley Hauerwas notes (1985), should be the goal of medical training.

For Hauerwas, "the physician's basic pledge is not to cure, but to share through being present to the one

in pain" (Hauerwas, 1985, p. 220). This pledge is difficult to carry out on a day-to-day basis. No individual has the resources to see so much pain without that pain hardening him or her. Pain, as Scarry notes, is destructive of human community; hence the prime directive of the healer to be present to those in pain carries with it an embodied threat to the ability to continue to be a healer (1985). She or he must not only be formed as a healer by a compassionate community, but must also be continually sustained and nurtured by such a community—the kind of community, Hauerwas notes, that the Christian church claims to be.

There is a rich and varied tradition of healing not only within the Christian church but also in virtually every religious tradition. In fact, the role of healer in early societies encompassed not only the people's health but their entire welfare, including their spiritual welfare. The specialization that has accompanied modern civilization, however, makes discussion of the relationship between healing and religious belief problematic in that it is no longer clear who is priest, who is healer, and whose authority should predominate. The relation of medicine to particular religious traditions (Numbers and Amundsen, 1986) and the relevance of theological ideas, particularly that of covenant, to medical ethics (May, 1983) have opened up areas of fruitful exploration for both medicine and religion. But it may be well to concentrate, as Hauerwas does, not on these theoretical relationships but on the practical relation between communities, between those who practice religion and those who practice healing (Hauerwas, 1985).

It is in this sense, Hauerwas says, that those who profess to heal need religion—not to provide miracles when there is a failure to cure, not even to supply a foundation for their moral commitments, but rather as a source of the habits and practices necessary to sustain them over the long haul as they care for those in pain. There needs to be a body of people who have learned the skills of presence to keep the world of the ill from becoming a separate world, both for the sake of the ill and for those who care for them. "Only a community that is pledged not to fear the stranger (and illness always makes us a stranger to ourselves and others) can welcome the continued presence of the ill in our midst" (Hauerwas, 1985, p. 223).

In the final analysis, healing is a communal action whose goal is the restoration not only of physical and mental wholeness to those who suffer illness but also of their integrity as persons, that is, as beings-in-relation to themselves and to other persons. It is a communal action in two senses: It reaches out to those isolated by illness to reconnect them to the human family; and it is sustainable only within a community that practices compassion as a virtue. The future of the healing professions everywhere depends as much on this nurture as on technical competence and the wise use of material resources. Those who profess to heal must know that no one is fully healed until all are healed.

J. PAT BROWDER
RICHARD VANCE

For a further discussion of topics mentioned in this entry, see the entries AUTHORITY; BODY, *especially the articles on* EMBODIMENT: THE PHENOMENOLOGICAL TRADITION, *and* SOCIAL THEORIES; CARE; COMPASSION; ETHICS, *article on* RELIGION AND MORALITY; FEMINISM; FRIENDSHIP; HEALTH AND DISEASE, *especially the article on* HISTORY OF THE CONCEPTS; INTERPRETATION; LIFE; LITERATURE; LOVE; MEDICAL ETHICS, HISTORY OF, *section on* EUROPE, *subsection on* ANCIENT AND MEDIEVAL, *article on* GREECE AND ROME; MEDICINE, ANTHROPOLOGY OF; MEDICINE, PHILOSOPHY OF; MEDICINE, SOCIOLOGY OF; NARRATIVE; PATERNALISM; PROFESSIONAL–PATIENT RELATIONSHIP; SOCIAL MEDICINE; TECHNOLOGY; *and* VIRTUE AND CHARACTER. *For a discussion of related ideas, see the entries* ALTERNATIVE THERAPIES; AUTONOMY; BENEFICENCE; CHRONIC CARE; COMPETENCE; CONSCIENCE; EMOTIONS; FAMILY; HARM; MEDICAL CODES AND OATHS; MEDICAL EDUCATION; MEDICAL MALPRACTICE; NURSING, THEORIES AND PHILOSOPHY OF; OBLIGATION AND SUPEREROGATION; PAIN AND SUFFERING; PASTORAL CARE; PATIENTS' RIGHTS; RESPONSIBILITY; RIGHTS; *and* TRUST. *See also the* APPENDIX (CODES, OATHS, AND DIRECTIVES RELATED TO BIOETHICS).

Bibliography

BISHOP, ANNE H., and SCUDDER, JOHN R., JR. 1991. *Nursing: The Practice of Caring.* New York: National League for Nursing Press.

BRODY, HOWARD. 1987. *Stories of Sickness.* New Haven, Conn.: Yale University Press.

———. 1992. *The Healer's Power.* New Haven, Conn.: Yale University Press.

CASSELL, ERIC J. 1976. *The Healer's Art: A New Approach to the Doctor–Patient Relationship.* New York: Penguin Books.

———. 1991. *The Nature of Suffering and the Goals of Medicine.* New York: Oxford University Press.

FOUCAULT, MICHEL. 1973. *The Birth of the Clinic: An Archaeology of Medical Perception.* Translated by Alan M. Sheridan Smith. New York: Pantheon.

GILLIGAN, CAROL. 1982. *In a Different Voice: Psychological Theory and Women's Development.* Cambridge, Mass.: Harvard University Press.

HAUERWAS, STANLEY. 1985. "Salvation and Health: Why Medicine Needs the Church." In *Theology and Bioethics: Exploring the Foundations and Frontiers,* pp. 205–224. Edited by Earl E. Shelp. Dordrecht, Netherlands: D. Reidel.

INGELFINGER, FRANZ J. 1976. "The Physician's Contribution to the Health System." *New England Journal of Medicine* 295, no. 10:565–566.

KASS, LEON R. 1985. *Toward a More Natural Science: Biology and Human Affairs.* New York: Free Press.

KATZ, JAY. 1984. *The Silent World of Doctor and Patient.* New York: Free Press.

KESTENBAUM, VICTOR. 1982. "Introduction: The Experience of Illness." In *The Humanity of the Ill: Phenomenological Perspectives,* pp. 3–38. Edited by Victor Kestenbaum. Knoxville: University of Tennessee Press.

LAÍN ENTRALGO, PEDRO. 1956. *Mind and Body: Psychosomatic Pathology: A Short History of the Evolution of Medical Thought.* Translated by Aurelio M. Espinosa, Jr. New York: P. J. Kenedy & Sons.

MAY, WILLIAM F. 1983. *The Physician's Covenant: Images of the Healer in Medical Ethics.* Philadelphia: Westminster.

NODDINGS, NEL. 1984. *Caring: A Feminine Approach to Ethics and Moral Education.* Berkeley: University of California Press.

NUMBERS, RONALD L., and AMUNDSEN, DARRELL W., eds. 1986. *Caring and Curing: Health and Medicine in the Western Religious Traditions.* New York: Macmillan.

ORTEGA Y GASSET, JOSÉ. 1963. *Meditations on Quixote.* Notes and introduction by Julian Marais. Translated by Evelyn Rugg and Diego Marin. New York: Norton.

PELLEGRINO, EDMUND D. 1982. "Being Ill and Being Healed: Some Reflections on the Grounding of Medical Morality." In *The Humanity of the Ill: Phenomenological Perspectives,* pp. 157–166. Edited by Victor Kestenbaum. Knoxville: University of Tennessee Press.

SCARRY, ELAINE. 1985. *The Body in Pain: The Making and Unmaking of the World.* New York: Oxford University Press.

SHERWIN, SUSAN. 1992. *No Longer Patient: Feminist Ethics and Health Care.* Philadelphia: Temple University Press.

WARREN, VIRGINIA L. 1989. "Feminist Directions in Medical Ethics." *Hypatia* 4, no. 2:73–89.

HEALTH, INTERNATIONAL

See INTERNATIONAL HEALTH. *See also* HEALTH POLICY, *article on* HEALTH POLICY IN INTERNATIONAL PERSPECTIVE.

HEALTH, MENTAL

See MENTAL HEALTH; *and* MENTAL ILLNESS.

HEALTH CARE, MENTAL-

See MENTAL-HEALTH SERVICES; *and* MENTAL-HEALTH THERAPIES. *See also* MENTAL HEALTH; *and* MENTAL ILLNESS.

HEALTH CARE, QUALITY OF

Quality of health care is a measure of the extent to which health services increase the likelihood of desired health outcomes and are consistent with current professional knowledge (Institute of Medicine, 1990). This idea applies to a broad range of services, many types of health-care professionals (such as physicians, nurses, dentists, and certain others), and all settings of care (from hospitals and nursing homes to physicians' offices and private homes). The definition covers populations as well as individual patients; it therefore emphasizes access to health care and suggests that the perspectives of both individuals and society are important.

The definition's stipulation of desired health outcomes draws attention to a link between the processes of health care and outcomes of that care, to patient well-being and welfare, to the importance of being well informed about alternative health-care interventions and their expected outcomes, and to the need for health-care professionals to take their patients' preferences and values into account. The emphasis on current professional knowledge underscores the need for health professionals to stay abreast of a dynamic knowledge base in health care and to take responsibility for clarifying for their patients the processes and expected outcomes of care.

By the sixth century C.E., quality of health care was already linked to the idea of profession. Notions about the responsibilities of the professions, such as the healing arts, date at least to St. Benedict (c. 480–547). The Rule of St. Benedict required new members of the order to make solemn profession of their intention to live the rule and to advance in that profession by way of their vows, in the manner of "continuous improvement." This Benedictine notion of profession—professing before peers—together with the attendant requirements of self-examination and self-regulation, provided a model for all the professions. According to this model, health care professionals would profess their responsibility for assuring the continued improvement of the quality of care they give.

The relationships of quality of care to ethical principles such as beneficence, nonmaleficence ("first, do no harm"), and patient autonomy are clear. The medical profession, as other professions, functions under a form of social contract in which it enjoys certain privileges, such as self-governance, in return for meeting certain obligations, such as stewardship of the public interest. In the nineteenth century, pioneers such as the nurse Florence Nightingale (for British troops in the Crimean War) and the surgeon Ernest A. Codman (for hospitalized patients in Boston, Massachusetts) led the way in studying outcomes of care. By the middle of the twentieth century, concerns about quality of care were more frequently voiced; concepts such as quality assessment and quality assurance, and ways to put them into practice, were being developed, most often under the leadership of physicians and nurses.

In the 1960s, the physician-philosopher Avedis Donabedian offered a unifying concept of "structure, process, and outcome" that became the primary framework to guide those concerned with quality of care in the latter part of the twentieth century. *Structural measures* are the characteristics of the resources in the health-care delivery system and are assumed to reflect the capacity of a practitioner or institutional health-care provider to deliver good-quality care. *Processes of care* consist of what is done to and for the patient, from screening and prevention of disease, through diagnosis and treatment of illness, to counseling and palliation of symptoms. A further distinction is sometimes made between the technical or skill-based aspects of care (the "science" of care) and the interpersonal, or humanistic, aspects of care (the "art" of care). *Outcomes* are the end results of care—that is, the effect of the care processes on the health and well-being of individuals and populations.

The notion of outcomes has evolved from a fairly narrow concern with death and disease to recognition that a much broader set of measures must be used as quality indicators. These concepts are sometimes referred to as health status or health-related quality of life. They include, in addition to survival, such dimensions of health as physical functioning, mental and emotional well-being, cognitive functioning (ability to think and reason), social and role functioning (ability to engage in social and other activities, such as work or school, that are usual for a person of a given age or other characteristics), activities of daily living (ability to perform at least simple activities to care for oneself and to live independently outside of an institution). Sometimes other measures—such as energy, vitality, pain, and satisfaction with life (or with health care)—are included in the broad concept of outcomes. Thus, quality of care implies that judgments are made both about how well health care has been handled technically and about how well from a standpoint of interpersonal exchanges; those judgments may be made using explicit, objective criteria or implicit, subjective criteria, or both.

Quality assessment is the act of measuring quality of care—that is, detecting problems with quality and finding examples of good performance and good outcomes. *Quality assurance* is a more complete cycle of assessment and intervention: detecting a problem, verifying that it truly exists and is important, identifying what might be correctable about the problem, intervening to correct it, studying further to ensure that the problem has been corrected, and making certain that no further problems have been generated as a side effect of the intervention. Quality assessment and assurance tend to be concerned with three major problems regarding quality of care—poor technical or interpersonal performance, overuse of unnecessary or inappropriate services, and underuse of needed or appropriate services—with most attention going to the first two.

Concerns about quality of care can relate to other health policy concerns, such as overly high expenditures on health care (for example, when unneeded, inappropriate, or ineffective services are provided) and poor access to care (for example, when people do not receive needed care at all or obtain it only after inappropriate delay or in unsuitable circumstances). In practice, traditional quality assessment and assurance efforts have tended to focus on individuals rather than systems and to emphasize identifying and correcting or disciplining poor performers rather than finding and rewarding superior performers.

In the 1980s in the United States, concepts of *continuous quality improvement* and *total quality management* began to be popular in the manufacturing and service sectors, and later in health care. These programs are based on statistical quality-control models designed for manufacturing industries by American statisticians such as W. Edwards Deming and applied mainly after World War II in Japan. Like traditional quality-assurance programs, they entail a cycle of system design, examination, action, and redesign. The underlying philosophy and analytic methods differ somewhat from the traditional approaches. They are oriented toward systems and organizations rather than individuals, emphasize "customer-supplier" relationships, focus on improving performance as a goal rather than simply on finding poor performers, and seek out excellence as a benchmark against which to measure performance. Also, they employ formal, although relatively simple, statistical concepts and methods for continuously collecting and analyzing data on processes and outcomes of care.

Monitoring the quality of care is typically seen as an endeavor of the professions and the private sector in the United States. This is reflected, for example, in specifications for education, training, and professional certification for members of the health-care professions that date to the early part of the twentieth century and continue to the present; in requirements for hospital accreditation that have been specified and refined by the Joint Commission on Accreditation of Healthcare Organizations for several decades; in professional peer review programs, such as Foundations for Medical Care, that emerged in the middle of the century; and in various committees and other programs of individual hospitals, health maintenance organizations, and other health-care delivery institutions. The regulatory aspects of quality assurance are seen most clearly in the establishment of Professional Standards Review Organizations (in the 1970s) and Utilization and Quality Control Peer Review Organizations (in the 1980s) for the Medicare program (which finances health care for the elderly in the United States). The many state and federal laws and regulations concerning accreditation, licensure, and certification for health-care professionals, facilities, and institutions also speak to governmental or public sector concern with quality of care.

Several trends in the late twentieth century may draw yet more attention to quality of care and make quality assurance and quality improvement far more complex to manage than in previous decades. These trends include efforts to control excessive costs and expenditures on health; new ways to pay hospitals and physicians; growth of hybrid health-care financing and organization schemes; malpractice litigation and efforts to reduce the risk of malpractice liability; movement of complex technologies outside institutions and into outpatient and home settings; and changing demographics of populations. Both professional and regulatory perspectives are likely to be reflected as quality assurance and improvement programs grow in number and in complexity. Because quality assurance and improvement are better developed for hospitals than for outpatient settings, and because more is known about how to identify good or poor care and performance than about how to change the attitudes, behaviors, and performance of individual clinicians or institutions, a considerable agenda of research and development is still needed.

The United States is seen as the world leader in organized quality-assessment, quality-assurance, and quality-improvement programs for health-care professionals and institutions. Some efforts outside the United States took hold in the late 1980s; these include programs in several postindustrial Western countries, especially the Netherlands, and the organization of the International Society of Quality Assurance in Health Care.

KATHLEEN N. LOHR

For a further discussion of topics mentioned in this entry see the entries AUTONOMY; BENEFICENCE; HEALTH-CARE DELIVERY; HEALTH-CARE FINANCING; HEALTH-CARE RESOURCES, ALLOCATION OF; HEALTH POLICY, *article on* POLITICS AND HEALTH CARE; LICENSING, DISCIPLINE, AND REGULATION IN THE HEALTH PROFESSIONS; MEDICAL MALPRACTICE; MEDICINE, ART OF; MEDICINE AS A PROFESSION; NURSING AS A PROFESSION; *and* PROFESSION AND PROFESSIONAL ETHICS. *For a discussion of related ideas see the entries* BIOETHICS EDUCATION; ECONOMIC CONCEPTS IN HEALTH CARE; *and* HOSPITAL, *article on* CONTEMPORARY ETHICAL PROBLEMS. *Other rel-*

evant material may be found under the entries LIFE, QUAL-
ITY OF, *article on* QUALITY OF LIFE IN HEALTH-CARE
ALLOCATION; PROFESSIONAL–PATIENT RELATIONSHIP,
article on ETHICAL ISSUES; *and* WHISTLEBLOWING.

Bibliography

BERWICK, DONALD M. 1989. "Continuous Improvement as an
    Ideal in Health Care." *New England Journal of Medicine*
    320, no. 1:53–56.
BERWICK, DONALD M.; GODFREY, A. BLANTON; and ROESS-
    NER, JANE. 1990. *Curing Health Care. New Strategies for
    Quality Improvement.* San Francisco: Jossey-Bass.
BROOK, ROBERT H. 1973. *Quality of Care Assessment: A Com-
    parison of Five Methods of Peer Review.* DHEW Publication
    no. HRA 74-2100. Rockville, Md.: Public Health Ser-
    vice, Health Resources Administration, Bureau of Health
    Services Research and Evaluation.
BROOK, ROBERT H., and APPEL, FRANCIS A. 1973. "Quality-
    of-Care Assessment: Choosing a Method for Peer Re-
    view." *New England Journal of Medicine* 288, no. 25:
    1323–1329.
DONABEDIAN, AVEDIS. 1966. "Evaluating the Quality of Med-
    ical Care." *Milbank Memorial Fund Quarterly* 44, no. 3,
    pt. 2:166–203.
———. 1980–1985. *Explorations in Quality Assessment and
    Monitoring.* 3 vols. Ann Arbor, Mich.: Health Adminis-
    tration Press.
FRY, TIMOTHY, ed. 1982. *RB1980: The Rule of St. Benedict in
    English.* Collegeville, Minn.: Liturgical Press.
GOLDFIELD, NORBERT, and NASH, DAVID B., eds. 1989. *Pro-
    viding Quality Care: The Challenge to Clinicians.* Philadel-
    phia: American College of Physicians.
INSTITUTE OF MEDICINE. 1990. *Medicare: A Strategy for Quality
    Assurance.* Edited by Kathleen N. Lohr. 2 vols. IOM Pub-
    lication nos. 90–92. Washington, D.C.: National Acad-
    emy Press.
LOHR, KATHLEEN N., ed. 1992. "Advances in Health Status
    Assessment. Fostering the Application of Health Status
    Measures in Clinical Settings. Proceedings of a Confer-
    ence." *Medical Care* 30, no. 5 (Suppl.):MS1–MS293.
LOHR, KATHLEEN N.; YORDY, KARL D.; and THIER, SAMUEL
    O. 1980. "Current Issues in Quality of Care." *Health Af-
    fairs* 7, no. 1:5–18.
PALMER, R. HEATHER; DONABEDIAN, AVEDIS; and POVAR,
    GAIL J. 1991. *Striving for Quality in Health Care. An In-
    quiry into Policy and Practice.* Ann Arbor, Mich.: Health
    Administration Press.
Quality Assurance in Health Care. 1989–. Official journal of the
    International Society of Quality Assurance in Health
    Care. Oxford: Pergamon Press.
WILLIAMSON, JOHN W. 1978. *Assessing and Improving Out-
    comes in Health Care: The Theory and Practice of Health
    Accounting.* Cambridge, Mass.: Ballinger.

HEALTH-CARE ALLOCATION

See HEALTH-CARE RESOURCES, ALLOCATION OF.

HEALTH-CARE DELIVERY

I. Health-Care Systems
    L. Gregory Pawlson
    Jacqueline J. Glover
II. Health-Care Institutions
    Roger J. Bulger
    Christine K. Cassel

I. HEALTH-CARE SYSTEMS

A health-care system can be defined as the means by
which heath care is financed, organized, delivered, and
reimbursed to a given population. It includes considerations of access (for whom and to what services), expenditures, and resources (health-care workers and
facilities). The goal of a health-care system is to enhance
the health of the population in the most effective manner possible, given a society's available resources and
competing needs. During the twentieth century, access to health care has come to be regarded by most
countries and the United Nations as a special good that
is necessary either as or pursuant to basic human rights.
An examination of health-care systems therefore reasonably includes consideration of how a particular system
addresses commonly held values.

The extent and form of a particular system is influenced by a variety of factors, including the unique culture and history of a population or country. What is
considered health care, as opposed to other types of social services, can vary markedly according to a particular
country's development. Some populations put far more
emphasis on prevention of disease, while others include
only the care for or cure of particular illnesses. Definitions of health and disease and of "appropriate" health-
care providers are also subject to cultural variability.

A second major influence derives from the priorities
given various ethical values. These values include respect for autonomy (of both patients and providers), the
maximization of benefit, and the promotion of justice or
fairness, understood as equality or liberty. Balancing
these values in health care poses a special problem in
the United States. Public opinion polls have revealed
that most Americans see access to health care as a fundamental right. Yet equally strong beliefs in individual
autonomy and responsibility, the market as a means of
distribution of goods and services, and fears about government interference create conflict and have led to a
fragmented health-care system.

A third obvious influence on the structure of a system is the level of economic resources available. There
is a strong positive correlation between economic resources, as measured by the per capita gross national

product (GNP), and both health-care expenditures and the proportion of the GNP that is spent on health care. This indicates that while health care is generally valued, populations with very limited resources may consider food, shelter, or in some instances, spending for the military, of greater importance. However, while the economic resources available to a country have a great effect on the overall expenditures on health care, there is nearly as much variation in the forms of the health-care systems in countries that are economically poor as there is in wealthy countries.

Public versus private control

All governments have some involvement in health care, since essentially all countries have a centrally funded agency concerned with public-health issues. The proportion of health-care expenditures spent on public health tends to be greater in developing countries, although the level of effort varies greatly from country to country. Government involvement usually includes communicable disease surveillance and interventions to prevent or curtail epidemics. Some countries have more extensive government involvement through direct service delivery (immunizations, well-child care, screening for developmental disabilities), treatment of communicable diseases, and health promotion programs. Public-health efforts in the United States are rather fragmented but have begun to receive more attention as the costs of personal, disease-oriented health care have rapidly increased.

· Beyond public-health measures, health-care systems vary dramatically according to the degree of public versus private control. In fact, the degree of government control is probably the single most distinguishing characteristic among systems.

In developed countries other than the United States, the health-care system is dominated by a publicly determined program, in many instances with a small but important private market. In the United States, the opposite is the case; the private sector of insurers, employers, and providers accounts for over 60 percent of health-care expenditures. While the United States spends a higher proportion of its GNP (about 14%) on health care than any other nation (the closest being Canada at 10%), the proportion of total spending by the public sector (40%) is the lowest of any economically developed country (the nearest being Austria at 68%). The public sector health-care systems of developed countries can be grouped into those with comprehensive programs and strong government control of virtually all aspects (financing, delivery, quality monitors) of the system (such as in Britain, the Scandinavian countries, and the countries of the former Soviet Union), and those systems in which the government role is usually limited to financing or guaranteeing enrollment for all citizens in a health-insurance plan (such as in Germany, Bel-

gium, France, and Canada). Both types of systems are characterized by public financing or mandates that guarantee universal coverage; reimbursement that is negotiated between the public sector and providers; and facility and health-care worker policies that are predominantly modulated by the public sector. The individual autonomy of patients to choose providers of insurance or services, or the autonomy of providers to determine their charges, is tempered by a strong sense of community and a relatively high degree of trust in government.

By contrast, patient and professional autonomy are dominant in the United States. Most individuals or employers are free to choose from multiple insurers and providers, and most provider groups are afforded a wide latitude in whom to serve, how much to charge, and what credentials are requisite to provide a given service. Especially notable has been the strong distrust of government intervention except where deemed necessary to guarantee access to a group that is seen as "entitled" by some special service they have rendered (retirees, veterans) or by special need (disability). It should be noted, however, that even in the United States there have been a number of occasions (as in 1910, 1935, 1948, 1965, 1972, and 1994) when a reasonably strong attempt has been made to provide a substantial increase in government involvement in the health-care system. Except in 1965 these attempts have failed due to a combination of factors, including provider opposition, a lack of public consensus, fears of increased government involvement, and the relatively comprehensive health-care benefits that most Americans receive from employment-based private insurance.

Financing

The means of financing health care, perhaps more than any other aspect of a health-care system, mirrors the values and priorities of a society. As noted above, the United States is the only nation with a highly developed economy to finance privately a majority of health care. South Africa, the Philippines, and Indonesia are examples of less well-developed countries with relatively little public financing for personal health care. Given the high cost of many interventions and the very unequal distribution among individuals of health-care costs, the lack of a broad-based system of public financing creates, de facto, a system in which health care is rationed on the ability to pay.

Beginning with Germany in 1883, most economically developed nations have implemented a government-coordinated or controlled system of financing for personal health-care services. This varies from those countries such as Great Britain and the former Soviet Union, in which virtually all health care is financed through revenues collected by the national government as general revenues; to systems, such as Canada's, that are financed from both state and national revenues; to those of Germany, France, Belgium, and the Netherlands, in which financing is mandated by the national government through requiring participation in a community- or employment-based insurance fund. In these latter systems most funds are obtained through required contributions (taxes) based on wages that are paid primarily by the employer. All countries have at least an underground market of privately financed health care used predominantly by the rich or politically connected. Those systems with strong central control tend to have a relatively small private market, while some countries with mixed systems have a substantial minority of persons with private insurance, such as Japan and Australia.

While the proportion of public financing of health care in the United States has been steadily increasing (from less than 10% in 1950 to nearly 40% in 1993), a key element that is lacking is government-guaranteed, compulsory health insurance. While employer-based or individually purchased private insurance is clearly the dominant means of financing, a variety of publicly financed programs also exist. They represent a spectrum of public financing from federal and local government revenues, including the use of income and employment-based taxes, and in some states, revenues from a lottery.

Financing for one of the largest single-delivery systems in the United States (for active duty military personnel) mirrors the most centrally controlled health-care systems of Great Britain and the former Soviet Union in that financing comes from the federal income tax. The health-care system for veterans and Native Americans is also derived from general tax revenues. The Medicare program (for elderly retirees and their dependents) is financed primarily from a wage tax, while the Medicaid system (for certain categories of low-income persons) is publicly financed from a combination of state and federal general tax revenues. Financing for some care of the poor who are not eligible for Medicaid comes from general tax revenues at the state or local level paid to city and county public hospitals and state mental hospitals. Only one state (Hawaii) has in place a system of financing of health care that approximates universal coverage. Hawaii requires employers to pay a specified proportion of the cost of private health insurance, with general tax financing for those not employed.

The dominance of a private system of financing in the United States is a reflection not only of its values but also of a number of historical events. While there were some examples of employment-based health insurance as early as 1900, the real spread of this form of health insurance occurred during World War II, when wages, but not fringe benefits, were frozen as a wartime price-control measure. This rapid spread was primed in the 1930s by hospitals' creation of Blue Cross insurance programs for hospital care. Doctors followed this lead with the development of Blue Shield plans for physician service coverage. As more firms began to offer health insurance as a benefit, private insurance companies saw potential for expanding their markets and encouraging those enrolled in health-insurance plans to buy their other insurance products. An even further impetus to the market was the decision by the federal government to exempt health-care benefits from federal income tax. The large number of insurance plans in the United States (each with its own marketing, benefit packages, premiums, deductibles or copayments, billing, and reimbursement requirements), together with thousands of private physicians, clinics, and hospitals, has given rise to an immense administrative bureaucracy that is estimated to cost over $50 billion per year.

Access and delivery

A second major characteristic of a health-care system is access. How do different groups in the population gain entry to health care and what specific services are made available? There are basically three approaches to access. The first, provided by systems with strong central control (as in Great Britain, the Scandinavian countries, and the countries of the former Soviet Union), is a single-payment system with most health-care providers as salaried government employees and a single government-defined set of benefits. There tends to be strong emphasis on primary care by general practitioners, and relatively tight controls on the number and distribution of providers and facilities that provide highly technical services. In some countries this degree of government control results in substantial waiting times for some services, and limited access to advanced technologies. Thus, while this approach produces an apparently high level of equal opportunity to obtain needed health services, it may deny some individuals access to lifesaving technologies and restrict both provider and patient choices.

Those countries with less centralized systems vary more in the level of access and in the delivery system. In some countries, access to health care for the poor is restricted when compared to those with employment-based programs. In some instances, lower reimbursement rates allow providers, who are free to choose their patients, to restrict access to services for persons with low incomes. In other countries, such as the United States, out-of-pocket expenses for copayments, deductibles, or premiums often create financial barriers for some individuals employed in low-paying jobs. Likewise, the limited control of health-care workers and facility location tends to result in geographic maldistribution of providers and, in some instances, a relative lack of generalists.

The degree of variation is most extreme in the predominantly private system of the United States. The financial barriers to access are substantial for the more than thirty-five million Americans who lack health insurance at any given time, and the estimated twenty million more who have inadequate insurance. Studies have shown that those who are poor and have no health insurance have a markedly lower use of almost all forms of health care, despite a tendency to a lower baseline health status. This lack is especially great in terms of primary care and preventive services. While the uninsured have some access to high-technology care, especially in urban areas through the emergency rooms and outpatient clinics of public hospitals, research has shown poorer outcomes of hospitalization (controlling for severity) and markedly lower use of high technology by those without insurance. There is also growing evidence that limited access to primary care results in not only poorer outcomes but also higher overall costs through delayed treatment, reduced patient adherence to therapeutic regimens, and increased emergency room and hospital admissions.

Reimbursement

The level and means by which providers of health care are reimbursed has a substantial effect on access, costs, and quality of care. In those countries that rely on a private health-care delivery system (the United States, Canada, France, and Belgium), the predominant mode of reimbursement for physicians providing ambulatory care is fee-for-service. In most instances, physicians bargain with insurers or the government over a fee schedule, often with some provision that physicians can charge patients more than the allowed fees in certain circumstances. There is concern that the financial incentives inherent in fee-for-service result in a general overutilization of services, especially of those services that are reimbursed at a high level relative to other services. However, the autonomy of providers is well preserved, and there is an incentive for increased productivity. Also, there is no conflict between the financial interests of providers and their duty to provide all services that are of benefit to patients. Cost- or charge-based reimbursement for institutions (hospitals, nursing homes, etc.) has similar risks and benefits.

A growing number of insurers in the United States are using capitation (a set payment per person per year) or a set payment per case to pay providers. Capitation payments provide an incentive for health-care workers and facilities to limit the volume of services and allow flexibility to providers to determine precisely what services are provided. At the same time, case-based payment and capitation create a conflict between the financial incentive of the provider and the interest of the individual patient in receiving all services that are of possible benefit. A study of health maintenance organizations in capitated systems, the Rand Health Insurance Study (Rand Corporation, 1978), did suggest that persons from low socioeconomic groups had some poorer outcomes of care in capitated systems.

In many countries, hospitals are paid on prospectively negotiated global budgets, and hospital-based providers, including physicians, are paid on a salaried basis. These methods of reimbursement have little apparent effect on the provision of services to individuals. However, the level of reimbursement may have a profound effect globally on what technology to acquire or on whether to expend the time and effort required to provide a given service in general.

Costs and cost controls

Since 1960, in virtually every country in the world, expenditures for personal health-care services have been rising in absolute terms and in relation to the GNP. Health expenditures have been increasing at a rate nearly double that of other major sectors of some national economies. Increasingly, concerns are being raised that medical-care spending is occurring at the expense of other socially desirable goods and services. This is especially true in the United States, where despite the highest per capita and GNP-adjusted health-care costs, health care is still not accessible to all, and there is growing concern about other social problems like deteriorating schools, homelessness, poverty, and crime. In addition, there is strong evidence that more health care is not necessarily better. Even more compelling is the growing evidence that a substantial number of medical-care services may provide, at best, only small marginal benefits. At the same time that small benefits and high cost are the norm in developed countries, many developing and economically disadvantaged countries cannot provide their populations with even basic public-health measures such as immunization and sanitation.

The response of different health-care systems to the growing problem of cost has in general reflected the basic organization and values within a particular country. In those countries with strong central control, there has been increasing pressure to create fixed budgets and tight control over the acquisition of advanced technologies. Access to basic health services for everyone has been maintained at the expense of not providing services that are potentially lifesaving for a few individuals.

By contrast, in the United States there are relatively fewer advocates for global budgeting and government set rates. Efforts to reduce costs have focused primarily on regulations and requirements developed by public and private insurers to limit utilization of health-care services ("managed" care) and on enhanced competition. Prospective and retrospective review of health-care services appear to have produced some one-time reductions in health-care spending and the shortest length of hospital stays in the world but has had a very modest effect on the rate of growth of expenditures.

Because of the seemingly inexorable rise in costs, employers have been shifting more of the cost of health care to employees by increasing employee-paid premiums, eliminating coverage for dependents, increasing copayments and deductibles, or eliminating coverage altogether. The response of private insurance companies to growing cost concerns has been to refuse to insure high-risk employees (medical underwriting), or to tie premiums directly to the previous year's expenditures by a particular group (experience rating). These two factors, along with a rise in employment in small, nonunion service industries that lack medical benefits and in the number of part-time workers, have been primary determinants in the growing number of persons in the United States who are without health insurance.

Resources

The most visible aspects of any health-care system are the facilities and personnel involved in the delivery of health care. Centralized systems have attempted to provide greater equality in the distribution of facilities and health-care workers by focusing on the needs of the community rather than on the autonomy of providers and patients. In some centralized systems, the national government may determine how many and what types (specialties) of physicians, nurses, and other health-care workers are produced; the location of hospitals and what technology they may purchase; and the location of both hospital-based and outpatient-care providers. There is greater use of health professionals other than physicians, such as public-health nurses and primary-care providers, who serve as "gatekeepers" to subspecialist services. Care is strongly regionalized, with easily accessible primary care for most common health-care problems, some specialty care available in the regional hospitals, and subspecialty and tertiary care confined to a few large teaching centers.

As in most aspects, the health-care system in the United States offers the greatest contrast to central control. There has been almost complete autonomy for providers, starting with a system of health-professional education having a substantial number of private schools and little or no restriction on specialty choice, practice, or hospital location, or on the availability of technology. Because of the prestige and generous reimbursement for new technology, nearly all hospitals provide a full array of technologies. This complements a strong trend toward subspecialization among health professionals. In the case of physicians, the proportion of generalists to subspecialty physicians declined from nearly 50 percent in 1950 to just over 30 percent in 1990. The abundance of subspecialists, and especially those who are trained to perform high-technology procedures, is felt to exacerbate the overutilization of some health-care services. Conversely, the decline in the number of generalists is believed to be a contributing factor in the poor access experienced by those in rural areas or in urban areas among those with low incomes.

Choices for the future

The health-care system of any country reflects not only the culture, history, and general wealth of the country, but most important, its values and traditions. Unless there is an unforeseen period of increased and sustained economic growth, every country will have to come to terms with the difficult task of placing limits on those health-care technologies that provide small marginal benefits to a few individuals at a great cost to the community.

Tensions will grow between the values of individual autonomy (reflected in the assumption by patients that the "right" to health care includes all interventions that are of possible benefit and by providers that they have the "right" to set prices and choose where and whom to serve), and concern for the good of the community and other societal needs. Attempts to achieve equality in the systems of financing, reimbursement, cost control, and delivery will have to face increasing competition for limited resources and the perceived infringement of personal freedoms. Balancing these competing claims will be especially difficult in the United States with its multiple systems and distrust of government involvement in human services.

A renewal of a sense of community and a careful balancing of values will be necessary in approaching a reasonable solution. While the future is unclear, the United States seems perched on the edge of great change. These changes may include some form of global budgeting to allow rational allocation between health care and other sectors of the economy; government regulation to require universal and equitable access to defined "basic" insurance policies; mandated employer-based insurance with a publicly financed safety net; reimbursement based on capitation with some adjustment for the severity of illness in a given group of patients; and incentives (including scholarships and loan forgiveness) for providers who choose to render primary care in shortage areas.

L. GREGORY PAWLSON
JACQUELINE J. GLOVER

Directly related to this article is the companion article in this entry: HEALTH-CARE INSTITUTIONS. *Also directly related are the entries* HEALTH POLICY; HEALTH-CARE RESOURCES, ALLOCATION OF, *article on* MACROALLOCA-

tion; and HEALTH-CARE FINANCING. *For a further discussion of topics mentioned in this article, see the entries* ECONOMIC CONCEPTS IN HEALTH CARE; HOSPITAL, *article on* MODERN HISTORY; JUSTICE; PUBLIC HEALTH, *article on* HISTORY OF PUBLIC HEALTH; RIGHTS; *and* UTILITY. *Other relevant material may be found under the entries* ADVERTISING; HEALTH CARE, QUALITY OF; PUBLIC POLICY AND BIOETHICS; *and* SOCIAL MEDICINE.

Bibliography

BLANK, ROBERT H. 1988. *Rationing Medicine.* New York: Columbia University Press.

BRECHER, CHARLES, ed. 1992. *Implementation Issues and National Health Care Reform: Proceedings of a Conference.* Washington, D.C.: Josiah Macy, Jr., Foundation Conference sponsored by the Robert F. Wagner Graduate School of Public Service, New York University, Washington, D.C., June 12.

BROWN, E. RICHARD. 1988. "Principles for a National Health Program: A Framework for Analysis and Development." *The Milbank Quarterly* 66, no. 4:573–617.

NEWHOUSE, JOSEPH P. AND THE INSURANCE EXPERIMENT GROUP. 1993. *Free for All? Lessons from the RAND Health Insurance Experiment.* Cambridge, Mass.: Harvard University Press.

PRIESTER, REINHARD. 1992. "A Values Framework for Health System Reform." *Health Affairs* 11, no. 1:84–107.

"Pursuit of Health Systems Reform." 1991. *Health Affairs* 10, no. 3. Special issue.

RAND CORPORATION. 1978. *Conceptualization and Measurement of Health for Adults in the Health Insurance Study.* 8 vols. Santa Monica, Calif.: Author.

ROEMER, MILTON I. 1991. *National Health Systems of the World.* New York: Oxford University Press.

WYSONG, JERE A., and ABEL, THOMAS. 1990. "Universal Health Insurance and High-Risk Groups in West Germany: Implications for U.S. Health Policy." *Milbank Quarterly* 68, no. 4:527–560.

II. HEALTH-CARE INSTITUTIONS

Health-care institutions are often overlooked in discussions of health-care policy, biomedical ethics, and the allocation of resources. Institutions, however, are major players within the ethical and policy arena of health care and should be considered when one examines the forces at work in any specific issue in health care.

A health-care institution usually has been thought of as a hospital, a nursing home, a rehabilitation facility, or another such single-site entity. Such an institution consists of the human beings who work in many different capacities within it, the leaders who direct and manage it, and its governing body—usually a board of directors or board of trustees that is responsible for hiring (and firing) the chief executive officer or president of the institution and for setting policy and direction in partnership with the employed leaders. Many institutions now, however, are much larger than a single facility. For example, there are integrated hospital health-care networks that include everything from physician group practices to long-term-care facilities. There are also networks that provide a single level of care, such as nursing-home chains and hospital chains. As the competitive environment of health care continues to drive efforts to reduce costs and capture market share, the institution made up of multiple components will become increasingly more common. Nonetheless, whether institutions are single units or made up of multiple units, they have important characteristics in common that must be considered.

One of the most important functions of leadership and governance in an institution is to establish and articulate that institution's mission. This is usually written in a mission statement. An academic health center may have a mission that includes research, education, and patient care as equally strong components of the mission. A community hospital may point to excellent patient care and improvement of community health as its mission. A for-profit hospital or hospital chain may articulate excellent patient care and optimal return to shareholders as its mission. As one can imagine, this latter bipartite mission can lead to troubling conflicts of interest, which have been examined now by ethicists in some detail (Gray, 1991).

The mission of an institution may also be articulated in the framework of its membership in a larger institution such as a church or religious network. Thus, some Catholic hospitals provide care to a large number of patients in the United States (who are not necessarily Catholic) and their mission specifically derives from values espoused by the Catholic church. Similarly, many other hospitals have emerged from religious systems because of the latter's commitment to helping the vulnerable and caring for the sick and suffering. Institutional missions may sometimes conflict with bedside ethical decisions, such as the decision to forgo life-sustaining therapy or to have an elective abortion. In these settings it is important for patients and providers alike to be clear about the underlying moral environment of the institution and the degree to which it may or may not be flexible on certain issues. Patients who feel strongly that they do not want care with those articulated standards should then have access to other institutions. Besides the question of abortion, the issue of forgoing life-sustaining treatment has been one of the most prominent in this kind of conflict. Often a patient's family member who makes a decision about discontinuing nutrition and hydration in a comatose or unresponsive patient with far advanced dementing illness will find that the institution housing that patient does not allow nutrition and hydration to be withdrawn. If the underlying reason is fear of malpractice or liability concerns, it is sometimes possible for the institution to figure out a way to work together with and respect the wishes of the patient and family. However, if the underlying reason is a moral or religious belief consistent with the underlying values of the governance of this institution, then it is less likely that a compromise can occur (Miles et al., 1989).

To generalize about these many and varied institutions—both secular and religious, for-profit and not-for-profit—is not a simple matter, but it is useful to explore certain issues relating to the value systems that undergird their several missions and roles in society. Many of the older institutions were launched on the bedrock principle of simply caring for the sick and suffering and many in the public still, quite unrealistically, think of all health-care institutions in this way. Because the United States as a nation has not yet realized the right of equal access for all its citizens to health care and embraced the concept of health care as a social good, there is no consistent underlying covenant between the society and these institutions. Social covenant would lead to some kind of centralized planning for health-care needs, and institutional missions would flow from this. Instead, the United States relies on marketplace values combined with a variable and often unreliable "safety net" of public institutions. It has proven to be very difficult for any of these institutions to live up to their traditional foundational institutional values and at the same time survive the economic and social realities of U.S. culture. The one shared ethical principle that all would espouse is the commitment to competence and excellence, values that have permeated Western medicine through its physicians since the time of Hippocrates. This is not always altruistic, however, since a minimum of quality is required for accreditation, and evidence of excellent quality gives some institutions a market edge in attracting paying patients.

The public institutions created by a county, city, or state for the purpose of delivering health services to a specific population have an unambiguous mission and foundational institutional ethic: to carry out the function for which they were created and for which they continue to receive operating funds from the public sector. The objective of these institutions is to provide care in an appropriate and highly competent fashion to the specified population, usually those who are poor and without access to other sources of care. The fact that, on paper, the goals and objectives of these institutions never change belies the fact that the public's commitment wavers from year to year with the obvious result that there is considerable variation in the level of financial support it is willing to provide; serious underfunding for many public hospitals thus significantly compromises the quality of care in many places. So there remains the paradox, despite an unambiguously consistent mission

statement: Compromised public commitment to provide services for the poor has translated in some of these institutions to a serious loss of quality. The profit motive seldom creates an untoward tension among workers at these institutions; the limits imposed by funding sources may, however, lead to the curtailing or closing of certain expensive services, perhaps to the detriment of the patients.

The private, not-for-profit institutions that were established for the purpose of serving the community may share a public-service vision with the public hospitals. Private, not-for-profit hospitals also, however, experience extreme pressures that run counter to their community-service mission. Since the early 1980s, in the United States, these institutions have often thrived financially by maximizing income from insurance and philanthropy, both of which have supported the enormous growth of specialty medicine and heroic high-technology care. Governed by boards of directors made up of citizens of the community, these institutions can be expected to have an awareness of community needs. On the other hand, the charity care these hospitals may provide generally must be paid for in one of two ways: (1) by using available reserve funds; or (2) by cost-shifting so as to overcharge those who can pay more, so as to make up for the losses in primary care, chronic care, and general care for the poor or uninsured.

The CEOs of the larger of these hospitals, especially those at the more prominent academic and tertiary-care institutions, are treated and paid as though they were corporate executives. This trend toward providing top-level management for these institutions came from the growing awareness beginning in the early 1970s that these institutions were administratively out of control or at the very least generally ill-prepared to fulfill their potential in a volatile marketplace. Few would argue that the majority of these institutions have become heavily bottom-line oriented. Balancing cross-subsidization among the various payers with issues of access for the poor is a fine art. Many of these hospitals, though losing money on each and every Medicaid and Medicare patient, continue to enjoy an overall surplus. An occasional institution will have a "profit" margin or annual surplus that comes closer to $75 million than to $1 million, an outcome that seldom triggers a similar-sized internal redistribution of dollars into care for the underserved. More often such bonanzas are used to implement programs aimed at increasing "market share" for the hospital, usually appealing to the more affluent sectors of society.

Some not-for-profit institutions have extraordinarily idealistic community-service orientations, expressed through their written missions and goals; these orientations have sometimes become so consumed by the direction provided by bottom-line oriented, high-priced management teams that a variety of less desirable and short-sighted practices have been implemented in order to produce a positive bottom line. These include: (1) salary incentives to unit managers based primarily upon the financial performance of their cost centers; (2) high-tech and manpower investment strategies determined primarily by their potential for high earnings; (3) transfer policies that favor keeping patients whose care will add to the bottom line ("cream-skimming"); (4) policies to reduce existing teaching programs because of uncompensated expenses and negative impacts upon marketing strategies designed to reach more desirable clienteles; and (5) different patterns of care based on whether or not patients possess ample insurance coverage or other financial resources. Whether or not one finds these practices appropriate or inappropriate, whether they are more or less typical of not-for-profit as compared with for-profit institutions, the main lesson from these examples is that the pressures and forces inherent in the competitive market-oriented environment that has become dominant since the early 1980s have served to overtake the charitable values and philosophies that were central to the creation of many of these institutions. There is a tendency for health-care institutions to believe that they are involved in a competitive fight for survival and they all, in various ways, try to combine that pressure as best they can with the imperative to serve the sick.

Even institutions sponsored by religious organizations charge paying patients more than cost in order to cover the costs of nonpaying patients. Financial stability is the key to survival and thus to carrying out an altruistic mission. It is therefore more realistic to stop envisioning Saint Francis of Assisi when we think of not-for-profit hospitals and think instead of "Saint Robin of Hood," robbing the rich to care for the poor.

Most observers see this behavior less as human frailty than as a system failure, the result of an environment that is filled with perverse incentives. A detailed analysis of the ethics of for-profit as compared to not-for-profit health-care institutions (Brock and Buchanan, 1986) concludes that there are no rationally compelling grounds upon which to find ethical fault with the profit motive in health care under the ground rules by which U.S. society now operates. Improvements can come only when the ground rules and societal expectations are altered; it is not enough simply to hope that institutions will take the lead in changing their behavior, in the face of existing incentives to the contrary.

The role of governance is very important in the character of institutions. In many health-care institutions, including the not-for-profit sector, the board of trustees may be made up largely of individuals who are prominent business people with a great deal of experience in running large and successful businesses, as well as otherwise wealthy and influential members of the local social circle who may themselves be important philanthropic supporters of the hospital and able to draw others into making major donations. Thus, it is often a minority of individuals on the board who have direct experience with health care, such as physicians or nurses, or whose major concerns are with education or research. Therefore it is not surprising that as health care has become a $1,000,000,000 business in the United States, even not-for-profit hospitals and health systems have looked at the success of the bottom line as a marker of how well they are doing. Even though there are no shareholders to pay, an excess of revenue over expenses allows the nonprofit institution to initiate new programs and, in many cases, to salt away substantial reserves that both provide interest income and allow for a cushion in case of adversity.

Because so much money is involved and because of the business orientation of much of hospital governance, it is not surprising that the investments in new programs or capital investments that are made when excess funds are available are not always, or even primarily, directed toward care of the poor and underserved but are often directed toward ensuring a continuing stream of revenue for the hospital. This usually means investing in additional high-technology medical care that will be marketed to insured patients. For this reason it is not hard to see why the Internal Revenue Service in recent years has begun to ask whether the not-for-profit hospital sector really ought to remain tax exempt. In order to maintain their tax exemption, these institutions must demonstrate that they are community-service organizations and that the educational research missions remain important to them, if not central.

Brock and Buchanan (1986) make an important distinction in their comprehensive treatise between for-profit chains, generally owned by investors and listed on the stock exchange, and individual for-profit institutions, usually owned by an individual or small group of individuals (frequently physicians from the community). These organizational differences create different incentives and different institutional behavioral responses. Here we are concerned with the latter subset of for-profit institutions, but this in no way ameliorates the validity of these conclusions. The thrust toward identifying health care as a commodity distributed according to business rules has, since the early 1980s, been the overwhelming ethical reality for private and not-for-profit private institutions. All of these factors have fueled the debate about the appropriateness of maintaining the tax-free status of not-for-profit hospitals (Gray, 1991). If the societal pendulum swings back toward the treatment of health care as a right, we may expect to see alterations in institutional behavior that, however, need not drive the individual for-profit institution out of business.

An important new dynamic for a subset of these institutions is the statement by the American Medical Association (AMA) that physician ownership of facilities to which they refer patients is professionally unethical. This overdue but laudatory and courageous position will have an impact on the aggregate cost of this sector within the total health-care bill.

It is probable that the implementation of national and regional policy decisions about health care (such as the trend toward capitation, community-rating of insurance, universal access to care, regional data bases capable of rendering comparative institutional quality-of-care estimates, and so on) will have more to do with affecting the behavior of these independent institutions than anything else. The most far-reaching impact may result from the pressure for these institutions to join effective consortia or networks of health-care providers; they may well need to become part of an organized delivery system in order to survive. Thus, by around the year 2005, their numbers may be severely depleted. Certainly, one already sees a trend in the direction of independents moving into organized systems, not only in the hospital industry but also in the traditionally "Mom and Pop" nursing-home arena.

A wide variety of individually governed institutions play a wide variety of roles in the inchoate patchwork quilt of health-care delivery in the United States. As the forces for systemic reform build, it seems clear that they will have a predominant influence on alterations in the behavior of these various entities. Until such changes occur, we can conclude that this independent sector will in general deliver the best health care it can under the vagaries of access and quality and cost that are in general dictated by the perverse organizational and fiscal incentives created by U.S. society. As a result of a wise reform movement, we can hope for an improved, more equitable, and more uniform performance from this sector of the health-care distribution system.

During the organizational upheaval inherent in our impending health system reform, it seems clear that the independent institutions should each revisit their charters, the values that govern their being, and the true nature of their missions, and seek to bring their organizational behavior into greater concordance with their highest institutional values. If it is true that the 1950s, 1960s, and 1970s saw the emergence of hospital administration as a mature profession, and if it is true that a growing army of professionals in turn raised the level of organization and effectiveness in U.S. hospitals, then we may similarly generalize about the 1980s as a decade that was dedicated to productivity and positive financial outcomes based upon market-based incentives. With our health-care engines having been so highly tuned through the past four decades, it may strangely be true that in the 1990s a new societal drive toward equity of access and efficiency of effort could provide the fiscal and moral support necessary to empower the nation's health-care institutions to recover, reconsider, reinvigorate, and recommit to their implicit social contract to care for those in need of help.

Roger J. Bulger
Christine K. Cassel

Directly related to this article is the companion article in this entry: HEALTH-CARE SYSTEMS. *Also directly related are the entries* HOSPITAL, *article on* MODERN HISTORY; HEALTH-CARE RESOURCES, ALLOCATION OF, *article on* MACROALLOCATION; *and* HEALTH-CARE FINANCING. *For a further discussion of topics mentioned in this article, see the entries* ECONOMIC CONCEPTS IN HEALTH CARE; JUSTICE; PUBLIC HEALTH, *article on* HISTORY OF PUBLIC HEALTH; RIGHTS; *and* UTILITY. *Other relevant material may be found under the entries* ADVERTISING; HEALTH CARE, QUALITY OF; HEALTH POLICY; PUBLIC POLICY AND BIOETHICS; *and* SOCIAL MEDICINE.

Bibliography

BROCK, DAN W., and BUCHANAN, ALLEN. 1986. "Ethical Issues in For-Profit Health Care." In *For-Profit Enterprise in Health Care*, pp. 224–249. Edited by Bradford H. Gray. Washington, D.C.: National Academy Press.
———. 1987. "The Profit Motive in Medicine." *Journal of Medicine and Philosophy* 12, no. 1:1–35.
GRAY, BRADFORD H. 1991. *The Profit Motive and Patient Care: The Changing Accountability of Doctors and Hospitals.* Cambridge, Mass.: Harvard University Press.
MILES, STEVEN H.; SINGER, PETER A.; and SIEGLER, MARK. 1989. "Conflict Between Patients' Wishes to Forgo Treatment and the Policies of Health Care Facilities." *New England Journal of Medicine* 321, no. 1:48–50.
WHITE, KERR L., and CONNELLY, JULIAN E., eds. 1992. *The Medical Schools' Mission and the Population's Health.* New York: Springer-Verlag.

HEALTH-CARE FINANCING

I. INTRODUCTION

In 1994 the United States was poised on the verge of major health-care reform. The political environment acknowledged alarm about rising health-care costs, combined with an increase in the number of uninsured people and widespread recognition of the inadequacy of coverage for those who were insured. President Bill Clinton and Hillary Rodham Clinton led an effort to propose a major health-care revision based on managed competition, while others promoted expanded government programs through Medicare or a single-payer approach such as that used in Canada. In single-payer models, like Medicare, the government provides insurance financed by general taxation to pay for health care provided by a diverse private delivery system. Other, more market driven approaches, such as managed competition, rely on employers to provide health insurance and promote larger alliances of insurance consumers to spread risk and provide purchasing power in relationship to insurance companies and health-care systems. During most of the year, some major reform that could achieve universal coverage seemed inevitable, but toward the end of the year doubts began to appear.

The major stumbling block for policymakers and legislators is the matter of how to finance health-care insurance. Most agree, at least theoretically, with the idea of universal coverage for all basic health-care services. But since the United States system currently does not have such coverage, any changes to achieve it would involve additional cost. The debate on financing is central to the issue of systems reform. Many have argued that greater efficiencies in a reformed system would produce funds that could pay for covering the uninsured, but all agree that systematic changes in financing will produce new economic winners and losers, and the losers would pose political obstacles to reform.

A description of the 1994 status quo and the ethical issues it raises follows in articles on health-care insurance, Medicare, Medicaid, and profit and commercialism. Most working Americans are covered by health-care insurance provided by their place of employment. This arrangement, somewhat unique to the United States, has led many employees to believe that their health-care coverage is "free." Employers, of course, do not see it as free; they recognize that because of rising health-care insurance costs, they must reduce wages, increase the cost of their products, or both. Health insurance is now a major issue in negotiations between unions and management. Medicare is a health-care insurance program for elderly and disabled people financed through payroll taxes within the Social Security system, beneficiary-paid premiums, and general taxation. Everyone who works is required to pay into Medicare and becomes eligible for Medicare coverage when they turn sixty-five. Medicaid is a program for poor people that is funded jointly by federal and state governments. Over time, Medicaid has also come to represent the major insurance function for long-term care; it covers elderly and disabled people who have become impoverished enough to qualify for poverty status to be eligible for Medicaid coverage for nursing home care. Private long-term care insurance does exist, but is too costly for most elderly people. The growth of the costs within the Medicaid program, and especially the growth of the long-term care segment, have led to reductions in the eligibility level for poor people and further increases in the number of uninsured.

In 1994 the prevailing approaches to health-care reform focused on maintaining the existing employment-based framework for health-care insurance and keeping Medicare as it is. Under various approaches to sharing risk by forming large groups to purchase insurance collectively, some proposals foresee folding poor people now covered by Medicaid into large purchasing pools. Others propose expanding Medicare to include the poor. Within most of these proposals, however, the major financing structure for the nonelderly remains the employer, with some degree of employee costs sharing. This has been one of the major factors leading to erosion of support for health-care reform in the United States. The business community—and small business in particular—has opposed a requirement that employers provide insurance for their employees. The only other potential source of financing, general taxation, is unpopular because of the sentiment of the public against any new taxes. As a result, policymakers face a "catch 22." In fact, the same amount of dollars would actually be involved in either case, with a somewhat different distribution. But given business's opposition and the American public's general fear of paying more for their health insurance, it is hard to make an acceptable case for financing through either employer mandate or general taxation. Some policymakers have proposed an "individual mandate," requiring individuals to purchase insurance for themselves and their families.

Important ethical issues—in particular, responsibility and fairness—underlie these questions of financing. Can we require individuals to be responsible for their health-care coverage, and if so, how such responsibility can be enforced? People who do not have health insurance, either because of personal choice or because their employer does not provide it, do sometimes get sick. When they do, they are cared for in emergency rooms or public hospitals; this adds to others' health-care costs, either because costs are shifted to insured patients' bills or because more tax dollars are spent to support public health-care facilities.

A responsible approach to sharing the cost of health care would be to require every individual to be insured so that his or her costs would not be transferred to others. The same argument can be made within the case for an employer-based health-care insurance system. If we reject general taxation or the individual mandate as a financing mechanism, turning to employers becomes the only remaining option. In the early 1990s, because of rising health-care costs, more and more employers were dropping health-care coverage or reducing it drastically. Among small business owners, approximately 30 percent provided no health-care coverage to their workers. Strictly speaking, these 30 percent are shifting their health-care costs to the 70 percent of businesses who do provide health-care insurance, inflating the rates due to cost shifting. Since most hospitals will care for uninsured people, especially in emergencies or critical illness, the costs of this care are included in the general rates charged to those patients who do pay for services. This is called "cost shifting." It also occurs when hospitals or other providers are reimbursed for less than their costs, for example, by Medicare, Medicaid, or some managed-care contracts, and transfer those costs to payers who are willing to pay more for the same services. From the perspective of the 70 percent of employers who do cover their employees, an approach that requires all employers to behave similarly is both more equitable and more efficient.

As these issues continue to be debated, more arguments may focus on these questions of responsibility and fairness in the distribution of costs of health-care coverage. What cannot be avoided is the reality that without financing it is impossible to expand coverage to the entire population. Consideration of private health-care insurance, Medicare, and Medicaid demonstrates that the structure of financing has a profound influence on the quality and effectiveness of the delivery of health care.

CHRISTINE K. CASSEL

Directly related to this article are the other articles in this entry: HEALTH-CARE INSURANCE, MEDICARE, MEDICAID, *and* PROFIT AND COMMERCIALISM. *Also directly related are the entries* ECONOMIC CONCEPTS IN HEALTH CARE; HEALTH-CARE RESOURCES, ALLOCATION OF; *and* LIFE, QUALITY OF, *article on* QUALITY OF LIFE IN HEALTH-CARE ALLOCATION. *For a further discussion of topics mentioned in this article, see the entries* HARM; JUSTICE; RISK; UTILITY; *and* VALUE AND VALUATION. *Other relevant material may be found under the entries* COMMERCIALISM IN SCIENTIFIC RESEARCH; CONFLICT OF INTEREST; HEALTH-CARE DELIVERY; HEALTH POLICY, *article on* POLITICS AND HEALTH CARE; LIFE, QUALITY OF, *article on* QUALITY OF LIFE IN CLINICAL DECISIONS; PUBLIC POLICY AND BIOETHICS; *and* TECHNOLOGY, *article on* TECHNOLOGY ASSESSMENT.

II. HEALTH-CARE INSURANCE

Ethical issues related to health insurance

From its origins in the nineteenth century, health insurance has been intimately associated with the social and economic vulnerability of wage laborers. For those whose household flow of resources depends on being able to work and earn wages, sickness for any prolonged period threatens the ability to secure food and shelter. The practice of organizing workers to contribute a portion of their wages to health (or sickness) insurance funds was a response to this vulnerability and set a social pattern in industrialized nations that has continued for more than a century. The two principal ethical concepts associated with health insurance are social solidarity and social justice.

Health insurance and social solidarity. The insurance compact expresses an underlying solidarity among insurance pool subscribers. Persons facing a common vulnerability organize into a group whose shared resources, built up from relatively small individual contributions, will assist members who suffer financial loss as a result of illness or injury. Since the anticipated harm is a matter of probability, the group that pools its resources must be large enough and composed of persons with sufficiently variable risk levels so that, in the period of time covered by the contributions (or premiums), only a minority of those at risk will actually experience illness or injury, while the majority will contribute without drawing on the pooled resources. Those who do not encounter harm stand in a relationship of fiscal solidarity with those who do. The smaller the group, the more vulnerable it is to being overwhelmed by a small number of very large claims. If the group includes a large number of persons with high probability of need, a high level of member contributions will be required to guarantee adequate resources to cover every claim.

In addition to the purely fiscal relationship among contributors, reigning social and political ideas affect the conscious feelings of solidarity they experience as members of an insured group. Compulsory sickness insurance for workers, providing for both lost wages and the cost of medical care, was first organized at a national level in 1883 in Germany by the conservative Chancellor Otto von Bismarck as a defensive maneuver against the rising influence of the German Social Democratic Party. Bismarck believed workers were less likely to demand more radical reforms if certain harsh realities of the industrial revolution could be tempered with benevolence flowing from the monarchy (Starr, 1982).

In the closing decades of the nineteenth century, several other European nations took similar actions to protect workers' vulnerability, but the United States showed little interest in the idea until the Progressive reformers began to press the issue in the early years of the twentieth century (Hirshfield, 1970). They promoted compulsory health insurance as a form of enlightened self-interest on the part of the middle class: The survival of individual freedoms essential to capitalism required taming the tendency of free enterprise to pursue profit without concern for the precarious circumstance of wage laborers. The vocabulary of individualism typical of the culture of private consumption (Bellah et al., 1985) has largely shaped public discourse about health insurance in the United States, and the concept of social solidarity is only faintly evident in the debate that has evolved since the early twentieth century.

In some societies, social consciousness about health insurance sees it as a component of the nation's system of social insurance, that is, a public guarantee that certain basic human needs will be met at some minimum level for all members of the community. This has typically been the meaning of health insurance in western Europe. Conversely, health insurance may be seen as a marketable service properly residing in the private sector, which has been the dominant, though not unanimous, social understanding in the United States.

The Progressives' compulsory insurance campaign had failed prior to 1920, and by the late 1930s, the idea of voluntary health insurance for workers as a fringe benefit of employment had taken over as the prevailing rationale for social change. The appeal of voluntary insurance, supported by tax subsidies for employers and workers, was fully compatible with the Progressives' individual freedoms argument. Indeed, the voluntary approach seemed capable of solving the solidarity problem as the percentage of the whole population with voluntary hospital insurance shot up from less than 10 percent in 1940 to 57 percent in 1950 and to nearly 90 percent by the early 1970s (Anderson, 1985). With health insurance spreading widely through the working community, yet systematically leaving those not in the workforce outside the fold, the idea of national health insurance based on explicit appeals to solidarity and social justice emerged periodically but failed in several attempts to pass into law (Hirshfield, 1970; Starr, 1982).

Health insurance, social justice, and rights. The concept of justice is the second major ethical theme associated with health insurance. Concerns about justice and health insurance derive from the question whether it is fair for some, but not all, citizens to have insured access to health care. Originally, health insurance was viewed as required by social justice not for everyone, but only for those made vulnerable by the conditions of wage labor. Compulsory insurance schemes were designed to help capitalism by making the working class more secure. The U.S. middle class broadly committed itself to the voluntary purchase of health insurance when, as a means of winning better fringe benefits through collective bargaining (intensified under wage

and price controls during the 1940s), getting health insurance as a benefit became a normative expectation of workers.

Once the idea of health insurance has taken hold in a society and is widely believed to give access to a fundamental benefit of social existence, it comes to be seen as the way members of the society purchase their health care, not merely the way they protect themselves from potential financial loss. Having insurance and getting needed health care become closely linked in the logic of justice. (For an account of how social expectations give rise to societal obligation, see Walzer, 1983.)

The idea of a right to health care is part of the justice dimension of collectively financed health care. The notion that health care might count among positive human rights is a function of the widespread belief that health care successfully meets fundamental human needs, such as security, relief from suffering, prevention of unnecessary death, and maintenance of functional capacity. (For a philosophical argument about the grounds and limits of universal entitlement, see Daniels, 1985.) Creating legal protections for that right becomes a problem of political will.

The injection of rights language into political arguments about health insurance is itself evidence of the evolution of the concept and expansion of its original limited goal of protecting wage laborers from the effects of major illness. In the absence of a constitutional or statutory declaration of a right to health care, opinion leaders use human rights language to motivate members of society and to provoke legislative action aimed at helping persons whose needs are being ignored. While specific contractual rights to health care exist between insured persons and their insurance carriers, that is not what advocates of a right to health care have in mind. When reformers argue for a right to health care, they mean that basic relationships of solidarity and interdependence among all members of society create a societal obligation to ensure access to health care for all. (For a discussion of issues raised by rights discourse in relation to health insurance and access to health care, see the U.S. President's Commission report, 1983, and Chapman, 1994.)

During the second half of the twentieth century, aggregate expenditures for health care rose at such a dramatic rate that by the 1980s, cost control in health care became a central issue for reformers. However, the question of setting limits makes debate about a right to health care politically difficult. Unlike rights to liberty or the pursuit of happiness, which entail noninterference by others, a right to health care entails paying someone to provide costly services. By 1990, the need to speak of a limited right was clear to many leaders, although negative reaction to the idea of rationing health care led many to deny its necessity, and how to define limits was hotly debated. In 1989, the state of Oregon intensified the debate when it organized a unique social experiment to guarantee coverage to uninsured persons while setting limits on what would be covered based on a prioritized list of health-care services (Garland, 1992, 1994).

Organization and financing of health insurance

The fundamental concept of any form of insurance is risk sharing: A large number of people who face a common threat of harm (auto accident, fire damage, costs of treatment for illness or injury) share their risks by paying premiums to an insurer who promises to finance payments to those who in the future actually suffer misfortune. All members of the risk-sharing group set security in return for their contributions even if they do not receive financial benefits as a result of being personally harmed.

Ethical issues in risk sharing through health insurance are shaped by the insurer's decisions about how to organize and finance the common fund that members of a group rely on to protect themselves against financial loss. For example, insurers may organize risk-sharing pools among individual subscribers, various age groups, business firms, or labor organizations. Financing might be done through a single, community-wide premium or through variable premiums tied to health-risk or ethnic group or age or gender. The European approach was to develop social insurance mechanisms, or sick funds, initiated by the public sector. In the United States, the free market casualty insurance model was adapted in a unique form to fulfill the social insurance function.

The major development in U.S. health insurance in the 1930s and 1940s was led not by government or business but by nonprofit corporations such as Blue Cross (hospital insurance service corporations), Blue Shield (physician insurance service corporations), and a variety of consumer and producer cooperatives that provided coverage for hospital and medical services. The corporate missions and characteristics of these organizations gave U.S. health insurance a strong social insurance tendency without fully incorporating the European approach.

Because they believed that the nonprofit organizations' approach to health insurance violated the basic tenets of casualty insurance, commercial insurers initially showed no interest in this market (Iglehart, 1992). Casualty insurance assumes that a hazard insured against is measurable and not something the insured person wants (such as checkups or preventive services), or can control (such as pregnancy).

From the beginning in the United States these characteristics were ignored. While health insurance protects a few subscribers from the financial impact of occasional high-cost medical services, plans also cover many low-cost services used every year by most members of the insured group. The typical health insurance plan provided to employees of large corporations includes coverage for some ambulatory care costs (physician, X-ray, and laboratory services) and most of the cost of emergency room and hospital services. About 80 percent of the population will use some ambulatory care services, while only 10 percent of the population will use hospital services in any given year.

By the time the commercial insurers overcame their suspicion of the field, the nonprofit insurers had already brought much social insurance philosophy into the market. Consequently, while the health insurance language includes many standard insurance terms ("adverse selection," "moral hazard," "product lines," "lives covered by plans"), leading the casual observer to conclude that the field is a traditional casualty insurance market, it is, in reality, a form of social insurance peculiar to the United States. However, the competitive practices of commercial insurers has led to widespread use of experience rating (see below), which tends to undermine the social insurance spirit by making health insurance more difficult to obtain for those in greatest need.

Health insurance plans use three basic methods to protect subscribers: indemnity benefits, service benefits, or direct provision of service. Indemnity insurance, typical of commercial insurers, reimburses a patient for a portion of incurred medical expenditures. Service benefits, typical of nonprofit insurers, pay physicians and hospitals directly on behalf of subscribers. Health maintenance organizations, by contrast, actually organize and deliver services directly to their members at clinics and hospitals that the plans usually own and operate, paying for professional services by salary or contract, not on a fee-for-service basis.

Six major tendencies characterize the way U.S. health insurance adapted casualty insurance concepts to serve a social insurance function: leadership by nonprofit corporations; a gradual shift from financing based on equal shares (community-rated premiums) to financing based on unequal shares (experience-rated premiums); consumer preference for comprehensive benefits; use of service and indemnity methods of benefit definition; carriers' preference for group rather than individual marketing of plans; and persistent ambivalence in the general public about the role of government in health insurance.

Nonprofit status of health insurance pioneers. Because the pioneers in U.S. health insurance were nonprofit, charitable organizations, they were developed to provide a social function beyond creating a profit for shareholders or syndicate owners. However, the social objective was not always to benefit consumers. Blue Cross was organized to provide for the financial survival of the American voluntary, nonprofit hospital system. Although organized medicine initially opposed the new insurance schemes as unwanted intrusions into the privacy of the patient–physician relationship, Blue Shield was eventually formed as a preventive measure to keep physician financing mechanisms under the direct control of organized medicine. Provider cooperative prepaid group practices, such as Kaiser Permanente, were formed because some physicians believed that prepaid group practice was a more satisfying and socially responsible way to practice medicine.

These nonprofit institutions were chartered in the public domain and were guided by boards of directors who were reminded that they represented society at large, rather than a group of stockholders. The corporate cultures that emerged under this influence generally produced organizational behavior different from that found in commercial insurance companies (Greenlick, 1988). The nonprofit corporations possessed a sense of mission to the community, a sense nurtured by their close ties to community hospitals and physicians' organizations. In the 1970s, pressured by their large corporate customers to contain costs, the nonprofit insurers began to behave like their competitors, the commercial insurance companies, and moved from community rating of premiums to experience-rating practices. Consequently, premiums increased for high-risk groups, making it difficult for the most needy to maintain health insurance coverage.

Community-rated versus experience-rated premiums. In an institutionalization of the concept of solidarity, the pioneer U.S. health insurance organizations originally used community-rating principles to fund their programs. In pure community rating, the premium is set by estimating the required budget for the covered population for the next year and dividing the total budget by the number of people expected to be covered. The result is the premium charged to each member of the population for the coming year. Thus, all employers in an insurer's service area would be charged the same per capita premium for their employees.

By contrast, in an experience-rated system, the approach traditionally used by commercial carriers, the most recent available claims experience is analyzed to define a risk profile for specific groups. These risk profiles are applied to the next year's expected total budget to calculate group-specific premiums. Experience rating increases the premiums for groups that include high-use subscribers and reduces premiums for groups that include infrequent users. Consequently, people who most need the risk-sharing of health insurance are forced to pay higher and higher premiums, until they can no longer afford the cost of coverage (Greenlick, 1989).

As experience rating became more common, people with preexisting health conditions found themselves effectively excluded from insurance coverage. This led many states during the 1980s to create special high-risk pools for "uninsurables." The practice also made health insurance too expensive for thousands of firms with small numbers of workers, especially those where even one worker had recently experienced a high-cost illness episode. The shift toward experience rating by nonprofit insurers has led to a disturbing social policy incongruity between the U.S. health insurance market and prevailing public expectation that private health insurance should fulfill a social insurance function.

Comprehensive benefit packages. Because pioneer health insurance organizations had among their objectives supporting the providers of care, they designed insurance plans based on comprehensive benefits that would cover not only infrequently needed high-cost services but also many low-cost services that might be used regularly by most subscribers. The idea of comprehensive benefits was very popular with the employees whose employers were paying most, or all, of the premiums for health insurance. This popularity was supported by the post–World War II belief that economic growth could permanently keep pace with new demands. During the 1960s and 1970s, most Blue Cross/Blue Shield and prepaid group practice plans covered, with little deductible or coinsurance cost to the insured, most of the costs of physician, laboratory, X-ray, emergency room, and hospital medical and surgical services. During the 1970s, insurers increasingly added coverage for prescription drugs. To keep pace, commercial insurance companies increased the breadth and depth of their coverage, particularly for low-risk groups.

The preference for comprehensive benefits contributed to the explosive rate of growth in the health services industry during the postwar era. In 1940, health care accounted for 4.1 percent of the Gross National Product. It had expanded to 7.2 percent by 1970, reaching 10.7 percent in 1985 (Eastaugh, 1987). By the late 1970s, a chronic sense of crisis afflicted business and government administrators of health insurance budgets. Cost-containment strategies successfully used deductibles and coinsurance to reduce the use of health services by insured persons. However, these typical casualty insurance mechanisms conflicted with the social insurance function of health insurance and were hotly debated among health insurance reformers in the early 1990s.

Service benefits versus indemnity benefits. A distinguishing characteristic of the Blue Cross/Blue Shield programs and the prepaid group practices is that they sell their customers a promise to provide medical care services (service benefits) rather than a promise to reimburse incurred expenses (indemnity benefits). Service benefit organizations concern themselves with issues of delivery of care more than indemnity insurers who cover only a specified portion of medical care expenses.

Preferred provider organizations (PPOs) and multiple forms of health maintenance organizations (HMOs) emerged from the cost-controlling strategies of the 1970s and 1980s. These service-delivery reforms sought cost savings through peer group review of practice patterns, favoring those that produced effective care while reducing frequency and length of hospitalizations, using fewer repeat visits, and increasing the use of outpatient care in place of costly hospital services. U.S. insurers took a hand in designing and administering these delivery system reforms, giving them a significant role in health care that went far beyond merely paying the bills.

Group enrollment versus individual marketing. Like the European social insurance movement, the development of health insurance in the United States was based on enrollment through employment groups. As more Americans left rural occupations and moved to the cities during and after the Great Depression of the 1930s, they found work in large industrial companies that increasingly offered comprehensive health insurance coverage as a fringe benefit of employment. The health insurance industry focused on enrolling members through work groups. As long as employment in these industries grew, so did the proportion of U.S. citizens covered by health insurance. Labor market forces seemed to be producing social insurance goals without the need of centralized decisions.

Employment-based group enrollment ultimately comes up short from the social insurance perspective, however, since many persons with significant health-care needs are not in the work force and will not have access to health insurance. This way of distributing health insurance leaves workers doubly vulnerable to fluctuations in the labor market: Low-wage jobs frequently do not include health insurance benefits, and business cycles or industry competition may cause work force reductions leading to loss of health insurance for employees and their dependents (homemakers and children).

Inequities in the labor market carry over to health insurance when employment is the basis for its distribution (Jecker, 1993). Women's groups argue that health-care services important to women, such as mammography, have tended not to be covered. Women who work are less likely than men who work to have employer or union contributions to their insurance. Women are also more likely to work part-time and receive no fringe benefits. Women are less likely to belong to a labor union and they change jobs more frequently than men, making them more vulnerable to preexisting condition exclusions from insurance. Women predomi-

nate in low-paying jobs where insurance is usually not offered as a benefit. Many of these distribution inequities also affect minorities, leading some reformers to argue for uncoupling health insurance from employment.

After a vigorous growth between 1940 and 1960, the employment-based system had generated health insurance coverage for nearly 70 percent of the population under sixty-five, while only slightly more than 40 percent of the elderly were covered, leading to the establishment of Medicare and Medicaid in 1965 (Anderson, 1985). These two programs brought health insurance protection to virtually all of the elderly, and to a significant proportion of those living in poverty, as well. They did not, however, provide coverage for everyone, so that the United States entered the 1990s with more than thirty million citizens having no health insurance. This fueled a vigorous revival of interest in a national health insurance program capable of guaranteeing coverage for every citizen.

During the 1980s, self-insurance emerged as a cost-control strategy among large corporations. These firms stopped buying health insurance for their workers and set themselves up as the at-risk entity for health-care costs incurred by their employees. The practice put these corporations beyond the reach of state insurance regulations because of a 1974 federal law, the Employee Retirement Income Security Act (ERISA). The intent of ERISA was to protect pension trust funds in companies with employees in several states from inconsistent and burdensome state regulations. The effect on health insurance, while not a primary goal of ERISA, so complicated health-insurance reform that, by the late 1980s, it became a critical element in all proposals that relied on employee benefits as the primary vehicle for distributing health insurance to citizens.

The government role in U.S. health insurance. The U.S. government has had a role in health insurance since the eighteenth century, when it accepted the responsibility to provide medical care for the U.S. Merchant Marine. During the growth period of private health insurance in the United States prior to Medicare and Medicaid (1940–1965), the federal government let the private market work, limiting itself to indirect involvement through tax incentives for employers and employees who favored the purchase of health insurance as a fringe benefit. State and local governments were expected to provide care to the indigent and to the mentally ill. As a large employer, the federal government became a major purchaser of health insurance for its employees.

Finally, the federal government is a major supplier of social insurance for medical care for Native Americans, active-duty military personnel and their dependents, and veterans. The total public expenditure for medical care services exceeded $312 billion during 1990, nearly 50 percent of the total national expenditure for health services and supplies during the year.

Government involvement in U.S. health insurance differs distinctly from paths followed by most other industrial nations. In Europe, several nations have made the direct delivery of health care a national government responsibility (e.g., the United Kingdom and the Scandinavian countries); others have taken up the role of coordination in mixed public-private systems (e.g., Germany, the Netherlands, Switzerland); others have assumed the role of providing health insurance to the citizenry, allowing hospitals and physicians to operate in a fee-for-service environment (France).

In the late 1960s, Canada adopted an approach similar to France's: Each province has a monopoly on health insurance for basic services, while the federal government plays a coordinating role. Canadian Medicare rests on five essential principles: universal entitlement, accessibility of services, comprehensive benefits, portability of benefits across provincial boundaries, and public administration of the system within each province.

Questions about the proper role of government in health insurance continue to be central issues in debates among U.S. health insurance reformers. Proposals put forward in the 1990s will succeed or fail on the basis of their ability to make the case that they have found an acceptable balance point on the public–private continuum where private markets (insurance carriers, providers, suppliers) come together under public policy constraints to produce an acknowledged common good.

Conclusion

As the 1990s dawned, the evolution of health insurance in the United States and elsewhere had reached a point where significant new public policy decisions were increasingly demanded by the consumer groups, business, politicians, and health professionals (see Fein, 1989). In all industrial nations, the rates of growth in total expenditures for health care were creating economic strains and social concern (see Government Committee on Choices in Health Care, 1992). Particularly in the United States, which has the highest percentage of Gross National Product devoted to health care, business, government, and consumer groups insisted on effective control of total health-care expenditures. Some argued that the solution had to come from submitting health care to a competitive market. Others preferred government regulation through global budgets, delivery system reforms, and limitations on services that qualify for collective financing. Both groups insisted that health insurance had to stop fueling uncontrolled growth in health-care spending.

Expenditure control has major consequences for the social insurance dimension integral to health insurance schemes. Many European nations and Canada have sought to control total expenditures without sacrificing the health-care component of their social insurance commitments. In the United States, many providers, social reformers, and the general public have demanded explicit commitment to the social insurance dimension of health insurance: a universal system that would guarantee a decent minimum of health care to every citizen. Reformers were particularly concerned to have the nation address the equity issue. During a thirty-two-month period in 1990–1992, one-fourth of the entire population outside of institutions were without health insurance for at least one month; but more than one-third of the African-American population and nearly one-half of the Hispanic population found themselves excluded from coverage (Pear, 1994).

Growing public awareness of the size of the uninsured population and the vulnerability of the middle class to loss of job-related health insurance have led to growing dissatisfaction with the system and sparked a renewed interest in health insurance reform. Dozens of proposals emerged in the late 1980s and early 1990s driven by several key questions. Should America continue its multiple payer, public-private system, or embark on a new path with a streamlined single-payer system? Should the single payer be the federal government or each state? If there were to be multiple payers, who would conduct the negotiations needed to coordinate their practices so that universal coverage would be achieved and maintained?

The multiple-payer approach continues the path of adapting casualty insurance and free-market forces to serve the social insurance function. President Bill Clinton proposed a market-structuring, multiple-payer solution (White House Domestic Policy Council, 1993; Zelman, 1994), and was immediately criticized by sponsors of competing market proposals for interfering too much with market forces and not trusting them to achieve efficient allocations (Enthoven and Singer, 1994). Single-payer advocates, arguing that Clinton was fundamentally mistaken and that the private health insurance market was simply the wrong vehicle for achieving universal coverage and cost control, invoked the social insurance model, abandoning market pluralism in favor of uncomplicated universality and administrative efficiency achievable through centralized financing.

Health insurance in the United States continues to evolve. The enduring challenge is to formulate policies that can control total expenditures while allocating resources both fairly and in service of the common good.

MICHAEL J. GARLAND
MERWYN R. GREENLICK

Directly related to this article are the INTRODUCTION *and other articles in this entry:* MEDICARE, MEDICAID, *and* PROFIT AND COMMERCIALISM. *For a further discussion of topics mentioned in this article, see the entries* AUTONOMY; FREEDOM AND COERCION; HARM; JUSTICE; RACE AND RACISM; RIGHTS; RISK; SEXISM; *and* WOMEN, *article on* HEALTH-CARE ISSUES. *For a discussion of related ideas, see the entries* ECONOMIC CONCEPTS IN HEALTH CARE; HEALTH CARE, QUALITY OF; HEALTH-CARE RESOURCES, ALLOCATION OF; MEDICAL ETHICS, HISTORY OF, *section on* EUROPE, *subsection on* CONTEMPORARY PERIOD, *and section on* THE AMERICAS, *article on* CANADA; PATIENTS' RIGHTS, *article on* ORIGIN AND NATURE OF PATIENTS' RIGHTS; *and* UTILITY.

Bibliography

ANDERSON, ODIN W. 1985. *Health Services in the United States: A Growth Enterprise Since 1875.* Ann Arbor, Mich.: Health Administration Press.

BELLAH, ROBERT N.; MADSEN, RICHARD; SULLIVAN, WILLIAM M.; SWINDLER, ANN; and TIPTON, STEVEN M. 1985. *Habits of the Heart: Individualism and Commitment in American Life.* New York: Harper & Row.

"Caring for the Uninsured and the Underinsured." 1991. *Journal of the American Medical Association* 265, no. 19. Special issue.

CHAPMAN, AUDREY, ed. 1994. *Health Care Reform: A Human Rights Approach.* Washington, D.C.: Georgetown University Press.

DANIELS, NORMAN. 1985. *Just Health Care.* Cambridge: At the University Press.

EASTAUGH, STEVEN R. 1987. *Financing Health Care: Economic Efficiency and Equity.* Dover, Mass.: Auburn House.

ENTHOVEN, ALAIN C., and SINGER, SARA J. 1994. "A Single-Payer System in Jackson Hole Clothing." *Health Affairs* 13, no. 1:81–95.

FEIN, RASHI. 1989. *Medical Care, Medical Costs: The Search for a Health Insurance Policy.* Cambridge, Mass.: Harvard University Press.

GARLAND, MICHAEL J. 1992. "Justice, Politics and Community: Expanding Access and Rationing Health Services in Oregon." *Law, Medicine and Health Care* 20, nos. 1–2: 67–81.

———. 1994. "From Manifesto to Enforceable Right: Oregon's Contribution to Defining Adequate Health Care." In *The Right to Health Care in the United States: Conceptualization, Policy Implications, and Measurement Standards.* Edited by Audrey Chapman. Washington, D.C.: Georgetown University Press.

GOVERNMENT COMMITTEE ON CHOICES IN HEALTH CARE. 1992. *Choices in Health Care: A Report.* Zoestermeyer, Netherlands: Author.

GREENLICK, MERWYN R. 1988. "Profit and Nonprofit Organizations in Health Care: A Sociological Perspective." In *In Sickness and In Health: The Mission of Voluntary Health Care Institutions,* pp. 155–176. Edited by J. David Seay and Bruce C. Vladeck. New York: McGraw-Hill.

———. 1989. "Health Care for Adults." In *Handbook of Medical Sociology.* 4th ed., pp. 381–399. Edited by Howard E. Freeman and Sol Levine. Englewood Cliffs, N.J.: Prentice-Hall.

HEALTH INSURANCE ASSOCIATION OF AMERICA. 1990. *Source Book of Health Insurance Data.* 30th ed. Washington, D.C.: Author.

HETHERINGTON, ROBERT W.; HOPKINS, CARL E.; and ROEMER, MILTON I. 1975. *Health Insurance Plans: Promise and Performance.* New York: Wiley.

HIRSHFIELD, DANIEL S. 1970. *The Lost Reform: The Campaign for Compulsory Health Insurance in the United States from 1932 to 1943.* Cambridge, Mass.: Harvard University Press.

IGLEHART, JOHN K. 1992. "The American Health Care System: Private Insurance." *New England Journal of Medicine* 326, no. 5:1715–1720.

JECKER, NANCY S. 1993. "Can an Employer-Based Health Insurance System Be Just?" *Journal of Health Politics, Policy and Law.* 18, no. 3, pt. 2:657–673.

PEAR, ROBERT. 1994. *New York Times.* March 29, p. D23. "Gaps in Coverage for Health Care."

STARR, PAUL. 1982. *The Social Transformation of American Medicine.* New York: Basic Books.

TAYLOR, MALCOLM G. 1990. *Insuring National Health Care: The Canadian Experience.* Chapel Hill: University of North Carolina Press.

U.S. PRESIDENT'S COMMISSION FOR THE STUDY OF ETHICAL PROBLEMS IN MEDICINE AND BIOMEDICAL AND BEHAVIORAL RESEARCH. 1983. *Securing Access to Health Care: A Report on the Ethical Implications of Differences in the Availability of Health Services.* Washington, D.C.: Author.

WALZER, MICHAEL. 1983. *Spheres of Justice: A Defense of Pluralism and Equality.* New York: Basic Books.

WHITE HOUSE DOMESTIC POLICY COUNCIL. 1993. *Health Security: The President's Report to the American People.* Washington, D.C.: Author.

ZELMAN, WALTER A. 1994. "The Rationale Behind the Clinton Health Reform Plan." *Health Affairs* 13, no. 1:9–29.

III. MEDICARE

At its inception in 1966, the Medicare program was understood as a way to assure the elderly a stable place in the mainstream of American medicine. Over the first quarter-century of its operation, Medicare came increasingly to be viewed as an instrument to influence the character and costs of doctors, hospitals, and health insurance. In 1986, Medicare marked its twentieth birthday with considerable fanfare. In 1991, along with American medicine, Medicare faced severe financial pressures, and its silver anniversary was not celebrated. This article briefly explains Medicare's origins, sketches its programmatic development since 1966, and reflects on the philosophical premises its founding and subsequent operation express.

The origins of Medicare

When the Great Depression made economic insecurity a pressing national concern, the social insurance reformers thought health insurance should be included in a comprehensive American scheme of social protection. From 1936 to the late 1940s, there were recurrent calls to incorporate universal health insurance within America's nascent welfare state. But despite the broad public support for national health insurance, the conservative coalition in Congress defeated this measure (Marmor, 1973).

By 1952, the original architects of Social Security, well aware of this frustrating opposition, had formulated a plan of incremental expansion of government health insurance. The proponents of what became known as Medicare restricted the category of beneficiaries to the retired while retaining the conceptual link to social insurance. Medicare would provide retirees with limited hospitalization insurance—a partial plan for part of the population whose financial fears of illness were as real as their difficulty in purchasing health insurance at affordable cost. So began the long battle to turn a national health-insurance proposal acceptable to the public into one passable by the Congress (Hirshfield, 1970; Starr, 1982; Numbers, 1978; Marmor, 1973).

These origins had much to do with the initial design of the Medicare program and the expectations of how it would develop over time. The incrementalist strategy assumed that hospitalization coverage was the appropriate first step in benefits and that wider benefits would be enacted later under a common pattern of Social Security financing. Likewise, the strategy's proponents assumed that eligibility would be expanded gradually to include most, if not all, of the population, extending first, perhaps, to children and pregnant women. All the Medicare enthusiasts took for granted that the rhetoric of enactment should emphasize the expansion of access to medical care, not its regulation and reform. The clear aim was to reduce the risks of financial disaster—for the elderly and their families—and the clear understanding was that Congress would demand a largely hands-off posture toward the doctors and hospitals providing the care Medicare would finance. Some twenty-five years after the program's enactment, it is taken for granted that how—or how much—one pays for medical care affects the care given. But in the buildup to enactment in 1965, no such presumption existed.

Once this incrementalist proposal was outlined, who and what shaped its fate? Medicare's principal antagonists and their adversarial methods illustrated a familiar American form of ideological politics. The most prominent opponents—national medical, business, and labor organizations—engaged in open, hostile communication and brought into their opposing camps many groups whose economic interests were not directly af-

fected by the Medicare outcome. Both the contest and the contestants remained remarkably stable from 1952 to 1964; two well-defined camps with opposing views reigned, and few groups remained impartial or uncommitted.

The particular features of the political environment in 1965 explain details of the original Medicare program that seem problematic decades later. The overwhelming Democratic victory of 1964 seemed to guarantee that hospitalization insurance for the aged would pass in 1965. President Lyndon B. Johnson's commitment to Medicare was plain in his presidential campaign, and the new Congress of 1965 acted to prevent further delays in the president's "Great Society" agenda. The result, however, was far more complex than expected. The certainty that a Medicare bill would be enacted transformed the struggle from a polemic over Medicare's wisdom to a complicated strategy game about exactly what the program would do. Out of that game came the benefits, financing, and administrative design of the operational Medicare program. Few participants had expected Medicare to pay physicians at all, let alone their "reasonable and customary" charges in a new Part B. And, while reimbursing hospitals (under Part A) by the Blue Cross formula of reasonable costs was anticipated, the Department of Health, Education, and Welfare hardly imagined the inflationary impact that would have.

Development of Medicare

In the first period, from roughly 1966 to 1972, Medicare's administrators accommodated the demands of medical providers for a largely hands-off stance by public regulators. Out of this period—described by Lawrence Brown as "consensual corporatism"—emerged rapid inflation in Medicare's expenditures and the fumbling efforts to find acceptable means to control its costs (Brown, 1985).

From 1972 to the beginning of the 1980s, Medicare's woes were masked by the national preoccupation with the mix of inflation and unemployment known as stagflation, with broader proposals to reform American medicine, and with the growing appeal of "pro-competitive" alternatives to public regulation of discrete programs like Medicare and Medicaid. This period was characterized by the growing dispersal of government regulation among federal and state agencies ("inverted corporatism" [Brown, 1985]). The frustrating experience with health planning, with experiments in hospital reimbursement, and with the rapid growth of costs prompted broader reform approaches. A striking illustration of both the problems and the frustration was the addition of a special disease program under Medicare: one for all Americans suffering from renal failure. Enacted with great fanfare in 1972, the end-stage renal-disease program grew rapidly—in beneficiaries, in costs, and in complexity. And it soon became a symbol of disappointment with traditional ideas of government health insurance (see Starr, 1982). Throughout the 1970s, health policy experts produced a bewildering array of reform proposals, but Medicare's reform remained a special world of policy specialists, congressional committees, and the responsible executive agency, Social Security's Bureau of Health Insurance, until the Health Care Finance Agency (HCFA) took over in 1977 (Marmor, 1988).

A third period of Medicare's administrative history—labeled "technocratic corporatism"—flowered in the 1980s (Brown, 1982). With universal health insurance dislodged from the national agenda, the attention of policymakers and technical experts returned to Medicare itself. Medicare and Social Security had been specially protected under the mantle of social insurance theories of entitlement and by the elderly population's reputed political clout. That protected status was what the budget and tax politics of the 1980s were to challenge (Ball, 1988).

Three developments exemplify this period, which extends to the mid-1990s. First, there were continuing efforts to reduce the rate of expenditure growth in Medicare, efforts that initially shifted costs to the elderly and later burdened hospitals and physicians. Second, there was the surprisingly rapid enactment in 1983 of a new form of hospital reimbursement within Medicare: the widely noted diagnosis-related group (DRG) method of prospective payment. Developed by technocrats in the academy and within HCFA, supported by policy experts within the Congress, and with some operational trials in New Jersey, DRGs dominated the hospital world of the 1980s and symbolized the faith in scientific, apolitical answers to Medicare's troubles. At this time, there was no specific provision for monitoring the quality of hospital care, though there was no question of the potential effects on patient care of changing hospital financial incentives so drastically (Smith, 1992). A new federal institution—the Prospective Payment Commission—became the monitor of DRGs and later in the decade spawned a similar institution for Medicare's Part B medical insurance, the Physician Payment Review Commission. It was assumed that the associated peer review organizations would take care of balancing Medicare's cost and quality.

The irony of the Reagan era is that an administration committed ideologically to "free markets" produced the most obvious examples of administered prices in American medicine. At the same time, increases in the medical expenses paid directly by the elderly prompted what came to be known as the "catastrophic debacle" of 1987–1989. The Reagan administration proposed, and the Congress more generously delivered, a complicated piece of legislation to cover the catastrophic expenses of the elderly. A firestorm of protest erupted over the financing of this benefit expansion (affecting largely the more affluent elderly) and, for the first time in Medicare's history, in 1989 the Congress repealed a benefit that had been regarded as a gift to the program's beneficiaries.

Twenty-five years after enactment of the Medicare program, its budget woes were part of the national preoccupation with increasing public deficits. The catastrophic debacle had symbolized and worsened the charges of "generational inequity," with "greedy geezers" caricatured as the enemies of America's children, future, and tradition of fairness. With deficits untamed, further cuts in Medicare's rate of expenditure growth remained on the policy agenda in 1992 and thereafter, even as the nation debated more comprehensive forms of medical-care reform.

Philosophical reflections

Most philosophical commentary on American medicine neglects Medicare's institutional details. Indeed, the focus of most medical ethics is the problematic case: the tragic choice where withholding of lifesaving technology is concerned (for example, kidney dialysis; see Whitbeck, 1985). Seldom have philosophers—or the philosophically minded—addressed the operating presumptions of large-scale medical programs or buttressed their observations with evidence about the costs, character, and political struggles of these major elements of the modern welfare state.

Yet, in a world where resources are understood to be scarce—the American world of social policy in the last two decades of the twentieth century—being clear about what one is after is an exceedingly useful guide to thought and action.

The striking fact about the origins of Medicare is not the surprising character of the 1965 legislation but the ambiguous commitment to a special program for the aged. Health insurance for the aged under Social Security was what reformers thought they could get from American politics, not what they really wanted. Medicare began with hospital insurance for the elderly, not with the benefits it ought to (or in the end did) include. Protection from the unbudgetable expenses of illness was Medicare's announced aim, but few of its backers imagined that the program's features in 1965 constituted reasonable provision of that protection (Bowler, 1987).

But appropriate standards of access and distribution of costs are not directly confronted in incremental, pragmatic adjustments to the political possibilities of the moment. America's guiding philosophy—to the extent one existed at all—was largely negative: specification of what Medicare was not, rather than what its aims and methods entailed.

Medicare's enactment had a political explanation, not a philosophical rationale. If Medicare's social-insurance provisions provided a statutory basis for the "right" to insurance coverage, precisely what was the character of that right and the extent of the protection it assured? It is here that the absence of a guiding philosophy becomes most apparent. For the elderly, circumstances of income, housing, illness, and family differ, sometimes profoundly. Protection from medical-care expenses, from this point of view, simply means that equally ill elderly should receive the same treatment, that their ability to pay for care should be irrelevant to the care they justly receive. The right to such treatment places a corresponding obligation on the guarantors of the right to make other considerations irrelevant to the treatment deemed appropriate. Note that this conception does not require heroic treatment of any particular class of ailments; it requires that whatever treatment is otherwise appropriate be provided free of the impediments of class, region, race, and the like. Equal opportunity in this context means equal treatment—not luxurious treatment, heroic treatment, or unlimited treatment. Ascetic equality of treatment is as justifiable as luxurious equality of treatment.

Our discussion has emphasized the relevance of philosophical reflection to current and future concerns about the access, financing, and quality of care that elderly Americans will receive under the Medicare program. It is over a quarter of a century and hundreds of billions of dollars too late to act as if Medicare were an aberration whose features we have just now noticed. Conceived as a prelude to national health insurance for all, Medicare is now one of America's largest social programs and remains in the 1990s one of its most controversial.

THEODORE R. MARMOR

Directly related to this article are the INTRODUCTION *and other articles in this entry:* HEALTH-CARE INSURANCE, MEDICAID, *and* PROFIT AND COMMERCIALISM. *For a further discussion of topics mentioned in this article, see the entries* AGING AND THE AGED, *article on* HEALTH-CARE AND RESEARCH ISSUES; HEALTH CARE, QUALITY OF; HEALTH-CARE DELIVERY; HEALTH-CARE RESOURCES, ALLOCATION OF, *article on* MACROALLOCATION; *and* HEALTH POLICY. *For a discussion of related ideas, see the entry* JUSTICE. *Other relevant material may be found under the entry* FUTURE GENERATIONS, OBLIGATIONS TO.

Bibliography

BALL, ROBERT M. 1988. "The Original Understanding on Social Security: Implications for Later Developments." In *Social Security: Beyond the Rhetoric of Crisis*, pp. 17–39. Edited by Theodore R. Marmor and Jerry L. Mashaw. Princeton, N.J.: Princeton University Press.

BOWLER, M. KENNETH. 1987. "Changing Politics of Federal Health Insurance Programs." *P.S.: Political Science and Politics* 20, no. 2:202–211.

BROWN, LAWRENCE D. 1985. "Technocratic Corporatism and Administrative Reform in Medicare." *Journal of Health Politics, Policy and Law* 10, no. 3:579–599.

HIRSHFIELD, DANIEL S. 1970. *The Lost Reform: The Campaign For Compulsory Health Insurance in the United States From 1932 to 1943*. Cambridge: At the University Press.

MARMOR, THEODORE R. 1973. *The Politics of Medicare*. Rev. ed. Chicago: Aldine.

———. 1988. "Coping with a Creeping Crisis: Medicare at Twenty." In *Social Security: Beyond the Rhetoric of Crisis*, pp. 177–199. Edited by Theodore R. Marmor and Jerry L. Mashaw. Princeton, N.J.: Princeton University Press.

NUMBERS, RONALD L. 1978. *Almost Persuaded: American Physicians and Compulsory Health Insurance, 1912–1920*. Baltimore: Johns Hopkins University Press.

SMITH, DAVID G. 1992. *Paying for Medicare: The Politics of Reform*. New York: Aldine de Gruyter.

STARR, PAUL. 1982. *The Social Transformation of American Medicine*. New York: Basic Books.

WHITBECK, CAROLINE. 1985. "Why the Attention to Paternalism in Medical Ethics?" *Journal of Health Politics, Policy and Law* 10, no. 1:181–187.

IV. MEDICAID

In the years preceding Medicaid's enactment, health care for the poor was outside the mainstream of the American medical system. The financing and provision of health care for the poor relied on charity and public hospitals and clinics, coupled with limited public welfare-based assistance. Segregation in health facilities and by practitioners further restricted access to care for poor minorities. Concerns over lack of health insurance for elderly Americans grew during the 1950s and 1960s, culminating in the passage of Medicare and its companion legislation, Medicaid, in 1965. Medicare provided basic hospital- and physician-care insurance for all elderly Americans entitled to Social Security benefits, while Medicaid replaced the Kerr-Mills program of medical assistance for the low-income aged, covering both the nonelderly and the elderly poor.

Initial goals and early challenges

Medicaid was designed, and remains primarily, a means-tested program for individuals who are within the welfare-based categories of assistance and meet state-determined income and assets tests for eligibility. It is not designed to provide social insurance to the full poverty population but, rather, to cover particular recipients of public aid, often referred to as the "deserving poor." Medicaid primarily assists children and families receiving Aid to Families with Dependent Children, and elderly, blind, and disabled persons receiving Supplemental Security Income. These programs' eligibility criteria exclude single individuals and childless couples, as well as most two-parent families, no matter how poor, leaving nearly half of the nonelderly poor without coverage.

The initial goals of the Medicaid program were to ensure that recipients obtained adequate care and that the burden of their medical costs was reduced. This meant both the reduction of differences in use of services between the poor and the nonpoor and the elimination of the two-class medical-care system.

States provide up to half of the financing for Medicaid; the remainder is paid by the federal government. Within federal guidelines and options, states determine who will be covered, what services will be paid for, how much providers will be paid, and how the program will be administered. Although sharing a common national framework, Medicaid in fact operates as fifty different state programs.

Within a few years of Medicaid's implementation, expenditures for the program became a major concern of state and federal officials, and the social concern for health-care equity was replaced with cost-containment apprehension. While the number of recipients grew slowly between 1975 and 1990 (twenty-two million in 1975 to twenty-six million in 1990), total government costs for Medicaid increased dramatically, from $12 billion to $72 billion. Medicaid has never been a popular program, largely because of its tie to the stigma of welfare, the high expenditures required, and the tensions generated by increased spending for the politically voiceless poor, nearly half of whom are children.

Growth in the Medicaid safety net

Since its inception in 1965, the Medicaid program has grown in unanticipated ways. Long-term care was added to mandated benefits in 1972. Given the paucity of long-term-care insurance coverage, middle-class Americans become impoverished due to nursing home costs and thereby qualify for Medicaid. Pressure to improve coverage of the disabled resulted in Medicaid's assuming an increased role in financing care of the mentally retarded. Now institutional benefits account for over 40 percent of Medicaid costs. Pressure to broaden Medicaid's role in long-term care remains as long as alternative means to cover nursing home costs are not available. Gradually, coverage of pregnant women and children has expanded through creation of more generous eligibility levels and broadening of coverage beyond welfare categories. As the health insurance program for the disabled poor, who must wait over two years before becoming eligible for Medicare, Medicaid now covers at least 40 percent of persons with AIDS, underscoring its value as the safety net for health crises.

Impact on America's health

Despite systematic problems, the fact that Medicaid can survive at all is a testament to the critical role it plays in financing indigent care. Today Medicaid serves one in ten Americans, paying one out of every eleven dollars spent on health care in the United States.

Medicaid has achieved significant advances in the health care of the poor. Studies of health-service utilization among the poor have shown that those with Medicaid use health services at the same rate as the nonpoor with similar health status, while poor persons without Medicaid continue to lag significantly behind those with Medicaid coverage. Beyond improving use of services, Medicaid has reduced the financial burden of medical costs for the poor and provides access to a broader service package that supplements physician care, such as dental care and prescription coverage.

Dependence on charity and free care has been replaced with financial access to both public and private providers, although access to care in private physicians' offices is an area where Medicaid's attempts have clearly fallen short. Eighty-five percent of Medicaid beneficiaries report a usual source of care, but they are more likely than the privately insured to list a hospital outpatient department or emergency room as this source. Physician participation in the Medicaid program has been a consistent problem. Some of the reasons cited for this include low payment levels, complex billing procedures, perceptions of increased exposure to malpractice claims associated with high-risk patients, and poor patient compliance. Access to prenatal care is better for those with Medicaid than for the uninsured, but a third of women with Medicaid rely on health departments and public clinics rather than on private physicians.

Despite improvements in health care for Medicaid beneficiaries, use of health services has not been equalized between the poor and the nonpoor because half of the poverty population is outside of the program's welfare-based reach. Given that the poor are in worse health, differences are even more notable when health status and needs are accounted for; accounting for these would provide the measure of an equitable health-care system.

The impact of Medicaid coverage on the health status of the poor is difficult to assess directly. It is clear, however, that the health of the poor has improved significantly in the post-Medicaid era with substantial declines in infant mortality, maternal mortality, and death rates for major diseases where medical intervention is effective. The gap in health status between blacks and whites also has narrowed.

What is perhaps more clearly documented is that the loss of Medicaid coverage and the absence of insurance can adversely affect health status. The termination of Medicaid coverage for chronically ill and poor adults in California has been shown to result in decreased access to care and worsened health status.

Major criticisms of the program

Tied as it is to the welfare system, Medicaid is not a "user-friendly" program. Many who are eligible for the program do not enroll because they are unwilling to apply to a welfare program or are turned away by procedural barriers to enrollment. Once a person is enrolled, eligibility status is periodically evaluated, as frequently as monthly in some programs. When income eligibility standards are no longer met, Medicaid coverage is denied, resulting in high turnover of the covered population.

The state-based nature of the program has resulted in variations in coverage and benefits across the states. State income eligibility levels for families of three in 1991 varied from 13 to 75 percent of the federal poverty level, and no two programs had identical benefit packages. State Medicaid waivers have added to the diversity by allowing states to experiment with provider payment and delivery systems.

Throughout its history, there have been repeated cycles of cutbacks in response to fiscal pressure in the states. Cutbacks in the 1980s eroded Medicaid coverage of the poor and began to reverse the progress in closing gaps in access to care across income groups.

Concerns about access to mainstream medical care have remained throughout Medicaid's history. Low payments for hospital and physician care contribute to the problem. Hospitals now are taking legal action to improve reimbursement, and 25 percent of physicians choose not to participate in the program. Several states are experimenting with managed-care systems for their Medicaid populations, contracting with capitated payment plans such as health maintenance organizations, hoping that by decreasing fragmentation of care and episodic treatment, a worthy goal in itself, costs will be controlled.

Issues for the future of Medicaid

The mounting pressure for health-care reform to expand coverage to over thirty million uninsured Americans has brought renewed interest in restructuring or replacing Medicaid. As the states and federal government grapple with double-digit cost increases in Medicaid spending, identifying and implementing new approaches for improved coverage while controlling costs takes on a greater sense of urgency.

Medicaid reform is charged with moral issues that frame the fundamental policy decisions. Who are the "deserving poor" in the 1990s? Can public health insurance be equitable when it is targeted only to the poor, or is the inevitable outcome a lesser program? What kinds of health care should the safety net provide? Can an equitable minimum benefit package be determined? In the interim, is rationing of services to the disadvantaged and poor morally acceptable?

Do managed-care systems impinge on beneficiaries' freedom of choice of providers any more than the current system of limited physician access? Do the benefits of diverse, state-run programs outweigh the disadvantages of their complexity and obvious inequities? How should society share the costs that a decent health-care safety net will incur?

New forces have emerged to influence the resolution of these issues, and a critical mass for reform has been achieved. Financially strapped state governments, corporations struggling with high health-insurance premiums, the families of working-class uninsured, an empowered senior citizen lobby, and disabled persons with AIDS have the potential to steer the course of public health insurance into the next century.

DIANE ROWLAND
CATHERINE HOFFMAN

Directly related to this article are the INTRODUCTION *and other articles in this entry:* HEALTH-CARE INSURANCE, MEDICARE, *and* PROFIT AND COMMERCIALISM. *For a further discussion of topics mentioned in this article, see the entries* AGING AND THE AGED, *especially the article on* OLD AGE; AIDS, *especially the article on* HEALTH-CARE AND RESEARCH ISSUES; CHILDREN, *articles on* RIGHTS OF CHILDREN, *and* HEALTH-CARE AND RESEARCH ISSUES; HOSPITAL, *article on* CONTEMPORARY ETHICAL PROBLEMS; *and* SOCIAL MEDICINE. *For a discussion of related ideas, see the entries* ADVERTISING; ECONOMIC CONCEPTS IN HEALTH CARE; FETUS, *article on* HUMAN DEVELOPMENT FROM FERTILIZATION TO BIRTH; HARM; HEALTH CARE, QUALITY OF; HEALTH-CARE RESOURCES, ALLOCATION OF; HEALTH POLICY, *article on* POLITICS AND HEALTH CARE; JUSTICE; MEDICAL ETHICS, HISTORY OF, *section on* EUROPE, *subsection on* CONTEMPORARY PERIOD, *article on* UNITED KINGDOM, *and section on* THE AMERICAS, *article on* CANADA; RACE AND RACISM; RESPONSIBILITY; *and* SEXISM.

Bibliography

AMERICAN MEDICAL ASSOCIATION. 1991. "Physician Participation in Medicaid." *Physician Marketplace Update* 2, no. 4.

BROWN, E. RICHARD. 1983. "Medicare and Medicaid: The Process, Value, and Limits of Health Care Reforms." *Journal of Public Health Policy* 4, no. 3:335–356.

DAVIS, KAREN. 1976. "Achievements and Problems of Medicaid." *Public Health Reports* 91, no. 4:309–316.

DAVIS, KAREN, and SCHOEN, CATHY. 1978a. "Health, Use of Medical Care, and Income." In their *Health and the War on Poverty: A Ten-Year Appraisal,* pp. 18–48. Washington, D.C.: Brookings Institution.

———. 1978b. "Medicaid: Successes and Problems." In their *Health and the War on Poverty: A Ten-Year Appraisal,* pp. 49–91. Washington, D.C.: Brookings Institution.

FREEMAN, HOWARD E.; BLENDON, ROBERT J.; AIKEN, LINDA H.; SUDMAN, SEYMOUR; MULLINEX, CONNIE F.; and COREY, CHRISTOPHER R. 1987. "Americans Report on Their Access to Care." *Health Affairs* 6, no. 1:6–8.

HEALTH CARE FINANCING ADMINISTRATION. 1990. *Financing Health Care for People with AIDS: The Role of the Health Care Financing Administration.* Washington, D.C.: U.S. Department of Health and Human Services, Health Care Financing Administration.

HOWELL, EMBRY M. 1988. "Low Income Persons' Access to Health Care: NMCUES Medicaid Data." *Public Health Reports* 103, no. 5:507–514.

JENCKS, STEVEN F., and BENEDICT, M. BETH. 1990. "Accessibility and Effectiveness of Care Under Medicaid." *Health Care Financing Review* (Ann. Suppl.):47–56.

LEVIT, KATHARINE R.; LAZEMBY, HELEN C.; COWAN, CATHY A.; and LETSCH, SUZANNE W. 1991. "National Health Expenditures, 1990." *Health Care Financing Review* 13, no. 1:29–54.

LURIE, NICOLE; WARD, NANCY B.; SHAPIRO, MARTIN F.; and BROOK, ROBERT H. 1984. "Termination from Medi-Cal: Does it Affect Health?" *New England Journal of Medicine* 311, no. 7:480–484.

LURIE, NICOLE; WARD, NANCY B.; SHAPIRO, MARTIN F.; VAGHAIWALL, RATI; and BROOK, ROBERT H. 1986. "Termination of Medi-Cal Benefits: A Follow-up Study One Year Later." *New England Journal of Medicine* 314, no. 19:1266–1268.

MITCHELL, JANET B. 1991. "Physician Participation in Medicaid Revisited." *Medical Care* 29, no. 7:645–653.

NEWACHECK, PAUL W. 1988. "Access to Ambulatory Care for Poor Persons." *Health Services Research* 23, no. 3: 401–419.

NEWACHECK, PAUL W., and HALFRON, NEAL H. 1986. "The Financial Burden of Medical Care Expenses for Children." *Medical Care* 24, no. 12:1110–1117.

REILLY, THOMAS W.; CLAUSER, STEVEN B.; and BAUGH, DAVID K. 1990. "Trends in Medicaid Payments and Utilization, 1975–89." *Health Care Financing Review* (Ann. Suppl.):15–33.

ROGERS, DAVID E.; BLENDON, ROBERT J.; and MOLONEY, THOMAS W. 1982. "Who Needs Medicaid?" *New England Journal of Medicine* 307, no. 1:13–18.

ROWLAND, DIANE; LYONS, BARBARA; and EDWARDS, JENNIFER. 1988. "Medicaid: Health Care for the Poor in the Reagan Era." *Annual Review of Public Health* 9:427–450.

STEVENS, ROSEMARY, and STEVENS, ROBERT. 1974a. "The Federal Role: An Aphilosophical Explanation." In their *Welfare Medicine in America: A Case Study of Medicaid,* pp. 42–56. New York: Free Press.

———. 1974b. "Public and Political Concern with Medical Care." In their *Welfare Medicine in America: A Case Study of Medicaid,* pp. 9–41. New York: Free Press.

U.S. BUREAU OF THE CENSUS. 1991. *Poverty in the United States: 1990.* Current Population Reports, Series P-60, no. 175. Washington, D.C.: U.S. Government Printing Office.

U.S. PHYSICIAN PAYMENT REVIEW COMMISSION. 1991. *Annual Report to Congress,* chapter 15. Washington, D.C.: Author.

U.S. PROSPECTIVE PAYMENT ASSESSMENT COMMISSION. 1991. *Report and Recommendations to the Congress.* Washington, D.C.: Author.

WILENSKY, GAIL R., and BERK, MARC L. 1982. "Health Care, the Poor, and the Role of Medicaid." *Health Affairs* 1, no. 4:93–100.

V. PROFIT AND COMMERCIALISM

The practice of medicine is clearly a profession, as usually defined. In some sense it is also a business. However, the extent to which the professional behavior of physicians ought to be influenced by business considerations is a matter of debate (Veatch, 1983). A more general but closely related question is the degree to which business values should control the health-care system (Gray, 1991).

Physicians in private practice must generate income to pay their costs and earn a livelihood. In this sense profit (the excess of gross revenues over costs) is as economically important in the fee-for-service practice of medicine as it is in the conduct of a business. But some have carried the analogy further and have maintained that the payment of a fee is an essential part of the professional relation between physicians and patients because this relation is in effect a commercial contract between the supplier of a service (the physician) and the purchaser of a service (the patient). Although the service is professional, and therefore involves more constraints and responsibilities for the supplier than does an ordinary market transaction, this interpretation of medical practice effectively blurs most of the distinction between medicine and business (Sade, 1971). This argument further asserts that physicians may choose to offer their services to indigent patients gratis or at reduced rates, but their professional status does not require them to do so. Nor are physicians required to ignore or minimize their own economic interests when making professional decisions, provided their treatment is medically appropriate (Engelhardt and Rie, 1988).

Opposed to this point of view is a different and perhaps more traditional interpretation that regards medical practice primarily as a ministering function—a commitment to serve the needs of patients without concern for self-interest (Relman, 1992). According to this interpretation, profit may be an economic necessity in fee-for-service practice, in the aggregate if not in each individual case, but a de facto contract binding all physicians establishes an overriding obligation to serve those in need of medical care regardless of their ability to pay. Furthermore, fee for service is not considered to be a critical, or even an important, feature of professional practice. The contract between doctor and patient is basically ethical, not commercial, and is seen as part of a broader commitment that physicians make to society in exchange for licensure, authority, and the many other benefits bestowed on them by the state.

Although there has always been an uneasy tension between these two perspectives, until recently the traditional view of the ethical obligations of the medical profession generally prevailed. Most people considered medical care to be a social good, not an economic commodity, and most physicians and medical professional organizations acted as if they agreed. For example, the version of the American Medical Association's (AMA) ethical code prevailing from 1957 to 1980 said: "The practice of medicine should not be commercialized nor treated as a commodity in trade" (AMA, 1969, p. 28). Advertising was discouraged, and physicians were advised to limit the source of their professional incomes to services to patients rendered by them or under their supervision (AMA, 1969).

A similar view of the role of hospitals as essentially not-for-profit social institutions was widely accepted. Although many small proprietary hospitals existed in the early part of the twentieth century, until fairly recently, virtually all hospitals larger than seventy-five beds were public or private, not-for-profit institutions that considered their primary mission to be public service. Most of the private, not-for-profit (voluntary) hospitals admitted patients—particularly those who were acutely or seriously ill—without regard to income, and many accepted less than full payment from patients with limited means. They often operated at a deficit and depended on philanthropy, public contributions, or other nonpatient-derived income to continue operation. The public hospitals, of course, were tax-supported and were not expected to meet their expenses from patient revenues.

Beginning in the late 1960s, however, a new commercial spirit began to permeate the health-care system (Relman, 1980; Gray, 1991). It started with the hospitals but soon spread rapidly to virtually every other part of the system. In response to the growing opportunities for profit resulting from the expansion of government-supported health insurance through Medicare and Medicaid in the 1960s, and employment-based private health insurance, large chains of investor-owned hospitals sprang up in many communities. Other types of for-profit medical facilities and services soon followed, attracted by the seemingly unlimited opportunities for financial gain. Today about 15 percent of all private general hospitals and the majority of private nursing homes, psychiatric hospitals, and free-standing ambulatory care and diagnostic facilities are owned by for-profit corporations. In addition, about two-thirds of all health maintenance organizations (HMOs), most private indemnity health insurance companies, and most health-care management and consulting services are in the investor-owned sector. Together with the new and rapidly growing biotechnology companies and the traditional pharmaceutical and medical supplies and equipment industries, these for-profit businesses constitute a vast commercial network with a pervasive and powerful influence on the U.S. health-care system. In no other country is so much of the health-care delivery system operated by investor-owned corporations, and in no other country does private business have so large a stake in health-care policy.

Even the not-for-profit voluntary hospitals have become infused with the entrepreneurial spirit. Overexpansion of hospital capacity and the advent of aggressive investor-owned health-care facilities, both inpatient and ambulatory, forced voluntary hospitals to become more competitive. As a result, their marketing and advertising efforts, and their preoccupation with the generation of revenue, are almost indistinguishable from those of their investor-owned competitors. Care of the indigent, once considered a prime responsibility of voluntary as well as public hospitals, has been increasingly shifted to public institutions as the voluntary hospitals struggle to maintain their economic viability in an increasingly hostile competitive market.

In the 1980s it was the practitioners' turn to feel the economic pressures that were forcing the voluntary hospitals into entrepreneurial behavior. The numbers of competing specialists were growing rapidly, while available fee-for-service patients were becoming more scarce and insurance companies were shifting from unquestioning payment of the doctor's bill to increasingly stringent efforts to control expenses. To protect their income, many physicians began to act like competing business-people seeking more customers and more ways to deliver profitable services (Relman, 1988). Physicians also became interested in opportunities to increase their revenues through partnership in, or ownership of, health-care facilities and through financial arrangements with companies supplying the drugs and devices they prescribe for their patients. In some parts of the country almost half of all practicing physicians were referring their patients to free-standing diagnostic facilities in which the physicians held financial interest—a practice called "self-referral."

In 1975 the U.S. Supreme Court had declared that the reach of antitrust law extended to the professions (*Goldfarb v. Virginia State Bar*, 1975), and shortly thereafter the AMA was legally enjoined from interfering with the advertising and marketing practices in which increasing numbers of physicians were engaged. In response to the growing view that health care was a competitive marketplace and physicians were essentially small independent entrepreneurs, the AMA retreated in the 1980s from its earlier proscriptions against commercialization. Its 1982 revised ethical code says nothing about the distinction between medical practice and trade; instead, there is a statement that competition is "not only ethical but is encouraged" (AMA, 1982, p. 22). Advertising was sanctioned provided it was not misleading, and the earlier restriction on sources of professional income was removed. Self-referral and other kinds of economic interests by physicians in the medical products they prescribe were said to be ethical, provided the financial interest was disclosed to patients and did not influence medical judgment. At the end of 1991, the AMA reconsidered this latter position and approved a recommendation from its Council on Ethical and Judicial Affairs that advised against such financial dealings (AMA, 1992). Six months later, in a close vote, this approval was rescinded, only to be supported at the next meeting. The hesitant and vacillating stance of the AMA on this question accurately reflects the current divisions within the profession on the ethics of entrepreneurship within the practice of medicine.

Ethical issues aside, does the commercialization of the health-care system bestow any special benefit on patients or on society in general? In most sectors of the economy, free market competition among suppliers of goods and services helps to control prices and encourages quality. Although suppliers promote consumption through marketing and advertising, the cost-conscious choices of consumers largely determine the number of units purchased and the total expenditures allotted to each product. Goods and services are distributed primarily according to consumers' desires, their judgments about price and quality, and their ability to pay.

But the health-care sector is quite different from most other parts of the economy, and the consequences of market competition are not the same. Consumers (patients) can make relatively few independent and informed purchasing decisions because they must rely so heavily on advice from their physicians. And because of third-party payment, neither the consumer nor the provider of services (the physician) is much constrained by cost. Physicians largely determine the distribution and use of services. Professional judgment of the patient's medical needs is the primary consideration, but the economic benefits to the physician also play a role, particularly when the medical needs are uncertain. Therefore, when health care paid by indemnity insurance becomes commercialized, competition serves not to limit but to increase expenditures, because providers have greater economic incentives to offer their services to patients who are, for the most part, dependent and unresisting consumers. Profit motives thus intensify inflation in a health-care system inherently deficient in cost-control mechanisms.

When payment for medical services is made in advance, as in HMOs and other kinds of prepaid managed care, economic incentives tend to force physicians to reduce, rather than increase, their allocation of services to patients. In such a system insurers and providers profit most when medical expenditures are kept to a minimum. Commercialization of managed care thus raises concerns about cutting corners and underserving patients' needs, just as the commercialization of fee-for-service care raised concerns about excessive and unnecessary services. In both cases, there is the risk that the profit motive may influence professional judgment and make it more difficult for physicians to act in the best interests of their patients.

Furthermore, a commercialized health-care system has little concern for the needs of the uninsured and the underinsured. Unless government intervenes, those without means to pay are denied access to all but emergency care. The steadily rising number of patients without ensured access to health care (estimated at the start of the 1990s to be more than 15 percent of the population) testifies to the social indifference of a profit-oriented medical marketplace and to the inability of tax-supported institutions to accept the growing burden of the medically indigent. Efforts by voluntary hospitals to remain economically viable require them not only to restrict charity but also to promote profitable services, which may not be those most needed by the community.

Proponents of commercialization in health care argue that it rewards innovation and technological development. They say that one of the benefits of an expanding medical marketplace is stimulation of applied research and development, leading to the more rapid introduction and dissemination of useful new products. However, there is no reason to believe that the pace of worthwhile innovation would be significantly slowed in a system that encouraged research and development but allowed industry to market only properly tested new products, and restrained entrepreneurialism in the delivery of medical care. The current dominance of the United States in the development of new medical technology is probably the result more of substantial public support of medical research than of the commercialization of the health-care system.

In any event, the worsening health-care crisis in the United States during the 1990s prompted many reform proposals in Congress and in state legislatures. Medical costs have to be controlled and universal access to good, affordable care ensured. Inasmuch as commercialism and entrepreneurial medical practices are partly to blame for the current problems of the health-care system, it is ironic that a more competitive market has been offered as a solution. One reform proposal, managed competition, envisions regulated price competition among managed-care plans offering a standard package of comprehensive medical benefits. Most of the plans would be owned by insurance companies that would hire or contract with physicians and take the financial risks, thus further expanding the commercialization of the health delivery system.

Probably the simplest and most effective way to reduce the commercialization of health care would be to encourage not-for-profit groups of physicians to form their own community-based plans that would manage care on a prepaid basis. This would require changes in the organization of medical care and in the way physicians are paid. Medical services would be provided through groups and the emphasis would be on salaries and capitation contracts rather than on fee-for-service solo practice.

It remains to be seen whether commercialism in medicine will continue to grow and ultimately dominate our health-care system. Those who believe medical care is a business like any other regard such an outcome as desirable and necessary for the achievement of optimal efficiency. On the other hand, those who believe medical care is primarily a social rather than an economic good hope that the present trend toward commercialism will be resisted and in the long run reversed. They believe the ultimate solution of our health-care problems will be found through social action and community responsibility.

ARNOLD S. RELMAN

Directly related to this article are the INTRODUCTION *and other articles in this entry:* HEALTH-CARE INSURANCE, MEDICARE, *and* MEDICAID. *For a further discussion of topics mentioned in this article, see the entries* ADVERTISING; ECONOMIC CONCEPTS IN HEALTH CARE; HARM; HEALTH-CARE DELIVERY, *especially the article on* HEALTH-CARE SYSTEMS; HEALTH-CARE RESOURCES, ALLOCATION OF; HOSPITAL; INTERPRETATION; MEDICAL CODES AND OATHS; MEDICINE AS A PROFESSION; PHARMACEUTICS; PROFESSIONAL–PATIENT RELATIONSHIP; RESEARCH POLICY; *and* VALUE AND VALUATION. *For a discussion of related ideas, see the entries* ACADEMIC HEALTH CENTERS; AUTHORITY; AUTONOMY; BENEFICENCE; CARE; COMMERCIALISM IN SCIENTIFIC RESEARCH; COMPASSION; LICENSING, DISCIPLINE, AND REGULATION IN THE HEALTH PROFESSIONS; LONG-TERM CARE; MEDICINE, PHILOSOPHY OF; *and* NURSING AS A PROFESSION. *See also the* APPENDIX (CODES, OATHS, AND DIRECTIVES RELATED TO BIOETHICS), SECTION II: ETHICAL DIRECTIVES FOR THE PRACTICE OF MEDICINE.

Bibliography

AMERICAN MEDICAL ASSOCIATION. Council on Ethical and Judicial Affairs. 1992. *Code of Medical Ethics: Annotated Current Opinions Including the Principles of Medical Ethics, Fundamental Elements of the Patient-Physician Relationship, and Rules of the Council on Ethical and Judicial Affairs.* Chicago: Author.

AMERICAN MEDICAL ASSOCIATION JUDICIAL COUNCIL. 1969. *Opinions and Reports of the Judicial Council.* Chicago: Author.

———. 1982. *Current Opinions of the Judicial Council of the American Medical Association: Including the Principles of Medical Ethics and Rules of the Judicial Council.* Chicago: Author.

ENGELHARDT, H. TRISTRAM, JR., and RIE, MICHAEL A. 1988. "Morality for the Medical-Industrial Complex: A Code of Ethics for the Mass Marketing of Health Care." *New England Journal of Medicine* 319, no. 16:1086–1089.

Goldfarb v. Virginia State Bar. 1975. 421 U.S. 773.

GRAY, BRADFORD H. 1991. *The Profit Motive and Patient Care: The Changing Accountability of Doctors and Hospitals.* Cambridge, Mass.: Harvard University Press.

RELMAN, ARNOLD S. 1980. "The New Medical-Industrial Complex." *New England Journal of Medicine* 303, no. 17:963–970.

———. 1988. "Medicine as a Profession and a Business." In Vol. 8 of *The Tanner Lectures on Human Values,* pp. 282–313. Edited by Sterling S. McMurrin. Salt Lake City: University of Utah Press.

———. 1992. "What Market Values Are Doing to Medicine." *Atlantic Monthly,* March, pp. 98–106.

SADE, ROBERT M. 1971. "Medical Care as a Right: A Refutation." *New England Journal of Medicine* 285, no. 23:1288–1292.

VEATCH, ROBERT M. 1983. "Ethical Dilemmas of For-Profit Enterprise in Health Care." In *The New Health Care for Profit: Doctors and Hospitals in a Competitive Environment,* pp. 125–152. Edited by Bradford H. Gray. Washington, D.C.: National Academy Press.

HEALTH-CARE RATIONING

See HEALTH-CARE RESOURCES, ALLOCATION OF.

HEALTH-CARE RESOURCES, ALLOCATION OF

I. Macroallocation
    John F. Kilner
II. Microallocation
    John F. Kilner

I. MACROALLOCATION

The allocation of health-care resources involves distributing health-related services among various people and uses. The concept of allocation can imply that a designated individual or group is responsible for each level of decision making within a system that is designed to distribute fixed amounts of resources. However, the degree to which such a system exists and such explicit allocation decisions occur varies widely. In the United States, for example, allocation of resources to and within health care has long been more the product of millions of individual clinical decisions and various market forces than the result of an overall social policy.

Health-care allocations are commonly classified in terms of two levels of decision making: microallocation and macroallocation. Microallocation focuses on decisions regarding particular persons. It often involves "patient selection": determining which patients among those who need a particular scarce resource, such as a heart transplant, should receive treatment. However, microallocation may instead entail deciding for an individual patient which of several potentially beneficial treatments to provide, particularly when only a limited time is available for treatment.

Macroallocation, on the other hand, entails decisions that determine the amount of resources available for particular kinds of health-care services. Macroallocation decisions include how a hospital budgets its spending as well as the amount of resources a nation devotes to primary and preventive care compared with high-technology curative medicine. The extent to which health is fostered through medical care as opposed to nonmedical interventions such as environmental regulation is also a matter of macroallocation, as is the amount of money, time, and energy a society allocates to the pursuit of health rather than to education, defense, and other activities.

The term "rationing" is a much less clearly defined term that appears in discussions of macroallocation and microallocation alike. Because the debate over rationing raises issues at the foundation of health-care allocation, it will be the focus of the opening section. The remainder of the article will then discuss substantive standards for judging macroallocation, under three headings: the individual's right to health care, the community's responsibility for health care, and the importance of efficiency in health care.

Rationing

Rationing involves leaving some people, at least temporarily and against their wishes, without particular forms of health care that might benefit them. Some use the label "rationing" only if a person is barred from treatment by an explicit policy or decision. Those operating from this definition often oppose rationing on the grounds that there are sufficient resources, if they are correctly managed and distributed, to address at least the most important health needs of all. Others view the unavailability of care as rationing, whether or not explicit policies or decisions are involved. While part of this group also holds that there are sufficient resources to avoid rationing for the most part, the majority see implicit or explicit rationing as unavoidable and tend to favor developing explicit, ethical criteria (Blank, 1988; Wikler, 1992).

A fundamental ambiguity then, attends the word "rationing." Moreover, the word's association with a short-term policy for handling a temporary crisis, such as shortage of goods in wartime, makes it a misleading word to designate society's long-term task of health-care provision. So the less ambiguous terminology of macroallocation and microallocation is probably more helpful in most discussions. Nevertheless, the debate over the term "rationing" has identified two important issues that should be examined before embarking on a more detailed consideration of macroallocation: 1) Is implicit allocation of desired and potentially beneficial health care occurring today? 2) Will some form of allocation be necessary in the future?

There is little dispute that implicit allocation of beneficial care is taking place today. For example, waiting lists for certain types of health care are commonplace in Canada and Europe. There the structure of the system (referral and reimbursement policies, acquisition and location of technologies), rather than the explicit exclusion of people or services from coverage, limits overall national spending on health care (Grogan, 1992). In less-developed countries, some resources are located only in major urban centers and are unavailable to most of the population (Attfield, 1990).

Even in the United States, where per capita spending on health care far exceeds that of any other country, many have not been able to obtain certain forms of beneficial health care. In recent decades, tens of millions annually have gone without any health insurance and at least as many more have been underinsured—predicaments that result in reduced access to health care and reduced health (U.S. Office of Technology Assessment,

1992). Employer decisions to limit employee health-benefits packages, as well as governmental decisions to omit services from the Medicaid and Medicare programs, have excluded certain people from potentially beneficial health care. So have health-facility decisions not to operate in the most accessible locations or at the most convenient times, and insurance company decisions to exclude from coverage people with preexisting conditions or other high-risk factors.

Greater controversy surrounds the second question, whether health-care resources can be allocated so that no one has to go without potentially beneficial health care (Kilner, 1990). The possibility of avoiding rationing in this sense of the term hinges on achieving sufficient cost containment. Proposed strategies include reducing expenditures on items less vital to society (e.g., potato chips and advertising); eliminating medical procedures with little health benefit; placing greater emphasis on preventive care that preempts the need for more expensive acute care; reforming tort law to reduce the need to practice defensive medicine; simplifying administration; imposing global budgets on the entire health-care system; and limiting the huge gap between the incomes of physicians and other full-time workers ($164,000 vs. $25,900, respectively, in the United States in 1990, after deducting office and malpractice-insurance expenses). Various forms of "managed care" arrangements pursue several of these strategies simultaneously by restricting patients to approved providers (e.g., in preferred provider organizations or health maintenance organizations) who agree to limit their charges or forgo fee-for-service entirely in exchange for a salary or at per-enrollee payment.

Some commentators contend that significant cost savings could be obtained through each of these strategies. Others disagree, adding that the scope and cost of potential health-care benefits are so vast that any savings will prove insufficient to fund needed benefits for everyone. Time will tell how effective various cost containment strategies can be in reducing the need for limiting the access to health care. However, the experience of other countries such as the Netherlands, with health-care systems more nationally coordinated than that of the United States, suggests the pragmatic limits of cost containment (The Netherlands, Government Committee on Choices in Health Care, 1992). Such experience underscores the importance of making allocation decisions explicit if allocation is not to be shaped by unknown factors and unethical considerations.

Macroallocation

Numerous people have proposed ways to prioritize the potential uses of limited resources. These proposals tend to be rooted in one or more of three major ethical concerns: the individual's claim to health care, the community's responsibility for health care, and the importance of efficiency in health care. Different understandings of justice are at work in all three, as are different weights attached to competing ethical considerations such as liberty, care, and utility.

The individual's claim to health care.   Those who are primarily concerned about the health care that is due to each individual often invoke the notion of a right to health care. When the World Health Organization in 1976 affirmed the "enjoyment of the highest attainable standard of health" to be one of the fundamental rights of every human being, it both reflected and fostered a growing debate over health-related human rights.

The concept of a human right promotes the idea that each person is entitled to have or to be free from something. It commonly reflects the basic conviction that each human being has special and great significance. While this conviction is not necessarily religious in nature, it receives special emphasis in theological traditions such as Christianity, Judaism, and Islam (Kilner, 1992; Rahman, 1989).

Negative and positive rights are frequently distinguished, as are moral and legal rights. Negative (or liberty) rights guarantee freedom from certain types of interference with the pursuit of one's interests. Positive (or material) rights guarantee access to important services and goods. Accordingly, a right to protection from anything that is seriously harmful to one's health is a negative right; a right to receive certain forms of health care is a positive right. Whereas moral rights involve claims about what one ought to have on ethical grounds, legal rights involve claims about what one is actually entitled to by law. Whether everyone has an ethically justifiable right to health care is debated in the United States, yet Medicare legislation confers a legal right to health care on elderly people in the United States.

In light of such distinctions and the conflicting conceptions of justice and freedom that underlie them, it is not surprising that people have fundamentally different views about the meaning and legitimacy of a "right to health care." Some hold that there is a right to health. The point of the right is to make sure that people actually have health itself, not just access to resources. Others insist on a right to health care. Because of the fundamental importance of health, people should have guaranteed access to resources that foster it. Still others reject both positions. While all of these claims represent worthwhile aspirations, they argue, such claims are not rights because no one has the obligation to satisfy them. Probing this last argument first provides useful entry into the debate.

The most prominent basis for rejecting a right to health care is a libertarian view of justice that emphasizes negative rights over positive rights (Engelhardt, 1991). According to this view, people ought to be free to pursue their own life plans, including their economic livelihood. Government should prevent others from interfering with that pursuit. A right to health care that forces health-care professionals to provide care—or that forces certain people to give up part of what they have earned to pay for other people's care—directly contradicts what justice requires. That some people lack (the ability to pay for) health care is simply unfortunate rather than unfair. No rights are violated in a market-based system where people are free to buy and sell as their resources permit.

Critics of this position argue that it is self-defeating and mistaken. It is self-defeating because, in its zeal to protect people's freedom to use their resources for health care and other desired goods, it effectively ensures that those with insufficient resources will not have the freedom to obtain health care. It is mistaken in three assumptions. First, some note the implausibility of assuming that the present distribution of general resources is fair. In their view, the vastly unequal distribution of the means by which people pay for health care is attributable to forces that have affected the fairness of the market over time.

Others doubt a second assumption, namely, that a free-market approach is appropriate for health care. Consumers in this case are frequently sick patients with limited knowledge about health care. For a free market to function well, consumers would have to be able to understand the costs and benefits of all the available medical options and be willing and able to trade health or even life for money. A free-market approach, then, unfairly discriminates against those who are uneducated as well as those who are poor due to social circumstances or genetic endowments beyond their control.

A third debatable assumption, most frequently questioned by those who operate from a theological perspective, is the understanding of liberty as autonomy. Autonomy, derived from the Greek words auto (self) + nomos (law), tends to emphasize people's separateness from others. According to a more relational understanding, freedom entails "freedom for"—the ability (and obligation) to help others—as much as it involves "freedom from" the interference of others.

Some of those who reject a libertarian approach instead affirm the right to health. They insist that health, like life itself, is something so fundamental to human existence that it must be fostered as much as possible. Precisely what the right to health entails, though, is not always clear. It may involve only the negative right that would protect one's freedom from actions that undermine health. This formulation of the right is compatible with the libertarian outlook already discussed. Alternatively, the right to health may entail that people have an entitlement to be healthy and that others have failed in their moral obligations toward individuals who are not healthy.

Those who find this outlook objectionable worry about the prospect of making one person's health another person's responsibility. Such a view tends to undermine people's responsibility for their own health. Opponents also note that it is not possible to maintain someone else's health indefinitely—everyone dies eventually—so it seems mistaken to suggest that anyone has an obligation to do so.

To avoid these problems some people advocate the right to health care. The right to health care is a positive right that holds that all people are entitled to receive some measure of health care. Whereas some others argue that people are entitled only to an amount of monetary resources that they can spend on whatever they deem important (Brody, 1991), supporters of the right to health care insist that people must be assured health care in particular. Rights, they maintain, do not involve the sort of discretionary items regarding which people's priorities differ. Rather, they concern goods that all people require in order to pursue their various life courses.

Sometimes the right to health care is formulated in comparative terms. According to this view, everyone should have access to whatever health care is necessary to provide for a level of access—or even of health itself—equal to that of others (Veatch, 1986). Many have resisted this egalitarian outlook because it tends to focus more on the value of equality than on the health care people receive. People with chronic illnesses or congenital disabilities may never achieve a level of health equal to that of others and so could claim an infinite amount of health-care resources by invoking an egalitarian right to health care. Alternatively, this right could justify leaving all at a relatively low level of access or health, as long as everyone was treated alike. If, on the other hand, this egalitarian approach requires that everyone be able to receive every treatment that may provide any benefit, then it seems hopelessly unsuited to a world of limited resources.

To correct these deficiencies, various people have proposed identifying the right to health care with some sort of achievable standard of health care that could be guaranteed to all. They often suggest that since health care is provided in response to need, some standard of need should determine the level of health care to which all people have a right.

Others would similarly root the individual's claim to health care in her or his need for that care, but would appeal to various understandings of justice rather than to the notion of rights. For example, a contractarian approach, which appeals to what all people would agree to in hypothetically fair positions, usually advocates people's access to basic goods that anyone must have in order to carry out a personal life plan. Health care is one such good, and whatever amount is essential to enable people to function at a normal level is mandated by justice (Daniels, 1985). Religious traditions that posit a divinely created world also tend to espouse a needs-based understanding of justice. However, they may view "normal" more in terms of how people were created to be than how they typically are (Mackler, 1991).

A utilitarian conception of justice might also undergird a right to health care, but the support is tenuous. Because classical (act) utilitarianism advocates acts that will produce the greatest good for the greatest number of people, it is often criticized for lacking any concept of justice that will protect individuals from oppressive majorities. On the other hand, rule utilitarianism, which supports standards that produce the greatest good for the greatest number if followed consistently, might well support a standard of justice (Beauchamp, 1989).

In light of the important place a standard of need commonly has in formulations of the right to health care and in conceptions of justice, it is essential to consider what this standard entails. Defining the standard and delineating its implications are not easy, for even marginal benefits can be considered "needs" (U.S. President's Commission for the Study of Ethical Problems in Medicine and Biomedical and Behavioral Research, 1983). One definitional approach is to think of meeting needs in terms of restoring normal functioning. Another ties the meeting of needs to providing "significant" health benefit. Establishing significance might involve a careful assessment of the quality and length of life that various forms of health care would likely provide in various situations, together with some individual or societal evaluation of those benefits.

A broad range of considerations is relevant to the delineation of health-care needs. In particular, needs less dramatic than the need for acute medical care must receive sufficient attention. Some non–health-care goods can make an important claim on whatever portion of its resources a society devotes to the pursuit of health. Food, education, and shelter, for example, all contribute directly to health (Tuckson, 1992). So do programs that encourage healthy lifestyles. Habits of eating, drinking, sleeping, and drug use can all have a dramatic impact on health, although they may not reduce total health-care expenditures over the course of an individual's lifetime (Russell, 1986).

Preventive medicine, supportive care, and medical research must similarly receive sufficient attention along with curative medicine. While preventive medicine is not necessarily less expensive or more effective than curative medicine, it can be both. Prenatal care for a mother as opposed to neonatal intensive care for her low-birth-weight infant is a case in point. Analyses of need must give due attention to the importance of sup-

portive care such as long-term care for elderly persons or effective pain relief for dying patients. Finally, fascination with current curative capabilities can all too easily siphon resources away from medical research. Without sufficient attention to research, there will be fewer new medical resources in the future, to the long-term detriment of society's health.

In the face of such a broad array of health-care needs, many people believe that everything that is needed cannot be provided for all. Accordingly, they conclude that justice or the right to health care must mandate only that each individual receive some reasonable level of health care—so-called "essential care" or a "decent minimum" (Eddy, 1991). Determining this exact level presents the same challenges as determining need, with the added task of tailoring the determination to the level of overall resources available at the time (Buchanan, 1989).

Moreover, people in different locations differ dramatically in their perceptions of "need" and "essential care." Those in European countries, for example, avoid the notion of a decent minimum altogether. Nevertheless, each country's effort to provide comprehensive care is unique in terms of the particular forms of care that receive emphasis (Grogan, 1992). Canada acknowledges differences by allowing each of its provinces to determine which health-related services will be included in the package of guaranteed benefits.

The United States, lacking the nationally coordinated financing system of Canada, has traditionally left its states to develop their own priorities and health-care systems (Moon and Holahan, 1992). For instance, Oregon has explicitly ranked all health-related services in terms of their funding priority. Hawaii has required all employers to provide health insurance to all employees working over twenty hours per week (Hawaii acted in 1974 before federal legislation barred this approach). Minnesota has linked improving health-care access with an array of measures to control costs.

The differences among these and other state initiatives underscore what an international comparison also illustrates: that varying perceptions of need call forth different health-care priorities and systems. Cross-cultural sensitivity will be essential if efforts to meet health-related needs are to cross national and international boundaries successfully (Attfield, 1990).

Employing need as a basis for allocation, then, presents various challenges. Challenges can be reasons for rejecting an idea. However, challenges may be no more than obstacles to overcome so that a good idea may be implemented effectively.

The community's responsibility for health care. The substantial disagreement over the idea of the individual's claim to health care has made many people doubt its usefulness as a basis for allocating health-care resources. Some reject the idea on more principled grounds as well. One prominent concern is the impact that a preoccupation with the rights of the individual can have on the well-being of the community as a whole (Churchill, 1987). A case in point is the United States, a highly individualistic culture where the use of the language of rights has been particularly prominent. The demand of U.S. taxpayers, patients, health professionals, and health-care financers for the rights to pursue and satisfy their own various interests may have inhibited the development of an integrated, comprehensive health-care system.

Those who would not jettison completely the notion of rights may argue—on theological or other grounds—that while people have rights, they have no "right to rights" (Kilner, 1992). According to this view, rights themselves (in the sense of freedoms and goods all people ought to have) are not the problem. The problem is people's preoccupation with their own (right to) rights—a preoccupation that undermines commitment to pursuing the rights of all. In this sense, group rights are as problematic as individual rights, since attention to the claims of one's own group tends to encourage the same kind of self-focus and neglect of others as the pursuit of individual rights.

Therefore, some favor deemphasizing or even replacing the notion of the individual's claim to health care—as well as rights language in general—with a more explicit conception of the community's responsibility for health care. Sensitivity to the needs of individuals and particular groups is not absent in this approach, but the driving concern is the community's obligation to ensure the well-being of the whole community.

In European societies such as Germany and the Netherlands, for example, discussions of health care often invoke social solidarity as a fundamental goal to be pursued through resource allocation (Netherlands, Government Committee on Choices in Health Care, 1992). In the United States, an increasing emphasis on community responsibility is reflected in the ethics literature (Dyck, 1994) and in the appearance of such interdisciplinary journals as *The Responsive Community*. Appeals to the common good are also becoming more frequent, especially in religious circles (Catholic Health Association, 1991). Increasingly, people are concluding that ethical macroallocation of health-care resources in the United States will probably require a different way of thinking about the relationship between the individual and society.

Accordingly, the 1983 U.S. President's Commission explicitly rejected the rights-oriented language of the 1952 U.S. President's Commission on the Health Needs of the Nation. Instead the 1983 Commission affirmed the community's ethical obligation to provide all with equitable access to an "adequate level" of health

care. Its report argued that a community must ensure that all of its members can obtain such care because health care is so important in relieving suffering, preventing premature death, restoring functioning, increasing opportunity, providing information, and strengthening relationships of caring (U.S. President's Commission, 1983). This approach affirms that ungenerous or uncaring health-care allocations are clearly as wrong as those that are unjust.

Caring in this context entails looking beyond what theoretical formulations of justice require. It means giving special consideration to those who have been marginalized in the allocation of health-care resources. Identified in certain religious and liberationist contexts as "the preferential option for the poor," this sensitivity toward disadvantaged persons is characteristic of much feminist analysis as well (Caes, 1992; Holmes and Purdy, 1992). It embraces the notion of the "common good," but not in the utilitarian or majority-rule sense of the term. It insists that there is no true common good if all do not have the good in common.

Emotional as well as rational, engaged as well as theoretical, a caring commitment to those who are least well-off may or may not justify a different health-care allocation than that which a rights- or justice-based approach to health-care allocation would advocate. However, its proponents maintain that such a commitment almost certainly will make a difference in the ways that allocation is implemented. For example, it may be widely acknowledged that justice requires directing more health-care resources toward African-Americans and other disadvantaged groups in the United States (LaVeist, 1993). However, reallocation is not likely to take place as long as people do not see others' health as their responsibility in any way.

Basing allocation on the community's responsibility for health care, then, differs from basing it on the individual's claim to health care. But attributing responsibility to the community does not absolve the individual from responsibility. Since individuals are part of the community and share in its well-being, they must share the burden of paying for the cost of the community's health care in an equitable manner. Moreover, they have some responsibility for their own health. However, the implications of this responsibility are controversial. In particular, does an apparently irresponsible person forfeit the community's care?

Both justice and respect for people's liberty may entail that those who voluntarily cause their own health problems should take responsibility for them, particularly under circumstances of insufficient resources to meet the health-care needs of all. Holding people responsible in this way might have the added benefit of reducing illness and injury resulting from risky behaviors, thereby lowering related health-care costs as well.

However, it is extremely difficult in most cases to prove that people caused their illnesses and did so voluntarily. Often there are many causes of an illness, few of which are within a person's control. Even if a person's behavior, such as smoking or overeating, does cause an illness, the voluntary nature of the behavior is difficult to demonstrate conclusively. The person may have engaged in the behavior without understanding that it could cause the resulting illness. Regardless of foreknowledge, other factors—advertising, peer pressure, cultural values, dietary deficiencies, psychological instabilities, or genetic predispositions—may have significantly impaired the ill person's ability to act freely.

Even if a society becomes sufficiently adept at identifying those who have voluntarily caused their own health problems, three further ethical considerations are relevant. First, fairness may require that an allocation policy based on personal responsibility not apply only to those engaging in the least socially desirable behaviors. In other words, the policy should apply not only to smokers and IV-drug abusers, but also to those who overwork or overeat if responsibility can be established in all four types of cases.

Second, the idea that a society would have a responsibility truly to care for its members may call for the provision of more health care than strict justice alone requires, even for those who voluntarily engage in risky behavior. The health-care professions have a longstanding tradition of offering care without making such offers depend on the extent to which ill people caused their own need. Finally, if caring with fairness requires some form of accountability for risky behaviors, requiring payment of a tax to engage in those behaviors, say on cigarettes and alcohol, would be more humane than denying needed health care.

The importance of efficiency in health care. Efficiency is also a central and disputed issue in ethical resource allocation. How best to eliminate health-related expenditures that are not truly beneficial in order to maximize funding for beneficial health care is only part of the efficiency problem. Even greater controversy surrounds proposed mechanisms for determining which forms of beneficial care are most worth their cost.

Two mechanisms for comparing costs and benefits have received particular attention as promising ways to pursue efficiency in health care: cost–benefit analysis and cost-effectiveness analysis (Sox et al., 1988). While both mechanisms typically involve assessing the costs of various forms of health care in monetary units, cost–benefit analysis also uses monetary units exclusively to assess the benefits of care, whereas cost-effectiveness analysis does not.

Cost–benefit analysis is well-suited in principle to a broad range of resource allocation decisions both within and outside of health care. It employs identical units, such as dollars, to measure all costs and benefits. Accordingly, it can subtract total costs from total benefits to determine if an expenditure is wasteful (i.e., its costs outweigh its benefits). When applied to alternative health-related and other uses for the same funds, cost–benefit analysis can also determine which use will provide the greatest net benefit. This approach has proven particularly attractive to economists and policy analysts who must prioritize diverse uses of limited funds. It has been identified by the U.S. Office of Management and Budget, for example, as one of the acceptable means agencies may use to justify their budgets (Emery and Schneiderman, 1989).

Since cost–benefit analysis is the more familiar efficiency mechanism of the two and it alone has the potential to compare all possible uses of available funds, it appears at first glance to be the superior mechanism for allocating health-care resources. However, it has a number of pragmatic and substantive weaknesses in its most common forms. Some of these difficulties are inherent in the overall way the mechanism operates. Identifying the numerous ways that people are affected by particular allocation decisions is difficult enough, but reducing the entire range of health-care outcomes (including continued life itself) to monetary value is virtually impossible. More substantively, while cost–benefit analysis helps to identify the allocation of resources that yields the greatest balance of benefit over cost for a society as a whole, it may fail to consider how fairly the benefits and burdens of that allocation are distributed throughout society. Programs targeting affluent suburbs, for example, can tend to have better cost–benefit ratios than programs in poor inner-city areas because of the bad health fostered by poor social and economic conditions. Ethics, though, must attend to more than economics.

Other difficulties concern the methods cost–benefit analysis uses to convert lives saved and other benefits of health care into monetary units. One approach is the "past decisions" approach, which compares how much money a society spent on selected programs to save lives in the past with how many lives were saved for that money. The unique funding and implementation context of each such program, however, renders generalizations risky.

Two more popular conversion methods involve future earnings (human capital) and willingness to pay. The future-earnings approach determines the monetary value of a health benefit by calculating how much more money patients will earn in the future if they receive treatment than if they do not. Fairness again is a major problem, for this approach implies that the life of a person making twice the income of another person is twice as valuable (i.e., important to save) as that of the other person. Since women and minorities tend to receive less pay than white males for comparable work, this approach devalues the lives of women and minorities. In fact, whatever employment-related discrimination already exists in a society becomes compounded when health-care allocation reflects salary level.

A willingness-to-pay approach, on the other hand, calculates the value of a health benefit on the basis of the amount of money people would pay to receive a specified increase in the likelihood of receiving that benefit over a particular length of time. This approach, like the previous one, tends to compound certain forms of discrimination. Since wealthy people are generally able to pay more for a program to reduce the risk of illness and death than are poor people, a willingness-to-pay approach systematically reproduces existing injustices in the distribution of wealth.

All forms of cost–benefit analysis, then, are vulnerable to the charges that they are inadequate measures of the value of lives and that they neglect some important ethical considerations in resource allocation. Accordingly, a better mechanism for maximizing the benefit of limited health care resources has been sought.

Cost-effectiveness analysis has generally been the favored alternative because it avoids a major difficulty that troubles cost–benefit analysis: the need to convert health outcomes, including continued life itself, to a monetary equivalent. Cost-effectiveness analysis typically calculates the cost of alternative health initiatives in monetary terms. But it can adopt a nonmonetary unit for comparing the health benefits of these initiatives, such as degree of mobility restored or years of life saved. If, for example, two treatments for hip problems claim to improve mobility, cost-effectiveness analysis can determine which one restores more mobility for the same cost or identical mobility for less cost. It can also determine which utilization of earmarked funds will produce the greatest health benefits. While this approach cannot determine if costs outweigh benefits or compare all benefits inside and outside of the health-care field, it can identify the cost per standardized unit of benefit for alternative health-related interventions.

Broad societal health-care allocations, however, necessitate a more generic measure of health benefit than mobility. Since increased quality and length of life are the two primary goals of health care, the standard of "quality-adjusted life years" (QALYs) seems to many to provide a suitable measure. To determine the number of QALYs that a health-related intervention will produce, the number of years people will likely live after the intervention is multiplied by a percentage reflecting the quality of life to be experienced during those years—0 percent (0.00) signifying death, and 100 percent (1.00) signifying perfect health with no disability.

While QALY-based cost-effectiveness analysis represents an improvement over cost–benefit analysis for the purpose of comparing health-related allocations, it,

too, has proven controversial (Harris, 1987; Menzel, 1990). For example, certain analysts, while affirming the approach in principle, note that studies to date have gathered only limited data on health-care outcomes, costs, and quality-of-life preferences. Much more is needed before cost-effectiveness can be consistently employed as a basis for making comprehensive health-care allocations.

The state of Oregon, for instance, originally intended to use a form of cost-effectiveness analysis during the early 1990s when it redesigned its approach to allocating public health-care funds. Through a telephone survey, the state asked people to rank various functional limitations and other symptoms on a quality-of-life scale. The goal was to ascertain a quality-of-life score and cost figure for every health-related intervention so that these interventions could be prioritized for budgetary purposes. Reliable cost data proved so difficult to acquire, though, that the quality-of-life information was employed essentially only to identify which interventions produced the most benefit, irrespective of costs (Garland, 1992). Moreover, some rankings had to be altered in the end. The state discovered that interventions producing relatively little health benefit—if inexpensive enough—could rank higher than much more beneficial (even lifesaving) interventions.

Another methodological debate over cost-effectiveness concerns who should assess quality of life (Fleck, 1992). The QALY approach determines the quality-of-life percentages for particular outcomes by interviewing large numbers of healthy people concerning the value they place on various qualities of life. Some insist that healthy people are the right ones to make these judgments because resource allocation is like purchasing health insurance. People will appropriately weigh alternative benefit packages before they contract a particular disease, but after contracting it they place disproportionate weight on covering that disease. Others cite studies documenting that healthy people frequently underestimate the quality of life of people who are ill or disabled. One inference drawn is that only those who have experienced such conditions can adequately assess the degree to which they render living more difficult (Lawton et al., 1990; Kaplan, 1993).

The most heated disputes over QALYs, however, involve problems of fairness similar to those attributed to cost–benefit analysis. Although QALY-based cost-effectiveness analysis does not intentionally discriminate against certain groups, it tends to disadvantage patients who are older or disabled—in fact, everyone whose future length or quality of life is comparatively limited. Because QALY calculations are based on precisely these two variables, the treatments most beneficial to such persons tend to receive lower QALY scores and so receive low funding priority. For many who believe in the sanctity of human life, this discrimination is typical of the devaluing of certain types of people that generally results when anticipated quality of life is employed as a basis for ranking patients rather than as a desirable outcome to be sought for each individual patient.

As it turned out, the U.S. government refused the state of Oregon's initial application, which sought legal permission to allocate the state's limited Medicaid funds by ranking health-related interventions based on public quality-of-life judgments. The government's controversial rationale was that the approach discriminated against persons with disabilities. Oregon successfully revised its proposal by eliminating reliance on quality-of-life data. While cost-effectiveness analysis, then, attends well to efficiency, like other efficiency mechanisms it can easily be insensitive to other ethical concerns such as degree of need and fairness.

The individual's claims, the community's responsibilities, and efficiency's importance all represent widely held ethical sensitivities to which resource allocation must attend. The ongoing challenge is to determine how to affirm the best elements of each, where they are not mutually contradictory, in a way that also minimizes their ethically objectionable features.

JOHN F. KILNER

Directly related to this article is the companion article in this entry: MICROALLOCATION. *Also directly related is the entry* HEALTH POLICY, *article on* POLITICS AND HEALTH CARE. *For a further discussion of topics mentioned in this article, see the entries* AGING AND THE AGED; AUTONOMY; ECONOMIC CONCEPTS IN HEALTH CARE; FEMINISM; FREEDOM AND COERCION; HEALTH CARE, QUALITY OF; HEALTH-CARE FINANCING; HEALTH AND DISEASE, *especially the article on* THE EXPERIENCE OF HEALTH AND ILLNESS; HOSPITAL, *article on* CONTEMPORARY ETHICAL PROBLEMS; INTERNATIONAL HEALTH; JUSTICE; LIFE, QUALITY OF; LIFESTYLES AND PUBLIC HEALTH; MEDICAL ETHICS, HISTORY OF, *section on* EUROPE, *subsection on* CONTEMPORARY PERIOD, *and section on* THE AMERICAS, *article on* CANADA; OBLIGATION AND SUPEREROGATION; RIGHTS; TECHNOLOGY, *especially the article on* HISTORY OF MEDICAL TECHNOLOGY; *and* UTILITY. *This article will find application in the entries* KIDNEY DIALYSIS; *and* ORGAN AND TISSUE TRANSPLANTS, *especially the article on* ETHICAL AND LEGAL ISSUES. *For a discussion of related ideas, see the entries* ADVERTISING; AIDS; BENEFICENCE; CARE; CHRONIC CARE; DISABILITY, *especially the article on* HEALTH CARE AND PHYSICAL DISABILITY; HEALTH PROMOTION AND HEALTH EDUCATION; ISLAM; JAINISM; LABORATORY TESTING; LONG-TERM CARE; MENTAL-HEALTH SERVICES; PAIN AND SUFFERING; PATIENTS' RIGHTS; PROTESTANTISM; RACE AND RACISM; RESPONSIBILITY; ROMAN CATHOLICISM; SEXISM; *and* WOMEN.

Bibliography

ATTFIELD, ROBIN. 1990. "The Global Distribution of Health Care Resources." *Journal of Medical Ethics* 16, no. 3:153–156.

BEAUCHAMP, TOM L. 1989. "Allocation and Health Policy." In *Contemporary Issues in Bioethics*, 3d ed., pp. 553–559. Edited by Tom L. Beauchamp and LeRoy Walters. Belmont, Calif.: Wadsworth.

BLANK, ROBERT H. 1988. *Rationing Medicine.* New York: Columbia University Press.

BRANSON, ROY. 1978. "Theories of Justice and Health Care." In *Encyclopedia of Bioethics*, pp. 630–637. Edited by Warren T. Reich. New York: Free Press.

BRODY, BARUCH A. 1991. "Why the Right to Health Care Is Not a Useful Concept for Policy Debates." In *Rights to Health Care*, pp. 113–131. Edited by Thomas Bole III, and William B. Bondeson. Dordrecht, Netherlands: Kluwer.

BUCHANAN, ALLEN. 1989. "Health-Care Delivery and Resource Allocation." In *Medical Ethics*, pp. 291–327. Edited by Robert M. Veatch. Boston: Jones and Bartlett.

CAES, DAVID, ed. 1992. *Caring for the Least of These: Serving Christ Among the Poor.* Scottdale, Pa.: Herald.

CATHOLIC HEALTH ASSOCIATION. 1991. *With Justice for All? The Ethics of Healthcare Rationing.* St. Louis, Mo.: Author.

CHURCHILL, LARRY R. 1987. *Rationing Health Care in America: Perceptions and Principles of Justice.* Notre Dame, Ind.: University of Notre Dame Press.

DANIELS, NORMAN. 1985. *Just Health Care: Studies in Philosophy and Health Policy.* Cambridge: At the University Press.

DOUGHERTY, CHARLES J. 1988. *American Health Care: Realities, Rights, and Reforms.* New York: Oxford University Press.

DYCK, ARTHUR J. 1994. *Rethinking Rights and Responsibilities: The Moral Bonds of Community.* Cleveland, Ohio: Pilgrim Press.

EDDY, DAVID M. 1991. "What Care Is 'Essential'? What Services are 'Basic'?" *Journal of the American Medical Association* 265, no. 6:782–788.

EMERY, DANIELLE D., and SCHNEIDERMAN, LAWRENCE J. 1989. "Cost Effectiveness Analysis in Health Care." *Hastings Center Report* 19, no. 4 (July–August):8–13.

ENGELHARDT, H. TRISTRAM, JR. 1991. *Bioethics and Secular Humanism.* London: SCM.

FLECK, LEONARD M. 1992. "Just Health Care Rationing: A Democratic Decisionmaking Approach." *University of Pennsylvania Law Review* 140, no. 5:1597–1636.

GARLAND, MICHAEL J. 1992. "Justice, Politics and Community: Expanding Access and Rationing Health Services in Oregon." *Law, Medicine, and Health Care* 20, nos. 1 and 2:67–81.

GROGAN, COLLEEN M. 1992. "Deciding on Access and Levels of Care: A Comparison of Canada, Britain, Germany, and the United States." *Journal of Health Politics, Policy and Law* 17, no. 2:213–232.

HARRIS, JOHN. 1987. "QALYfying the Value of Life." *Journal of Medical Ethics* 13, no. 3:117–123.

HOLMES, HELEN B., and PURDY, LAURA M., eds. 1992. *Feminist Perspectives in Medical Ethics.* Bloomington: Indiana University Press.

JONSEN, ALBERT R. 1978. "Right to Health-Care Services." In *Encyclopedia of Bioethics*, pp. 623–630. Edited by Warren T. Reich. New York: Macmillan.

KAPLAN, ROBERT M. 1993. *The Hippocratic Predicament: Affordability, Access, and Accountability in American Medicine.* San Diego, Calif.: Academic Press.

KILNER, JOHN F. 1990. *Who Lives? Who Dies? Ethical Criteria in Patient Selection.* New Haven, Conn.: Yale University Press.

———. 1992. *Life on the Line: Ethics, Aging, Ending Patients' Lives, and Allocating Vital Resources.* Grand Rapids, Mich.: W. B. Eerdmans.

LAVEIST, THOMAS A. 1993. "Segregation, Poverty, and Empowerment: Health Consequences for African Americans." *Milbank Quarterly* 71, no. 1:41–64.

LAWTON, M. POWELL; MOSS, MIRIAM; and GLICKSMAN, ALLEN. 1990. "The Quality of the Last Year of Life of Older Persons." *Milbank Quarterly* 68, no. 1:1–28.

MACKLER, AARON L. 1991. "Judaism, Justice, and Access to Health Care." *Kennedy Institute of Ethics Journal* 1, no. 2:143–161.

MENZEL, PAUL T. 1990. *Strong Medicine: The Ethical Rationing of Health Care.* New York: Oxford University Press.

MOON, MARILYN, and HOLAHAN, JOHN. 1992. "Can States Take the Lead in Health Care Reform?" *Journal of the American Medical Association* 268, no. 12:1588–1594.

MOONEY, GAVIN, and MCGUIRE, ALISTAIR. 1988. "Economics and Medical Ethics in Health Care: An Economic Viewpoint." In *Medical Ethics and Economics in Health Care*, pp. 5–22. Edited by Gavin Mooney and Alistair McGuire. Oxford: Oxford University Press.

NETHERLANDS, GOVERNMENT COMMITTEE ON CHOICES IN HEALTH CARE. 1992. *Choices in Health Care.* Rijswijk, Netherlands: Ministry of Welfare, Health and Cultural Affairs.

RAHMAN, FAZLUR. 1987. *Health and Medicine in the Islamic Tradition: Change and Identity.* New York: Crossroad.

RUSSELL, LOUISE. 1986. *Is Prevention Better Than Care?* Washington, D.C.: The Brookings Institution.

SOX, HAROLD C.; PLATT, MARSHAL A.; HIGGINS, MICHAEL C.; AND MARTON, KEITH I. 1988. *Medical Decision Making.* Boston: Butterworths.

TUCKSON, REED. 1992. "A Question of Survival: An Interview with Tuckson Reed." *Second Opinion* 17, no. 4:48–63.

U.S. OFFICE OF TECHNOLOGY ASSESSMENT, CONGRESS OF THE UNITED STATES. 1992. *Does Health Insurance Make a Difference?* Washington, D.C.: U.S. Government Printing Office.

U.S. PRESIDENT'S COMMISSION FOR THE STUDY OF ETHICAL PROBLEMS IN MEDICINE AND BIOMEDICAL AND BEHAVIORAL RESEARCH. 1983. *Securing Access to Health Care: A Report on the Ethical Implications of Differences in the Availability of Health Services*, vol. 1. Washington, D.C.: U.S. Government Printing Office.

VEATCH, ROBERT M. 1986. *The Foundations of Justice: Why the Retarded and the Rest of Us Have Claims to Equality.* New York: Oxford University Press.

WIKLER, DANIEL. 1992. "Ethics and Rationing: 'Whether,' 'How,' or 'How Much?'" *Journal of the American Geriatrics Society* 40, no. 4:398–403.

II. MICROALLOCATION

When the need or demand for health-care resources exceeds the available supply, resources must be distributed on some basis. The more explicit the criteria, the more likely the term "rationing" is to be applied, although the meaning of the term varies considerably in the bioethical, health-care, economic, and public-policy literature. Rationing often refers to general limitations placed on the availability of certain types of health care, but it may also encompass specific treatment decisions for particular patients. Distribution of health care at a broad institutional or societal level is referred to as "macroallocation." Macroallocation includes the way a hospital budgets its spending, as well as the amount of resources a nation devotes to primary and preventive care compared with high-technology curative medicine and nonmedical activities such as education and defense.

Microallocation, on the other hand, focuses on treatment decisions regarding particular persons. It may entail deciding which of several potentially beneficial treatments to provide an individual patient, particularly when only a limited time is available for treatment. Caregivers most commonly employ various medical criteria in order to make such decisions. However, these decisions take place in institutional and societal contexts of limited resources. Accordingly, the relative merits of devoting particular resources to one patient rather than to others may exert at least an unconscious influence on treatment decisions, and nonmedical considerations may become involved. Patients' values and beliefs often play a role here as well.

Other microallocation decisions, sometimes referred to as "patient selection decisions," more explicitly involve choices among patients. In the less developed countries of the world, large numbers of people die for lack of vaccines to prevent disease, antibiotics to cure infections, oral rehydration therapy to replenish fluids lost through severe diarrhea, and the health-care personnel to administer such interventions (UNICEF, 1993). Microallocation decisions constantly determine who will receive the limited care that is available. Some countries not only continue to wrestle with these low-technology scarcities but also face the high-technology microallocation dilemmas commonly encountered in the more developed countries of the world, where expensive medical technologies have proliferated.

Organ transplantation and hospital intensive care are two primary examples of such technologies. The expense of heart, liver, and other types of organ transplantation keep some patients from even considering such operations. Of those seeking transplantation, over 1,000 patients in the United States alone die each year while waiting for a suitable organ to be donated (United Network for Organ Sharing). Microallocation of hospital intensive care, meanwhile, must occur whenever more patients could benefit medically from access to it than the available space can accommodate—a common occurrence even in the more developed countries of the world (Truog, 1992).

Scarcities of vital health-care resources are not likely to disappear in the future. The degree of scarcity in the less developed countries will likely decrease through worldwide cooperative efforts. Nevertheless, social, political, and economic constraints will continue to hamper such efforts. Even in the more developed countries, the need for microallocation will persist (and probably grow) for at least three reasons. First, many emerging technologies such as artificial organs and brain imaging techniques are so expensive that the cost of making them available to all who could benefit from them is prohibitive. Second, the scarcity of some treatments (e.g., organ transplantation) is not simply a matter of funding but reflects the limited supply of the critical resource itself (e.g., the donated organ). Third, technological development will continue to yield new resources that only a limited number of patients can obtain until the capacity to produce those resources expands sufficiently. The history of health care is filled with examples of such scarcity, including the early years of the polio vaccine, the antibiotic streptomycin, the hormone insulin to treat diabetes, the iron lung to enable patients with polio to breathe, and the dialysis machine to filter people's blood when their kidneys fail (Mehlman, 1985).

Those responsible for microallocation decisions have adopted a wide range of criteria for determining which patients receive available resources. Sometimes a "triage" model has been used, drawing on the experience of prioritizing the treatment of casualties/patients on the battlefield or in the emergency room (Rhodes et al., 1992; Bell, 1981). At other times these criteria have only been implicit, as was common during the early years of kidney dialysis in the United States, prior to universal funding by the federal government in 1972. Many dialysis centers employed an ad hoc approach, in which particular patients were selected from eligible pools without any set of guidelines developed in advance. The resulting decisions were widely criticized as arbitrary. Of greater concern is the tendency of ad hoc

decision making to reflect the biases and preferences of the decision makers (Fox and Swazey, 1978).

Ad hoc decision making continues to take place when individual caregivers, ethics committees, or health-care institutions make microallocation decisions without first developing an explicit set of allocation criteria to guide them. Nevertheless, significant attention in practice and theory has been devoted to formulating a more ethically acceptable decision-making approach. Overall approaches will be discussed in the closing section of this article.

Allocation criteria

Before examining such approaches, this article will address the justifications and weaknesses of the major allocation criteria from which implemented or proposed approaches have been constructed to date. As one nationwide questionnaire study of microallocation criteria favored by selected medical directors has documented (Kilner, 1990—hereafter, "U.S. Study"), these criteria can be clustered into four major types: social, sociomedical, medical, and personal criteria.

Social criteria. The characteristic feature of social criteria is that they seek to promote some particular or general social good as a result of the allocation decisions made. There are five such criteria, the most basic of which is a social value criterion. Given some place in microallocation decisions by 56 percent of the U.S. Study participants, this criterion gives preference to patients judged to be of greatest value to society, according to whatever standards of value the decision makers decide to employ. While the criterion may be explicitly invoked, it can also operate covertly to influence treatment decisions. One result in the United States has been that socially privileged groups such as whites and males have received scarce treatments disproportionately often (Council on Ethical and Judicial Affairs, 1990 and 1991).

The primary attraction of employing a social value criterion is that it helps to maximize the amount of benefit derived from health-care resources. Since society has invested its resources in a patient's treatment—or at least in developing the possibility of that treatment—it is understandably interested in a good return on its investment. Absent this criterion, there might well be an undesirable loss of some of society's most gifted people. A social value criterion usually employs a utilitarian calculus, according to which the patients judged most likely to be most valuable to society in the future are favored. However, past contributions to society may also enter the calculus on the basis of just reward or gratitude for a patient's past.

In any form, the criterion is highly controversial. Conscientiously ranking people according to social value is a virtually impossible task. Agreeing on a ranking of all possible social contributions—based on an accurate understanding of future as well as present needs—is extremely problematic even in a setting much more homogeneous than the United States. Assessing how particular individuals rank on this scale requires a virtually unobtainable level of knowledge about people's lives. The omniscience and wisdom required has led critics to label the use of this criterion "playing God." The criterion is also criticized for unfairly discriminating against individuals or groups who cannot contribute as much to society as others. Their relative inability may be due to unchangeable genetic factors or uncontrollable social circumstances (e.g., past discrimination that has undermined either their ability or society's appreciation of their contributions). Moreover, the toll on the caregiver–patient relationship can be severe. Patients can no longer be sure that confidential information about embarrassing symptoms or lifestyle habits, which caregivers often must know in order to treat patients effectively, will not be used to deny them treatment in deference to another more socially promising patient.

The second social criterion, progress of science, is closely related to a social value criterion and receives roughly the same support in the U.S. Study (58 percent of the participants). It gives priority to patients whose treatment will yield the most scientifically useful information. For example, during the years when kidney dialysis was still scarce in the United States, a hypothesis surfaced that dialysis might alleviate the mental disorder schizophrenia as well as replace kidney function. Under such circumstances, a progress of science criterion favors treating patients who have both medical needs. Since the same number of people will be treated with or without the criterion, it is arguably best to learn as much as possible, through careful patient selection, about the full beneficial potential of a scarce resource.

On the other hand, many of the shortcomings of a social value criterion also apply to a progress of science criterion. For example, the pragmatic difficulties of identifying precisely which (groups of) patients, if treated, will yield the most important scientific information loom large. So does the coercion inherent in the experimentation (with possible added tests or procedures) the criterion entails. Those eligible for priority treatment must either consent or risk a lower priority of being treated—which could mean substantial suffering or even death. Ultimately the criterion may not really be necessary, since patients with scientifically interesting conditions are usually selected through the application of other criteria. Such patients can volunteer for any special tests or procedures and data on those patients can be pooled in a central location.

A favored group criterion is the third of the social criteria. According to this criterion, people of a certain type (e.g., children or military veterans) or who live within certain geographic boundaries receive priority. Much of health care operates on this basis, both for the sake of convenience and in order to enhance the quality of care for particular groups. Such justifications become problematic, however, when resources are limited and people who are denied care at a particular facility on the basis of this criterion cannot necessarily obtain it in a different location. Accordingly, only 27 percent of the participants in the U.S. Study support it.

On the other hand, some rationales for the criterion are more strictly medical and may apply to any patient. For example, when perishable resources such as transplantable organs or patients receiving treatment and follow-up care must travel long distances, medical outcomes may suffer considerably. If medical considerations are central, though, then at issue is really some form of medical criterion, not one's group identity per se. Moreover, it is arguably better to try to remedy barriers to treatment—e.g., by relocating people nearer to a treatment facility—than to employ barriers as grounds for denying treatment.

In certain cases, a very different favored-group justification is at work. A group, even an entire state or country, should arguably have the freedom to produce special resources available only to its own members, as long as the resources available to others are not thereby limited. In practice, though, such is rarely the case. Consider organ transplantation. Since the supply of organs itself is limited, giving some people special access means less access for others. Moreover, neither a particular U.S. state nor the country as a whole can claim all the credit for developing every aspect of the technology required. Accordingly, some have proposed eliminating geographic boundaries or at least implementing regional or national quota systems that would establish priorities without completely excluding any group (U.S. Task Force on Organ Transplantation, 1986).

The fourth social criterion, a resources required criterion, receives somewhat more support (66% of the participants in the U.S. Study). It prioritizes treating those who need less of a given resource before patients who need more of it, though it is usually restricted to situations in which its application will likely increase the number of lives saved. Saving lives is a central task of health care and a praiseworthy goal from most philosophical and religious perspectives. The requirement of a greater lifesaving potential most clearly distinguishes the criterion from a more general social value criterion. Usually only patients requiring substantially fewer resources than other patients are favored by the criterion. For instance, patients needing temporary rather than long-term use of a scarce drug receive priority, as do patients needing a single-organ rather than multi-organ transplant. The criterion is not designed to bias patient selection automatically against patients who have previously been treated for the same problem, such as those whose failing organ transplants must be replaced.

A resources required criterion can be criticized as too attentive, or not attentive enough, to maximizing good results from treatment. It is too attentive if the life-threatening needs of each patient requiring a particular treatment should receive equal weight regardless of the overall number of lives saved. It is not attentive enough if many characteristics of people should be considered other than whether or not they will survive. From this latter perspective, saving the life of one outstanding person could be preferable to saving two who are not.

The final social criterion, a vital responsibilities criterion, has a legitimate role in microallocation decisions according to 69 percent of the participants in the U.S. Study. Intended for exceptional situations only, this criterion accords special priority to patients on whom others depend. The broadest form of the criterion favors any patient who has "family dependents." Generally, though, there must be some sort of unusual social need that requires special treatment for particular people. In a disaster situation, for example, treating those with medical expertise first may make it possible for them in turn to save additional lives. As in the case of a resources required criterion, the strictest form of the criterion requires more than producing general social value: Additional lives must be saved every time the criterion is applied.

Without this lifesaving requirement, the criterion is merely a specific type of social value criterion and therefore open to all of the critiques to which that criterion is vulnerable. Invoking the criterion to favor patients with family dependents is particularly problematic since not everyone has equal access to having children. In some cultures, moreover, sustaining the life of one who has not yet maintained the family name by having children is more important than treating one who already has children. On the other hand, if the pursuit of general social value in microallocation decisions is ethically legitimate, then allowing a vital responsibilities criterion to apply only when additional lives are saved by it is unduly restrictive.

Sociomedical criteria. Three other microallocation criteria are similar to the social criteria, in that they generally seek to promote some social good. However, they are distinctive in that their stated justifications are often medical in nature. The first such sociomedical criterion is age.

Old age has long been employed as a reason for limiting medical treatment on the basis that elderly people do not sufficiently benefit from it due to their weakened physical condition. At issue may be the likelihood of benefit, the length of benefit, or the quality of benefit. So it is not surprising that 88 percent of the participants in the U.S. Study support the criterion to some degree.

In response to book-length justifications of an age criterion that addresses far more than aspects of medical benefit (e.g., Callahan, 1987; Daniels, 1988), a wide body of literature has emerged (e.g., Homer and Holstein, 1990; Winslow and Walters, 1993). Some supporters of the criterion favor younger candidates for treatment over older candidates in order to give all an equal opportunity to live. A health-care system, first of all, should keep people from dying "early." Others argue that whereas all people may have an equal claim upon available health-care resources, that claim diminishes once people have achieved their so-called natural life span (perhaps 75 or 80 years). Furthermore, were people themselves given the choice, they might prefer to concentrate life-sustaining resources in their earlier years if that would make possible better long-term and supportive care in their elderly years.

Those who reject an age criterion find all such justifications unconvincing. Medical justifications arguably support medical criteria rather than a criterion based on age per se. Equal regard for persons appropriately focuses on persons as a whole—persons who should receive needed health care whenever that need occurs—rather than on persons as accumulations of life years, the number of which is to be maximized in the name of equal opportunity. Limiting equal access to people who have not yet lived their natural life span, meanwhile, relies on the debatable notion that there is a fixed natural life span. Moreover, it imposes on older people the judgment that, relatively speaking, their lives are not worth living, even if they disagree. (At least such is the case if age per se, rather than quality or length of life, is at issue.) Finally, if given a choice, people might well prefer criteria other than age for allocating limited resources. They would likely recognize that in people's actual experience, they would not be denying certain forms of health care to their own older selves, but rather the rest of the community would be denying needed life-sustaining care to a certain group of its members. This denial is more discriminatory than it may at first appear, for the group denied is not only old but also largely female (Jecker, 1991).

In the end, all rationales for limiting health care for elderly persons are often suspected of being fueled, at least unconsciously, by a utilitarian preference for the achievement and economic productivity more characteristic of younger persons. Not only is the unbounded pursuit of social value itself controversial but also the economic productivity orientation of that pursuit reflects the questionable bias of Western culture toward productivity even at the expense of personal relationships (Kilner, 1992).

A second sociomedical criterion is that of psychological ability. Acknowledged to play at least some legitimate role in allocation decisions by 97 percent of the participants in the U.S. Study, the ability of patients to cope emotionally and intellectually with treatment is commonly assumed to be essential to effective health care. Without it, patients are unable to follow medical instructions and may even reject treatment or life itself after considerable resources have been expended. Such patients are the most difficult to treat and tend to be the least valuable to society.

These justifications also constitute arguments against the criterion. Rationales that are medical in nature actually support medical criteria rather than a psychological ability criterion per se. When psychological ability per se is invoked, the convenience of the staff or the presumed social value of the patient is problematically allowed to override the patient's claim to equal access. Moreover, caregivers' judgments about the coping abilities and cooperativeness of patients are much more subjective than the physical assessments they conduct and are therefore vulnerable to personal bias. Like everyone else, caregivers find that they can work best with those most like themselves, and many question the appropriateness of ranking human lives based on how well matched patients are to caregivers.

A supportive environment criterion favoring those patients who will have the most supportive living environment during and following treatment constitutes the final sociomedical criterion. Considered potentially valid by 61 percent of the participants in the U.S. Study, this criterion favors patients with the best access to personal and professional caregivers as well as facilities and other material resources relevant to effective treatment. Without sufficient postoperative care, for example, not only may scarce resources be wasted, but a treatment such as a heart transplant may result in a worse death than if the patient had received no treatment at all. Alternatively, the absence of a supportive environment may indicate that the patient warrants low priority on social value grounds.

A supportive environment criterion per se, however, is unnecessary if the concerns it addresses are already accounted for by medical benefit and social value criteria. Even as a form of another criterion, supportive environment is a problematic consideration, since the connection between people's environment and their medical outcomes or social value is far from precise. Helpful supports are not always necessary for a satisfactory medical outcome, and personal bias easily intrudes when assessing lifestyles or home situations quite different from one's own. In fact, the criterion by its very nature can be unjust when it denies treatment to patients (e.g., children with an inadequate home environment) on the basis of the irresponsibility of others (e.g.,

parents) or society at large. Arguably, the special needs of such situations call for extra care, not less.

Medical criteria.   The third cluster of criteria are explicitly medical in nature, having to do with health-related outcomes of treatment. The most basic of these is a medical benefit criterion, acknowledged as a legitimate allocation criterion by 95 percent of the participants in the U.S. Study. Unlike many other medical criteria that compare and rank candidates for treatment, this criterion includes for further consideration everyone with a reasonable likelihood of receiving a significant length and quality of medical benefit from treatment. The criterion casts a wide net: any degree of likelihood, length, and quality that can reasonably be considered minimally significant is sufficient. Treatments not offering such benefit are commonly excluded as futile, though futility itself is a concept that requires careful definition (Jecker and Schneiderman, 1992).

The requirement that patients benefit medically from scarce medical resources is rooted in ethical standards of efficiency and justice. Without the requirement, precious resources would be wasted on patients who would receive no benefit from them. Moreover, according to many theological and philosophical traditions, need constitutes the major exception to the egalitarian presumption generally built into concepts of justice. The notion of need includes the ideas that some disease or injury condition is present (or will be, where the need for preventive care is in view), and that a person's life is thereby undesirably altered. A need for a lifesaving resource, for example, implies that a person's life is in jeopardy without it; no preferable alternatives remain.

The major difficulty with this criterion is the way in which standards of need can be manipulated. A classic illustration is the provision of kidney dialysis in Great Britain (Aaron and Schwartz, 1984). Resources allocated for dialysis by the government-run health-care system have been insufficient to treat all who could benefit medically from dialysis, according to normal standards of need. Yet many have claimed that all who need treatment receive it. Matching of available resources and need has been achieved by tightening standards of need in sections of the country where resources are particularly scarce. Also, general practitioners do not even refer certain patients to kidney specialists for dialysis when practitioners know that sufficient resources are not available.

The second medical criterion, imminent death, takes the standard of need a step farther. Sometimes called an "urgency" criterion, it accords special priority to patients who will die soon without treatment. While the term "imminent" is not precise—generally ranging from a few days to a few weeks—it has been found workable by many in clinical and legal contexts alike (Kilner, 1990).

Not only does this criterion recognize situations of special need, it also results in more lives saved. (A necessary stipulation, though, is that it be applied together with the medical benefit criterion, so that priority will not be accorded to patients for whom treatment is futile.) Since patients whose death is not imminent can survive for a period of time while imminently dying patients receive priority care, a new treatment may become available in the interim, enabling patients in both categories to live. Alternatively (and more likely), additional resources may be made available at any point as the life-threatening situation becomes better known. In fact, the scarcity itself may be only intermittent, as is often the case with intensive-care space.

An imminent death criterion, though, is more problematic in practice than it may appear to be in theory. In many situations it is impossible to determine with precision whether or not a patient's death is imminent. In others, caregivers can overstate the urgency of their patients' conditions in order to give them priority access to lifesaving resources. While doing so may be unfair, it may represent an understandable attempt to avoid another problem with the criterion. By making patients wait until they have deteriorated almost to the point of death before they receive priority access to treatment, the criterion ensures that resources will be devoted to the sickest patients. Worse medical outcomes for those treated and greater suffering for those who might wait are bound to result. Moreover, additional resources may never become available for those not prioritized by the criterion.

Each of the three remaining medical criteria addresses a particular aspect of medical effectiveness. The first of these, likelihood of benefit, is affirmed by 96 percent of the participants in the U.S. Study. The criterion assumes that more than a minimal likelihood of medical benefit is a necessary prerequisite for receiving scarce medical resources. Those with the greatest likelihood should be favored to ensure the most productive use of available resources. While this justification resembles the rationale underlying a social value criterion, the benefits in view here are limited to medical benefits experienced by the persons receiving the scarce resources. Moreover, more lives may ultimately be saved if this criterion is applied, although such will not be the case in every situation where the criterion is applied.

Several obstacles attend this criterion. Precisely quantifying the probabilities of every patient's benefiting from a particular treatment so that all can be comparatively ranked is quite difficult. Furthermore, while a productive use of resources may be applauded, the cost of achieving it is arguably too great. Many patients have significant (albeit lesser) likelihoods of benefiting from treatment; yet the criterion leaves them with no realistic prospect of receiving lifesaving care if enough patients

with better prospects are waiting for the same treatment. Patients can no longer trust caregivers with essential information that suggests their cases may be complicated, since caregivers must steer resources to the patient with the best prospects rather than simply attending to the needs of each patient. Ultimately, the criterion tends to discriminate against whichever groups in society have the poorest health in general and thus the lowest likelihood of having optimal outcomes from any treatment. Poor persons, disabled persons, and members of racial minorities are particularly vulnerable on this score.

Another medical criterion, length of benefit, ranks all patients according to the length of time, rather than the likelihood, that they will benefit medically from treatment. As in the case of other comparative medical criteria, the underlying concern is to achieve as much medical benefit as possible from the available limited resources. Specifically in this case, the criterion helps to maximize the success of treatment by maximizing the length of time patients live following treatment. Of the participants in the U.S. Study, 96 percent indicated that a length of benefit criterion should have some place in microallocation decisions.

Several of the difficulties with this criterion parallel those of a likelihood of benefit criterion. Accurately predicting the length of time patients will survive following treatment is extremely hard. The criterion also tends to discriminate against the same groups of people disadvantaged by a likelihood of benefit criterion, since these typically less-healthy groups on average do not live as long as others following many treatments. This discriminatory effect extends to elderly patients as well, since they tend to have fewer years of life remaining regardless of the treatment in view. However, the significance of this concern is as debatable as the age criterion itself. The most fundamental problem with a length of benefit criterion may be its presumption that length of life rather than persons per se is the appropriate focus of allocation decisions. Each person's life is uniquely important to that person. Those who argue that all people have a right to life (including life-sustaining resources) add that rights do not diminish the sicker one gets.

The final medical criterion, quality of benefit, shares the wide support expressed for other medical criteria, including acknowledgment by 97 percent of the U.S. Study participants. Like the two previous criteria, it ranks patients on a scale, in this case a scale of quality of life following treatment. The criterion rejects the common preoccupation with merely keeping patients alive and insists that health care is also responsible for producing lives with as high a quality as possible. Good quality of life is important to patients because it contributes substantially to their happiness as well as to their autonomy (their ability to make uncoerced decisions concerning their own lives). From a social standpoint, higher quality lives have a tendency to be more socially productive lives.

Quantifying all qualitative considerations in order to compare patients on the same scale, however, may be impossible. Even if it were possible, predicting the quality of life that will follow treatment sufficiently precisely to distinguish most patients remains problematic. So does achieving agreement as to what factors characterize a good quality of life and how these factors should be ranked. While such measures as QALYs (quality-adjusted life years) have been developed to assist macroallocation decision making, they have not proven as helpful in distinguishing individual patients at the microallocation level. Another difficulty arises when some people (usually caregivers) must assess the quality of others' lives. People judge others' quality of life on the basis of objective, observable quality of life indicators. Unfortunately, evidence has long suggested that such objective indicators do not correlate well with patients' subjective experience of their own lives (U.S. Congress, 1987). In fact, what is unacceptable to the well may be quite acceptable to the sick. When some people impose their standards of quality on others, moreover, biases against such groups as disabled, poor, and elderly persons can easily intrude.

Personal criteria. The final four criteria may be designated as "personal" because their justifications are rooted in personal values such as liberty and the worth of the individual. The first such criterion is willingness. Supported to some degree by 89 percent of the participants in the U.S. Study, this criterion ensures that only patients who genuinely want treatment receive it. The criterion respects patients' rights to bodily integrity, as well as their autonomy, or freedom, to make vital decisions that primarily concern their own lives. People have unique life plans and values, and only they can accurately assess the balance between the benefits and burdens of their own treatment. For many, a right to the free exercise of religion is at stake. When resources are allocated to willing recipients, the recipients themselves are happier and the resources are less likely to be ineffective or rejected mid-course. Even if people choose to forgo treatment because other qualified patients need the same treatment, the choice can be applauded as an act of giving rather than simply branded as a typical suicide.

Nevertheless, a willingness criterion can also be problematic. For it to be employed ethically, patients must have complete information concerning the health care in question, including the costs and benefits of receiving it; they must understand this information; they must be free from the (sometimes subtle) coercion of family, professional, or other caregivers who might want them to accept or reject treatment; and they must have the mental capacity, despite their current health predic-

ament, to make and communicate decisions that reflect their values. A willingness criterion can also easily become a cover for patients' selfish behavior—for example, suicidal rejection of life-sustaining treatment with no regard for others who in some way depend on them.

The second personal criterion, responsibility, is actually a willingness criterion of a different sort. It steers resources away from people who willingly engage in unhealthy lifestyles or risky activities that result in the need for treatments. Most commonly invoked as a macroallocation criterion, this criterion has provoked significant debate. Proving responsibility in specific cases is particularly controversial (Wikler, 1987).

The third personal criterion, ability to pay, receives support from 43 percent of the participants in the U.S. Study. People with insufficient funds or other necessary resources are explicitly excluded by this criterion from access to certain forms of health care. The criterion functions in many indirect ways as well. The uninsured, in fact, use health services only about half as much as the insured and are more likely to die from treatable conditions as a result (Evans, 1989). The inability of some patients to pay for the support services that necessarily accompany certain treatments—such as travel expenses and postoperative care—has also in effect excluded some patients from treatment. When transplantable organs have been the scarce resource, those with the ability to mobilize the media or key politicians have occasionally gained special access to the necessary organs. The ethical considerations here are essentially those attending a market approach to macroallocation.

When all other ethically justifiable criteria have been applied, and there remain more eligible candidates for resources than there are resources to provide, caregivers sometimes invoke an impartial selection criterion. Affirmed by 31 percent of the participants in the U.S. Study, this criterion mandates a random selection from among eligible candidates. Its rationale is that each person who has an equal moral claim on a scarce resource should have an equal opportunity to receive it. The apparent arbitrariness of the selection helps to keep the tragedy of the situation clearly in view. It focuses more attention on the need for additional resources to be made available at the macroallocation level, if possible. There is no comforting illusion that the "best" candidates are being treated.

Some forms of impartial selection, though, may be better than others. One option is a first-come, first-served approach. Since the time that each person is stricken with a medical condition and seeks treatment is more or less random, this approach functions as a sort of natural lottery. Its appeal stems from the familiarity of waiting lines inside and outside the realms of health care, and the way that this approach does not seem as starkly random as an explicit lottery. However, true randomness is the whole point of an impartial selection criterion. First-come, first-served is inferior to a genuine lottery on this score. Patients with the greater power, mobility, information, and confidence associated with the relatively wealthy have better access to health care generally and to referral networks in particular. Accordingly, they tend to get on the waiting lists for scarce resources sooner than those who are less wealthy and empowered.

Some weaknesses of an impartial selection criterion, though, are not unique to a particular form of the criterion but are inherent in the criterion itself. For instance, many of the social benefits that other criteria generate are lost when an impartial selection criterion is applied. Socially destructive persons such as dangerous criminals are sometimes selected instead of people who have made great positive contributions to society. Rather than respecting human dignity, impartial selection may demean it by not considering the unique features of each person. Admittedly, people cannot make infallible decisions. In the eyes of some, however, human judgments are arguably better than blind chance.

Allocation approaches

Allocation criteria, the building blocks of microallocation, must be prioritized and arranged into some sort of basic approach if microallocation decisions are to be ethically consistent. This approach can then serve as a framework for designing specific allocation procedures tailored to particular resources and settings. Approaches tend to be justified ethically by appeals to norms such as productivity, equality, and freedom, but relatively little grounding is typically provided for these norms in the context of allocation discussions. Such norms have long had broad intuitive appeal in Western culture. However, increasing ethical pluralism together with the tensions among the norms themselves underscore the need for a larger frame of reference (religious, rationalistic, or otherwise) within which such norms can be justified (Palazzani, 1994).

The many approaches to microallocation that have been advocated sort ethically into two groups. One group of approaches is oriented primarily toward making the most productive use of resources; the other, toward ensuring that suitable candidates have equal access to treatment through some form of impartial, or random, selection. Impartial selection may play a minor role in productivity-oriented approaches, but usually only to break ties. Furthermore, all approaches generally affirm or assume some sort of willingness criterion because of the importance of respecting people's freedom.

Productivity.   Three forms of productivity-oriented approach can be distinguished. One form focuses

exclusively on medical considerations (e.g., Leenen, 1988). Employing only medical criteria, along with sociomedical criteria whenever they are essential to good medical outcomes, this approach seeks to allocate resources to those most likely to benefit medically. Medical criteria, particularly when rooted in the notion of meeting needs, can be defended on the basis of ethical concerns other than productivity: for example, a principle of justice. However, when all (or virtually all) decision making depends on comparative medical judgments among patients, a more utilitarian concern to maximize productivity is typically at work. The strengths and weaknesses of such approaches will vary depending on which of the three comparative medical criteria (likelihood, length, and quality of benefit) are employed.

A second, related form of productivity-oriented approach attempts to enhance the productivity of an exclusively medical orientation by allowing special exceptions on the basis of value to society. The concern may be to ensure treatment for particularly valuable individuals (e.g., Langford, 1992) or to exclude particularly unworthy candidates (e.g., Bayles, 1990). In the former case, the relevant rationales are those supporting social value and/or vital responsibilities criteria; in the latter, rationales undergirding a responsibility criterion also apply.

The third form of productivity-oriented approach takes this concern about social value one step further. It makes social considerations primary, combining whatever criteria are necessary to yield the most productive use of scarce resources. The ethical justifications and weaknesses of this form of approach are fundamentally those of the social value criterion itself—most obviously when such approaches affirm social value per se as the overarching consideration (e.g., Basson, 1979). When social criteria such as social value and progress of science are combined with comparative medical criteria and/or sociomedical criteria (e.g., Rescher, 1969), the additional justifications and weaknesses of those criteria come into play secondarily.

Impartiality.   The major alternative to productivity-oriented approaches seeks to give suitable candidates equal access to treatment through some form of impartial selection. The pool of suitable candidates typically includes all who meet the medical benefit criterion. Priority groups within this pool are identified on the basis of nonutilitarian criteria: vital responsibilities alone (e.g., Childress, 1981), vital responsibilities plus resources required (e.g., Winslow, 1982), or both of these criteria plus imminent death (e.g., Kilner, 1990). (A priority may also be given to any group of people whose likelihood of benefit is substantially higher than that of all others, though the productivity-oriented nature of this priority creates ethical tension within an impartiality-oriented approach.) Finally, candidates are ordered within each priority group through impartial (usually random) selection.

In contrast to the explicit or implicit utilitarian bent of productivity-oriented approaches, in which benefit to society is the primary goal, the justification of this last type of approach is more egalitarian in nature. Within certain limitations designed to save as many lives as possible, all potential recipients of scarce resources are insured an equal opportunity to receive them. This commitment to life and equality may simply be intuitive or reflect popular sentiment. Alternatively, respect for life and equality may be grounded in a philosophical or religious understanding of ethics. One philosophical example would be social contract theory, in which such respect may be seen as something to which all people would agree, if they had to decide upon ethical standards to govern society under certain ideal conditions (Winslow, 1982; Rawls, 1971). A religious example would be the biblical accounts of God's exemplary commitment to even the poorest, foundational to Christianity and Judaism (Kilner, 1991; Ramsey, 1970; Mackler, 1991).

Particular settings. Implementing any approach requires tailoring it to particular settings. For instance, medical assessments are handled differently when allocating intensive care (Zoloth-Dorfman and Carney, 1991) as opposed to transplantable organs (Caplan, 1992) or kidney dialysis (Cummings, 1993). In the intensive-care setting, a common tool is the APACHE (Acute Physiology and Chronic Health Evaluation) System. Through laboratory tests and bodily measurements, the APACHE System is able to predict patient death rates and length of intensive-care stay when patients are first admitted to intensive care (Knaus et al., 1993). A different quantitative system has been developed for assessing both medical and nonmedical considerations in organ transplantation. UNOS (United Network for Organ Sharing) has developed a national point system to prioritize patients needing transplants. In the case of kidney transplants, for instance, candidates whose blood type is compatible with that of the donated organ are ranked according to point totals. These totals represent the sum of points given for medical considerations such as antigen matching and for nonmedical considerations such as time on the waiting list (United Network for Organ Sharing, 1993). Methods of quantifying social value rankings in particular geographic settings have also been developed (Charny et al., 1989).

Numerical systems are helpful to facilitate consistent comparisons among potential recipients of health care. However, the need for judgment in microallocation is unavoidable (Council on Ethical and Judicial Affairs, 1993). Caregivers must help identify medically appropriate courses of action, assess the likely outcomes of those courses, and assist potential recipients in their decision making. Potential recipients must evaluate the benefits and burdens of all available courses of action in light of their own sets of values and beliefs. Interdisciplinary committees and health-care teams in public policy and institutional settings must not only craft ethically sound allocation criteria into workable allocation approaches; they must also determine what shape such approaches take in specific settings and discern how they apply to particular people. Microallocation, like health care itself, remains an art as well as a science.

JOHN F. KILNER

Directly related to this article is the companion article in this entry: MACROALLOCATION. *Also directly related are the entries* ECONOMIC CONCEPTS IN HEALTH CARE; HEALTH-CARE DELIVERY; HEALTH-CARE FINANCING, *the* INTRODUCTION *and article on* HEALTH-CARE INSURANCE; HEALTH POLICY, *article on* POLITICS AND HEALTH CARE; HOSPITAL, *article on* CONTEMPORARY ETHICAL PROBLEMS; *and* LIFE, QUALITY OF, *article on* QUALITY OF LIFE IN HEALTH-CARE ALLOCATION. *This article will find application in the entries* ARTIFICIAL HEARTS AND CARDIAC-ASSIST DEVICES; ARTIFICIAL ORGANS AND LIFE-SUPPORT SYSTEMS; CLINICAL ETHICS, *article on* ELEMENTS AND METHODOLOGIES; DEATH AND DYING: EUTHANASIA AND SUSTAINING LIFE, *article on* ETHICAL ISSUES; ORGAN AND TISSUE TRANSPLANTS, *article on* ETHICAL AND LEGAL ISSUES; *and* PUBLIC POLICY AND BIOETHICS. *Other relevant material may be found under the entries* BIOETHICS; CONFLICT OF INTEREST; HEALTH-CARE FINANCING; HEALTH POLICY, *article on* HEALTH POLICY IN INTERNATIONAL PERSPECTIVE; RIGHTS; *and* UTILITY.

Bibliography

AARON, HENRY J., and SCHWARTZ, WILLIAM B. 1984. *The Painful Prescription: Rationing Hospital Care.* Washington, D.C.: Brookings Institution.

BASSON, MARC D. 1979. "Choosing Among Candidates for Scarce Medical Resources." *Journal of Medicine and Philosophy* 4, no. 2:313–333.

BAYLES, MICHAEL D. 1990. "Allocation of Scarce Medical Resources." *Public Affairs Quarterly* 4:1–16.

BELL, NORA K. 1981. "Triage in Medical Practices: An Unacceptable Model?" *Social Science and Medicine* 15F, no. 4:151–156.

CALLAHAN, DANIEL. 1987. *Setting Limits: Medical Goals in an Aging Society.* New York: Simon and Schuster.

CAPLAN, ARTHUR L. 1992. *If I Were a Rich Man Could I Buy a Pancreas? and Other Essays on the Ethics of Health Care.* Bloomington: Indiana University Press.

CHARNY, M. C.; LEWIS, P. A.; and FARROW, S. C. 1989. "Choosing Who Shall Not Be Treated in the NHS." *Social Science and Medicine* 28, no. 12:1131–1138.

CHILDRESS, JAMES F. 1981. *Priorities in Biomedical Ethics.* Philadelphia: Westminster Press.

COUNCIL ON ETHICAL AND JUDICIAL AFFAIRS. AMERICAN MEDICAL ASSOCIATION. 1990. "Black-White Disparities in Health Care." *Journal of the American Medical Association* 263, no. 17:2344–2346.

———. 1991. "Gender Disparities in Clinical Decision Making." *Journal of the American Medical Association* 266, no. 4:559–562.

———. 1993. "Ethical Considerations in the Allocation of Organs and Other Scarce Medical Resources Among Patients," Report 49. Chicago: American Medical Association.

CUMMINGS, NANCY B. 1993. "Ethical Considerations in End-Stage Renal Disease." In *Diseases of the Kidney,* 5th ed., pp. 3097–3128. Edited by Robert W. Schrier and Carl W. Gottschalk. Boston: Little, Brown.

DANIELS, NORMAN. 1988. *Am I My Parents' Keeper?* New York: Oxford University Press.

EVANS, ROGER W. 1989. "Money Matters: Should Ability to Pay Ever Be a Consideration in Gaining Access to Transplantation?" *Transplantation Proceedings* 21, no. 3:3419–3423.

FOX, RENÉE C., and SWAZEY, JUDITH P. 1978. *The Courage to Fail.* 2d ed. Chicago: University of Chicago Press.

HOMER, PAUL, and HOLSTEIN, MARTHA, eds. 1990. *A Good Old Age? The Paradox of Setting Limits.* New York: Simon and Schuster.

JECKER, NANCY S. 1991. "Age-Based Rationing and Women." *Journal of the American Medical Society* 266, no. 21:3012–3015.

JECKER, NANCY S., and SCHNEIDERMAN, LAWRENCE J. 1992. "Futility and Rationing." *American Journal of Medicine* 92, no. 2:189–196.

KILNER, JOHN F. 1990. *Who Lives? Who Dies? Ethical Criteria in Patient Selection.* New Haven, Conn.: Yale University Press.

———. 1992. *Life on the Line: Ethics, Aging, Ending Patients' Lives, and Allocating Vital Resources.* Grand Rapids, Mich.: W. B. Eerdmans.

KNAUS, WILLIAM A.; WAGNER, DOUGLAS P.; ZIMMERMAN, JACK E.; and DRAPER, ELIZABETH A. 1993. "Variations in Mortality and Length of Stay in Intensive Care Units." *Annals of Internal Medicine* 118, no. 10:753–761.

LANGFORD, MICHAEL J. 1992. "Who Should Get the Kidney Machine?" *Journal of Medical Ethics* 18, no. 1:12–17.

LEENEN, H. J. J. 1988. "Selection of Patients: An Insoluble Dilemma." *Medicine and Law* 7, no. 3:233–245.

MACKLER, AARON L. 1991. "Judaism, Justice, and Access to Health Care." *Kennedy Institute of Ethics Journal* 1, no. 2:143–161.

MEHLMAN, MAXWELL J. 1985. "Rationing Expensive Lifesaving Medical Treatments." *Wisconsin Law Review* 1985, no. 2:239–303.

PALAZZANI, LAURA. 1994. "Personalism and Bioethics." *Ethics and Medicine* 10, no. 1:7–11.

RAMSEY, PAUL. 1970. *The Patient as Person: Explorations in Medical Ethics.* New Haven, Conn.: Yale University Press.

RAWLS, JOHN. 1971. *A Theory of Justice.* Cambridge, Mass.: Harvard University Press.

RESCHER, NICHOLAS. 1969. "The Allocation of Exotic Medical Lifesaving Therapy." *Ethics* 79, no. 3:173–186.

RHODES, ROSAMIND; MILLER, CHARLES; and SCHWARTZ, MYRON. 1992. "Transplant Recipient Selection: Peacetime vs. Wartime Triage." *Cambridge Quarterly of Healthcare Ethics* 1, no. 4:327–331.

TRUOG, ROBERT D. 1992. "Triage in the ICU." *Hastings Center Report* 22, no. 3:13–17.

UNICEF. 1993. *Annual Report.* New York: UNICEF.

UNITED NETWORK FOR ORGAN SHARING. 1993. "Bylaws and Policies." November 4. Richmond, Va.: United Network for Organ Sharing.

U.S. CONGRESS. OFFICE OF TECHNOLOGY ASSESSMENT. 1987. *Life-Sustaining Technologies and the Elderly.* Washington, D.C.: U.S. Government Printing Office.

U.S. TASK FORCE ON ORGAN TRANSPLANTATION. 1986. *Organ Transplantation: Issues and Recommendations.* Rockville, Md.: U.S. Dept. of Health and Human Services.

WIKLER, DANIEL. 1987. "Who Should Be Blamed for Being Sick?" *Health Education Quarterly* 14, no. 1:11–25.

WINSLOW, GERALD R. 1982. *Triage and Justice.* Berkeley: University of California Press.

WINSLOW, GERALD R., and WALTERS, JAMES W., eds. 1993. *Facing Limits: Ethics and Health Care for the Elderly.* Boulder, Colo.: Westview Press.

ZOLOTH-DORFMAN, LAURIE, and CARNEY, BRIDGET. 1991. "The AIDS Patient and the Last ICU Bed: Scarcity, Medical Futility, and Ethics." *QRB/Quality Review Bulletin* 17, no. 6:175–181.

HEALTH-CARE SYSTEMS

See HEALTH-CARE DELIVERY, *article on* HEALTH-CARE SYSTEMS.

HEALTH-CARE TEAMS

See TEAMS, HEALTH-CARE.

HEALTH AND DISEASE

I. History of the Concepts
   Dietrich von Engelhardt
II. Sociological Perspectives
   Charles L. Bosk
III. Anthropological Perspectives
   Allan Young

IV. Philosophical Perspectives
    H. Tristram Engelhardt, Jr.
    Kevin Wm. Wildes
V. The Experience of Health and Illness
    Drew Leder

I. HISTORY OF THE CONCEPTS

Health and disease are among the fundamental experiences of human life. The concepts that people in various cultures have used in an attempt to understand and respond to those experiences have to do with the way humans relate to nature and culture. The concepts of health and disease have far-reaching consequences for diagnosis and therapy, the attitude and behavior of physicians, how patients deal with disease, social attitudes and structures, the shape of moral choices, and the cultural significance of sickness and wellness behaviors.

Health and disease are not merely medical terms; they are also vital themes in art, philosophy, theology, sociology, and psychology. In fact, these very disciplines remind medicine again and again of its distinctly "anthropological" character, in the sense that medicine deals with the nature and destiny of humans. Neither medicine nor the concepts of health and disease with which it deals can be properly understood by using the starkly contrasting categories of natural sciences and human sciences as a framework. Just as medicine cannot be reduced to either of the two, so also it is necessary to connect nature and culture if we are to understand health and disease.

A universally valid definition of health has been as hard to formulate as a universally valid definition of disease. Health and disease are physical, social, psychological, and spiritual phenomena that can be represented in concepts that are both descriptive and normative, although these two sorts of concepts have not always been clearly distinguished in the historical development of these ideas. Humans not only determine what will be regarded as health and disease; at the same time they also interpret these experiences and decide how to respond to them.

Concepts of disease and health are especially important because they influence the manner and goal of medical treatment. Thus a mechanical or technologically structured understanding of disease (that views the human as a defective machine) requires a mechanical or technologically structured therapy (regarded as repair) and therapeutic relationship (a relationship of technician to defective machine). More personal or holistic concepts urge corresponding types of therapy and healer–patient relationship.

Contemporary medicine increasingly faces the task not only of overcoming sickness but also of preserving health. Prevention and rehabilitation play increasingly important roles alongside curative therapies. Treatment is understood to include attentive caring and support. Chronic suffering and death place different demands on the doctor–patient relationship than do acute illnesses. In light of such developments, concepts of health and disease require new definitions. A historical retrospective may assist in arriving at those definitions.

This article does not attempt to offer a thorough cross-cultural analysis of concepts of health and disease; rather, it presents essential dimensions and changes in these concepts in the general course of history, their relationships with sociocultural backgrounds, and their practical and ethical consequences (Diepgen et al., 1969; Riese, 1953; Rothschuh, 1975; Schipperges et al., 1978; Temkin, 1973). A consideration of these historical developments can stimulate new reflections and initiatives, but history differs from any theoretical system. History has its own rules and logic. A progressionist explanation of the gradual development of notions of health and disease is inadequate. There are continuities and discontinuities, progress and regress, even within a single event or movement. This complex nature of history in general characterizes the history of medicine and specifically the history of the concepts of health and disease.

Health and disease suggest a variety of meanings from psychological, social, and spiritual perspectives. The word "illness" in the English language refers to the subjective or personal side of disease whereas "disease" refers to the medical conception of pathological abnormality. It is possible for a person to feel ill without having a disease, and conversely, to have a disease without feeling ill. The term "sickness" transcends both of these concepts by focusing on social consequences. The concept of the "sick role" corresponds to the social nature of disease. The way in which societies vary in their interpretations of physical and mental disorders and in their treatment of and symbolic reactions to them reflects the cultural dimension of disease.

Nonetheless, some basic categories will be useful in the following discussion. One category is the explanation of disease, illness, and sickness. From a physical perspective, the different approaches of the past attribute disease to either liquid or solid components of the body, or to the relationship between the body and the soul. Other distinctions refer to whether diseases should be regarded as existing entities (ontological notion of disease) or as phenomena affecting individual persons in a variety of ways (symptomatic notion of disease); and whether and to what extent the constitution and disposition of the individual (endogenous) and/or external factors (exogenous) play a significant role in determining health and disease.

A second category concerns response to disease, illness, and sickness. These responses were frequently shaped by the explanation of disease, illness, and sickness. These two categories evolved into the science and clinical practice of medicine.

Primitive peoples

There is no life without disease and pain; their ubiquitous nature is demonstrated by history. The skeletons of the first humans (500,000 B.C.E.) display bone disturbances and fractures. It is difficult to offer accurate descriptions of the health and disease of historically primitive peoples, because claims must depend on limited and problematic archaeological, paleopathological, and written sources (Clements, 1932).

At the dawn of human history, medicine had a magicomystical, demonic-religious character. Exogenous factors such as spirits, spells, and gods were responsible for disease. Personified living entities, spirits, took over a healthy body and made off with the soul of the person, or allowed foreign elements to invade the body. Spirits, dead or living, could exercise fateful effects, acting out of revenge for breaches of taboos. Disease, directly related to sin and wrongdoing, represented not only an individual but also a social destiny. What befell one person befell the whole family, group, or tribe.

The diagnostic and healing powers of the healer or priest-doctor were supernatural. The healer had to be able to recognize which forces were at work in any given case. He did this by reading the stars, or by drawing meaning from minerals, plants, and animals. Amulets and magic spells, oracles, atonement and confession, exorcism, bloodletting, and ceremonies of purification functioned as both preventive measures and cures. The whole community took part in the healing process; even pets were brought into it. Primitive peoples exhibited great cleanliness for the sake of prevention and strictly observed their cultural taboos.

There are remnants of these primitive notions of disease in today's lay language. For example, in English slang menstruation is sometimes called "the curse"; the German word for lumbago, *Hexenschuss*, means witch's wound. To what extent one can observe these assumptions about sickness and health, and the social structures that correspond to them, among the primitive peoples of today is hard to say. Modern civilization and medicine have left their impact in every part of the world. Primitive peoples, too, change over time.

Ancient cultures

Precursors to medical systems and theories of disease were found in the ancient cultures of Mesopotamia and Egypt between the fourth millennium B.C.E. and the first, which established connections between concepts of nature and religion, on the one hand, and views of sickness and health on the other. Parallels between Chinese, Tibetan, Indian, and Greek perceptions of sickness and health indicate that these cultures may have derived these ideas from the same sources. Ancient American cultures also shared similar perceptions.

For these cultures health and disease were physical as well as religious phenomena. Sickness was still associated with sin, even as empirical interpretation of health and disease began to spread. Egyptian papyri (2000–1500 B.C.E), for example, describe the courses of various diseases and categorize them according to regions of the body. The papyri list causes, symptoms, and prognoses, as well as empirical interventions. Putrefaction within the body in the form of spoiled material (*materia peccans*) caused sickness; these substances had to be removed if the patient were to be cured. The Greek historian Herodotus (5th century B.C.E.) describes monthly purifications in Egypt.

Dietetic, medicinal, and surgical interventions were used, and much attention was given to public health. The medicine of ancient cultures combined religious ritual with empirical treatment. The Babylonian Code of Hammurabi (ca. 1700 B.C.E.) contained the first list of surgical fees and penalties in the case of failure; each varied according to the social status of the patient.

The explanatory dimensions of medicine, such as symptomology, nosology, diagnosis, etiology, as well as clinical dimensions such as prognosis, therapy, and prevention, began to establish themselves in these centuries. The traditional healer became the professional doctor; specialization developed. In this era, empirical observation, causal explanation, magic, and faith coexisted in medical theory and practice.

Greece and Rome

More extensive and reliable historical sources exist for ancient Greece and Rome. The ancient Greeks (500 B.C.E.) explained health and disease cosmologically and anthropologically, that is, in close relation to nature in general and to human nature in particular. Medicine sought not only to cure disease, but also to maintain health. The pre-Socratic philosophers, who were the physicians of this time, developed a universal model of health, whose outlines can be found in the medical texts of Hippocrates (ca. 460–ca. 375 B.C.E.) and other physicians of the Corpus Hippocraticum (400 B.C.E.–200 C.E.). These pre-Socratic physicians must be distinguished from magicoreligious healers, who still existed at that time (Kudlien, 1968).

The great physician Galen (130–199 C.E.) elaborated a model of health and disease as a structure of elements, qualities, humors, organs, temperaments, times of day, and times of year (Schöner, 1964). Health was understood in this perspective to be a condition of harmony or balance (*isonomia*) among these basic components that make up both nature in general and the individual body. Disease, on the other hand, was regarded as discordance, or the inappropriate dominance (*monarchia*) of one of the basic components. Disease in the perspective of humoral (pathology determined by bodily fluids) was interpreted as the disproportion (*dyscrasia*) of bodily fluids or humors: phlegm, blood, and yellow and black bile. Solidistic pathology traced disease to disturbances among the solid components of the body (shape, consistency, distance, etc.). The pneumapathological (spirit) approach attributed disease to a failed relationship between body and soul. Health (*eucrasia*) was characterized by equilibrium in the body.

Dietetics was considered of primary importance to the therapeutic process, followed by medication and lastly by surgery, a hierarchy exactly opposite to ours today. In the ancient perspective, dietetics involved much more than a health-conscious regulation of food and drink. Rather, it entailed a broad concept of how one should live a healthy life. It was concerned with six aspects of life that, although natural, did not regulate themselves, as did such physiological functions as respiration and digestion. Because they required human manipulation, these six aspects of life were called "nonnatural" (*sex res non naturales*). These areas included how humans deal with (1) air and light; (2) food and drink; (3) sleep; (4) motion and rest; (5) secretions; and (6) passions of the mind (Rather, 1968).

According to Galen, and in contrast to contemporary views, health and sickness were not the only states of existence. Rather, there was a third condition, an intermediate state of "neutrality" that existed between health and sickness: Medicine was therefore conceived as the science of health, sickness, and neutrality. In this notion of medicine, the overcoming of sickness was secondary to the preservation of good health or the aid of living with impediments and handicaps. Galen said that since both in time and in esteem health precedes illness, we should try first to preserve health and only second to cure the illness as far as possible.

Philosophy and medicine mutually influenced one another in antiquity, although Hippocrates is said to have separated medicine from philosophy. Health and disease are not only empirical descriptions. They always have philosophical implications and practical effects. Plato (ca. 428–ca. 348 B.C.E.) defined medicine as the theory of health, and in the perspective of his ethical concept of health, he legitimized the active euthanasia of the physically handicapped and the mentally ill. Plato and Aristotle (384–322 B.C.E.) developed a typology of three physicians with corresponding types of relationship with the patient. The "slave doctor" commands, and the patient has to obey; the "doctor for freemen" explains

the treatment to the patient and the patient's family. The doctor understood as "medically educated layman" signifies the individual who takes responsibility for his or her own health, sickness, and death.

While abortion and active euthanasia were forbidden as therapeutic acts for the Hippocratic physician, the Stoics justified these practices in situations where the patient had lost or was in danger of losing moral autonomy and rational awareness. Harmony of the mind was placed above health and disease, above wealth and poverty. For the Stoic philosopher Seneca (4 B.C.E.–40 C.E.), disease meant physical pain (*dolor corporis*), the suspension of joy (*intermissio voluptatum*), and the fear of death (*metus mortis*); i.e., disease combines physical, psychological, social, and mental dimensions. While being persecuted by Nero, Seneca ended his own life through active euthanasia with the help of his friend and doctor Statius Annaeus.

The Middle Ages

The Christian Middle Ages (500–1300) interpreted health and sickness in a theological perspective. Cosmological (or natural) and anthropological (or human) approaches were subordinated to, without being supplanted by, the supernatural notion of transcendence. Christian beliefs and natural causes for health and disease were not mutually exclusive. Sicknesses could be described simultaneously as physical entities and as acts of God's intervention. The Christian, Arabic, and Jewish traditions all viewed health or "quality of life" as the outcome of a good relationship with God.

Medicine consisted of theory and practice, each of which was further divided. Medical practice consisted of dietetics, medicaments, and surgery. Galen's humoral pathology prevailed throughout the Middle Ages, and dietetics in antiquity's broad sense of the term continued to function as the most important form of treatment. The emphasis on spirituality did not run counter to medical aid and health education. As the vessel of the soul, the body warranted careful attention.

During the Middle Ages, a variety of specific health rules (*Regimina sanitatis*) were developed for people of various ages, occupations, and classes, as well as for both sexes. One famous example, the *Regimen Sanitatis Salernitanum* from the thirteenth century, has survived in various medical customs, and was published in all major European languages.

According to the medieval Christian viewpoint, the figure of Christ as healer (*Christus medicus*) stood behind every doctor, and behind every patient was the figure of the suffering Christ. Health, disease, and healing gained their meaning from this perspective: They were related intimately to the idea of salvation history, seen as a progression of the world starting with its establishment in paradise (*constitutio*), through its earthly existence (*destitutio*), and finally to resurrection (*restitutio*).

These concepts also had their practical consequences, manifested in biographies and other documents of arts and literature. Each transition from health to sickness and from sickness to health represented this eschatological process on an individual level. Even though sickness, suffering, and death had salvific significance or were essential traits of human life, they were fought with dietetics and medical therapy. But they were also to be accepted, for earthly life is different from paradise. In this regard, Saint Augustine (345–430) remarked that we have to say yes to some forms of pain but are not forced to love them.

The Graeco-Roman link between health, beauty, and morality was abandoned during the Middle Ages. Every sick, suffering, or handicapped individual had the right to receive medical treatment. Hospitals, first founded during the Middle Ages, were open to all suffering and helpless people, based on Jesus' words: "I was sick, and you cared for me" (Matthew 25:26). At the same time, however, the Bible was used to justify excluding lepers from society.

The classical and Christian concept of the seven cardinal virtues (prudence, temperance, fortitude, justice, faith, hope, and love) applied to healthy people as well as to the sick, doctors, and the community. Suicide and euthanasia were regarded as sins because they were deliberate attempts to shorten life. Therefore the ancient Hippocratic Oath was continuously accepted in this epoch. The art of dying (*ars moriendi*) was considered a central part of the art of living (*ars vivendi*). Sickness could be traced to inherited sin, personal guilt, demonic possession, or a test from God. Job of the Old Testament represented a classic example of this sort of test by God.

In contrast to present-day attitudes, health was also viewed as negative in the moral and religious sense ("corrupting health": *sanitas perniciosa*) and sickness as positive ("a healing sickness": *infirmitas salubris*). Coping with illness was believed to manifest a person's fortitude; furthermore, a life without physical or psychical damage or pain was thought to produce a false image of earthly life and the human condition. A contemporary biographer, writing about the constant illness of the saintly abbess Hildegard of Bingen (1098–1179), who was also a prominent naturalist and physician, said that her whole life could be compared to a "precious dying."

The modern era

With the coming of the modern era at the time of the Renaissance (1300), an emphasis on this world, nature, and the individual replaced the medieval focus on the hereafter. The secularization of paradise—or the hope of realizing beauty, youth, and health in an earthly life—has influenced human thought and action and the course of medicine up to the present. Empirical observation, causal explanation, and rational therapy became the ideals of education, research, and practice in medicine. However, magic, astrology, and alchemy continued to play a role in medicine for quite some time.

At the transition from the Middle Ages to the modern era, the physician and philosopher Paracelsus (1493–1541) designed an all-encompassing system of medicine. Along with philosophy, astronomy, and alchemy, ethics acquired a fundamental role. Paracelsus replaced the ancient humoral pathology with three rudiments from alchemy: salt, mercury, and sulphur. Dominance of one of these biochemical components over the others led to different types of diseases. Disturbances in the spiritual principle also led to disease. According to Paracelsus, the general factors that contributed to disease belonged to nature as well as culture: (1) cosmic influences (*ens astorum*); (2) material influences (*ens veneni*); and (3) individual constitution (*ens naturale*), spirit (*ens spirituale*), and God (*ens Dei*). Paracelsus's concept of disease is ontological or essentialistic: Disease is a "thing," which he compared with a parasite, a separate organism. This notion contrasts with the Hippocratic concept, which explained sickness as an individual, symptomatic phenomenon.

The utopian writings of Thomas More (1478–1535), Francis Bacon (1561–1626), and Tommaso Campanella (1568–1639) include basic categories for determining health and disease as well as guiding principles for eugenic public health policies. Their concepts justified suicide and euthanasia—but only under the condition that it be done freely (at the decision of the individual). During the Renaissance the different types of euthanasia, still relevant in the discussions of the subject today, were already established. Not everyone supported active euthanasia as a social reaction to sickness. The theologian Johann Valentin Andreae (1586–1654), unlike More and Bacon, expressly rejected euthanasia in his work *Christianopolis* (1619). He stated that "reason commands that human society should be more gently disposed toward those who have been less kindly treated by nature" (Andreae, 1916, p. 274).

The philosophy of René Descartes (1596–1650) with its mechanical model of health and disease became highly important for the concepts of disease and therapy. According to Descartes, the body is a perfect clockwork mechanism set in motion by God to function mechanically. The soul, also divinely created, acts independently from the body. This dualistic system of body (*res extensa*) and soul (*res cogitans*) was widely accepted in medicine, and produced a mechanistic view of physiology, still accepted in the present, that existed also in lay interpretations of health and disease. Scientific explanation concerned the discovery of the fixed rules of mechanistic structures and their processes. Clinical medicine concerned the detection of damaged structure, malfunction, and departure from these rules, and restoration of proper anatomic structures and physiology.

During the Enlightenment (eighteenth century), the real beginnings of a public-health movement began to take shape. The philosopher Gottfried Wilhelm Leibniz (1646–1716) made numerous recommendations for public health. A characteristic phrase of that time was formulated by Benjamin Franklin (1706–1790): "Health is wealth." The physician Johann Peter Frank (1775–1821) and the philosopher Jean-Jacques Rousseau (1712–1778) represented the opposition between state policies and individual agendas. According to Rousseau, civilization and the state had ruined human health in its natural state. Frank, in contrast, believed that social reforms lead to progress. Several books were published primarily on prevention and rehabilitation. Christoph Wilhelm Hufeland (1762–1836), author of the widespread *Makrobiotik* (1797), manifested again the relationship between concepts of health and disease—especially as normative categories—with therapy and society in its attitudes and reactions. He believed that physicians should not be allowed to engage in active euthanasia, pointing out that physicians who start to decide which sick persons are worthy of living become "the most dangerous people in the state."

The concepts of health and disease vacillate between anatomy and physiology. John Brown's (1735–1788) definitions of disease and health received great recognition in medicine, philosophy, and literature of his time. His 1780 work *Elementa Medicinae* defined health and disease in terms of the relationship of opposing forces within a person: of organic excitability and external and internal stimuli, resulting in an excited or irritated condition of the organism. According to Brown, disease is the result of overstimulation (*sthenie*) or insufficient stimulation (*asthenie*). Health, on the other hand, is characterized by equilibrium between the capacity to be stimulated, and internal and external stimuli. Treatment, therefore, functioned either to strengthen or subdue stimuli. Bloodletting and diet calmed a condition of overstimulation, whereas ether, camphor, and opium had the opposite effect. Equally important for the further progress of medicine was the anatomical foundation of pathology by Giovanni Battista Morgagni (1682–1771) with his fundamental work *De sedibus et causis morborum* (*On the Seats and Causes of Disease*), published in 1761.

Romanticism and idealism, around 1800, introduced interpretations of health, disease, and death that are of general importance and transcend substantially the limits of medicine (Leibbrand, 1956). These three states were regarded as dialectically connected with one another and interpreted as the main stages of the genesis of Spirit out of nature, a Hegelian theme (Engelhardt, 1984). According to Novalis, or Friedrich von Hardenberg (1772–1801), there is always disease in health and health in disease; illness or sickness is given a central value: "Medicine should be an elementary science of every cultivated person" (Novalis, 1981, p. 474). Illness can be an experience or medium of personal growth. The personhood of the patient becomes a central claim: "Human being = person; that is the point of unity," categorically announced the physician Johann Heinroth (1773–1843). The philosopher Joseph Schelling (1775–1854) held that health is the harmonious relationship of the basic organic functions of sensibility, irritability, and reproduction. The philosopher Georg Hegel (1770–1831) argued that life would be impossible without disease; each organism contains the "germ of death" from birth, all therapy presupposes that disease is not a total loss of health but rather a conflict within physical or psychical forces. Only through disease and death of the individual does the universal and eternal world of the spirit come into being. "Above this death of Nature, from this dead husk, proceeds a more beautiful Nature, proceeds Spirit" (Hegel, 1970, p. 443).

Medicine and the natural sciences. Medicine in the remainder of the nineteenth century followed the model of the natural sciences and not of natural philosophy and philosophical anthropology of the romantic-idealistic era.

This increasingly self-conscious scientific medicine concentrated on curing disease, and neglected the maintenance of good health. It also neglected the contributions of the arts, literature, and theology. The patient became more and more an object. His subjectivity or personality was disregarded, and the history of the patient was reduced to the history of the disease. Anatomy and physiology were connected; the cell replaced tissue as the center of attention. Experimentation, statistics, and causal thinking became the basis for medical research. A Cartesian concern for mechanistic structure and function according to discernible rules became paramount.

Rudolf Virchow's (1821–1902) definition of disease was widely accepted: "Disease begins at that moment when the regulatory system of the body is not sufficient to overcome a disturbance. It is not life under abnormal circumstances, nor the disturbance as such which produces a disease, rather the disease begins with the insufficiency of regulatory mechanism" (Virchow, 1869, p. 193). According to Virchow, the body's regulatory ability varied from person to person. The healthy body is capable of bringing an abnormal situation back into equilibrium. Disease was an observable phenomenon in the living body, caused by internal and external factors. The cell became the basis of disease, and—using a political metaphor—it deserves recognition, along with blood and nerves, as the "third estate." The infection of cells, and thus the body, by external infectious agents became the dominant explanation of disease. The clinical response was to eradicate the infection.

In the nineteenth century, dietetics lost its broader or anthropological meaning, and came to refer simply to the intake of food and drink. Thus a 2000-year-old tradition, already limited in the eighteenth century, reached its end. However, the tradition of dietetics survived longer in the area of hygiene than in pathology. Scientific medicine in its modern form considered heredity, psychical, and social factors relatively unimportant to the etiology of disease. Infection was the decisive explanatory factor; therapeutic results from the period substantiated their theory. Thus, the development of concepts of health and disease and of clinical responses to them was synergistic, a historical process that continues into the present.

At the beginning of the twentieth century, constitutional pathology and anthropological medicine began to counteract the one-sided approach of infectious disease modules of medicine. Medicine recovered the importance of the individual and social circumstances in health and disease—constitutional pathology on the physical level, anthropological medicine on the psychical or mental level. Human beings were conceived as participating in nature as well as in culture. The physician Viktor von Weizsäcker (1886–1957) reintroduced in his anthropological medicine "the person as subject," in regard to the patient, the doctor, and science (1951).

In medicine as well as in biology, the concept of finality (causa finalis) regained attention; diseases have not only a physical cause (causa efficiens) but manifest also sense of meaning. The controversy between monocausal thinking ("causalism") and multifactorial thinking ("conditionalism") influenced medicine during those decades around 1900 and is still lively: Can disease be deduced from one cause or is it necessary to take different causes of different areas of reality into consideration? The concept of cause not only has consequences for the theory of disease origin and disease process, but also affects medical therapy, prevention, and rehabilitation, all of which in turn shape the individual and social situation of the sick person.

Philosophers and theologians, as well as writers and artists, hoping to give people assistance the natural sciences and medicine were unable to provide, continued to produce valuable interpretations of health and disease that took the spiritual or cultural nature of human experience into account, problematizing the established normative equation of health as positive and disease as negative. The writer Marcel Proust (1871–1922) states that humankind owes its major cultural accomplishments to sick and suffering people: "They alone founded

religions and created masterpieces" (Proust, 1975, p. 405). Increasingly, arts and literature have been acknowledged as helpful in coping with disease, pain, and death.

The philosopher Martin Heidegger (1889–1976) claimed that he wrote his analysis of death in Being and Time especially for doctors; only the human has the consciousness of death and of his own death. The physician and philosopher Karl Jaspers (1888–1969) defined disease and health in the perspective of his philosophical position. Neurosis being "a failure in the marginal situations (Grenzsituationen) of life," he visualizes the goal of its therapy "as a self-realisation or as a self-transformation of the individual through the marginal situation, in which he is revealed to himself and affirms himself in the world as it is" (Jaspers, 1973). Jaspers views psychiatry as sharing two major methodologies: that of "explanation," which characterizes the natural sciences (disease), and that of "understanding," which is typical of the human sciences (illness). The ethical and practical consequence of his concept of disease in the objective, subjective, and cultural sense is outlined in his concept of the existential communication between the physician and the patient. Existential communication combines the subjective and cultural dimensions in an ethical perspective.

In the twentieth century, psychology and sociology expanded the scientific understanding of health and disease, emphasizing the difference between "disease" as objective and physical, and "illness" and "sickness" as subjective and social. According to this general perspective, contemporary people associate disease with the following interpretations: (1) challenge; (2) enemy; (3) punishment; (4) weakness; (5) relief; (6) strategy; (7) loss or damage; and (8) value (Lipowski, 1970). Medicine concentrates on weakness, loss, and damage, i.e., the physical components of this model.

In the sociological perspective the role of the sick person is characterized by: (1) freedom from daily duties, (2) freedom from the responsibility for the sick condition, (3) the obligation to want to become well again, and (4) the obligation to seek medical help (Parsons, 1973; Schaefer, 1976). Descriptive and normative aspects permeate this sociological definition of the role of the sick person. Disease is not only described in its social causes and consequences; demands and expectations are formulated. Recent studies revealed further processes of different levels (age, sex, socioeconomic state, type of diseases, etc.) of defining a person as sick. Also important are the differentiation between "bad" and "ill," or criminal behavior and sickness, and the negative or stigmatizing consequences of diagnostic acts.

The 1947 World Health Organization definition of health—"a state of complete physical, mental, and social wellbeing and not merely the absence of disease or infirmity"—has to be interpreted in its social and political context and purposes. These included attempts to justify international involvement in the internal affairs of countries. Whether medicine could offer explanations and therapies to achieve "complete," multifunctional wellbeing is another matter. This definition includes social and spiritual as well as medical aspects. It was used as the starting-point for intense bioethical debates, on the moral and political responsibilities of the international community for health care—especially for corresponding projects in developing countries. But this definition, taken generally, is limited in its sharp contrast between health and disease and its exaggerated estimation of health. With good reason, health can also be regarded as the ability to bear injury, handicaps, and the anticipation of death, and to successfully integrate them into one's life. Integration is the capacity to cope with death; death is a part of life and not only its contrary or end.

The history of concepts of health and disease is the history of concepts that explain and direct response to disease, illness, sickness, and health. These concepts are deeply rooted in physical and psychical experiences and have medical and social consequences. The importance of scientific explanations, with their roots in Cartesian medicine and developments in the nineteenth century is obvious. Of equal importance, perhaps, are attempts to counterbalance an excessive emphasis on scientific medicine with anthropologic, social, ethical, and political dimensions of the concepts of health and disease. After all, for much of its history medicine has not been confined solely to disease but also took responsibility for health. Therapy in the past meant more than just curing; it also meant prevention or preservation of health and assistance in chronic disease and in dying. Disease was interpreted as a disturbance of the organism, the sick person and his or her social situation. Furthermore, medicine did not have sole domain over health and disease; a multitude of important interpretations originated from the arts, theology, and philosophy. In this holistic perspective people of the present also expect medical and social aid.

Sickness and health, in their natural and cultural breadth, remind medicine of its fundamentally scientific and humanistic nature. Health and disease are concerned with life and death, and are closely connected to the physical, social, psychic, and spiritual nature of humans.

Today, disease and health are conceived as more closely connected (Canguilhem, 1984; Engel, 1960). The transitions and parallels are seen more strongly, and the interplay of the body, soul, spirit, and environment is more carefully observed. Attention is shifting from infectious diseases to chronic illness and death, though the experience of the acquired immunodeficiency syndrome (AIDS) and other diseases proves the continuity of those events. The emergence of molecular medicine, with its reliance on genetic concepts of health and disease, may lead to a reintegration of the scientific and humanistic dimensions of the concepts of health and disease. The global scientific as well as economic limitations of medicine have made the concepts of health and disease a central topic in theory as well as in practice, for science as well as for everyday life.

Developing countries have special problems to overcome that stem from their own cultural changes as well as their reception of Western medicine. The Western world must be critical of its own normative position in regard to these developing countries as in regard to its own concept of life. Disease should not be understood merely as a limitation or a loss, but also as a challenge. Coping with illness can manifest courage and compassion; meeting this challenge strengthens self-confidence, causes social reform, and enriches the world of culture.

DIETRICH VON ENGELHARDT

Directly related to this article are the other articles in this entry: SOCIOLOGICAL PERSPECTIVES, ANTHROPOLOGICAL PERSPECTIVES, PHILOSOPHICAL PERSPECTIVES, *and* THE EXPERIENCE OF HEALTH AND ILLNESS. *Also directly related are the entries* PROFESSIONAL–PATIENT RELATIONSHIP, *article on* HISTORICAL PERSPECTIVES; BODY, *articles on* EMBODIMENT: THE PHENOMENOLOGICAL TRADITION, *and* SOCIAL THEORIES; *and* DISABILITY, *articles on* ATTITUDES AND SOCIOLOGICAL PERSPECTIVES, *and* PHILOSOPHICAL AND THEOLOGICAL PERSPECTIVES. *For a discussion of related ideas, see the entries* BIOLOGY, PHILOSOPHY OF; DEATH, ATTITUDES TOWARD; GENDER IDENTITY AND GENDER-IDENTITY DISORDERS; GENETICS AND HUMAN SELF-UNDERSTANDING; INTERPRETATION; LIFE, QUALITY OF, *article on* QUALITY OF LIFE IN CLINICAL DECISIONS; MEDICINE, SOCIOLOGY OF; PAIN AND SUFFERING; *and* VALUE AND VALUATION.

Bibliography

ANDREAE, JOHANN VALENTIN. 1916. *Christianopolis.* Edited and translated by Felix Emil Held. New York: Oxford University Press.

CANGUILHEM, GEORGES. 1984. *Le normal et le pathologique.* 5th ed. Paris: Presses universitaires de Paris.

CLEMENTS, FOREST EDWARD. 1932. "Primitive Concepts of Disease." *American Archeology and Ethnology* 32:185–243.

DIEPGEN, PAUL; GRUBER, GEORGE B.; and SCHADEWALDT, HANS. 1969. "Der Krankheitsbegriff, seine Geschichte und Problematik." In *Handbuch der Allgemeinen Pathologie,* vol. 1, pp. 1–50. Edited by Franz Büchner. Berlin: Springer-Verlag.

ENGEL, GEORGE L. 1960. "A Unified Concept of Health and Disease." *Perspectives in Biology and Medicine* 3, no. 4: 459–485.

ENGELHARDT, DIETRICH VON. 1984. "Der metaphysische Krankheitsbegriff des Deutschen Idealismus. Schellings und Hegels naturphilosophische Grundlegung." In *Medizinische Anthropologie*, pp. 17–31. Edited by Eduard Seidler. Berlin: Springer-Verlag.

HEGEL, GEORG WILHELM FRIEDRICH. 1970. *Philosophy of Nature*. Oxford: At the Clarendon Press.

JASPERS, KARL. 1973. [1913]. "Die Begriffe Gesundheit und Krankheit." In *Allgemeine Psychopathologie*, 9th ed., pp. 651–711. Berlin: Springer-Verlag.

KUDLIEN, FRIDOLF. 1968. "Early Greek Primitive Medicine." *Clio Medica* 3, no. 4:305–336.

LEIBBRAND, WERNER. 1956. *Die spekulative Medizin der Romantik*. Hamburg: Classen.

LIPOWSKI, ZBIGNIEW JERZY. 1970. "Physical Illness, the Individual and the Coping Processes." *Psychiatry in Medicine* 1, no. 2:91–102.

NOVALIS. 1981. *Schritten*. Vol. 3. Darmstadt: Wissenschaftliche Buchgesellschaft.

PARSONS, TALCOTT. 1973. "Definition von Gesundheit und Krankheit im Lichte der Wertbegriffe und der sozialen Struktur Amerikas." In *Der Kranke in der modernen Gesellschaft*, 4th ed., pp. 57–87. Edited by Alexander Mitscherlich, Tobias Bruchner, Otto von Mening, and Klaus Horn. Cologne: Klepenheuer & Witsch.

PROUST, MARCEL. 1975. *Auf der Suche nach der verlorenen Zeit*. Frankfort: Suhrkampf.

RATHER, LELLAND J. 1968. "The 'Six Things Non-Natural': A Note on the Origins and Fate of a Doctrine and Phrase." *Clio Medica* 3, no. 4:337–347.

RIESE, WALTHER. 1953. *The Conception of Disease: Its History, Its Versions and Its Nature*. New York: Philosophical Library.

RISSE, GÜNTER B. "Health and Disease. I. History of the Concepts." In *Encyclopedia of Bioethics*, pp. 579–585. Edited by Warren T. Reich. New York: Macmillan.

ROTHSCHUH, KARL ERNST, ed. 1975. *Was ist Krankheit? Erscheinung, Erklärung, Sinngebung*. Darmstadt: Wissenschaftliche Buchgesellschaft.

SCHAEFER, HANS. 1976. "Der Krankheitsbegriff." In *Handbuch der Sozialmedizin*, pp. 15–31. Edited by Maria Blohmke, Christian von Ferber, Karl Peter Kisker, and H. Schaefer. Stuttgart: Erike.

SCHIPPERGES, HEINRICH; SEIDLER, EDUARD; and UNSCHULD, U. PAUL, eds. 1978. *Krankheit, Heilkunst, Heilung*. Freiburg: Alber.

SCHÖNER, ERICH. 1964. *Das Viererschema der antiken Humoralpathologie*. Wiesbaden: Steiner.

TEMKIN, OWSEI. 1973. "Health and Disease." In *Dictionary of the History of Ideas*, vol. 2, pp. 395–407. Edited by Philip P. Wiener. New York: Charles Scribner's Sons.

VIRCHOW, RUDOLF. 1869. "Über die heutige Stellung der Pathologie." *Tageblatt der 43. Versammlung deutscher Naturforscher und Ärzte*:185–195.

WEIZSÄCKER, VIKTOR VON. 1951. *Der kranke Mensch. Einführung in die medizinische Anthropologie*. Stuttgart: Koehler.

II. SOCIOLOGICAL PERSPECTIVES

The sociology of health and disease has two distinct traditions, each with somewhat different implications for the field of bioethics. The first tradition is socioepidemiologic in nature, which is to say it focuses on understanding how the distribution of death and illness is influenced by such factors as age, gender, race, and social class. The second tradition is oriented to the doctor–patient relationship and is concerned with the meanings of illness for patients and practitioners, and with how these meanings reflect the nature of power and authority in the society.

The social epidemiology of illness

Origins. Origins are, of course, difficult to track with precision, but sociological perspectives on health and disease can be traced to the French sociologist Emile Durkheim's classic treatise, *Suicide* (1951). In this work, Durkheim looks at the impact on the suicide rate of such variables as residence (urban or rural), marital status, and religious affiliation.

Durkheim's basic assumption is that if suicide were purely an individual phenomenon, these variables would have no impact on group rates. Using public-health statistics, Durkheim finds that the suicide rate is higher among urban dwellers than among those who live in rural areas, the rate of the unmarried exceeds that of the married, and that of Protestants exceeds that of Catholics. The theory that he develops to explain these results is that social ties linking individuals to society inhibit suicidal impulses, while the absence of such ties does not. Much subsequent socioepidemiology of illness echoes Durkheim's findings that those with a greater stake in society fare better than those with a lesser stake.

Since Durkheim, sociologists have dedicated themselves to showing that who becomes ill is not just a matter of individual constitutions but is heavily influenced by the standard variables of sociological explanation—gender, race, and class.

Gender. Despite their greater life expectancies, women report more morbidity and utilize health services more frequently than do men (Verbrugge, 1989). Explanations advanced for the higher rates of illness among women include less satisfying, more conflictual social and economic roles; greater stress; more cultural permission for reporting discomfort; and biological differences.

Class. The relationship between class and mortality and morbidity is well documented. At all age levels in the United States, there is an inverse relationship between morbidity and social class (Syme and Berkman, 1976). This means that as class standing increases, the prevalence of illness decreases or, conversely, as class standing decreases, the prevalence of illness increases.

Similar relationships have been demonstrated for other countries in the industrialized West.

Although the link between social class and the prevalence of illness is not disputed, the reasons for it are. A number of competing and complementary explanations have been advanced to account for this relationship, including lack of access to health-care resources; lifestyle (there is an inverse relationship between obesity, as well as tobacco and alcohol consumption, and social class); and increased exposure to economic and social stress. Work has been indicted as a causal factor in the relationship between social class and heart disease (Siegrist et al., 1986; Marmot and Theorell, 1988). Lower-class jobs provide less autonomy, more constraint, and less opportunity for expression than more middle-class occupations. In addition, the causal direction of the link between class and illness has been questioned, with some analysts suggesting that since the less well are unable to compete in the economic system, they have their class standing lowered as a result. This is known as the "downward drift hypothesis."

Race. Race is another variable that affects mortality and morbidity. Vincente Navarro argues that once class is taken into account, differentials between whites and blacks disappear (1991). This may be so, but at a pragmatic level there is a very real association of urban poverty and race. This association accounts for morbidity and mortality associated with violence, infant mortality, and HIV infection associated with intravenous drug use and prostitution. The problems of the urban poor in gaining access to health-care services such as adequate prenatal care have also been well documented. Compliance with treatment regimens (e.g., hypertension medications) is an issue for inner-city populations—the most common explanation usually being the cultural distance between providers and patients.

Stress. Stress has been used as a variable to explain relationships among gender, social class, race, and illness. Stress seems to better account for variations in rates of mental rather than physical illness (Lin and Ensel, 1989). Despite the widespread agreement on how to measure it, there is nonetheless some confusion about what stress is. There is also widespread agreement that social supports and networks buffer stress but there is some confusion about exactly how (Kessler et al., 1985). Moreover, stress does not have an equal impact on men and women. Marriage, for example, buffers stress better for men than for women.

Social epidemiology and bioethics

The social epidemiology of illness demonstrates that sickness does not fall alike upon rich and poor, men and women, black and white. Distributional inequities are more than simple political and economic problems. They have an ethical dimension as well.

Bioethicists will need to pay greater attention in the future than they have in the past to issues of justice and equity at a political level—to the ethical dimensions of political decisions. As the allocation of scarce resources becomes a public issue of greater salience, the underserved will need advocates. The championing of individual patient rights that marked bedside bioethics in its formative years may be extended to the class of uninsured and underinsured patients as health care grows in importance on the national political agenda.

As its scope of inquiry and moral concerns expands, bioethics may have the opportunity to play a greater role in policy making. Bioethics has taken philosophers from the ivory tower to the bedside (Rothman, 1991); the next arena of problems promises to extend their horizons from bedside to the legislature. However, there is a danger here as well. So long as bioethics is focused on the bedside, both its subject matter and the texts appropriate to it are limited. Once the links between class, race, gender, and illness are illuminated, the boundaries of bioethics become murky. The doctor–patient relationship may be fraught with moral complexity, but it is a rather neatly defined, bounded whole. This is not so for the entire distributive system of society. Moreover, as the link between lifestyle and illness becomes more firmly established, there is an implicit challenge to autonomy as a fundamental value in bioethics.

The social construction of illness

The second tradition in the sociology of illness is less concerned with the distribution of illness by race, class, and gender and more concerned with the social meanings attached to illness. It is more concerned with the roles of health-care provider and patient and with what these roles say about the distribution of power and authority in society. The social epidemiological tradition is involved in the analysis of large data sets such as national samples for structural regularities expressed in statistical terms as correlations between health status and a social trait such as gender, class, or race. The social constructionist approach is more likely to involve first-hand observation of behavior in a limited number of settings. These observations of behavior then provide a basis for drawing conclusions about the nature of health care more generally. Favored themes in the social constructionist approach include the management of uncertainty, the difficulties of lay–professional communication, and the use and misuse of professional authority.

The sick role. Sociological speculation about the nature of the doctor–patient relationship begins with Talcott Parsons's discussion of the sick role (1951).

Although Parsons's unique insight is so commonplace today that we do not appreciate its originality, he was among the first to focus on the doctor–patient dyad as a role relationship with a set of reciprocal rights, duties, and obligations.

Parsons begins with a discussion of the basic social situation in which patients and physicians find themselves. Patients are not to blame for their condition, are powerless, and are technically incompetent. Physicians' existential position is one beset with uncertainty about what ails the patient and how to treat it best, impotence to cure so many of the ills of patients, and unusual access to both patients' bodies and the intimate details of their lives.

Each role consists of four interlocking imperatives that grow out of the social assumptions made about each actor. The patient is granted a temporary exemption from normal social responsibilities. He or she is not expected to carry on as usual while sick. In exchange for this exemption, the patient must seek technically competent help, must be motivated to get well, and must comply with treatment regimens. The passivity of the patient stems from what has been called the power asymmetry, which Parsons says characterizes the relation of doctor and patient. The only positive action Parsons ascribes to the patient is to seek help. By imposing help-seeking from a technically competent other as a role obligation, Parsons ignores the complexities of help-seeking behaviors. Such complexities include the recognition of a condition as "illness"; of the cultural and economic barriers to access; and of the nature of lay networks. In addition, with his stricture on technically competent help, Parsons invalidates any and all alternatives to allopathic medicine.

Physicians, according to Parsons, occupy roles whose demands are dictated by their existential situation. First, physicians achieve their roles by mastering basic areas of knowledge. Some physicians are smarter than others, some know more; but all have completed the same core medical curriculum and passed the same tests. Parsons calls this "universal achievement." Second, physicians limit their ministrations to areas of competence. They are expert in areas of health and illness, and their advice is limited to these areas. Parsons identifies this as "functional specificity." The limits of functional specificity have widened as the links among lifestyle, stress, and illness have been documented. Nonetheless, there are limits. Next, in their work physicians maintain an attitude of affective neutrality. Renée Fox and Harold Lief (1963) identify this as "detached concern." Physicians are involved with the problems of their patients but not so involved as to interfere with rational decision making. Finally, physicians act from a stance that Parsons identifies as "collective neutrality." The physician is not guided, as the ordinary commercial actor is, by self-interest or the profit motive. Rather, physicians' actions are guided by altruism, by what will restore health, whatever the sacrifice or cost to the physician, patient, or collectivity.

Parsons's analysis describes normative patterns rather than empirical occurrences. His physicians live in a world in which they share values with patients and always act in the best interests of the patient. At the same time, his physicians act as agents of social control. The physician provides legitimate excuses from work, directs treatment, and controls access to healing resources. Tension may arise because the interests of the social system in social control and of the patient may not coincide.

The social construction of illness.   Parsons's "sick role" is the first sociological theory to recognize that the experience of illness is determined by social factors. Many sociologists accept Parsons's basic insights but differ with him on exactly how the experience of illness is shaped by values and beliefs that are implicit, tacit, unexamined, and variable across cultural groupings. Conflict theorists, for example, emphasize that society is made up of competing groups with different values rather than, as Parsons argued, cooperating groups with shared values (Freidson, 1970). For these sociologists, the physician's role as a fiduciary whose actions express the interests of patients is disputed; the physician is seen instead as a "moral entrepreneur" who cloaks in a neutral scientific language either his or her self-interest or the interests of his or her social class.

Conflict or "labeling" theorists share with Parsons the understanding that physicians act as agents of social control; they differ about who benefits from these gatekeeping activities and what the consequences of these activities are. For Parsons, the physician's actions certifying illness serve the entire society by promoting an environment in which the individual designated "sick" can later return to productive social and economic roles. There are no long-term consequences to the labeling of individuals.

Labeling, the labeling theorists contend, is used by the dominant classes to protect their interests, suppress the less fortunate, and reinforce established hierarchies (Becker, 1963; Freidson, 1970). Casting an individual in the sick role stigmatizes him or her and spoils life chances (Goffman, 1963; Scheff, 1966). Susan Sontag (1978) has argued that the vocabulary of illness leads those who are sick to blame themselves. Those who are vulnerable to labeling engage in a variety of social strategies to avoid it. Joseph Schneider and Peter Conrad (1980) have described how those with epilepsy, for example, attempt to stay "in the closet" with their condition rather than suffer the discrimination that attends candor.

Much of the work of labeling theorists depends on the contention that the locus of social control in the modern state has shifted. Peter Conrad and Joseph Schneider (1980) observe that our explanations of deviance now rely on madness instead of badness. The dominant agents of social control are no longer clergy but physicians. Social problems become medicalized, and the targets of therapeutic activity are more likely than not to be the socially disadvantaged. For example, in a study of Riverside, California, Jane Mercer (1973) found that the label "mentally retarded" was significantly more likely to be applied to members of minority populations.

In labeling theory a key variable of interest is social power. Labels are used to depress the social chances of the disadvantaged and are also manipulated to aid the powerful. New categories of pathology emerge that create opportunities for health-care professionals who use the newly discovered syndromes to expand their power. The social and structural conditions that generate problems remain or become invisible. For example, Stephen Pfohl (1977) views the discovery of the "battered-child syndrome" as a boon to pediatric radiologists and other pediatric professionals. The beating of children is not new; rather, its treatment as a medical problem is novel. Entire diagnostic classification systems may be viewed this way. Joel Kovel (1988) has criticized the American Psychiatric Association's *Diagnostic and Statistical Manual* (*DSM-III*), the official diagnostic system of mental-health professionals, for hiding social and political meanings in apparently neutral language. The purpose of the *DSM-III*, in this view, is to enable the psychiatric profession to control the institutions of mental health.

Individuals may actively seek some labels and avoid others, based on a calculation of the advantages or disadvantages of labeling. Tsunetsugu Munkata (1989) points out that in Japan the label "neurasthenia" is widely adopted to avoid the stigmatizing term "schizophrenia." Peter Conrad (1975) shows how both parents and school professionals embraced the label of "hyperkinesis" to describe unruly children. Parents accepted the label because it absolved them of blame for their children's conditions; school officials accepted the term because it offered an individual-level explanation for restive behavior, allowing them to overlook deficiencies in school organization. Many illness designations—ranging from "hypoglycemia" to "chronic fatigue syndrome" to "premenstrual syndrome" to "total allergy syndrome"— signify entities whose precise, objective markers of disease are unclear; sufferers, however, seek the legitimation of the disease label. Suffering is a powerful determinant of self-labeling; the proper label serves to excuse and explain behavior that would otherwise be unacceptable. The early labeling theorists concentrated on labeling as a top-down phenomenon, stressing the repressive features of labels while ignoring the benefits some labels conferred.

The fact that the powerful resist as well as discover, create, or construct disease classification should also not be overlooked. Phil Brown and Edward Mikkelsen (1990) describe how the inherently conservative bias of epidemiological methods that depend on population-based measures retarded the identification of an environmentally generated cancer cluster in Woburn, Massachusetts, a small community. In another case, scientific medicine and organized mining interests retarded the recognition of "black lung" as an occupational disease (Smith, 1981). Both cases illustrate how the alliance of organized science with corporate interests burdened and delayed eventually successful efforts to discover or construct disease or its cause.

Social construction and bioethics

Two key points of contention distinguish Parsons's theory of the sick role from labeling theory. The first point centers on the question of whether physicians have patients' interests reliably at heart. Parsons, in claiming that physicians have a "collectivity orientation," signals his confidence that they do. Labeling theorists' claim that physician altruism in interaction cloaks self-interested action suggests a distrust of physicians. This difference in attitude is very apparent in the writing from each orientation on the role uncertainty plays in medicine. From a Parsonsian orientation, uncertainty is a problem to be overcome and a psychological burden to physicians, who deploy a variety of coping strategies (Fox, 1959). From a labeling orientation, uncertainty is a ploy that physicians magnify in order to control patients (Davis, 1960).

The second key difference between Parsons and the labeling theorists concerns patient autonomy. For Parsons, the only autonomous decision made by the patient is the one to seek care. After that, patients simply—and appropriately—follow the doctor's orders. Since the physician has the patient's best interest in mind, there is no reason for the patient to balk or to question. For labeling theorists, on the contrary, there is no reason for the patient to follow medical regimes without question, since there is no guarantee that the physician has the patient's best interest in mind.

Informed consent is based on the principles of autonomy and self-determination. Sociological description of the doctor–patient relationship, whether from Parsons or from the labeling theorists, illuminates the absence of autonomy and self-determination. Sociologists differ on the necessity and value of such principles.

The earliest sociological studies of death and dying (Glaser and Strauss, 1965) described how much autonomy and self-determination were missing in the doctor–patient relationship. Physicians operated in what Barney Glaser and Anselm Strauss called a "closed awareness context." Physicians knew of fatal conditions but routinely did not pass this information to patients. Often they colluded with family members to keep this information from patients. These practices were rationalized by both physicians and family members as kinder than being candid.

Because of informed consent, a veritable revolution occurred in the doctor–patient relationship. Candor replaced evasion. With informed consent, patients are more than ever the masters of their own treatment. The paternalism that marked Parsons's description of the doctor–patient relationship has given way to a more egalitarian, more formally contractual relationship. While there is much to celebrate in these changes, it is also possible that something may have been lost. There are costs involved with a fuller patient autonomy. Under the banner of autonomy physicians may hide behind their role as technical experts and leave weighty matters to patients. There are new possibilities for the psychological abandonment of patients.

CHARLES L. BOSK

Directly related to this article are the other articles in this entry: HISTORY OF THE CONCEPTS, ANTHROPOLOGICAL PERSPECTIVES, PHILOSOPHICAL PERSPECTIVES, *and* THE EXPERIENCE OF HEALTH AND ILLNESS. *Also directly related is the entry* MEDICINE, SOCIOLOGY OF. *For a further discussion of topics mentioned in this article, see the entries* AGING AND THE AGED; AIDS; ALTERNATIVE THERAPIES; AUTHORITY; AUTONOMY; BODY; HEALING; HEALTH CARE, QUALITY OF; HEALTH-CARE RESOURCES, ALLOCATION OF; HOMICIDE; INFORMATION DISCLOSURE; INFORMED CONSENT; LIFESTYLES AND PUBLIC HEALTH; MARRIAGE AND OTHER DOMESTIC PARTNERSHIPS; OBLIGATION AND SUPEREROGATION; PATERNALISM; PATIENTS' RESPONSIBILITIES; PATIENTS' RIGHTS; PROFESSIONAL–PATIENT RELATIONSHIP; PROSTITUTION; RACE AND RACISM; RIGHTS; SELF-HELP; SEXISM; SOCIAL MEDICINE; SUBSTANCE ABUSE; SUICIDE; VALUE AND VALUATION; VIRTUE AND CHARACTER; *and* WOMEN. *For a discussion of related ideas, see the entries* ABUSE, INTERPERSONAL, *article on* CHILD ABUSE; ADVERTISING; CARE; DEATH; DEATH, ATTITUDES TOWARD; DISABILITY, *article on* ATTITUDES AND SOCIOLOGICAL PERSPECTIVES; MENTAL ILLNESS; HEALTH POLICY, *article on* POLITICS AND HEALTH CARE; *and* PUBLIC POLICY AND BIOETHICS.

Bibliography

BECKER, HOWARD S. 1963. *Outsiders: Studies in the Sociology of Deviance.* New York: Free Press.

BROWN, PHIL, and MIKKELSEN, EDWARD. 1990. *No Safe Place: Toxic Waste, Leukemia, and Community Action.* Berkeley: University of California Press.

CONRAD, PETER J. 1975. "The Discovery of Hyperkinesis: Notes on the Medicalization of Deviant Behavior." *Social Problems* 23, no. 1:12–21.

CONRAD, PETER J., and SCHNEIDER, JOSEPH W. 1980. *Deviance and Medicalization: From Badness to Sickness.* St. Louis, Mo.: Mosby.

COOPER, CARY L., and MARSHALL, JUDI. 1979. "Occupational Sources of Stress: A Review of the Literature Relating to Coronary Heart Disease and Mental Ill Health." *Journal of Occupational Psychology* 49, no. 1:11–28.

DAVIS, FRED. 1960. "Uncertainty in Medical Prognosis: Clinical and Functional." *American Journal of Sociology* 66, no. 1:41–47.

DURKHEIM, EMILE. 1951. [1897]. *Suicide: A Study in Sociology.* New York: Free Press.

FOX, RENÉE C. 1959. *Experiment Perilous: Physicians and Patients Facing the Unknown.* Glencoe, Ill.: Free Press.

FOX, RENÉE C., and LIEF, HAROLD I. 1963. "Training for Detached Concern in Medical Students." In *The Psychological Basis of Medical Practice.* Edited by Harold I. Lief, Victor Lief, and Nina Lief. New York: Harper & Row.

FREIDSON, ELIOT. 1970. *The Profession of Medicine: A Study in the Sociology of Applied Knowledge.* New York: Harper & Row.

GLASER, BARNEY G., and STRAUSS, ANSELM L. 1965. *Awareness of Dying.* Chicago: Aldine.

GOFFMAN, ERVING. 1963. *Stigma: Notes on the Management of Spoiled Identity.* Englewood Cliffs, N.J.: Prentice-Hall.

KESSLER, RONALD C.; PRICE, RICHARD H.; and WORTMAN, CAMILLE B. 1985. "Social Factors in Psychopathology: Stress, Social Support, and Coping Processes." *Annual Review of Psychology* 36:531–572.

KOVEL, JOEL. 1988. "A Critique of the DSM-III." *Research in Law, Deviance and Social Control* 9:127–146.

LIN, NAN, and ENSEL, WALTER M. 1989. "Life Stress and Health: Stressors and Resources." *American Sociological Review* 54, no. 3:382–399.

MARMOT, MICHAEL, and THEORELL, TORES. 1988. "Social Class and Cardiovascular Disease: The Contribution of Work." *International Journal of Health Services* 18, no. 4:659–674.

MERCER, JANE R. 1973. *Labeling the Mentally Retarded: Clinical and Social System Perspectives on Mental Retardation.* Berkeley: University of California Press.

MUNKATA, TSUNETSUGU. 1989. "The Socio-Cultural Significance of the Diagnostic Label 'Neurasthenia' in Japan's Mental Health Care System." *Culture, Medicine, and Psychiatry* 13, no. 2:203–213.

NAVARRO, VINCENTE. 1991. "Race or Class or Race and Class: Growing Mortality Differentials in the United States." *International Journal of Health Services* 21, no. 2:229–235.

PARSONS, TALCOTT. 1951. *The Social System.* New York: Free Press.

PFOHL, STEPHEN J. 1977. "The 'Discovery' of Child Abuse." *Social Problems* 24, no. 3:310–323.

ROTHMAN, DAVID J. 1991. *Strangers at the Bedside: A History of How Law and Bioethics Transformed Medical Decision Making.* New York: Basic Books.

SCHEFF, THOMAS J. 1966. *Being Mentally Ill: A Sociological Theory.* Chicago: Aldine.

SCHNEIDER, JOSEPH W., and CONRAD, PETER J. 1980. "In the Closet with Illness: Epilepsy, Stigma Potential and Information Control." *Social Problems* 28, no. 1:32–44.

SIEGRIST, JOHANNES; SIEGRIST, KARIN; and WEBER, INGBERT. 1986. "Sociological Concepts in the Etiology of Chronic Disease: The Case of Ischemic Heart Disease." *Social Science and Medicine* 22, no. 2:247–253.

SMITH, BARBARA. 1981. "Black Lung: The Social Production of Disease." *International Journal of Health Services* 11, no. 3:343–359.

SONTAG, SUSAN. 1978. *Illness as Metaphor.* New York: Farrar, Straus & Giroux.

SYME, S. LEONARD, and BERKMAN, LISA F. 1976. "Social Class, Susceptibility and Sickness." *American Journal of Epidemiology* 104, no. 1:1–8.

THOITS, PEGGY A. 1985. "Self-Labeling Processes in Mental Illness: The Role of Emotional Deviance." *American Journal of Sociology* 91, no. 2:221–242.

VERBRUGGE, LOIS M. 1989. "The Twain Meet: Empirical Explanations of Sex Differences in Health and Mortality." *Journal of Health and Social Behavior* 30, no. 3:282–304.

III. ANTHROPOLOGICAL PERSPECTIVES

Medical anthropologists focus on people's life worlds (the subjective experience or phenomenology of sickness and healing), their cultural systems of meaning (e.g., ideas about what causes disease and how it is diagnosed), and the material conditions in which experiences and beliefs are situated (e.g., local disease ecology). Medical anthropologists are interested in understanding and describing the medical beliefs and practices of people whose cultures and life worlds are often very different from their own. They are routinely confronted with the problem of translating unfamiliar meanings and experiences into familiar (Western) terms and concepts without tearing them out of context or subordinating them to specifically Western assumptions about sickness, health, efficacy, autonomy, and so on (Lock and Gordon, 1988; Kleinman, 1988; Gaines, 1992).

The anthropological perspective makes it possible to examine and clarify bioethical issues from multiple cultural points of view. Current debate over the bioethics of "organ harvesting"—the surgical removal of transplantable body parts such as the heart, liver, and kidneys—illustrates why it is important to have a clear understanding of cultural points of view. For transplantation to succeed, organs must be removed either (1) from a living donor, in cases where the organ is not vital to the donor's own survival (e.g., a single kidney), or (2) immediately after a donor's death, before the organs have begun to decompose. In most Western societies, the line between life and death, in the context of organ harvesting, is identified with "brain death," the irreversible loss of higher-brain functions. The decision to identify death with "brain death" is consistent with Western cultural notions: Selfhood is identified with the mind, and the mind is, by convention, located in the brain. This arrangement has the practical advantage of leaving a working heart in a harvestable body, thus facilitating the collection of transplantable organs. Japanese culture, in contrast, recognizes a different relation between selfhood and the body: The self is not identified with a single body region. From this perspective, a "brain dead" body with a functioning heart has not crossed the line from life to death, and the body is not yet a harvestable resource.

Orientations to the body

The history of medical anthropology is in no small part a history of scrutinizing and challenging Western assumptions about sickness, beginning with the distinction between biomedicine and traditional medicine. (Most medical anthropologists prefer the term "biomedicine" over the alternative terminology: "scientific," "modern," and "Western" medicine. For an explanation, see Leslie, 1976.) At first glance, the distinction appears to be a common-sense way of classifying medical systems. In practice, classification brings with it a set of problematic assumptions. First, it implies that "traditional" medical systems have something fundamental in common. In reality, so-called traditional systems are highly diverse in both their medical theories and practices, and share little as a category, other than being different from biomedicine. Some of them, notably the systems associated with classic Asian medicines—Ayurveda (Indian) and Unani (Greco-Islamic) in south Asia, and Chinese medicine farther east—have more in common with biomedicine than with the other systems in the traditional category. (For anthropologists' accounts describing the epistemologies of Asian medical systems, see Leslie and Young, 1992). A second limitation of juxtaposing "traditional" medical systems with biomedicine is its implication that "biomedicine" is a monolithic system, beyond the reach of culture. Social scientists have demonstrated significant variation in biomedical notions and clinical practices, both within communities and across cultures (Hahn and Gaines, 1985; Lock, 1993; Wright and Treacher, 1982).

A more edifying way of comparing medical systems across cultures is to start with the question, "How do the beliefs and practices of this or that medical system orient healers and patients to their bodies?" An answer from the Western perspective might be that since the body is the site of the pain and suffering that are associated with sickness, the body must be the focus of attention for patients and healers everywhere. In reality, medical systems are not equally interested in the body. Rather, these systems and their perspectives are distributed along a continuum that includes the biomedical perspective, among many others.

At one end of the continuum are the systems whose orientation to the body can be called "externalizing," in that their diagnostic and therapeutic ideas and techniques direct people's attention away from the sufferer's body. In these systems, the medical gaze looks outward, scanning networks of people and beings (ancestral spirits, possession spirits, demons, and so on) for morally significant encounters and events involving the sick person or close relatives. The diagnostic goal is to construct a useful etiology, that is, a string of circumstances and events that lead to the onset of suffering and distress, and that identify the ultimate source of the sickness. The therapist's goal in these systems is to insert himself or herself into the patient's sickness narrative and, once there, to persuade or coerce the pathogenic agents to stop afflicting the patient. The classic account of diagnosis and treatment in an externalizing system is E. E. Evans-Pritchard's *Witchcraft, Oracles and Magic Among the Azande,* published in 1937. (For commentaries on epistemological and ethical issues raised by this book, see Wilson, 1987, and Hollis and Lukes, 1982).

The sick person's body is a site of discomfort and distress and, in this sense, sickness is the same all along the continuum. At the externalizing end, however, the patient's bodily experiences and transformations are mute. Typically, the body is a black box, in that, though people may have names for certain of body parts and organs, they can posit no functions or systemic connections for them. Pain, suffering, and the visible transformations that accompany sickness and disease signify only themselves. They reveal nothing about processes and events that biomedicine knows are taking place inside. While practitioners may give patients medicaments to take, these medicines are characteristically anodynes, or substances that are intended to make the patient more comfortable while the actual cure is being pursued elsewhere. In short, in externalizing systems medical meanings and experiences are created and connected by discrete socio-logics, rather than a universal bio-logic (Lock and Gordon, 1988).

Anthropologists describe three broad types of therapeutic strategies operating in externalizing medical belief systems: *agonistic* strategies, where the goal is to eliminate or neutralize pathogenic agents; *initiatory* strategies, where the goal is to initiate the patient and pathogenic agent into a permanent and manageable relationship (e.g., Boddy, 1989); and strategies of *persuasion*, where the goal is to convince the pathogenic agent, through offerings or appeals, to cease afflicting the patient (e.g., see Lewis, 1975, for a detailed account of sickness associated with intergenerational tensions in New Guinea). Beyond these generalizations, externalizing systems are highly heterogeneous.

Biomedicine is located at the opposite end of the continuum, among the "internalizing" systems, where diagnosis and therapy orient patients and healers toward the body. Here, sickness coincides with the limits of the body, and the goal of diagnosis and therapy is to get inside the body, to take control of its internal parts and processes. Circumstances and events outside the body are interesting only to the degree that they lead to inferences about pathological processes taking place inside. It is in these systems that we find theories of pathophysiology, the grammars that enable people to read bodily changes symptomatically.

Medical efficacy

Common sense inclines us to suppose that because internalizing systems are able to read embodied symptoms, they are more empirical and realistic than externalizing systems. Ethnographic research, however, indicates that all medical systems, externalizing as well as internalizing, are generally empirical and realistic. That is, they are capable of routinely producing self-vindicating outcomes, evidence that demonstrates their efficacy. Medical efficacy can be demonstrated by two different kinds of results. First, efficacy is sometimes a capacity for producing "hoped-for results," such as the amelioration of pain or the remission of symptoms. In practice, it is not difficult for either externalizing or internalizing systems to produce hoped-for results, given that the majority of medical problems consist of either (1) transient or recurrent symptoms that are perceived as being discrete disorders or (2) self-limiting diseases, episodes that end in either spontaneous remissions or death. In these circumstances, medical practices acquire a reputation for hoped-for efficacy when three conditions are met: An intervention routine occurs between onset and outcome, remissions predominate over deaths and other unwanted outcomes, and superior alternative interventions are absent or inaccessible. (For an account that examines other conditions favoring hoped-for efficacy, see Young, 1976.)

Second, efficacy can take the form of producing "expected results." This occurs when practices and procedures are able to produce evidence that affirms the line of reasoning and underlying assumptions that persuaded patients and practitioners to select these particular interventions. Expected results can be produced without also producing hoped-for results. Thus the grim joke that the operation succeeded but the patient died: The patient's body, once opened up, reveals a pathology that affirms the correctness of the assumptions and choices that have led from diagnosis to surgery, but the intervention is unsuccessful, because of circumstances beyond the clinician's control. All medical systems, whether internalizing or externalizing, appear capable of distinguishing between hoped-for and expected results.

In addition, serious sickness is a source of distressing feelings that are only incidentally connected to the pain and suffering of the sick person. Medical practices may have the effect of reducing such distress by connecting sickness events to local systems of moral and cosmological meaning. This power to give meaning and impose moral order on chaotic and threatening events may be sufficient to perpetuate certain medical practices, even when the practices have no great reputation for producing cures. These practices are sometimes called "healing rituals" by anthropologists.

The mind–body problem

One of the current debates in biomedicine surrounds the "mind–body" problem, which has arisen from the observation that sickness is simultaneously an objective and subjective phenomenon. In the language of the social sciences, the objective (or bodily) component is called "disease," and refers to abnormalities and dysfunctions in organs and organ systems. The subjective component is called "illness," and refers to the patient's unique and holistic experience of either disease-related distress or certain other socially disvalued states, such as psychogenic mental disorders, that are conventionally bracketed together with diseases. Disease can occur in the absence of illness, as in the case of undiagnosed and asymptomatic hypertension, and illness can occur without disease, as in adjustment disorder and somatization disorder.

Anthropologists have critiqued the mind–body distinction in two ways. The first critique asks for a reconceptualization of the relationship between mind and body. The argument is that we need to free ourselves from the objective/subjective comparison and to take account of the interaction that continuously flows between mind and body: the capacity of the mind to affect bodily states positively and negatively, the mind's predilection for using bodily states as idioms of distress, and so on.

The second, more radical, critique refers back to anthropology's task of translating unfamiliar meanings and experiences into intelligible concepts without subordinating them to Western assumptions about sickness, healing, agency, and so on. Both Western culture and biomedicine assume the existence of a "mind," located in the brain. In practice, the mind is one of our ways of talking about the "self"—the body's seat of consciousness, the subject of its experiences, the initiator of the body's purposeful actions, the repository of its memories, and the locus of moral agency. To the anthropologist, the Western mind/self is a cultural artifact; it exists because we have practices that make it exist, in the same way that possession spirits exist in the Sudanese zar cult. Indeed, there are many cultures and systems of medicine that are "mindless," in the sense that they have no cor-

responding network of mental and moral meanings, and they constitute people and experiences in fundamentally different ways. Thus, the mind–body distinction has been criticized not because we need more effective concepts for connecting the psyche (mind) to soma (body), but rather because the notion of "mind" itself, and the practices through which this notion emerges, subordinate non-Western cultures and realities to a distinctively Western ontology (Good and Kleinman, 1985; Kleinman, 1988).

Patterns of resort

The idea that, in any community, an individual's medical behavior is congruent with a unitary set of meanings concerning sickness and its causes, diagnosis, and treatment is an obstacle to translating medical realities between cultures. Anthropologists make a series of distinctions between medical traditions, sectors, and systems in order to compare cultural norms of medical behavior:

1. A medical *tradition* is a set of practices and technologies organized around historically situated ideas about etiology, symptomatology, and treatment. Biomedicine, Ayurvedic medicine, and the *zar* cult are examples of medical traditions. Traditions are simultaneously vocabularies for interpreting the world and plans of action and technologies for producing facts that confirm their interpretations of the world.

2. The actual forms that a tradition takes in a given community make up its medical *sector*. A given medical tradition can be put into action in various ways. It can be used to justify a range of practices, technologies, and routines, and it can be adapted to a variety of institutional settings. For example, in many less developed countries, the biomedical tradition is practiced in four sectors: licensed professionals (physicians, nurses, etc.), fee-for-service injectionists (who inject clients with substances from the biomedical pharmacopeia), pharmacists (who can diagnose symptoms as well as prescribe treatments), and domestic settings (where the biomedical tradition is employed mainly to diagnose problems). Although the four sectors share a single tradition, they comprise different sets of options. In the first sector, clinicians monopolize diagnosis and treatment choice, and it is they rather than their patients who decide which etiologies will be tested and confirmed, and which sets of cultural meanings and socioeconomic implications will be realized through these practices. The injectionist and pharmacist represent patron-dominated sectors of biomedicine, in the sense that patients (or members of their families) make their diagnoses prior to consulting the practitioner. Practitioners may be asked for alternative diagnoses, but the ultimate decision is the patient's.

3. A medical *system* is equivalent to the collection of traditions and sectors that are available to people liv-

ing in a particular community. Medical beliefs and practices are useful to patients and their families because they know how to incorporate them into *patterns of resort*. These are the paths that people create in the course of actual sickness episodes, as they navigate their way from one medical sector to another, picking and choosing from among their options.

The ethnographic literature suggests two main patterns of resort. In the first, the patient or a surrogate simultaneously consults alternative traditions. People have various motives for following this strategy. In some cases patients believe the effects of multiple interventions are cumulative; in other cases, they are unsure which, if any, of the available traditions will provide an effective cure. In some communities, notably in south Asia, the simultaneous pattern of resort reflects a therapeutic division of labor. Biomedicine is prized for its quick effects against causal agents, such as "microbes," and its ability to treat symptoms such as high fevers. The Ayurvedic tradition is valued for its ability to counter the perceived side-effects of biomedicines, especially antibiotics, and for its ability to restore an equilibrium among the body's organs and humors, that is, the state synonymous with health. The alternative strategy consists of a sequential pattern of resort, in which the individual exhausts the resources of a given tradition or sector before moving on to an alternative tradition in the medical system (Young, 1983).

The paths that individuals follow through their medical systems are determined by a variety of factors. For example, patients who want to avoid stigmatizing etiologies (that would contaminate or spoil the individual's social identity) or diagnoses with poor prognosis are likely to compare the range of diagnoses and etiologies that belong to the various traditions in their medical system, and then start off with the tradition that offers the most favorable outcomes. Choice may be influenced by cost–benefit calculations. That is, a practitioner's or sector's economic and geographic accessibility are weighed against the perceived seriousness of the patient's sickness and the value of the patient to his or her family. This is a significant consideration in communities whose members value the survival of female children less than the survival of males. The characteristics of particular practitioners may also influence a patient's strategy, as, for example, when a patient believes that a healer's medicines have a unique affinity for him or her. (For detailed case studies relating to these issues, see Nichter, 1989.)

Conclusion

A community's medical beliefs, then, do not correspond to a homogeneous set of meanings. Both in complex societies and in "traditional" and "tribal" societies individuals are drawn by sickness into multiple and often contradictory systems of meanings and action. The appearance of unity and homogeneity within a given community is not accidental, however. Usually, it is an expression of power, of the capacity of one segment of the community—its medical experts, political leaders, moral authorities, and others—to define and control which of the alternative sets of medical meanings will be carried over into public discourse. In this sense, power is the ability to convince people that the socially dominant meanings of sickness are also the authentic meanings (Young, 1982).

ALLAN YOUNG

Directly related to this article are the other articles in this entry: HISTORY OF THE CONCEPTS, SOCIOLOGICAL PERSPECTIVES, PHILOSOPHICAL PERSPECTIVES, *and* THE EXPERIENCE OF HEALTH AND ILLNESS. *Also directly related is the entry* MEDICINE, ANTHROPOLOGY OF. *For a further discussion of topics mentioned in this article, see the entries* BODY, *articles on* SOCIAL THEORIES, *and* CULTURAL AND RELIGIOUS PERSPECTIVES; DEATH, *especially the article on* ANTHROPOLOGICAL PERSPECTIVES; DEATH, ATTITUDES TOWARD; DEATH, DEFINITION AND DETERMINATION OF; HEALING; HEALTH-CARE DELIVERY, *article on* HEALTH-CARE SYSTEMS; ORGAN AND TISSUE PROCUREMENT; ORGAN AND TISSUE TRANSPLANTS; PAIN AND SUFFERING; *and* VALUE AND VALUATION. *For a further discussion of related ideas, see the entries* ALTERNATIVE THERAPIES; *and* BIOETHICS.

Bibliography

BODDY, JANICE P. 1989. *Wombs and Alien Spirits: Women, Men, and the Zar Cult in Northern Sudan.* Madison: University of Wisconsin Press.

EVANS-PRITCHARD, E. E. 1937. *Witchcraft, Oracles, and Magic Among the Azande.* Oxford: At the Clarendon Press.

GAINES, ATWOOD, ed. 1992. *Ethnopsychiatry: The Cultural Construction of Professional and Folk Psychiatries.* Albany: State University of New York.

GOOD, BYRON. 1994. *Medicine, Rationality, and Experience: An Anthropological Perspective.* Cambridge: At the University Press.

GOOD, BYRON, and KLEINMAN, ARTHUR, eds. 1985. *Culture and Depression: Studies in the Anthropology and Cross-Cultural Psychiatry of Affect and Disorder.* Berkeley: University of California Press.

HAHN, ROBERT A., and GAINES, ATWOOD D., eds. 1985. *Physicians of Western Medicine: Anthropological Approaches to Theory and Practice.* Dordrecht, Netherlands: D. Reidel.

HOLLIS, MARTIN, and LUKES, STEVEN, eds. 1982. *Rationality and Relativism.* Cambridge, Mass.: MIT Press.

KLEINMAN, ARTHUR. 1980. *Patients and Healers in the Context of Culture: An Exploration of the Borderland Between Anthropology, Medicine, and Psychiatry.* Berkeley: University of California Press.

———. 1988. *Rethinking Psychiatry: From Cultural Category to Personal Experience.* New York: Free Press.

LATOUR, BRUNO, and WOOLGAR, STEVE. 1986. *Laboratory Life: The Construction of Scientific Facts.* Princeton, N.J.: Princeton University Press.

LESLIE, CHARLES M. 1976. "Introduction." In *Asian Medical Systems: A Comparative Study*, pp. 1–12. Edited by Charles M. Leslie. Berkeley: University of California Press.

LESLIE, CHARLES M., and YOUNG, ALLAN, eds. 1992. *Paths to Asian Medical Knowledge.* Berkeley: University of California Press.

LEWIS, GILBERT. 1975. *Knowledge of Illness in a Sepik River Society: A Study of the Gnau, New Guinea.* London: Athlone.

LOCK, MARGARET M. 1993. *Encounters with Aging: Mythologies of Menopause in Japan and North America.* Berkeley: University of California Press.

LOCK, MARGARET M., and GORDON, DEBORAH R., eds. 1988. *Biomedicine Examined.* Dordrecht, Netherlands: Kluwer.

NICHTER, MARK. 1989. *Anthropology and International Health: South Asian Case Studies.* Dordrecht, Netherlands: Kluwer.

WILSON, BRYAN R., ed. 1987. *Rationality.* Oxford: Basil Blackwell.

WRIGHT, PETER, and TREACHER, ANDREW, eds. 1982. *The Problem of Medical Knowledge: Examining the Social Construction of Medicine.* Edinburgh: University of Edinburgh Press.

YOUNG, ALLAN. 1976. "Some Implications of Medical Beliefs and Practices for Social Anthropology." *American Anthropologist* 78, no. 1:5–24.

———. 1982. "The Anthropologies of Illness and Sickness." *Annual Review of Anthropology*, 1982:257–285.

———. 1983. "The Relevance of Traditional Medical Cultures to Modern Primary Health Care." *Social Science and Medicine* 17, no. 16:1205–1211.

IV. PHILOSOPHICAL PERSPECTIVES

Concepts of health and disease, as well as of sickness, wellness, deformity, disability, dysfunction, and disfigurement, direct social energies. They inform medicine and health-care policy regarding what is wholesome, to be avoided, or to be treated, all else being equal. Concepts of health and disease either directly or indirectly describe, evaluate, and explain reality and assign social roles. Decisions about the meaning and scope of concepts of health and disease profoundly influence the character of health care (e.g., if alcoholism, homosexuality, menopause, and aging are considered diseases, then medical treatment, resources, and research will be focused on treating them). These concepts therefore become the focus of public-policy debates and may conceal value judgments that should be treated more explicitly as bioethical issues.

Diseases and sicknesses are usually distinguished from sins, crimes, and social problems as not directly under the control of the will and as explainable, predictable, and/or treatable by an appeal to somatic or psychological laws, generalizations, and associations. Pains that are directly under one's own control or that of others (e.g., the pain from standing on one's own foot), difficulties of a moral sort (e.g., being blameworthy), problems of a spiritual sort (e.g., refusing to repent for one's sins or being in the possession of a devil), or legal disabilities (e.g., being a convicted felon) are contrasted with states of disease or illness. This contrast discloses a boundary between disparate human practices: blaming the immoral, convicting felons, exorcising demons, and treating diseases. The criteria used to distinguish between any of these practices will vary from culture to culture, and they will shift within the history of a particular culture. In part, the line between medical and other problems is a function of the competencies of those making the judgment. Diseases and illnesses are what medicine treats.

Illnesses and diseases are generally identified because they involve a failure of function, a pain that is considered abnormal (compare the pain of teething with that of migraine [King, 1981]), a deformity, or the threat of premature death. Insofar as judgments regarding proper function, normal pain, correct human form, and normal span of life can be made without reference to culture-dependent values, concepts of disease will not depend on social norms of proper human function. The same can be said with regard to concepts of health. Though much is said regarding health care, health, and wellness, one may question whether such notions can be understood only in positive terms. The positive concepts of health must be understood in relation to the absence of particular dysfunctions, pains, or deformities. There may be numerous concepts of health corresponding to different absences of disease or deformity or to different positive views of human well-being and exemplary function (Boorse, 1975). It is also difficult to provide a positive account of health and well-being that will not have such ill-defined boundaries so as to include economic, political, and social health. The World Health Organization's 1958 definition of health as a "state of complete physical, mental, and social well-being" (WHO, 1958, p. 459) has been criticized for being too broad and ill defined (e.g., Callahan, 1990) to guide the formation of health policy. The philosophical literature, aside from addressing these difficulties with concepts of health, has focused mainly on concepts of disease and illness.

Philosophical concerns regarding the nature of concepts of health and disease can be organized under six questions: (1) Are disease entities to be discovered or are they and their classifications instrumental constructs that are created to achieve certain ends? (2) How do explanatory models shape the boundaries between health and disease and determine the meaning of disease? (3) What values shape concepts of health and disease, and to what extent are these culturally determined? (4) Is the definition of mental disease and health different from that of somatic (or physical) disease and health? (5) Do concepts of animal disease function in the same way as concepts of human disease? (6) How can concepts of health and disease be used for overt political and social ends?

The *ens morbi* (disease entity)

The history of medicine is replete with talk of clinical findings constituting an *ens morbi*, a disease entity. Disease entities have been conceived of as metaphysical entities, clinical entities, pathological entities, etiological entities, and genetic entities. These ways of considering diseases (i.e., as disease entities) generated a significant dispute in the nineteenth century between those who held that disease entities, and the classifications within which they are understood, identify realities in the world and those who held that disease classifications are at best distinctions imposed on reality to achieve certain goals (e.g., of diagnosis, therapy, and prognosis). The first were termed "ontologists." Those who took a more conventionalist, instrumentalist, or nominalist position were termed "physiologists." This distinction appears to have been articulated in 1828 by François-Joseph-Victor Broussais (1772–1838), who denounced ontological accounts of disease (1821). Carl Wunderlich (1815–1877), Ernst Romberg (1865–1933), Alasdair MacIntyre, Samuel Gorovitz, and others have, in various ways, taken positions in sympathy with Broussais.

Ontological theories have held that "disease" terms or classifications name things in the world. Though Broussais had directed his criticisms against only clinical classifications, ontologists of disease can be taken to include any who perceived diseases as entities, including metaphysical views advanced by individuals such as Paracelsus (1493–1541). Paracelsus (1941) held that diseases are specific entities that arise outside the body.

Disease entities have also been understood not as things in the usual sense but as clinical realities, as recurring constellations of findings. Thomas Sydenham (1624–1689), in classifying disease entities, construed them as enduring types and patterns of symptoms. "Nature in the production of disease is uniform and consistent; so much so, that for the same disease in different persons the symptoms are for the most part the same; and the selfsame phenomena that you would observe in the sickness of a Socrates you would observe in the sickness of a simpleton" (Sydenham, 1848, p. 15). It is within such a view of disease that one can speak of "Jones" being (having) a typical case of typhoid. Such language expresses the view that there is a certain, central identity for a disease that is its essence or "type." In this way one can classify diseases by type, and one can

also speak of instances of a disease as approximating a "typical" case. Within this understanding, one can also talk of typical cases as rare: "One rarely sees a typical case of secondary syphilis." Patients embody clinical realities where the typical is the full, complete expression of a disease, not necessarily its usual expression. The typical is an ideal type. It was against this genre of account that Broussais spoke.

Etiological accounts, like metaphysical views, focused on the cause of the disease as the disease entity, but regarded disease entities as empirical, usually infectious agents. Rudolf Virchow (1821–1902) characterized this view as "ontological in an outspoken manner" (1958, p. 192). Virchow considered this understanding of disease entities to rest on a confusion between a disease and its cause. "The parasite," he wrote, "was therefore not the disease itself but only its cause" (1958, p. 192). The confusion of the disease with its cause led to a "hopeless, never-ending confusion, in which the ideas of being (*ens morbi*) and causation (*causa morbi*) have been arbitrarily thrown together, [and] began when microorganisms were finally discovered" (1958, p. 192). The mature Virchow had embraced a view of disease entities grounded in pathological findings. Virchow himself held that a disease entity is "an altered body-part, or, expressed in first principles, an altered cell or aggregate of cells, whether tissue or organ" (p. 192). "This conception is expressly ontological. That is its merit, not its deficiency. There is in actuality an ens morbi, just as there is an ens vitae (life force); in both instances a cell or cell-complex has the claim to be thus designated" (p. 207).

Genetic accounts can also interpret the disease entity as an empirical reality. The disease entity is to be found in genetic abnormalities (Anderson, 1989; Fowler et al., 1989). The promise of somatic-cell gene therapy raises the question of a disease entity once again. That is, does the disease exist in the genetic structure, or is the structure the cause of the disease?

Current uses of "disease" in standard nomenclatures and nosologies, or classifications, have a predominantly non-ontological character. A conventionalist view of concepts of disease allows one to choose on pragmatic grounds whether one wishes, for example, to treat tuberculosis as an infectious, genetic, or environmental disease (recognizing that all three sorts of factors contribute to the development of tuberculosis) on the basis of which variables are most easily manipulated. One may decide, because little is known about the inheritance of resistance against tuberculosis, and because any eugenic programs to eliminate tuberculosis would be very slow in taking effect, that it would be best to treat tuberculosis as an infectious disease (or as an environmental disease, as a disease depending on socioeconomic conditions such as housing, food, etc.). It is meaningless to ask whether a definition of disease is true or false, only whether it is useful (Wulff, 1981).

Diseases as clinical findings and explanatory accounts

Many people take the term "illness" to identify a subjective experience, an experience of failed function, pain, distress, or unwellness. "Disease," in contrast, is then an explanatory concept or part of an explanatory account (Boorse, 1975). Or one might distinguish illnesses from diseases where illness identifies constellations of signs and symptoms, and disease identifies illnesses joined to disease models or explanations, where the content of the illness is augmented by the phenomena found on the basis of a disease model. But to recognize a state of unwellness as a state of disease is already to have begun to explain it and to recast the meaning of the findings within an interpretive context. A constellation of phenomena is held to be recurrent. If such a constellation of phenomena is encountered again in the future, it can be identified, for example: "That is a case of chronic fatigue." Diagnoses of syndromes, of recurrent patterns of signs and symptoms, allow predictions to be made (prognoses) as well as management of outcomes (therapy). Such predictions and attempts at therapy can succeed even in the absence of causal explanations.

During much of its history, medicine has been concerned with classifying patterns of signs and symptoms so that they can be recognized in the future with greater ease. Thomas Sydenham's classic *Observationes Medica* (1676) suggested classifying diseases in definite species, following the methods of botanists in classifying plants. His work was followed by Carolus Linnaeus's (1707–1778) *Genera Morborum in auditorum usum* (1759), François Boissier de Sauvages de la Croix's (1706–1767) *Nosologia Methodica sistens Morborum Classes Juxta Sydenhami mentem et Botanicorum ordinem* (1763), and William Cullen's (1712–1790) *Synopsis Nosologiae Methodicae* (1769). These classifications functioned without causal explanations, though these were also given. Such medical descriptions and explanations at a clinical, phenomenological level are still employed whenever a new illness is identified for which a causal explanation is not yet forthcoming. For example, when at first no causal explanation was available, acquired immunodeficiency syndrome (AIDS) was identified as a clinical, phenomenological entity.

Medicine also explains by relating what is observed via general laws of physiology, anatomy, psychology, genetics, and so forth to other phenomena. The result is a two-tier account of diseases. The first tier is that of the observed constellations of phenomena, for example, a clinical description of yellow fever. The second tier is that of a model advanced within the laboratory medical sciences to explain the observed clinical phenomena, for example, an explanation of the clinical findings in yellow fever in terms of the effects of a group B arbovirus (a group of viruses transmitted by mosquitoes and ticks) that causes the death of essential cells in the liver.

The laws of pathophysiology (the physiology of disordered function) and pathopsychology (the psychology of mental disease) relate new phenomena to the original clinical constellations of signs and symptoms. Some of these phenomena are then recognized as the causes of the illness. The concept of disease thus comes to identify disease models, supporting the search for unnoticed causal factors and expressions of disease. For example, Giovanni Battista Morgagni (1682–1771) in his *De Sedibus et Causis Morborum per anatomen indagatis* (1761) correlated clinical observations with postmortem findings, and Philippe Pinel (1755–1826) incorporated anatomical considerations into his *Nosographie philosophique* (1798), producing nosologies that embraced not only clinical observations, but anatomical considerations as well. This change in focus was strengthened when Xavier Bichat (1771–1802) argued that constellations of symptoms and signs could be explained in terms of underlying pathological processes. According to Bichat, the way to medical advance is through autopsies (Foucault, 1973). This shift to the study of pathological findings as a way to explain clinical observations was then supplemented by accounts drawn from microbiology, endocrinology, biochemistry, genetics, and so on, producing contemporary explanations of illnesses.

In the process of moving from accounts of illness that were predominantly clinical observations to pathoanatomical accounts of illnesses that were based on observable illnesses of the anatomy, the meanings of diseases were altered. Individuals who once were thought to die of acute indigestion were now understood to die of a myocardial infarction. The meanings of the phenomena observed (e.g., illnesses with their clinical signs and symptoms) were reinterpreted in terms of disease models. As a result of this recasting, medical complaints often came to be considered legitimate only to the extent that they had a demonstrable, underlying pathophysiological or pathoanatomical lesion.

Health and diseases: Discoveries or cultural inventions?

If certain physiological and psychological functions can be identified as natural or essential to humans, then their absence can be used to define disease states. Leon Kass (1975) and Christopher Boorse (1976) have argued that one can specify those functions integral to being human, and thus secure accounts of disease that are not relative to a particular culture or set of values. Such understandings of health and disease could then be used to sort out essential from nonessential, if not proper from improper, applications of medicine. Such views may depend on particular understandings of what is "natural" to humans as such. Others appeal to an evolutionary account of what should count as species-typical levels of species-typical functions appropriate for age and gender (Boorse, 1976).

In contrast, Joseph Margolis, H. Tristram Engelhardt, and others have argued that definitions of disease and health depend on sociological, culturally determined value judgments and, as a result, these definitions can be understood only in terms of particular cultures and their ideologies (Margolis, 1976). The view that the concepts of health and disease are culturally determined has been supported by feminist writings on health care. Many authors have pointed out that the practice of medicine has had an androcentric focus in defining what constitutes medical problems. Some authors argue that women's issues largely have been ignored, and experiences that have been reported by women that could not be documented by the experimenter have been treated as invalid (Rosser, 1989; Oakley, 1993).

Partisans of the view that social and cultural ideas influence concepts of health and disease stress that a definition of disease tied to evolution makes disease concepts dependent on particular past environments and past adaptations. Successful adaptation must always be specified in terms of a particular environment, including a particular cultural context and particular goals. Definitions of disease can then be regarded in instrumental terms (Wulff, 1981). Norms for "better" or "worse" can be constituted within the practice of medicine (Wartofsky, 1975). A culture-dependent account of concepts of health and disease need not deny that there will be great similarities as to what will count as diseases across cultures. Certain states of affairs, for slightly different reasons, will probably be understood as diseases across most environments and in most cultures. Supporters of a value-infected, culture-dependent account of disease have argued that those who would attempt a purely evolutionary account of disease have not reconstructed the practice of medicine, but some practice of characterizing individuals as members of particular biological species (Engelhardt, 1975). The practice of medicine depends on culturally constructed understandings of health and disease.

How one understands health and disease will in turn influence how one conceptualizes medical practice. Henrik Wulff has argued that an exclusively biological or empirical model of illness contributes to paternalistic medical practice. If concepts of health and disease can be fully understood in biological terms, then there may be no need to assign the patient an active role in the decision process (Wulff, 1981). If, however, determinations of health and disease are not just empirical concepts, but concepts that are also related to cultures and values, the patient will have a more active role in determining the burden of the disease and the extent of treatment.

The conceptualization of medicine will be influenced by developments in genetic research, which hold the promise not only to correct diseases in patients but to prevent them in future generations of patients (Anderson, 1989; Zimmerman, 1991). As the capacities of genetic medicine increase, our understanding of preventive medicine will expand since diseases will be prevented in future generations as well as in individuals. Somatic and germ-line therapies further illustrate the relationship of culture to concepts of health and disease as choices are made about which genetic variances should be treated as disease abnormalities (e.g., homosexuality, alcoholism, shortness of stature).

Physical, mental, and social diseases

It has been argued that only somatic diseases are legitimately diseases, while those states of affairs usually termed "mental diseases" are problems with living (Szasz, 1974). Such arguments may require a Cartesian assumption that disease predicates are somatic and can only be predicated of bodies, while problems with living, states of affairs similar to moral vices, can be predicated of minds. Following similar lines of argument, individuals have contended that enterprises such as psychotherapy are tantamount to applied ethics (Breggin, 1971), or that the cure of somatic disease constitutes the prime end of medicine (Kass, 1975).

Against such views, it has been responded that such stark dichotomies or dualisms usually fail to offer satisfactory accounts of reality. If mental life is dependent on brain function, then all mental diseases can, in some sense, be tied to physical pathology or abnormal anatomy; for example, depression can be presumed to be dependent on a neurophysiological substrate and thus, in principle, open to pharmacological treatment. If one views diseases as explanatory models for the organization of signs and symptoms, then it does not matter whether the signs and symptoms identify physiological states of affairs ("I have a rash") or psychological states of affairs ("I feel depressed"). Nor does it matter whether models employed to correlate these phenomena are pathophysiological or psychological. Most accounts of disease will, in fact, mingle physical and psychological observables, as well as pathophysiological and pathopsychological causal constructs, in order to explain the patterns of phenomena identified as illnesses. As a consequence, one may come to view distinctions among somatic, psychological, or social models of disease in terms of pragmatic needs, of accenting the usefulness of particular modes of therapeutic intervention. One may even advance sociological models of disease, construing diseases primarily in terms of social variables and giving secondary place to the pathophysiological.

Distinctions between medical and nonmedical models of therapy, unlike somatic, psychological, and sociological accounts of disease, are often meant to contrast the autonomy of clients in nonmedical therapeutic models with the dependence of patients on health-care practitioners in medical models. Talcott Parsons characterized the "sick role" as (1) excusing ill individuals from some or all of their usual responsibilities; (2) holding them not responsible for being ill (though they may be responsible for becoming sick); as well as (3) holding that they should attempt to become well (a therapeutic imperative); and (4) seek out experts to treat their illness. Medical models tend to support paternalistic interventions by health-care practitioners who are experts and to relieve patients of responsibility for directing their own care and cure. Nonmedical models, in contrast, tend to accent individual, client responsibility.

Somatic models of disease may be employed within both medical and nonmedical models of therapy: for example, compare treating hypertension with antihypertensive agents versus enjoining the afflicted individuals to find ways to change their lifestyles with regard to stress, eating patterns, and so on. The same is true of psychological models of disease: for example, compare treating depression chemotherapeutically versus enjoining individuals to make changes in their ways of living.

As predisposing factors toward particular diseases become better known and easier to control or avoid, individuals are held increasingly responsible for becoming ill, even though they will remain nonresponsible for being ill. One is not responsible for being a person with bronchogenic carcinoma as one is responsible for being a willful malingerer; one cannot be told to stop having cancer, but one can be held responsible for having developed cancer through one's smoking habits. As the impact of lifestyle on the development of diseases becomes clearer, the responsibility of individuals for their health may increase the possible scope of nonmedical models of therapy.

Animals and disease

If concepts or notions of human illness, disease, and health are, in part, social constrictions, there will be differences between the ways in which diseases are identified for humans and the ways they are identified for other animals. Illnesses and diseases in animals will be judged through the social or cultural criteria of human beings. Nonhuman animals will tend to be regarded in terms of human cultures and societies. Pets or domestic animals may be regarded as having disease or being healthy depending on how they are viewed through hu-

man purposes and constructs. Along with those of plants, the diseases or illnesses of those animals that are not pets may be understood less in terms of human social or cultural criteria and more in terms of generalized knowledge about the species. In the case of animals in the wild, there may not be concern for individual suffering, disability, or deformity, but rather with the general health of the species. Identifying the role human values play in the concepts of animal disease and illness expands the discussions of the ethical treatment of nonhuman animals in bioethics.

The social force of diagnosis

Concepts of disease have been used to impose political judgments. For example, in the United States prior to the Civil War, there was the proposal to regard the flight of a slave to the North ("drapetomania") and the absence of a wholesome inclination to do effective plantation work ("dysaesthesia aethiopis" or "hebetude of mind and obtuse sensibility of body") as diseases for which explanatory accounts and treatments could be provided (Cartwright, 1851). Masturbation was also appreciated as a serious disease for which castration, excision of the clitoris, and other invasive therapies were employed. Individuals were even determined to have died of masturbation, and postmortem findings "substantiated" this cause (Engelhardt, 1974). In the case of the diseases of slaves, the motivation may have been to protect slaves from punishment. In the case of masturbation, the influence of cultural values on the psychology of discovery was not appreciated.

Historical perspective can increase our awareness that medical practitioners and researchers have tended to "discover" what already was assumed. More recent political uses of disease concepts (e.g., in psychiatry) have been closely connected with repressive goals and political agendas of certain governments. Much social employment of disease definitions is meant to be benevolent, such as advocating a view of alcoholism and drug addiction as diseases so as to recruit the forces of medicine in their control. Moreover, such conditions may be termed diseases in order to relieve alcoholics and drug addicts of the social opprobria that attend what is understood as immoral behavior.

Summary

Concepts of health and disease shape descriptions of medical reality, convey explanations, advance value judgments, and structure social reality. They influence not only the scope of medicine but health-care policy as well. Because they may involve not only moral values but values associated with human bodily and mental excellence, they raise questions pertinent to both bioethics and the philosophy of medicine. As they are tied to moral and cultural values, the concepts of health and disease, as well as their application, will be the subject of debate in societies that are morally and culturally pluralistic.

H. TRISTRAM ENGELHARDT, JR.
KEVIN WM. WILDES

Directly related to this article are the other articles in this entry: HISTORY OF THE CONCEPTS, SOCIOLOGICAL PERSPECTIVES, ANTHROPOLOGICAL PERSPECTIVES, *and* THE EXPERIENCE OF HEALTH AND ILLNESS. *Also directly related is the entry* MEDICINE, PHILOSOPHY OF. *For a further discussion of topics mentioned in this article, see the entries* AGING AND THE AGED, *article on* THEORIES OF AGING AND LIFE EXTENSION; ANIMAL WELFARE AND RIGHTS, *articles on* ETHICAL PERSPECTIVES ON THE TREATMENT AND STATUS OF ANIMALS, WILDLIFE CONSERVATION AND MANAGEMENT, *and* PET AND COMPANION ANIMALS; DEATH; EUGENICS; EVOLUTION; ENDANGERED SPECIES AND BIODIVERSITY; FEMINISM; GENE THERAPY; GENETIC ENGINEERING; HOMOSEXUALITY; MENTAL HEALTH; MENTAL ILLNESS; NATURE; PATERNALISM; PATIENTS' RESPONSIBILITIES; PSYCHIATRY, ABUSES OF; SUBSTANCE ABUSE; VALUE AND VALUATION; *and* WOMEN, *article on* HEALTH-CARE ISSUES. *For a further discussion of related ideas, see the entries* DEATH, ATTITUDES TOWARD; HEALING; MEDICINE, ANTHROPOLOGY OF; MEDICINE, SOCIOLOGY OF; PSYCHOPHARMACOLOGY; REPRODUCTIVE TECHNOLOGIES; *and* SEXUAL DEVELOPMENT. *Other relevant material may be found under the entries* PSYCHOANALYSIS AND DYNAMIC THERAPIES; *and* PSYCHOSURGERY.

Bibliography

ANDERSON, W. FRENCH. 1989. "Human Gene Therapy: Why Draw a Line?" *Journal of Medicine and Philosophy* 14, no. 6:681–693.

BOORSE, CHRISTOPHER 1975. "On the Distinction Between Disease and Illness." *Philosophy and Public Affairs* 5, no. 1:49–68.

———. 1976. "Wright on Functions." *Philosophical Review* 85, no. 1:70–86.

BREGGIN, PETER ROGER. 1971. "Psychotherapy and Applied Ethics." *Psychiatry* 34, no. 1:59–74.

BROUSSAIS, FRANÇOIS-JOSEPH-VICTOR. 1821. *Examen des doctrines médicales et des systèmes de nosologie*, 2 vols. Paris: Mequignon-Marvis.

CALLAHAN, DANIEL. 1990. *What Kind of Life: The Limits of Medical Progress.* New York: Simon and Schuster.

CARTWRIGHT, SAMUEL A. 1851. "Report on the Diseases and Physical Peculiarities of the Negro Race." *New Orleans Medical and Surgical Review* 7:691–715.

ENGELHARDT, H. TRISTRAM, JR. 1974. "The Disease of Masturbation: Values and the Concept of Disease." *Bulletin of the History of Medicine* 48, no. 2:225–248.

———. 1975. "The Concepts of Health and Disease." In *Evaluation and Explanation in the Biomedical Sciences*, pp. 125–141. Edited by H. Tristram Engelhardt, Jr., and Stuart F. Spicker. Dordrecht, Netherlands: Reidel.

FOUCAULT, MICHEL. 1973. *The Birth of the Clinic: An Archeology of Medical Perception.* New York: Pantheon Books.

FOWLER, GREGORY; JUENGST, ERIC T.; and ZIMMERMAN, BURKE K. 1989. "Germ-Line Gene Therapy and the Clinical Ethos of Medical Genetics." *Theoretical Medicine* 10, no. 2:151–165.

KASS, LEON R. 1975. "Regarding the End of Medicine and the Pursuit of Health." *Public Interest* 40:11–42.

KING, LESTER. 1981. "What Is Disease." In *Concepts of Health and Disease: Interdisciplinary Perspectives*, pp. 107–108. Edited by Arthur L. Caplan, H. Tristram Engelhardt, Jr., and James McCartney. Reading, Mass.: Addison-Wesley.

MARGOLIS, JOSEPH. 1976. "The Concept of Disease." *Journal of Medicine and Philosophy* 1, no. 3:238–255.

OAKLEY, ANN. 1993. *Essays on Women, Medicine, and Health.* Edinburgh: Edinburgh University Press.

PARACELSUS. 1941. *Four Treatises of Theophrastus von Hohenheim, Called Paracelsus.* Edited by C. Lillian Temkin, George Rosen, G. Zilboorg, and Henry E. Sigerist. Baltimore: Leidecker.

PARSONS, TALCOTT. 1971. *The System of Modern Societies.* Englewood Cliffs, N.J.: Prentice-Hall.

ROSSER, SUE V. 1989. "Re-Visioning Clinical Research—Gender and the Ethics of Experimental Design." *Hypatia* 4, no. 2:125–139.

SYDENHAM, THOMAS. 1848. *The Works of Thomas Sydenham.* Vol. 1. *Medical Observations Concerning the History and Cure of Acute Diseases*, pp. 11–27. Translated from the Latin by Dr. Greenhill. London: Sydenham Society.

SZASZ, THOMAS. 1974. *The Myth of Mental Illness: Foundations of a Theory of Personal Conduct.* Rev. ed. New York: Harper & Row.

VIRCHOW, RUDOLF LUDWIG KARL. 1958. *Disease, Life, and Man: Selected Essays.* Translated by Lelland J. Rather. Stanford, Calif.: Stanford University Press.

WARTOFSKY, MARX W. 1975. "Organs, Organisms, and Disease: Human Ontology and Medical Practice." In *Evaluation and Explanation in the Biomedical Sciences*, pp. 67–83. Edited by H. Tristram Engelhardt, Jr., and Stuart F. Spicker. Dordrecht, Netherlands: Reidel.

WORLD HEALTH ORGANIZATION (WHO). 1958. "Constitution." *The First Ten Years of the World Health Organization.* Geneva: Author.

WULFF, HENRIK R. 1981. *Rational Diagnosis and Treatment: An Introduction to Clinical Decision-Making.* 2d ed. Oxford: Blackwell Scientific Publications.

ZIMMERMAN, BURKE K. 1991. "Human Germ-Line Therapy: The Case for Its Development and Use." *Journal of Medicine and Philosophy* 16, no. 6: 593–612.

V. THE EXPERIENCE OF HEALTH AND ILLNESS

This article will address not only the experience of health and illness but also the significance of this experience for clinical medicine and bioethics. Some people would argue that given the wide range of historical, cultural, and individual differences that shape people's experience of health and illness, little could be said on this topic that would have universal validity. Others would point toward certain invariant features of the human body, psyche, or society that could ground cross-cultural commonalities. This article will not take a position on this debate. It will present a description of health and illness as experienced within a contemporary Western context. While this description may not be universalizable, it can nonetheless provide a starting point for elucidating similarities and differences among cultures and individuals.

The experience of health

In setting out to portray the experience of health, one is struck by how little we are used to focusing upon it. This ordinary tendency to overlook health, to take it for granted, is also reflected in the paucity of descriptive literature on the subject. In many ways this is precisely the point: To be healthy is to be freed from some of the limitations and problems that promote self-reflection. The healthy woman or man need not pause before heading off for work, scheduling a dinner for later in the week, or grabbing a shovel to clear the driveway of snow. The workday, the social occasion, the snow, are themselves the objects of attention. The state of health, bodily and psychic, that allows for such engagements usually remains the tacit background. This is not always the case. One may revel in the good health one feels after getting over the flu, or appreciate the vigor that suffuses one after running. But usually these contrasting experiences that make health stand forth sooner or later fall away. Health returns to its status as the great forgotten.

Yet this experiential absence remains an implicit presence in our daily lives. It is the background of what Maurice Merleau-Ponty, drawing on the work of Edmund Husserl, calls the bodily "I can" (Merleau-Ponty, 1962). *I can* get out of bed, move across the room, brush my teeth, prepare my breakfast, drive my car to work, and so forth, all because of the taken-for-granted horizon of sufficient health that enables these actions. I need not think about my body (Leder, 1990), or of its mortality (Heidegger, 1962). But my cheerful obliviousness is not simply an existential evasion; it also frees me to engage the outer world.

The word "health" comes from the same root as the word "whole." To be healthy is to be in a state of relatively unproblematic wholeness. The body is operating harmoniously and is therefore able to meet the demands of its world and carry out the self's intentions. The healthy person, able to integrate into his or her social surroundings, feels "a part of things." In this integration of self and body, self and world, self and others, we live

as fish in water, inhabiting our all-embracing and invisible milieu.

Disease and illness

Illness teaches us of the precariousness of this world; like fish we can also be cast onto dry land, flopping and gasping for breath. To capture the profound dislocations caused by illness, it is useful first to distinguish between "illness" and "disease" (Cassell, 1985; Engelhardt, 1982). Modern medicine has been largely concerned with understanding and treating diseases such as acute myelocytic leukemia or rheumatoid arthritis. To diagnose an individual as having a disease is already to overleap that particular individual: One notes a cluster of signs and symptoms that have repeatedly presented in a range of cases. The disease label also frequently and ideally invokes an explanatory etiology, a prognostic picture, and a set of treatment options, all drawing upon the theories and knowledge base of medical science. Since the eighteenth century, disease classifications have progressively moved from a basis in the patient's reported symptoms to one grounded on the pathological lesions and processes exposed after death or, by medical technologies, in the living (Engelhardt, 1986; Foucault, 1973). Hence "dyspepsia" is gradually replaced by reference to "peptic ulcer disease," uncovered by endoscopy or other such techniques (Baron, 1985). This shift has greatly advanced the explanatory and therapeutic powers of modern medicine. However, it has also diminished the attention paid to the patient's experience.

In contrast to the medical characterization of disease, we can use the term "illness" to refer to the experience of the sick person. To fall ill is to undergo a series of transformations, often involving modes of discomfort, dysfunction, and/or disfigurement that distinguish this state from health. In a sense, any illness is inescapably individual. Even if one shares the same disease with another—for example, juvenile-onset diabetes—the challenges, limitations, and suffering involved can radically vary from person to person. Yet just as the physician-researcher can uncover the repeated patterns typical of a disease, so one can describe certain features that commonly accompany the illness experience.

This topic has been addressed within the school of philosophy known as phenomenology. The phenomenologist seeks to set aside ("bracket") any scientific, theological, or other metaphysical assumptions concerning the nature of the phenomenon under investigation. The phenomenon, be it that of memory or perception, space or time, religion or mathematics, is then described insofar as it surfaces within human experience. For example, while Newtonian time may flow evenly, time as experienced runs at a variable rate. It may speed up when we are absorbed in our tasks; slow down when we are stuck with an interminable bore; all but stop in its tracks as we anxiously await a coming event. The phenomenologist seeks to describe a domain of experience, in this case that of lived time, and clarify its essential features. In such a way, this article will set aside the scientific understanding of disease to better chart the illness experience. (Here the focus will be on so-called physical illness, for an investigation of the many and varied "mental illnesses" would take us too far afield [see Straus, 1966]).

Illness and the experience of the body. If health is a kind of wholeness, an accomplished integration along a number of dimensions, illness involves a set of experienced dis-integrations. We can see this first in relation to the body. Ordinarily the body operates as a seamless whole (Merleau-Ponty, 1962); in response to my perceptions I move through and act upon the surrounding world, my internal organs supplying the needed life energy. In illness the body can split into problematic parts and functions. An aching stomach or a pulled muscle suddenly stands out from the rest of the body, demanding attention. As my organic harmony is disrupted, so too is my integration with the world. I want to reach out for a cup of tea—ordinarily no problem—but a slipped disk pulls me back in pain; or blurred vision causes me to knock it over; or the pervasive lassitude of the flu leaves me without the strength. My ill body is no longer at home in its world but awkward and limited, a stranger in a strange land.

This dis-integration of the body within itself and vis-à-vis its world also brings about a felt split between my body and *me*. Ordinarily, I move through the world in an embodied way. The body is not simply something I have, but an inseparable part of *who I am*; it grounds all my interactions with the environment. When I fall ill, this body becomes something alien (Leder, 1990; Zaner, 1981). It is what is causing me pain, limiting my movement, humiliating me with an unpleasant look or odor. At such moments I realize how deep my ties are to the flesh. However, this flesh I am seems also what I am not—the "other," capable of thwarting and opposing me in a way health had never fully revealed.

This experience presents a severe challenge to our usual sense of the autonomous self. The ill person may neither understand nor control what is happening within the body, though his or her life may depend upon it. One's relationship to one's own body often must be mediated through others: the physician who probes it and informs the ill person of the diagnosis; the surgeon who opens it up, scrutinizing organs the patient has never seen. In the face of this mysterious and recalcitrant flesh turned inside out for others, one's experience of lived autonomy ("self-rule") can be undermined.

Illness and the experience of space and time. These modes of embodied dis-integration typical of illness also suffuse space and time as experienced. When healthy, the "here" I inhabit opens onto a variety of beckoning "theres." I look up a flight of steps I know I can climb. I gaze across an open street I can cross. Even though I hold back from many options, space unfolds as a field of possible movement, activity, desires to be fulfilled (Straus, 1963).

With many forms of illness this spatial field is disrupted. I remain confined in my bed, floating like an island in a vast sea separating me from the workaday world (Berg, 1966). Or I look up the flight of stairs and know that, due perhaps to arthritis or a neuromuscular disease, I cannot reach the top. That region remains cut off, a kind of Mount Olympus accessible only to those empowered by health. They are heedless of the glories of their capable flesh, but the sick person knows.

As space is thus altered by illness, so too is time. Ordinarily, human beings dwell largely in the future (Heidegger, 1962). Our present activities are geared toward the future accomplishment of desired goals. One goes to the paint store but is already envisioning and pointing toward the finished room with its redone walls. If I should fall sick I would find that my way toward that future was blocked—lying in bed, unable to paint, tethered annoyingly to the present. Illness often pins us like a captured specimen to the here and now of insistent discomfort and fluctuating symptoms. The claustrophobic world of concern closes in on the sufferer; the energetic traveler and the soaring intellectual can both become unendurable bores as their focus is seized by present nausea and aches. There are avenues of escape. One can "lose oneself" in a good book or the virtual world of the hospital television. One can dwell in past nostalgia or dream of a future restored to health. But these wanderings never fully lose their character as modes of escape from the confinement of illness.

Illness and the experience of others. This dis-integration of our spatiotemporal world is often matched by a felt dis-unity with others. When healthy, we are a part of the mainstream, involved with work, family, and socializing. We tend to share with those around us a common context of activity and experience. Yet as simple a sensation as pain can suddenly open a profound distance (Scarry, 1985). Inches away and sympathetic, the other person cannot experience my pain, nor can they relieve it. I may not even find the words needed to communicate my pain; this most private of experiences is notoriously resistant to our common language.

Illness can sever or render problematic our social relations in a variety of ways. In addition to its pains, the disability of illness may cut us off from the world. We linger in bed while everyone goes to their tasks, friends and family absorbed in their busy lives. We may not even have the energy for socializing, or we may wish to hide. "I don't want you to see me like this" is a frequent refrain of the person reduced by illness to sallow skin and problematic bowels. And the healthy may be more than willing to accommodate; we often wish to avoid the world of the sick, who remind us of our own vulnerability.

Loneliness can contribute greatly to the suffering of the ill. There is a sense of exile—from one's body, suddenly hostile; from one's activities and goals, now distant, unattainable; and from one's fellows, caught up in their own world of which one was recently a part. In the face of this exile, social connection often takes on heightened importance for the sick person. The compassion (etymologically, "to suffer with") that grounds another's willingness to listen to, touch, and take care of the sick person often does a great deal to alleviate suffering.

Illness and the experience of the cosmos. The term "cosmos" refers to the world discerned as an ordered and harmonious whole. This is precisely what illness can bring into question. Serious maladies often fracture one's sense of meaning and order. One might discover in the midst of an ordinary day a growth that is subsequently diagnosed as malignant. Questions scream forth: "Why has this happened?" "Why now?" "Why to me?" The possibility arises that these questions have no good answers. The meanings one has taken for granted shatter. We say, "his universe fell apart"—it lost its unity.

This experience of meaninglessness can prove intolerable. Any meaning may be preferable, even a negative one: "I have done wrong and this illness is my punishment" (Kopelman, 1988). The ill often search for their offending infractions, be it smoking, eating fatty foods, having a "cancer-prone personality," or transgressions against God. This association of sickness and sin preserves the coherence of a just universe, as well as the sense of one's own power. If I have brought this on myself, I may be able to repair it. However, this reading of illness brings its own sense of painful exile. Sickness remains a scarlet letter, branding the individual's moral failings. The healthy, eager to strengthen their own illusions of invulnerability and superiority, may concur with this judgment.

Illness, then, is not simply a biological event; it is also an existential transformation. One may be stripped of one's trust in the body, reliance on the future, taken-for-granted abilities, professional and social roles, even one's place in the cosmos.

Of course, this need not always be the case. The experience of illness varies a great deal; it depends on the nature of the attacking disease, the vagaries of individual psychology, and the social milieu. Some of this diversity is captured in the growing literature on medical phenomenology and so-called pathographies—accounts of illness written by or about the sufferers (Brody, 1987; Hawkins, 1993). One can ultimately imagine textbooks of illness, as there are now for diseases, that would describe experiences typically associated with, for example, severe psoriasis, heart attacks, or neurological

diseases (Sacks, 1985). This article will seek but to highlight a few differences between broad types of acute and chronic illnesses.

Acute illnesses and inflicted traumas. In the common phenomena of acute, but passing, illnesses—the flu, for example, or even a bout with pneumococcal pneumonia, serious but treatable with antibiotics—discomfort and disability shrink one's world and distance it from that shared by others, but the horizon of health remains visible. One is buoyed by the assurance that this illness is temporary, that after this brief visit to a foreign land one will surely return home. The sense of suffering and cosmic dislocation are thus greatly diminished.

Then there are illnesses and traumas of acute onset but more catastrophic consequences. One may be severely burned, for example, or suffer a serious heart attack that even after recovery throws one's life into jeopardy. The sudden and unpredictable nature of such events leaves its own psychic scars. The world and one's body are no longer safe places but a kind of horror house in which danger can leap forth at any moment and from any quarter. This sense may be especially acute when trauma is inflicted by another, as through a gunshot wound or a sexual assault (Brison, 1993). The embodied self is revealed as profoundly vulnerable to disruption, penetration, or violation by others.

In the face of acute catastrophe, William F. May suggests the individual experiences something of an existential obliteration. As Dax Cowart calls out after suffering severe burns covering two-thirds of his body, "Don't you see, I am a dead man" (May, 1991, p. 16). The old self lies in ruins. However, this death can be followed by rebirth. The painful period of reconstruction may involve not simply reclaiming one's previous identity but forging a new one that in some ways may be stronger (Brison, 1993).

This is an especially difficult task for those subject to traumas inflicted by others, as in cases of child molestation or spousal battering. Here, the confinements imposed by illness take on new dimensions. The victim is entrapped not only within physical suffering but by a double imprisonment—external and internal—to which May refers. There are external barriers to breaking free of the violence: the dominion of adults over children in the case of molestation; the difficulty in attaining employment, financial independence, shelter, and/or child care in the case of a battered wife contemplating escape. There are internal barriers as well: The victim often feels guilty, tainted, or shamed by his or her participation, and may thus comply with secrecy. Victims may also fear that exposing the truth or leaving will cause harm and compound their guilt. A sense of inferiority and powerlessness can set in from repeated abuse: "This will never change. There's nothing I can do. I'm not worth it anyway." Finally, as awful as this abusive world is, it is familiar, it is home, and the victim may cling to it for security amid the fear. Many break free, but psychological forces may pull victims back, making escape an arduous struggle.

Chronic illness.   Many illnesses are neither transitory nor based on acute events: Instead, they are chronic, lifelong, and involve relatively stable or progressive patterns of disability. Forms of arthritis, bronchitis-emphysema, kidney disease, diabetes, Alzheimer's disease, colitis, and autoimmune diseases, for example, fall into this category. The onset may come early in life; however, the elderly often suffer from such degenerative conditions, and with the aging of the overall population, along with advances in the prevention and cure of acute disease, chronic illness is increasingly the staple of medical practices and hospital care.

Chronic illness can bring with it all of the dis-integrations described above: within and from one's body, from the spatiotemporal world, from others, and from the cosmos. Unlike acute and treatable illness, there may be no horizon of health that allows one to look beyond present suffering. The day-in-and-day-out persistence of pain and disability, without hope of relief, can bring about a sort of existential fatigue. On the other hand, the chronicity of the condition may enable reconstruction and habituation. With severe arthritis, for example, tying one's shoe can become a trying task, walking to the store an impossibility. But the chronic nature of arthritis also gives one time to work through its meanings and accustom oneself to this new body and world. Modes of limitation and dependency need to be recognized, along with the possibilities for self-fulfillment that are still available.

This process of habituation is particularly difficult in the case of chronic illness with a downhill course. S. Kay Toombs (1992a) discusses her multiple sclerosis in this light. The disease is typified by sudden exacerbations and remissions (e.g., of visual disturbance or bowel and bladder incontinence), but with a gradual buildup over time of neurological deficits. There is thus a continual need to redefine the self in the face of new incapacities. Adjusting to muscle weakness, one becomes accustomed to using a walker and the consequent restrictions and possibilities. But even this achievement is unpredictably impermanent. As the disease advances, one becomes wheelchair-bound. The dignity associated with the upright posture is lost, together with passage to regions now inaccessible. The ill person faces the Sisyphean task of repeated readjustment without promise of rest.

Medical treatment and healing

This survey of the illness experience raises the question of the impact of contact with the medical profession upon the sufferer (Toombs, 1992b). When illness results from a curable disease, medical treatment plays a powerful role in restoring the individual to wholeness. However, such a remedy is not always possible or immediate, nor are the experiential impacts of health care always benign.

Just as we speak of "iatrogenic disease"—disease caused by medical intervention—so we could speak of "iatrogenic illness." Many of the experiential dis-integrations associated with illness can also be brought about or exacerbated by the process of medical treatment. When illness fragments the body into problematic parts and functions and renders this body alien to the self, that process is often intensified in the doctor's office. The physician has the patient disrobe, probes and palpates different organs, investigating the body as if it were a malfunctioning machine. The patient learns to internalize this distancing and objectifying gaze on the body.

Similarly, treatment can exacerbate the disruption of ordinary space and time and of social relations. Hospitalization provides a vivid example. One's clothes, a mark of personal identity, are replaced with a hospital gown that is embarrassingly open at the back. One is displaced from the routines of everyday life, leaving friends, family, home, and community for a strange world of rules and protocols, frightening technologies, and authorities who loom and then disappear. Just when one's world most needs shoring up, it is further challenged.

Medical talk also effects subtle but pervasive displacements. Struggling to make existential sense of "What is happening?" "Why me?" and "How can I rise to the occasion?" the patient may find little help in diagnostic labels. In Leo Tolstoy's story "The Death of Ivan Ilych," Ivan grapples with the profound issue of his life and death, but for the doctor "the real question was to decide between a floating kidney, chronic catarrh, or appendicitis" (Tolstoy, 1960, p. 121). The exclusive focus on disease leaves the illness unaddressed. Loneliness is intensified when one most needs communion; the search for meaning is truncated by a heap of scientific words.

Some of these deficiencies so characteristic of contemporary medicine emerge from its basis in a mechanistic worldview. The seventeenth-century philosopher René Descartes, who helped lay the groundwork of modern science and medicine, took a dualist position. The human being, he argued, is a complex of two very different parts—the "mind," imbued with rationality and free will, and the "body," a mechanism governed by the same physical laws as the rest of nature. Bodily disease can then be understood according to the model of machine breakdown. Doctors become scientists/technicians whose task it is to fix or replace the broken part. This Cartesian paradigm has generated the search for precision drugs and surgical procedures, the emphasis on scientific (rather than humanistic) training for the physician, and the hospital conceived as a temple to technology. Much of the efficacy of modern medicine rests on its dualist and mechanist foundations. But this focus on the body-as-machine has led to a relative neglect of the person-as-ill and of the theater of suffering in which he or she dwells (Leder, 1992).

However, many sensitive clinicians do seek to be healers of illness, not only treaters of disease. To "heal" is to begin reweaving into wholeness the tapestry of life shredded by illness. Even when disease is not curable, the practitioner can seek to relieve pain and preserve physical function. The practitioner can explain in understandable terms what is happening within the patient's body and encourage him or her to be an active participant in decision making and treatment. Thus, the ill person regains a measure of knowledge and control vis-à-vis the recalcitrant body.

Cut off from others by the privacy of pain and the loss of function, the sick person may reach out to the provider with the longing of a shipwrecked castaway who spies a sail on the horizon. Here is someone who can hear my story, someone who may offer me transport home. The sensitive practitioner can do this to an extent simply through listening. When the patient is permitted to tell his or her story, voice fears, ask questions, and hear genuine responses, a social reconnection is forged. The practitioner furthers this process by informing and mobilizing the patient's support system. The participation of family and friends is invited, and isolating modes of treatment such as hospitalization can, when possible, be avoided.

Just as the body seeks to heal itself, so individuals seek an interpretive healing by trying to make sense of what has occurred (Kleinman, 1988). Anne Hawkins, studying written accounts of illness, charts out the mythic motifs the sick often use: They may see themselves in heroic struggle against a dangerous foe, or journeying to the underworld to retrieve a great prize (Hawkins, 1993). These myths can sometimes turn disabling—for example, the battle metaphor provides little guidance or solace when the disease finally emerges the victor. Susan Sontag focuses on such negative effects of understanding disease metaphorically (Sontag, 1990); and the practitioner may need to challenge a patient's unhelpful fantasy. But these mythic interpretations can also serve a healing role, helping the ill person to render events coherent, rise to the occasion, and extract what is good (Hawkins, 1993). The practitioner who resists the temptation to rely on reductionist "medicalese" or on metaphors foreign to the needs of the patient can support the ill person's own healing narrative.

Ultimately, healing is not just a reconstruction of a prior life but the building of something new. For many, illness serves as the oyster grit from which a pearl is formed: a deeper compassion for others, perhaps, or a greater intimacy with loved ones; an attentiveness to the joys of ordinary living, or a reordering of lifestyle and priorities; the development of virtues such as courage or patience; an acceptance, perhaps, of the vulnerability and dependence of all human life and the need for powers beyond the self. The suggestion that illness can be a grace is not a license to grow callous to the suffering it involves. Few seriously ill people wish to be told, "Cheer up, this is the best thing that could have happened!" But the patient and practitioner alike can remain open to the healing gifts that illness itself may bring.

Bioethical implications

The illness experience has implications not only for clinical practice but for the field of bioethics. Bioethical reflections need not be "top-down"—starting from overarching theories and principles that then are applied to cases. They can be "bottom-up," that is, commencing with the concrete situation of the ill and drawing out the needs and moral claims that follow. Indeed, some suggest that bioethics is undergoing a "paradigm shift," with a new openness toward methodologies that pay close attention to the experience of illness and caregiving (DuBose et al., 1994). Several consequences might ensue for the field.

First, taking lived experience more seriously may shed new light on the traditional issues of bioethics. For example, "truth-telling" and "informed consent" are often supported by reference to a Kantian framework of "respect for persons." Within this framework, emphasis is placed on preserving the individual's autonomy. When we move from this abstraction to the concrete situation of the ill, however, new features come into view. It is not simply the "autonomous individual" of ethical theory who comes to the doctor's office in pain. By this time the person's sense of lived autonomy may already be compromised by uncertainty and confusion, emotional turmoil, a threatened future, and a body run amok. In this light, informed consent becomes not simply a way to preserve autonomy prior to treatment; rather it becomes a part of the treatment itself, a way to restore autonomy through enhancing knowledge, control, and trust in others. The patient, to the extent possible, regains the position of decision maker and is empowered by truth.

Or is he? Much depends on how the "truth" is conveyed. Medical jargon that conveys "the facts of the case" can disempower the ill person. As with Ivan Ilych's doctor, the physician's terms may obliterate the patient's narrative. Moreover, the theater in which this conversation is enacted—private office or hospital—is the physician's domain. He or she is in a position of power: an "agent" as opposed to a "patient," the healthy person as opposed to the sick one—the physician is the one with privileged knowledge, authority, and professional status (Zaner, 1988). To really understand "informed consent" we must attend to these features that structure "truth" and power relations.

Starting from lived experience rather than theory can thus reshape our ethical sensitivities toward current issues. For example, discussions of abortion, organ transplantation, and termination of life support call out for the contributions of a rich phenomenology of the lived body. However, an experience-based bioethics could do more than reformulate traditional issues; the very topics taken as paradigmatic could shift. Bioethical discourse has typically focused on particular quandaries brought about by new technologies and conflicting moral intuitions. When should we "pull the plug"? Who has the right to refuse treatment? When can we breach confidentiality? While such issues are real, they often leave unquestioned the general context of medical practice, as if only special dilemmas called for bioethical thought. But the experience of illness and treatment is intrinsically a moral theater. The ill person is confronted with the dis-integration of his or her world and must grapple to restore "the good" or forge a new vision. The individuals and institutions involved in health care participate in this drama in myriad ways; the language used, the texture of personal relations, the fees exacted, and the structuring of space and time all have ethical significance.

One promising topic for an experience-based bioethics is the "moral ecology" of health-care institutions. An example is George Agich's study of long-term care, detailing how the lived experience of autonomy is enhanced or diminished by environmental patterns. Are schedules set for the convenience of a nursing home bureaucracy or with the client's needs in mind? Are there spatial cues to orient the elderly resident, or does the layout of the home contribute to confusion, powerlessness, and isolation? Is infantilizing baby talk the everyday language, or is there an atmosphere that enhances dignity? Such issues are not as dramatic as those that make bioethics headlines, but they are at least as significant to the lives of many. One can imagine the day when institutional ethics committees attend to such issues of moral ecology, not simply the quandary cases.

An experience-based bioethics would also look at the calls placed upon the individual practitioner by the special situation of the ill. This is not simply a matter of "What action do I take?" (the focus of deontological and utilitarian ethics), but of "What kind of person should I be?" (the focus of virtue ethics). For example, the isolation and incapacity of the ill underscore the importance of correlative virtues in the practitioner—compassion, for example, and trustworthiness (Pellegrino and Thomasma, 1993).

In addition, an experience-based bioethics shows us that it is not simply the practitioner who is a moral actor but also the ill person. Though defined as "patient" vis-à-vis the medical bureaucracy, he or she is also an agent wrestling with a profound existential challenge (May, 1991). In the face of the dis-integrations described above, the sick person cannot evade responsibility—that is, the "ability to respond." Depending upon the qualities of this response, the individual can forge a good life even in the face of suffering, or may cave in to bitterness and despair. Special virtues are called for in meeting well the challenge of illness—for example, courage, patience, humility, proper assertiveness, and hope. Sickness is an arena that calls us to test and reforge who we really are and who we wish to be. For too long the ill person as agent has been absent from bioethical reflection just as from much of clinical practice. Close attention to the illness experience can help remedy this lack.

DREW LEDER

Directly related to this article are the other articles in this entry: HISTORY OF THE CONCEPTS, SOCIOLOGICAL PERSPECTIVES, ANTHROPOLOGICAL PERSPECTIVES, *and* PHILOSOPHICAL PERSPECTIVES. *For a further discussion of topics mentioned in this article, see the entries* ABUSE, INTERPERSONAL; AGING AND THE AGED; AUTONOMY; BODY; CASUISTRY; CHRONIC CARE; COMPASSION; DEATH; IATROGENIC ILLNESS AND INJURY; INTERPRETATION; METAPHOR AND ANALOGY; NARRATIVE; PAIN AND SUFFERING; REHABILITATION MEDICINE; SURGERY; *and* VIRTUE AND CHARACTER. *For a discussion of related ideas, see the entries* ACADEMIC HEALTH CENTERS; HEALING; INFORMATION DISCLOSURE; INFORMED CONSENT; LONG-TERM CARE; MENTAL ILLNESS; *and* MENTALLY ILL AND MENTALLY DISABLED PERSONS.

Bibliography

AGICH, GEORGE J. 1993. *Autonomy and Long-Term Care.* New York: Oxford University Press.

BARON, RICHARD J. 1985. "An Introduction to Medical Phenomenology: I Can't Hear You While I'm Listening." *Annals of Internal Medicine* 103, no. 4:606–611.

BERG, JAN HENDRIK VAN DEN. 1966. *The Psychology of the Sickbed.* Pittsburgh: Duquesne University Press.

BRISON, SUSAN J. 1993. "Surviving Sexual Violence: A Philosophical Perspective." *Journal of Social Philosophy* 24, no. 1:5–22.

BRODY, HOWARD. 1987. *Stories of Sickness.* New Haven, Conn.: Yale University Press.

CASSELL, ERIC J. 1985. *The Healer's Art.* Cambridge, Mass.: MIT Press.

———. 1991. *The Nature of Suffering and the Goals of Medicine.* New York: Oxford University Press.

DuBose, Edwin R.; Hamel, Ronald P.; and O'Connell, Laurence J., eds. 1994. *A Matter of Principles? Ferment in U.S. Bioethics.* Valley Forge, Pa.: Trinity Press International.

Engelhardt, H. Tristram, Jr. 1982. "Illnesses, Diseases, and Sicknesses." In *The Humanity of the Ill: Phenomenological Perspectives,* pp. 142–156. Edited by Victor Kestenbaum. Knoxville: University of Tennessee Press.

———. 1986. *The Foundations of Bioethics.* New York: Oxford University Press.

Foucault, Michel. 1973. *The Birth of the Clinic.* Translated by Alan M. Sheridan Smith. New York: Vintage.

Hawkins, Anne Hunsaker. 1993. *Reconstructing Illness: Studies in Pathography.* West Lafayette, Ind.: Purdue University Press.

Heidegger, Martin. 1962. *Being and Time.* Translated by John Macquarrie and Edward Robinson. San Francisco: Harper San Francisco.

Kleinman, Arthur. 1988. *The Illness Narratives: Suffering, Healing and the Human Condition.* New York: Basic Books.

Kopelman, Loretta M. 1988. "The Punishment Concept of Disease." In *AIDS: Ethics and Public Policy,* pp. 49–55. Edited by Christine Pierce and Donald Van DeVeer. Belmont, Calif.: Wadsworth.

Leder, Drew. 1990. *The Absent Body.* Chicago: University of Chicago Press.

———. 1992. "A Tale of Two Bodies: The Cartesian Corpse and the Lived Body." In *The Body in Medical Thought and Practice,* pp. 17–35. Edited by Drew Leder. Dordrecht, Netherlands: Kluwer.

May, William F. 1991. *The Patient's Ordeal.* Bloomington: Indiana University Press.

Merleau-Ponty, Maurice. 1962. *Phenomenology of Perception.* Translated by Colin Smith. London: Routledge & Kegan Paul.

Pellegrino, Edmund D., and Thomasma, David C. 1993. *The Virtues in Medical Practice.* New York: Oxford University Press.

Sacks, Oliver W. 1985. *The Man Who Mistook His Wife for a Hat and Other Clinical Tales.* New York: Summit.

Scarry, Elaine. 1985. *The Body in Pain: The Making and Unmaking of the World.* New York: Oxford University Press.

Sontag, Susan. 1990. *Illness as Metaphor and AIDS and Its Metaphors.* New York: Doubleday Anchor Books.

Straus, Erwin W. M. 1963. *The Primary World of Senses: A Vindication of Sensory Experience.* Translated by Jacob Needleman. New York: Free Press.

———. 1966. *Phenomenological Psychology: The Selected Papers of Erwin M. Straus.* Translated in part by Erling Eng. New York: Basic Books.

Tolstoy, Leo. 1960. *The Death of Ivan Ilych and Other Stories.* New York: New American Library.

Toombs, S. Kay. 1992a. "The Body in Multiple Sclerosis: A Patient's Perspective." In *The Body in Medical Thought and Practice,* pp. 127–137. Edited by Drew Leder. Dordrecht, Netherlands: Kluwer.

———. 1992b. *The Meaning of Illness: A Phenomenological Account of the Different Perspectives of Physician and Patient.* Dordrecht, Netherlands: Kluwer.

Zaner, Richard M. 1981. *The Context of Self: A Phenomenological Inquiry Using Medicine as a Clue.* Athens: Ohio University Press.

———. 1988. *Ethics and the Clinical Encounter.* Englewood Cliffs, N.J.: Prentice-Hall.

HEALTH EDUCATION

See Health Promotion and Health Education.

HEALTH INSURANCE

See Health-Care Financing, *article on* health-care insurance.

HEALTH AS AN OBLIGATION

See Patients' Responsibilities.

HEALTH OFFICIALS AND THEIR RESPONSIBILITIES

Health officials are responsible for organizing health services, for administering policies and regulations that protect the health and safety of communities and nations, for preparing and distributing information aimed at reducing risks to health, and for the provision of adequate health care for all. High-ranking health officials, such as the surgeon general in the United States and the chief medical officer in the United Kingdom, may have to make decisions affecting the health of millions of people. Health officials include staff of the World Health Organization, the United States Public Health Service, and many other agencies at international, national, state or provincial, and local levels. Health officials come from diverse professional and scientific backgrounds: medicine, nursing, dentistry, social and behavioral sciences, sanitary and environmental sciences, health education, nutrition, statistics, epidemiology, administration, and so on. They differ from health workers, who provide personal medical care, in that they are responsible for groups or communities rather than individuals: The community is their patient. This is particularly true of local public-health officials, although many of these are also responsible for aspects of individual personal care.

In addition to their primary duty to protect the health needs of communities, health officials have general duties and obligations to individuals; to colleagues; to science; to the traditions, standards, and codes of conduct of their profession; and to their employers (e.g., members of legislatures, hospital management committees, local boards of health).

Individual rights and community needs

In public health, concern for the collective good may take precedence over respect for the dignity, rights, or freedom of individuals. This concern has deep historical roots: In medieval Europe, belief in the concept of contagion led to customs such as the distinctive clothing worn and warning bell carried by lepers, to the establishment of prisonlike lazarettos where contagious cases could be isolated, and to the practice of quarantine. These and many other actions aimed at protecting community health were codified by Johann Peter Frank in *System einer vollständigen medicinischen Polizey* (1779). Much modern public-health legislation requires limits to liberty and property, such as laws requiring motorcycle riders to wear helmets or drivers and passengers to buckle their seat belts while riding in automobiles, measures that do not evoke punitive or stigmatizing responses. Yet stigmatization and loss of freedom as social penalties can result from public-health regulations: As the HIV epidemic powerfully reminds us, a sanction can arise from the mere suspicion that a person or family has a contagious disease.

Insensitive disclosure of information about the health status of persons, communities, or socially distinct groups by health officials can stigmatize these persons, communities, or groups. One responsibility of health officials such as health statisticians and epidemiologists, therefore, is to exercise tact in conveying information about high-risk persons or groups. Health officials have a duty to avoid harm to members of the population whose health they safeguard while ensuring that no individual or group is publicly identified as a "case," "contact," "carrier," or "high-risk" person, or receives any other pejorative label that exposes such person or group to scorn, derision, ostracism, persecution, needless segregation, or other discriminatory behavior.

Successful efforts to eliminate infectious diseases (smallpox, diphtheria, poliomyelitis, etc.) and to ensure safe drinking water have engendered the respect and admiration of the general public. Most people approve of efforts to reduce and ultimately eliminate tobacco addiction. Lingering traces of antagonism to health officials still persist, however, and are attributable to their image as "medical police" who punish sick people by isolating them, prevent them from working, and force them to submit to unpleasant treatments. Allan Brandt (1987) described the extremes to which health officials in the United States went in their efforts to contain the spread of venereal diseases during World War I: Prostitutes (and other "loose" women) were imprisoned on the mere suspicion that they might infect soldiers. During the polio-

myelitis epidemic of 1916, health officials in New York City searched private homes and forcibly removed children believed to have been in contact with paralytic cases (Paul, 1971). Similar coercive measures have been discussed as options in efforts to prevent the spread of HIV infection.

Sometimes the regulatory function of health officials has been perceived as opposing the interests of large numbers of people in a community. Mining and processing of asbestos in the Eastern Townships of Quebec endangered the health of all the people living there. To close the mines and factories meant much economic hardship—a variation on the theme of Henrik Ibsen's play *An Enemy of the People,* with health officials acting like Dr. Stockmann (who was reviled by townspeople, even his own family, when he recommended closing a spa that was the economic mainstay of his town to control an epidemic of typhoid fever). Health officials may have to invoke laws or regulations to close restaurants, food-handling facilities, swimming pools, and so forth because these are a danger to the health of people who use them. Such actions cannot be lightly undertaken if they threaten anyone's livelihood. Health officials have an obligation to ensure that their actions are not needlessly heavy-handed. A restaurant need not be closed because an outbreak of food poisoning is traced to it, though such action would be appropriate if repeated outbreaks have the same focus of infection.

Distributive justice and public-health advocacy

An important responsibility of health officials, congruent with their obligation to give first priority to the needs of communities, is to advocate equitable resource allocation. This means seeking a fair share of resources and expenditure for public-health actions that will benefit all, such as providing safe drinking water and sanitation services, immunization and family-planning programs; and ensuring that all, including especially the most disadvantaged, have access to necessary health-care services. Health officials have long recognized this responsibility and have been identified as advocates of fiscally sound plans for universal coverage (Roemer, 1986). They also have a duty to discourage excessive investment in expensive high-technology treatment facilities that will serve relatively few people or add only minimally, if at all, to the duration of life without enhancing the quality of life (Callahan, 1987).

Health officials and the media: Education or censorship?

Health officials collaborate with representatives of the media (press, radio, television) to develop and disseminate educational messages on a wide range of health-related issues: diet and nutrition, safe driving practices, the benefits of exercise, and so on. Since epidemiologic studies clarified the methods of spread of the HIV epidemic, health officials have been in the forefront of education aimed at effective control measures, notably advocacy of "safe sex" through use of condoms and avoidance of promiscuous sexual encounters (U.S. Presidential Commission, 1988). Former Surgeon General C. Everett Koop played a prominent leadership role in energizing such efforts despite opposition from more conservative cabinet colleagues in the Reagan administration.

Sometimes health officials seek to restrict or ban advertising and promotion of products that can harm health—in particular, to limit tobacco advertising, on the grounds that the public interest justifies censorship of advertisements for this harmful addictive substance (U.S. Department of Health and Human Services, 1989). Tobacco companies and their advertising agencies argue that this infringes on free speech and is unjustifiable in a democratic society. The moral and ethical issues here are challenging and are probably best decided at the local level. Smoking-control measures are often introduced in local government jurisdictions after approval by local surveys. As social values have shifted away from tolerance of smoking, the decision has tended to favor smoke-free environments, but restrictions on advertising are sometimes viewed as censorship and are less often approved.

Other aspects of censorship in the public interest are more controversial. There is circumstantial evidence that portrayal of violence on television encourages acts of violence, especially among impressionable young viewers. Many experts in behavioral aspects of public health, in the media and in the entertainment industry, believe that even if the evidence were more persuasive, it would be wrong to censor such programs with the aim of reducing the incidence of violent behavior. Nevertheless, the evidence does justify attempts to develop collaborative strategies that involve health officials and creative artists in a partnership aimed at promoting the presentation of programs that demonstrate values of caring and compassion rather than the notion of problem solving by resort to force.

Health officials have occasionally used health education and supporting regulations in an overly zealous, even authoritarian, manner, in efforts to control a wide variety of public-health problems, for example, seeking to restrict the freedom of pregnant women to smoke or drink alcohol, or regulating the dietary intake of foods incriminated as risk factors for coronary heart disease. They must beware that their quest for improved health does not deteriorate into paternalism. The risk may be greatest when their motives are highest, as when they seek to reduce and ultimately eliminate tobacco addiction among girls and pregnant women. Advocacy of this cause can sometimes overstep the bounds of scientific objectivity.

Personal health services and the public health

The problem of reconciling individual human rights, dignity, and freedom with the role and responsibility of the health official is nowhere more difficult than when family-planning programs are organized and provided as part of public-health services. The decision to begin or continue with a pregnancy is personal and very private. Physicians, nurses, and others who work in publicly funded family-planning programs may be obliged to adhere to government policies that are at variance with the aspirations of individual clients or patients. To whom are health officials answerable—the political decision makers who set the policy or individual clients? The law may urge them one way while their consciences pull them in another direction. Ethics and moral values may well count for more than bad law, but in the matter of reproductive freedom there is no consensus on what is right and what is wrong.

Public health includes many other personal services: maternal and infant care; treatment and surveillance aimed at control of conditions such as tuberculosis and sexually transmitted diseases; dental and medical care of indigent persons; and comprehensive care of certain disadvantaged and other groups such as recent immigrants. Often persons in such categories are vulnerable and easily stigmatized; many belong to socially and economically disadvantaged groups who may be unaware of their basic human rights. Such people are sometimes referred to as an underclass that exists outside the organized structure of society. Health officials have an obligation to respect the dignity and autonomy of these people, for instance, by adhering to procedures for obtaining informed consent before initiating preventive or therapeutic procedures. There is no excuse for shameful episodes such as the Tuskegee experiment—the prolonged observation of untreated syphilis among uneducated black men who were kept in ignorance of their condition and of modern methods to treat it, so that the investigators could study the natural history of the disease (Jones, 1981).

Conflicts of interest

Conflict of interest is defined as compromise of a person's objectivity when that person has a vested interest in the outcome of a situation. Conflicts of interest can arise in public-health practice. Boards of health can become politicized and require health officials to act in politically expedient ways that are contrary to their professional judgment, or face the threat of dismissal and replacement with others who will be more compliant.

The first loyalty of health officials is to the public whose health they are committed to safeguard; but it can be easy to rationalize a wrong decision or to submit to political pressure reinforced by the economic threat of loss of one's job. This form of conflict of interest may be considered a particular problem in industrial health services, but it can occur in local and even in national health departments, for example, if it is politically inconvenient to reveal the health hazards associated with an industry of national importance. This might apply to defense-related industries or to the nuclear power industry.

Codes and guidelines

Health officials have such diverse responsibilities and come from so many scientific and professional backgrounds that it is difficult to formulate all-embracing guidelines or codes of conduct that would enunciate appropriate standards of practice and behavior for all. Physicians and nurses have clearly defined ethical codes. Health officials who work in some areas of specialization, for example, compilers of official statistics, have developed codes of conduct (International Statistical Institute, 1986); others, such as epidemiologists, have done or are doing the same. Locally compiled rules or regulations in many departments of health include statements formally defining the rules of procedure to be followed in given circumstances. While such edicts are useful, they do not cover all possible contingencies. Many ambiguous situations arise in everyday practice, and the range and complexity of these situations continue to increase. This makes it essential for health officials to be constantly cognizant of the moral and ethical dimensions of their work.

JOHN M. LAST
MICHAEL D. PARKINSON

Directly related to this entry are the entries PUBLIC HEALTH; *and* PUBLIC HEALTH AND THE LAW, *especially the article* LEGAL MORALISM AND PUBLIC HEALTH. *For a further discussion of topics mentioned in this entry, see the entries* ABORTION, *section on* CONTEMPORARY ETHICAL AND LEGAL ASPECTS; ADVERTISING; AIDS, *article on* PUBLIC-HEALTH ISSUES; BEHAVIOR CONTROL; COMMUNICATION, BIOMEDICAL, *article on* MEDIA AND BIOETHICS; CONFLICT OF INTEREST; ECONOMIC CONCEPTS IN HEALTH CARE; EPIDEMICS; HEALTH-CARE RESOURCES; ALLOCATION OF; HEALTH PROMOTION AND HEALTH EDUCATION; HEALTH SCREENING AND TESTING IN THE PUBLIC-HEALTH CONTEXT; INFORMED CONSENT; JUSTICE; LIFESTYLES AND PUBLIC HEALTH; PATERNALISM; SUBSTANCE ABUSE, *article on* ALCOHOL AND OTHER DRUGS IN A PUBLIC-HEALTH CONTEXT; *and* UTILITY. *Other relevant material may be found under the entries* AUTHORITY; BENEFICENCE; HEALTH POLICY, *article on* POLITICS AND HEALTH CARE; LAW AND BIOETHICS; *and* OCCUPATIONAL SAFETY AND HEALTH.

Bibliography

BRANDT, ALLAN M. 1987. *No Magic Bullet; A Social History of Venereal Disease in the United States Since 1880.* Expanded ed. New York: Oxford University Press.

CALLAHAN, DANIEL. 1987. *Setting Limits: Medical Goals in an Aging Society.* New York: Simon and Schuster.

FRANK, JOHANN PETER. 1779–1829. *System einer vollständigen medicinischen Polizey.* 9 vols. Translated into English by Erna Lesky as *A System of Complete Medical Police: Selections from Johann Peter Frank.* Baltimore: Johns Hopkins University Press, 1976.

INTERNATIONAL STATISTICAL INSTITUTE. 1986. "Declaration on Professional Ethics." *International Statistical Review* 54, no. 2:227–242.

JONES, JAMES H. 1981. *Bad Blood: The Tuskegee Syphilis Experiment, a Tragedy of Race and Medicine.* New York: Free Press.

PAUL, JOHN R. 1971. *A History of Poliomyelitis*, pp. 148–152. New Haven, Conn: Yale University Press.

ROEMER, MILTON I. 1986. "Comparative Health Care Systems." In *Maxcy-Rosenau Public Health and Preventive Medicine*, pp. 1747–1792. 12th ed. Edited by John M. Last. Norwalk, Conn.: Appleton-Century-Crofts.

U.S. DEPARTMENT OF HEALTH AND HUMAN SERVICES. 1989. *Reducing the Health Consequences of Smoking: 25 Years of Progress.* DHHS Publication no. (CDC) 89-8411. Washington, D.C.: Author.

U.S. PRESIDENTIAL COMMISSION ON THE HUMAN IMMUNODEFICIENCY VIRUS EPIDEMIC. 1988. *Report.* Washington, D.C.: Author.

HEALTH POLICY

I. Politics and Health Care
  Nancy E. Gin
  Howard Waitzkin
II. Health Policy in International Perspective
  Gerard F. Anderson
  Stephanie L. Maxwell

I. POLITICS AND HEALTH CARE

At the heart of the health-policy debate in the United States has been the question of health care as a basic human right. The concept of a right to needed services is not new to America; for instance, the constitutional right to legal representation establishes that all individuals are entitled to at least some basic services. However, the Constitution does not provide for a clear right to health care, in contrast to the constitutions of many other countries (Fuenzalida-Puelma and Connor, 1989).

The United States and the Republic of South Africa are the only two economically developed countries in the world without a national policy that accepts the principle of universal entitlement to basic medical care. Many observers believe, however, that the American system has become ethically intolerable. This article analyzes American health policy and some proposed directions of policy change.

Gaps in public coverage

Medicaid and Medicare were created in 1965 to improve the accessibility of medical services to the poor and the elderly. However, major problems have remained. Federal Medicaid payments go to limited categories of the poor and therefore exclude about one-third of American citizens with incomes below the poverty level; provisions vary from state to state. The elderly, on the other hand, have experienced erosion in Medicare coverage, with increasing copayments and deductibles on covered services, as well as continued noncoverage for nursing-home care and prescription drugs. Historically, individuals with Medicare have paid out of pocket for more than half of all medical expenses, a higher proportion than before the inception of Medicare (Minkler and Robertson, 1991).

The number of uninsured rose steeply after 1980, reflecting changes in the labor force, as more people were employed without benefits in service industries and many companies eliminated benefits due to the escalating cost of health insurance. Indeed, by the early 1990s, more than 37 million people were without insurance. During the 1980s, 13 percent of the American population, representing more than 11 million individuals, lost private insurance. African-American and Hispanic populations have remained disproportionately uninsured. Employed people and their dependents comprise approximately three-quarters of the uninsured. More than half of these employed uninsured earn middle-income or high-income wages but have no health benefits provided by their employer, nor do they purchase health insurance on their own. Working-age persons with private insurance face deductible provisions and limited coverage that frequently create major financial difficulties as well as frustrating complexities in obtaining benefits (Himmelstein et al., 1992).

Because there is no universal entitlement to basic health care, the availability, quality, and utilization of services depend on local conditions. In some geographical regions, there is a surplus of health professionals; in others, a shortage. Access differs according to patients' personal finances, initiative, and linguistic abilities.

Mechanisms to ensure quality of care are insufficient, and malpractice litigation is extensive. In different localities, the utilization of expensive medical procedures varies widely, indicating wasteful practice patterns (National Leadership Commission on Health Care, 1989). A laissez-faire approach to planning and organization has created a situation in which very high-quality medicine is available for part of the population, while others cannot receive the most basic services. Patients frequently face the frustrations of high costs, complex administrative procedures, inaccessible services, and variablequality. Due to cutbacks at the federal, state, and county levels, practitioners frequently cannot arrange for needed hospitalization, diagnostic procedures, or treatments when patients are uninsured or underinsured. As a result, patients frequently utilize emergency rooms for primary health-care needs at substantially higher cost to hospitals and society than if they were treated in less costly outpatient clinics.

Policy options

Competitive strategies.   Since the 1980s, competitive strategies have achieved prominence in health-policy circles. Such proposals aim to foster competition among providers, and thus to lower costs (Enthoven and Kronick, 1991). Competitive strategies culminated in "managed competition," a policy option favored initially by the Clinton administration (elected in 1992). The basic assumption of managed competition is that allowing competitive forces of the market to control health-care delivery will result in a high-quality, cost-effective system. Under such a system, two or three large managed-care providers operated by insurance companies would provide a government-determined basic package of health care to a specified region.

Competitive strategies have received major criticism. Forces of competition historically have not controlled health-care costs, as illustrated by the rise in overall costs at a rate higher than general inflation and by higher costs in regions with keen competition among health-care providers (Robinson and Luft, 1988). Further, medical services never have shown the characteristics of a competitive market, since government pays for more than 40 percent of health care and since the insurance, pharmaceutical, and medical-equipment industries all manifest monopolistic tendencies that inhibit competition. Hospitals and physicians maintain political-economic power through professional organizations that reduce the impact of competitive strategies. Physicians also affect the demand for services through recommendations about referrals, diagnostic studies, and treatment. Analytically, the effects of competition on costs are difficult to separate from other important changes, especially the effects of general inflation, the requirement of major copayments by patients, and the impact of prepayment (Siminoff, 1986).

Such competitive strategies also have led to major dislocations and gaps in services. For example, competitive contracting and prospective reimbursement under Medi-Cal (California's Medicaid system) have worsened the financial crises of hospitals with a large proportion of indigent clients. The resultant disruption in services due to underfunding of Medicaid has led to a measurable worsening of some patients' medical conditions (Lurie et al., 1986). In other states, competitive health plans have suffered severe and unpredicted financial problems, and patients have encountered major barriers to access, including direct refusal of care by providers (Freeman and Kirkman-Liff, 1985).

Several ethical issues also arise with "managed competition." On an individual level, autonomy may be compromised through elimination of a consumer's free choice of physicians and hospitals. Increased out-of-pocket costs may further impair autonomy by restricting access to care, especially among the poor. On the societal level, a two-tiered system remains in place, with the working poor and unemployed receiving minimum health care compared with more extensive coverage enjoyed by a relative few in the upper classes who can afford to pay out of pocket for additional coverage. Furthermore, managed competition does not curtail administrative waste, which has been estimated at approximately 15 percent of health-care expenditures, or about $120 billion annually (Woolhandler and Himmelstein, 1991).

Corporate involvement in health care. Various policies have encouraged corporate expansion in the medical field. By the mid-1970s, private insurance companies, pharmaceutical firms, and medical-equipment manufacturers had achieved prominent positions in the medical marketplace. In the 1980s, multinational corporations took over community hospitals in all regions of the country, acquired and/or managed many public hospitals, bought or built teaching hospitals affiliated with medical schools, and gained control of ambulatory-care organizations (Gray, 1991; Relman, 1980).

Despite concerns about cost containment, corporate profitability in health care has encountered few obstacles. In the early 1990s, after-tax profits for corporations with direct activities in health care ranked the third highest among American industrial groups ("Forty-Fifth Annual Report," 1993). Nationally, for-profit chains control about 15 percent of all hospitals, but in some states (for example, California, Florida, Tennessee, and Texas) the chains operate between one-third and one-half of hospitals. Ownership of nursing homes by corporate chains has increased by more than 30 percent. For-profit corporations have enrolled about 70 percent of all health-maintenance organization subscribers throughout the country.

While proponents perceive several economic advantages of corporate involvement in health care, substantiation of such claims is limited. For example, it is argued that tough-minded managerial techniques increase efficiency and decrease costs, although several studies have shown that for-profit health-care organizations are no more efficient than nonprofit ones (Watt et al., 1986). Similarly, research on corporate management has not supported the claim that corporate take-over can alleviate the financial problems of hospitals serving indigent clients (Lewin et al., 1988).

Corporate involvement in health care also has raised ethical questions. There is concern that corporate strategies lead to reduced services for the poor. While some corporations have established endowments for indigent care, the ability of such funds to ensure long-term access is doubtful, especially when cutbacks occur in public-sector support (Feder and Hadley, 1985). Other ethical concerns have focused on physicians' conflicting loyalties to patients and corporations, the implications of physicians' referrals of patients for services to corporations in which the physicians hold financial interests, the unwillingness of for-profit hospitals to provide unprofitable but needed services, and similar issues (Mitchell and Scott, 1992). These observations lead to doubts about the wisdom of policies that encourage corporate penetration of health care.

Public-sector programs. Policies enacted between 1980 and 1992 greatly reduced public-sector health programs. Cutbacks occurred in the national Medicaid program; Medicare; block grants for maternal and child health, migrant health services, community health centers, and birth-control services; health planning; educational assistance for medical students and residents (affecting especially minority recruitment); the National Health Service Corps; the Indian Health Service; and the National Institute of Occupational Safety and Health. Many federally sponsored research programs also have been cut.

During this same time period, measures of health and well-being in the United States either stopped improving or actually became worse. For example, a marked slowing in the rate of decline in infant mortality coincided with cutbacks in federal prenatal and perinatal programs; in several low-income urban areas, infant mortality increased (U.S. Department of Health and Human Services, 1987). Among African-Americans, postneonatal and maternal mortality rates stopped falling, after decades of steady decline, and a growing proportion of African-American women have not been able to receive adequate prenatal care (Hughes et al., 1988). These reversals in health status and health services, emerging as direct manifestations of changes in federal policies, have been unique among economically developed countries (World Bank, 1993; Cereseto and Waitzkin, 1986).

Alongside these programmatic cutbacks, bureaucratization and regulation in the health-care system have grown rapidly (Stern and Epstein, 1985). A distinction between the rhetoric of reduced government and the reality of greater government intervention is nowhere clearer than in the Medicare diagnosis-related group (DRG) program. Intended as a cost-control device, DRGs introduced unprecedented complexity and bureaucratic regulation. By providing reimbursement to hospitals at a fixed rate for specific diagnoses, DRGs encouraged hospitals to limit the length of stay, since the hospital receives the same amount whether a patient stays one day or five days. The same disincentive exists for providing services during the hospitalization, since fewer services translate into higher income for the institution. Hospitals responded to DRG regulations with an expansion of their own bureaucratic staffs and data-processing operations, more intensive utilization review, and a tendency to discharge patients with unstable conditions when DRG payments are exhausted. Private hospitals admitting a small proportion of indigent patients profited under DRGs; public and university hospitals that serve a higher percentage of indigent and multi-problem patients faced an unfavorable case mix within specific DRGs and thus fared poorly. The extensive utilization review that DRGs encouraged focused on cost cutting rather than on ensuring quality of care. Moreover, DRGs' contribution to cost controls remains unclear, in comparison with other factors, such as reduced inflation in the economy as a whole.

A national health program for the United States

History of prior proposals. Although advocacy for a national health program (NHP) dates back to the mid-1920s, with the proposal of the Committee on the Costs of Medical Care (an independent body funded by private foundations), the most intense efforts occurred during the 1970s, when Congress considered at least eighteen separate proposals. The supporters of these measures ranged across a wide political spectrum, including the Nixon administration, the American Medical Association, and both liberal and conservative legislators. During the Carter administration of the late 1970s, conflicts within the Democratic Party over reforms in health care helped prevent enactment of an NHP. Later, during the Reagan and Bush administrations (1981–1993), the support for an NHP from the legislative and executive branches of government seen during the 1970s was replaced by a policy of cutbacks in health and welfare programs, effectively eliminating the possibility of enactment. An NHP again emerged as a priority during the 1992 presidential campaign.

Within the range of NHP proposals considered during the late 1970s, several problems became clear. First, the NHP would have changed payment mechanisms rather than the organization of the health-care system. Under these proposals, the federal government would have guaranteed payment for most health services. However, the NHP would not have ensured that practitioners would work in different ways, in different areas, or with different patients.

Most of these plans for the NHP would not have covered all needed medical services. Copayment provisions would have required out-of-pocket payment by each person for some fixed percentage of health costs. While such copayments might have helped control costs, coinsurance predictably would have had a detrimental impact on the poor and other vulnerable groups, for whom such out-of-pocket payments are deterrents to obtaining needed care.

New and compulsory taxation, usually as fixed payroll deductions, would have paid for the NHP. The financing arrangements therefore would have been regressive; that is, low-income people would have paid a proportionately higher part of their income for health care than would the wealthy. Although various tax mechanisms could relieve the burden of health insurance for low-income persons, legislators devoted little attention to this issue (Mitchell and Schwartz, 1976).

In most NHP plans, private insurance companies would have served as the fiscal intermediaries. They would have received compensation for distributing NHP payments from the government to health providers. Such provisions thus would have assured continued profits for the private insurance industry and would have done little to reduce the administrative waste that has characterized this industry (Woolhandler and Himmelstein, 1991). Administrative costs account for approximately 25 cents of every health-care dollar spent in America, compared with approximately 10 cents in countries with NHPs. That translates to 15 percent less money available for direct patient care in America.

Regarding accessibility, NHP proposals would have contained few provisions for improving geographical maldistribution of health professionals. Fee schedules might have been higher in some proposals for doctors who practiced in underserved areas, but such incentives could not ensure that physicians actually would work in these areas.

Perspectives from other countries. Planning for an NHP in the United States would require open-minded consideration of the strengths and weaknesses of existing NHPs around the world. For instance, most countries in western Europe have initiated NHP structures permitting private practice in addition to a strong public sector. Canada has achieved universal entitlement to health care through an NHP that depends on private practitioners, private hospitals, and strong planning and coordinating roles for the national and provincial governments (Evans et al., 1991).

NHPs vary widely in the degree to which the national government employs health professionals and owns health institutions. For example, the NHPs of Great Britain, Denmark, and the Netherlands contract with self-employed general practitioners for primary care; Canadian private practitioners receive insurance payments mainly on a fee-for-service basis; in Finland and Sweden a high proportion of practicing doctors work as salaried employees of government agencies. In the United Kingdom, the national government owns most hospitals; regional or local governments own many hospitals in Sweden, Finland, and other Scandinavian countries; and Canada's system depends on governmental budgeting for both public and private hospitals.

The Canadian system is very pertinent to the United States, because of geographical proximity and cultural similarity. Canada assures universal entitlement to health services through a combination of national and provincial insurance programs. Doctors generally receive public insurance payments through fee-for-service arrangements. Hospitals obtain public funds through annually negotiated contracts based on projected costs, eliminating the need to bill for specific services. Progressive taxation finances the Canadian system, and the private insurance industry does not play a major role in the program's administration. Most Canadian provinces have initiated policies that aim to correct remaining problems of access based on geographical maldistribution. Cost controls in Canada depend on contracted global budgeting with hospitals, limitations on reimbursements to practitioners, and markedly lower administrative expenses because of reduced eligibility, billing, and collection procedures.

Since the structure of the economy in the United States is very similar to that of Canada and western European countries, which have established and comparatively successful NHPs, the feasibility of implementing such a program in America is high. As in these other countries, private hospitals, private practitioners, pharmaceutical companies, and other corporations involved in health care would remain in place. The systems in Canada and several European countries achieve their cost savings through drastic reductions in administrative activities, made possible by the use of a government agency as the only payer for needed health services. This type of monopsony financing allows private insurance for nonessential services and amenities, like cosmetic surgery or a private hospital room, but does not permit duplicating private insurance coverage for essential services. Curtailing the role of private insurance companies in health care could become the most important modification, under a single-payer system, of current financing policies in the United States.

Because of the commonly expressed concern about costs in the United States, the experiences of existing NHPs are instructive. American health-care expenditures, already the highest in the world, account for (as of 1993) approximately 14 percent of the gross national product. The presumption that an NHP would increase costs is not necessarily correct; depending on how an NHP is organized, costs might well fall below their prior level. First of all, major savings would come from reduced administrative overhead for billing, collection procedures, eligibility determinations, and other bureaucratic functions that no longer would be necessary. In the Canadian NHP, for instance, global budgeting for hospitals has greatly reduced administrative costs, and a much smaller role for the private insurance industry has lowered costs even further by restricting corporate profit. An analysis by the U.S. General Accounting Office (1991) showed that, due to savings from reduced administrative functions and entrepreneurism, a single-payer NHP like Canada's, if introduced in the United States, would lead to negligible added costs despite achieving universal access to care. For comparison, the cost of instituting a single-payer NHP is one order of magnitude less than expenditures on military systems like the Stealth bomber or government support for the financial sector in the savings and loan bailout.

Principles and prospects for a U.S. national health program. NHP proposals can be appraised against several basic principles (Waitzkin, 1989):

1. The NHP would provide for comprehensive care, including diagnostic, therapeutic, preventive, rehabilitative, environmental, and occupational-health services; dental and eye care; transportation to medical facilities; social work; and counseling.
2. These services generally would not require out-of-pocket payments at the point of delivery. While carefully limited copayments for certain services might be appropriate (as in Canada), copayments would be implemented in such a way as to ensure that they do not become barriers to access.
3. Coverage would be portable, so that travel or relocation would have no effect on a person's ability to obtain health care.
4. Financing for the NHP would come from a variety of sources, including continued corporate taxation, "health taxes" on cigarettes and alcoholic beverages, "conservation taxes" on fossil fuels and other energy sources, "pollution taxes" on known sources of air and water pollution, and a restructured individual tax. Taxation would be progressive, in that individuals and corporations with higher incomes would pay taxes at a higher rate.
5. The NHP would reduce administrative costs, private profit, and wasteful procedures in the health-care system. A national commission would establish a generic formulary of approved drugs, devices, equipment, and supplies. A national trust fund would disburse payments to private and public health facil-

ities through global and prospective budgeting. Profit to private insurance companies and other corporations would be closely restricted.

6. Professional associations would negotiate the fee structures for health-care practitioners regionally. Financial incentives would encourage cost-control measures through health-maintenance organizations, community health centers, and a plurality of practice settings.

7. To correct geographical maldistribution of health professionals, the NHP would subsidize education and training, in return for required periods of service by medical graduates in underserved areas.

8. The NHP would initiate programs of prevention that would emphasize individual responsibility for health, risk reduction (including programs to reduce smoking, alcoholism, and drug abuse), nutrition, maternal and infant care, occupational and environmental health, long-term services for the elderly, and other efforts to promote health.

9. Elected community representatives would work with providers' groups in local advisory councils. These councils would participate in quality-assurance efforts, planning, and feedback that would encourage responsiveness to local needs.

There is and has been wide support for an NHP in the United States. Public opinion polls consistently have shown that a majority of the American population favors an NHP that assures universal entitlement to basic health-care services (Blendon and Edwards, 1991). Major professional organizations, including the American Medical Association (Todd et al., 1991), the American College of Physicians (Scott and Shapiro, 1992), the American Public Health Association, and a major physicians' organization favoring a single-payer option (Himmelstein and Woolhandler, 1989), have called for an NHP. Leaders and members of corporations, senior citizens' groups, and a large number of civic organizations have pressed Congress to create an NHP, although specific proposals have varied. Likewise, many state legislatures have considered setting up state health programs to provide universal access to care.

Strong opposition to an NHP will come from the corporations that currently benefit from the lack of an appropriate national policy: the private insurance industry, pharmaceutical and medical-equipment firms, and the for-profit chains. While corporate resistance should not be underestimated, there is also growing support for an NHP from the corporate world. The costs of private-sector medicine have become a major burden to many nonmedical companies that provide health insurance as a fringe benefit to employees. Corporations that do not directly profit from health care have influenced public policy in the direction of cost containment. In western Europe, corporations have come to look kindly on the

cost controls and services that NHPs provide, even when corporate taxation contributes to NHP financing.

Conclusion

Ultimately, policies for health care are shaped by a multitude of forces, including ethical, economic, and political forces. Through research and analysis, the intellectual discipline of health policy contributes to national debates. There is no assurance, however, that the views of health-policy experts based in academia, government, or foundations will prevail. Knowledge generated from research and analysis enters a political process in which health-policy decisions are determined by political power as well as rational deliberation (Waitzkin and Hubbell, 1992).

With increasing discontent among the general public and practitioners, health-policy debates take on a certain urgency. While an ethical perspective tells us that basic health care for all is an individual right and a societal obligation, the burgeoning costs of the American health-care system hamper domestic economic growth and stability. Meanwhile, millions of people face major access barriers. Change in health policies to address these problems doubtless will occur during the 1990s, but the specifics of change remain difficult to predict with certainty in the complex political terrain of the United States.

NANCY E. GIN
HOWARD WAITZKIN

Directly related to this article is the companion article in this entry: HEALTH POLICY IN INTERNATIONAL PERSPECTIVE. *Also directly related are the entries* HEALTH-CARE FINANCING; HEALTH-CARE DELIVERY; HEALTH CARE, QUALITY OF; *and* SOCIAL MEDICINE. *For a further discussion of topics mentioned in this article, see the entries* CONFLICT OF INTEREST; HEALTH-CARE RESOURCES, ALLOCATION OF; HOSPITAL, *article on* CONTEMPORARY ETHICAL PROBLEMS; MEDICAL MALPRACTICE; MENTAL-HEALTH SERVICES; PUBLIC POLICY AND BIOETHICS; *and* RIGHTS. *For a discussion of related ideas, see the entry* ACADEMIC HEALTH CENTERS. *Other relevant material may be found under the entries* CHRONIC CARE; COMMERCIALISM IN SCIENTIFIC RESEARCH; LONG-TERM CARE; MEDICAL INFORMATION SYSTEMS; *and* VALUE AND VALUATION.

Bibliography

BLENDON, ROBERT J., and EDWARDS, JENNIFER N. 1991. "Caring for the Uninsured: Choices for Reform." *Journal of the American Medical Association* 265, no. 19:2563–2565.
CERESETO, SHIRLEY, and WAITZKIN, HOWARD. 1986. "Economic Development, Political-Economic System, and the

Physical Quality of Life." *American Journal of Public Health* 76, no. 6:661–666.

ENTHOVEN, ALAIN C., and KRONICK, RICHARD. 1991. "Universal Health Insurance Through Incentives Reform." *Journal of the American Medical Association* 265, no. 19:2532–2536.

EVANS, ROBERT G.; BARER, MORRIS L.; and HERTZMAN, CLYDE. 1991. "The 20-Year Experiment: Accounting for, Explaining, and Evaluating Health Care Cost Containment in Canada and the United States." *Annual Review of Public Health* 12:481–518.

FEDER, JUDITH, and HADLEY, JACK. 1985. "The Economically Unattractive Patient: Who Cares?" *Bulletin of the New York Academy of Medicine* 61, no. 1:68–74.

"Forty-fifth Annual Report on American Industry." 1993. *Forbes*, January, p. 244.

FREEMAN, HOWARD E., and KIRKMAN-LIFF, BRADFORD L. 1985. "Health Care Under AHCCCS: An Examination of Arizona's Alternative to Medicaid." *Health Services Research* 20, no. 3:245–266.

FUENZALIDA-PUELMA, HERNÁN L., and CONNOR, SUSAN SCHOLLE, eds. 1989. *The Right to Health in the Americas: A Comparative Constitutional Study.* Washington, D.C.: Pan American Health Organization.

GRAY, BRADFORD H. 1991. *The Profit Motive and Patient Care: The Changing Accountability of Doctors and Hospitals.* Cambridge, Mass.: Harvard University Press.

HIMMELSTEIN, DAVID U. and WOOLHANDLER, STEFFIE. 1989. "A National Health Program for the United States: A Physicians' Proposal." *New England Journal of Medicine* 320, no. 2:102–108.

HIMMELSTEIN, DAVID U.; WOOLHANDLER, STEFFIE; LEWONTIN, JAMES P.; TANG, TERRY; and WOLFE, SIDNEY M. 1992. *The Growing Epidemic of Uninsurance: New Data on the Health Insurance Coverage of Americans.* Cambridge, Mass.: Center for National Health Program Studies, Harvard Medical School/Cambridge Hospital.

HUGHES, DANA; JOHNSON, KAY; ROSENBAUM, SARA; BUTLER, ELIZABETH; and SIMONS, JANET. 1988. *The Health of America's Children: Maternal and Child Health Data Book.* Washington, D.C.: Children's Defense Fund.

LEWIN, LAWRENCE S.; ECKELS, TIMOTHY J.; and MILLER, LINDA B. 1988. "Setting the Record Straight: The Provision of Uncompensated Care by Not-for-Profit Hospitals." *New England Journal of Medicine* 318, no. 18: 1212–1215.

LURIE, NICOLE; WARD, NANCY B.; SHAPIRO, MARTIN F.; GALLEGO, CLAUDIO; VAGHAIWALLA, RATI; and BROOK, ROBERT H. 1986. "Termination of Medi-Cal Benefits: A Follow-up Study One Year Later." *New England Journal of Medicine* 314, no. 19:1266–1268.

MINKLER, MEREDITH, and ROBERTSON, ANN. 1991. "Generational Equity and Public Health Policy: A Critique of 'Age/Race/War' Thinking." *Journal of Public Health Policy* 12, no. 3:324–344.

MITCHELL, BRIDGER M., and SCHWARTZ, WILLIAM B. 1976. "Strategies for Financing a National Health Insurance: Who Wins and Who Loses." *New England Journal of Medicine* 295, no. 16:866–871.

MITCHELL, JEAN M., and SCOTT, ELTON. 1992. "New Evidence for the Prevalence and Scope of Physician Joint Ventures." *Journal of the American Medical Association* 268, no. 1:80–84.

NATIONAL LEADERSHIP COMMISSION ON HEALTH CARE. 1989. *For the Health of a Nation: A Shared Responsibility.* Ann Arbor, Mich.: Health Administration Press.

RELMAN, ARNOLD S. 1980. "The New Medical-Industrial Complex." *New England Journal of Medicine* 303, no. 17:963–970.

ROBINSON, JAMES C., and LUFT, HAROLD S. 1988. "Competition, Regulation, and Hospital Costs, 1982 to 1986." *Journal of the American Medical Association* 260, no. 18:2676–2681.

SCOTT, H. DENMAN, and SHAPIRO, HOWARD B. 1992. "Universal Insurance for American Health Care: A Proposal of the American College of Physicians." *Annals of Internal Medicine* 117, no. 6:511–519.

SIMINOFF, LAURA. 1986. "Competition and Primary Care in the United States: Separating Fact from Fancy." *International Journal of Health Services* 16, no. 1:57–69.

STERN, ROBERT S., and EPSTEIN, ARNOLD M. 1985. "Institutional Responses to Prospective Payment Based on Diagnosis-Related Groups: Implications for Cost, Quality, and Access." *New England Journal of Medicine* 312, no. 10:621–627.

TODD, JAMES S.; SEEKINS, STEVEN V.; KRICHBAUM, JOHN A.; and HARVEY, LYNN K. 1991. "Health Access America—Strengthening the U.S. Health Care System." *Journal of the American Medical Association* 265, no. 19:2503–2506.

U.S. DEPARTMENT OF HEALTH AND HUMAN SERVICES. 1987. *Health: United States, 1986: And Prevention Profiles.* DHHS publication no. (PHS) 87-1232. Hyattsville, Md.: National Center for Health Statistics.

U.S. GENERAL ACCOUNTING OFFICE. 1991. *Canadian Health Insurance: Lessons for the United States.* GAD-HRD-91-90. Washington, D.C.: Author.

WAITZKIN, HOWARD. 1989. "Why It's Time for a National Health Program in the United States." *Western Journal of Medicine* 150, no. 1:101–107.

WAITZKIN, HOWARD, and HUBBELL, F. ALLAN. 1992. "Truth's Search for Power in Health Policy: Critical Applications to Community-Oriented Primary Care and Small Area Analysis." *Medical Care Review* 49, no. 2:161–189.

WATT, J. MICHAEL; DERZON, ROBERT A.; RENN, STEVEN C.; SCHRAMM, CARL J.; HAHN, JAMES S.; and PILLARI, GEORGE D. 1986. "The Comparative Economic Performance of Investor-Owned Chain and Not-for-Profit Hospitals." *New England Journal of Medicine* 314, no. 2: 89–96.

WOOLHANDLER, STEFFIE, and HIMMELSTEIN, DAVID U. 1991. "The Deteriorating Administrative Efficiency of the U.S. Health Care System." *New England Journal of Medicine* 324, no. 18:1253–1258.

WORLD BANK. 1993. *World Development Report 1993: Investing in Health.* New York: Oxford University Press.

II. HEALTH POLICY IN INTERNATIONAL PERSPECTIVE

The health policies of international agencies and individual countries reflect choices involving diverse ethical issues, including the rights and responsibilities of individuals versus society, choices over who benefits and who pays for health-care services, trade-offs between saving identifiable lives and statistical lives, and choices involving interpersonal and intergenerational equity. This article begins by examining ethical issues that have shaped international agencies' and countries' policies involving traditional public-health activities. It then outlines four generic health-care financing and delivery models for acute-care services that many countries have adapted to their unique circumstances. These four health-care financing and delivery models reflect different choices about an individual's right to basic health-care services, views about whether ability to pay should influence access to certain services, perspectives on how progressive the method of financing health care should be, methods for allocating scarce resources, and perspectives on whether and how to control provider behavior.

Public-health and preventive services

International agencies play a critical role in health policy, first by setting public-health and health-status goals, and then by monitoring an individual country's progress toward these goals. For example, the World Health Organization (WHO) has established goals and thirty-eight specific targets for an initiative titled "Health for All by the Year 2000." A fundamental objective of this initiative is equity in health—ensuring an equal opportunity for everyone in the world to obtain and maintain good health. A specific goal of this objective is to reduce the differences in health status among and within countries. In order to monitor this objective, Health for All by the Year 2000 has identified specific targets that each country should meet by 2000, such as eliminating certain infectious diseases through childhood immunization and providing safe water systems (WHO, 1981).

In most countries, public-health agencies have primary responsibility for developing programs that will achieve these targets. International agencies, such as the World Bank and the United Nations, and some of the most affluent countries have programs to assist developing countries. The U.S. Agency for International Development (USAID), for example, operates programs that help developing countries establish and operate a variety of public-health activities.

While there is generally a consensus that government agencies should finance and provide public-health and disease-prevention services, policy differences and financial commitments affect the success of specific programs. For example, the childhood immunization rate for six major infectious diseases (diphtheria, pertussis, tetanus, measles, poliomyelitis, and tuberculosis) varies greatly from country to country. The immunization rate in 1987 ranged from less than 40 percent of five-year-old children immunized in Africa and Southeast Asia to over 80 percent of five-year-old children immunized in Europe (Keja et al., 1988). WHO's target rate for the year 2000 is 90 percent coverage. Immunization rates typically are highest in countries that provide universal access to immunizations, as in most European nations, and in nations that require and enforce immunization before entering elementary school, such as the United States.

Another public-health activity, the testing and approval of drugs, highlights conflicting ethical values. Beneficence, in terms of concern for public welfare, is reflected when nations employ comprehensive, time-consuming approval processes in order to ensure a safe and efficacious drug supply. The U.S. Food and Drug Administration, for example, has adopted strict regulatory standards that delay the domestic adoption of new drugs and devices until their safety and efficacy are established beyond a reasonable doubt. In contrast, liberty, in terms of individual access to health care, is obstructed when the length of a drug-approval process delays access to potentially lifesaving treatments—particularly for patients who have exhausted current treatment options and are willing to take experimental drugs.

Recently, people with acquired immunodeficiency syndrome (AIDS) have been the most vocal and effective proponents of allowing individuals greater access to unproven medical treatments. Advocates of placing greater weight on beneficence, on the other hand, point to the approval of thalidomide by the United Kingdom in the 1960s, while it was still in testing stages in other countries. The drug was never approved in other countries, and was pulled from the British market after it became apparent that severe congenital deformations resulted from maternal use of the drug (Burger, 1976).

Many developing nations have used drugs not approved in industrialized countries, in part because bans severely reduce the demand for these drugs, leading pharmaceutical companies to turn to developing nations as markets for them, and because drug therapy is a relatively affordable medical treatment option for poorer nations. In some cases, the interests of individuals in developing nations are benefited by access to various drugs, while in other cases individuals are harmed by access to unsafe or inefficacious therapies. In order to assist the efficient purchase of safe and efficacious drugs by developing nations, WHO and other international agencies have established "essential drug lists" that identify key and complementary drugs (Thrupp, 1984).

Acute-care services

Particular attention should be paid to ethical choices in the financing and delivery of acute-care services, since these services account for about 30 percent of many countries' total health care spending (Schieber et al., 1991). The provision of acute-care services requires policymakers to resolve myriad ethical values and conflicts, and each country's acute-care delivery and financing system reflects its choices about underlying ethical matters.

Unlike public-health activities, which are considered to benefit all members of society, acute-care services are generally considered as private goods, since it is the individual who benefits directly from them. Some countries consider acute care a merit good—a good that, although private, benefits society as well. The concept of merit good is reflected in the financing and delivery system of many countries, such as the United Kingdom, where coverage for most acute-care services is available to all inhabitants, regardless of ability to pay. Other countries are willing to use ability to pay as a method to allocate acute-care services. The United States, for example, uses ability to pay as a major determinant in access to acute-care services. As a result, 15 percent of its citizens, mostly low-income, lacked health insurance in 1992 (U.S. Department of Commerce, 1993).

Similar value choices are exemplified by the scope of services that countries' health systems offer. Some countries' health systems cover only hospital and physician care, while others include items such as long-term care, drugs, dental care, home health services, and eyeglasses. In addition, many European countries incorporate housekeeping and other social services into their provision of health-care services. Some countries restrict the use of expensive technologies to patients with certain demographic characteristics, or who have a certain level of health status (Aaron and Schwartz, 1984). Cultural norms also affect a country's system of health benefits. Japan, for example, has not established a formal system of long-term care, in part because of the tradition that the eldest son and his wife have responsibility for the son's parents.

Countries' decisions about government involvement in provider issues can highlight conflicts between individual liberty of providers and patient access to care. Some countries, such as Israel, have adopted policies that restrict providers' ability to practice in areas that exceed a certain physician-to-population ratio, and have developed policies that encourage them to operate in underserved locations (Anderson and Antebi, 1991). Other policies may limit the total income that can be generated by health professionals, either through restrictions on the salaries that physicians can earn or by limiting the number of patients the physician may treat. In addition, some countries, such as the United Kingdom, permit providers to operate both publicly (through a national health program) and privately (through fee-for-service arrangements). Other countries, such as Canada, require a provider to work completely in the public or completely in the private system (Glaser, 1991).

Countries use three basic mechanisms, in addition to out-of-pocket payments, to finance acute-care services. One option is to use general tax revenues. With this method, citizens pay for medical services based on the structure of the overall tax system. This option is considered to be the most progressive because most countries' tax systems are progressive—their income tax rate increases as the taxpayer's income rises. A second basic method to generate funds for acute-care services is through a payroll tax earmarked for the health system. This is referred to as a proportional tax, since the tax rate does not vary with income. The third basic method to finance acute-care services is through health-insurance premiums. This method is considered to be regressive because the rate falls as income rises.

A related financing and access issue is that of cost sharing by individuals. Cost sharing is introduced when countries want to give patients a financial incentive not to use certain health services—especially services they believe to by only marginally beneficial. The health-care systems of some countries, such as the United Kingdom, Canada, and Germany, operate with no or nominal deductibles and coinsurance (Glasier, 1991; U.S. General Accounting Office, 1991a, 1991b). Other countries have varying cost-sharing requirements. For example, 10 to 20 percent coinsurance requirements are typical in the United States and France, and 20 to 30 percent coinsurance requirements are typical in Japan (U.S. General Accounting Office, 1991b). Korea has used even higher coinsurance rates to direct ambulatory patients away from teaching hospitals and primary health clinics, in order to make their health-care system more cost effective (Anderson, 1989). Cost sharing is generally considered a regressive financing mechanism, since poorer individuals are more likely to forgo visits to primary-care providers, and generally delay medical care, when faced with cost sharing.

Four health-care financing and delivery models

As individual countries design their own health-care financing and delivery systems, they make a number of policy decisions that are based upon ethical considerations. These decisions involve choices regarding who is included in the national system, the method of financing the medical-care delivery system, how much individuals must pay out of pocket for the specific care they receive, how the delivery system is organized, and whether the delivery system is public or private. We now categorize health-care financing and delivery systems into four models, and identify specific countries that exemplify each type of model. It is important to recognize, however, that no country fits any model precisely, and that health-care systems are dynamic. The four generic models are national health services, national health insurance, social insurance, and private voluntary health insurance.

National health service. National health service systems usually collect revenues from general taxation, employ public facilities, and have limited cost sharing. As a result, countries with national health services generally offer the greatest equality in access to care and employ the most progressive financing methods. However, a recent concern is that they may be relatively inefficient and unresponsive to individuals' health-care service preferences (Iglehart, 1984).

The United Kingdom's National Health Service (NHS) is the archetypal example of this model. Since its creation in 1948, the guiding principal of the NHS has been equity—equal access to health-care services for all inhabitants. The NHS offers a comprehensive array of government-provided services and is financed by general tax revenues. Recently, rising costs and concerns about inefficiencies in the NHS have led to the development of a system of competition within the NHS, where some providers now compete for patients and funds (Graig, 1993).

National health-insurance program. National health-insurance systems usually generate revenues from general taxation, have private facilities, allow the government to set payment rates for health-care providers, and have limited cost sharing. The major difference between national health insurance and national health services is the ownership of facilities.

The Canadian health system is an example of a national health-insurance system. Revenues are generated from general taxation, the government sets payment rates for the providers who participate in the system, and there is no cost sharing. Health-care professionals must choose between participating in the national health-insurance system and opting out of the system entirely (U.S. General Accounting Office, 1991a).

Social insurance. In social insurance systems, revenues are generated from payroll taxes, the private sector provides insurance, private facilities are common, and the government sometimes sets payment rates for providers. Although insurance is compulsory, and thus accessible to all, the scope of health-care benefits may vary by plan.

Social insurance, the first type of health insurance to be developed, was introduced in Germany by Otto von Bismarck in 1883. Germany has continued to use a social insurance system, and several European nations and other countries, such as Japan and Korea, have modified the basic social insurance model to meet their own needs (Glaser, 1991; Powell and Anesaki, 1990; Anderson, 1989).

Private voluntary health insurance. In this model, revenues come from a variety of sources, including premiums, payroll taxes, and general taxation; pri-

vate facilities are the norm; the government may or may not set provider payment rates; and coinsurance is common. This system is likely to have the greatest disparity in access to health-care services, since access is based upon ability to pay. In addition, it is common for a proportion of the population to be uninsured. In theory, this system should be more efficient than government-run health systems, because the free-market competition that should characterize private voluntary systems should result in greater efficiency (Enthoven and Kronick, 1989). However, it is believed by many that free-market principles, such as a free flow of product information and price sensitivity among consumers, do not fully apply to the health-care sector, and consequently competition and greater efficiency do not always occur (Rice et al., 1993). The United States and many developing countries use a system of voluntary private health insurance.

Summary

Health policies are influenced by divergent views on a number of ethical issues. The variety of health-care financing and delivery systems in the world reflect choices made by individual countries on these issues. Ethical issues influencing health policy include the allocation of scarce resources between the old and the young, between the ill and the relatively healthy, between acute care and public health or preventive care, and between health care and other social needs. Illustrations of such conflicts include decisions that societies must make about disseminating medical technology that benefits the few versus providing preventive or low-technology services to vast numbers. The choice is frequently between providing services to those who are basically healthy and undertaking heroic efforts to save individuals likely to die or have profound disabilities. As the burdens on health systems grow and countries explicitly examine the ways they ration and allocate health-care resources, the similarities and divergences in countries' values and priorities will become even more apparent.

GERARD F. ANDERSON
STEPHANIE L. MAXWELL

Directly related to this article is the companion article in this entry: POLITICS AND HEALTH CARE. *For a further discussion of topics mentioned in this article, see the entries* AIDS; BENEFICENCE; CHILDREN, *article on* HEALTH-CARE AND RESEARCH ISSUES; ECONOMIC CONCEPTS IN HEALTH CARE; FREEDOM AND COERCION; FUTURE GENERATIONS, OBLIGATIONS TO; HEALTH-CARE FINANCING; INTERNATIONAL HEALTH; MEDICAL ETHICS, HISTORY OF, *section on* SOUTH AND EAST ASIA, *articles on* JAPAN, *and* SOUTH EAST ASIAN COUNTRIES; *section on*

EUROPE, *subsection on* CONTEMPORARY PERIOD, *articles on* SOUTHERN EUROPE, UNITED KINGDOM, *and* GERMAN-SPEAKING COUNTRIES AND SWITZERLAND; *and section on* THE AMERICAS, *article on* CANADA; PHARMACEUTICS, *article on* PHARMACEUTICAL INDUSTRY; PUBLIC HEALTH; *and* RIGHTS. *For a discussion of related ideas, see the entries* FOOD POLICY; HEALTH-CARE DELIVERY; *and* HEALTH SCREENING AND TESTING IN THE PUBLIC-HEALTH CONTEXT.

Bibliography

AARON, HENRY J., and SCHWARTZ, WILLIAM B. 1984. *The Painful Prescription: Rationing Hospital Care.* Washington, D.C.: Brookings Institution.

ALTMAN, STUART H., and RODWIN, MILTON A. 1988. "Halfway Competitive Markets and Ineffective Regulation: The American Health Care System." *Journal of Health Politics, Policy and Law* 13, no. 2:323–339.

ANDERSON, GERARD F. 1989. "Universal Health Care Coverage in Korea." *Health Affairs* 8, no. 2:24–34.

ANDERSON, GERARD F., and ANTEBI, SHLOMI. 1991. "A Surplus of Physicians in Israel: Any Lessons for the United States and Other Industrialized Countries?" *Health Policy* 17, no. 1:77–86.

BURGER, EDWARD J. 1976. *Protecting the Nation's Health: The Problems of Regulation.* Lexington, Mass.: Lexington Books.

CALLAHAN, DANIEL. 1990. *What Kind of Life: The Limits of Medical Progress.* New York: Simon and Schuster.

ENTHOVEN, ALLEN, and KRONICK, RICHARD. 1989. "A Consumer-Choice Health Plan for the 1990s: Universal Health Insurance in a System Designed to Promote Quality and Economy." *New England Journal of Medicine* 320, no. 1:29–37 and no. 2:94–101.

GLASER, WILLIAM A. 1991. *Health Insurance in Practice: International Variations in Financing, Benefits, and Problems.* San Francisco: Jossey-Bass.

GRAIG, LAURENE A. 1993. *Health of Nations: An International Perspective on U.S. Health Care Reform.* 2d ed. Washington, D.C.: Congressional Quarterly.

IGLEHART, JOHN K. 1984. "The British National Health Service Under the Conservatives—Part II." *New England Journal of Medicine* 310, no. 1:63–67.

KEJA, KO; CHAN, CAROLE; HAYDEN, GREGORY; and HENDERSON, RALPH H. 1988. "Expanded Programme on Immunization." *World Health Statistics Quarterly* 41, no. 2: 59–63.

MORONE, JOHN A. 1990. "American Political Culture and the Search for Lessons from Abroad." *Journal of Health Politics, Policy and Law* 15, no. 1:129–143.

ORGANIZATION FOR ECONOMIC COOPERATION AND DEVELOPMENT. 1990. *Health Care Systems in Transition: The Search for Efficiency.* Social Policy Studies no. 7. Paris: Author.

POWELL, MARGARET, and ANESAKI, MASAHIRA. 1990. *Health Care in Japan.* London: Routledge.

RICE, THOMAS; BROWN, RICHARD; and WYN, ROBERTA. 1993. "Holes in the Jackson Hole Approach to Health Care Reform." *Journal of the American Medical Association* 270, no. 11:1357–1362.

SCHIEBER, GEORGE J.; POULLIER, JEAN-PIERRE; and GREENWALD, LESLIE M. 1991. "U.S. Health Expenditure Performance: An International Comparison and Data Update." *Health Care Financing Review* 13, no. 4:1–87.

THRUPP, LORI ANN. 1984. "Technology Policy and Planning in the Third World Pharmaceutical Sector: The Cuban and Caribbean Community Approaches." *International Journal of Health Services* 14, no. 2:189–216.

U.S. DEPARTMENT OF COMMERCE. BUREAU OF THE CENSUS. 1993. *SIPP: Survey of Income and Program Participation.* Washington, D.C.: Author.

U.S. GENERAL ACCOUNTING OFFICE. 1991a. *Canadian Health Insurance: Lessons for the United States.* Pub. no. GAO/HRD-91-90. Washington, D.C.: Author.

———. 1991b. *Health Care Spending and Control: The Experience of France, Germany and Japan.* Pub. no. GAO/HRD-92-9. Washington, D.C.: Author.

U.S. PRESIDENT'S COMMISSION FOR THE STUDY OF ETHICAL PROBLEMS IN MEDICINE AND BIOMEDICAL AND BEHAVIORAL RESEARCH. 1983. *Securing Access to Health Care: A Report on the Ethical Implications of Differences in the Availability of Health Services.* Washington, D.C.: Author.

WALT, GILL. 1993. "WHO Under Stress: Implications for Health Policy." *Health Policy* 24, no. 2:125–144.

WORLD HEALTH ORGANIZATION. 1981. *Global Strategy for Health for All by the Year 2000.* Geneva: Author.

HEALTH PROMOTION AND HEALTH EDUCATION

Governments promote health by financing medical research and care, by ensuring safe and clean workplaces and environments, and by encouraging healthy behavior. The last (and not necessarily the most important) of these is the focus of this entry.

On the surface, health promotion and health education would seem to pose few ethical problems. Governments that draw on research in medicine and public health have knowledge to impart to the population about the health effects of particular behaviors; members of the public value their health and welcome attempts to provide this information.

Health education and promotion is a beneficial and necessary element of national health policy. Nevertheless, health promotion has always engendered controversy. Those who urge changes in behavior, such as quitting smoking or reducing alcohol consumption, implicitly condemn chosen ways of living. The ascription of personal responsibility can be understood as an insult—and perhaps, if the target is a member of a particular class or ethnic group, a deeply resented insult. The behavior in question may be highly personal, as with sexually transmitted diseases. Health promotion can thus conflict with other deeply held values. In the guise of promoting health, moreover, the authorities may resort to coercion, setting up a conflict between the values of good health and personal liberty.

The politics of health promotion

Health promotion may be engaged in for purely benevolent reasons, but other motivations may be present. By singling out the individual as an agent of change, health promotion may become a substitute for government action on other determinants of ill health.

For example, "wellness" initiatives at the workplace, which involve such interventions as drug counseling and exercise and are marketed to employers as enhancing productivity and reducing costs, are conducted in isolation from traditional occupational safety and health programs that typically call for remedial action by the employer as well as the worker. Seen in the worst light, wellness programs generally call upon workers to adapt to unhealthy environments; the employees, not the employer, bear the burden of protection.

Health promotion can substitute for effective action in response to public pressure for governmental responses to health risks. In place of instituting product-safety regulations, government can coach consumers to be careful in using the products; instead of restricting toxic substances, such as tobacco, government may simply warn the public not to abuse them. Reliance on health education permits the government to claim that it is taking action to preserve health, even while refraining from any genuinely effective action that would impinge on the interests of those who may be profiting from the unhealthy behavior. The very fact that health education is compatible with freedom of choice can camouflage this strategy: For many years, American automobile manufacturers successfully opposed regulations mandating such safety equipment as seatbelts and airbags, while driver education programs in the schools encountered little opposition.

Health promotion and health education can run afoul of persistent class and racial divisions. The newspaper of America's educated elite, the *New York Times*, in 1966 called cholera "the curse of the dirty, the intemperate, and the degraded." The beneficiaries of health education, on the other hand, are likely to be those who have access to it and who have the psychological disposition and practical opportunity to take advantage of it. In many cases, this has meant that public-health ed-

ucation campaigns have benefited mainly the middle and upper classes, who are healthier to begin with. Poor Americans are almost three times more likely than rich Americans to smoke, although the numbers were equal in 1960, before the antismoking campaigns began in earnest. Urgent public-health advice on avoiding AIDS has largely been heeded by well-educated gays, but has had much less impact on poor drug abusers. Correction of this class bias may require that the authorities choose between expending much greater sums to reach the poor, who may be difficult to reach, and diverting existing funds from education of the better-off, where results per dollar would have been greater.

Health education and personal liberty

Insofar as health promotion and health education are understood as alternatives to coercive regulation of behavior, they uphold rather than threaten the goal of self-determination. Indeed, education increases autonomy, for it points out consequences of one's behavior and the possible alternatives to it. There is a gray zone, however, between the innocuous provision of information and blatant coercion, and in this category are some of the tools used by health educators.

There may be no such thing as the neutral presentation of "facts," for some selection must be made among the facts, and this will be done with a goal in mind. Health education campaigns, however, differ in the extent to which neutrality is an ideal. Health educators may frequently manipulate the public

- by designing "education" programs that produce behavioral changes by inducing individuals to feel shame when contemplating the unhealthy behavior (as when smoking is paired with being a social outcast responsible for endangering others with passive smoke);
- by overestimating the risk faced by individuals in order to promote healthy behavior, as with attempts to secure voluntary vaccinations even where those who are not vaccinated are generally protected by the vast majority of individuals who are;
- by concealing the degree of behavioral change necessary to promote good health if full candor seems likely to result in total noncompliance (e.g., by recommending a reduction of fat consumption to 30 percent of daily caloric intake instead of a healthier 10 to 15 percent of intake).

Manipulative health promotion might be defended, sometimes successfully, on any number of grounds: the individual's benefit; the fact that the pressure is mild and easily resisted by those determined to take risks; and the fact that the behavior in question may not be voluntary to begin with. Nevertheless, recourse to manipulation forfeits the claim of being purely informative, and stands in need of justification.

Health promotion and other values

The central objective of health promotion and health education is health, but the behavior targeted for change might be serving other valued ends. Indeed, the behavior promoted by health authorities may be offensive in its own right.

In the present era, the chief conflicts occur with AIDS. Provision of sterile needles for drug abusers can prevent the spread of AIDS in this vulnerable population, but to the extent that the difficulty of obtaining needles inhibits drug use, providing free needles may conflict with national drug policy; even if distributing free needles does not appear to increase drug abuse, some shrink from the alleged symbolic acceptance of drug use that providing needles may signal.

Promotion of safe sex, the key AIDS strategy (other than research toward a cure) of public-health authorities, has faced strong opposition. Supporters of traditional sexual mores dislike promotion of any sexual behavior other than that in marriage, even if the educators mention the superiority of abstinence. Condom use is specifically condemned by the Roman Catholic church, and in Latin America, where the church's influence is strong, public-health officials have had to fight AIDS in other ways. Even in the United States, squeamishness about sex has inhibited candid and direct public education on safe sexual practice; condom advertisements, for example, are still rare on television.

Ideologies of health promotion

Health promotion is a heterogeneous field, and there is no single ideology underlying its many manifestations. Perhaps the common element in all health promotion is the incontestable premise that health is valuable in its own right. No further motivation need be cited to explain the dedication and enthusiasm of health educators for their work.

Throughout its long history, however, health promotion has often been married to ideologies and fads of the day. Nineteenth-century American health promotion was linked to social Darwinism, while today it is often packaged with near-mystical faith in the power of attitudes and diet and the enshrinement of healthful living as a moral virtue.

The belief that individual beliefs, efforts, and attitudes can overcome nearly all threats to health, implicit in some contemporary health promotion, carries both the promise of freedom from disease and the burden of guilt and blame for those who do succumb. Although many authors who promote the concept of personal responsibility for health disavow any intent to penalize or stigmatize those who cannot or will not adopt healthful living habits, the promotion of "wellness" is coincident with increased resentment of those whose lifestyles impose financial and other costs on others. The individual who tries but fails to lose weight or stop smoking risks being burdened not only by increased risk of serious illness but also with a loss of sympathy and support. Eventually, the illness might incur resentment and, as in Butler's *Erehwon*, even punishment. Health educators face the challenge of pointing out the individual's contribution to his or her own disease and disability without unduly diverting attention from the contributions of both nature and the social environment.

DANIEL WIKLER
DAN E. BEAUCHAMP

Directly related to this entry are the entries HEALTH SCREENING AND TESTING IN THE PUBLIC-HEALTH CONTEXT; LIFESTYLES AND PUBLIC HEALTH; PUBLIC HEALTH, *articles on* HISTORY OF PUBLIC HEALTH, *and* PHILOSOPHY OF PUBLIC HEALTH; SEXUALITY IN SOCIETY, *article on* SOCIAL CONTROL OF SEXUAL BEHAVIOR; SUBSTANCE ABUSE, *articles on* SMOKING, *and* ALCOHOL AND OTHER DRUGS IN A PUBLIC-HEALTH CONTEXT; *and* TRUST. *For a further discussion of topics mentioned in this entry, see the entries* AIDS, *article on* PUBLIC-HEALTH ISSUES; FERTILITY CONTROL; *and* SUBSTANCE ABUSE, *articles on* ADDICTION AND DEPENDENCE, *and* ALCOHOLISM. *Other relevant material may be found under the entries* BEHAVIOR MODIFICATION THERAPIES; CLINICAL ETHICS, *article on* ELEMENTS AND METHODOLOGIES; ENVIRONMENTAL HEALTH; INJURY AND INJURY CONTROL; ORGAN AND TISSUE PROCUREMENT; PATIENTS' RESPONSIBILITIES; *and* SELF-HELP.

Bibliography

CONRAD, PETER. 1987. "Wellness in the Work Place: Potentials and Pitfalls of Work-site Health Promotion." *Milbank Quarterly* 65, no. 2:255–275.

CRAWFORD, ROBERT. 1977. "You Are Dangerous to Your Health: The Ideology and Politics of Victim Blaming." *International Journal of Health Services* 7, no. 4:663–680.

LEICHTER, HOWARD M. 1991. *Free to Be Foolish: Politics and Health Promotion in the United States and Great Britain.* Princeton, N.J.: Princeton University Press.

MORENO, JONATHAN D., and BAYER, RONALD. 1985. "The Limits of the Ledger in Public Health Promotion." *Hastings Center Report* 15, no. 6:37–41.

WHORTON, JAMES C. 1982. *Crusaders for Fitness: The History of American Health Reformers.* Princeton, N.J.: Princeton University Press.

WIKLER, DANIEL. 1985. "Holistic Medicine: Concepts of Personal Responsibility for Health." In *Examining Holistic Medicine*, pp. 137–148. Edited by Douglas Stalker and Clark N. Glymour. Buffalo, N.Y.: Prometheus.

———. 1987. "Who Should Be Blamed for Being Sick?" *Health Education Quarterly* 14, no. 1:11–25.

HEALTH SCREENING AND TESTING IN THE PUBLIC-HEALTH CONTEXT

Health screening, used predominantly to detect potential diseases in asymptomatic people, came into practice in the nineteenth century, when progressive reformers promoted the idea that adults should have regular precautionary medical examinations. Later the growing use of the automobile, which needed regular checkups, suggested that the human "machine," too, could benefit from regular inspection (Reiser, 1978).

The military employed health screening on a large scale during World War I to discover who should be disqualified from the draft (Yerkes, 1921). Tests were administered to establish both the medical suitability and the intellectual competency of potential draftees. Of the 2.7 million men called into service, 47 percent were found to have previously undetected physical impairments. Since many of these impairments could have been prevented, preventive health examinations became a major objective of public-health organizations in the 1920s, when syphilis was a major concern (Brandt, 1985). The initiative came primarily from consumers, but physicians, too, took an interest in mass screening programs, and the American Medical Association endorsed regular examinations for those "supposedly in health."

Interest in preventive health declined after the 1920s when the control of disease through mass screening appeared economically impractical, especially during the Great Depression. It revived again in the late 1950s and 1960s, when the federal government supported multiphasic screening programs that would identify a variety of conditions. These programs consisted of routine urine and blood tests and, in some circumstances, X rays and electrocardiograms. They became possible on a large scale with the introduction of efficient automated laboratory analyzers in the late 1960s (Rushmer and Huntsman, 1970). Subsequently, in the context of growing concern about national health-care costs, preventive screening has become increasingly important and, indeed, the basis for a burgeoning industry.

The screening of targeted groups has become a major aspect of predictive medicine, and the range of tests has expanded with technological advances. Adults believed to be vulnerable are routinely tested for their predisposition to diseases such as breast, colon, cervical, and prostate cancer and diabetes; for risk factors such as hypertension, cholesterol level, and HIV status; and for genetic diseases such as Tay-Sachs disease and sickle-cell anemia. Despite the expansion of testing, however, there has been limited development of tests for the specific conditions of women and minorities.

The growing availability of computers and automated diagnostic systems has encouraged the expansion of screening in many nonclinical contexts: for example, in the military, to test for drug abuse; in prenatal clinics, to test for genetic disease; in schools, to discover learning disabilities; and in the workplace, to define the health status of prospective employees. In these settings, however, tests have often focused on intelligence and personality traits, where indicators are less precise and predictions unreliable. The tests have included ALPHA, used in the military to test intelligence (Anastasi, 1976; Gould, 1981); the Minnesota Multiphasic Personality Inventory, used in industry for personality assessment (Friedman et al., 1989); and instruments such as the Statistical Assessment of Diagnostic Syndromes, for detecting psychopathology (Kaplan et al., 1991).

Individuals may benefit from the identification of a hidden health risk if there are available preventive strategies. But it is mainly institutions such as schools, employers, and insurers that stand to gain from better understanding of the present and future health status and behavioral syndromes of their clients. In these contexts, diagnostic screening is a means to facilitate planning and reduce costs by predicting future risks. Tests can provide predictive parameters for insurance companies designing premiums, for schools attempting to assess the potential of students before admitting them to lengthy and costly special-education programs, for health-maintenance organizations seeking to anticipate the possible development of disease among their clients—indeed, for any organization concerned with problems of health and behavior that might contribute to future costs (Nelkin and Tancredi, 1989).

Assumptions underlying screening practices

The expansion of screening from clinical to nonclinical contexts is a source of growing controversy that must be understood in terms of the nature and purpose of tests. Health screening differs from clinical diagnosis in significant ways. A clinical test is intended to obtain data about an individual's health status in response to a specific complaint. Accuracy of diagnosis is the primary goal. In contrast, health screening is intended to identify from a large population those individuals who in some way deviate from a statistically derived norm (Morton and Hebel, 1979). Individuals with latent conditions are identified as problematic because in the future they may be at risk for developing a serious condition (Thorner and Remein, 1961).

The use of diagnostic tests for public-health screening is directly linked to social or medical intervention through therapy, prevention, or exclusion. For example, genetic screening of potential carriers of Tay-Sachs disease (a hereditary disorder resulting in serious retardation and early death) is a way to identify those who may perpetuate the trait, in order to provide genetic counseling prior to pregnancy. Prenatal screening for genetic disorders is a way of providing parents with the option of terminating a pregnancy if the predicted condition is sufficiently serious (Elias and Annas, 1987). Genetic screening in the workplace is a way of identifying those predisposed to illness from exposure to toxic chemicals so as to prevent potential harm to the individual, which could lead to legal actions and compensation (Draper, 1991).

There are many public-health benefits to be gained by the expansion of screening of targeted groups with a suspected predisposition to specific diseases. Such screening may point the way to particular preventive or therapeutic measures. It can provide families with the opportunity to avoid the anxiety and cost of bearing a child with an untreatable disease. It can identify potential health or behavioral problems for remedial or preventive action through diet. It can help in the early recognition of learning-disabled children. It can protect vulnerable workers from exposure to toxic substances.

Nevertheless, screening has become increasingly controversial. This reflects, in part, discomfort regarding the significant possibilities for error—especially in screening programs involving large numbers of people, where there are many areas ripe for interpretive bias (Tversky and Kahneman, 1974). Interpreting tests involves assumptions about the accuracy and reliability of the instruments and about the validity of the theories relating biological conditions to their expression in disease. For example, screening for mental illness—in particular, schizophrenia—would be especially problematic in view of changing diagnostic criteria. Correlations can easily be misperceived as causation and exploited to meet economic or policy agendas. Some tests are so sensitive that they pick up indicators that may in fact have no predictive relevance, while others may miss relevant indicators.

Such questions of uncertainty have different meanings in screening than they do in individual diagnosis. Because cost and administrative efficiency are essential in the effective screening of large populations, certainty

is necessarily compromised, and the extent of compromise will depend on the purposes of a test. A high degree of false positives may be tolerated if the goal is to detect all cases of a condition—for example, in the early efforts of some companies to screen for drug abuse. In calibrating the level of acceptable diagnostic certainty, the goals of institutions may override the interests of affected individuals. This is the source of many of the ethical dilemmas inherent in screening practices.

Ethical issues

The problems of diagnostic uncertainty are greatest when a technology developed in the context of clinical care is transferred to another setting for use as a screening tool. This is the case when tests are used by the institutions that oversee health-care financing, education, or work. Genetic tests, such as those for sickle-cell anemia, were developed to help carriers of the disease make informed family-planning choices. But some of these tests have been used in the workplace to identify those susceptible to illness resulting from exposure to chemicals (U.S. Congress, Office of Technology Assessment, 1983). In this context they can limit opportunities, as when identified carriers are excluded from the military. Genetic information, mainly intended as a basis for genetic counseling, can be used to identify those at risk for a condition that may be too costly for an insurance plan (Karjala, 1992).

In a clinical situation, inconsistencies and errors are easily discovered because the purpose of a test is to discover the abnormalities underlying a single individual's overt symptoms. But when tests are used for screening purposes, or when the objective is to deduce statistical levels of disease in a large population, individual inconsistencies can remain undetected and the potential for misdiagnosis, with all its problematic consequences, is far greater. Moreover, the pressures for efficiency and cost control that encourage efforts to predict the potential diseases of a client population can overshadow the uncertainties of screening techniques. For example, test results that detect very small deviations, such as a minor amount of blood in urine or slightly high blood pressure, may have minimal consequences for a person's health but can be used to exclude that person from insurance or employment.

For the institution carrying out the screening test, a low level of reliability may be adequate to meet its needs for long-term planning or for the allocation of resources. But for the individual being screened, errors may have very high costs. A false positive diagnosis of AIDS, for example, would be devastating, since persons falsely diagnosed as seropositive would experience not only emotional and psychological distress but also the social stigma attached to the disease. A test that identifies those with genetic vulnerability to heart disease may encourage a preventive lifestyle, but the prediction itself could affect a person's career. Tests have often been abused, serving not only as a basis for preventing harm but also as a means to justify racial or gender biases, to legitimate arbitrary exclusionary practices, and to enhance institutional power with little regard for the rights or personal fates of individuals (Duster, 1990).

The expansion of screening techniques and their extension outside the clinical context introduce a host of ethical dilemmas that are currently under debate: What is the institutional obligation to inform a person that his or her body fluids may be used for screening? Who has a right to know the information available from test results, and what is the bearing of such information on racial and gender discrimination? What are the obligations of an institution to inform the screened person of a positive result? Does the obligation extend to family members or other affected persons? How much reliance should be placed on screening for emotional and personality characteristics when indicators are relatively subjective? Is the use of blind screening for epidemiological studies ethically appropriate? Such questions will have to be addressed with the expansion of screening programs.

The potential abuses of public-health screening are beginning to generate legislative initiatives to assure the confidentiality of medical records and the protection of individual privacy (Westin, 1993); and there is increased awareness of the need to control institutional uses that would infringe on individual rights. Meanwhile, improvements in diagnostic predictability allow detection of very early biological changes, expanding the number of people defined as vulnerable, predisposed, or at risk. Measures to protect the public health are inextricably connected to the search for efficiency and cost-effective practices. Advances in screening technologies and their increasing use by diverse social institutions may expand the number of people considered uninsurable and unemployable. This could, in effect, create a genetic underclass—a class of individuals excluded from critical social benefits on the basis of their predicted biological characteristics.

DOROTHY NELKIN
LAURENCE TANCREDI

For further discussion of topics mentioned in this entry, see the entries CONFIDENTIALITY; GENETIC COUNSELING; GENETIC TESTING AND SCREENING; HEALTH-CARE FINANCING, *especially the article on* HEALTH-CARE INSURANCE; LABORATORY TESTING; MEDICAL ETHICS, HISTORY OF, *section on* EUROPE, *subsection on* NINETEENTH CENTURY, *and section on* THE AMERICAS, *articles on* COLONIAL NORTH AMERICA, *and* UNITED STATES IN

THE TWENTIETH CENTURY; RACE AND RACISM; *and* SEXISM. *This entry will find application in the entry* AIDS. *For a further discussion of related ideas, see the entries* HEALTH OFFICIALS AND THEIR RESPONSIBILITIES; HEALTH PROMOTION AND HEALTH EDUCATION; LIFESTYLES AND PUBLIC HEALTH; OCCUPATIONAL SAFETY AND HEALTH, *article on* TESTING OF EMPLOYEES; PUBLIC HEALTH; *and* PUBLIC HEALTH AND THE LAW.

Bibliography

ANASTASI, ANNE. 1976. *Psychological Testing.* 5th ed. New York: Macmillan.
BRANDT, ALLAN M. 1985. *No Magic Bullet: A Social History of Venereal Disease in the United States Since 1880.* New York: Oxford University Press.
DRAPER, ELAINE. 1991. *Risky Business: Genetic Testing and Exclusionary Practices in the Hazardous Workplace.* Cambridge: At the University Press.
DUSTER, TROY. 1990. *Backdoor to Eugenics.* New York: Routledge.
ELIAS, SHERMAN, and ANNAS, GEORGE J. 1987. "Routine Prenatal Genetic Screening." *New England Journal of Medicine* 317, no. 22:1407–1408.
FRIEDMAN, ALAN F.; WEBB, JAMES T.; and LEWAK, RICHARD W. 1989. *Psychological Assessment with MMPI.* Hillsdale, N.J.: Lawrence Erlbaum.
GOULD, STEPHEN J. 1981. "A Critique of the Army Mental Tests." In his *The Mismeasure of Man,* pp. 199–226. New York: W. W. Norton.
KAPLAN, HAROLD I.; SADOCK, BENJAMIN J.; and GREBB, JACK A. 1991. *Synopsis of Psychiatry: Behavioral Sciences, Clinical Psychiatry.* 6th ed. Baltimore: Williams & Wilkins.
KARJALA, DENNIS S. 1992. "A Legal Research Agenda for the Human Genome Initiative." *Jurametrics* 32, no. 2:121–311. See especially "Special Legal Problem Areas: D. Insurance," pp. 172–183.
MORTON, RICHARD F., and HEBEL, J. RICHARD. 1979. *A Study Guide to Epidemiology and Biostatistics.* Baltimore: University Park Press.
NELKIN, DOROTHY, and TANCREDI, LAURENCE R. 1989. *Dangerous Diagnostics: The Social Power of Biological Information.* New York: Basic Books.
REISER, STANLEY JOEL. 1978. *Medicine and the Reign of Technology.* Cambridge: At the University Press.
RUSHMER, ROBERT F., and HUNTSMAN, LEE L. 1970. "Biomedical Engineering." *Science* 167, no. 3919:840–844.
THORNER, ROBERT M., and REMEIN, QUENTIN R. 1961. *Principles and Procedures in the Evaluation of Screening for Disease.* Public Health Monograph 67. Washington, D.C.: U.S. Government Printing Office.
TVERSKY, AMOS, and KAHNEMAN, DANIEL. 1974. "Judgment Under Uncertainty: Heuristics and Biases." *Science* 185, no. 4157:1124–1131.
U.S. CONGRESS. OFFICE OF TECHNOLOGY ASSESSMENT. 1983. *The Role of Genetic Testing in the Prevention of Occupational Disease.* Washington, D.C.: Author.
WESTIN, ALAN. 1993. "Privacy and Confidentiality: Legal Implications." In *The Genetic Frontier: Ethics, Law, and Pol-*

icy. Edited by Mark S. Frankel and Albert H. Teich. Washington, D.C.: American Association for the Advancement of Science.

YERKES, ROBERT M. 1921. *Psychological Examining in the United States Army.* Washington, D.C.: National Research Council.

HEART TRANSPLANTATION

See ORGAN AND TISSUE PROCUREMENT; ORGAN AND TISSUE TRANSPLANTS; *and* ARTIFICIAL HEARTS AND CARDIAC-ASSIST DEVICES.

HEMODIALYSIS

See KIDNEY DIALYSIS.

HERMENEUTICS

See INTERPRETATION; LITERATURE; *and* NARRATIVE. *See also* ETHICS, *article on* MORAL EPISTEMOLOGY.

HINDUISM

The following is a revision and update of the first-edition entry "Hinduism" by A. L. Basham. Portions of the first-edition entry appear in the revised version.

Hinduism is a religious system that has grown and developed from the Vedic religion identified with Aryans who invaded the Indian subcontinent over a period of centuries in the second millennium B.C.E. It is rooted in an oral tradition that gave rise to four groups of sacred texts during a period that is difficult to pinpoint more precisely than 1500 to 900 B.C.E. Based on this informal collection of traditions, beliefs, and practices and the corpus of formal written treatises, which together provided a context for development of the medical system known as *Ayurveda,* Hinduism encompasses a range of values and codes of conduct highly relevant to a study of Indian bioethics.

Hinduism as we might recognize it today took shape in the Gupta Period (c. 300–500 C.E.), often regarded as the classical age of Hindu India. This entry will identify and briefly discuss basic concepts, which clarify the setting for analysis of bioethics in Hindu India, before focusing on medical ethics in *Ayurveda.* Just as they do now, social and cultural values defined standards of medical education and practice, ideas about ethical behavior as a determinant of health and disease, the balance of commercial and altruistic motives of clinicians, access to care and humane treatment, and the rights and responsibilities of patients and physicians.

Hindu worldview

The doctrine of transmigration is a definitive concept for Hinduism. It postulates the existence of an innermost self (*ātman*) for all beings, ranging from the highest god to the meanest insect, that is essentially immutable. By becoming incarnate, this self becomes further involved with matter, which some philosophical systems hold to be fundamentally illusory and others regard as the primordial source of intellect, ego, elements, and the material world. According to the conduct of the embodied being, the soul or self is carried at death to another body, in which it flourishes or suffers according to previous behavior (the law of *karma*). This process is called *samsāra.* From an outsider's perspective, the force of *karma* operates as a tangible manifestation of an ethical system associated with principles of righteous conduct and moral values inherent in the concept of *dharma,* a difficult-to-translate term that embodies cosmic order, sacred law, and religious duty. Within the system, however, the effects of *karma* are typically conceived more as the operation of natural law governing the effects of behavior than a statement of moral and ethical values.

Transmigration links all living beings in a single system. Unlike the Judaeo-Christian and Islamic religious systems, Hinduism makes no sharp distinction between human and animal. *Dharma* as a guide to proper behavior is relative, not the same for different people or different beings. The ideas of *karma* and *samsāra* motivate values of nonviolence (*ahimsā*) and vegetarianism. Nonviolence, which was never so prominent a value in Hinduism as it was in Jainism and Buddhism, has less stringent implications for laypersons than for ascetics, and it does not interfere with righteous warfare, punishment of criminals, or self-defense.

The process of transmigration is considered painful, and the main quest of classical Hinduism has been to find "release" (*moksa*) from the cycle of birth and death and thereby enter a state of timeless bliss. For the orthodox schools of Hindu philosophy and systems of Buddhism and Jainism that sprang from them, knowledge provides a means of escaping this repetitive cycle of birth, death, and rebirth. Each of these schools has a somewhat different interpretation of the problem and the solution. Both the *Sāmkhya* school, identified with yoga practice and once very influential, and the heterodox sect of Jainism, define release as the complete separation of the individual soul from matter. The *Advaita*

Vedānta system, which exerts the greatest influence on intellectual Hinduism, interprets it as a full realization of the illusory character of the material world, the speciousness of individual personality, and the recognition of the soul's identity with an underlying impersonal world spirit, often called *Brahman*. Theistic Hinduism of the *Viśiṣṭādvaita* school, which has had the greatest influence on popular ideas, interprets release as union with the personal God not through knowledge but through devotion to *Viṣṇu*, who is identified with *Brahman*, the ultimate reality of the universe and out of whom the world repeatedly emerges in the course of cosmic cycles.

Ideally, release is the aim of all striving, but Hinduism recognizes the validity of other aims, which for laypersons are fully legitimate. The ascetic (*sannyāsi*), on the other hand, "who has given up the world," should pursue only release. Ordinary people approach this goal through gradual stages over many lives. For them there are three legitimate aims: *dharma*, adherence to religious and ethical norms in order to ensure a happier rebirth; *artha*, amassing wealth for the benefit of oneself and one's family; and *kāma*, seeking pleasure and the satisfaction of personal desires. These three aims are valued in descending hierarchical order, but each is fully acceptable for different persons at a particular stage of life and for caste-based communities, which may emphasize one of them.

The Hindu pantheon begins with one primeval being, or God, and innumerable supernatural beings, all of whom are endowed with individual volition. Some of these beings adhere to the will of the higher gods, but others oppose the work of creation. Battles between gods and demons, light and darkness, and good and evil were important features of the earliest Hindu literature, and these themes are widely represented in popular beliefs and practices. Complementing more intellectual naturalistic explanations that are also a prominent feature of Hinduism, some look upon the world as a place full of demons, which are normally at war with gods, and which can be potent factors in causing misfortune and disease.

Hindu cosmology refers to four ages (*yuga*) over the period of a great cycle (4,320,000 years). The current cycle, the *Kali yuga*, is the worst, but fortunately the shortest, lasting 432,000 years, about 5,100 of which have elapsed. Looking backward to better times provides a guide in this troubled age. Neither the doctrine of *karma* nor that of cosmic decline, however, implies fatalism. Human effort may influence the process, and it holds potential for gaining release from the personal cycles of birth and rebirth. Hindu texts emphasize the virtue of human effort (*puruṣakāra*), rather than passive acceptance of adversity that may follow from destiny or chance.

Social norms

The four great classes (*varṇa*), constituting an eternal hierarchical social order, were believed to have emerged at the beginning of time from the body of the Creator as the fundamental basis of society. The *Brahman* (priest), the *Kṣatriya* (warrior and ruler), the *Vaiśya* (merchant), and the *Śūdra* (worker) formed these four classes, each with different roles, responsibility, and status. Maintaining differences that distinguish each of them was a prerequisite of the social order, and any effort to violate the boundaries of social organization and behavior was an affront to nature and the gods, degrading for those at the top and punishable for those at the bottom. Below the four great classes were the untouchables, theoretically outside, but operating at the bottom of the social order. They performed important social functions that others considered polluting, such as removing garbage, cremating corpses, working in leather, and so forth. Contact between them and the other classes was strictly limited.

Although aspects of this class structure persist in Hindu society today, social conditions rarely operated according to textbook norms. More important and more complex in everyday life was the caste (*jāti*), a group of families generally following the same profession and theoretically contained within one of the four classes, though not always recognizably so in practice, especially in South India. Castes were also hierarchically graded and normally endogamous. Local councils of elders exerted great power over their members.

Family

Social research in recent years has emphasized the primacy of the family over the individual in Hindu and other societies outside North America and western Europe. Hindu individuals were more likely to define themselves with reference to the extended family (*kula*) as a corporate unit. Social responsibilities, which constitute underpinnings for the concept of *dharma*, rather than individual rights, were clearly the priority among ethical concerns. Except in some parts of South India, primarily Kerala, the family was patrilinear, patriarchal, and patrilocal, though the authority of the patriarch was limited by traditional law. He did not have the right to dispose of family property arbitrarily, nor did he have complete control over the lives of family members.

The ritual of *śrāddha*, whereby dead ancestors retained a presence, sustained by the living, was a powerful force in shaping the character of Hindu family life. A male descendant to perform the *śrāddha*, a ritual offering of rice balls (*piṇḍa*), was needed not only to sustain the ancestral lineage but also to avoid one's own suffering in the afterlife. In view of heavy child mortality, it was incumbent upon families to produce as many children as possible, in the hope that at least one surviving son would maintain the lineage, attend to the spiritual needs of the ancestors, and contribute to the economic well-being of the family.

A Hindu wife was integrated into her husband's family, and theoretically (though not always in practice) completely subordinate to him. In many communities it was considered indecent to leave a girl unmarried after her first menstruation, and marriage normally required the payment of a heavy dowry. Thus, the birth of a daughter was often looked on as a misfortune. Although female infanticide has been practiced and persists in some parts of India, the practice is completely without foundation in the Hindu scriptures, which look upon abortion and infanticide as grave forms of murder.

Prospective parents employed various techniques to increase their chances of bearing a male, rather than female, child. Diet and activities of a pregnant woman were believed to influence the sex, physical features, and character of the offspring. Treatises of *Ayurveda* advise that intercourse on even days after the onset of menstruation produces sons, and on odd days it produces daughters (Caraka, 1949, iv. 8. 5). *Puṃsavana* rites to alter the sex of a recently conceived embryo and ensure the birth of a male child are discussed in the texts of *Ayurveda*. They are also discussed in religious treatises of the Veda and other texts that detail proper Hindu codes of conduct (*dharmaśāstra*) (Kane, 1968–).

In recent years profitable ultrasound clinics have proliferated in India, in some states illegally, to make use of modern technology to identify and abort female fetuses. Responding to a culturally based gender bias and a persisting dowry system that taints perceptions of female children as economic liabilities, this ultrasound technology challenges the viability of *puṃsavana* clinics previously established in some *Ayurvedic* hospitals and employing traditional Hindu medical methods for assuring the birth of male children.

Individual conduct

Within the framework of the three aims of life (*puruṣārtha*) acceptable for the high-caste individual were a series of ritual observances and taboos throughout life. Sacraments beginning before birth and continuing after death marked the progress of life. The *Brahman* was expected to devote a considerable amount of time each day to prayer and ritual, and members of other castes were encouraged to imitate him.

The aim of many of these sacraments and taboos was to maintain ritual purity. Although conceived with reference to another conceptual framework, many practices also maintained a hygienic standard contributing to health in a tropical climate. Notable examples include insistence on a daily bath, the custom of eating

with the right hand and washing the anus and sexual organs with the left, the ban on eating cooked food left overnight, and a strict taboo against contact with human corpses and animal carcasses. The bodily fluids of others, such as saliva and mucus, are considered polluting, and contact with anything contaminated by them, such as used dishes or drinking glasses, was to be avoided.

Social values and a conflicting emphasis in various texts of classical Hinduism portray an ambivalent attitude that both exalts and denies sexuality. *Vedic* texts regard sexuality as a metaphor for a ritual sacrifice. The *Bṛhadāraṇyika Upaniṣad* (vi. 2. 13), among the best known of this speculative genre of Hindu scriptures (*Upaniṣad*), identified woman as a sacrificial fire fueled both by her own and her male partner's genital organs in the act of sexual intercourse. Semen is an offering to this fire, which may generate a person.

In later texts, however, sex is affirmed as a valid source of gratification, a legitimate pursuit among the three aims of life: righteousness, wealth, and pleasure. Erotic temple art and texts devoted to the details of enhancing sexual gratification, such as the *Kāma Sūtra*, document a cultural sanction of pleasure seeking for men. These texts acknowledge female sexuality but consider it primarily from a male perspective—how to attract and please a man. Hindu texts concerned with moral codes of conduct (*Dharmaśāstra*) emphasize chastity and procreation more from the classical period onward than previously (Bhattacharyya, 1975).

Even for men, classical Hinduism confines sexual activity to one stage of a man's life. An initiation ceremony (*upanayana*) that preceded a long period of celibate studentship was a milestone for upper-caste boys. Afterwards, a young man was married, normally to a bride chosen by his parents, and raised a family. According to the ideal, he was expected to give up family cares in late middle age to devote the rest of his life to religion and to strive for liberation. Ascetic values discouraged sexual activity, which not only distracts the individual from a quest for release from the cycle of rebirth but also results in the loss of physical and spiritual power.

In addition to the emphasis on a moral code of religious practices, Hinduism also emphasizes ethical principles of social relations. The principle of nonviolence has often been interpreted in a positive sense, as actively benefiting others. Though subject to the constraints of conflicting values in a comprehensive social order, Hindu texts and practices encourage virtues of honesty, hospitality, and generosity. Explicit codes detailing how guests are to be received, fed, and looked after emphasize hospitality as a social value (see chap. 21 on receiving guests in Kane, 1968–). The *Taittirīya Upaniṣad* (i. 11. 2) admonishes students to treat parents, teachers, and guests as gods.

Hindu medicine

A complex medical system, known as *Ayurveda*, "the science of (living to a ripe old) age," developed in India over the first millennium B.C.E. The theory of health and disease according to *Ayurveda* refers to a humoral physiology based on the balance of three substances (*doṣas*): wind (*vāta*), bile (*pitta*), and phlegm (*kapha*). They are recognizable indirectly by their impact on health and illness. The excess of one or another and their locus in the body or among bodily elements (*dhātu*) determines the nature of specific physical and mental diseases, their manifestations, and subtypes. Although *karma*, demons, and deities may also play a role in producing ill health, it is a relatively minor role in the medical texts and more of a concern in other settings. The role of a physician practicing *Ayurveda* is to restore the harmony of humoral balance with medicines, purification, massage, diet, and directives for appropriate lifestyle. Experience with an exceptionally wide pharmacopoeia and careful observations of the symptomatology, clinical course, and treatment response of various diseases—especially chronic conditions for which Western medicine does not provide a clearly superior alternative—have enabled practitioners of the system to maintain the respect of a large number of South Asians who continue to use it.

Health, disease, and morality

Ayurveda, despite its emphasis on the humoral basis of health and disease, also recognized external (*āgantu*) causes that provided a better account than endogenous (*nija*) causes—that is, humoral imbalance—to explain some medical conditions. *Karma* referred to the impact of misdeeds in a previous life. Irreverent, unethical behavior and other violations of codes of conduct (*prajñā-aparādha*) in one's current life were not limited to effects on that individual; they could also affect offspring (Caraka, 1949, iv. 8. 21, 30). Serious transgressions of the king might also produce epidemic disease and disasters (*janapadoddvamsana*) in his kingdom (Caraka, 1949, iii. 3). Moral conduct, affecting individuals, distinct from epidemics affecting populations, operated through the all-embracing doctrine of *karma*; in some instances, *karma* explained health or disease if the humoral theory or demonic possession could not, and in other instances, it provided a complementary explanation.

Illnesses might be caused by the sins or shortcomings of a previous existence; longevity was also explained by this idea of *karma*. The doctrine encouraged inner acceptance of disease and gave a ready-made explanation of its cause, but nowhere is a person advised to submit to illness without attempting its cure. *Karma* could explain otherwise mysterious congenital defects. Someone born with a deformed hand, for example, could be said to have incurred this misfortune as a result of an evil deed (for instance, striking a *Brahman*) committed by the same hand in a previous life. This did not necessarily discourage efforts to improve the condition by surgery, since the duration of the punishment through *karma* was not known, and the trouble might be only temporary. Since the evil brought about by *karma* cannot be estimated with certainty, and the bad effects of sins can be offset by the merit gained by good deeds, there was every reason why a sick person should seek all available medical help to achieve health.

Other factors besides *karma* were believed to promote health or disease. Devotion (*bhakti*) to God, who might set aside the law of *karma* for the faithful, promoted longevity and health. Neglect of religious duties and lack of faith, on the other hand, might lead to the withdrawal of divine protection, increasing the risk that demons might exert their influence, leading to disease or madness.

More closely linked with ethics was the general view in the medical treatises that equanimity and kindness are therapeutic in their effects. Excess in every respect is looked on with disfavor by the medical texts. An impressive emphasis on the values of moderation, altruism, and love to promote health and longevity is found in the seventh-century text of the Buddhist physician Vāgbhata, the *Astāṅgahrdayasamhitā* (1965, i. 2). This work, along with the *Caraka Samhitā* and the *Suśruta Samhitā*, is among the so-called great-three (*brhat-trayī*) texts of classical *Ayurveda*. After reviewing the benefits of exercise and symptoms resulting from overexercise, it enjoins the physician to support those who are sick, poor, or needy and to treat them with respect.

Mental and spiritual training in concentration and meditation, commonly known as yoga, was also believed to promote health and longevity. Yoga is still widely practiced both as treatment for clinical problems in yoga clinics of some Indian hospitals and more generally to promote health and well-being. Different forms of yoga practice involve physical postures and exercises (*hatha-yoga*), meditation (*rāja-yoga*), or both. These produce not merely health and longevity; they also provide a way for the most advanced adepts to attain liberation from the cycle of rebirth, and hence immortality.

Ethics of medical practice

The activities of the physician (*vaidya*) were closely linked with the doctrine of the three aims of Hindu life (Caraka, 1949, i. 30. 29; Vāgbhata, 1965, i. 2. 29). Viewed as complementary, rather than contradictory, they guide appropriate behavior. By relieving suffering and adding to the sum of human happiness, a physician (assumed in the texts to be a man) fulfills the first aim, carrying out his religious duty; from the generous fees of his wealthy patients he achieves the second aim, riches; while the third aim, pleasure, is achieved by the satisfaction he obtains, first, from a high reputation as a healer and, second, from the knowledge that he has cured many people whom he loves and respects.

The last two aims were not to be disparaged. The few famous physicians described in story and tradition were not selfless servants of humanity but very wealthy men—in that regard resembling successful practitioners of modern times. There appears to have been no ban to keep a physician from advertising his skill. As the example of Vāgbhaṭa indicates, Hindu and Buddhist medical traditions were closely linked. A Buddhist text, the *Mahāvagga*, provides more biographical detail than the Hindu sources about medical practice in the same society. It refers to the material interests of a renowned doctor in his youth, Jīvaka, recently qualified and in search of patients. As he entered an ancient Indian city, to earn money for his onward journey, he walked through the streets inquiring, "Who is ill here? Who wants to be cured?" (Mahāvagga, 1881–1882, viii. i. 8–13).

Although Jīvaka's concern for his fees was matched by qualifications and skill, it appears that quackery was also rampant in ancient India; charlatans would come canvassing as soon as they heard that a well-to-do person was sick (Caraka, 1949, i. 29. 8–12). Recognizing such problems, Suśruta (1947, i. 10. 3) referred to a system of licensing qualified medical practitioners. Texts on politics and statecraft suggested punishments for doctors whose ineffective treatment resulted in injury or death (*Kauṭilya*, 1969, iv. 1; Kane, 1968–). Caraka also advocated a high moral standard for a proper physician, based on religious duty (*dharma*). At the outset, a physician's training began with a solemn initiation, at which his teacher (*guru*) instructed him that he was to live a frugal and ascetic life, celibate and vegetarian, while undergoing training. He must obey his teacher implicitly "unless instructed to commit a mortal sin." The prescribed instruction continues:

> When you have finished your studies, if you want to have a successful, wealthy, and famous practice, and to go to heaven when you die, you must pray every day, when you get up and go to sleep, for the welfare of all beings, especially cattle and brahmans, and you must strive with all your power to heal the sick. You must not betray your patients, even at the risk of your own life. . . . You must always be pleasant of speech . . . and always strive to improve your knowledge. . . . Having entered a patient's home, a physician's speech, mind, intellect, and senses should be devoted to nothing other than caring for the patient. Any peculiarities of the household you may learn about should not be disclosed outside. (Caraka, 1949, iii. 8. 13. 4–5, 7)

This well-known passage has been compared with the Hippocratic oath. The text also addressed other persisting dilemmas of medical practice. If it becomes clear that a patient in treatment has a fatal condition, the matter of whether or not a doctor should disclose this information was left largely to the doctor's discretion. Caraka advised that if a physician concludes that the condition of the patient is hopeless and if he believes that it might shock the patient or others, he should keep this knowledge to himself.

The same chapter of the *Caraka Saṃhitā* also contains advice about when a physician should refuse to provide treatment. He should not treat the king's enemies, women unattended by a husband or guardian, or patients for whom a request for treatment comes as they are about to die (Caraka, 1949, iii. 8. 13.6). Accepting a terminal case might damage his reputation.

The Hindu medical tradition is based on a relatively stable theory of health and illness, but it advocates a policy of openness to new ideas about treatments. Although the theoretical basis rooted in the doctrine of the three humors has always guided *Ayurveda* and undergone little modification over the course of time, the *vaidya* was advised to be constantly on the lookout for new drugs and treatment methods. Compared chronologically, the texts show a steady increase in the number of items in the pharmacopoeia. Even after his long apprenticeship was over, the physician was counseled to continue to improve his knowledge by studying his patients and inquiring about unusual but potentially useful remedies from hermits, cowherds, and hillmen (Suśruta, 1947, i. 36. 10).

Professional gatherings of physicians were regarded as valuable opportunities for the exchange of knowledge that could enhance a clinician's skills. The descriptions of these colloquiums distinguish friendly discussions from hostile debates, and the exchange of information was not necessarily free and open. Many physicians guarded proprietary knowledge not recorded in professional textbooks, knowledge they might reveal to prove a point in the heat of impassioned debate. Entering into professional discussions, the clinician is advised not to boast, embarrass others, or fear discomfort. In the company of knowledgeable colleagues, he is advised to listen attentively and speak freely. The text also advises how to handle hostile discussions with superiors, inferiors, and equals. "The wise never applaud a person engaging in hostile discussion with a superior . . . but the following methods help in quickly overpowering an inferior disputant . . ." (Caraka, 1949, iii. 8. 15–21; see also the remainder of chap. iii. 8).

The texts encouraged the physician, though he might be wealthy and unfettered by any rules of an ascetic character, to consider himself a sort of secular priest with a special, almost supernatural charisma bestowed on him by the initiation ceremony at the beginning of his studies. The high-caste man who had undergone the normal Hindu initiation (*upanayana*) was "twice-born" (*dvija*), and thus superior to the Śūdra or woman, who had only one birth. The *vaidya* was even a step beyond, "thrice-born" (*trija*). As the prescribed words of his teacher show, this exalted status required a high standard of fortitude and conduct. The student was taught that as a physician he should always be "of calm mind, pleasant speech, . . . the friend of all beings" (Suśruta, 1947, i. 10. 3). To some extent professional identity relieved him of the burden of caste taboos. He could enter the homes of people of a lower caste than his, handle their bodies, and even taste their urine when making a diagnosis.

Notwithstanding vegetarian cultural values, treatment employed animal products to compound drugs, and they appear to have been prescribed freely. The taboo that proscribed handling a corpse, however, may have applied to most physicians. Most medical texts do not advocate the actual dissection of a cadaver; *Suśruta Saṃhitā* (1947, iii. 5), however, is an exception. It advises that for a surgeon to study the position of internal organs, a carefully selected dead body should be placed in a cage after removing excrement from the entrails, positioned in a stream with a swift current, and examined after seven days as it begins to decompose. In that way the body might be studied in each anatomical layer, beginning with the skin.

Although concerns about ritual pollution and principles of nonviolence inhibited anatomical study and surgery in *Ayurveda*, in recent years they appear to have had surprisingly little influence on modern medicine in India, known as allopathy, with respect to the burgeoning surgical practice of organ transplantation. Concern about the adverse impact on the transmigration of souls has had a negligible effect on the transmigration of vital organs from one person to another. Bombay has acquired a dubious distinction as a world center for transplants from unrelated live donors, spawned by a profitable private-practice medical industry, an impoverished subpopulation willing to donate organs for a fee, and enterprising brokers whose activities reflect little concern for the ethics of these practices.

Access to health care

The provision of free medical care to the poor was looked on as part of a king's duty to protect his subjects, which was generally interpreted in a positive sense (Caraka, 1949, i. 30.29; see also the background essay in vol. 1, pp. 254–264 of P. M. Mehta's translation). From the days of the benevolent Buddhist emperor Aśoka in the third century B.C.E., the better rulers of India responded in some measure to this responsibility. Medical clinics of one kind or another, where professional doctors provided free services to the poor, existed in many cities. These were sometimes supported by the states, but others were often financed by private charity. In South India especially, hospitals and dispensaries were often attached to the great temples. Medical services might have been subsidized by doctors themselves, for they were encouraged to treat the poor, learned *Brahmans*, and ascetics without charge (Suśruta, i. 2. 8; vi. 11. 12–13). Free medical services in South and Southeast Asia, however, were more extensive in Buddhist Sri Lanka and Cambodia.

Reasoned suicide and mental health

The aim of the idealized ascetic to attain release and end the cycle of rebirth provided an acceptable rationale for suicide in highly selected circumstances. *Sallekhanā* is a Jain practice sanctioned for elderly mendicants involving ritual fasting that ends in death; its aim is for the individual to meet the final moment with utmost tranquillity (Settar, 1990). The *Dharmaśāstra* literature, which outlines Hindu codes of conduct, also refers to another form of religious suicide, the "great journey," justified by incurable disease or great misfortune (Kane, 1968–). Those who undertake this ultimate renunciation in the final stage of life proceed in a northeasterly direction, "subsisting on water and air, until his body sinks to rest" (*The Laws of Manu*, 1988, 6. 31). Other means of accomplishing religiously motivated suicides include jumping from a height (*bhṛgupāta*), often associated with pilgrimage sites where these suicides were most frequent, such as Śravaṇa Belgola, west of Bangalore in South India, and Prayāga (modern Allahabad) in the North.

Questions about these carefully reasoned suicides, usually sanctioned only for the elderly, were framed in religious rather than medical contexts, unlike current debates about euthanasia and assisted suicide in the West. Nevertheless, issues identified as appropriate justification by those who advocate these practices in both settings are comparable, especially the role of terminal illness and functional disability. Whether one regards these socially sanctioned self-willed deaths as suicide or something else is a debatable matter. Some scholars avoid the stigmatized English term (Settar, 1990), although more commonly suicide is used descriptively, regardless of whether it is proscribed.

Although Hindu texts were very much concerned about ethical questions that ultimately lead to sanctioning or condemning suicides, based on their circumstances, the context of the discourse was strikingly different from that of present-day debates about physician-assisted suicides. Suicide in the West typically raises questions about deviance and mental disorder. Concerns for victims are framed in clinical terms with a focus on prevention and cure of psychopathology associated with suicidal impulses. Hindu traditions that consider suicide are concerned with a different set of questions, which focus not on deviance but on cultural values. Religious suicides of ascetics and pilgrims and the self-immolation of a widow on the funeral pyre of her husband (*anumaraṇa*)—an act that has come to be known as *sati*, after the Sanskrit term for the "righteous woman" who undertakes it—were not discussed in medical contexts. Modern criticism of *sati* proceeds from social, economic, and feminist perspectives; it focuses on questions about the deviance and disorder not of the victims but of societies that disvalue women, especially widows.

Suicide was regarded neither as a defining feature nor an important symptom of mental disorder. Mental disorders (*unmāda*), however, were recognized and classified according to threatening, disorganized, and disordered behaviors, and by disturbing emotional states. The classification of some of these mental disorders fit the characteristic humoral framework, but others did not. Like some childhood diseases discussed in the texts (but few other health problems), they were explained by the influence of demons and deities. The texts prescribe a mix of gentle, humane treatment, as well as not-so-gentle efforts to restrain and shock patients into normalcy with threats of harm and false reports of the death of loved ones. Offerings to demons and deities (*bali*) and medicines to correct a humoral imbalance of excessive wind, bile, or phlegm were also prescribed for mental illnesses attributed to these respective causes.

Conclusion

Many issues that remain concerns in modern medical practice were recognized and addressed by Hindu religious texts, codes of conduct, and Sanskrit treatises of *Ayurveda.* The medical texts discussed responsibilities of the physician to society, patients, and colleagues in terms that recognized the professional nature of these interactions, distinctive social values, and political forces. Medical theory, which was primarily humoral, incorporated a moral basis for explaining health and illness of individuals. Some questions that have become major concerns for medical ethics in the West, such as the status of rational suicide, were considered in the context of Hindu traditions other than medicine.

Recent developments in biotechnology have placed controversial questions about bioethics and cultural values near the top of an agenda for equitable social policy in South Asia. The ongoing debate that follows from the impact of new technologies should be informed by an appreciation of the cultural and historical contexts in which these questions emerge.

MITCHELL G. WEISS

Directly related to this entry are the entries DEATH, *article on* EASTERN THOUGHT; EUGENICS AND RELIGIOUS LAW, *article on* HINDUISM AND BUDDHISM; MEDICAL ETHICS, HISTORY OF, *section on* SOUTH AND EAST ASIA, *article on* INDIA; *and* POPULATION ETHICS, *section on* RELIGIOUS TRADITIONS, *article on* HINDU PERSPECTIVES. *For a further discussion of topics mentioned in this entry, see the entries* CHILDREN, *article on* HISTORY OF INFANTICIDE; *and* SUICIDE. *Other relevant material may be found under the entries* BUDDHISM; CONFUCIANISM; ETHICS, *article on* RELIGION AND MORALITY; HEALING; HEALTH AND DISEASE; JAINISM; SIKHISM; TAOISM; *and* WOMEN, *article on* HISTORICAL AND CROSS-CULTURAL PERSPECTIVES.

Bibliography

BASHAM, ARTHUR LLEWELLYN. 1967. *The Wonder That Was India: A Survey of the History and Culture of the Indian Sub-Continent Before the Coming of the Muslims.* 3d rev. ed. London: Sidgwick and Jackson.

BHATTACHARYYA, NARENDRA NATH. 1975. *History of Indian Erotic Literature.* Delhi: Munshiram Manoharlal.

CARAKA. *Caraka Saṃhitā.* 1949. 6 vols. Edited by P. M. Mehta with translations in Hindi, Gujarati, and English by the Shree Gulabkunverba Ayurvedic Society. Jamnagar, India: Gulabkunverba Ayurvedic Society.

COWARD, HAROLD G.; LIPNER, JULIUS J.; and YOUNG, KATHERINE K. 1989. *Hindu Ethics: Purity, Abortion, and Euthanasia.* Albany: State University of New York Press.

DESAI, PRAKASH N. 1988. "Medical Ethics in India." *Journal of Medicine and Philosophy* 13, no. 3:231–255.

DOSSETOR, JOHN B., and MANICKAVEL, V. 1991. "Ethics in Organ Donation: Contrasts in Two Cultures." *Transplantation Proceedings* 23, no. 5:2508–2511.

FILLIOZAT, JEAN F. 1949. *La doctrine classique de la médecine indienne: Ses origines et ses parallèles grecs.* Paris: P. Geuthner & Imprimerie nationale. Translated by Dev Raj Chanana under the title *The Classical Doctrine of Indian Medicine: Its Origins and Its Greek Parallels.* Delhi: Munshiram Manoharlal, 1964.

GEORGE, SABU; ABEL, RAJARATNAM; and MILLER, BARBARA D. 1992. "Female Infanticide in Rural South India." *Economic and Political Weekly* 27, no. 22:1153–1156.

JEFFERY, ROGER; JEFFERY, PATRICIA; and LYON, ANDREW. 1984. "Female Infanticide and Amniocentesis." *Social Science and Medicine* 19, no. 11:1207–1212.

JOLLY, JULIUS. 1901. *Medicin.* Strasbourg: K. J. Trubner. Translated and edited by Chintaman Ganesh Kashikar under the title *Indian Medicine.* Poona, India: C. G. Kashikar, 1951.

KANE, PANDURANG VAMAN. 1968–. *A History of Dharmasastra: Ancient and Mediaeval Religious and Civil Law in India.* 2d rev. ed. Poona, India: Bhandarkar Oriental Research Institute.

KAUTILIYA. 1969. *The Kautiliya Arthasāstra.* 2d ed. 2 vols. Edited and translated by R. P. Kangle. Bombay: University of Bombay. Text and translation.

LANNOY, RICHARD. 1971. *The Speaking Tree: A Study of Indian Culture and Society.* London: Oxford University Press.

The Laws of Manu. 1988. Translated by Georg Buhler. Delhi: Motilal Banarsidass.

Mahāvagga [The Great Division]. 1881–1882. Translated by T. W. Rhys Davids and Hermann Oldenberg. Edited by Friedrich Max Müller. Oxford: At the Clarendon Press.

MAJUMDAR, R. C. 1971. "Medicine." In *A Concise History of Science in India,* 213–273. Edited by D. M. Bose, S. N. Sen, and B. V. Subbarayappa. New Delhi: Indian National Science Academy.

MENON, I. A., and HABERMAN, H. F. 1970. "The Medical Students' Oath of Ancient India." *Medical History* 14, no. 3:295–299.

MONIER-WILLIAMS, MONIER. 1883. *Religious Thought and Life in India: Vedism, Brāhmanism and Hinduism.* London: John Murray.

REDDY, D. V. SUBBA. 1941. "Medical Relief in Medieval South India: Centres of Medical Aid and Types of Medical Institutions." *Bulletin of the History of Medicine* 9:385–400.

———. 1961. "Medical Ethics in Ancient India." *Journal of the Indian Medical Association* 37, no. 16:287–288.

SETTAR, SHADAKSHARI. 1990. *Pursuing Death: Philosophy and Practice of Voluntary Termination of Life.* Dharwad, India: Institute of Indian Art History, Karnatak University.

SHARMA, PRIYA VRAT, ed. 1992. *History of Medicine in India: From Antiquity to 1000 A.D.* New Delhi: Indian National Science Academy.

SUŚRUTA. *Suśruta Samhitā.* 1947. 3 vols. Translated by Kaviraj-Kunja Lal Bhishagratna. Varanasi, India: Chowkhamba Sanskrit Series.

VĀGBHATA. 1965. *Astāṅgahrdayasamhitā. The First Five Chapters of Its Tibetan Version.* Edited and translated by Claus Vogel. Deutsche Morgenländische Gesellschaft. With original Sanskrit text. Wiesbaden: Franz Steiner.

WEISS, MITCHELL G. 1980. "*Caraka Samhitā* on the Doctrine of *Karma.*" In *Karma and Rebirth in Classical Indian Traditions,* 90–115. Edited by Wendy Doniger O'Flaherty. Berkeley: University of California Press.

WILLIAMS-MONIER, MONIER. 1883. *Religious Thought and Life in India: Vedism, Brāhmanism and Hinduism.* London: J. Murray.

ZYSK, KENNETH G. 1991. *Asceticism and Healing in Ancient India: Medicine in the Buddhist Monastery.* New York: Oxford University Press.

HIPPOCRATIC OATH

See MEDICAL CODES AND OATHS. See also the APPENDIX (CODES, OATHS, AND DIRECTIVES RELATED TO BIOETHICS), SECTION II: ETHICAL DIRECTIVES FOR THE PRACTICE OF MEDICINE.

HISTORY OF MEDICAL ETHICS

See MEDICAL ETHICS, HISTORY OF.

HIV

See AIDS; *and* EPIDEMICS. See also BLOOD TRANSFUSION; *and* IATROGENIC ILLNESS AND INJURY.

HOME HEALTH CARE

See LONG-TERM CARE, *article on* HOME CARE.

HOMEOPATHY

See ALTERNATIVE THERAPIES; *and* UNORTHODOXY IN MEDICINE.

HOMICIDE

Homicide is the "killing of one human being by the act, procurement, or omission of another" (Black, 1951, p. 867). It is an extreme act: the ultimate and fatal extreme in the categories of intentional injury and assaultive violence, the moral extreme in terms of relations between people. In the United States, unfortunately, homicide is losing its extreme character and is becoming more commonplace. It has become the tenth leading cause of death in the United States. For ages one to fourteen it is the fourth leading cause of death; for ages fifteen to twenty-four, the second. Overall, homicide is the fourth leading cause of premature mortality. The number of people who die each year in the United States as the result of homicide has surpassed 22,000. For black males fifteen to thirty-four years of age, homicide has become the leading cause of death (Rosenberg and Mercy, 1992; Baker et al., 1992; Fingerhut and Kleinman, 1990). According to a Centers for Disease Control and Prevention report, "Much of the disparity in the burden of death and illness experienced by blacks relative to the majority white population is attributable to rates of black homicide that are 5 to 6 times higher than those for whites" (U.S. Department of Health and Human Services, 1989, p. 17).

It was not always so. In 1930 the U.S. homicide rate was 9 per 100,000 population; in 1957 it had fallen to 4 per 100,000; by 1980 it had climbed to 11 per 100,000; and in 1988 it stood at 9 per 100,000 (Baker et al., 1992). The United States has the highest homicide rate of all developed countries, and one of the highest rates among all countries that report homicide statistics to the World Health Organization (Rosenberg and Mercy, 1992). A large part of this high rate seems to be related to firearms.

For years homicide was viewed simply as a criminal justice problem, with emphasis on using criminal law to deter violent acts by individual lawbreakers. From this conceptual perspective, homicides appeared as random, unpredictable acts. Neither general nor specific deterrence seemed to hold out much hope of significantly reducing homicide rates. "Regarding violence in our society as purely a sociologic matter, or one of law enforcement, has led to unmitigated failure" (Koop and Lundberg, 1992, p. 3076).

U.S. Surgeon General Antonia Novello warned that "Violence in the United States is a public health emergency" (Novello et al., 1992, p. 3007). Most violent injuries are not the result of criminal activity but are closely tied to social ills, ranging from poverty and racism to alcohol abuse and family dysfunction. Thus both the magnitude and the nature of the problem make it sensible for homicide and nonfatal assaultive violence to be approached as public-health problems. Violent injuries are not random but in fact are predictable; they are amenable to public-health techniques for surveillance, epidemiological analysis, and interdisciplinary primary prevention. This approach recognizes multicausal explanations and emphasizes environmental factors while eschewing concentration on victim fault. Scientists from the National Center for Injury Prevention and Control note the following:

> The public health approach consists of health-event surveillance, epidemiologic analysis, and intervention design and evaluation, focused unwaveringly on a single, clear outcome—the prevention of a particular illness or injury. This approach was originally developed to combat infectious diseases, when such diseases were the leading causes of death. It has been successfully applied, however, to many causes of premature death and preventable physical illness including lung cancer, coronary heart disease, and, more recently, motor vehicle crashes. (Rosenberg et al., 1992, p. 3071)

Viewed solely as a criminal justice issue, homicide may not be a subject of bioethical concern. But the public-health approach to homicide, focusing as it does on predictability and preventability, underscores why homicide and its prevention are indeed bioethical issues. The class and racial biases of homicide add to its significance as a bioethical concern.

Epidemiology

A standard way of dealing with public-health problems is to identify specific risk factors and then to intervene in ways tailored to dealing with these factors. Various factors seem to be associated with the alarming epidemic of violent deaths in the United States. The most notable factors are firearm availability, unemployment and poverty, racism and sexism, alcohol and drug use, and media emphasis on violence. Other risk factors include male gender, young age, mental illness, history of previous abuse, history of violent behavior by parents, and an obsession with physical prowess (Rosenberg and Mercy, 1985; Hawkins, 1989). An important interactional risk factor is the relationship between homicide victim and perpetrator. FBI figures for 1986 show that 40 percent of reported homicides involved friends and acquaintances, 15.1 percent involved family members, and 12.5 percent involved strangers. Rosenberg and Mercy speculate that much of the remaining 32.4 percent "unknown relationship" homicides may involve strangers (Rosenberg and Mercy, 1992). These differences underscore the fact that most homicides do not arise out of criminal activities, and suggest that interventions and prevention strategies may need to vary according to the relationship between homicide victim and perpetrator.

Susan Baker and her colleagues note that homicide rates are highest for males, especially those twenty-five to twenty-nine, and are two-and-a-half times as high in low-income areas as in high-income areas for all races combined, with this becoming a tenfold disparity in central cities. "When socioeconomic status is controlled for, racial differences in homicide rates decrease markedly. . . . The inverse correlation between homicide rates and income is most pronounced for firearm homicides" (Baker et al., 1992, p. 83). Such correlations are reminders that (a) increased homicide risk is yet another disadvantage of poverty, and (b) stereotypes based on race are as unhelpful as they are wrong.

Alcohol and drug use have been associated with all homicides other than child homicide. Researchers continue to debate whether the disinhibiting effect of alcohol may be more psychological than physiological. Drugs can affect behavior in the same way as alcohol. In addition, they play a critical role in homicide because of their illegal nature; criminal activities mean high monetary stakes combined with a violent private enforcement system. "It has been estimated . . . that a minimum of 10% of homicides nationwide are related to illicit drug use" (U.S. Department of Health and Human Services, 1989, p. 19; Goldstein et al., 1989; Goldstein, 1990).

Finally, and most critically, firearms play a key role in homicides. Rosenberg and Mercy report that in 1986, three-fifths of all homicides were committed with firearms; three-quarters of the victims were killed with handguns (Rosenberg and Mercy, 1992). Firearm-associated assaults by family members and other intimates are three times more likely to result in death than those involving knives or other cutting instruments, and 23.4 times more likely to result in death than those involving other weapons or the use of bodily force (Saltzman et al., 1992). The greater lethality of firearms is exacerbated by the fact that they have become more plentiful and more readily available throughout the United States since the early 1960s. The dramatic increase in gun ownership seems to be related to fear of crime and civil disorder combined with a mistaken belief that guns provide self-defense advantages and heightened safety. The draft position paper on violence prevention prepared for the federal government's Third National Injury Control Conference in 1991 stated: "Trends in our overall rates of violent death are largely determined by firearm violence. . . . Most developed countries report near-negligible numbers of firearm deaths, and their rates of overall violence are far lower than ours" (Panel on Violence Prevention, 1991, p. I-15).

This represents a dramatic escalation of gun violence in the United States. "Between 1960 and 1980 the death rate from firearm homicide increased by 160 percent (from 2.6 to 6.8 per 100,000), while the rate for all other homicides increased by 100 percent (from 1.9 to 3.8)" (Baker et al., 1992, p. 86). As a dramatic symbol of the change that has been occurring, a *New York Times* headline reported, "1990 Gun Deaths Top Auto Fatalities in Texas" (Lewin, 1991).

Data sources

A problem in exploring the epidemiology of homicide is that complete information is hard to collect (although it is much easier to acquire homicide data than data on nonfatal assaultive violence). Sources of national data include the Federal Bureau of Investigation Uniform Crime Report, the National Crime Survey, and the National Center for Health Statistics Mortality Data. Unfortunately, all of these have serious limitations; dependable data on weapons employed, circumstances, and relationships of perpetrator and victim are often incomplete, especially as to weapon type (Ryan et al., 1990; Rokaw et al., 1990).

Approaches to solutions

Despite limitations in available data, it is relatively clear which preventive approaches are most likely to reduce homicide rates. The three most critical interventions would be

1. Increases in social support spending
2. Restrictions on the availability of firearms
3. Limitations on alcohol consumption.

More extensive and detailed recommendations for reducing homicide and other types of assaultive violence were developed for the 1985 Surgeon General's Workshop on Violence and Public Health (Surgeon General's Workshop, 1985). Similar recommendations are included in a 1992 review article by Rosenberg and Mercy. These recommendations for intervention include (1) so-

cial and cultural changes, such as decreasing the cultural acceptance of violence and reducing racial discrimination, gender inequality, and the consumption of alcohol and other drugs; (2) health and related social-service changes, such as developing education programs to teach conflict resolution skills and increasing education for family life, family planning, and child rearing; and (3) environmental and other changes, such as developing strategies to reduce injuries associated with firearms (Rosenberg and Mercy, 1992). The lead recommendation of the 1985 Surgeon General's Workshop on Violence and Public Health was that there "should be a complete and universal federal ban on the sale, manufacture, importation and possession of handguns (except for authorized police and military personnel); and regulation of manufacture, sale and distribution of other lethal weapons . . ." (Surgeon General's Workshop, 1985, p. 1).

Although the United States has more gun laws than any other country, most are local place-and-manner restrictions that do not affect the proliferation of firearms. The United States has little experience with bans, and research on the effectiveness of such laws has been limited. However, recent studies suggest that governmental restrictions can be effective in reducing homicide (Sloan et al., 1988; O'Carroll et al., 1991; Loftin et al., 1991). For example, Colin Loftin and colleagues found a statistically significant association between the adoption of restrictive licensing of handguns and a prompt decline in homicides and suicides by firearms in the District of Columbia. They estimated that restrictions on access to guns there prevented "an average of 47 deaths each year after the law was implemented" (Loftin et al., 1991, p. 1615).

Despite the magnitude of the homicide problem in the United States and the identification of promising interventions by the research and public-health communities, policymakers have followed a course almost opposite to these proposed interventions. They have underfunded social-support programs, all but guaranteeing increased social crises, including increased homicide.

During the 1980s, in particular, politicians embraced an ideology that promoted individual accrual of wealth while ignoring the increasing number of people in poverty and the loss of community social supports. Government programs that might have decreased some of the factors associated with homicide, such as drug and alcohol abuse, dysfunctional family relationships, and poverty in and of itself, were significantly eroded. Minority citizens in the United States, especially African-Americans and Hispanics, were the major victims of this increasing disparity of wealth and this erosion of important social programs, since they are disproportionately represented among the poor. Many leaders of minority groups have expressed the belief that the neglect of poor inner-city communities stems from a racist bias within government.

Most tragically, a majority of politicians opposed all efforts to restrict the availability of firearms, even though the U.S. Supreme Court has made it clear that the Second Amendment to the U.S. Constitution has no significant limiting impact on efforts by government to control (and even ban) firearms. In *Presser* v. *Illinois* (116 U.S. 252 [1886]), the Court ruled that the Second Amendment applies to congressional action only, and has no effect on state and local gun restrictions. In *United States* v. *Miller* (307 U.S. 174 [1939]), the Court held that the Second Amendment applies only to a *collective* right having "some reasonable relationship to the preservation or efficiency of a well regulated [state] militia," and creates no *individual* "right" to keep and bear arms. These two Supreme Court decisions remain the definitive interpretation of the meaning of the Second Amendment, yet politicians have hidden behind a mythical individual "right" to guns to avoid offending a powerful gun lobby. In short, the political leadership of the nation has facilitated homicide even as the public-health and medical communities have geared up to reduce intentional violence. Perhaps this situation will improve. Legislative actions in New Jersey and Virginia, where gun-control laws have been strengthened, suggest that politicians are beginning to get the message that ready access to guns can no longer be tolerated.

TOM CHRISTOFFEL

For a further discussion of topics mentioned in this entry, see the entries PUBLIC HEALTH, *articles on* DETERMINANTS OF PUBLIC HEALTH, *and* PUBLIC-HEALTH METHODS: EPIDEMIOLOGY AND BIOSTATISTICS; PUBLIC HEALTH AND THE LAW, *article on* LEGAL MORALISM AND PUBLIC HEALTH; RACE AND RACISM; SEXUAL IDENTITY; *and* SUBSTANCE ABUSE, *especially the articles on* ADDICTION AND DEPENDENCE, *and* LEGAL CONTROL OF HARMFUL SUBSTANCES. *For a discussion of related ideas, see the entry* ABUSE, INTERPERSONAL, *especially the article on* ABUSE BETWEEN DOMESTIC PARTNERS. *Other relevant material may be found under the entries* JUSTICE; NARRATIVE; *and* VALUE AND VALUATION.

Bibliography

BAKER, SUSAN P.; O'NEILL, BRIAN; GINSBURG, MARVIN J.; and LI, GUOHUA. 1992. *The Injury Fact Book.* 2d ed. New York: Oxford University Press.

BLACK, HENRY CAMPBELL. 1951. *Black's Law Dictionary.* 5th ed. St. Paul, Minn.: West Publishing.

FINGERHUT, LOIS A., and KLEINMAN, JOEL C. 1990. "International and Interstate Comparisons of Homicides Among Young Males." *Journal of the American Medical Association* 263, no. 24:3292–3295.

GOLDSTEIN, PAUL J. 1990. "Drugs and Violent Crime." In *Pathways to Criminal Violence,* pp. 16–48. Edited by Neil A. Weiner and Marvin E. Wolfgang. Newbury Park, Calif.: Sage.

GOLDSTEIN, PAUL J.; BROWNSTEIN, HENRY H.; RYAN, PATRICK J.; and BELLUCCI, PATRICIA A. 1989. "Crack and Homicide in New York City, 1988: A Conceptually Based Event Analysis." *Contemporary Drug Problems* 16, no. 4:651–687.

HAWKINS, DARNELL, F. 1989. "Intentional Injury: Are There No Solutions?" *Law, Medicine, and Health Care* 17, no. 1:32–41.

KOOP, C. EVERETT, and LUNDBERG, GEORGE D. 1992. "Violence in America: A Public Health Emergency: Time to Bite the Bullet Back." *Journal of the American Medical Association* 267, no. 22:3075–3076.

LEWIN, TAMAR. 1991. "1990 Gun Deaths Top Auto Fatalities in Texas." *New York Times,* November 9, p. A4.

LOFTIN, COLIN; MCDOWALL, DAVID; WIERSEMA, BRIAN; and COTTEY, TALBERT J. 1991. "Effects of Restrictive Licensing of Handguns on Homicide and Suicide in the District of Columbia." *New England Journal of Medicine* 325, no. 23:1615–1620.

NOVELLO, ANTONIA C.; SHOSKY, JOHN; and FROEHLKE, ROBERT. 1992. "From the Surgeon General, U.S. Public Health Service: A Medical Response to Violence." *Journal of the American Medical Association* 267, no. 22:3007.

O'CARROLL, PATRICK W.; LOFTIN, COLIN; WALLER, JOHN B.; MCDOWALL, DAVID; BUKOFF, ALLEN; SCOTT, RICHARD O.; MERCY, JAMES A.; and WIERSEMA, BRIAN. 1991. "Preventing Homicide: An Evaluation of the Efficacy of a Detroit Gun Ordinance." *American Journal of Public Health* 81, no. 5:576–581.

PANEL ON VIOLENCE PREVENTION. 1991. Draft Position Paper on Violence Prevention. Atlanta: U.S. Centers for Disease Control.

ROKAW, WILLIAM M; MERCY, JAMES A.; and SMITH, JACK C. 1990. "Comparing Death Certificate Data with FBI Crime Reporting Statistics on U.S. Homicides." *Public Health Reports* 105, no. 5:447–455.

ROSENBERG, MARK L., and FENLEY, MARY ANN, eds. 1991. *Violence in America: A Public Health Approach.* New York: Oxford University Press.

ROSENBERG, MARK L., and MERCY, JAMES A. 1985. *Homicide and Assaultive Violence: Background Paper Prepared for the Surgeon General's Workshop on Violence and Public Health.* Atlanta: U.S. Centers for Disease Control.

———. 1992. "Assaultive Violence." In *Public Health and Preventive Medicine,* pp. 1035–1039. 13th ed. Edited by John M. Last, Robert B. Wallace, Elizabeth Barrett-Connor, Jonathan E. Fielding, Arthur L. Frank, F. Douglas Scutchfield, Carl W. Tyler, Jr., and Richard P. Wenzel. Norwalk, Conn.: Appleton & Lang.

ROSENBERG, MARK L.; O'CARROLL, PATRICK W.; and POWELL, KENNETH E. "Let's Be Clear: Violence Is a Public Health Problem." *Journal of the American Medical Association* 267, no. 22:3071–3072.

RYAN, PATRICK J.; GOLDSTEIN, PAUL J.; BROWNSTEIN, HENRY H.; and BELLUCI, PATRICIA A. 1990. "Who's Right: Different Outcomes When Police and Scientists View the

Same Set of Homicide Events, New York City, 1988." In *Drugs and Violence: Causes, Correlates, and Consequences,* pp. 239–264. Edited by Mario De La Rosa, Elizabeth Y. Lambert, and Bernard Gropper. NIDA Research Monograph 103. Rockville, Md.: U.S. Department of Health and Human Services; Public Health Service; Alcohol, Drug Abuse, and Mental Health Administration; National Institute on Drug Abuse.

SALTZMAN, LINDA E.; MERCY, JAMES A.; O'CARROLL, PATRICK W.; ROSENBERG, MARK L.; and RHODES, PHILIP H. 1992. "Weapon Involvement and Injury Outcomes in Family and Intimate Assaults." *Journal of the American Medical Association* 267, no. 22:3043–3047.

SLOAN, JOHN HENRY; KELLERMANN, ARTHUR L.; REAY, DONALD T.; FERRIS, JAMES A.; KOEPSELL, THOMAS; RIVARA, FREDERICK P.; RICE, CHARLES; GRAY, LAUREL; and LOGERFO, JAMES. 1988. "Handgun Regulations, Crime, Assaults, and Homicide: A Tale of Two Cities." *New England Journal of Medicine* 319, no. 19:1256–1262.

SURGEON GENERAL'S WORKSHOP ON VIOLENCE AND PUBLIC HEALTH. 1985. "Recommendations from the Working Groups." Leesburg, Va.: Author.

U.S. DEPARTMENT OF HEALTH AND HUMAN SERVICES. PUBLIC HEALTH SERVICE. CENTERS FOR DISEASE CONTROL. CENTER FOR ENVIRONMENTAL HEALTH AND INJURY CONTROL. DIVISION OF INJURY EPIDEMIOLOGY AND CONTROL. 1989. *Year 2000 Health Objectives for the Nation: Reduce Violent and Abusive Behavior.* Draft Report of the Interagency Workgroup, April 11, 1989. Atlanta: U.S. Centers for Disease Control.

HOMOSEXUALITY

I. Clinical and Behavioral Aspects
   Eli Coleman
II. Ethical Issues
   Louis Tietje
   James Harrison

I. CLINICAL AND BEHAVIORAL ASPECTS

In order to understand the clinical and behavioral aspects of homosexuality, it is important to recognize that terms such as homosexual, bisexual, and heterosexual are constructed within a sociopolitical and cultural climate. As this climate changes, our understanding of the meaning of such labels changes, too. This point is important for clinicians to keep in mind when assessing an individual's sexual orientation and in choosing the terms to describe it. Historically, clinicians have assessed sexual orientation (e.g., Kinsey et al., 1948) based upon the assumption that sexual orientation is determined by one's sex or genitalia and the sex or genitalia of the

individual to whom one is erotically attracted. Many clinicians have also assumed that a person's sexual orientation is fixed and immutable.

Recent research, however, has challenged these assumptions. We now recognize that biological sex is only one of the many components of the attraction or orientation two individuals experience in relation to one another. Sexual orientation must be understood as multidimensional, incorporating the various components of a person's sexual identity (male or female physical characteristics, male or female gender identification, traditional masculine or feminine sex-role characteristics) and various dimensions of sexuality (behavior, fantasies, and emotional attachments). Recognizing this multidimensional complexity, clinicians and their clients are finding that sexual orientation identities (homosexual, bisexual, and heterosexual) are no more important than any other single aspect of overall identity.

Theories on the cause of homosexuality

Many theories of the development of sexual orientation have been articulated, but no current one prevails. Traditional psychoanalytic theorists have believed that homosexuality is a result of childhood trauma that causes intrapsychic conflict and an arrested psychosexual development (e.g., Socarides, 1968, 1988); many psychoanalysts still hold this view. This traditional view of the cause of homosexuality has been challenged by many sexual scientists and by gay-identified and some other psychoanalysts. For example, the psychoanalyst Richard Isay (1989) believes that homosexuality is innate and influenced by prenatal biological influences.

Learning theorists and behavior therapists have traditionally seen homosexuality as a maladaptive learned behavior. Behaviorists hold the belief that sexual deviations are learned through operant and classical conditioning mechanisms.

Both psychoanalytic and behavioral theories have held that homosexuality is an illness or a maladaptive behavior. In contrast, John Money (1988), a sexologist who has studied the origins of sexual attractions for over forty years, believes that homosexuality is a normal variation of sexual expression and develops along a nature/critical period/nurture pathway (i.e., prenatal influences interact with environmental events at critical periods)—although the exact mechanisms are still unknown. In a major study of the development of sexual orientation, Alan Bell, Martin Weinberg, and Sue Hammersmith (1981) were unable to confirm any of the psychoanalytic or behavioral theories among their large sample of participants. While unable to find an environmental influence, the authors suggested that research might focus on biological factors to find the etiology of heterosexuality and homosexuality.

In the 1980s and 1990s, a few studies focused on biological correlates (hormonal, neuroanatomical, genetic) of adult sexual orientation (Gladue et al., 1984; Swaab and Hoffman, 1990; LeVay, 1991), and a few studies identified a substantial genetic component (Bailey and Pillard, 1991; Bailey et al., 1993). These studies attracted significant media attention and have promoted a belief in biological factors as the basis of sexual orientation.

Without solid replication studies, the relative influence of biological factors is still unclear (Coleman et al., 1989). If these recent findings follow other biological research in the complex area of human sexuality, William Byne and Bruce Parsons have argued, answers regarding a biological cause of homosexuality are unlikely in the near future (Byne and Parsons, 1993).

Apart from the contributions such biological studies may make to our understanding of how we come to be the sexual persons we are—whether hetero-, bi-, or homosexual—their findings have significant implications for how society treats persons identified as homosexual. Some argue that if "biology made them do it," homosexual men and women cannot be held responsible for their behavior, should not be seen as morally depraved, and should be given the same legal and social rights as heterosexual individuals. But some people fear that evidence of a biological basis will strengthen the hand of those who would use medical or psychological treatment to correct the biological "mistake" of homosexuality.

Beyond the illness paradigm

Since Alfred Kinsey's pioneering work in the 1940s and early 1950s, the association of homosexuality with illness has been gradually but thoroughly refuted by scientific research (see Gonsiorek, 1991, for a review of these studies). This scientific evidence led to the American Psychiatric Association's 1973 decision to declassify homosexuality per se as an illness in their diagnostic manual of mental disorders (DSM-II). Some psychiatrists still dispute whether this decision was based upon science or politics. The concept of illness was nevertheless retained (American Psychiatric Association, 1973) by the introduction of the disorder "ego-dystonic homosexuality" to describe individuals who had persistent homosexual desires but were troubled by them and desired a change in sexual orientation. This category was finally eliminated in DSM-III-R (American Psychiatric Association, 1987) and DSM-IV (American Psychiatric Association Task Force, 1991), but a vestige of the illness notion could still be found as an example of "Sexual Disorders Not Otherwise Specified" (DSM-IV, p. 538). Nevertheless, the fundamental change declassifying homosexuality per se as a mental disorder has been upheld in recent revisions of the DSM.

In spite of these changes in scientific opinion and the removal of homosexuality as a mental disorder, there is no complete consensus on this matter. Some professionals and laypeople still view homosexuality as the result of an abnormal process of development that is driven by some type of pathology (e.g., Aardweg, 1986; Society of Medical Psychoanalysts, 1988; Socarides, 1988).

The development of sexual identity and sexual identification

While the process of developing sexual identity is most probably a complex interaction of biopsychosocial influences of which we have very little understanding, theorists have developed various models that suggest that individuals acquire a homosexual identity in stages (e.g., Cass, 1979; Coleman, 1981–1982). The developmental stages illustrate how individuals who are predominantly homosexual construct their identity in a positive, self-affirming manner, despite living in a society that stigmatizes homosexuality.

After a period of confusion and a sense of "differentness," an individual adopts a homosexual label and begins a process of exploring his or her sexual identity and sexual relationships, learning about intimacy, and finally reaching a stage of self-acceptance and integration (Coleman, 1981–1982). Adopting the label "gay," "lesbian," or "bi" is often a means of developing more positive attitudes about one's homosexual behavior and identity. These labels are positively construed and help counteract negatively construed labels such as "faggot," "dyke," and "queer." Although this process of identity formation is similar for men and women, sex-role socialization makes for gender differences. Men are likely to experience more sexual relationships during their exploration stage and women are more likely to define their identity based upon awareness of their emotional attachments (Coleman, 1981–1982).

The psychological problems that homosexual men and women face result from social stigma rather than from their sexual orientation. The effects of stigmatization on psychological well-being are well understood. As long as homosexuality is stigmatized in a society, homosexual men and women are at risk for psychological maladjustment, impaired psychosocial development, family alienation, inadequate interpersonal relationships, alcohol and drug abuse, and depression and suicidal ideation, in addition to the inevitable anxiety about AIDS and other sexually transmitted diseases (Coleman, 1988). Conversely, affirming sexual diversity is linked to psychological and physical health. Social attitudes profoundly affect individuals with same-sex attractions either by assisting them in the development of a positive and integrated sexual identity or by thwarting such development. Psychotherapy is often needed to help individuals whose development has been thwarted by negative societal attitudes.

Medical and social attitudes toward homosexuality

Medical professionals have participated in the widespread discrimination against individuals who identify themselves as gay or lesbian. In one study of 1,000 physicians, three-quarters acknowledged that knowing that a male patient was homosexual would adversely affect their medical management (Pauly and Goldstein, 1970). More recent studies are lacking, but there is anecdotal evidence that irrational fears of homosexuality and negative attitudes toward homosexuality among physicians compromise comprehensive and quality health care of homosexual men and women. On the other hand, as more and more physicians acknowledge their homosexuality to their colleagues, it becomes increasingly difficult for the latter to maintain discriminatory attitudes and irrational fears, at least openly. It is more difficult to hold these attitudes and views about people one knows and respects than about a class of people or abstractions of people portrayed in the media. Some professional medical organizations have taken active responsibility to help dispel prejudice. The American Academy of Pediatrics (1983), for example, has provided a positive policy statement:

> Teenagers, their parents, and community organizations with which they interact may look to the pediatrician for clarification of the medical and social issues involved when the question or fact of adolescent homosexual practices arises. . . . The American Academy of Pediatrics recognizes the physician's responsibility to provide health care for homosexual adolescents and for those young people struggling with the problems of sexual expression. (pp. 249–250)

These changes in the medical world reflect societal changes. Numerous social, political, and religious organizations have legitimized homosexual behavior. New laws in some cities and states of the United States and in other Western countries prohibit discrimination based on homosexual behavior or sexual orientation. Personnel policies of many corporations prohibit discrimination on the basis of sexual orientation. Public and private institutions provide health-care and other personnel benefits to the partners of gay men and lesbians (Jefferson, 1994). At the same time, antihomosexual prejudice and discriminatory practices persist. Even as the civil rights of gay and lesbian persons are explicitly guaranteed, there has been an escalation in the number of "hate crimes" against people identified as gay or lesbian. Unfortunately, society still struggles with accept-

ing its diversity. However, the overall social trend indicates less fear, prejudice, bigotry, and discrimination and greater understanding and respect for individual differences.

Ethical issues in psychological or psychiatric treatment

The ethical issues in the treatment of gay men and lesbians are for the most part no different from the ethical issues a psychotherapist encounters in treating those who seek his or her help. The issue of "conversion" to heterosexuality remains an ethical issue principally for those who view homosexuality as an illness. There is no evidence that adults sustain long-term change in sexual orientation through therapy (Coleman, 1978). Behavior modification, for example, has had limited success and is generally not sustainable over time. Still, some individuals who have homosexual attractions seek a "conversion" to heterosexuality. Parents who are concerned that their children might be gay or lesbian often will encourage them to seek psychotherapy to ensure a heterosexual outcome. And some therapists continue to accept patients into therapy with the goal of changing their sexual orientation. But authorities have rejected pursuit of these goals of treatment as unscientific, unjustified, unethical, and psychologically scarring (Gonsiorek, 1988; Isay, 1989). Nevertheless, some psychoanalysts still consider it possible to change a person's sexual orientation and see pursuing this goal as ethical as long as the individual desires this change (Aardweg, 1986; Society of Medical Psychoanalysts, 1988; Socarides, 1988). This issue remains controversial.

In reviewing this ethical controversy, Gerald C. Davidson, one of the pioneers of "conversion therapy" who used behavior therapy approaches, concluded:

> Change of orientation therapy programs should be eliminated. Their availability only confirms professional and societal biases against homosexuality, despite seemingly progressive rhetoric about its normalcy. Forsaking the reorientation option will encourage therapists to examine the life problems of some homosexuals, rather than focusing on the so-called problem of homosexuality. (1982, pp. 97–98)

Consequently, most therapists focus upon improving the psychological and interpersonal functioning of homosexual men and women rather than on changing their sexual orientation (e.g., Coleman, 1988; Friedman, 1988; Isay, 1989).

But the issue of sexual orientation is not moot. Because sexual orientation is still salient to overall identity, psychotherapists can and do help people define themselves in terms of their sexual orientation, recognize and value the complexity of that sexual orientation, and further their overall sexual identity development and satisfaction.

Health professionals can create for their patients an atmosphere in which sexuality can be discussed openly. By raising the issue of sexual orientation, related problems and concerns can be addressed and resolved. Health professionals' attitudes toward homosexuality greatly influence their ability to be helpful. They, too, are affected by societal attitudes and values concerning homosexuality. And, while some health professionals hold intellectually positive attitudes, their emotional responses can hinder them from conveying full acceptance and from encouraging the exploration of a positive and integrated homosexual identity.

Psychotherapists are sometimes called upon to offer opinions to clients or to appear as expert witnesses in family courts that are assessing whether homosexual men and women are fit parents. Most of the research in this area pertains to lesbian mothers and their children and has been extrapolated to gay men. There has been no evidence that children develop sexual orientation conflict, intra- or interpersonal conflict, or any other significant mental-health concern when raised by their lesbian mothers in the absence of the biological father (see Kirkpatrick, 1988, for a review of these studies). Given the continued societal stigma of homosexuality, however, these children, like gay and lesbian individuals, are especially vulnerable to societal stressors. Further research (especially longitudinal) is needed in this area because of the growing number of gay, lesbian, and bisexual individuals who are choosing to become parents through adoption and foster care or through retaining custody of their biological children.

Another ethical issue involves the objectivity and the capacity for empathy and understanding of a clinician having a certain sexual orientation. Should the sexual orientation of the clinician be a factor in selecting a health-care provider? Further, should a clinician disclose his or her sexual orientation as part of the therapeutic process? There is little scientific research on which to base consideration of these questions. Training and experience should probably be the most salient variables in selecting a clinician—regardless of the client's sexual orientation. Self-disclosure is a therapeutic intervention and should be applied when it seems to be in the client's best interest and to have potential therapeutic value. By following these general ethical principles of health care, the clinician can resolve these ethical dilemmas.

ELI COLEMAN

Directly related to this article is the companion article in this entry: ETHICAL ISSUES. *Also directly related are the entries* SEXUAL IDENTITY; SEXUALITY IN SOCIETY; SEXUAL ETH- ICS; *and* SEXUAL DEVELOPMENT. *For a further discussion of topics mentioned in this article, see the entries* BEHAVIOR MODIFICATION THERAPIES; CONFIDENTIALITY; GENDER IDENTITY AND GENDER-IDENTITY DISORDERS; GENETICS AND HUMAN SELF-UNDERSTANDING; HEALTH AND DISEASE, *especially the articles on* SOCIOLOGICAL PERSPECTIVES, ANTHROPOLOGICAL PERSPECTIVES, *and* PHILOSOPHICAL PERSPECTIVES; HUMAN NATURE; LIFESTYLES AND PUBLIC HEALTH; MARRIAGE AND OTHER DOMESTIC PARTNERSHIPS; PRIVACY IN HEALTH CARE; PROFESSIONAL–PATIENT RELATIONSHIP, *article on* ETHICAL ISSUES; *and* PSYCHIATRY, ABUSES OF. *Other relevant material may be found under the entires* AUTONOMY; EMOTIONS; HEALTH CARE, QUALITY OF; JUSTICE; MEDICINE, SOCIOLOGY OF; OBLIGATION AND SUPEREROGATION; RESPONSIBILITY; *and* RIGHTS.

Bibliography

AARDWEG, GERALD J. M. VAN DEN. 1986. *On the Origins and Treatment of Homosexuality.* New York: Praeger.

AMERICAN ACADEMY OF PEDIATRICS COMMITTEE ON ADOLESCENCE. 1983. "Homosexuality and Adolescence." *Pediatrics* 72, no. 2:249–250.

AMERICAN PSYCHIATRIC ASSOCIATION. 1973. *Diagnostic and Statistical Manual of Mental Disorders (DSM-II).* 2d ed. Washington, D.C.: Author.

———. 1980. *Diagnostic and Statistical Manual of Mental Disorders (DSM-III).* 3d ed. Washington, D.C.: Author.

———. 1987. *Diagnostic and Statistical Manual of Mental Disorders—Revised (DSM-III-R).* 3d ed. Washington, D.C.: Author.

———. 1994. *Diagnostic and Statistical Manual of Mental Disorders (DSM-IV).* 4th ed. Washington, D.C.: Author.

AMERICAN PSYCHIATRIC ASSOCIATION TASK FORCE ON DSM-IV. 1991. *DSM-IV Options Book: Work in Progress, 7-1-91.* Washington, D.C.: Author.

BAILEY, JAMES M., and PILLARD, RICHARD C. 1991. "A Genetic Study of Male Sexual Orientation." *Archives of General Psychiatry* 48, no. 12:1089–1096.

BAILEY, JAMES M.; PILLARD, RICHARD C.; NEALE, MICHAEL C.; and AGYEI, YVONNE. 1993. "Heritable Factors Influence Sexual Orientation in Women." *Archives of General Psychiatry* 50, no. 3:217–223.

BELL, ALAN P.; WEINBERG, MARTIN S.; and HAMMERSMITH, SUE K. 1981. *Sexual Preference: Its Development in Men and Women.* Bloomington: Indiana University Press.

BYNE, WILLIAM, and PARSONS, BRUCE. 1993. "Human Sexual Orientation: The Biologic Theories Reappraised." *Archives of General Psychiatry* 50, no. 3:228–239.

CASS, VIVIENNE C. 1979. "Homosexual Identity Formation: A Theoretical Model." *Journal of Homosexuality* 4, no. 3:219–235.

COLEMAN, ELI. 1978. "Toward a New Model of Treatment of Homosexuality: A Review." *Journal of Homosexuality* 3, no. 4:345–359.

———. 1981–1982. "Developmental Stages of the Coming

Out Process." *Journal of Homosexuality* 7, nos. 2–3:31–43.

———, ed. 1988. *Psychotherapy with Homosexual Men and Women: Integrated Identity Approaches for Clinical Practice.* New York: Haworth Press.

COLEMAN, ELI; GOOREN, LOUIS; and ROSS, MICHAEL. 1989. "Theories of Gender Transpositions: A Critique and Suggestions for Further Research." *Journal of Sex Research* 26, no. 4:525–538.

DAVIDSON, GERALD C. 1982. "Politics, Ethics, and Therapy for Homosexuality." In *Homosexuality: Social, Psychological and Biological Issues*, pp. 89–98. Edited by William Paul, James D. Weinrich, John C. Gonsiorek, and Mary Hotvedt. Beverly Hills, Calif.: Sage Publications.

FRIEDMAN, RICHARD C. 1988. *Male Homosexuality: A Contemporary Psychoanalytic Perspective.* New Haven, Conn.: Yale University Press.

GLADUE, BRIAN A.; GREEN, RICHARD; and HELLMAN, RONALD E. 1984. "Neuroendocrine Response to Estrogen and Sexual Orientation." *Science* 225, no. 4669:1496–1499.

GONSIOREK, JOHN C. 1988. "Mental Health Issues of Gay and Lesbian Adolescents." *Journal of Adolescent Health Care* 9, no. 2:114–122.

———. 1991. "The Empirical Basis for the Demise of the Illness Model of Homosexuality." In *Homosexuality: Research Implications for Public Policy*, pp. 115–136. Edited by John C. Gonsiorek and James D. Weinrich. Newbury Park, Calif.: Sage Publications.

ISAY, RICHARD A. 1989. *Being Homosexual: Gay Men and Their Development.* New York: Farrar Strauss Giroux.

JEFFERSON, DAVID J. 1994. "Family Matters: Gay Employees Win Benefits for Partners at More Corporations." *Wall Street Journal*, March 18, pp. A1–A2.

KINSEY, ALFRED C.; POMEROY, WARDELL B.; and MARTIN, CLYDE E. 1948. *Sexual Behavior in the Human Male.* Philadelphia: W. B. Saunders.

KIRKPATRICK, MARTHA. 1988. "Clinical Implications of Lesbian Mother Studies." In *Psychotherapy with Homosexual Men and Women: Integrated Identity Approaches for Clinical Practice*, pp. 201–211. Edited by Eli Coleman. New York: Haworth Press.

LEVAY, SIMON. 1991. "A Difference in Hypothalamic Structure Between Heterosexual and Homosexual Men." *Science* 253, no. 5023:1034–1037.

MONEY, JOHN. 1988. *Gay, Straight, and In-Between: The Sexology of Erotic Orientation.* New York: Oxford University Press.

PAULY, IRA B., and GOLDSTEIN, STEVEN G. 1970. "Physicians' Attitudes in Treating Male Homosexuals." *Medical Aspects of Human Sexuality* 4, no. 12:26–45.

SOCARIDES, CHARLES W. 1968. *The Overt Homosexual.* New York: Grune and Stratton.

———. 1988. *Preoedipal Origin and Psychoanalytic Therapy of Sexual Perversions.* Madison, Conn.: International University Press.

SOCIETY OF MEDICAL PSYCHOANALYSTS. 1988. *Homosexuality: A Psychoanalytic Study.* Northvale, N.J.: Aronson.

SWAAB, DICK F., and HOFFMAN, MICHEL A. 1990. "An Enlarged Suprachiasmatic Nucleus in Homosexual Men." *Brain Research* 537, nos. 1–2:141–148.

II. ETHICAL ISSUES

Scientists and historians have produced a large body of research that has significantly improved our understanding of all aspects of homosexuality. Despite this research, the precise definition of homosexuality is still controversial. One approach to the problem of definition distinguishes four components of sexual identity: biological sex, gender identity, social sex role, and sexual orientation (Gonsiorek and Weinrich, 1991). (For alternative definitions of sexual identity, gender identity, or gender identity/role, and discussion of terminological divergence; see Pleck, 1981; Weinrich, 1987; Money, 1986, 1988; Friedman, 1988.)

Sex researchers generally agree that no necessary relationship exists among the components of sexual or gender identity. Homosexuals as a group are unique only in their sexual orientation; they are erotically attracted to members of their own sex. Strong evidence that erotic attraction is relatively permanent after a critical period early in a person's life has led scientists to adopt the term "sexual orientation." The term "sexual preference" implies greater volitional capacity to change erotic disposition than seems to exist (Green, 1988).

Although the bipolar distinction between homosexuality and heterosexuality has heuristic value in describing behavior, it is not adequate to understand the complexity of sexual orientation. There are some persons who are bisexual in the sense that they are able to respond erotically to qualities in their partners regardless of biological sex. Current thinking recognizes that sexual orientation is multidimensional and specific to the person (Money, 1986).

Moral disagreement about homosexuality can be traced to different interpretations of the facts, different definitions of the meaning and scope of concepts, and different assumptions in ethical theory about what constitutes good sexuality and right sexual conduct. Disagreements are often difficult to clarify and resolve because of unacknowledged differences in factual interpretation, the meaning of concepts, and ethical theory. Many moral disagreements might be resolved by information if the reason for the disagreement is only factual or conceptual. But no amount or kind of information will resolve a disagreement if the reason for the disagreement is a fundamental difference in ethical assumptions.

In evaluating homosexuality, moral philosophers assume that the questions we are trying to answer are moral questions. We make many judgments that do not seem to be morally significant: For example, "That is a good television." Or, "You should tie your right shoe before your left." Such judgments may have practical importance in our daily lives, but they do not necessarily involve moral matters. Our task, then, is to determine why and under what circumstances homosexuality is a moral matter.

The distinction between homosexual orientation and behavior implies two general questions, one concerning the quality of being and the other the quality of action: Is homosexuality morally good sexuality? What kinds of homosexual activity, if any, are morally right? We cannot simply assume that all judgments about homosexual orientation and behavior are moral judgments. An ethical theory is required in order to decide which judgments about homosexuality are moral judgments.

These general questions involve the good and the right, two basic ethical concepts. Ethical theories provide a structural definition of the relationship between value (the good) and obligation (right and wrong conduct). How the basic concepts of good and right are defined and related determines the structure of an ethical theory. Structurally, ethical theories can be divided into either teleological or deontological types. In teleological theories, some nonmoral good or value (e.g., pleasure, health, or happiness) is defined independently of the right. Right is based on the good, that is, the promotion or maximization of this value. In deontological theories, the good is not defined independently of the right. Right depends on some characteristic of an action itself (e.g., that it can be universalized or that it involves appropriate treatment of persons).

Premodern approaches

Premodern European society did not evaluate the goodness or badness of homosexuality in terms of sexual orientation. People may have recognized that categories of persons with a homosexual orientation exist, but they did not attach moral significance to the categories or their mutability. Sexuality was evaluated in terms of its expression in prescribed social roles and behaviors.

In ancient Greece, various patterns of same-sex intimacy were permitted and in some cases prescribed. For example, in the city-state of Athens, during the classical period and among the educated, good homosexuality was defined as a tutorial relationship between an older and a younger male citizen of equal status, expressed through intercrural (between the thighs) "intercourse." Sexual activity between persons of the same age was sometimes cause of laughter. In Sparta, however, pairs of soldiers were often lovers (Dover, 1980; Lewis, 1983; Halperin, 1989).

The early Christian approach did not depart from the Greek and Roman practice of evaluating sexuality in terms of social role and not in terms of the biological sex of the persons in a relationship. Christian criticisms were directed at promiscuous forms of sexual expression or ones that involved participation in idolatrous cultic practices. Christian constraints on sexuality probably were related to the assumption, also present in Hellenistic culture, that sex is a potentially dangerous force requiring careful control. Celibacy was seen either as an ideal or as the best option for those who could not control their sexuality. For others, regardless of erotic disposition, sexuality should be confined to relationships marked by permanence and fidelity.

The history of Christian sexual ethics can be understood as a development of restrictions on the role of sexuality and not as a radical departure from previous views. The most restrictive position, that only a sexual act with procreative purpose could be sinless, existed early in Christian thought. The development is toward a gradual elimination of all other possibilities. This position "gradually spread throughout the Christian world and became the favored position of ascetics in the West since it both limited sexuality to the smallest possible arena and appealed to an easily articulated and understood principle. Ultimately, it became the standard of Catholic orthodoxy, although hardly inevitably: Not for a millennium after it first appeared did it sweep all other approaches before it" (Boswell, 1990, pp. 18–19. See also Boswell, 1980, for a detailed historical analysis).

Natural-law theory

Thomas Aquinas (1225–1274) gave the restrictive position its most systematic theoretical formulation. His argument rests on two assumptions. His implicit assumption is that good sexuality cannot be determined by asking what social role sexuality plays in human affairs. His explicit theological assumption is that the world was created and is governed by divine reason. Human beings participate in divine reason through their own reason, which gives them access to the eternal law, the natural law, or God's plan for the world.

We can uncover God's sexual plan by asking what the purpose, goal, or function of sexuality is. Aquinas argued that the purpose of sexuality is reproduction or procreation. Sexual activities are natural if they fulfill this purpose and thus accord with the eternal or natural law. All nonprocreative sexual activities are unnatural (Aquinas, 1980).

The argument from natural law has faced two major challenges. The first is a challenge to the idea that procreative purpose is disclosed in the design of the sexual organs. Skeptics point out that most organs of the body have multiple purposes. A mouth is used for the purpose of speaking, eating, and tasting. Which of these is its proper function? The design of the sexual organs includes a large concentration of nerve endings that provide pleasurable sensations. Why is the production of pleasure not a proper function of the sexual organs? A second challenge concerns the implication that interpersonal purposes of sexuality are not proper purposes. Why should the purpose of expressing affection, nurturance, or love of one person for another be excluded as proper purposes?

Modern traditional Roman Catholic theologians have responded to these challenges by expanding the range of proper purposes to cover interpersonal love as well as procreation. They have not conceded, however, that the expanded range of purposes extends beyond the context of fidelity in heterosexual marriage or to persons of the same sex. Homosexuals are excluded because their sexual relationships cannot include physical complementarity, "the structural and systemic receptivity of the female vagina for the male sexual organ," and biological complementarity, "the mutual contribution of male and female to the procreation of new life" (Hanigan, 1988, p. 87). That persons of the same sex do express love for each other in a sexual act and do have committed relationships is not given moral significance because these are not relationships of physical and biological complementarity. Physical and biological differences are given moral significance because they have been interpreted in a theological framework of complementarity. These modes of complementarity disclose to human reason God's purposes for sexuality. Celibacy is the only moral option for homosexuals, even if sexual orientation is immutable (Hanigan, 1988).

Critics of natural-law theory do not challenge the view that procreation and interpersonal love are purposes of sexuality or deny that these purposes are good. Rather, they challenge limiting good sexuality to these purposes. A theological commitment to physical and biological complementarity is the only justification for the limitation. This limitation disavows the spiritual dimension of a loving relationship that may be possible for all persons, regardless of sexual orientation (McNeill, 1976, 1988. See Batchelor, 1980, for a selection of traditional Roman Catholic and Protestant positions and critiques based on various moral norms in the scriptural tradition.)

In sum, premodern European ethical thought appears to begin with the question, "What is good sexuality?" Sexual orientation probably did not exist as a concept. The goodness or badness of sexuality was evaluated according to prescribed social roles. The biological sex of persons in a sexual relationship was not a primary consideration until Aquinas shifted the focus of evaluation from social role to an account of natural purpose. It was assumed that all individuals could participate in prescribed social roles and voluntarily control their sexual behaviors. The question of the mutability of sexual orientation, therefore, did not arise. Premodern ethical thought was teleological in structure. Right or wrong

sexual conduct depended on an answer to the prior question of good sexuality. Aquinas did not change the structure of ethical reasoning in premodern Europe. He only changed the basis for the answer.

Modern approaches

Modern ethical theories emerged in a context of social instability and religious intolerance and warfare. John Locke (1632–1704) suggested a solution to religious and moral disagreement that became the foundation of constitutional democracies in the West. Locke believed that, as a moral minimum, rational people agree that individuals have rights to life, liberty, and property. He proposed that the rules of social and political life be based on this consensus. His solution means that, in the course of their cooperative endeavors, individuals must be willing to exercise considerable tolerance of religious and moral opinions outside this minimal consensus (Locke, 1980).

The theoretical assumption of Locke's proposal is that liberty is the fundamental moral characteristic of individuals. Individual liberty is natural, since it exists prior to and independent of particular social laws and customs. Individual rights to life, liberty, and justly obtained property are grounded in this moral assumption. The existence of individual rights implies the existence of obligations to respect these rights. Rights entail obligations to refrain from interfering with individual liberty. The conviction that individuals have a right to live as they choose, compatible with the same right of all other individuals, is central to all natural-rights theories.

In the natural-rights approach, individuals are free to choose the sexual activities in which they want to participate. A wide variety of these activities is morally right, or at least morally neutral. Only those activities that are coercive or injurious to others are morally wrong. Coercive or injurious sexual activities violate the rights of others. Sexual conduct that violates individual rights, not an evaluation of good sexuality, is morally significant. Natural-rights theories are deontological. Right and wrong homosexual conduct depends on free consent and respect for the rights of others.

The natural-rights perspective has been called "libertarian," not to be confused with "libertine." In this tradition, it is not as if anything goes. It is true that libertarians define a wide zone of permissible sexual behavior. For libertarians, the normative question of good sexuality is important, although the answer is left to individual choice. Homosexual activities that violate individual rights, however, are clearly wrong. The major problem for libertarians is how and under what circumstances to limit sexual conduct between consenting adults. (An example of a contemporary libertarian approach to homosexuality is Mohr, 1988, 1994.)

The theory of Immanuel Kant (1724–1804) is also deontological in structure and coincides with the libertarian supposition that right and wrong sexual conduct does not depend on an independent evaluation of good sexuality. Kant, however, did not argue from the primacy of individual rights. Rather, he argued that moral judgments depend on a maxim of action determined by the categorical imperative: "Act only according to that maxim by which you can at the same time will that it should become a universal law" (Kant, 1959, p. 39).

Kant concluded that homosexual conduct is morally wrong because it cannot be universalized without contradiction. Perhaps he reached this conclusion by reasoning that the universalization of homosexual conduct involves the exclusion of heterosexual intercourse. If all persons were homosexual, the human species would not survive (Kant, 1963).

Many Kantian philosophers think that Kant's reasoning in condemnation of homosexuality is flawed and that the universalization formula does not support his conclusion. They maintain that the distinctive content of Kantian ethics is contained in another formulation: "Act so that you treat humanity, whether in your own person or in that of another, always as an end and never as a means only" (Kant, 1959, p. 47).

According to this formulation, respect for autonomy is the standard of moral evaluation. Sexual orientation in itself is not a moral issue. For either heterosexuals or homosexuals, the danger is that a person in an erotic relationship will be objectified and will be used merely as a means to another's end. The end might include a desire to control, manipulate, dominate, or simply to experience sexual pleasure. In any of these instances, persons are not treated as ends in themselves. The Kantian understanding is expressed in the judgment that sexual relationships ought to be characterized by mutual respect, trust, and love. Another judgment—that using persons as sex objects is dehumanizing and morally wrong—expresses the same Kantian position on how persons ought to be treated.

The Kantian and natural-rights approaches concur that voluntary, free consent in sexual relationships is a moral minimum, but, for Kantians, free consent is not sufficient. The way in which persons treat each other is also morally significant. A Kantian could not sanction a mutual agreement between persons to use each other only as a means to sexual pleasure, even if the agreement were entered into freely. Kantians are therefore inclined to see permanence, stability, and commitment as conditions of the proper treatment of persons in sexual relationships. Anonymous sex is suspect. (See O'Neill, 1985 for a contemporary Kantian interpretation.)

Since modern utilitarian theories are teleological in structure, they must answer the question of what nonmoral value defines good sexuality. Jeremy Bentham (1724–1832) undoubtedly imagined that this question is not difficult to answer. He thought that pleasure is a value everyone accepts. Sexual activities that promote pleasure are right; those that promote pain are wrong. Bentham's approach suggests that homosexuality cannot be bad sexuality because many people take pleasure in homosexual activities. He would agree with libertarians and Kantians that sexual orientation itself is not a morally significant issue (Bentham, 1984).

Even in his own time, Bentham's simple answer to the question of right conduct was met with criticism. The value of pleasure may be a sufficient criterion for animals, but not for human beings. Bentham's concept of sensuous pleasure seemed too narrow. John Stuart Mill (1806–1873) agreed that elementary sensuous pleasures such as eating, drinking, and sexuality are valuable to humans. But he noted that, as creatures with higher-order faculties, they also take pleasure in a variety of intellectual, aesthetic, and social activities. Mill argued that happiness, defined in terms of both lower- and higher-order pleasures, is the inclusive norm of the good for humans on the basis of which right and wrong conduct ought to be evaluated (Mill, 1979). Mill's amendment, however, does not alter Bentham's apparent position on the moral significance of sexual orientation.

Mill believed that freedom is a constituent element of happiness. He was antipaternalistic, arguing that, as a matter of law and public policy, government should not limit what might be considered behavior harmful to self. He argued that only behavior harmful to others is the basis for limiting individual liberty (Mill, 1978). In affirming Mill's harm principle, libertarians and utilitarians are classical liberals. Either can support the recommendation of the English Wolfenden Report in the 1950s to lift the legal ban on homosexual activities between consenting adults in private.

Utilitarians, however, confront a major problem in defining what counts as harm. This difficulty is illustrated in English judge Patrick Devlin's famous response to the Wolfenden Report. Lord Devlin did not dispute Mill's harm principle, but he argued that society's deeply felt moral revulsion is also a valid reason for the legal restriction of homosexual behavior, even between consenting adults in private. Disagreement over the definition of harm has been repeated in a number of court cases. The United States Supreme Court case of *Bowers* v. *Hardwick* (1986), in which the Court upheld Georgia's sodomy statute, is a good example. In this case, the Court supported its majority ruling by appealing to an alleged consensus in the Judeo-Christian tradition on the immorality of homosexuality and its presumed threat to the American family as the legitimate basis of legal restriction. (For a critical analysis of the issues raised by Lord Devlin's response to the Wolfenden Report, see Feinberg, 1990, Chapter 30; see also Mohr, 1988, especially Chapters 2 and 3.) Seidman (1992) outlines a "pragmatic formalistic sexual ethic" based on moral criteria of consent and responsibility for the consequences of sexual acts. Seidman's proposal begins with minimal libertarian and utilitarian criteria of individual free choice and harm to other individuals but expands their meaning and scope to take account of the interrelational, social-communitarian context in which individuals act. His proposal is designed for what has been called the "postmodern" situation, in which a plurality of moral approaches exists and moral disagreement prevails.

The medical model

The advance of modern science and medicine opened the possibility of evaluating homosexuality in nonreligious and nonmoral terms. In the nineteenth century, physicians such as Sigmund Freud, Magnus Hirschfeld, and Carl Westphal thought that this new evaluation would help rather than hurt persons whose sexual practices departed from accepted norms (McWhirter et al., 1990; Bullough and Bullough, 1993). The terms changed from "good," "bad," "right," and "wrong" to "health," "disease," "illness," and "pathology." This change created a new debate over the value-neutrality of medical categories.

The debate has been conducted theoretically and in the context of scientific research. Theoretically, the burden of proof seems to be on those who advocate that categories of health and disease are objective and value-neutral in light of modern historical awareness of cultural and cross-cultural diversity. Christopher Boorse is often cited as one of the most articulate recent spokespersons for the value-free position (Boorse, 1987). His position resembles natural-law theory in that what appears to be a value-neutral, descriptive state of affairs is grounded in an answer to the question of purpose or function.

In Boorse's account, the natural and the normal are associated with health, and abnormality and pathology are associated with disease. For Boorse, definite standards of health can be identified by reference to the full number of biological capacities members of the human species possess on average. These capacities are defined by their functional contribution to survival and reproduction. Diseases represent some deficiency in, or lack of, functional capacity. Boorse advises us to distinguish between disease and illness. Disease is a descriptive biological concept; illness is a value judgment of desirabil-

ity. A person whose reproductive organs are deficient has a disease. Classifying this person as ill is a value judgment.

Boorse concludes that exclusive homosexuality is probably a form of pathology, which apparently means a functional disease, because of reproductive failure. This conclusion, however, is difficult to understand. Although sexual orientation is not chosen, homosexuals, heterosexuals, and celibates may choose their reproductive behavior. Heterosexuals may choose not to have children without a diagnosis of functional incapacity.

Some contemporary heterosexual couples choose not to be married because they want to avoid state intervention into their interpersonal relationship, not because they lack commitment to each other or an intention to parent. Similarly, many lesbians and gay men choose committed relationships that at this time are not sanctioned by the state. Some lesbians and gay men also choose to become surrogate parents or to parent through adoption or alternative insemination. In addition, numerous married persons of both sexes who are already effective parents realize their homosexual orientation later in life and redefine their conjugal relationships while continuing to affirm their parental responsibility. It seems that in the final analysis, Boorse's distinction between disease and illness, at least concerning homosexuality, collapses into a subjective judgment of desirability. (For a positive, sociobiological interpretation of the ways in which gay men and lesbians may have contributed to survival, reproduction, and parenting in the human species, see Weinrich, 1987. See also Ruse, 1985, 1988.)

Researchers, using accepted measures of mental disorder, have not found valid evidence that homosexuality per se is related to psychopathology or psychological adjustment. (For a review of the evidence, see Gonsiorek, 1991.) This does not mean that there are no psychologically disturbed homosexuals or that no homosexuals are disturbed by their sexual orientation. It would be unusual if some homosexuals did not experience psychological distress in an environment of negative stigma and social prejudice. Research has uncovered more alcohol and drug abuse, attempted suicides, use of mental health services, and troubled adolescent years in a subgroup of gay and lesbian people. Nevertheless, those who survive the stigma may demonstrate a trend toward superior adjustment (Hooker, 1957; Harrison, 1987; Gonsiorek and Rudolph, 1991).

Developmental issues

Although scientific research does not support a connection between homosexual orientation and psychopathology or psychological adjustment, many people continue to believe that homosexuality is a problem. As parents, they hope that their children will grow up to be heterosexual and worry about why they might not. At the same time, many parents think that sexuality is a topic children should not be aware of until they mature enough to understand and manage it. Paradoxically, it is not assumed that heterosexuality develops naturally, but its development is precarious and may be derailed by minimal interference (Pleck, 1981).

In our society, therefore, all the developmental questions are related to a single concern about how sexual identity and orientation are influenced. The first question involves the influence of homosexual parents on their biological or adopted children. There is reason to believe that the biological children of homosexual parents are more likely to be homosexual than children whose parents are heterosexual (Kirsch and Weinrich, 1991). However, the sexual orientation of adoptive children raised by homosexual parents seems to reflect the same distribution rates as sexual orientation in the population (Green and Bozett, 1991). Children of any sexual orientation raised in happy and secure environments tend to share the values and beliefs of their parents. Children raised in unhappy homes either identify with or develop reaction formations against violent parental behavior and negative or prejudicial parental values and opinions.

Another question involves the influence of teachers on the sexual orientation of their children. Teachers may be competent, benevolent, and heterosexual, but, despite great respect and admiration, students do not emulate the sexual orientation of their teachers. There is no known instance of a student's becoming homosexual because of identification with a teacher.

However, the needs of young people who have emerging homosexual identities are rarely considered. Instead of receiving sympathetic attention and accurate information about how to live responsible lives with homoerotic desire, they are often given inaccurate information, encouraged to feel ashamed of their emotions, and expected to take responsibility for sexual desire, which is not under their conscious control. Most homosexual teachers are so fearful of the accusation of inappropriate conduct that they are likely to abandon the perceived needs of some of their students to avoid the accusation.

Another question frequently asked is, "Does seduction by an adult influence the sexual orientation of a young person?" Since one of the terms for intergenerational sex in our language is "pederasty," the background of this question may be some awareness of the educational context of homosexual expression in Classical Athens. There is no evidence to support the view that seduction alone affects sexual orientation. Clinicians re-

port that many young people say they would like to be seduced by an admired adult, and some say they initiated sexual activity with an older person (Silverstein, 1977, 1981).

People also wonder if influencing the "feminine" or "masculine" characteristics of children might alter sexual orientation. Developmental research indicates that most "feminine" boys grow up to be homosexual men. Similar studies on women are not available, perhaps because greater tolerance of "tomboy" behavior in girls exists in our society (Green, 1987; Friedman, 1988). Research does not support the efficacy of early intervention to influence the development of a heterosexual orientation in "feminine" boys. However, clinical evidence suggests that early intervention with "feminine" boys who are having difficulty in social adjustment is effective in helping them develop self-esteem, a wide range of coping skills, and satisfactory peer relationships (Coates, 1992; Coates and Wolf, 1994).

In ordinary cases, all moral theories assume that moral agents are normal, competent adults who are able to deliberate rationally about alternative courses of action and control their behavior in a way that is typical for members of the society as a whole. Decisions and control shift to surrogates for individuals who do not meet typical standards. Moral theories cannot tell us when, in fact, individuals are rational and capable of controlling their behavior. For this reason, the age of consent is in some sense arbitrary and has changed historically.

In the case of children, and young people before the age of consent, parents are usually the surrogates. In our society, the natural-rights tradition is the origin of the minimal moral criterion of individual free choice for competent adults and surrogates. By extension, the autonomy of the family, for practical purposes, is considered to be a sacrosanct zone. We are reluctant to authorize the state to interfere in family affairs except in extreme cases of neglect or harm. Short of neglect or harm, parents should have the right to raise their children in the way they choose, transmit the values they uphold, decide how their children should be educated, and decide how and when children should be treated medically and psychotherapeutically.

Kantians, utilitarians, and natural-law theorists support the minimal criterion of free choice. These theorists, however, do not believe that the minimal criterion is sufficient. They add an additional moral criterion of respect or some concept of the good. The problem is what additional moral criteria can be imposed, and under what circumstances, on all members of a democratic society. This problem becomes acute and a matter of dispute in public institutions such as education because parents fear that the values they want to transmit or the ways in which they have parented their children in the home will be negatively influenced by teachers and other adults who are surrogate role models.

Most of the influences that some parents fear are not supported by scientific evidence. For healthy development, children require loving and supportive environments, at home and in public institutions with surrogates. Beyond this, scientists cannot tell us how to ensure that children become heterosexual or homosexual, even if one outcome or another is desired by the parent. What scientists do know, however, is that neglectful, violent, or punitive parental behavior—that is, behavior most people consider harmful to any person—is likely to damage the psychosexual development of children and deny a child the possibility of loving, intimate interpersonal adult relationships, regardless of sexual orientation.

"Diagnosis" and "treatment"

Recognizing a need to amplify the World Health Organization's *International Classification of Diseases* for the practice of psychiatry in the United States, the American Psychiatric Association began production of a series of diagnostic manuals. The first edition of its *Diagnostic and Statistical Manual of Mental Disorders* (DSM, 1952) was essentially a compilation of diagnostic categories used by practicing psychiatrists at the time. The second edition was a more comprehensive and better-organized manual based on psychoanalytic theory, broadly defined. (See Friedman, 1988, for a sympathetic critique of the psychoanalytic tradition informed by social science research.)

The association was challenged by gay activists and some psychiatrists and psychologists such as George Weinberg, Judd Marmor, Richard Pillard, and Charles Silverstein to recognize that categorizing homosexuality as a personality disorder or sexual deviation in the first two editions of its manual had no scientific basis. In the third edition, the association attempted to circumvent the debate over the value-neutrality of concepts of health and disease by developing a phenomenological, atheoretical, nosological system. Homosexuality was declassified as a mental disorder, but, in order to account for the experience of persons who have difficulty affirming their sexual orientation, the concept of ego-dystonic homosexuality was retained and defined as "a sustained pattern of overt homosexual arousal that the individual explicitly states has been unwanted and a persistent source of distress" (DSM-III, 1980, p. 281). In this edition, the remaining sexual deviations were called "paraphilias," in which "unusual or bizarre imagery or acts are necessary for sexual excitement" (DSM-III, 1980,

p. 266). For an historical account of the highly politicized classification debates, see Bayer, 1987; see also Conrad and Schneider, 1992. In a revision of the third edition (DSM-III-R), ego-dystonic homosexuality was removed as a diagnostic category. In the fourth edition (DSM-IV), homosexuality is not mentioned under any diagnostic category.

Without a theory of health and disease, however, it is not clear what the criterion of inclusion or exclusion should be. The difficulty of formulating a value-neutral nosology has convinced many that categories of mental disorder are only a codification of prevalent social mores. In this view, the list of paraphilias retained in the *Diagnostic and Statistical Manual* cannot be justified and should also be removed (Suppe, 1984).

The codification view of the categories of mental disorder is called "social constructionist." Social constructionists believe that all categories of human understanding, even categories of moral judgment and the category of sexual orientation, develop and have meaning only within particular historical constellations of power. In contrast, those who are labeled "essentialists," and are often classified under "the medical model," hold that the objective validity of categories across historical periods and cultures can be established scientifically. The postmodern debate between social constructionists and essentialists has been conducted under various banners in all scholarly disciplines. (See Stein, 1992, for a survey of the debate on sexual orientation. See Boswell, 1983, who interprets the debate in terms of the nominalist–realist controversy in philosophy.)

Proponents of the constructionist perspective argue that diagnostic categories are relative to social rules and function to maintain conformity and to prevent and control nonconformist sexual behavior. Therapists construct both what is to be understood as a psychological problem and what is to constitute a cure. Therapeutic interventions are therefore also guidelines for how clients ought to shape their lives in a moral sense. The therapeutic objective for gay people should be the alleviation of shame and low self-esteem due to social stigma. Therapists should assist the integration of gay people into society (Silverstein, 1991, and Davison, 1991).

These proponents believe that the value of a new egalitarianism, reflected in the black civil rights and women's liberation movements, contributed to social change in the 1960s and 1970s. Social, economic, and political conditions did not support the value of conformity and the need for strong social control. Conditions changed in the 1980s with the emergence of the AIDS crisis and resurgence of conservative religious ideas. Anonymous sex with a large number of partners became problematic for both individuals and society; it represented a threat to life for individuals and a public health disaster of unprecedented magnitude.

In this threatening environment, it is not surprising that some mental-health practitioners "discovered" the new pathologies of sexual addiction and compulsivity. The need for individual self-control seemed urgent. Advocates of the constructionist perspective claim that the clinical entities of pathological addiction and compulsivity were invented to support moral judgments. These "value-neutral" clinical entities only conceal the judgment that nonrelational sex is bad and that individuals should exercise more control over their sexual behavior (Levine and Troiden, 1988).

Sex researcher John Money, a psychologist working within the medical model, has been critical of the view that categories of mental disorder are only a codification of social mores. Money supports the movement to secure civil rights for gay people, but he argues that prior medical mistreatment of persons does not invalidate biomedical research that is conducted with fully informed and knowledgeable consent and with independent protection of individual rights. The scientific search for criteria to differentiate conditions that produce individual suffering and are potentially dangerous to others is essential. Money's research indicates that paraphilia occurs among both heterosexuals and homosexuals and that sexual compulsivity is a real, though rare, clinical entity.

A paraphilia entails an individually or socially unacceptable obligatory stimulus, for example, types of clothing, an amputated limb, or activity such as receiving an enema, which must be present for sexual arousal and orgasm and over which individuals often have little control. It is not addiction to sex in general but dependence on a unique stimulus that is the problem. Individuals with paraphilias may suffer from loneliness because idiosyncratic erotic objects and activities and not relationships with persons predominate in their lives. If the stimulus is an activity such as rape, paraphilic compulsion obviously becomes a threat to society.

Money admits that what is defined as sexuoerotically normal and acceptable varies historically according to ideological norms. Who is to say, then, what is good sexuality and right and wrong sexual conduct? Money is not reluctant to say that good sex is sex that leads to the integration of lust (erotic desire) and love in a reciprocal, mutually responsive, pairbonded relationship between persons. Loving, pairbonded relationships are possible for homosexuals. People with restrictive paraphilic conditions have disorders of love, not sex. They experience a cleavage between lust and love that resists integration in therapy and usually results in a failure to achieve personally satisfying sexuoerotic relationships.

Money's attention to the quality of sexual relationships, not sexual orientation, is reminiscent of the Kantian approach to moral evaluation of sexual conduct. Money's thesis that paraphilia inevitably leads to sexual objectification suggests a formulation of the Kantian injunction not to treat persons as mere means. Persons with paraphilias are compelled to seek sexual satisfaction in unique objects and activities and not in pairbonded relationships.

Money, however, does not attribute moral significance to the inability to form a pairbond; he calls this inability an "unfortunate affliction." Instead, he recommends libertarian criteria of "personal inviolacy" and "subjective discontent." According to the first criterion, "no one has the right to infringe upon someone else's personal sexual inviolacy by imposing his or her own private ideological version of what is or is not erotic and sexual, without the other person's informed consent" (Money, 1988, p. 140). The second criterion is "the personal and subjective discontent with having one's life dictated by the commands of a paraphilic lovemap" (Money, 1988, p. 142). Money defers here to the moral minimum of the natural-rights tradition. He believes that these are the only criteria possible that guarantee both societal rights and equal sexual rights for everyone in a "sexual democracy."

Many kinds of therapy, even sexual orientation conversion therapies, are permissible under libertarian criteria. Some critics charge that conversion therapies do not support human dignity, may involve consumer fraud, and potentially harm clients because there is no evidence that they are effective (Haldeman, 1991). These charges presuppose the moral criteria of respect and harm endorsed by modern ethical theories.

An important question is whether it is morally wrong for therapists to offer treatments of dubious efficacy and safety. Libertarians and utilitarians would not morally disapprove of the provision of conversion therapy if individuals are adequately informed about the unlikely prospect of success and potential harms. Kantians might be more hesitant. They would be fearful that informed consent is not sufficient to protect individuals from improper treatment by therapists. Natural-law theorists would be the most willing to approve of conversion therapy for homosexuals because a change in sexual orientation means that a moral alternative to celibacy becomes available in heterosexual marriage.

Conclusion

All the traditions of ethical thought coexist in modern liberal societies. Some moral disagreements about homosexuality derive from the teleological or deontological structure of ethical theories. In natural-law and utilitarian theories, moral judgments of right and wrong conduct are based on an account of good sexuality. The problem is that people do not agree on whether good sexuality should be defined in terms of the purposes of procreation, interpersonal love, pleasure, or happiness. Utilitarians approve of homosexual activities that promote pleasure and happiness, whereas natural-law theorists disapprove of these activities because they do not have a procreative purpose. Libertarians and Kantians do not confront the problem of defining good sexuality because they base their moral judgments on respect for individual rights and autonomy. Kantians, however, disagree that respect for individual rights is a sufficient moral criterion.

Other moral disagreements derive from differences in factual interpretation. Libertarians, Kantians, and utilitarians agree that the biological sex of a partner is not morally significant. The morally relevant facts involve free consent, harmful conduct, and the treatment of persons. Their disagreements are over what counts as free consent, harmful conduct, and the proper treatment of persons in sexual relationships. They also disagree about what kinds of sexual behavior ought to be legally sanctioned. For natural-law theorists, however, facts about the harmlessness of homosexual behavior or even the proper treatment of persons are not the only relevant facts. For them, physical and biological complementarity have normative implications that are morally significant. Natural-law theorists are bound to complain that the tolerance of what some regard as harmless homosexual behavior in modern liberal societies encourages what they believe is immoral conduct.

Louis Tietje
James Harrison

Directly related to this article is the companion article in this entry: clinical and behavioral aspects. *Also directly related is the entry* sexual identity. *For a further discussion of topics mentioned in this article, see the entries* aids; autonomy; ethics, *article on* task of ethics; family; human nature; marriage and other domestic partnerships; natural law; protestantism; rights; roman catholicism; sex therapy and sex research; sexual ethics; sexuality in society; *and* utility. *For a discussion of related ideas, see the entries* freedom and coercion; harm; interpretation; love; *and* value and valuation. *Other relevant material may be found under the entries* behavior control; behavior modification therapies; children, *article on* health-care and research issues; genetics and human behavior; lifestyles and public health; *and* public health and the law, *article on* legal moralism and public health.

Bibliography

American Psychiatric Association. 1952. 1980. 1987. 1994. *Diagnostic and Statistical Manual of Mental Disorders.* 1st ed. 3d ed., revised. 4th ed. Washington, D.C.: American Psychiatric Association Press.

Aquinas, Thomas. 1980. *Summa Theologica,* 2a2ae, 153 & 154. In *Homosexuality and Ethics,* pp. 39–47. Edited by Edward Batchelor, Jr. Translated by Mortimer Downing. New York: Pilgrim Press.

Batchelor, Edward, Jr., ed. 1980. *Homosexuality and Ethics.* New York: Pilgrim Press.

Bayer, Ronald. 1987. *Homosexuality and American Psychiatry: The Politics of Diagnosis.* Princeton, N.J.: Princeton University Press.

Bentham, Jeremy. 1984. [1978]. "An Essay on 'Paederasty.'" In *Philosophy and Sex,* rev. ed., pp. 353–369. Edited by Robert Baker and Frederick Elliston. New York: Prometheus Books.

Boorse, Christopher. 1987. "Concepts of Health." In *Health Care Ethics: An Introduction,* pp. 359–393. Edited by Donald VanDeVeer and Tom Regan. Philadelphia: Temple University Press.

Boswell, John. 1980. *Christianity, Social Tolerance, and Homosexuality: Gay People in Western Europe from the Beginning of the Christian Era to the Fourteenth Century.* Chicago: University of Chicago Press.

———. 1982–1983. "Revolutions, Universals and Sexual Categories." *Salmagundi* (58–59):88–113.

———. 1990. "Sexual and Ethical Categories in Premodern Europe." In *Homosexuality/Heterosexuality: Concepts of Sexual Orientation,* pp. 15–31. Edited by David P. McWhirter, Stephanie A. Sanders, and June Machover Reinisch. New York: Oxford University Press.

Bowers v. Hardwick. 1986. 478 U.S. 186, 92 L. Ed. 2d. 140, 106 S.Ct. 2841.

Bullough, Vern L., and Bullough, Bonnie. 1993. *Cross Dressing: Sex and Gender.* Philadelphia: University of Pennsylvania Press.

Coates, Susan. 1992. "The Etiology of Boyhood Gender Identity Disorder: An Integrative Model." In *Interface of Psychoanalysis and Psychology,* pp. 245–265. Edited by James W. Barron, Morris N. Eagle, and David L. Wolitzky. Washington, D.C.: American Psychological Association.

Coates, Susan, and Wolfe, Sabrina. October, 1994. "The Treatment of Gender Identity Disorder in Boys." Paper presented at the annual meeting of the American Academy of Child and Adolescent Psychiatry, New York.

Conrad, Peter, and Schneider, Joseph. 1992. "Homosexuality: from Sin to Sickness to Life-Style." In *Deviance and Medicalization: From Badness to Sickness,* expanded ed., pp. 172–214. Philadelphia: Temple University Press.

Davison, Gerald C. 1991. "Constructionism and Morality in Therapy for Homosexuality." In *Homosexuality: Research Implications for Public Policy,* pp. 137–148. Edited by John C. Gonsiorek and James D. Weinrich. Newbury Park, Calif.: Sage.

DOVER, KENNETH JAMES. 1980. *Greek Homosexuality.* New York: Vintage Books.

FEINBERG, JOEL. 1990. *Harmless Wrongdoing.* New York: Oxford University Press.

FRIEDMAN, RICHARD C. 1988. *Male Homosexuality: A Contemporary Psychoanalytic Perspective.* New Haven, Conn.: Yale University Press.

GONSIOREK, JOHN C. 1991. "The Empirical Basis for the Demise of the Illness Model of Homosexuality." In *Homosexuality: Research Implications for Public Policy,* pp. 115–136. Edited by John C. Gonsiorek and James D. Weinrich. Newbury Park, Calif.: Sage.

GONSIOREK, JOHN C., and RUDOLPH, JAMES R. 1991. "Homosexual Identity: Coming Out and Other Developmental Events." In *Homosexuality: Research Implications for Public Policy,* pp. 161–176. Edited by John C. Gonsiorek and James D. Weinrich. Newbury Park, Calif.: Sage.

GONSIOREK, JOHN C., and WEINRICH, JAMES D. 1991. "The Definition and Scope of Sexual Orientation." In *Homosexuality: Research Implications for Public Policy,* pp. 1–12. Edited by John C. Gonsiorek and James D. Weinrich. Newbury Park, Calif.: Sage.

GREEN, G. DORSEY, and BOZETT, FREDERICK W. 1991. "Lesbian Mothers and Gay Fathers." In *Homosexuality: Research Implications for Public Policy,* pp. 197–214. Edited by John C. Gonsiorek and James D. Weinrich. Newbury Park, Calif.: Sage.

GREEN, RICHARD. 1987. *The "Sissy Boy Syndrome" and the Development of Homosexuality.* New Haven, Conn.: Yale University Press.

———. 1988. "The Immutability of (Homo)sexual Orientation: Behavioral Science Implications for a Constitutional (Legal) Analysis." *Journal of Psychiatry & Law* 16, no. 4:537–575.

HALDEMAN, DOUGLAS C. 1991. "Sexual Orientation Conversion Therapy for Gay Men and Lesbians: A Scientific Examination." In *Homosexuality: Research Implications for Public Policy,* pp. 149–160. Edited by John C. Gonsiorek and James D. Weinrich. Newbury Park, Calif.: Sage.

HALPERIN, DAVID M. 1989. "Sex Before Sexuality: Pederasty, Politics, and Power in Classical Athens." In *Hidden from History: Reclaiming the Gay and Lesbian Past,* pp. 37–53. Edited by Martin Bauml Duberman, Martha Vicinus, and George Chauncey, Jr. New York: New American Library.

HANIGAN, JAMES P. 1988. *Homosexuality: The Test Case for Christian Sexual Ethics.* New York: Paulist Press.

HARRISON, JAMES. 1987. "Counseling Gay Men." In *Handbook of Counseling and Psychotherapy with Men,* pp. 220–231. Edited by Murray Scher, Mark Stevens, Glenn Good, and Gregg A. Eichenfield. Newbury Park, Calif.: Sage.

HOOKER, EVELYN. 1957. "The Adjustment of the Male Overt Homosexual." *Journal of Projective Techniques* 21:18–31.

KANT, IMMANUEL. 1959. [1785]. *Foundations of the Metaphysics of Morals, and What Is Enlightenment?* Translated by Lewis White Beck. New York: Liberal Arts Press.

———. 1963. [1775–1781]. *Lectures on Ethics.* Translated by Louis Infield. New York: Harper & Row.

KIRSCH, JOHN A. W., and WEINRICH, JAMES D. 1991. "Homosexuality, Nature, and Biology: Is Homosexuality Natural? Does It Matter?" In *Homosexuality: Research Implications for Public Policy,* pp. 13–31. Edited by John C. Gonsiorek and James D. Weinrich. Newbury Park, Calif.: Sage.

LEVINE, MARTIN P., and TROIDEN, RICHARD R. 1988. "The Myth of Sexual Compulsivity." *Journal of Sex Research* 25:347–363.

LEWIS, THOMAS S. W. 1982–1983. "Brothers of Ganymede." *Salmagundi* (58–59):147–165.

LOCKE, JOHN. 1980. [1689]. *Second Treatise of Government.* Edited by C. B. Macpherson. Indianapolis, Ind.: Hackett.

McNEILL, S. J., and JOHN J. 1976. *The Church and the Homosexual.* Kansas City: Sheed Andrews and McMeel.

———. 1988. *Taking a Chance on God.* Boston: Beacon Press.

McWHIRTER, DAVID P.; SANDERS, STEPHANIE A.; and REINISCH, JUNE MACHOVER, eds. 1990. *Homosexuality/Heterosexuality: Concepts of Sexual Orientation.* New York: Oxford University Press.

MILL, JOHN STUART. 1978. [1859]. *On Liberty.* Edited by Elizabeth Rapaport. Indianapolis, Ind.: Hackett.

———. 1979. [1859]. *Utilitarianism.* Edited by George Sher. Indianapolis, Ind.: Hackett.

MOHR, RICHARD D. 1988. *Gays/Justice: A Study of Ethics, Society, and Law.* New York: Columbia University Press.

———. 1994. *A More Perfect Union: Why Straight America Must Stand Up for Gay Rights.* Boston: Beacon Press.

MONEY, JOHN. 1986. *Lovemaps.* New York: Irvington.

———. 1988. *Gay, Straight, and In-Between: The Sexology of Erotic Orientation.* New York: Oxford University Press.

O'NEILL, ONORA. 1985. "Between Consenting Adults." *Philosophy & Public Affairs* 14:252–277.

PLECK, JOSEPH H. 1981. *The Myth of Masculinity.* Cambridge, Mass.: MIT Press.

RUSE, MICHAEL. 1985. [1981]. "Are There Gay Genes? Sociobiology and Homosexuality." In *Philosophy and Homosexuality,* pp. 5–34. Edited by Noretta Koertge. New York: Harrington Park Press.

———. 1988. *Homosexuality: A Philosophical Inquiry.* New York: Basil Blackwell.

SEIDMAN, STEVEN. 1992. *Embattled Eros: Sexual Politics and Ethics in Contemporary America.* New York: Routledge.

SILVERSTEIN, CHARLES. 1977. *A Family Matter: A Parents' Guide to Homosexuality.* New York: McGraw-Hill.

———. 1981. *Man to Man: Gay Couples in America.* New York: William Morrow.

———. 1991. "Psychological and Medical Treatments of Homosexuality." In *Homosexuality: Research Implications for Public Policy,* pp. 101–114. Edited by John C. Gonsiorek and James D. Weinrich. Newbury Park, Calif.: Sage.

STEIN, EDWARD, ed. 1990. *Forms of Desire: Sexual Orientation and the Social Constructionist Controversy.* New York: Garland.

SUPPE, FREDERICK. 1984. "Classifying Sexual Disorders: The *Diagnostic and Statistical Manual* of the American Psychiatric Association." *Journal of Homosexuality* 9, no. 4: 9–28.

WEINRICH, JAMES D. 1987. *Sexual Landscapes: Why We Are What We Are, Why We Love Whom We Love.* New York: Scribner's.

HOSPICE AND END-OF-LIFE CARE

While the hospice has medieval roots as a service to pilgrims and other travelers, the modern hospice movement began during the late 1960s as a response to the complex needs of persons who were terminally ill and close to death. The first contemporary hospices were founded in England, including the well-known St. Christopher's Hospice in London, which was established in 1966 by Cicely Saunders, M.D. (Stoddard, 1990).

The success of the hospice movement in England and the publication of Elisabeth Kübler-Ross's findings about the dying person's experience (Kübler-Ross, 1969) gave rise to the hospice movement in the United States. The Connecticut Hospice, established in 1974, was the first hospice program in the United States. The number of persons using hospice programs has increased every year since. The 1,935 programs in the United States provided services to over 246,000 persons in 1992 (National Hospice Organization [NHO] *Newsline*, 1993). In the United States, cancer patients account for 78 percent of hospice admissions; AIDS patients, 4 percent; those with cardiac diseases, 10 percent; those with Alzheimer's-type dementia, 1 percent; those with renal disease, 1 percent; and patients with all other diagnoses, 6 percent (National Hospice Organization, 1993). Eighty-nine percent of hospices in the United States are non-profit organizations (NHO, 1993).

In the United States, the hospice has gained widespread acceptance, both as a program of health services and as a change agent in the dominant health-care system. The health-care systems of most European countries have integrated hospice care as an option, and hospices are slowly emerging in Latin American, African, and Asian countries.

The philosophy of hospice care

Hospice care is ordinarily perceived as an alternative to hospital-based, conventional health care. Hospice is not defined by the locus of care, however. The goal of hospice care is to ensure that dying persons live as fully and comfortably as possible, a goal that can be achieved in a variety of settings, including the patient's place of residence and in-patient hospice units.

Hospice is a concept that embraces a philosophy of caring, combined with the best medical knowledge and clinical skills to provide care that is both compassionate and competent. In selecting hospice care, a dying person chooses health care that focuses on comfort and function rather than on cure or prolongation of life. Hospice care does not aim to shorten life nor to prolong dying.

Its providers realistically deal with grief and death, but with a focus on quality living. Hospice care seeks to advance the patient's goals and to provide support and assistance for family and friends during the patient's dying and the bereavement period thereafter.

Since the outcomes to be valued or avoided vary greatly among dying patients, hospice providers must be as familiar with the patient's values and priorities as they are with clinical medicine. The success of hospice care depends on the ongoing commitment to provide the kind of comfort and caring that is supportive of the patient's goals and values. An array of services is necessary to meet the physiological, emotional, social, and spiritual needs of the dying, including medical care, nursing, social services, pastoral care, volunteers, therapists, nursing assistants, homemakers, and bereavement counselors. Effectiveness of the hospice team requires collaboration and substantial cross-disciplinary expertise.

Hospices originally depended entirely upon the efforts of volunteers, but that has changed. Although most of the care and support is now provided by paid professionals, volunteers still offer an important element of community commitment and solidarity, as well as an array of concrete services.

Hospice programs in the United States have had to work within a complex and often uncertain reimbursement system. Although the number of insurance companies and managed-care systems that offer payment for hospice services has increased, many do not have a specific hospice benefit and all vary greatly. A great deal of time and effort is required to estimate likely payments for prospective hospice patients. Dying patients often discover that their hospice coverage is too thin or uncertain to provide the services they will need.

Following several years of an experimental program at twenty-six hospices, Medicare was restructured in 1986 to provide a hospice benefit alternative for most U.S. citizens over sixty-five years of age. Patients choosing the Medicare hospice option are obligated to forfeit most benefits for hospitalization and other aggressive therapies that might require hospitalization. Approximately 35 percent of all hospices in the United States are authorized Medicare providers. The Medicare hospice program pays the hospice provider on a per diem capitated basis, with four rates of pay that depend upon service intensity (though almost all payments have been at the lowest rate). This effectively makes the hospice program the "at risk" insurer, since costly patients must be balanced by inexpensive ones. This financial structure has substantial conflicts of interest for providers and serious barriers to enrollment for potential patients.

Perversely, the advent of a Medicare hospice program and ensuing acceptance of some hospice benefits in most private insurance and managed-care programs in the United States has diminished the availability of philanthropic funds and volunteers to provide charitable care. Along with the popularity of hospice services and the constraints imposed on access, a major problem for hospice staffs and administrators has been to find creative and equitable responses to the mandate to limit access even in the face of obvious patient need.

Symptom management

Hospice has made its best known contributions in the area of effective symptom management. The judicious use of pharmacological agents for pain and effective treatment for the other discomforts associated with terminal disease allow the patient to die with comfort and dignity. Because of the complex nature of symptoms, especially pain, symptom management includes technologically intensive nonpharmaceutical approaches, such as radiation and nerve blocks, as well as more interactive methods, such as relaxation techniques, imagery, acupuncture, and therapeutic touch. A combination of therapies can result in comfort for nearly all patients. Most estimates hold that fewer than 5 percent of dying patients must be substantially sedated in order to be comfortable.

These treatment strategies have given rise to serious ethical concerns (Gibson, 1984). Specific practices aimed at relieving suffering may also shorten life. For example, the use of substantial amounts of narcotics to relieve the physical pain of advanced cancer might hasten debilitation; morphine administered to those dying from respiratory insufficiency effectively sedates those struggling to breathe but also predictably hastens death. The careful evaluation of all alternatives by a trained clinical team, together with a well-informed patient or surrogate who understands the implications of treatment, usually makes it possible to negotiate such difficult decisions. However, efforts must continue to clarify and define acceptable standards of practice. There is a real risk of inattentive overmedication. Patient comfort and control, not physiological imbalances or habitual responses to abnormalities, must be the guide to service delivery.

Ethical issues in patient care

Although hospice care is preferable to conventional care for many who are dying, changes in the health-care system—indeed, in hospice care itself—have created some difficult ethical issues. Advances in medical science continue to generate new and expanded technologies to prolong life, seeming to call into question the wisdom of forgoing treatment. Proponents of the right to life and of assisted suicide engage in heated debate, with each agreeing only that hospice offers too limited a set of treatment options. Society has become increasingly focused on inexpensive care, rather than quality care, for the dying.

The complexity of information that must now be given to the patient regarding services available and financial implications, at a time when he or she is experiencing the impact of death coming close, often makes it unrealistic to expect a patient to make an informed decision about hospice. When a patient does not have decision-making capacity, hospice regulations and state laws in the United States are often unclear about what would constitute appropriate surrogate decision making.

A hallmark of hospice care has been its focus on the patient and family as the "unit of care." Although the patient's interests are of primary concern, the life of a patient necessarily affects the lives of those closest to him or her. Most patients will consider family interests when making decisions. Family-focused care works well as long as there is agreement, but difficulty arises when family preferences conflict with patient choices. What happens when a family wants artificial feeding started, but the patient has clearly refused such intervention? If a patient has asked to go home to die, and the family is physically and emotionally unable to comply, how should the care proceed? Patient autonomy cannot supersede all other considerations, but the balance is, as yet, not clear.

Killing versus letting die.   One of the more controversial ethical issues involved in hospice care focuses on the distinction between active euthanasia and allowing death to occur as a result of the disease process, without intervention. In the context of hospice care, a well-informed patient (or surrogate, acting in the patient's best interest) can refuse treatment and accept a plan of care that is focused on comfort rather than life extension. Some people thereby may die sooner then they would otherwise. The deliberate act of inducing death in order to terminate hopeless suffering or a meaningless existence has been distinguished, in medical ethics, from allowing a terminally ill patient to die with peace of mind and his or her symptoms relieved (Crowley, 1988; U.S. President's Commission, 1993, Hastings Center, 1987). Nevertheless, in practice the delineation of wrongful killings from acceptable practice is challenged by cases requiring exceedingly high doses of narcotics to ease pain, or by forgoing a treatment that might well grant many more months of life.

Hospice supports the patient's right to choose to end his or her life naturally, and perhaps earlier than necessary, by forgoing life-prolonging medical intervention. If a patient is strongly pressured to accept hospice care (e.g., if it is the only course of care paid for by his or her health insurance), he or she may not be exercising a truly free choice for an earlier, "natural" death; for such a person, who may have preferred medical care in a more aggressive setting, the pressure to accept hospice care may well convey a weakness in the societal commitment to sustain life. On the other hand, the refusal of hospice providers to offer assistance in deliberate suicide also acts as a constraint on self-determination, one whose justification is currently involved in controversy.

Artificial nutrition and hydration. Providing food and water to those who are unable to feed themselves is ordinarily seen as a fundamental societal obligation. Failure to treat the malnutrition and dehydration that often accompanies the dying process creates an apparent ethical conundrum for the hospice care provider, especially since tube feeding and intravenous hydration seem so simple. Clearly, some patients are harmed by the artificial provision of food and water, since such interventions can cause suffering by inducing fluid overload, requiring restraints, and occasioning other complications. Patients often die more comfortably without artificial hydration and nutrition, and those who are able to communicate rarely want artificial feeding. Patients and their surrogates must be aware of alternatives regarding the provision of nutrition and hydration and the likely effects of choices to use or to forgo artificial support (Lynn, 1986).

Access to hospice care

The decision to enter a hospice program usually follows the patient's choice to forgo life-sustaining treatment, or the recognition that there is no treatment offering life extension. What sorts of life-extending treatment should remain available in hospice care has been quite controversial. The decision to use hospice requires the patient (or surrogate) to understand the services that will be provided, and hospice has traditionally required a substantial standard of consent. The patients must usually acknowledge that the illness is in its final stage, life expectancy is limited, and death will occur within approximately six months. Life expectancy is difficult to predict. Prognosticating life span for terminal illness relies upon woefully inadequate data, is quite imprecise in most circumstances even if substantial data is collected, and is an uncomfortable challenge to physicians' usual professional experience and practice. Patients are often denied access to hospice because their physicians are too uncertain about prognosis. Only with cancer is there regularly a discernible terminal phase of a month or less, so uncertainty with prognosis acts to deny access to those dying of most organ system failures or dementia.

Another limitation upon access has been the requirement under most U.S. financing strategies to provide most services in the home. While this comports with the dominant image of hospice, it also is insensitive to the presence of large numbers of persons in need who do not have homes, or do not have adequate homes, or do not have available unpaid family caregivers to serve them at home.

Conclusion

Hospice care as an organized and recognized part of the health-care delivery system is a relatively recent phenomenon that has become institutionalized in Great Britain and the United States and is growing in most other parts of the world. The commitment to comprehensiveness in care plans, patient preferences as arbiters of the course of care, and effective symptom management have made hospice care a desirable alternative choice for care at the end of life for many patients, though hospice programs have focused upon those dying of cancer.

Hospice care regularly encounters the problems of decision making about the treatment of dying persons, and thus regularly confronts conventional issues of medical ethics such as the distinction between killing and letting die, the uncertain obligation to provide nutrition and hydration, and the problem of informed consent. Resolution of these problems is complicated by a commitment to serve the family as well as the patients.

Finally, hospice as a program of health services in the United States has had troubling problems induced by having administrative reasons to exclude many persons who would benefit greatly from hospice care and by having to provide services more efficiently than conventional health care. Access to hospice has been arbitrarily limited by policies aiming to constrain costs, but utilization of hospice has also been un   ifiably encouraged by the same considerations.

JOANNE LYNN
MONICA KOSHUTA
PHYLLIS SCHMITZ

For a further discussion of topics mentioned in this entry, see the entries AIDS, *article on* HEALTH-CARE AND RESEARCH ISSUES; ALLIED HEALTH PROFESSIONS; DEATH; DEATH, ATTITUDES TOWARD; DEATH AND DYING: EUTHANASIA AND SUSTAINING LIFE; HEALTH-CARE FINANCING; HEALTH-CARE RESOURCES, ALLOCATION OF, *article on* MACROALLOCATION; LIFE, QUALITY OF; LONG-TERM CARE; *and* TEAMS, HEALTH-CARE. *For a discussion of related ideas, see the entries* CARE; COMPASSION; PAIN AND SUFFERING; *and* VALUE AND VALUATION. *Other relevant material may be found under the entries* AGING AND THE AGED, *article on* HEALTH-CARE AND RESEARCH ISSUES; *and* HOSPITAL.

Bibliography

Aroskar, Mila A. 1985. "Access to Hospice—Ethical Dimensions." *Nursing Clinics of North America* 20, no. 2:299–309.

Crowley, Margaret A. 1988. "The Hospice Movement: A Renewed View of the Death Process." *Journal of Contemporary Health Law and Policy* 4, no. 4:295–320.

Gibson, Donald E. 1984. "Hospice: Morality and Economics." *Gerontologist* 24, no. 1:4–8.

Hagerman, Audrey Sander. 1988. "Hospice: An Alternative of Care for the Terminally Ill." *Pace Law Review* 8, no. 1:115–157.

Hastings Center. 1987. *Guidelines on the Termination of Life-Sustaining Treatment and the Care of the Dying.* Bloomington: Indiana University Press.

Koshuta, Monica A.; Schmitz, Phyllis J.; and Lynn, Joanne. 1991. "Development of Institutional Policy on Artificial Hydration and Nutrition." *Kennedy Institute of Ethics Journal* 1, no. 2:133–140.

Kübler-Ross, Elisabeth. 1969. *On Death and Dying.* New York: Macmillan.

Lynn, Joanne, ed. 1986. *By No Extraordinary Means: The Choice to Forgo Life-Sustaining Food and Water.* Bloomington: Indiana University Press.

Mor, Vincent; Greer, David S.; and Kastenbaum, Robert, eds. 1988. *The Hospice Experiment.* Baltimore: Johns Hopkins University Press.

Rhymes, Jill. 1990. "Hospice Care in America." *Journal of the American Medical Association* 264, no. 3:369–372.

Stoddard, Sandol. 1990. "Hospice: Approaching the 21st Century." *American Journal of Hospice and Palliative Care* 7, no. 2:27–30.

U.S. President's Commission for the Study of Ethical Problems in Medicine and Biomedical and Behavioral Research. 1983. *Deciding to Forego Life-Sustaining Treatment: A Report on the Ethical, Medical, and Legal Issues in Treatment Decisions.* Washington, D.C.: Author.

HOSPITAL

I. Medieval and Renaissance History
    Timothy S. Miller
II. Modern History
    Günter B. Risse
III. Contemporary Ethical Problems
    Corrine Bayley

I. MEDIEVAL AND RENAISSANCE HISTORY

Hospitals have become the primary theaters of modern medical practice. The early history of these institutions dates from about 400 to 1600, and includes these developments: (1) the origins of hospitals; (2) their development in the Byzantine and Islamic worlds; (3) their history in medieval western Europe; and (4) their flowering in Renaissance Italy. For purposes of this discussion, the term "hospital" refers to an institution that focused on caring for patients and, if possible, curing them. "Hospice" describes an institution that offered food and shelter to the poor, travelers, and the homeless sick but did not maintain specific services, such as the attentions of physicians, to treat those who were ill.

Hospital origins

Several early cultures developed institutions to care for the sick. Ancient Indian sources describe centers that dispensed medicines and engaged specially trained personnel to care for the ill. Classical Greek society produced the *asklepieia,* the temples of the god of medicine, where the sick sought divine and natural cures. The Roman Empire supported *valetudinaria* (infirmaries) providing medical care to legionaries stationed on the barbarous northern frontier. None of these institutions, however, was strong enough to survive the upheavals that destroyed much of ancient civilization in Eurasia between 200 and 600. Modern hospitals trace their origins, and even their name, not to Indian treatment centers, Greek *asklepieia,* or Roman *valetudinaria* but to the hospices and hospitals established by the Christian church during the late Roman Empire.

From its earliest days, Christianity demanded that its adherents aid sick and needy people. Christians believed that on the Last Day, God would judge according to the love one had shown those in need. Had one fed the hungry, sheltered the homeless, visited the sick (Matt. 25:31–46)? By the early second century, bishops such as Polykarp of Smyrna expected Christian clergy to take care of the sick, orphans, and widows.

Local Christian clergy assisted the unfortunate without any formal charitable institutions until the fourth century. Thereafter, in the eastern Greek-speaking provinces of the Roman Empire, the demand for charity became so great, especially in the larger cities, that specialized institutions called *xenodocheia* (hospices) appeared. By the 320s the church in Antioch operated a hospice to feed and shelter the poor of Syria. By the mid-fourth century, the pagan emperor Julian referred to hospices as common Christian institutions.

Before 360, Christian hospices did not focus attention on the sick; but during the 370s Basil, bishop of Caesarea in Asia Minor, opened an institution where physicians and nurses treated patients. Two decades later, Bishop John Chrysostom supervised hospitals in Constantinople where doctors tended the sick. By about 410, the monk Neilos of Ankyra considered the hospital physician a common figure in the Greek Christian world. These early hospitals thus evolved from simpler hospices by expanding their services to include free medical care for needy guests.

Christian bishops built hospices during the fourth century and subsequently created more specialized hospitals for the sick, not only because they wished to follow Christ's command to practice charity but also because they sought support for the new religion among the urban lower classes. During the fourth century the cities of the Eastern provinces experienced an influx of rural poor who migrated to towns in search of food and employment. Classical civic institutions could not feed, house, and care for these new residents. The local bishops used the expanding resources of the Christian church to build hospices and hospitals for these migrants, and thereby won support both from the many poor and from the urban aristocrats. When Emperor Julian (361–363) tried to halt the spread of Christianity, he emphasized that the "Galilaeans" had succeeded in part because of their charitable institutions.

Early hospitals met their expenses from the revenue of lands that local bishops had donated. Subsequently, wealthy aristocrats and the emperors augmented these resources. As Christianity expanded it destroyed some aspects of classical civilization, but others it simply reoriented. For example, Christianity wholeheartedly accepted the classical obligation of aristocrats to benefit local cities, but the Christian church encouraged donors to endow institutions such as hospitals rather than traditional theaters, baths, and ornamental colonnades. By supporting hospitals a Christian aristocrat not only acted charitably but also fulfilled the classical duty toward the city. Moreover, such benefactions cemented local political support. This same combination of Christian morality, classical traditionalism, and political realism motivated emperors in their benefactions (Miller, 1985).

Hospitals of the Byzantine and Muslim worlds

Hospitals developed most rapidly where they had first appeared, in the eastern half of the Roman Empire. The large cities of the eastern Mediterranean and the stable political conditions of the eastern Roman, or Byzantine, Empire fostered their hospitals' further evolution. By the late sixth century, Christian hospitals such as the Sampson Xenon (hospital) of Constantinople maintained specialized wards for surgery patients and those with eye diseases. Moreover, the premier physicians (archiatroi) of the Byzantine capital were assigned monthly shifts to treat patients in the Sampson and in other hospitals of the city. By the twelfth century the hospitals of Constantinople had evolved into relatively sophisticated medical centers. The Pantokrator Xenon maintained five specialized wards, seventeen physicians, thirty-four

nurses, eleven servants, and a store of medicines supervised by six pharmacists. The Pantokrator treated outpatients as well as those who were hospitalized. Emperor John II (1118–1143), the founder of the Pantokrator, reminded the hospital's staff that the sick were God's special friends and that caring for patients was more important than maintaining buildings (Volk, 1983).

From their beginnings, the Christian hospitals of Byzantine cities were designed for the poor, but as these institutions became increasingly sophisticated medical centers served by the best physicians, some middle-class and a few wealthy patients began to use them. In this regard Byzantine practice differed markedly from the medieval West, where the bourgeoisie and nobility shunned hospitals as institutions solely for the destitute.

Medieval Islamic society maintained hospitals (in Persian, bimaristani) that equaled those of Byzantium. The first Islamic hospitals were founded in Baghdad during the reign of the caliph Harun al-Rashid (786–809). According to a governor of the caliph, Islamic hospitals had become common by the 820s; subsequently Muslims considered support of hospitals a mark of true piety.

Like Byzantine hospitals, bimaristani had evolved from earlier Christian philanthropic institutions in large cities of the Byzantine Empire. When Emperor Zeno expelled Nestorian Christians from Syria in 489, many sought refuge in Persia, where they established institutions, including hospitals, modeled on those in Byzantine cities such as Antioch. After the Muslims conquered Sassanid Persia in the seventh century, they came in contact with Nestorians. Impressed by Nestorian medical skills, they adopted many Syrian medical traditions—teaching methods, scientific texts, and hospitals—as models for shaping Islamic institutions.

Although Islamic hospitals evolved from Christian institutions, they experienced a unique development. They differed strikingly from their Byzantine counterparts by including separate sections for mental patients. Gradually these psychiatric wards became the most prominent features of bimaristani. Neither Byzantine nor medieval Western hospitals had wards for mental patients (Dols, 1987).

Medieval western Europe

Hospitals developed more slowly in the western Roman Empire. Saint Jerome (ca. 331–420) mentioned two small hospitals near Rome about 400. During the early Middle Ages, however, social conditions retarded hospital development in western Europe. Barbarian invasions from the north and Muslim advances in Africa inhibited political, economic, and social life. Few towns of the size and complexity that could support medical centers such as the Byzantine and Muslim hospitals survived. In the domains of Charlemagne (768–814), hospitals did not evolve beyond simple hospices. As late as the thirteenth century, hospitals were rare in Europe. None of the 112 houses for the sick in medieval England provided physicians for their patients, nor did they stock any medicines (Carlin, 1989).

In the twelfth century, a new religious order, the Knights of the Hospital of Saint John of Jerusalem (known today as the Knights of Malta) reintroduced into Europe specialized medical care for the sick when they organized their renowned hospital in Jerusalem. Under Byzantine influence, the Knights' rule for this hospital mandated a permanent medical staff of four physicians and four surgeons to treat patients. Moreover, the Knights developed a unique philanthropic ethic by adapting feudal notions to the traditional Christian command to aid those in need. The Knights were to treat the sick in the Jerusalem hospital as vassals served their overlords. As the Knights expanded, they built many smaller hospitals in the towns of Europe where they introduced practices they had established in Jerusalem (Sire, 1994).

The Knights' hospital in Jerusalem inspired many similar institutions throughout western Europe. Using its rule as a model, Pope Innocent III established in 1200 the famous Hospital of the Holy Spirit in Rome. In 1217 the church in Paris reorganized its ancient hospice, the Hôtel-Dieu, by drafting a new constitution based on the regulations of the Jerusalem hospital (Miller, 1978).

The Knights of Saint John had such a wide-ranging effect not only because their rule inspired western Europeans to help the needy, especially the sick, but also because Latin Christendom was entering a new phase of urban growth. As country dwellers migrated to the towns in growing numbers, these newcomers were exposed to a wider range of diseases. Hospitals became necessary to treat the rapidly growing number of sick among the urban poor. In fact, the economic and social conditions in the expanding towns of thirteenth-century Europe were remarkably similar to those in the fourth-century Byzantine cities where hospitals had first appeared.

An examination of the rule for the Roman Hospital of the Holy Spirit, however, indicates one important difference between the new institutions of the West and the Jerusalem hospital. The Roman rule mandated many of the Knights' practices, but it omitted any reference to physicians or surgeons. The same is true of the rule for the Hôtel-Dieu of Paris. Only gradually did physicians come to serve in these hospitals. The records of the Hôtel-Dieu do not mention a permanent staff physician until 1328. As late as the eighteenth century a physician visited Saint Bartholomew's Hospital in London only once a week. That trained doctors did not assume a major role in caring for patients in Western medieval hospitals distinguishes them from Byzantine *xenones* and Moslem *bimaristani*, where doctors not only treated the sick but supervised hospital administration.

It is also clear that some of the Western medieval hospitals did not provide care on the same level as did the Eastern medical facilities. The twelfth-century hospital at Saint-Pol in northern France maintained only six nurses (or nursing sisters) for sixty patients. Iconographic evidence indicates that at the Hôtel-Dieu in Paris patients sometimes shared beds. The wards of many medieval hospitals were also poorly heated. Conditions such as these no doubt made it difficult for hospitals to heal the sick and provided some support for the charges of later Enlightenment reformers that all medieval hospitals had in fact been death traps (Miller, 1985).

Renaissance Italy

Inspired by the Jerusalem hospital, the communes of Tuscany began building hospitals during the thirteenth century. Before 1300, for example, the town of Siena built an institution that differed from the Hôtel-Dieu of Paris in that it maintained on its staff a physician, a surgeon, and a pharmacist. In 1288 Folco Portinari, the father of Dante's Beatrice, founded the Hospital of Santa Maria Nuova in Florence; by the fifteenth century, this institution had developed into an elaborate center for medical treatment. A document dated 1500, but reflecting earlier arrangements, reveals that Santa Maria paid six of the best physicians of Florence to visit patients each morning. In addition, three young interns lived permanently at the hospital. In return for room and board and a valuable opportunity to gain experience in medical practice, they served the hospital's 300 patients by monitoring their conditions and making daily reports to the senior physicians.

Santa Maria Nuova was not a death trap, as were some less well-organized hospitals, nor was it a hospice where poor sick people were simply nourished. It provided its patients access to society's best physicians and boasted an excellent rate of cure. Hospital records reveal that about 85 percent of the patients recovered from their ailments (Park, 1985; Henderson, 1989).

At Santa Maria Nuova, the interns were willing to serve patients for free not only because such service was virtuous but also because it offered them an unparalleled opportunity to observe the course of many diseases. During the sixteenth century, the medical professors of Padua (in Venetian territory) established formal clinical instruction at the Hospital of San Francesco. Many students from northern Europe came to study at Padua because of its excellent empirical training (Bylebyl, 1982).

Conclusion

Modern scholars have not been inclined to examine medieval hospitals because of the prevailing view that these were poorly equipped asylums that offered the sick only minimal medical care. Such institutions supposedly had nothing in common with today's hospitals. This view has its origins in Enlightenment skepticism concerning religious institutions. Eighteenth-century intellectuals contrasted the efficacy of science in curing human ills, including disease, with the helplessness of Christian charity, which at best provided only comfort, not true remedies.

However, hospitals in Renaissance Italy, as well as those in medieval Constantinople and Baghdad, demonstrate that philanthropic institutions were not necessarily isolated from scientific medicine. In fact, hospital service in Italy came to form a vital part of medical training, first in Florence and then at the University of Padua. In hospitals such as Santa Maria Nuova, the Christian command to aid the needy interacted with a sense of civic pride and with a concept of professional ethics on the part of physicians to create institutions that were both truly philanthropic and efficient in curing the sick.

TIMOTHY S. MILLER

Directly related to this article are the other articles in this entry: MODERN HISTORY, *and* CONTEMPORARY ETHICAL PROBLEMS. *Also directly related are the entries* MEDICAL ETHICS, HISTORY OF, *section on* NEAR AND MIDDLE EAST, *and section on* EUROPE, *subsections on* ANCIENT AND MEDIEVAL, *and* RENAISSANCE AND ENLIGHTENMENT; PROFESSIONAL–PATIENT RELATIONSHIP, *article on* HISTORICAL PERSPECTIVES; *and* PUBLIC HEALTH, *article on* HISTORY OF PUBLIC HEALTH. *For a discussion of religions that sponsored hospitals, see* EASTERN ORTHODOX CHRISTIANITY; ISLAM; *and* ROMAN CATHOLICISM. *Other relevant material may be found under the entries* HEALTH AND DISEASE, *article on* HISTORY OF THE CONCEPTS; HOSPICE AND END-OF-LIFE CARE; *and* MEDICAL CODES AND OATHS, *article on* HISTORY.

Bibliography

AMUNDSEN, DARREL W. 1986. "The Medieval Catholic Tradition." In *Caring and Curing: Health and Medicine in the Western Religious Traditions*, pp. 65–107. Edited by Ronald L. Numbers and Darrel W. Amundsen. New York: Macmillan.

BYLEBYL, JEROME J. 1982. "Commentary." In *A Celebration of Medical History: The Fiftieth Anniversary of the Johns Hopkins Institute of the History of Medicine and the Welch Medical Library*, pp. 200–211. Edited by Lloyd G. Stevenson. Baltimore: Johns Hopkins University Press.

CARLIN, MARTHA. 1989. "Medieval English Hospitals." In *The Hospital in History*, pp. 21–39. Edited by Lindsay P. Granshaw and Roy Porter. London: Routledge.

DOLS, MICHAEL W. 1987. "The Origins of the Islamic Hospital: Myth and Reality." *Bulletin of the History of Medicine* 61, no. 3:367–390.

HENDERSON, JOHN. 1989. "The Hospitals of Late-Medieval and Renaissance Florence: A Preliminary Survey." In *The Hospital in History*, pp. 63–92. Edited by Lindsay P. Granshaw and Roy Porter. London: Routledge & Kegan Paul.

MILLER, TIMOTHY S. 1978. "The Knights of Saint John and the Hospitals of the Latin West." *Speculum* 53, no. 4: 709–733.

———. 1985. *The Birth of the Hospital in the Byzantine Empire.* Baltimore: Johns Hopkins University Press.

PARK, KATHARINE. 1985. *Doctors and Medicine in Early Renaissance Florence.* Princeton, N.J.: Princeton University Press.

SCHREIBER, GEORG. 1948. "Byzantinisches und Abendländisches Hospital." In his *Gemeinschaften des Mittelalters: Recht und Verfassung, Kult und Frömmigkeit*, pp. 3–80. Münster: Regensberg.

SIRE, H. J. A. 1994. *The Knights of Malta.* New Haven, Conn.: Yale University Press.

THOMPSON, JOHN D., and GOLDIN, GRACE. 1975. *The Hospital: A Social and Architectural History.* New Haven, Conn.: Yale University Press.

VOLK, ROBERT. 1983. *Gesundheitswesen und Wohltätigkeit im Spiegel der byzantinischen Klostertypika.* Munich: Institut für Byzantinistik und Neugriechische Philologie der Universität.

II. MODERN HISTORY

Although a few Renaissance institutions supplemented charitable assistance with professional medical care, the hospital's gradual "medicalization" occurred from the seventeenth century onward, within changing social and scientific frameworks. Three distinct periods can be identified within this development: (1) the early shift of the hospital from welfare to medical establishment, 1650–1870; (2) the evolution of a successfully medicalized institution for all social classes, 1870–1945; and (3) the creation of a specialized showcase of scientific medicine, 1945 to the present.

From welfare to medicine: 1650–1870

During the early modern period, hospitals in Europe's urban centers were charitable shelters for the poor and working classes, functioning primarily as instruments of religious charity and social control with minimal involvement of the medical profession. Whether the patients were Catholic or Protestant, hospitalization continued to be an opportunity for physical comfort as well as moral rehabilitation. However, in time of epidemics such as plague and syphilis, specialized hospitals were created to ensure the isolation of the sick and thus avoid the spread of contagion. Given the expanding institutionalization of charity, the decline of religious institutions, and new roles in the preservation of public health, hospitals increasingly came under lay control, including municipal governments, fraternal organizations, and private patrons.

After 1650, new geopolitical agendas designed to increase the power and prosperity of the emerging national states pressed hospitals into new roles. Human life was given greater financial value as population policies were aimed at increasing the number of inhabitants as a base for state power, economic development, and military strength. Proponents of emerging European mercantilism viewed labor as the key source of wealth and urged that the nation's workforce be mobilized and kept at an optimum state of productivity. Within such a framework, the desire to promote the health of citizens inspired new programs of public health, hygiene, and medical care.

At the same time, more optimistic visions of health preservation and rehabilitation elaborated by Enlightenment thinkers suggested that sickness, instead of an inevitable, sinful, and often long-term human burden, could be controlled and eliminated. In addition to their traditional moral and physical aims, hospitals were now envisioned as institutions for physical rehabilitation and cure, places of early rather than last resort, especially for military personnel and the labor force. This agenda implied a greater involvement of the health-care professions with large sectors of the population hitherto without such contacts.

To implement their new health policies, national governments, local authorities, and corporate professional bodies organized efforts to reform the existing medical and surgical professions. Physicians and surgeons were granted new forms of access to hospitals and given new rules to guide their institutional activities. Early models for the medicalization process came from military and naval establishments that provided for the sick and wounded members of Europe's expanding military forces. Later, medical professionals working in civil hospitals also began to argue successfully that their management of patients provided a valuable addition to the rest and food traditionally furnished to inmates in religious shelters. During the late eighteenth and early nineteenth centuries, medical objectives dramatically reshaped hospital routines from admission to the discharge or death of the patient. Acute rather than chronic illnesses were preferred; young rather than old patients were accepted. Rehabilitation and cure were the new goals.

Hospitals as training institutions. At the same time, surgeons—and later physicians—recognized the great opportunities hospitals offered to improve their clinical skills and thus increase their power and status. By the eighteenth century, shifts in scientific ideology emphasized the importance of empirical studies and the construction of knowledge based on observed facts. Sur-

geons in France and Great Britain were especially keen to acquire practical knowledge of anatomy, pathology, and clinical management. After the French Revolution, physicians in that country initiated a new strategy of professional and social advancement under the banner of what was generically called the "medicine of observation." With significant numbers of sick people assembled in hospital wards, doctors could observe at the bedside the evolution of individual diseases and their diagnoses on a much larger scale than they could in private practice. Postmortem dissections performed on former hospital inmates provided further information on the pathology responsible for the symptoms. Moreover, patient management offered unequaled opportunities to check the usefulness of the traditional medical regimens, especially the effects of older remedies. Efforts to upgrade the preparation and uses of drugs involved clinical trials and statistical analysis. Hospitals became the focal points of comprehensive bedside research programs.

Finally, the expanding medical and surgical presence in European hospitals made such institutions increasingly attractive as places for education and training of rank-and-file practitioners. Hospitals were seen as "great nurseries" that could "breed some of the best physicians and chirurgeons because they may see as much there in one year as in seven any where else" (Bellers, 1714). In certain establishments, the authorities created special teaching wards where professors and attendants, followed by their students, made regular rounds of the patients. Instruction varied greatly, from passive observation to supervised and even independent, hands-on examination and management of the patients by students and apprentices.

Reorganization of the hospital structure. How did the hospital as an institution adapt to these new agendas? France possessed several types of organizations, including massive *hôpitaux générales*, or hospices, for the elderly poor, beggars, vagrants, incurables, and prostitutes. There were also small welfare establishments at the parish level for similar cases. In larger urban areas, the traditional *Hôtels-Dieux* now limited admissions to the sick but excluded incurables, the insane, and venereal cases. All original ward layouts were based on medieval principles, providing in a shelter as many beds as possible and still crowding three to four individuals into each bed. Hospital size was fiercely debated, with advocates of medicalization arguing for smaller institutions to prevent cross-infections.

In Great Britain and the young American republic, major population centers possessed a number of "voluntary infirmaries," or private hospitals, founded and operated by local philanthropists and often financed by a system of yearly subscriptions solicited from local merchants and professionals. Except for accident cases, these establishments admitted only a very restricted number of the sick poor. These persons, recommended for admission by the subscribers, were judged by the community to be willing to work and thus "deserving" of hospital care and rehabilitation. In addition, there were a number of private special hospitals, especially in London after 1800, supported by contributions and patient fees and operating under the direction of medical professionals. By contrast, English "poor law" infirmaries were supported financially by parish taxes and linked to local workhouses, which provided free care to the sick poor deemed able bodied, or vagrant, and thus "undeserving" of other charitable assistance. Later, in the nineteenth century, many of these workhouse infirmaries evolved into municipal hospitals and were placed under the direction of salaried medical superintendents. At the same time, and with financial support from leading local citizens, Great Britain also created a string of small cottage hospitals, providing paid medical care to those who could afford it.

To support expanding medical services and teaching activities, nineteenth-century hospitals required more money and changes in their physical plants and administrative organizations. By the 1870s, hygienic principles had come to dominate the construction and functioning of new establishments, now equipped with single beds for the sick and providing ample ventilation in their pavilion-type wards. Isolation chambers, surgical amphitheaters, emergency rooms, morgues, libraries, and outpatient facilities became indispensable adjuncts. Medical control also shifted power from patients and caregivers to attending physicians, thereby creating conflicts between traditional charitable practices and scientific goals of disease identification and management. Medicalization implied a shift from the primary focus on shelter and food for the needy to the diagnosis and treatment of diseases exhibited by sick patients.

A hospital for all social classes: 1870–1945

Thanks in part to advances in medical knowledge and technology, the medicalization process of Western society was significantly advanced before the end of World War II. By 1900, upper- and middle-class patients in Europe and the United States were seeking and paying for medical care in hospitals. Staffed by competent medical and nursing professionals, and equipped with clinical laboratories and other diagnostic tools, hospitals became the preferred destination of those who were acutely sick and in need of surgical and medical care. The newly created demand for hospital care, spurred by urbanization and industrialization, expanded further to include the needs of birthing and child care.

In the United States, such requirements were eagerly met by the establishment of a vast, decentralized system of voluntary hospitals fiercely competing for community resources, physicians, and their patients. Local private citizens provided the necessary funds and volunteer service required to create general community hospitals. Alongside schools, police stations, and firehouses, U.S. general hospitals became emblems of community life, the pride of Main Street. In Europe, many hospitals became governmental facilities managed by paid professionals.

The new hospital mission was a result of converging ideologies, policies, and needs, some traditional, others new. Religious values and charitable donations still played an important role in the early 1900s, while developing economic tenets based on capitalism suggested that the health of workers in the industrial world was of great importance both to the state and to the private sector. In the United States, new social conditions favored the creation and utilization of more hospitals. Urbanization was accelerating at a rapid pace, bringing an ever-increasing number of adults into crowded city quarters. Among them were waves of new immigrants with multiple health-care needs and few resources. Industrialization, in turn, created a new panorama of occupational diseases and accidents. Without the means or family networks to get the necessary help, many sick or injured individuals were thus forced to seek medical care in hospitals.

Under the new banner of scientific medicine, hospitals became the institutions of first rather than last resort. Thanks to the increasingly sophisticated diagnostic and therapeutic procedures offered in hospitals after 1900, optimistic Enlightenment notions of physical rehabilitation and cure were becoming a reality. Radiology, electrocardiography, and the clinical laboratory greatly improved the ability of hospital personnel to refine diagnoses. In addition to providing rest and a healthier diet, hospitals focused increasingly on managing acute diseases, especially life-threatening conditions that required intensive and highly technical care. A new generation of chemotherapeutic agents and vaccines improved the odds of success in the battle against certain diseases. Following the adoption of anesthesia and antisepsis, hospitals became the primary centers for surgical operations. Surgeons recognized the advantage of centralizing their new and expensive equipment within the "surgical suites" of a hospital.

The changing status of nurses, physicians. For patient care, hospitals relied increasingly on a new generation of nurses, drawn from the middle class and trained in professional education programs based on the model established by Florence Nightingale (1820–1910). Shedding their previous low-status role of cleaning women and servants, these new hospital nurses gradually displaced the dwindling number of religious staff members who had traditionally performed patient services. In time, the Nightingale nurses became valuable assistants to the medical profession in patient management.

By the 1910s, more physicians joined hospital staffs, staking their professional reputations on the achievements of scientific medicine such institutions seemed to make possible. In U.S. voluntary hospitals, medical staff organizations remained flexible, bestowing admission privileges on both local general practitioners and specialists who could deliver paying patients. In Great Britain, however, traditional social and professional barriers between general practitioners, on the one hand, and hospital-appointed physicians and surgeons, on the other, created insurmountable barriers in voluntary establishments. Although referring their patients to hospitals, the former were not allowed to practice within them. As so-called consultants, the latter operated small units and exclusively took care of a specific number of patients.

Since the hospital was rapidly becoming the physician's primary workshop in the 1920s, medical goals, including specialization, education, and research, needed to become top institutional priorities. Twentieth-century hospitals witnessed a dramatic growth of specialized care through the creation of clinical departments, an increase in student doctors, called "house staff," and the performance of clinical research. Such activities became central to educational and licensing requirements, and conferred prestige and higher professional status on those allowed to work in the most preeminent institutions.

The changing focus of hospitals.   Once again the hospital as an institution adapted to these new agendas. Some new hospitals were associated or affiliated with medical and nursing schools. Others, especially in the United States, sprouted between 1890 and 1920 in ethnic urban neighborhoods, or strategic suburban locations, their creation influenced by state and local governments, population, philanthropy, or industry. Sectarian Jewish, Catholic, and Protestant institutions, German- and French-speaking clinics, municipal and state hospitals, private establishments sponsored by railroads and universities—all formed a constellation of autonomous units across the U.S. landscape.

In Europe, governments became increasingly involved in sponsoring and managing hospitals. In Great Britain, the Public Health Act of 1875 encouraged municipalities to establish isolation hospitals for persons suffering from infectious diseases. The poor law infirmaries were gradually taken over by local health departments and converted to general hospitals. The National Health Insurance Act of 1911 eliminated the charitable character of the voluntary hospitals and brought their services under the umbrella of regional health-care schemes.

In the United States, hospital organizations in the 1920s changed to serve the new medical objectives and compete for paying patients, an ever-greater source of needed revenue. The rapid growth of medical technology generated further budgetary pressures, forcing voluntary hospitals to redouble their fundraising efforts and use endowment income for capital expenditures. As they became individual corporations in a competitive health-care market, demands for greater efficiency prompted hospitals to bolster their administrations and institute stringent financial measures. Institutional care became a commodity, a product to be furnished mostly to those willing to pay for it directly or through health-insurance policies.

By the 1930s, economic conditions stemming from the Depression forced the creation of new funding systems, such as the Blue Cross health-insurance companies, organized by physicians. As competition for philanthropic support and patient revenue accelerated, accountability and public relations dominated the hospitals' administrative agendas. Since each U.S. institution was the proud product of individual community efforts, cooperation among hospital administrations was resisted.

As the hospital became the preferred locus for the application of scientific principles to medicine, new ethical problems appeared. The medicalization of life processes expanded the range of life experiences now addressed as medical problems by health professionals in hospital settings: Birth and death, formerly events that occurred in the home, now took place in the hospital. Since the early nineteenth century, a depersonalized, disease- and organ-centered approach had already replaced earlier holistic notions of sickness. As hospital routines became increasingly technical and standardized, patients came to be seen as merely embodiments of diseases that were the primary objects of inquiry and treatment. This approach affected the nature of the physician–patient relationship, as professionals focused primarily on successful problem solving in diagnosing and arresting human pathology. The physician's moral authority, hitherto based on personal qualities, now became grounded in scientific competence. Clinical experimentation became rampant, sometimes abusive, with few safeguards provided for the patients.

The hospital as biomedical showcase: 1945 to the present

Following World War II, the hospital rapidly consolidated its position as the embodiment of scientific and technologically sophisticated medicine. An explosion in medical knowledge led to the expansion of diagnostic and therapeutic services at hospitals. This development had far-reaching implications for institutional access, cost, and quality of care as delivered to a broad spectrum of the public under various private and state-sponsored health plans. The hospital's mission continued to reflect converging agendas, including the religious, political, economic, and scientific goals set in preceding decades.

In the United States, the federal government's involvement in sponsoring hospital care gradually expanded as the demand for institutional beds and services multiplied. Beginning with the Hill Burton Act in 1946, the federal authorities supported the existing system of decentralized, private hospitals—first, through the provision of construction subsidies, and later, through reimbursement schemes for services, such as the Medicare and Medicaid programs in 1966. This supportive rather than regulatory role preserved a network of independent and competing municipal, sectarian, and academic hospitals in each community. In marked contrast with events in Europe, the 1950s through the 1970s witnessed an impressive growth in U.S. hospital facilities, including neonatology and intensive-care units, imaging facilities, and transplantation services. Individual hospitals continue to operate as independent business organizations within a burgeoning health-care "industry." Periodic institutional accreditation by a joint commission of the American Medical Association and the American Hospital Association ensures compliance with a number of performance standards.

To work in hospitals of their choice, all practicing physicians in the United States must secure admission "privileges" in such institutions. Most hospital care is indeed rendered by private practitioners who briefly visit the hospital to check on the status of their patients. This system allows the establishment of larger and more mobile medical staffs whose authority remains diffuse. To exert some measure of control, medical staffs usually create a number of committees to deal with the issues of credentials, admissions, education, and quality control. (Hospital ethics committees grapple with a host of issues, from informed consent and patient autonomy to advance directives and the definition of death.) The resulting administrative complexity and instability require a great deal of consensus building, achieved through frequent meetings and written communications. This record keeping effort is especially important among the attending physicians and more permanent hospital personnel to achieve a necessary degree of internal standardization of medical and administrative procedures.

Hospitals in Europe, even those owned by municipalities or private bodies, continue to be closely supervised by central governments. All hospital planning, construction, management, and recruitment of medical personnel remains subject to state control. In Great Britain, the government has assumed responsibilities for ensuring free access to hospital care as a social right. The implementation of the National Health Service Act of 1946 brought about the outright nationalization of all hospitals and placed them under the authority of regional boards appointed by the government and responsible to the Ministry of Health. In many European communities, the larger municipal and voluntary hospitals erected more than a century earlier remain in full operation. Greater administrative uniformity has allowed for smaller staff requirements. Given these hospitals' outdated physical plants, limited technology, and often a lingering stigma from their charitable past, well-to-do patients still prefer smaller, privately owned hospitals or clinics, many of which are still owned or managed by religious orders.

European hospitals operate with closed, full-time medical staffs hierarchically organized within smaller, autonomous divisions, each of which operates its own clinical, diagnostic, and rehabilitative services. While such internal arrangements reduce administrative overhead and foster more stable relationships among patients, physicians, and nurses, the schism between hospital and private practice remains. In Great Britain, this decentralized staffing framework follows the traditional, voluntary models of allocating a specific block of beds to each hospital physician or consultant, who is assisted by a stratified junior medical staff in training for specialist status.

Financial difficulties of hospitals

Although outpatient facilities are quickly becoming an integral component of professional education, hospital-based training continues to be the backbone of all medical education programs. Given the range of diagnostic and therapeutic options available, hospital practice remains at the center of biomedicine, providing the specialized clinical experience and technical proficiency required for today's professional status. With medical specialization and subspecialization on the rise, U.S. hospitals have expanded dramatically and have extended their residency training programs. As a result, physicians in training exercise greater management responsibility and are better remunerated than ever before.

Due to restrictive reimbursement schemes instituted by government and the private insurance industry, and the escalating costs of technologically assisted medical care, together with a gradual fragmentation of the medical marketplace, many U.S. hospitals find themselves increasingly under siege, victims, in part, of their previous success. Excessively bureaucratized and inefficient, their physical facilities overexpanded, hospitals are struggling to maintain their patient volumes as costs continue to increase. Unable to survive in a highly competitive environment, some institutions have already merged while others are closing wards or their doors altogether, thus forcing a major restructuring of the entire medical-care delivery system. Many hospitals are being reorganized into for-profit corporations, extending their services into networks of clinics and practitioners, and offering health insurance and service plans.

Conclusion

Ultimately, the evolution of the hospital in recent centuries poses the central question of whether care is still the primary function of this institution. While subjected to competing agendas—including religious beliefs, social control, secular philanthropy, scientific curiosity, communal pride, and economic autonomy—the hospital's original purpose was to shelter and comfort all sufferers in need. To a great extent, hospitals now restrict admission to seriously ill patients who require the most sophisticated diagnostic and therapeutic measures. The tilt toward acute episodes of physical illness, complex technological interventions, and the increasing costs of confinement have made hospital stays episodic and brief. Bureaucratization, financial constraints, and the pervasive presence of instrumentation only accentuate the essential impersonality of institutional care. The trade-offs are clear. Three centuries of medicalization transformed the hospital from a caring shelter for the poor into a disease-oriented machine for the sick who can afford to be cured.

GÜNTER B. RISSE

Directly related to this article are the other articles in this entry: MEDIEVAL AND RENAISSANCE HISTORY, *and* CONTEMPORARY ETHICAL PROBLEMS. *Also directly related are the entries* HEALTH-CARE DELIVERY; HEALTH CARE, QUALITY OF; *and* HEALTH-CARE RESOURCES, ALLOCATION OF, *article on* MACROALLOCATION. *For a further discussion of topics mentioned in this article, see the entries* ACADEMIC HEALTH CENTERS; HEALTH POLICY, *article on* HEALTH POLICY IN INTERNATIONAL PERSPECTIVE; MEDICINE AS A PROFESSION; NURSING AS A PROFESSION; PUBLIC HEALTH, *article on* HISTORY OF PUBLIC HEALTH; *and* TECHNOLOGY, *article on* HISTORY OF MEDICAL TECHNOLOGY. *Other relevant material may be found under the entries* HEALTH-CARE FINANCING; IATROGENIC ILLNESS AND INJURY; MEDICAL INFORMATION SYSTEMS; PROFESSIONAL–PATIENT RELATIONSHIP, *article on* HISTORICAL PERSPECTIVES; STRIKES BY HEALTH PROFESSIONALS; *and* SURGERY.

Bibliography

ABEL-SMITH, BRIAN. 1964. *The Hospitals in England and Wales, 1800–1948: A Study in Social Administration.* Cambridge, Mass.: Harvard University Press.

ACKERKNECHT, ERWIN H. 1967. *Medicine at the Paris Hospital 1794–1848.* Baltimore: Johns Hopkins University Press.

BELLERS, JOHN. 1714. *Essay Towards the Improvement of Physick.* London: J. Sowle.

DOWLING, HARRY F. 1982. *City Hospitals: The Undercare of the Underprivileged.* Cambridge, Mass.: Harvard University Press.

FOUCAULT, MICHEL. 1973. *The Birth of the Clinic: An Archeology of Medical Perception.* Translated by Alan M. Sheridan Smith. New York: Pantheon.

FREIDSON, ELIOT, ed. 1963. *The Hospital in Modern Society.* New York: Free Press.

HOLLINGSWORTH, J. ROGERS, and HOLLINGSWORTH, ELLEN J. 1987. *Controversy About American Hospitals: Funding, Ownership and Performance.* Washington, D.C.: American Enterprise Institute for Public Policy Research.

HONIGSBAUM, FRANK. 1979. *The Division in British Medicine: A History of the Separation of General Practice from Hospital Care, 1911–1968.* London: Kogan Page.

LONG, DIANA E., and GOLDEN, JANET L., eds. 1989. *The American General Hospital: Communities and Social Contexts.* Ithaca, N.Y.: Cornell University Press.

PROCHASKA, F. K. 1992. *Philanthropy and Hospitals of London: The King's Fund, 1897–1990.* Oxford: At the Clarendon Press.

RISSE, GÜNTER B. 1986. *Hospital Life in Enlightenment Scotland: Care and Teaching at the Royal Infirmary of Edinburgh.* New York: Cambridge University Press.

RIVETT, GEOFFREY. 1986. *The Development of the London Hospital System, 1823–1982.* London: King Edward's Hospital Fund.

ROEMER, MILTON I. 1962. "General Hospitals in Europe." In *Modern Concepts of Hospital Administration,* pp. 17–37. Edited by Joseph K. Owen. Philadelphia: W. B. Saunders.

ROSEN, GEORGE. 1974. "The Hospital: Historical Sociology of a Community Institution." In his *From Medical Police to Social Medicine: Essays on the History of Health Care,* pp. 274–303. New York: Science History Publications.

ROSENBERG, CHARLES E. 1987. *The Care of Strangers: The Rise of America's Hospital System.* New York: Basic Books.

STEVENS, ROSEMARY. 1989. *In Sickness and in Wealth: American Hospitals in the Twentieth Century.* New York: Basic Books.

VOGEL, MORRIS J. 1980. *The Invention of the Modern Hospital, Boston, 1870–1930.* Chicago: University of Chicago Press.

WOODWARD, JOHN H. 1974. *To Do the Sick No Harm: A Study of the British Voluntary Hospital System to 1875.* London: Routledge & Kegan Paul.

YAGGY, DUNCAN, and HODGSON, PATRICIA, eds. 1985. *Physicians and Hospitals: The Great Partnership at the Crossroads: Based on the Ninth Private Sector Conference, 1984.* Durham, N.C.: Duke University Press.

III. CONTEMPORARY ETHICAL PROBLEMS

Hospitals are complicated institutions that bring together technological innovations and social services, salaried and unsalaried personnel, private and public funding, a charitable mission and a business orientation. Hospitals are accountable to patients, physicians, board members, employees, the local community, third-party payers, business partners, and other providers. It is no wonder that hospitals encounter ethical issues and problems. Some are carryovers from those faced by hospitals in the past, while others are quite new.

Ethical concerns confronting hospitals in the United States are discussed in the following categories: identity and mission; clinical issues; relationships with physicians; and special sponsorship.

Identity and mission

Perhaps the most fundamental ethical issue has to do with identity and mission. Is a hospital a business like any other, subject to the pressures of the marketplace, and primarily motivated by commercial interests and incentives? Or is it a social institution, primarily responsible for serving the health needs of the community and sometimes suffering financial loss in the process? Rosemary Stevens's book *In Sickness and in Wealth* (1989) elaborates on these questions and shows how hospitals experience tensions between their role as community servants and their role as entrepreneurs. These roles can coexist, as for-profit hospitals have tried to show. However, the public has come to expect more from the non-profits—for example, that they provide unreimbursed care, support unprofitable services, and be alert to community health-care needs.

Hospitals in the United States face more difficult questions of identity and mission than do hospitals in countries where health care is typically regarded as an essential service, not subject to the usual marketplace forces. A confluence of factors—including the growth of scientific medicine, the alliance of physicians and hospitals, the phenomenon of specialization, enormous capital investments, commercial ventures, and the payment system—has caused U.S. hospitals to behave much like businesses. Public policy has encouraged this by endorsing antitrust laws that discourage hospitals' collaboration with one another; by inadequate government-reimbursement programs; and by the failure to ensure universal entitlement to health care. These factors create financial incentives for hospitals that conflict with their stated mission, namely, to serve all people and to meet the needs of their communities.

Most hospitals remain not-for-profit and therefore tax-exempt. Voluntary hospitals, whose boards of trustees receive no pay because they are understood to serve the community, believe that this community orientation is the most effective way to deliver care. In their rhetoric, they cultivate an image of benevolence and moral worth that obscures their business orientation, seeking government subsidies but eschewing government control. Some business practices adopted by both for-profit and not-for-profit hospitals have tarnished this image of benevolence. These practices include aggressive marketing, advertising, and competition for paying patients; the creation of for-profit ventures, often with physicians, thus creating the potential for conflict of interest; resistance or refusal to care for the indigent; and expensive duplication of services to compete with other hospitals.

Until the latter part of the twentieth century, hospitals could count on the public's trust and support. The special nature of health care and the religious affiliation of many hospitals fostered this trust. Contemporary hospitals, however, face skepticism and criticism from patients and the public at large. This dissatisfaction with hospitals' behavior arises from an expectation that hospitals will behave differently from ordinary businesses, that they have a "higher purpose."

Thus, one of the most pressing ethical issues facing hospitals is whether to rededicate themselves to a mission based on altruism and community service. Their decision will be shaped in part by the nature of health-care reform at the end of the twentieth century, and the incentives it creates. Whether there will be more emphasis on collaboration or competition remains to be seen. However it turns out, hospitals will still have fundamental ethical choices about whom they serve, how they allocate their resources, and what sort of leadership and vision they will bring to providing quality health care.

Clinical issues

With advances in medical technology, hospitals have encountered a number of new and perplexing ethical questions, some of the most contentious of which arise in relation to the use of life-sustaining treatment. When is it appropriate to withhold or withdraw medical treatment from a critically ill patient? Who should make the decision if the patient cannot? What are the rights and obligations of nurses, physicians, family members? What role should the hospital play in disputes among these groups? What policies should the hospital have in place to deal with these questions?

From the 1970s to the 1990s, patients' (or their surrogates') right to refuse even life-sustaining treatment became well established in legal and medical ethics, largely due to several well-publicized court cases dealing with the forgoing of life-sustaining treatment, perhaps the most well known of these being the Karen Ann Quinlan case (*Quinlan*, 1975). In this and other cases, there was a departure from decision making based more on physician preferences than on patient preferences. The popularity of advance directives, such as living wills and durable powers of attorney, soon symbolized this shift and emphasized newly empowered patients' determination that their decisions be respected. Many hospitals created interdisciplinary ethics committees and used ethics consultants to aid physicians and hospital staff in applying this new social consensus to hospital practices, primarily in cases involving forgoing life-sustaining treatment. Hospital ethics committees were available to discuss individual cases as well as to recommend new policies on forgoing treatment that incorporated the preeminence of patient choices. Resuscitation, ventilation, tube and intravenous feeding, renal dialysis, and antibiotic therapy were some of the treatments discussed. But, whatever the treatment, the principle was clear: Patients were entitled to full disclosure about the risks, benefits, and alternatives of treatment, and they, or surrogates on their behalf, had the ethical and legal right to accept or refuse any treatment. Many, but not all, physicians and hospitals changed their policies and developed new practices to reflect this situation.

It was a matter of time before the newly elevated principle of patient autonomy would cause yet another set of ethical dilemmas for hospitals. In the early 1990s, some well-publicized cases arose in which patients' surrogates wanted life-sustaining interventions, but physicians and hospitals did not want to provide them. A claim of medical futility was the usual reason for this reluctance, although disputes about whether research had shown the desired treatment, such as cardiopulmonary resuscitation (CPR), to be reasonably effective also arose. Patients and surrogates invoked the principle of autonomy to justify their demands for treatment. These demands were particularly strong if the patient, or the patient's insurer, was willing to pay for the treatment.

Physicians and hospitals thus faced new issues: What are the limits of patients' or surrogates' rights to medical treatment? Are there situations in which physicians are justified in refusing to provide it? Is it ethical for physicians to have in mind scarce hospital resources when treating individual patients? What is the meaning, and what are the ethical implications, of medical futility? What are the economic and/or ethical conflicts of interest for hospitals in these cases?

These questions come at a difficult time for hospitals. If insurance companies pay on a per diem or fee-for-service basis, it is to the hospital's advantage that patients have extensive treatment and long hospital stays, particularly if the insurance pays close to the actual cost of caring for the patient. In the late 1980s, many insurers changed the method of payment to capitation. Under this method, hospitals are "at risk" and receive a predetermined reimbursement for each patient, regardless of the actual costs of caring for the patient. Capitation creates very different economic incentives for physicians and hospitals than they have under a fee-for-service system. Thus, money becomes a factor in responding to the ethical question of who should decide when treatment is to be provided. If the public thinks it is not receiving the medical care it needs because hospitals and/or physicians are afraid of losing money, trust between health-care providers and those they serve will be further eroded. This underscores how important it is that hospitals demonstrate their commitment to community service and educate the public about the importance of cost control. In order for trust to be renewed, the public will need to understand the connection between limiting expensive treatments for some patients and providing more basic care for others. They will need to agree that such changes are not primarily for the economic benefit of health-care providers but are for the benefit of society as a whole.

Relationships with physicians

Hospitals and physicians have always had an uneasy alliance: They need each other but often do not trust each other. For the first half of the twentieth century, hospitals were referred to as the "physicians' workshop." Hospitals provided the beds, equipment, nurses, and other personnel, and physicians provided the patients. Except in teaching institutions, hospitals and physicians had few common goals and mutual responsibilities beyond providing a place to care for patients. Physicians directed all aspects of patient care, and expected hospitals and their personnel to provide whatever the physicians deemed necessary. Until the middle of the twentieth century, hospitals themselves were not legally responsible for the care provided by physicians. At that time, courts began finding hospitals and their employees liable for not intervening to protect the patient when physicians provided inferior care. Since that time, hospitals have instituted mechanisms to monitor and intervene when necessary in physicians' care of patients.

This change was good for patients, but strained the relationship between hospitals and physicians. It created ethical conflicts for hospitals when, for example, physicians who admitted large numbers of patients were questioned or disciplined regarding quality of care. Some of these physicians left the hospitals, taking a large source of revenue with them. Accountability to patients required that hospitals and their organized medical staffs be vigilant about monitoring and intervening in the quality of care practiced by physicians. Economic self-interest, however, tempted hospitals to be more lenient with physicians.

Toward the end of the twentieth century, relationships between hospitals and physicians began to change again. Integrated delivery systems, through which health-care providers and payers (such as insurance companies) collaborate to deliver care to patients in a particular geographic region, align the economic incentives affecting both physicians and hospitals. Capitation, a fixed fee paid to a group of providers to provide care for a fixed number of patients, resolves some of the ethical problems of the past related to hospital reimbursement. But capitation creates new ethical issues due to economic incentives to provide the least expensive care to patients. This change is good for some patients, but may not be good for others. Hospitals will continue to face ethical dilemmas of conflicting loyalties to patients and physicians.

The introduction of integrated delivery systems changes the relationships between hospitals and physicians in other ways. Managed care requires that primary-care physicians be the "gatekeepers," seeing patients first and referring them to specialists only if absolutely necessary. This, combined with capitation systems, creates incentives for hospitals and primary-care physicians to offer their services as one unit. Many hospitals that purchase physicians' medical practices manage the business side of the practices. This is extremely difficult to accomplish with ethical integrity on both sides, because physicians and hospitals have historically operated independent of one another—both psychologically and practically—even though they are in the same building.

A related problem is that, after having courted specialists for years, hospitals now need primary-care physicians because of their gatekeeper role. Ethical issues of loyalty and integrity are raised, as physicians in specialty practices find themselves in professional and economic jeopardy when their interests no longer match those of their hospital.

Special sponsorship

Hospitals under religious sponsorship—Catholic, Jewish, Episcopal, Lutheran, Adventist, Presbyterian, Methodist, Jehovah's Witness—have special concerns. They were founded by traditions having particular beliefs and aspirations, yet they provide care in a pluralistic society. They neither employ nor provide care solely for persons of their own faith. Like other hospitals, they are heavily dependent on state and federal payment for services rendered. In some cases, a hospital under religious sponsorship may be the only hospital serving a particular community. Ethical conflicts may arise between their allegiance to their religious sponsors and their obligation to provide needed services to the community.

Identity and mission are of particular concern here. In the United States, the majority of hospitals are "private," that is, they are free to follow their own moral mission in religious matters. A hospital may therefore choose, on religious grounds, to offer different services from others in the community, for example, to follow certain dietary practices; not to perform blood transfusions, abortions, or sterilizations; or not to allow the termination of life-sustaining treatment.

Thus far, the policies of hospitals with religious affiliations have not been proscribed by law, and arguably should not be proscribed ethically, unless they create undue hardship for patients. This would occur if patients could not gain reasonable access to needed services in any other way. The definition of what is reasonable will be interpreted variously, of course, depending on whether the perspective adopted is that of the sponsor and its adherents or of those who desire the service. In any event, sponsored hospitals occasionally find themselves with conflicting loyalties, as they strive to be faithful to both their religious tradition and their constituents.

The growth of managed care and alliances among hospitals of different sponsorships creates another set of ethical conflicts for religious hospitals. If they are part of the new system of health-care delivery, they will be closely associated with those who practice differently from them. This will result in their cooperating with and financially profiting from the very practices they prohibit in their own hospitals. How they work this out will require careful consideration of their several ethical commitments.

Relationships with employees

The ethical requirements of all employers apply in the hospital, for example, fairness in wages, benefits, and other employment policies; the assurance of a safe environment; respect for privacy and confidentiality; the right to organize; job assignments in accordance with employees' abilities. These are mentioned because their importance should not be overlooked. They are not elaborated on because they are not unique to hospitals.

Contemporary hospitals encounter many ethical concerns and problems. All constituents—patients, physicians, employees, board members, volunteers, the community at large, payers, business partners—have a stake in the way these ethical issues are considered and resolved.

CORRINE BAYLEY

Directly related to this article are the other articles in this entry: MEDIEVAL AND RENAISSANCE HISTORY, *and* MODERN HISTORY. *Also directly related are the entries* CLINICAL ETHICS; HEALTH-CARE DELIVERY; HEALTH OFFICIALS AND THEIR RESPONSIBILITIES; *and* TEAMS, HEALTH-CARE. *For a further discussion of topics mentioned in this article, see the entries* CONFIDENTIALITY; DEATH AND DYING: EUTHANASIA AND SUSTAINING LIFE, *article on* PROFESSIONAL AND PUBLIC POLICIES; *and* INFORMED CONSENT, *articles on* CLINICAL ASPECTS OF CONSENT IN HEALTH CARE *and* LEGAL AND ETHICAL ISSUES OF CONSENT IN HEALTH CARE *(with its* POSTSCRIPT*). For a discussion of hospital economics, see the entries* ECONOMIC CONCEPTS IN HEALTH CARE; HEALTH-CARE FINANCING; HEALTH-CARE RESOURCES, ALLOCATION OF; *and* HEALTH POLICY, *article on* POLITICS AND HEALTH CARE. *Other relevant material may be found under the entries* ALLIED HEALTH PROFESSIONS; MEDICINE AS A PROFESSION; OCCUPATIONAL SAFETY AND HEALTH, *article on* OCCUPATIONAL HEALTH-CARE PROVIDERS; *and* STRIKES BY HEALTH PROFESSIONALS.

Bibliography

AMERICAN HOSPITAL ASSOCIATION. 1992. *Management Advisory: Ethics—Ethical Conduct for Health Care Institutions.* Chicago: American Hospital Association.

BULGER, RUTH ELLEN, and REISER, STANLEY JOEL. 1990. *Integrity in Health Care Institutions: Humane Environments for Teaching, Inquiry and Healing.* Iowa City: University of Iowa Press.

BURKE, MARYBETH. 1991. "Hospitals Tackle Image Problems at Many Levels." *Hospitals* 65, no. 5:24–31.

GRAY, BRADFORD H., ed. 1986. *For-Profit Enterprise in Health Care.* Washington, D.C.: National Academy Press.

———. 1991. *The Profit Motive and Patient Care: The Changing Accountability of Doctors and Hospitals.* Cambridge, Mass.: Harvard University Press.

HASTINGS CENTER. 1987. *Guidelines on the Termination of Life-Sustaining Treatment and the Care of the Dying: A Report.* Briarcliff Manor, N.Y.: Author.

JONSEN, ALBERT R.; SIEGLER, MARK; and WINSLADE, WILLIAM J. 1986. *Clinical Ethics: A Practical Approach to Ethical Decisions in Clinical Medicine.* 2d ed. New York: Macmillan.

MARTY, MARTIN E., and VAUX, KENNETH L., eds. 1982. *Health/Medicine and the Faith Traditions: An Inquiry into Religion and Medicine.* Philadelphia: Fortress Press.

McCORMICK, RICHARD A. 1984. *Health and Medicine in the Catholic Tradition.* New York: Crossroad.

Quinlan, in re. 1975. 348 A.2d 801 (N.J. Ch. Div.); 355 A.2d 647 (N.J. 1976).

ROSENBERG, CHARLES E. 1987. *The Care of Strangers: The Rise of America's Hospital System.* New York: Basic Books.

SEAY, J. DAVID, and VLADECK, BRUCE C. 1987. *Mission Matters: A Report on the Future of Voluntary Health Care Institutions.* New York: United Hospital Fund of New York.

STARR, PAUL. 1982. *The Social Transformation of American Medicine.* New York: Basic Books.

STEVENS, ROSEMARY. 1989. *In Sickness and in Wealth.* New York: Basic Books.

U.S. PRESIDENT'S COMMISSION FOR THE STUDY OF ETHICAL PROBLEMS IN MEDICINE AND BIOMEDICAL AND BEHAVIORAL RESEARCH. 1983. *Deciding to Forgo Life-Sustaining Treatment.* Washington, D.C.: Author.

HOSPITAL ETHICS COMMITTEES

See CLINICAL ETHICS, article on INSTITUTIONAL ETHICS COMMITTEES.

HUMAN NATURE

Theories of human nature offer systematic and comprehensive accounts of human beings' most significant distinguishing characteristics. Such accounts are central in people's perennial attempts to organize their understandings of the cosmos; to figure out their relation to God, to nature, and to each other; and to uncover the possibilities, meanings, and purposes of human life.

Western understanding of human nature

Modern Western theories of human nature, which will be the focus of this essay, typically differ from their classical and medieval predecessors in appealing to the findings of a variety of life and social sciences, including anthropology, medicine, physiology, psychology, economics, sociology, and even ethology. Nevertheless, although these sciences undeniably help us to understand specific aspects of human life, even contemporary theories of human nature are never simply summaries of the results of empirical research—despite their frequent claims to scientific authority.

One reason that theories of human nature are not simply generalizations from the conclusions of scientific study is that they enter into empirical investigations not only as conclusions but also as presuppositions, structuring the conceptual frameworks within which research programs are conducted. Contemporary psychological investigation, for instance, proceeds with a variety of models of the human mind, including the Freudian, the behaviorist, the existentialist or humanist, and the computer models. Empirical research cannot fully evaluate the adequacy of its own framework relative to others; determining the adequacy of an entire framework requires reference to considerations beyond empirical data, including how the framework coheres with other respected theories and even its moral and political implications.

A related reason that theories of human nature go beyond ordinary scientific claims is that typically they aspire to provide a comprehensive conceptual framework that will render coherent the contributions of all those disciplines and discourses that investigate various aspects of human life. These often represent human beings in ways that, at least on the surface, appear quite incompatible with each other; for instance, lawyers assume that people ordinarily are responsible for their actions, while psychologists may suggest that people's behavior is determined ultimately by factors outside their control. Theories of human nature endeavor to resolve these incompatibilities in a variety of ways, ranging from reinterpreting the meaning of a discourse, such as the religious, to setting limits on the domain within which its claims are accepted; occasionally, a theory of human nature may even proclaim the invalidity of a whole realm of discourse, such as the parapsychological. Rather than simply summarizing the conclusions of the various life and social sciences, therefore, theories of human nature typically perform a regulatory function, authorizing some methodological approaches while delegitimating others.

Yet another respect in which theories of human nature differ from scientific theories, at least as science is ordinarily understood, is in the prominence of their normative or evaluative component. Even if one contends that all knowledge is to some degree value-laden, the evaluative element is far more evident in theories of human nature than it is, for instance, in modern theories of the physical universe. All theories of human nature provide a general account of human capacities and human needs, human potentialities and human well-being, and thus contain at least an implicit, and often an explicit, diagnosis of human malaise and a prescription for human flourishing.

Like all theoretical constructions, theories of human nature are developed in specific historical circumstances and are designed to address specific conceptual puzzles or practical concerns; consequently, they shift their emphasis according to the scientific, moral, and political preoccupations of the time. Despite variations in focus and emphasis, however, the Western project of understanding human nature historically has centered on two questions. The first of these addresses the human aspect of "human nature": How can human be distinguished from nonhuman nature? The second addresses the natural aspect: How can what is natural for humans be distinguished from what is unnatural, abnormal, or artificial? The concerns inherent in these two questions constitute continuing themes that link the variety of Western inquiries into the nature of human beings.

Reflection on these themes reveals that the Western project of providing a systematic theory of human nature has been predicated historically on certain assumptions. They include the following: (1) that it is possible to discover specific qualities or features that characterize human beings universally and transhistorically; (2) that these characteristics decisively distinguish humans from all other beings, notably nonhuman animals; and (3) that, from the discovery of these characteristics, it is possible to derive specific prescriptions about the proper conduct of human life. In other words, the Western project of understanding human nature generally has been motivated by a desire to derive from it universal and unchanging values.

These assumptions went unquestioned and often unarticulated throughout most of Western history. Once they are made explicit, however, it is easy to see that they are all contestable; and we shall see how, in the nineteenth and twentieth centuries, each of them was contested. For instance, Karl Marx (1818–1883) and John Dewey (1859–1952) challenged the first assumption; Charles Darwin (1809–1882) and the twentieth-century sociobiologists challenged the second; and the theorists of positivism and neopositivism challenged the third.

Since the 1970s not only these assumptions but the whole project of developing a comprehensive theory of human nature has been subjected to more fundamental critiques, launched by poststructuralist or postmodern French writers such as Michel Foucault (1926–1984), Jacques Derrida (1930–), and Jean-François Lyotard (1924–). While these authors differ on many points, they are united in rejecting the possibility of any overarching philosophical framework capable of unifying and legitimating the specific disciplines. Such totalizing frameworks or discourses, they claim, reflect unrealizable aspirations to discover universal and absolute truths in morals, politics, or science. These authors deny that any genuinely universal truths can be found, and assert that claims to them typically are propounded by groups who wish to use them for promoting their own political agendas. Truth, they argue, is relative to specific discursive practices that are historically contingent and self-justifying. Consequently, there is no need for, as well as no possibility of, a "master" discourse designed to be the ground or foundation of these more specific discourses.

As described so far, the dominant tendency in Western thought has been to conceptualize human nature as both *universal* and *transhistorical*. Its conceptualizations typically take the form "All human beings throughout history have characteristics x, y, z," implying that x, y, and z are necessary, as well as universal, characteristics of human nature. However, the Western tradition also includes conceptions of human nature that are not universalistic although they are transhistorical. These *relational* theories take the form "Group x is inferior to group y with respect to characteristics x, y, z"; typically, relational theories are used to justify the dominance of one group over another. Finally, some Western conceptions of human nature are *historical* rather than transhistorical, used within theories that claim that as human cultures change, so do certain important human characteristics. Some theories contain elements both universal and relational—for example, the theories of Aristotle and the sociobiologists—or both transhistorical and historical—for example, the theories of Karl Marx and John Dewey.

Three classic Western approaches

Aristotle. The origins of Western philosophy, in the sense of systematic and rational inquiries into the nature of reality, knowledge, and value, are often traced to the reflections of ancient Greek thinkers in the fifth and fourth centuries B.C.E. Plato (ca. 428–347) and Aristotle (384–322), two of the three philosophical giants of this period (the third being Socrates, ca. 470–399), developed systematic theories of human nature. Aristotle's view has been particularly influential on the Western tradition because it was incorporated into the Scholastic philosophy that dominated Europe in the Middle Ages and early Renaissance, and continues to shape the thinking of the Roman Catholic Church.

Aristotle (1947) conceptualized human beings as complexes of soul and body. The soul was the distinctively human element—the essence or form or intelligible principle of the body—but it existed only in conjunction with a living human body. Aristotle's conceptualization of the soul as inseparable from its body contrasted with Plato's view that human beings were souls united only temporarily with bodies, but Aristotle also acknowledged the possibility of the actively knowing and thinking part of the soul, the mind or intellect, being "set free from its present conditions . . . immortal and eternal." When this happened, however, Aristotle asserted that the mind remembered nothing of its former embodied activity and, because all connection with a specific human body was thus lost, he did not regard the human soul as personally or individually immortal.

Aristotle's view of human nature, like Plato's, was *teleological,* which is to say that he regarded human beings, like other things in the world, as having a "function" or activity peculiar to them. He further assumed, again like Plato, that the good life, or *eudaimonia,* consisted in the successful or efficient performance of that function. For Aristotle, the distinctive function of human beings was reasoning, or "an active life of that which possesses reason," and so he inferred that the good life was one in which the rational part of the soul governed the appetitive or desiring part, thus avoiding excess and living in accordance with virtue.

For Aristotle, human beings were, by nature, political animals who needed to live in a community: "He who is unable to live in society, or who has no need of it because he is sufficient to himself, must be either a beast or a god." Within human communities, however, not everyone was capable of citizenship: The nature of some was to rule and of others to be ruled. Among those whose nature was to be ruled were children, barbarians, and Greek women; thus, while Aristotle posited a universal standard for human nature, he simultaneously asserted that some groups of humans were less than fully human. The theme of dominance and subordination runs not only through Aristotle's account of the relations between human beings but even through his account of the nature of individual humans. He compared the controlling relation between form and matter with the relation between male and female, and he asserted that the proper relation between mind and body was like that of master to slave.

Aquinas. The dominant philosophical figure of the Middle Ages was Thomas Aquinas (1226–1274), later Saint Thomas, who synthesized Greek thought and church doctrine into a Christian philosophy (1962). He conceptualized human nature in terms that were basically Aristotelian, with some (often Platonic) modifications made in order to adapt Aristotelian views to church doctrine.

Aquinas believed, like Aristotle, that there was a distinctive and essential human nature that could be understood teleologically; he also shared the Aristotelian belief that the good life or *eudaimonia* was action in accordance with this function. A proper understanding of the ends or purposes of human life was therefore essential to morality and should be achieved by discovering the precepts of *natural law.* Natural law, as Aquinas conceptualized it, was universal and unchanging. It described supposedly universal human tendencies, such as preserving life, but presented them not simply as empirical facts about human nature but also as manifestations of God's design for humanity. For Aquinas, therefore, natural law simultaneously described how things were and prescribed how they should be. It was discoverable by reason, which, because it gave insight into God's purposes, provided guidance on how humans should live.

Like Aristotle, Aquinas saw humans as combinations of soul and body, with the soul as the form of the body. To allow for the possibility of personal or individual immortality, however, Aquinas diverged from Aristotle, declaring that the soul was a "substantial" form, capable of existing separately from matter. Not only was personal immortality conceptually possible, according to Aquinas; it was humans' destiny. God would not have implanted the universal—and therefore natural—human desire to live forever unless this desire had an object.

While Aquinas shared the Aristotelian view that human nature had an end or purpose, he believed, in accordance with church doctrine, that this end was supernatural rather than natural: It was to spend eternity united with God in heaven, where alone perfect happiness might be enjoyed. Human life as we know it was no more than a preparation for life after death, and this world was simply a testing ground for the next. So long as humans inhabited this world, however, they should strive to live in accordance with natural law, which provided a test for the moral validity of the laws of the state.

Descartes. The thought of René Descartes (1596–1650) is generally considered to mark the beginning of modern philosophy. Refusing to accept the authority of tradition, Descartes developed "rules for the direction of the understanding" and a "method for rightly conducting reason" designed to enable each individual to establish certain truth in science and philosophy (1931). He wrote in the vernacular (French) as well as in Latin, in order to reach lay as well as clerical readers.

Descartes's conception of human nature was even more *dualistic* than that of Aristotle and Aquinas. Living human beings, for Descartes, were composed of two entirely different kinds of entities: souls, which were active, intellectual substances, immaterial and immortal; and bodies, which were unthinking, passive mechanisms, spatially extended and temporally finite. Individual humans were to be identified not with their bodies but with their souls, which were able to survive the death of the body. While Descartes's model allowed for the soul's separation from the body after death, it rendered problematic the relation of the soul to the body during life, since it was unclear how material and immaterial substances could have a causal influence on each other. Descartes never succeeded in providing a satisfactory explanation of mind–body interaction.

As a scientist, Descartes wanted his theory of human nature to be compatible with both the new developments in physical science and the doctrines of the Roman Catholic Church. He attempted to reconcile these two worldviews by postulating two spheres of reality, each governed by entirely different laws or principles. The laws of God governed spiritual or mental reality; the laws of science governed physical reality, understood by Descartes in mechanical terms. Although Descartes never developed a systematic moral philosophy, his assertion that all "men" were potentially equal in their capacity to reason laid the foundation for later egalitarian moves in ethics and politics. Simultaneously, his conceptualization of animals as mere stimulus–response mechanisms, lacking consciousness because they lacked souls, justified the exclusion of animals from moral consideration. Cartesian biologists, in defense of vivisection, have compared the howls of cut-up dogs to the squeaks of unlubricated machines.

Shared features of dominant pre-Darwinian conceptions of human nature.   There are at least six common features of pre-Darwinian conceptions of human nature:

1. Human nature is the same transhistorically.
2. It is distinguished primarily by possession of a soul.
3. Human souls are characterized by their capacity to reason. This capacity exists, perhaps in varying degrees, as a potential innate in all humans, sharply distinguishing them from all other beings, including animals.
4. Humans' possession of a rational soul gives them special moral worth.
5. Lacking such a soul, animals lack comparable moral worth or value. Those biological features that are similar in humans and animals comprise humans' "lower" nature, which humans should strive to rise above.
6. Developing our potential to reason is a key to the good life for humans. Reasoning not only tells us how to live well but actualizes our distinctively human potential. Thus, the concept of human nature is clearly normative: Our task is to realize our humanness by fulfilling our potential for rationality; those who are incapable of fulfilling this potential are less than human.

The materialist tradition and the Darwinian pivot

The features listed above as characterizing pre-Darwinian conceptions of human nature represent the dominant Western tradition prior to the nineteenth century. Running counter to this *rationalist* and dualist tradition, however, Western thought also includes a less prominent *materialist* or naturalist tradition.

Anaximander (ca. 500 B.C.E.), an early pre-Socratic philosopher, developed a speculative theory of evolution in which human beings were descended from lower forms of animal life. Democritus (460–370 B.C.E.), a contemporary of Socrates, developed a speculative atomic theory in which even the human soul was composed of atoms. The English philosopher Thomas Hobbes (1588–1679) assimilated individual behavior and politics to the laws of mechanics, regarding desire as motion toward an object, and human beings as motivated entirely by self-interest. The French philosopher Julien de La Mettrie (1709–1751) accepted Descartes's assertion that animals were like machines but insisted that so, too, were human beings. The German philosopher Baron Paul Henri d'Holbach (1723–1789) argued that thinking could be reduced to the functioning of the brain and explicitly denied the existence of a soul. Another of the French philosophes, Claude-Adrien Helvétius (1715–1771), argued that all mental faculties were ultimately reducible to physical sensation and that all humans were motivated by the desire to achieve physical pleasure and reduce pain. This latter idea was developed into an elaborate ethical calculus by the nineteenth-century British utilitarians, Jeremy Bentham (1748–1832), James Mill (1773–1836), and the latter's more famous son, John Stuart Mill (1806–1873). Collectively, these philosophers suggested an alternative understanding of human nature—one that focused more on the body than on the soul, on the emotions and desires more than on reason, and on the similarities rather than the differences between humans and animals. It remained for Charles Darwin to give this materialist tradition a scientific basis by providing a naturalistic analysis of the relations between humans and animals.

In his landmark work, *On the Origin of Species* (1859), Darwin argued that the distinctive features of human nature were not divinely created in an instant but had evolved over many millennia through a process he called "natural selection" (Darwin, 1936). Although the word "selection" suggested conscious purpose, Darwin's use of it was metaphorical, since nature "selects" only in the sense that certain new traits or mutations that appear accidentally are sufficiently adaptive to the environmental conditions within which the organism lives for the new organism to survive. The view that human beings had evolved through accidental mutations implied that there was no preordained nature, no ultimate meaning or cosmic purpose for human life to fulfill. In an attempt to escape this conclusion and reconcile science with Christianity, some later theorists postulated a direction and a goal in evolution, characterizing more recently evolved species as "higher" or otherwise superior; but such teleological and evaluative interpretations were ultimately alien to the basically antiteleological spirit of the concept of natural selection.

When Darwin first proposed his theory of evolution, the wife of the canon of Worcester Cathedral was said to have remarked, "Descended from the apes! My dear, we will hope it is not true. But if it is, let us pray that it may not become generally known." Indeed, the church denounced Darwin, recognizing that his theories challenged not only the beliefs in divine creation and a radical discontinuity between humans and animals but also the idea of an immortal soul with special moral worth. Darwin argued that morality had developed from the social instincts of animals; and he construed the uniquely human capacity for rationality, which Aristotle had seen as the telos of human existence, as the outcome of natural selection operating on accidental mutations.

Biological determinism: A critique

Once Darwin had demonstrated an evolutionary continuity between humans and other animals, questions arose about the causal role of human biology in relation to other aspects of human life. For many scientists, the project became the *reductionist* one of showing how the various psychological and social characteristics of human beings were causally determined by human biology.

Many *biological determinist* theories have negative social implications because they present human characteristics like aggression and dominance as biologically determined and therefore inescapable. For instance, Sigmund Freud (1856–1939), the founder of psychoanalysis, insisted that all human motivation could be reduced to two basic drives—the sexual drive, or libido; and the aggressive drive, an ineradicable instinct to hurt, torture, or kill other human beings (Freud, 1962). The German ethologist Konrad Lorenz (1903–1989) also posited an aggressive instinct in humans similar to that he found in his study of various animal species in their natural habitats. In each species, the instinct had evolved to serve one or more life-preserving functions, such as territorial dispersion, selection of the strongest for reproduction, defense of the young, and the establishment of a hierarchy that could provide the group with social cohesion. In species armed with sharp teeth, claws, or beaks, the aggressive instinct was generally coupled with an inhibitory mechanism preventing fighting animals from killing each other; Lorenz argued that

there had been no need for such an inhibitory mechanism to evolve in humans because they were not naturally armed. With the development of weaponry, however, the absence of such a mechanism was often lethal, and the advent of nuclear weapons made it a threat to the survival of the species (Lorenz, 1974).

More recent studies of animal behavior have generated a new form of biological determinism called *sociobiology.* Two precursors of sociobiology, anthropologists Lionel Tiger (1937–) and Robin Fox (1913–1971), proposed the concept of a "biogram," a code or program genetically "wired" into the brain that produced certain forms of social behavior, including patterns of dominance and submission—hierarchy among males and dominance of males over females. Both of these were assumed to be the evolutionary heritage of the hunting life of early hominids (Tiger and Fox, 1974). The same general line of thinking was employed by entomologist Edward O. Wilson (1929–), who first coined the term "sociobiology." Wilson insisted that "genes hold culture on a leash" and play a significant role in determining such human social behavior as altruism toward kin, communal aggression, nationalism, racism, homosexuality, and the dominance of males over females. Wilson has conceded that these biologically based tendencies might be counteracted through extreme social measures, but he argues that humans would pay a high price for doing so (Wilson, 1977).

While Wilson's assertion of a universal genetic tendency toward ethnocentric and racist attitudes was not an attempt to justify racism, there is a long Western tradition of using evolutionary theory to denigrate certain racial or ethnic groups. In the nineteenth century, some scientists in this tradition asserted that Caucasians and Orientals had crossed the *Homo sapiens* threshold before "Negroes," or that *Homo sapiens* had begun in Asia and migrated to Africa, where the original stock had degenerated. Others sought to prove racial, ethnic, and class inequalities in intelligence through the use of IQ (intelligence quotient) theory. Frances Galton (1822–1911), a cousin of Darwin who coined the term "eugenics," attempted to show that the upper classes had superior intellectual capacities and that blacks were "two grades" below whites. Many of the early IQ theorists in the United States made similar claims about various immigrant groups.

After World War II, when the Nazis had shown the possible social consequences of eugenic ideas, such theories fell into disrepute. They were revived in 1969 when educational psychologist Arthur Jensen (1923–) published an article in the *Harvard Educational Review* arguing as follows: Intelligence testing has demonstrated that whites score on average about fifteen IQ points above blacks; IQ is 80 percent "heritable"; therefore, the mean difference between the scores proves a hereditary difference in innate intelligence between the two groups (Jensen, 1969). Shortly after Jensen's article appeared, Harvard psychologist Richard Herrnstein (1930–) made a similar argument concerning the difference in IQ scores between "upper-class" and "lower-class" people. He concluded that humans should give up any aspirations to democratic equality and accept the idea of a natural meritocracy (Herrnstein, 1973).

Biological determinist theories were highly controversial in the late 1960s and 1970s, but in the 1980s and 1990s they became increasingly fashionable—claiming, for instance, genetic factors in alcoholism; locating homosexuality in the structure of the brain; and asserting that men with XYY chromosomes have a tendency toward criminal violence. However, biological determinist theories of human nature are problematic in a number of respects.

Empirically, the evidence for such theories is at best inconclusive. Even within the psychoanalytic tradition, some theorists have argued against Freud that aggressive desires may be explained as derivative manifestations rather than primary instincts, resulting from situations that frustrate other, nonaggressive desires. Ethologists and sociobiologists typically move incautiously from observations of certain animal species or conjectures about early hominids to claims about modern human beings. Sometimes, like Lorenz, they focus on the behavior of fish, birds, and other animals considerably removed from humans—while they ignore studies indicating that many higher mammals, especially primates, display almost no hierarchical organization or intraspecies aggression, being instead peaceful and cooperative. Finally, regardless of how nonhuman species behave, similarities in behavior between humans and nonhuman animals do not establish that the human behavior in question is biologically determined; it may still be a learned response.

Claims for the universality of human aggression, hierarchy, and male dominance also are not confirmed by anthropological evidence. Many hunter–gatherer societies are reported to be remarkably lacking in aggressive behavior, and some enjoy an exceptionally high degree of social equality. Assertions of women's "natural" dependence on men are undermined by evidence that gathering, a task often performed predominantly by women, is a more reliable food source than hunting in many hunter–gatherer societies. The sexual division of labor varies widely cross-culturally, and even where certain constants are observed, such as a tendency for women rather than men to care for young children, this may be a social adaptation to prevailing conditions rather than a biological predetermination.

Claims about the genetic basis of racial and ethnic differences in IQ are equally suspect. The idea of different evolutionary paths for different races is contradicted by the paleontological evidence; indeed, the concept of

race itself is now widely discredited, with anthropologists preferring instead to talk about the statistical frequency of certain characteristics within a geographical population. Further, the idea that IQ tests measure innate intelligence is undermined by the recognition that all tests are culturally biased, since they all require prior learning, and that learning experience can significantly raise IQ. Finally, the very concept of "heritability" is a technical one, designating a ratio of the contribution of heredity to environment within a given population; it cannot be used, therefore, to compare one population against another.

Biological determinist theories of human nature are not just empirically unconfirmed; they also fail to acknowledge what is most distinctive of our species. The human genetic constitution determines highly developed learning and cognitive capacities that allow humans to respond flexibly rather than instinctively to environmental problems, as well as to develop a range of distinctively human cultural characteristics. The implications of this were noted by one of the world's foremost geneticists, Theodosius Dobzhansky (1900–1975), who wrote, "In a sense, human genes have surrendered their primacy in human evolution to an entirely new, nonbiological or superorganic agent, culture. However, it should not be forgotten that human culture is not possible without human genes" (Dobzhansky, 1966, p. 113). In short, what has developed in the human evolutionary process is a primate with a genetic structure capable of a new kind of evolution, cultural evolution.

Biological determinist theories of human nature contrast sharply in content with their pre-Darwinian counterparts, but they are often inspired by the same motivation of discovering universal and unchanging social values. Typically, they describe as "natural" aspects of behavior thought to be biologically determined; though few would assert that natural behavior is always to be encouraged or even permitted, characterizing some behavioral tendencies as natural provides a certain legitimation for them. Because they are understood as resulting from natural selection, such tendencies are regarded as having been necessary at least at some time for human survival; in consequence, they cannot be entirely deplored, and they may even be romanticized as clues to a more "natural" way of life. Thus, biological determinist approaches to understanding and evaluating human nature may be seen as secular analogues of Aquinas's theory of natural law.

It may be the social function of biological determinist theories of human nature, rather than their scientific credentials, that accounts for their continuing popularity. Put simply, these theories tend to rationalize existing manifestations of aggression and inequality: Biological determinist analyses of violence, war, and crime tend to deflect attention from the social and economic causes of these phenomena, just as theories about the biological determinants of male and female behavior distract us from the ways in which men and women are socialized for their respective roles. The implication often drawn from biological determinist theories is that significant social movement in the direction of peaceful cooperation and equality is impossible because it is alleged to go against "human nature." Clearly, those in power benefit from such an assumption and are likely to encourage the development of such theories.

Behaviorism: Another form of post-Darwinian reductionism

The Western materialist or naturalist tradition has not always moved in a biological determinist direction. It also includes thinkers who claim that environmental or cultural factors are the primary determinants of the human mind or behavior. The philosopher John Locke (1632–1704) saw the human mind as a kind of blank tablet to be written upon by sensory impressions, while Enlightenment figures like Helvétius assumed that education could shape human beings into almost any form.

In the first part of the twentieth century, environmentalist ideas became popular in the United States through a psychological movement known as behaviorism. John B. Watson (1878–1958), who first systematically developed the theory, insisted that in order for psychology to become a rigorous experimental science, it must give up its introspective orientation. It should no longer take its task to be analyzing private mental states, such as feelings, desires, and thoughts, but instead should study the relation between publicly observable behavior and the environment. For Watson, the two basic forms of this relation were the *unconditioned* and the *conditioned reflex*. The former was the basic human physiological endowment, consisting of automatic responses to environmental stimuli, such as salivating in the presence of food and contracting pupils in the presence of light. Watson based his analysis of the conditioned reflex on the work of the Russian experimental psychologist Ivan Petrovich Pavlov (1849–1936), who had demonstrated that a hungry dog, repeatedly presented with both food and the ringing of a bell, would eventually salivate at only the bell-ringing. The sound of the bell had become a *substitute stimulus*, and the salivation was now a *conditioned response*. For Watson, all human behavior could be reduced to these two kinds of reflexes (Watson, 1925).

Watson's version of behaviorism was superseded by that of B. F. Skinner (1904–1990), who argued that reflex action could account for only a small part of human behavior. For Skinner, human behavior was primarily shaped by what he called *operant conditioning*, which *reinforced* certain spontaneous movements of the organism. For example, when a pigeon raised its head above a certain height and food was released into its cage, the result was a higher frequency of that behavior. Unlike the stimulus in Watson's model, the "reinforcer" (the food) was introduced *after* the "response" (the raising of the head to the desired height) occurred. For Skinner, most human behavior other than automatic reflex action, even human language, could be explained as the result of *positive* or *negative reinforcement*, which, by adding something to the situation (food, sex, money, praise, etc.)—or by removing something from it—increased the frequency of some behavior. While not denying that feelings and thoughts existed, Skinner refused to characterize them as residing in a special mental domain, consciousness, and claimed that they had no causal effect on human behavior (Skinner, 1953).

Both Watson and Skinner believed that human beings could be conditioned to develop almost any pattern of behavioral responses. Watson boldly declared that he could take almost any infant "at random and train him to become . . . doctor, lawyer, artist, merchant-chief, and, yes, even a beggar man and thief." Skinner insisted that operant conditioning "shapes behavior as a sculptor shapes a lump of clay." One evident consequence of the behaviorist program was that human freedom was an illusion. For Skinner, in particular, such concepts as freedom, moral responsibility, and human dignity were the conceits of a prescientific age (Skinner, 1973).

Behaviorism, just as much as biological determinism, is heir to the evolutionary paradigm because human behavior is still explained in terms of genetic dispositions regarded as having survival value. For behaviorism, however, these predispositions are not instincts or drives. Instead, specific unconditioned reflexes have evolved in the human species because they have survival value, while the human organism's susceptibility to conditioning helps it survive by allowing it to adapt to environmental changes more rapidly than its genetic structure could.

There are a number of difficulties with the behaviorist conception of human nature. First are the primary data of consciousness, such as desires, feelings, reflection, and decision making; it is hard to believe that these do not have at least some causal influence on human activity. Second, the fact that pigeons, rats, and human beings can sometimes be controlled by operant conditioning does not mean that all human behavior can be understood in this way. Linguist Noam Chomsky (1928–), for example, has argued against Skinner that linguistic competence requires creativity that goes beyond responses to prior conditioning because we are constantly constructing sentences that we have never before encountered (Chomsky, 1959). Finally, there is no room in the behaviorist model for human agency: The environment acts, human beings merely react. In this, behaviorism may be seen as ideologically reflecting a world in which people are continually managed and manipulated by technocratic and bureaucratic elites.

Social and historical conceptions of human nature

Social and historical conceptions of human nature offer an alternative to seeing human beings either as primarily determined by their biological drives or as passive clay to be molded by their physical and social environment. These approaches, while not ignoring human biology or the role of social conditioning, emphasize the importance of human social activity within specific historical contexts. The work of the revolutionary social theorist Karl Marx, together with his collaborator Friedrich Engels (1820–1895), and of the U.S. pragmatist philosopher John Dewey, provides two examples of this approach.

Marx and Engels's view of human nature (Schmitt, 1987) was embedded in their more general theory of human history, *historical materialism.* Human history, they contended, began with humans' attempt to satisfy their basic biological needs through producing their means of subsistence, so that human beings were, first and foremost, producers. Human production differed from that of nonhuman animals in that it was deliberate rather than instinctive, involving imagination, planning, and tool use. It was also inherently social, not only in requiring the coordination of human effort but also in utilizing skills and knowledge transmitted from one individual, group, or generation to another. In societies producing a surplus beyond that needed for immediate survival, human production typically involved a division of labor going beyond a division into separate tasks, to a division between intellectual and physical work and between work considered appropriate for men and for women. Most important for Marx and Engels was the class division of labor between those groups who owned the means of production and those who had to work for them, a division generating the class struggles regarded by Marx and Engels as the motor force in history.

Different economic systems, or what Marx and Engels called modes of production, established forms of social life through which human beings individuated and understood themselves. Peasants and artisans, "ladies" and "gentlemen," merchants and professionals, corporate capitalists and industrial workers would tend to think and act differently from each other. Changes in the mode of production would generate new forms of social life, new ways of understanding the world, and new ways of thinking and acting—in effect, new kinds of "individuals." Thus, human nature itself would change. Since human beings were active in the class struggle that caused these social and economic changes, however, it could also be said that human beings actively changed their own natures over the course of history.

For John Dewey, as for Marx and Engels, human beings were neither governed by instincts nor passive recipients of environmental forces; rather, they were social agents who changed their own natures in the process of changing their societal conditions. However, in contrast to Marx and Engels, Dewey regarded the motor force of social change not as class struggle but as the product of reflective intelligence (Dewey, 1957, 1963).

Dewey acknowledged that human beings had instincts—or impulses, as he preferred to call them in order to discourage associations of inflexibility. Impulses, in his view, were extremely flexible in that they could take on a variety of meanings, depending on the social context. Thus, the impulse of fear might become cowardice, caution, reverence, or respect; while the impulse of anger might become rage, sullenness, annoyance, or indignation. Impulses took on these meanings as habits, predispositions to certain kinds of thinking and acting, ultimately embodied in social customs and institutions. The content of these habits constituted our historical nature. However, when the habits proved inadequate to new social problems, humans could employ their reflective intelligence to redirect their impulses into new habits. For example, as war became increasingly problematic or as certain economic institutions become increasingly outmoded, human impulses could be rechanneled, creating new institutions embodying new habits.

To make sense of the claim that human nature changes, we need to remember the distinction between transhistorical and historical conceptions of human nature. For both Dewey and Marx, it is precisely because a certain transhistorical human nature exists—socially productive and reflectively intelligent—that the content of human nature can be changed historically. To put this point in a more contemporary idiom: Our distinctively human capacity to transform social institutions transforms social roles and, in so doing, transforms historically specific character structures.

Giving more weight to the social and historical aspects of human nature offers a new model of the relation between genetic determination and social conditioning, on the one hand, and social behavior, on the other. What is determined by our genes is our capacity to learn, reflect, and work for change. Humans can, thus, be agents of their own history. Biology determines certain potentialities, but it is only through concrete historical activities that humans develop certain specific cultural and psychological characteristics. Genes dictate the ability to develop general modes of response, such as learning languages, engaging in productive labor, and developing forms of social relatedness; but they do not dictate that humans learn English, produce nuclear weapons, or become selfish and competitive as opposed to altruistic and cooperative. Thus, historical and social conceptions of human nature do not deny biology but refuse to privilege it as the primary cause of human action. Similarly, they do not deny conditioning but equally refuse to privilege it in explaining human action. Certain social conditions undoubtedly encourage the development of certain habits, but these are not merely behavioral responses; instead, they are social patterns of meaning that connect thought to action. Furthermore, human beings do not merely react to social conditions but individuate themselves within them and can reflect intelligently on them. Thus, both individually and collectively humans can decide to change their habits and work to transform the social conditions from which they arose.

A social and historical conception of the human body

Although many theorists are willing to acknowledge that people's character or personality or behavior is socially shaped, at least to some degree, the biological constitution, the body, is often viewed as a presocial given, the universal and unchanging foundation on which elaborate cultural edifices are erected. According to this way of thinking, the body constitutes the most natural aspect of human nature. Itself a product of natural selection, the body sets the "natural," that is, biologically determined, limits of social variability.

While it may be true that there is less systematic cross-cultural and transhistorical variation in people's bodies than there is in their personalities and social institutions, it is too simple to regard the human body as a presocial given. Although the human body may sometimes be experienced as a given, in fact, like the mind or the personality, bodies are socially and historically shaped on several levels.

It is not difficult to recognize some of the ways in which human bodies are influenced by their social context. Different kinds of work and living conditions develop or distort the body in various ways. For instance, scarcity of food results in stunted growth, so that body size and development vary systematically not only between cultures but often also between social classes. While many of these bodily marks are unintended side effects of social practices, others are deliberately induced. Social norms are consciously inscribed on the body in a variety of ways, ranging from foot-binding and circumcision to diet clinics and cosmetic surgery. The varying social meanings assigned to bodily characteristics and functions influence a person's experience of his or her body, which, depending on the social context,

may become a source of pride, joy, pain, or embarrassment.

Social influences on the human body operate not only on the level of observable physical structure, the phenotype; in the past, they have also influenced the genotype, our genetic inheritance, and they continue to do so. While human prehistory is highly speculative, it seems likely that some genetically heritable characteristics have been selected not only "naturally," as adaptive to such nonsocial circumstances as climate and food availability; but also socially, as adaptive to certain forms of social organization or perhaps even as the results of conscious social preferences. For instance, the average size difference between human males and females may have been a consequence as much as a cause of male dominance: If the dominant males fed first and most, only smaller-framed women could survive on the leftover food. Even today, the human gene pool continues to be influenced by social factors. For instance, exposure to environmental pollutants sometimes leads to genetic mutations, and modern medicine now makes it possible for people to survive and reproduce with genetic conditions that otherwise would have led to their early deaths. Finally, genetic engineering is rapidly becoming a real possibility.

The recognition that even the genetic constitution is influenced by social factors has far-reaching consequences for understanding human nature. The point is not simply that most versions of biological determinism are false because they fail to give sufficient weight to the social determinants of human characteristics. It is, rather, that the usefulness of the whole nature–culture distinction as an analytical framework for understanding human beings comes into question. Just as we cannot identify any cultural or social phenomena uninfluenced in some way by human biology, neither can we identify any human biological or "natural" features that are independent of social influence. The biological and the social are so intertwined in the human past and present that it becomes impossible in principle to distinguish the natural from the social or cultural components in the constitution of human beings. As far as human beings are concerned, the relation between nature and culture is mutually constitutive: To oppose one to the other is incomprehensible. Everything that we are and do is revealed as simultaneously cultural and natural.

Ethical implications for the life sciences: A cautionary tale

What are the bioethical implications of these various conceptions of human nature? First, a cautionary note. Practical ethics reflects on a host of considerations in practical contexts and cannot simply deduce specific moral conclusions from general ethical principles, let alone from some general conception of human nature. Thus, the relation between the various conceptions of human nature and any specific bioethical position is unlikely to be one of logical entailment. This does not mean, however, that concepts of human nature have no relevance to bioethical issues. They may serve as starting points for bioethical analysis, raise suspicions about certain bioethical claims, or even rule out certain bioethical positions. In general, certain conceptions of human nature may be said to cohere, or provide a better "fit," with certain bioethical stances than with others.

The dominant pre-Darwinian conceptions of human nature view physical nature, including the human body, as the realm of the material, the immanent, and the profane, and identify God with the spiritual, the transcendent, and the sacred. It is only because human beings are endowed with a soul that they are regarded as capable of partaking in the sacred, and their mission is to transcend their bodies and realize their spiritual nature. Insofar as they are part of God's creation, nonhuman animals are sometimes assigned a degree of moral worth, but the view that they lack souls typically rationalizes the claim that nonhuman animals are merely resources to serve human purposes. Saint Francis of Assisi notwithstanding, the dominant view of the Judeo-Christian tradition is that God created nonhuman animals and, indeed, all of nonhuman nature, primarily for the use of human beings. This sharp bifurcation between human and nonhuman nature not only permits but even legitimates the human subjugation and exploitation of all nonhuman nature, and may therefore contribute to the contemporary ecological crisis.

Within this ontology, the human body occupies a unique and somewhat ambiguous moral status. Although material, and therefore a source of temptation, the body is nevertheless sacrosanct because it is indispensable to human life. God is thought to have a divine plan for humanity, and any attempt to subvert this plan by tinkering with the human body is regarded as at least prima facie wrong. When applied to humans as opposed to nonhuman animals, therefore, reproductive technology, genetic engineering, and euthanasia are viewed with suspicion, if not censure; and "brain death" may not be considered sufficient reason to switch off a life-support system, depending on when the soul is believed to leave the body. If, for example, the soul is thought to remain in the body until the last breath of life, then euthanasia can never be justified: Even the suffering and dying body must be revered as the house of the soul. Finally, because humans are morally distinguished by the possession of a soul, abortion is condemned at whatever point the fetus is believed to acquire a soul. It is interesting to note that the Catholic Church has not always held that fetal ensoulment occurs at the moment of conception: Saint Thomas Aquinas (1962), for instance, argued as an Ar-

istotelian that the fetus did not have a soul until it assumed human form, which he thought occurred after three months' gestation for the male fetus and six months' for the female.

In contrast with the pre-Darwinian dichotomies between human and nature, spiritual and material, sacred and profane, post-Darwinian conceptions of human nature posit an evolutionary continuity between human and nonhuman animals. This continuity is sometimes used as a basis for moral challenges to the human exploitation and domination of animals, especially animals that are close to human beings in evolutionary terms. It is precisely those nonhuman animals most like humans, however, that are most useful for many purposes, such as medical experiments and organ transplants; in consequence, some philosophers have sought to undercut moral challenges to the human exploitation of nonhuman animals by arguing that beings "lower" on the evolutionary scale may be sacrificed for the good of "higher" species. Opposing this position is a growing minority in the bioethics community which argues that such a position is an example of unwarranted human chauvinism or "speciesism," a term invoked to suggest parallels with racism and sexism.

Although post-Darwinian assumptions of an evolutionary continuity between humans and nonanimals may be used to challenge the view that animals are simply a resource for human use, they have also been used to justify radical interventions in human life processes. If it is legitimate to experiment on nonhuman animals, for instance, it may be equally legitimate to experiment on human beings. If *Homo sapiens* is the accidental outcome of natural selection, if there is no inherent purpose for which we are created, then there is no a priori reason to assume that further modifications in human biological processes should not be made via reproductive technologies or even genetic engineering. Since the human nervous system is a defining component of human life, the fetus at an early stage of brain development is likely to have a different moral status than it does once the brain has developed. Certainly, the post-Darwinian conception of human nature would generally assume that "brain dead" means dead.

These conclusions reflect the absence of the concept of a soul in post-Darwinian views of human nature, since it was the soul that, in earlier conceptions, provided the philosophical grounding for human dignity. Unless an adequate substitute for the concept of the soul can be found, post-Darwinian conceptions of human nature may permit the drastic manipulation of human beings. Behavior regarded as undesirable may be treated either as a biological abnormality or as a failure of social conditioning. Biological determinists may regard alcoholism, addictive gambling, violent criminal behavior, schizophrenia, depression, and even homosexuality as candidates for treatment with a variety of biological techniques: psychosurgery, shock therapy, hormonal therapy, psychopharmacological interventions, and perhaps, in the future, even genetic manipulation. Behaviorists, of course, emphasize the use of various conditioning techniques to modify human behavior, raising the prospect of a *Clockwork Orange* world. Skinner, in fact, wrote a utopian novel, *Walden Two* (1948), in which behavioral managers conditioned people from birth to make choices in accord with the goals and institutions of that society. Both biological and behavioral interventions often work toward the same goal—direct control of human behavior.

But who will control the controllers, and how far will such control be allowed to extend? There are already biological determinists who advocate the use of genetic manipulation to raise IQ or to alter certain "undesirable" tendencies in the human species, perhaps to create a Superman. Others would clone the embryo and store it for future use, perhaps in case of some failure of the original stock. Brave New World may be just around the corner unless we can reclaim the concept of human dignity. Social and historical conceptions of human nature offer a secular basis for doing so.

Although people who accept a social and historical conception of human nature may still utilize some concept of naturalness in describing various human activities, such as conceiving or giving birth, they recognize that what is taken to be natural or unnatural changes historically and culturally, so that ethical decisions cannot be grounded in some unchangeable concept of human nature. However, this does not prevent us from ethically evaluating various attempts to manipulate and control human nature. Indeed, those who accept social and historical conceptions of human nature are likely to urge caution in the use of biological interventions and conditioning techniques for the purposes of altering human behavior. They will be suspicious of all treatment and research modalities that fail to respect human agency, reflective intelligence, and decision-making capabilities, since it is precisely these transhistorical capacities that make possible the continuous transformation of our historical natures. In short, social and historical conceptions of human nature will tend to reaffirm the concept of human dignity. In the sphere of medicine, for instance, they are likely to insist on the dignity of medical subjects and emphasize informed consent and coparticipation in physician–patient relationships.

The recognition that human beings individuate themselves within and through social processes may also have implications for the abortion controversy; at the very least, it suggests that women and fetuses cannot have the same moral status. Moreover, social and historical conceptions of human nature emphasize that consideration of bioethical problems must be sensitive to concrete social and political contexts; in a society with an expressed commitment to human equality, for example, questions like procreative technology or contract parenting must be evaluated with special reference to their implications for people of different classes, genders, abilities, races, and ethnicities. Finally, social and historical conceptions regard human beings as transhistorically creative, productive, social, and capable of reforming their habits through reflective intelligence; and people who accept these conceptions are likely to valorize those capacities and seek to develop social institutions—including health-care, psychiatric, and research institutions—through which they would be enhanced.

The open-ended nature of these last implications serves as a reminder that ethical conclusions are not strictly entailed by any general conception of human nature, especially by social and historical conceptions. In addressing particular bioethical problems, therefore, the values implicit in these conceptions must be supplemented by explicitly ethical criteria, such as historically specific understandings of justice, freedom, and human well-being.

ALISON M. JAGGAR
KARSTEN J. STRUHL

Directly related to this article are the entries PERSON; NATURE; BODY; EMOTIONS; *and* FEMINISM. *For a further discussion of topics mentioned in this article, see the entries* ACTION; BEHAVIORISM; EUGENICS; GENETICS AND HUMAN BEHAVIOR; GENETICS AND HUMAN SELF-UNDERSTANDING; NATURAL LAW; RACE AND RACISM; *and* ROMAN CATHOLICISM. *For a discussion of related ideas, see the entries* BIOLOGY, PHILOSOPHY OF; DEATH, *articles on* WESTERN RELIGIOUS THOUGHT, *and* DEATH IN THE WESTERN WORLD (*with its* POSTSCRIPT); EVOLUTION; INTERPRETATION; SCIENCE, PHILOSOPHY OF; *and* VALUE AND VALUATION.

Bibliography

AQUINAS, THOMAS. 1962. [1272]. *Summa Theologiae.* Turin: Marietti.

ARISTOTLE. 1947. "Metaphysics." In *Introduction to Aristotle,* pp. 243–296. Translated by W. D. Ross. Edited by Richard P. McKeon. New York: Modern Library. Includes Books 1 and 12.

———. 1947. "Poetics." In *Introduction to Aristotle,* pp. 553–617. Translated by W. D. Ross. Edited by Richard P. McKeon. New York: Modern Library. Includes Books 1 and 3.

BLOCK, NED J., and DWORKIN, GERALD, eds. 1976. *The I.Q. Controversy: Critical Readings.* New York: Pantheon.

BLUM, JEFFREY M. 1978. *Pseudoscience and Mental Ability: The Origins and Fallacies of The IQ Controversy.* New York: Monthly Review Press.

CHOMSKY, NOAM. 1959. "Review of B. F. Skinner, *Verbal Behavior.*" *Language* 35:26–58.

DARWIN, CHARLES. 1936. [1859; 1871]. *On the Origin of Species by Means of Natural Selection; or, The Preservation of Favoured Races in the Struggle For Life;* and *The Descent of Man and Selection in Relation to Sex.* New York: Modern Library.

DESCARTES, RENÉ. 1931. [1637–1650]. "Rules for the "Direction of the Mind," "Discourse on the Method of Rightly Conducting the Reason," and "Meditations on First Philosophy." In vol. 1 of *Philosophical Works of Descartes.* Translated by Elizabeth S. Haldane and George R. T. Ross. Cambridge: At the University Press.

DEWEY, JOHN. 1957. *Human Nature and Conduct: An Introduction to Social Psychology.* New York: Modern Library.

———. 1963. *Freedom and Culture.* New York: Capricorn.

DOBZHANSKY, THEODOSIUS G. 1966. *Heredity and the Nature of Man.* New York: New American Library.

FREUD, SIGMUND. 1962. [1930]. *Civilization and Its Discontents.* Translated by James Strachey. New York: W. W. Norton.

HERRNSTEIN, RICHARD J. 1973. *I.Q. in the Meritocracy.* Boston: Little, Brown.

JENSEN, ARTHUR R. 1969. "How Much Can We Boost IQ and Scholastic Achievement?" *Harvard Educational Review* 39, no. 1:1–123.

LEE, RICHARD BORSHOY. 1979. *The !Kung San: Men, Women, and Work in a Foraging Society.* New York: Cambridge University Press.

LEWONTIN, RICHARD C.; ROSE, STEVEN P. R.; and KAMIN, LEON J. 1984. *Not in Our Genes: Biology, Ideology, and Human Nature.* New York: Pantheon.

LORENZ, KONRAD. 1974. *On Aggression.* Translated by Marjorie Kerr Wilson. New York: Harcourt Brace Jovanovich.

MONTAGU, ASHLEY, ed. 1970. *The Concept of Race.* London: Collier.

———. 1978. *The Nature of Human Aggression.* New York: Oxford University Press.

PASSMORE, JOHN A. 1970. *The Perfectibility of Man.* London: Duckworth.

REITER, RAYNA R., ed. 1975. *Toward an Anthropology of Women.* New York: Monthly Review Press.

SCHMITT, RICHARD. 1987. *Introduction to Marx and Engels: A Critical Reconstruction.* Boulder, Colo.: Westview.

SKINNER, B. F. 1948. *Walden Two.* New York: Macmillan.

———. 1953. *Science and Human Behavior.* New York: Macmillan.

———. 1972. *Beyond Freedom and Dignity.* New York: Bantam.

TIGER, LIONEL, and FOX, ROBIN. 1974. *The Imperial Animal.* New York: Dell.

TUCKER, ROBERT C., ed. 1972. *The Marx–Engels Reader.* New York: W. W. Norton.

WATSON, JOHN B. 1925. *Behaviorism.* New York: W. W. Norton.

WILSON, EDWARD O. 1977. *Sociobiology: A New Synthesis.* Cambridge, Mass.: Harvard University Press.

———. 1979. *On Human Nature.* New York: Bantam.

HUMAN RESEARCH

See INFORMED CONSENT, *article on* CONSENT ISSUES IN HUMAN RESEARCH; RESEARCH, HUMAN: HISTORICAL ASPECTS; RESEARCH, UNETHICAL; RESEARCH BIAS; RESEARCH METHODOLOGY; *and* RESEARCH POLICY. *See also the entries on various research subjects, such as* ADOLESCENTS; AGING AND THE AGED, *article on* HEALTH-CARE AND RESEARCH ISSUES; AUTOEXPERIMENTATION; CHILDREN, *article on* HEALTH-CARE AND RESEARCH ISSUES; FETUS, *article on* FETAL RESEARCH; INFANTS, *article on* ETHICAL ISSUES; MILITARY PERSONNEL AS RESEARCH SUBJECTS; MINORITIES AS RESEARCH SUBJECTS; MULTINATIONAL RESEARCH; PRISONERS, *article on* RESEARCH ISSUES; SEX THERAPY AND SEX RESEARCH; STUDENTS AS RESEARCH SUBJECTS; *and* WOMEN, *article on* RESEARCH ISSUES.

HUMAN RIGHTS

See PATIENTS' RIGHTS; *and* RIGHTS. *See also* CHILDREN, *article on* RIGHTS OF CHILDREN; PRISONERS; *and* WARFARE, *article on* PUBLIC HEALTH AND WAR.

HUNGARY

See MEDICAL ETHICS, HISTORY OF, *section on* EUROPE, *subsection on* CONTEMPORARY PERIOD, *article on* CENTRAL AND EASTERN EUROPE.

HUNGER, WORLD

See FOOD POLICY.

HUNTING AND FISHING

See ANIMAL WELFARE AND RIGHTS, *article on* HUNTING, *and also the articles on* ETHICAL PERSPECTIVES ON THE TREATMENT AND STATUS OF ANIMALS, *and* WILDLIFE AND CONSERVATION MANAGEMENT. *See also* ENDANGERED SPECIES AND BIODIVERSITY.

HYPNOSIS

Hypnosis induces a natural state of deeply focused inner attention familiar to anyone who daydreams, reflects, or imagines. However, its depth, intensity, and level of self-absorption create a unique trance state that has therapeutic value. Medical and psychological uses of hypnosis rely on these altered states of consciousness to help people change perception of pain, feelings, or memories. Hypnosis is a function of the subject and, contrary to popular belief, cannot be induced without the person's willingness to participate. However, different degrees of inherent hypnotizability characterize each person's ability to experience trance depth and the phenomena experienced in the laboratory, legal, or clinical setting. Fortunately, for clinical work, subjects in either light or deep trances may benefit from the use of medical and psychological hypnosis when it is used as an adjunct to their treatment.

History

The modern uses of hypnosis in therapy have historical antecedents. Early Greek sleep temples used hypnotic trance states for medical and psychological healing. In western Europe, Franz Anton Mesmer (1734–1815) treated psychosomatic illnesses and hysteria, using the concept of animal magnetism to account for his success. In 1843, James Braid (1795–1860), a Scottish physician, coined the term "hypnotism," derived from the Greek *hypnos* ("sleep"). James Esdaile (1808–1859), an English surgeon practicing in India from 1840 to 1850, reported his surgical use of hypnosis in leg amputations and removal of large scrotal tumors, commonly weighing as much as 80 pounds. He noted decreased operative mortality due to blood loss, shock, and infection—benefits still reported today in surgical procedures around the world using hypnosis as the sole anesthetic agent. Jean-Martin Charcot (1825–1893), the leading nineteenth-century French neurologist, treated patients with hysterical states at the Salpêtrière Hospital in Paris and taught that hypnosis was a pathological somatic condition derived from hysteria. Hippolyte Bernheim (1840–1919), professor of clinical medicine at the University of Nancy, argued that hypnotic phenomena were not a function of psychopathology but, rather, that hypnotic trance states were entirely normal and resulted from the individual's own suggestibility. Sigmund Freud (1856–1939), having studied first with Charcot and then with Bernheim, initially used hypnosis in uncovering repressed memories during psychotherapy. He soon embarked on his own scientific study of the mind using free association. His rejection of clinical hypnosis delayed its further development for nearly another half-century.

In 1899, Pierre Janet (1859–1947), working at Salpêtrière Hospital, proposed that patients could segregate memories of severe trauma into separate ego states by *désagrégation psychologique*, a process loosely translated into English as "dissociation." Since these memories were often kept out of awareness, Janet postulated that hypnosis might be useful in memory retrieval, resulting in psychological integration of memories of past traumas and perhaps more adaptive mental functioning.

In 1933, Clark Hull of Yale University published the first book about hypnosis from an experimental laboratory. Subsequent advances in the scientific understanding of the mechanisms of hypnosis and the role played by the context in which it occurs in science, law, and medicine have resulted in many new applications and ethical controversies surrounding its use.

Therapeutic uses

Hypnosis finds many uses by clinicians in dentistry, medicine, pediatrics, surgery, psychiatry, psychology, and social work. Its primary therapeutic use today is in the management of anxiety and stress. However, hypnosis also finds applications in providing pain relief to surgical and cancer patients during medical procedures and chemotherapy, and some reports document success in controlling blood loss in hemophiliacs during dental extractions. Hypnosis is a learned skill, not "an alternative therapy." Clinicians have successfully taught self-hypnotic skills to help in obstetrical deliveries and in treating various dermatological disorders. Psychotherapeutic uses include treating phobias, conversion disorders, multiple-personality disorders, and some forms of psychosis. People with posttraumatic stress disorders, including those resulting from physical and sexual abuse in childhood, sometimes benefit from hypnotic interventions. Smoking, obesity, and many psychosomatic disorders often respond to hypnosis when other approaches fail.

Numerous theories attempt to explain how hypnosis works. Hypnosis is a natural skill available in varying degrees to most people. All hypnosis is essentially self-hypnosis taught to the subject by the clinician for clinical, forensic, or research purposes. By creating a trusting alliance, the clinician teaches internal focusing, self-absorption, and the creation of images for the purpose of changing perceptions of pain, feelings, or memory. State-dependent theorists, those who view hypnotic phenomena as largely shaped by a person's internal events, such as images, self-absorption, and dissociation, understand hypnotic trances as altered states of consciousness, psychological age regressions, and nonpathological hallucinations. Non-state theorists, those who view hypnotic phenomena as largely shaped by external events such as beliefs, attitudes, and contextual clues of either the subject or the hypnotist, see hypnosis as a special type of interpersonal communication involving symbols and metaphors and enhancing the acceptance of suggestions. Monotonous, repetitive words timed with slowing spontaneous body movements usually lead to the trance state, yet little is actually known about how the mere exchange of words and images between two people in a suitable context brings about the impressive responses in hypnotherapy. However hypnosis works, it certainly affects the basic biochemistry of pain perception, mood maintenance, and memory storage in ways only faintly discernible at this time.

Ethical controversies

While there appears to be no danger in entering a hypnosis trance per se, credentialed clinicians are concerned that many hypnotherapists around the world are laypersons who use hypnosis to treat medical and psychological ailments without adequate training or licensure. Laws restricting the use of hypnosis to licensed health professionals have been passed successfully only in the Australian states (except New South Wales) and the province of Ontario in Canada. Most other countries, including the United States, have not passed such laws. One major difficulty in establishing such laws is the absence of a satisfactory definition of "hypnosis" for legislative purposes. As a result, nearly any layperson can open an office for the practice of hypnotherapy and remain beyond the reach of the law if he or she treats physical or mental illnesses. While hypnotherapy for better athletic performance, smoking cessation, and weight control might seem innocent, not requiring of legal regulation to protect the public, it seems apparent that lay practitioners should have some training in client selection and follow-up care. Under the shingle of hypnotherapy, such persons could easily practice medicine and psychology without proper training, credentials, and licensure. The risks to the public seem obvious.

Sometimes hypnosis is used to attempt tumor regression. While there is some evidence to suggest that the length and quality of life can be enhanced by hypnotic interventions in metastatic breast cancer, there is a risk that the patient will not seek proper medical treatment in concert with the hypnotherapy. As in all uses of hypnosis, it is best used by practitioners credentialed and licensed in their health fields; in addition, they should be required to employ this technique according to the principles and practices of their professions.

The potential for undue manipulation of patients experiencing heightened suggestibility presents a problem for psychotherapists concerned with contaminating patients' hard-won insights with direct or indirect suggestions of hypnosis. On the other hand, therapists who do not rely on patients' gaining insight into their problems and who consider change the first prerequisite for growth believe that symptom reduction through hypnosis is the preferred goal of treatment. Thus, ethical dilemmas depend in part on how the therapist understands the nature of psychotherapy and the purpose of the hypnotic intervention.

The use of hypnosis can have a great impact on due process and the Constitutional rights of defendants when hypnotically "refreshed" memories of crimes are introduced as direct evidence. However, guidelines exist to aid practitioners using hypnosis in obtaining such memories for forensic purposes to ensure fairness and respect for the need for corroborating evidence.

Hypnosis is often used to recover memories of forgotten traumas in adults suffering from dissociative disorders. It can frequently soften the dissociative defenses that block awareness of suspected trauma. Some therapists believe that once awareness of the original trauma is achieved, integration of these recovered memories can enhance full recovery. On the other hand, controversy surrounds whether the memories recovered, often decades after the incident, are accurate and true.

Memory is a complicated process. While some believe it is stored on a mental "videotape recorder," accessible in full and accurate detail by hypnosis several months or even decades later, memory researchers believe it to be much more malleable. Memory seems to be reconstructed as new perceptual, sensory, and cognitive inputs are subsequently processed. In fact, much current scientific evidence demonstrates an individual's ability in hypnosis to fabricate stories explaining his or her past. For example, leading questions by a therapist or the desire to please and cooperate in police interrogations can contribute to the reshaping of memories. Whereas any hypnotic procedure enhances the conviction that recovered material is true, this increased certainty and the emotional sincerity with which it is reported are not decisive in sorting fact from fantasy. In forensic settings, independent evidence corroborating the recovered memory is essential for court convictions in light of the malleability of memories. It is important to remember, however, that such corroboration is often unnecessary in the conduct of psychotherapy, where useful insights can be gleaned from recovered memories in the process of enhancing personal growth and meaning. Nonetheless, hypnosis can bring forth greater detail of memories, even those that are not true—so-called false memories. This issue is not benign if these memories are taken out of the office setting. In 1692, the Salem witch trials in Massachusetts Bay Colony cost many people their freedom and even their lives; today, families can be destroyed by allegations of child abuse based on false memories of adults in psychotherapy.

Finally, it is prudent for clinicians using hypnosis to recover memories of abuse to establish careful ethical guidelines governing its use and practice. Such guidelines have been proposed and include doing no harm; not jumping to the conclusion that abuse occurred merely because it seems plausible; never assuming that patients who cannot remember much from childhood are repressing traumatic memories or are in denial; avoiding the suggestion that patients cut off communication with their families; tolerating ambiguity; respecting the malleability of memory; and pursuing alternative diagnoses to account for presenting symptoms. When all is said and done, hypnosis is a powerful adjunct when used to alleviate human suffering, promote personal growth, and enhance creativity.

PETER B. BLOOM

For a further discussion of topics mentioned in this entry, see the entries ALTERNATIVE THERAPIES, *especially the article on* SOCIAL HISTORY; DENTISTRY; LICENSING, DISCIPLINE, AND REGULATION IN THE HEALTH PROFESSIONS; PAIN AND SUFFERING; PSYCHOANALYSIS AND DYNAMIC THERAPIES; SOCIAL WORK IN HEALTH CARE; SUBSTANCE ABUSE, *articles on* ADDICTION AND DEPENDENCE, SMOKING, *and* ALCOHOLISM; SURGERY; *and* TRUST. *For a discussion of related ideas, see the entries* ABUSE, INTERPERSONAL, *article on* CHILD ABUSE; ALLIED HEALTH PROFESSIONS; BEHAVIOR MODIFICATION THERAPIES; FAMILY; *and* PSYCHIATRY, ABUSES OF.

Bibliography

BLOOM, PETER B. 1994. "Clinical Guidelines in Using Hypnosis in Uncovering Memories of Sexual Abuse: A Master Class Commentary." *International Journal of Clinical and Experimental Hypnosis* 42, no. 3:173–178. A commonsense approach to using hypnosis in patients recovering memories of abuse in the course of their psychotherapy.

BOWERS, KENNETH S. 1976. *Hypnosis for the Seriously Curious.* New York: W. W. Norton. An excellent overview of the scientific understanding of hypnosis from its beginnings to 1976—still relevant.

COUNCIL ON SCIENTIFIC AFFAIRS, AMERICAN MEDICAL ASSOCIATION. 1985. "Scientific Status of Refreshing Recollection by the Use of Hypnosis." *Journal of the American Medical Association* 253, no. 13:1918–1923. The first forensic guidelines; now used in most states.

CRASILNECK, HAROLD B., and HALL, JAMES A. 1985. *Clinical Hypnosis: Principles and Applications.* 2d ed. Orlando, Fla.: Grune and Stratton. A standard, modern reference to most clinical uses of hypnosis in dentistry, medicine, psychiatry and psychology, and surgery.

FRANKEL, FRED H. 1990. "Hypnotizability and Dissociation." *American Journal of Psychiatry* 147, no. 7:823–829. A major discussion of the relationship and clinical utility of the ability to go into trance and the likelihood of experiencing dissociative defenses.

GANAWAY, GEORGE K. 1989. "Historical Versus Narrative Truth: Clarifying the Role of Exogenous Trauma in the Etiology of MPD and Its Variants." *Dissociation* 2, no. 4:205–220. A seminal discussion of the differences between narrative truth, useful for psychotherapy, and historical truth, useful for forensic purposes.

HULL, CLARK LEONARD. 1933. *Hypnosis and Suggestibility: An Experimental Approach.* New York: Appleton-Century. The first laboratory investigation in the United States of hypnotic phenomena.

LAURENCE, JEAN-ROCH, and PERRY, CAMPBELL W. 1988. *Hypnosis, Will and Memory: A Psycho-legal History.* New York: Guilford. An interesting narration taken from original French historical documents and current North American judicial cases, providing background for the use of hypnosis in modern-day forensic issues.

ORNE, MARTIN T., and BAUER-MANLEY, NANCY K. 1991. "Disorders of Self: Myths, Metaphors, and the Demand Characteristics of Treatment." In *The Self: Interdisciplinary Approaches,* pp. 93–106. Edited by Jaine Strauss and George R. Goethals. New York: Springer-Verlag. A forceful discussion of the controversies surrounding multiple-personality disorders.

PETTINATI, HELEN M., ed. 1988. *Hypnosis and Memory.* New York: Guilford. A modern compendium on what is known about how memory works.

SPENCE, DONALD P. 1982. *Narrative Truth and Historical Truth: Meaning and Interpretation in Psychoanalysis.* New York: W. W. Norton. The original discussion of the difference between perceived truth, useful in therapy, and factually corroborated truth, useful in legal settings.

SPIEGEL, DAVID; BLOOM, JOAN R.; KRAEMER, HELENA C.; and GOTTHEIL, ELLEN. 1989. "Effect of Psychosocial Treatment on Survival of Patients with Metastatic Breast Cancer." *Lancet* 2, no. 8668:888–891. The first controlled study suggesting the valid use of hypnosis in breast cancer patients.

VAN DER KOLK, BESSEL A., and VAN DER HART, OTTO. 1989. "Pierre Janet and the Breakdown of Adaptation in Psychological Trauma." *American Journal of Psychiatry* 146, no. 12:1530–1540. An excellent historical presentation of the ideas of Pierre Janet and their application in understanding dissociative disorders.

WEITZENHOFFER, ANDRE M., and HILGARD, ERNEST R. 1959. *Stanford Hypnotic Susceptibility Scale, Forms A and B.* Palo Alto, Calif.: Consulting Psychological Press. The original standardization of hypnotizability and how to measure it in different individuals.